10 0598738 7
KU-626-007

RADIOBIOLOGY FOR THE RADIOLOGIST

SIXTH EDITION

RADIOBIOLOGY FOR THE RADIOLOGIST

Eric J. Hall, D.Phil., D.Sc., F.A.C.R., F.R.C.R.
Higgins Professor of Radiation Biophysics
Professor of Radiation Oncology and Radiology
Director, Center for Radiological Research
College of Physicians & Surgeons
Columbia University
New York, New York

Amato J. Giaccia, Ph.D.
Professor of Radiation Oncology
Director, Division of Radiation and Cancer Biology
Stanford University School of Medicine
Stanford, California

Acquisitions Editor: Lisa McAllister
Developmental Editor: Louise Bierig
Managing Editor: Kerry Barrett
Project Manager: Fran Gunning
Senior Manufacturing Manager: Benjamin Rivera
Marketing Manager: Angela Panetta
Design Coordinator: Terry Mallon
Compositor: TechBooks
Printer: Courier-Westford

530 Walnut Street
Philadelphia, PA 19106 USA
LWW.com

Printed in the USA

Library of Congress Cataloging-in-Publication Data

Hall, Eric J.
Radiobiology for the radiologist / Eric J. Hall and Amato J. Giaccia.—6th ed.
p. ; cm.
Includes bibliographical references and index.
ISBN 0-7817-4151-3 (alk. paper)
1. Radiology, Medical. 2. Radiobiology. 3. Medical physics.
I. Giaccia, Amato J. II. Title.
[DNLM: 1. Radiation Effects. 2. Radiobiology. 3. Radiotherapy.
WN 600 H175r 2006]
R895.H34 2006
616.07′57—dc22

2005031128

Care has been taken to confirm the accuracy of the information presented and to describe generally accepted practices. However, the authors, editors, and publisher are not responsible for errors or omissions or for any consequences from application of the information in this book and make no warranty, expressed or implied, with respect to the currency, completeness, or accuracy of the contents of the publication. Application of this information in a particular situation remains the professional responsibility of the practitioner.

The authors, editors, and publisher have exerted every effort to ensure that drug selection and dosage set forth in this text are in accordance with current recommendations and practice at the time of publication. However, in view of ongoing research, changes in government regulations, and the constant flow of information relating to drug therapy and drug reactions, the reader is urged to check the package insert for each drug for any change in indications and dosage and for added warnings and precautions. This is particularly important when the recommended agent is a new or infrequently employed drug.

Some drugs and medical devices presented in this publication have Food and Drug Administration (FDA) clearance for limited use in restricted research settings. It is the responsibility of health care providers to ascertain the FDA status of each drug or device planned for use in their clinical practice.

10 9 8 7 6

To purchase additional copies of this book, call our customer service department at (800) 638-3030 or fax orders to (301) 223-2320. International customers should call (301) 223-2300.

Visit Lippincott Williams & Wilkins on the Internet: http://www.LWW.com. Lippincott Williams & Wilkins customer service representatives are available from 8:30 am to 6 pm, EST.

Contents

Preface to the First Edition

This book, like so many before it, grew out of a set of lecture notes. The lectures were given during the autumn months of 1969, 1970, and 1971 at the Columbia-Presbyterian Medical Center, New York City. The audience consisted primarily of radiology residents from Columbia, affiliated schools and hospitals, and various other institutions in and around the city.

To plan a course in radiobiology involves a choice between, on the one hand, dealing at length and in depth with those few areas of the subject in which one has personal expertise as an experimenter or, on the other hand, surveying the whole field of interest to the radiologist, necessarily in less depth. The former course is very much simpler for the lecturer and in many ways more satisfying; it is, however, of very little use to the aspiring radiologist who, if this course is followed, learns too much about too little and fails to get an overall picture of radiobiology. Consequently, I opted in the original lectures, and now in this book, to cover the whole field of radiobiology as it pertains to radiology. I have endeavored to avoid becoming evangelical over those areas of the subject which interest me, those to which I have devoted a great deal of my life. At the same time I have attempted to cover, with as much enthusiasm as I could muster and from as much knowledge as I could glean, those areas in which I had no particular expertise or personal experience.

This book, then, was conceived and written for the radiologist—specifically, the radiologist who, motivated ideally by an inquiring mind or more realistically by the need to pass an examination, elects to study the biological foundations of radiology. It may incidentally serve also as a text for graduate students in the life sciences or even as a review of radiobiology for active researchers whose viewpoint has been restricted to their own area of interest. If the book serves these functions, too, the author is doubly happy, but first and foremost it is intended as a didactic text for the student of radiology.

Radiology is not a homogenous discipline. The diagnostician and therapist have divergent interests; indeed it sometimes seems that they come together only when history and convenience dictate that they share a common course in physics or radiobiology. The bulk of this book will be of concern, and hopefully of interest, to all radiologists. The diagnostic radiologist is commended particularly to Chapters 11, 12, and 13 concerning radiation accidents, late effects, and the irradiation of the embryo and fetus. A few chapters, particularly Chapters 8, 9, 15, and 16, are so specifically oriented towards radiotherapy that the diagnostician may omit them without loss of continuity.

A word concerning reference material is in order. The ideas contained in this book represent, in the author's estimate, the consensus of opinion as expressed in the scientific literature. For ease of reading, the text has not been broken up with a large number of direct references. Instead a selection of general refernces has been included at the end of each chapter for the reader who wishes to pursue the subject further.

I wish to record the lasting debt that I owe my former colleagues at Oxford and my present colleagues at Columbia, for it is in the daily cut and thrust of debate and discussion that ideas are formulated and views tested.

Finally, I would like to thank the young men and women who have regularly attended my classes. Their inquiring minds have forced me to study hard and reflect carefully before facing them in a lecture room. As each group of students has grown in maturity and understanding, I have experienced a teacher's satisfaction and joy in the belief that their growth was due in some small measure to my efforts.

E. J. H.
New York
July 1972

Preface

This Sixth Edition has been completely revised and substantially rewritten. The format introduced in the Fifth Edition received many favorable comments and has been retained. Part I, the first 15 chapters, represents both a general introduction to radiation biology and a complete self-contained course in the subject, suitable for residents in diagnostic radiology and nuclear medicine. It follows the format of the Syllabus in Radiation Biology prepared by the Radiological Society of North America (RSNA) in 1999, and its content reflects the questions appearing in recent years in the written examination for diagnostic radiology residents given by the American Board of Radiology. Part II consists of more in-depth material designed primarily for residents in radiation oncology; in particular, it includes additional material in molecular biology.

In the preface to the Fifth Edition, the prediction was made that it was certainly the last, since the days of a single-authored text in a field as complex as radiation biology are numbered. This prediction did not turn out to be correct, and a Sixth Edition was made possible by the simple expedient of inviting a coauthor with complementary expertise and interests.

Times change, fashions are modified, and the relative emphasis of different topics needs to be revised. Chapters 16 and 17, "Molecular Techniques in Radiobiology" and "Cancer Biology," have been completely rewritten and expanded to take into account a rapidly changing field. Chapters 2, 5, and 6 have also been expanded to include the newer information on the molecular mechanisms involved in DNA repair and the oxygen effect.

Most of the other chapters have simply been revised and updated to reflect current thoughts and ideas. For example, the importance of hereditary effects has been downplayed in recent years, and this is reflected in reduced risk estimates for this end point by UNSCEAR and ICRP. On the other hand, doses in diagnostic radiology have increased substantially owing to the popularity of helical CT and interventional procedures.

For some time, we considered omitting the chapters on gene therapy and predictive assays, since these areas have yet to justify their early promise. In the end, we decided to leave them in because both are still a tantalizing dream that would revolutionize cancer therapy if only the problems could be worked out.

The ideas contained in this book represent, we believe, the consensus of opinion as expressed in the scientific literature. We have followed the precedent of previous editions, in that the pages of text are unencumbered with flyspeck-like numerals referring to footnotes or original publications, which are often too detailed to be of much interest to the general reader. On the other hand, there is an extensive and comprehensive bibliography at the end of each chapter for those readers who wish to pursue the subject further.

We commend this new edition to residents in radiology, nuclear medicine, and radiation oncology, for whom it was conceived and written. If it serves also as a text for graduate students in the life sciences or even as a review of basic science for active researchers or senior radiation oncologists, the authors will be doubly happy.

Eric J. Hall
Columbia University, New York

Amato J. Giaccia
Stanford University, California

Acknowledgments

We would like to thank the many friends and colleagues who generously and willingly gave permission for diagrams and illustrations from their published work to be reproduced in this book.

While the ultimate responsibility for the content of this book must be ours, we acknowledge with gratitude the help of a number of friends who read chapters relating to their own areas of expertise and made invaluable suggestions and additions. With each successive edition, this list grows longer and now includes Drs. Ged Adams, Philip Alderson, Sally Amundson, Joel Bedford, Roger Berry, Max Boone, Victor Bond, J. Martin Brown, Ed Bump, Denise Chan, Julie Choi, James Cox, Bill Dewey, Frank Ellis, Peter Esser, Stan Field, Greg Freyer, Charles Geard, Eugene Gerner, Julian Gibbs, George Hahn, Simon Hall, Ester Hammond, Tom Hei, Robert Kallman, Richard Kolesnick, Adam Krieg, Howard Lieberman, Philip Lorio, Edmund Malaise, Gillies McKenna, Mortimer Mendelsohn, George Merriam, Noelle Metting, Jim Mitchell, Anthony Nias, Ray Oliver, Stanley Order, Tej Pandita, Marianne Powell, Simon Powell, Julian Preston, Elaine Ron, Harald Rossi, Robert Rugh, Robert Sutherland, Roy Tishler, Len Tolmach, Liz Travis, Lou Wagner, John Ward, Barry Winston, Rod Withers, and Basil Worgul. Of particular note are Dr. Chris Schultz, who helped so much with Chapter 27, on chemotherapy agents, and Drs. Mark Dewhirst, Dennis Leeper, and Chang Song, who advised on the content of Chapter 28, on hyperthermia. Without their help, this volume would be much the poorer.

The principal credit for this book must go to the successive classes of residents in radiology, radiation oncology, and nuclear medicine that we have taught over the years at Columbia and Stanford, as well as at ASTRO and RSNA refresher courses. Their perceptive minds and searching questions have kept us on our toes. Their impatience to learn what was needed of radiobiology and to get on with being doctors has continually prompted us to summarize and get to the point.

We are deeply indebted to the United States Department of Energy, the National Cancer Institute, and the National Aeronautical and Space Administration, which have generously supported our work, and indeed much of the research performed by numerous investigators, that is described in this book.

We owe an enormous debt of gratitude to Moshe Friedman, who not only typed and formatted the chapter revisions, but played a major role in editing and proofreading.

Finally, we thank our wives, Bernice Hall and Jeanne Giaccia, who have been most patient and have given us every encouragement with this work.

RADIOBIOLOGY FOR THE RADIOLOGIST

SIXTH EDITION

Milestones in the Radiation Sciences

Now that the centennials of all of the major events involved with the genesis of both diagnostic radiology and radiation oncology have well and truly passed, it seems appropriate to compile a list of "milestones" of the principal events that have brought us to where we are today. The principal motive for doing so is that we need the constant reminder that each generation stands on the shoulders of the one that went before. As Sylvanus Thompson, the first president of the Röntgen Society, put it so eloquently soon after the discovery of x-rays:

> In the history of Science, nothing is truer than that the discoverer, even the greatest discoverer, is but the descendant of his scientific fore-fathers; he is always essentially the product of the age in which he is born.

1859—Changes in populations of organisms: Darwin.
1865—Traits inherited by individual organisms: Mendel.
1895—Röntgen discovers x-rays.
1896—Becquerel presents to the Paris Academy of Sciences the results of his discovery of radiations emitted by uranium compounds.
—First biologic effects of x-rays reported includes skin "burns," epilation, and eye irritation.
—Treatment of a hairy nevus by Freund.
1897—Rutherford examines the radiations from uranium after Becquerel's discovery of radioactivity and finds two types, which he calls α- and β-rays. Later he finds that α-particles consist of nuclei of helium and that β-particles consist of electrons discovered by Thomson.
—Rival claims of first use of x-rays to treat cancer: Grubbe, Despeignes, Williams, Voigt.
1898—Marie and Pierre Curie announce the discovery of "polonium" in July and of "radium" in December.
1902—Cancer in x-ray ulcer reported: Frieben.
—Chromosome theory of heredity.
1903—"Law of Bergonie and Tribondeau"; radiosensitivity related to mitotic activity.
—First suggestion to treat cancer by implanting radium: Bell.
1911—Leukemia in five radiation workers reported: Jagic.
1913—Bohr suggests a model of the atom with a central nucleus and electrons moving in orbits around it.
—Coolidge builds the first successful röntgen-ray tube with hot filament and tungsten target. Coolidge invents the hot-cathode x-ray tube.
1915—British Röntgen Society introduces proposals for radiation protection.
1919—Rutherford bombards nitrogen atoms with α-particles and finds that the nuclei of these atoms disintegrate, giving off hydrogen; oxygen atoms are left. The particles given off are found to be positively charged, and Rutherford names them *protons*. This is the first experiment in which one element is transformed artificially into another element, namely nitrogen into oxygen.
1920s—Barium contrast studies.
1922—Compton discovers the "Compton effect," namely the change in wavelength of scattered x-rays.
1923—Eugene Petry discovers the oxygen effect with plant roots.
1927—Rabbit testes experiments suggest the value of fractionation in radiotherapy: Regaud and Ferraux. Regaud carries out animal sterilization experiments.
—First observation of mutations by x-rays in *Drosophila:* Müller.
1928—Wilderöe suggests the principle of the cyclotron.
—Coutard reports superiority of fractionated treatment for human cancer.
—Unit of x-ray intensity proposed by Second International Congress of Radiology.
—International Committee on X-ray and Radium Protection established.
—First international recommendations on radiation protection adopted by Second International Congress of Radiology.

1929—Advisory Committee on X-ray and Radium Protection established (United States).
1930—First survival curve for bacteria exposed to radiation: Lea.
1930s—Intravenous contrast media.
1931—The roentgen adopted as the unit of exposure for x-rays.
1932—Lawrence invents the cyclotron.
—Chadwick announces the discovery of the neutron, a neutral nuclear particle of about the same mass as the positively charged proton. This experimental proof of the existence of the neutron confirms speculations made by Rutherford in 1919.
1933—Collaborating with M. S. Livingston, Lawrence builds a cyclotron capable of producing 5,000,000-V deuterons.
—Oxygen affects radiosensitivity of tumor "slices"; importance of oxygen in radiotherapy postulated: Crabtree and Cramer.
1934—Joliot and Irene Joliot-Curie produce artificial radioactivity by bombarding aluminum with α-particles and observe that neutrons and positively charged particles are emitted from the aluminum during this process.
—Paterson and Parker introduce their dosage system for γ-ray therapy.
1935—Mottram notes the effect of oxygen on radiosensitivity of *Vicia faba* roots and postulates its importance to radiotherapy.
1937—The Fifth International Congress of Radiology accepts the roentgen as an international dosage unit for x- and γ-radiation.
1938—Robert Stone uses 37-inch cyclotron at Berkeley to treat first patient with neutrons.
1940—Lea and Catcheside propose the linear-quadratic formalism for biologic response to radiation.
—Gray measures first quantitative oxygen enhancement ratio; published 1952.
—Zirke introduces the concept of linear energy transfer.
1940s—Angiography.
1941—The principle of "one gene–one enzyme" established.
1942—First self-maintaining nuclear chain reaction in a uranium graphite pile or reactor initiated in Chicago: Fermi and colleagues.
1943—First use of radioactive isotopes to label compounds in biology and medicine: Hevesy.
1944—Relation between dose and overall time for skin reaction proposed as dose $\alpha(\text{time})^{0.33}$: Strandquist.
1945—Atomic bombs explode July 16 in New Mexico, August 6 in Hiroshima, and August 11 in Nagasaki.
1946—Advisory Committee on X-ray and Radium Protection reorganized to the National Committee on Radiation Protection (United States).
—H. J. Muller wins a Nobel Prize for demonstrating that radiation can induce heritable mutations in fruit flies (*Drosophila melanogaster*).
1947—Atomic Bomb Casualty Commission (ABCC) formed to study the biologic effects of radiation on Japanese A-bomb survivors.
1949—Discovery of cysteine as a radioprotector: Patt.
1950—International Commission on Radiological Protection and International Commission on Radiological Units reorganized from prewar committees.
—Erwin Chargaff discovers a consistent one-to-one ratio of adenine to thymine and guanine to cytosine in DNA.
1950s—Fluoroscopic image intensifiers; catheter techniques.
1951—First clinical cobalt-60 unit, London, Ontario, Canada.
—Hereditary effects of radiation in mice reported: Russell.
—First patient treated with boron neutron-capture therapy: Sweet.
—Linus Pauling obtains precise measurements of a helical polypeptide structure.
1952—First quantitative measurement of the oxygen effect published: Gray.
—DNA identified as the molecule of heredity.
—International Commission on Radiological Units introduces concept of absorbed dose.
—Development of autoradiography and elucidation of the phases of the cell cycle: Howard and Pelc.
—First linear accelerator to treat patients, Hammersmith Hospital, United Kingdom.
—Structure of DNA discovered: Crick and Watson.
1954—Iridium-192 introduced into brachytherapy.
1955—Chronic hypoxia resulting from limitation of oxygen diffusion described: Thomlinson and Gray.
1956—The first *in vitro* radiation survival curve for mammalian cells: Puck.
1957—The K-curve for oxygen published: Howard-Flanders and Alper.
1959—Repair demonstrated by split-dose experiment with mammalian cells: Elkind.
—First *in vivo* survival curve for tumor cells: Hewitt and Wilson.
1960—Survival curve shape change with linear energy transfer: Barendsen and colleagues.
—Concept of growth fraction in tumors: Mendelsohn.
1961—Remote afterloading for brachytherapy: Henscke.

1962—First demonstration of the dose-rate effect in cells *in vitro*: Hall and Bedford.

1963—Relation between electron affinity and radiosensitizing potential: Adams and Dewey.

—First observation of variation of radiosensitivity through the cell cycle: Terasima and Tolmach.

—First demonstration that hypoxic cells limit curability of a mouse tumor by x-rays: Powers and Tolmach.

1966—Potentially lethal damage repair described: Tolmach.

—First patient treated in hyperbaric oxygen: Churchill Davidson.

—Genetic code solved.

—Dependence of oxygen enhancement ratio on linear energy transfer: Barendsen and colleagues.

1967—Concept of cell loss factor in tumors: Steel.

—First survival curve for cells *in vivo*—skin colonies: Withers.

1968—Classification of tissue radiosensitivity: Casarett.

—Description of the nominal standard dose system: Ellis.

1969—Accelerated repopulation shown in animal tumors: Hermens and Barendsen.

1970— Alice Stewart and George Kneale publish study on children in England and Wales showing increased cancer risk due to radiation they received from obstetric x-rays.

1970s—Computed tomography (CT).

1971—First cell survival curves for hyperthermia.

—Development of assay for crypt cells in mouse jejunum: Withers.

—Survival curve for bone-marrow stem cells: Till and McCulloch.

—Sensitivity to heat through the cell cycle: Westra and Dewey.

—Two-hit model to explain the paradigm of retinoblastoma: Knudsen.

1972—First computed tomographic scanner by EMI installed in a hospital in London.

—First recombinant DNA molecules produced.

—The term *reoxygenation* coined by Kallman.

—Discovery of apoptosis by Kerr and colleagues.

1973—Time course of proliferation in normal tissues following irradiation: Denekamp.

1974—First clinical trial with neutrons: Catterall.

—First cancer patients treated with negative π-mesons at Los Alamos: Kligerman.

1975—First cancer patients treated with heavy ions at Berkeley.

—The Radiation Effects Research Foundation (RERF) created to replace the Atomic Bomb Casualty Commission (ABCC).

—Positron emission tomography (PET) developed.

1976—Fowler and Douglas derive linear-quadratic parameters from fractionation experiments.

—First randomized clinical trial of neutrons, Hammersmith Hospital.

—Development of spheroids: Sutherland.

—First clinical trial of a hypoxic-cell radiosensitizer (metronidazole): Urtason and colleagues.

—Suppressor genes described in cultured cells: Stanbridge.

1979—Acutely hypoxic cells described: Brown.

—Three Mile Island nuclear power station accident.

1980—Difference in survival curve shape for early- and late-responding tissues: Withers.

—First repair gene in human cells: Rubin.

—First description of apoptosis: Kerr.

—First commercial magnetic resonance unit.

—Multileaf collimators developed.

1980s—Magnetic resonance imaging (MRI); digital radiology.

1981—Estimation of hereditary effects of radiation in humans: Schull, Otaka, Neel.

1982—Concept of biologically effective dose described: Barendsen.

—The first human oncogenes described: Bishop.

1983—Virtual colonoscopy suggested.

1985—First computer-controlled afterloader: Nucletron.

—Estimation of T_{pot} (potential doubling time) in patients from a single biopsy: Begg.

1986—Development of bioreductive drugs: Brown, Adams.

—The meltdown of a nuclear reactor in Chernobyl, resulted in the release of radioactive material in massive quantities.

1988—Intensity-modulated radiotherapy developed.

1989—Measurement of oxygenation status in human tumors with labeled nitroimidazoles: Chapman, Urtason, and colleagues.

—Polymerase chain reaction developed.

1990—Discovery of importance of mismatch repair genes in human colon cancer: Vogelstein.

—The Committee on the Biological Effects of Ionizing Radiation report (BEIR V) on Health Effects of Exposure to Low Levels of Ionizing Radiation.

1990s—Interventional radiologic techniques; picture archive and communications systems (PACS); teleradiology.

1991—Single-strand conformal polymorphism technique developed to detect mutations.

—First use of gene therapy in animals.

—First correlation of SF_2 (surviving fractions at 2 Gy) and tumor control: West.

1992—First clinical trial of WR2721 as a radioprotector: Kligerman.

—Radiation-induced "bystander effect" discovered.

1994—*BRCA1* discovered.

—Angiostatin and anti-angioangenic therapy conceptualized.

1995—*ATM* gene sequenced.

—*BRCA2* discovered.

—Functional imaging, dose painting, and dose sculpting developed.

—A microarray for gene expression first described.

—Stereotactic radiosurgery used extracranially to treat patients.

1996—p53 named as the molecule of the year—the guardian of the genome.

—A microarray with human genes was first used.

—Discovery that hypoxia modifies the malignant progression of tumor cells.

1998—Helical CT introduced.

—At the direction of Congress, the DOE creates the Low Dose Radiation Research Program to support research needed to establish science-based risk assessment standards and guidelines for exposures to low levels of low-LET ionizing radiation.

1999—First application of microarray to radiobiology.

2000—Draft sequence of the human genome completed.

2002—FDA approves a radiolabeled antibody for low-grade lymphoma.

2003—Virtual colonoscopy becomes a potential option for mass screening.

2004—Cetuximab and radiotherapy used to increase the survival of patients with squamous cell carcinoma of the head and neck.

—Avastin combined with radiotherapy phase I in rectal cancer.

2005—Keratinocyte growth factor approved as a protector against mucositis.

—BEIR VII report on Health Risks from Exposure to Low Levels of Ionizing Radiation.

CHAPTER 1

Physics and Chemistry of Radiation Absorption

In 1895, the German physicist Wilhelm Conrad Röntgen discovered "a new kind of ray," emitted by a gas discharge tube, that could blacken photographic film contained in light-tight containers. He called these rays "x-rays" in his first announcement in December 1895—the x representing the unknown. In demonstrating the properties of x-rays at a public lecture, Röntgen asked Rudolf Albert von Kölliker, a prominent Swiss professor of anatomy, to put his hand in the beam and so produced the first publicly taken radiograph (Fig. 1.1).

The first medical use of x-rays was reported in the *Lancet* of January 23, 1896. In this report, x-rays were used to locate a piece of a knife in the backbone of a drunken sailor, who was paralyzed until the fragment was removed following its location. The new technology spread rapidly through Europe and the United States, and the field of diagnostic radiology was born. There is some debate about who first used x-rays therapeutically, but by 1896, Leopold Freund, an Austrian surgeon, demonstrated before the Vienna Medical Society the disappearance of a hairy mole following treatment with x-rays. Antoine-Henri Becquerel discovered radioactivity emitted by uranium compounds in 1896, and two years later, Pierre and Marie Curie isolated the radioactive elements polonium and radium. Within a few years, radium was used for the treatment of cancer.

The first recorded biologic effect of radiation was due to Becquerel, who inadvertently left a radium container in his vest pocket. He subsequently described the skin erythema that appeared two weeks later and the ulceration that developed and required several weeks to heal. It is said that Pierre Curie repeated this experience in 1901 by deliberately producing a radium "burn" on his own forearm (Fig. 1.2). From these early beginnings, at the turn of the century, the study of radiobiology began.

Radiobiology is the study of the action of ionizing radiations on living things. As such, it inevitably involves a certain amount of radiation physics. The purpose of this chapter is to present, in summary form and with a minimum of mathematics, a listing of the various types of ionizing radiations and a description of the physics and chemistry of the processes by which radiation is absorbed.

TYPES OF IONIZING RADIATIONS

The absorption of energy from radiation in biologic material may lead to *excitation* or to *ionization*. The raising of an electron in an atom or molecule to a higher energy level without actual ejection of the electron is called **excitation**. If the radiation has sufficient energy to eject one or more orbital electrons from the atom or molecule, the process is called **ionization**, and that radiation is said to be **ionizing**

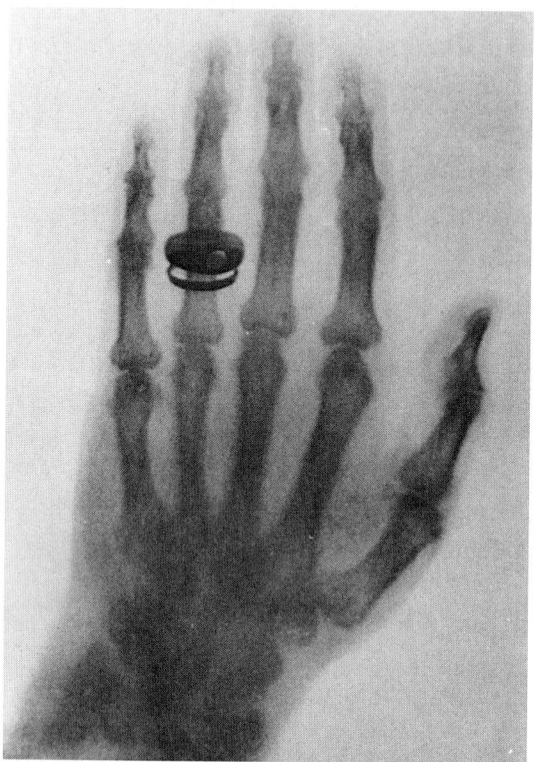

FIGURE 1.1 ● The first publicly taken radiograph of a living object, taken in January 1896, just a few months after the discovery of x-rays. (Courtesy of Röntgen Museum, Würzburg, Germany.)

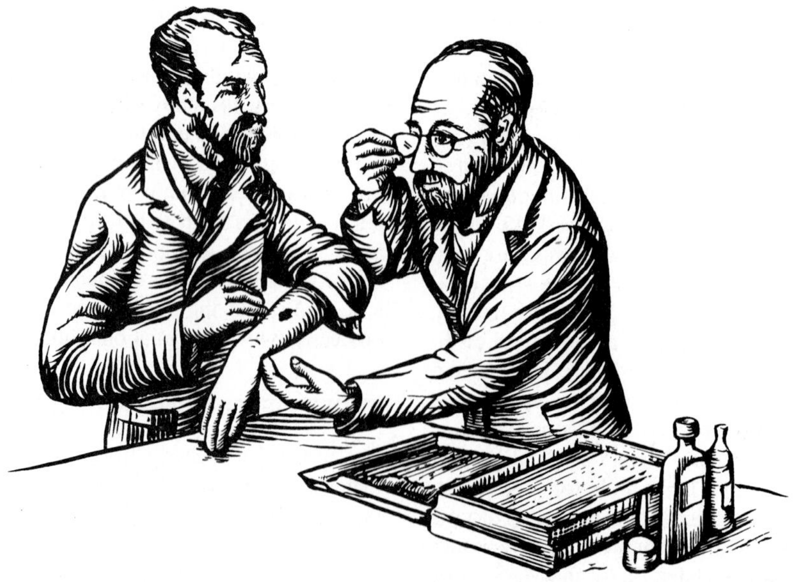

FIGURE 1.2 ● Based on Becquerel's earlier observation, Pierre Curie is said to have used a radium tube to produce a radiation ulcer on his arm. He charted its appearance and subsequent healing.

radiation. The important characteristic of ionizing radiation is the localized release of large amounts of energy. The energy dissipated per ionizing event is about 33 eV, which is more than enough to break a strong chemical bond; for example, the energy associated with a C=C bond is 4.9 eV. For convenience, it is usual to classify ionizing radiations as either **electromagnetic** or **particulate**.

Electromagnetic Radiations

Most experiments with biologic systems have involved x- or γ-rays, two forms of electromagnetic radiation. X- and γ-rays do not differ in nature or in properties; the designation of x- or γ-rays reflects the ways they are produced. X-rays are produced *extranuclearly*; γ-rays are produced *intranuclearly*. In practical terms, this means that x-rays are produced in an electrical device that accelerates electrons to high energy and then stops them abruptly in a target, usually made of tungsten or gold. Part of the kinetic energy (the energy of motion) of the electrons is converted to x-rays. On the other hand, γ-rays are emitted by radioactive isotopes; they represent excess energy that is given off as the unstable nucleus breaks up and decays in its efforts to reach a stable form. Natural background radiation from rocks in the earth also includes γ-rays. Everything that is stated about x-rays in this chapter applies equally well to γ-rays.

X-rays may be considered from two different standpoints. First, they may be thought of as waves of electrical and magnetic energy. The magnetic and electrical fields, in planes at right angles to each other, vary with time, so that the wave moves forward in much the same way as ripples move over the surface of a pond if a stone is dropped into the water. The wave moves with a velocity, c, which in a vacuum has a value of 3×10^{10} cm/s. The distance between successive peaks of the wave, λ, is known as the wavelength. The number of waves passing a fixed point per second is the frequency, ν. The product of frequency times wavelength gives the velocity of the wave; that is, $\lambda\nu = c$.

A helpful, if trivial, analogy is to liken the wavelength to the length of a person's stride when walking; the number of strides per minute is the frequency. The product of the length of stride times the number of strides per minute gives the speed, or velocity, of the walker.

Like x-rays, radio waves, radar, radiant heat, and visible light are forms of electromagnetic radiation. They all have the same velocity, c, but they have different wavelengths and therefore different frequencies. To extend the previous analogy, different radiations may be likened to a group of people, some tall, some short, walking together at the same speed. The tall walkers take long measured strides but make few strides per minute; to keep up, the short walkers compensate for the shortness of their strides by increasing the frequencies of their strides. A radio wave may have a distance between successive peaks (i.e., wavelength) of 300 m; for a wave of visible light, the corresponding distance is about 500 thousandths of a centimeter (5×10^{-5} cm). The wavelength for x-rays may be 100 millionths of a centimeter (10^{-8} cm). X- and γ-rays, then, occupy the short-wavelength end of the electromagnetic spectrum (Fig. 1.3).

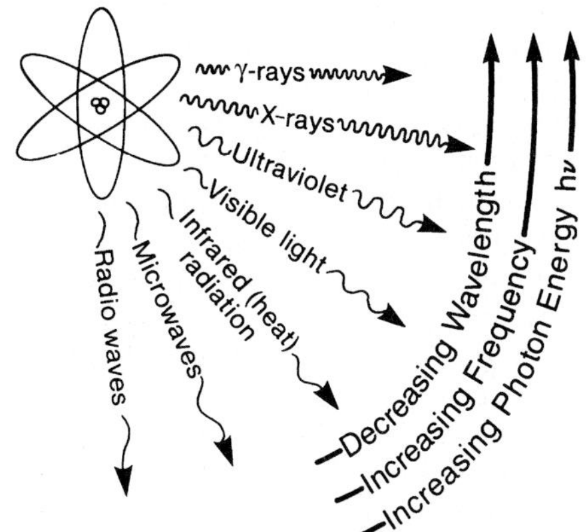

FIGURE 1.3 • Illustration of the electromagnetic spectrum. X-rays and γ-rays have the same nature as visible light, radiant heat, and radio waves; however, they have shorter wavelengths and consequently a larger photon energy. As a result, x- and γ-rays can break chemical bonds and produce biologic effects.

Alternatively, x-rays may be thought of as streams of photons, or "packets" of energy. Each energy packet contains an amount of energy equal to hν, where h is known as Planck's constant and ν is the frequency. If a radiation has a long wavelength, it has a small frequency, and so the energy per photon is small. Conversely, if a given radiation has a short wavelength, the frequency is large and the energy per photon is large. There is a simple numeric relationship between the photon energy (in kiloelectron volts*) and the wavelength (in angstroms†):

$$\lambda \text{Å} = 12.4/\text{E(keV)}$$

For example, x-rays with wavelengths of 0.1 Å correspond to a photon energy of 124 keV.

The concept of x-rays being composed of photons is very important in radiobiology. If x-rays

**The kiloelectron volt (keV) is a unit of energy. It is the energy possessed by an electron that has been accelerated through 1,000 volts (V). It corresponds to 1.6×10^{-9} ergs.*

† The angstrom (Å) is a unit of length equal to 10^{-8} cm.

are absorbed in living material, energy is deposited in the tissues and cells. This energy is deposited unevenly in discrete packets. The energy in a beam of x-rays is quantized into large individual packets, each of which is big enough to break a chemical bond and initiate the chain of events that culminates in a biologic change. The critical difference between nonionizing and ionizing radiations is the size of the *individual* packets of energy, not the *total* energy involved. A simple calculation illustrates this point. It is shown elsewhere (Chapter 8) that a total-body dose of about 4 Gy (400 rad)* of x-rays given to a human is lethal in about half of the individuals exposed. This dose represents an absorption of energy of only about 67 cal, assuming the person to be a "standard man" weighing 70 kg. The smallness of the amount of energy involved can be illustrated in many ways. Converted to heat, it would represent a temperature rise of 0.002°C, which would do no harm at all; the same amount of energy in the form of heat is absorbed in drinking one sip of warm coffee. Alternatively, the energy inherent in a lethal dose of x-rays may be compared with mechanical energy or work: It would correspond to the work done in lifting a person about 16 inches from the ground (Fig. 1.4).

Energy in the form of heat or mechanical energy is absorbed uniformly and evenly, and much greater quantities of energy in these forms are required to produce damage in living things. The potency of x-rays, then, is a function not so much of the total energy absorbed as of the size of the individual energy packets. In their biologic effects, electromagnetic radiations are usually considered ionizing if they have a photon energy in excess of 124 eV, which corresponds to a wavelength shorter than about 10^{-6} cm.

Total-Body Irradiation

X-ray

Mass = 70 kg
$LD_{50/60}$ = 4 Gy
Energy absorbed =

$$70 \times 4 = 280 \text{ joules} = \frac{280}{4.18} = 67 \text{ calories}$$

A

Drinking Hot Coffee

Excess temperature (°C) = 60° − 37° = 23°
Volume of coffee consumed to equal the energy in the $LD_{50/60}$ $= \frac{67}{23}$ = 3 mL = 1 sip

B

Mechanical Energy: Lifting a Person

Mass = 70 kg
Height lifted to equal the energy in the

$$LD_{50/60} = \frac{280}{70 \times 9.81} = 0.4 \text{ m (16 inches)}$$

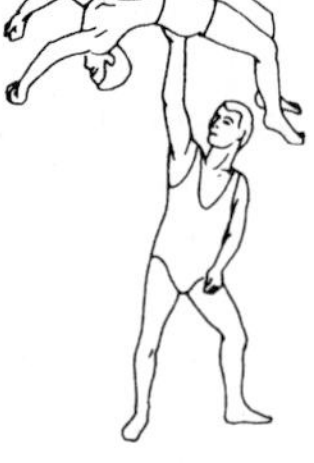

C

FIGURE 1.4 • The biologic effect of radiation is determined not by the amount of the energy absorbed but by the photon size, or packet size, of the energy. **A:** The total amount of energy absorbed in a 70-kg human exposed to a lethal dose of 4 Gy (400 rad) is only 67 cal. **B:** This is equal to the energy absorbed in drinking one sip of hot coffee. **C:** It also equals the potential energy imparted by lifting a person about 16 inches.

Particulate Radiations

Other types of radiation that occur in nature and also are used experimentally are electrons, protons, α-particles, neutrons, negative π-mesons, and heavy charged ions. Some also are used in radiation therapy and have a potential in diagnostic radiology not yet explored.

Electrons are small, negatively charged particles that can be accelerated to high energy to a speed close to that of light by means of an electrical device, such as a betatron or linear accelerator. They are widely used for cancer therapy.

Protons are positively charged particles and are relatively massive, having a mass almost 2,000 times greater than that of an electron. Because of their mass, they require more complex and more expensive equipment, such as a cyclotron, to

**Quantity of radiation is expressed in röntgen, rad, or gray. The röntgen (R) is the unit of exposure and is related to the ability of x-rays to ionize air. The rad is the unit of absorbed dose and corresponds to an energy absorption of 100 erg/g. In the case of x- and γ-rays, an exposure of 1 R results in an absorbed dose in water or soft tissue roughly equal to 1 rad. ICRU recommended that the rad be replaced as a unit by the gray (Gy), which corresponds to an energy absorption of 1 J/kg. Consequently, 1 Gy = 100 rad. Although Gy is now commonly used in Europe, its adoption in everyday practice in the United States has been slow; instead, the centigray is often used; thus, 1 cGy = 1 rad.*

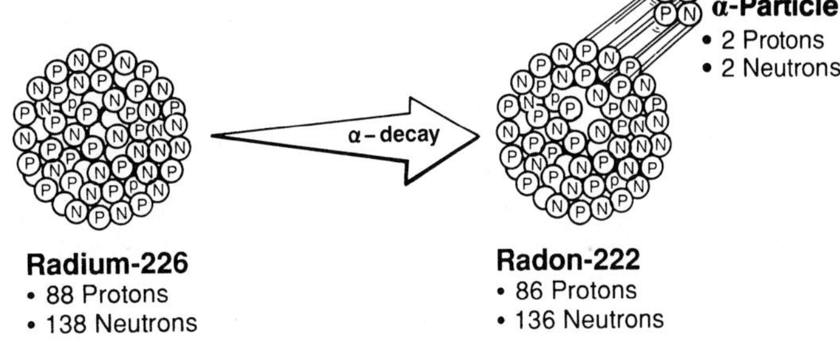

FIGURE 1.5 • Illustration of the decay of a heavy radionuclide by the emission of an α-particle. An α-particle is a helium nucleus consisting of two protons and two neutrons. The emission of an α-particle decreases the atomic number by 2 and the mass number by 4. Note that the radium has changed to another chemical element, radon, as a consequence of the decay.

accelerate them to useful energies, but they are used for cancer treatment in a few specialized facilities.

In nature, the earth is showered with protons from the sun, which represent part of the natural background radiation. We are protected on earth to a large extent by the earth's atmosphere and the magnetic field around the earth, which deflect charged particles. Protons are a major hazard to astronauts on long-range space missions.

α-Particles are nuclei of helium atoms and consist of two protons and two neutrons in close association. They have a net positive charge and therefore can be accelerated in large electrical devices similar to those used for protons.

α-Particles also are emitted during the decay of heavy naturally occurring radionuclides, such as uranium and radium (Fig. 1.5). α-Particles are the major source of natural background radiation to the general public. Radon gas seeps out of the soil and builds up inside houses, where, together with its decay products, it is breathed in and irradiates the lining of the lung. It is estimated that 10,000 to 20,000 cases of lung cancer are caused each year by this means in the United States, mostly in smokers.

Neutrons are particles with a mass similar to that of protons, but they carry no electrical charge. Because they are electrically neutral, they cannot be accelerated in an electrical device. They are produced if a charged particle, such as a deuteron, is accelerated to high energy and then made to impinge on a suitable target material. (A **deuteron** is the nucleus of deuterium and consists of a proton and a neutron in close association.) Neutrons are also emitted as a by-product if heavy radioactive atoms undergo fission, that is, split to form two smaller atoms. Consequently, neutrons are present in large quantities in nuclear reactors and are emitted by some artificial heavy radionuclides. They are also an important component of space radiation and contribute significantly to the exposure of passengers and crews of high-flying jetliners.

Heavy charged particles are nuclei of elements such as carbon, neon, argon, or even iron that are positively charged because some or all of the planetary electrons have been stripped from them. To be useful for radiation therapy, they must be accelerated to energies of thousands of millions of volts and therefore can be produced in only a few specialized facilities. There is no longer any such facility operational in the United States, but heavy-ion therapy is used increasingly in Europe and in Japan.

Charged particles of enormous energy are encountered in space and represent a major hazard to astronauts on long missions, such as the proposed trip to Mars. During the lunar missions of the 1970s, astronauts "saw" light flashes while their eyes were closed in complete darkness, which turned out to be caused by high-energy iron ions crossing the retina.

ABSORPTION OF X-RAYS

Radiation may be classified as *directly* or *indirectly* ionizing. All of the charged particles previously discussed are **directly ionizing**; that is, provided the individual particles have sufficient kinetic energy, they can disrupt the atomic structure of the absorber through which they pass directly and produce chemical and biologic changes. Electromagnetic radiations (x- and γ-rays) are **indirectly ionizing**. They do not produce chemical and biologic damage themselves, but when they are absorbed in the material through which they pass, they give up their energy to produce fast-moving charged particles that in turn are able to produce damage.

The process by which x-ray photons are absorbed depends on the energy of the photons concerned and the chemical composition of the absorbing material. At high energies, characteristic of a cobalt-60 unit or a linear accelerator used for radiotherapy, the **Compton process** dominates. In this process, the photon interacts with what is usually referred to as a "free" electron, an electron whose binding energy is negligibly small compared with the photon energy. Part of the energy of the photon is given to the electron as kinetic energy; the photon, with whatever energy remains, continues

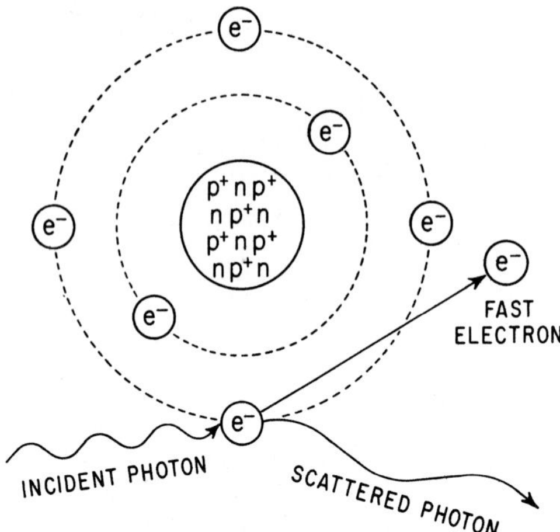

FIGURE 1.6 • Absorption of an x-ray photon by the Compton process. The photon interacts with a loosely bound planetary electron of an atom of the absorbing material. Part of the photon energy is given to the electron as kinetic energy. The photon, deflected from its original direction, proceeds with reduced energy.

on its way, deflected from its original path (Fig. 1.6). In place of the incident photon, there is a fast electron and a photon of reduced energy, which may go on to take part in further interactions. In any given case, the photon may lose a little energy or a lot; in fact, the fraction lost may vary from 0 to 80%. In practice, if an x-ray beam is absorbed by tissue, a vast number of photons interact with a vast number of atoms, and on a statistical basis, all possible energy losses occur. The net result is the production of a large number of fast electrons, many of which can ionize other atoms of the absorber, break vital chemical bonds, and initiate the change of events that ultimately is expressed as biologic damage.

For photon energies characteristic of diagnostic radiology, both Compton and photoelectric absorption processes occur, the former dominating at the higher end of the energy range and the latter being most important at lower energies. In the photoelectric process (Fig. 1.7), the x-ray photon interacts with a bound electron in, for example, the K, L, or M shell of an atom of the absorbing material. The photon gives up all of its energy to the electron; some is used to overcome the binding energy of the electron and release it from its orbit; the remainder is given to the electron as kinetic energy of motion. The kinetic energy (KE) of the ejected electron is therefore given by the expression

$$KE = h\nu - E_B$$

in which $h\nu$ is the energy of the incident photon and E_B is the binding energy of the electron in its orbit. The vacancy left in the atomic shell as a result of the ejection of an electron then must be filled by another

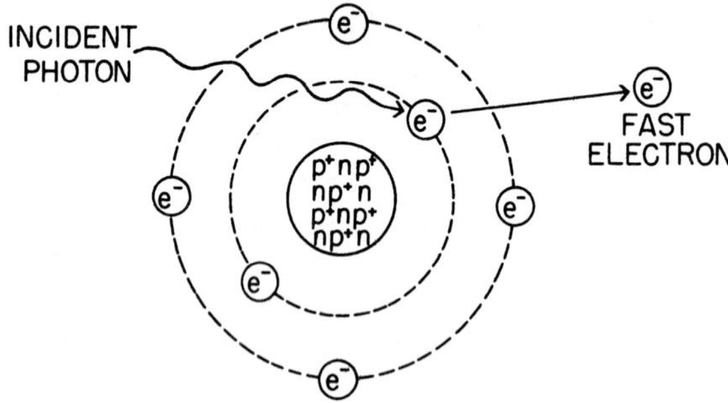

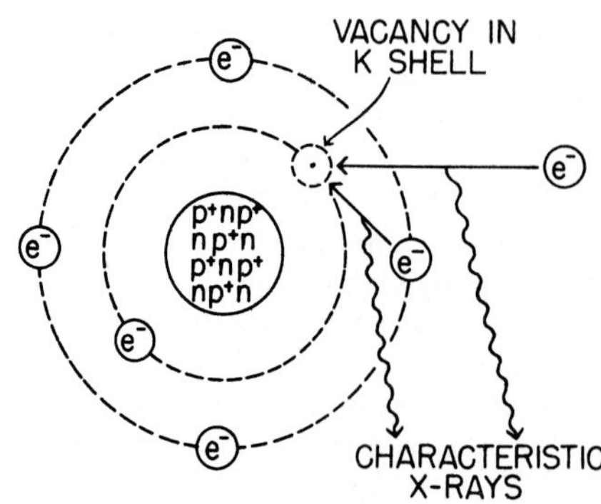

FIGURE 1.7 • Absorption of a photon of x- or γ-rays by the photoelectric process. The interaction involves the photon and a tightly bound orbital electron of an atom of the absorber. The photon gives up its energy entirely; the electron is ejected with a kinetic energy equal to the energy of the incident photon less the binding energy that previously held the electron in orbit (**top**). The vacancy is filled either by an electron from an outer orbit or by a free electron from outside the atom (**bottom**). If an electron changes energy levels, the difference in energy is emitted as a photon of characteristic x-rays. For soft tissue these x-rays are of very low energy.

electron falling in from an outer shell of the same atom or by a conduction electron from outside the atom. The movement of an electron from one shell to another represents a change of energy states. Because the electron is negatively charged, its movement from a loosely bound to a tightly bound shell represents a decrease of potential energy; this energy change is balanced by the emission of a photon of "characteristic" electromagnetic radiation. In soft tissue, this characteristic radiation has a low energy, typically 0.5 kV, and is of little biologic consequence.

The Compton and photoelectric absorption processes differ in several respects that are vital in the application of x-rays to diagnosis and therapy. The mass absorption coefficient for the Compton process is independent of the atomic number of the absorbing material. By contrast, the mass absorption coefficient for photoelectric absorption varies rapidly with atomic number (Z)* and is, in fact, about proportional to Z^3.

For diagnostic radiology, photons are used in the energy range in which photoelectric absorption is as important as the Compton process. Because the mass absorption coefficient varies critically with Z, the x-rays are absorbed to a greater extent by bone because bone contains elements with high atomic numbers, such as calcium. This differential absorption in materials of high Z is one reason for the familiar appearance of the radiograph. For radiotherapy, however, high-energy photons in the megavoltage range are preferred because the Compton process is overwhelmingly important. As a consequence, the absorbed dose is about the same in soft tissue, muscle, and bone, so that differential absorption in bone, which posed a problem in the early days when lower-energy photons were used for therapy, is avoided.

Although the differences among the various absorption processes are of practical importance in radiology, the consequences for radiobiology are minimal. Whether the absorption process is the photoelectric or the Compton process, much of the energy of the absorbed photon is converted to the kinetic energy of a fast electron.

DIRECT AND INDIRECT ACTION OF RADIATION

The biologic effects of radiation result principally from damage to DNA, which is the critical target, as described in Chapter 2.

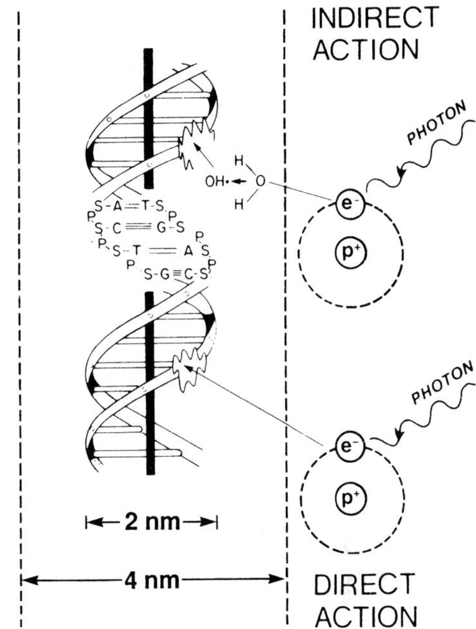

FIGURE 1.8 • Direct and indirect actions of radiation. The structure of DNA is shown schematically. In direct action, a secondary electron resulting from absorption of an x-ray photon interacts with the DNA to produce an effect. In indirect action, the secondary electron interacts with, for example, a water molecule to produce a hydroxyl radical (OH·), which in turn produces the damage to the DNA. The DNA helix has a diameter of about 20 Å (2 nm). It is estimated that free radicals produced in a cylinder with a diameter double that of the DNA helix can affect the DNA. Indirect action is dominant for sparsely ionizing radiation, such as x-rays. S, sugar; P, phosphorus; A, adenine; T, thymine; G, guanine; C, cytosine.

If any form of radiation—x- or γ-rays, charged or uncharged particles—is absorbed in biologic material, there is a possibility that it will interact directly with the critical targets in the cells. The atoms of the target itself may be ionized or excited, thus initiating the chain of events that leads to a biologic change. This is called **direct action** of radiation (Fig. 1.8); it is the dominant process if radiations with high **linear energy transfer (LET)**, such as neutrons or α-particles, are considered.

Alternatively, the radiation may interact with other atoms or molecules in the cell (particularly water) to produce free radicals that are able to diffuse far enough to reach and damage the critical targets. This is called **indirect action** of radiation.†

---

* *Z, the atomic number, is defined as the number of positive charges on the nucleus; it is therefore the number of protons in the nucleus.*

† *It is important to avoid confusion between directly and indirectly ionizing radiation, on the one hand, and the direct and indirect actions of radiation on the other.*

A **free radical** is an atom or molecule carrying an unpaired orbital electron in the outer shell. An orbital electron not only revolves around the nucleus of an atom but also spins around its own axis. The spin may be clockwise or counterclockwise. In an atom or molecule with an even number of electrons, spins are paired; that is, for every electron spinning clockwise, there is another one spinning counterclockwise. This state is associated with a high degree of chemical stability. In an atom or molecule with an odd number of electrons, there is one electron in the outer orbit for which there is no other electron with an opposing spin; this is an unpaired electron. This state is associated with a high degree of chemical reactivity.

For simplicity, we consider what happens if radiation interacts with a water molecule, because 80% of a cell is composed of water. As a result of the interaction with a photon of x- or γ-rays or a charged particle, such as an electron or proton, the water molecule may become ionized. This may be expressed as

$$H_2O \rightarrow H_2O^+ + e^-$$

H_2O^+ is an ion radical. An **ion** is an atom or molecule that is electrically charged because it has lost an electron. A free radical contains an unpaired electron in the outer shell, making it highly reactive. H_2O^+ is charged and has an unpaired electron; consequently, it is both an ion and a free radical. The primary ion radicals have an extremely short lifetime, on the order of 10^{-10} second. They decay to form free radicals, which are not charged but still have an unpaired electron. In the case of water, the ion radical reacts with another water molecule to form the highly reactive hydroxyl radical (OH·):

$$H_2O^+ + H_2O \rightarrow H_3O^+ + OH\cdot$$

The hydroxyl radical possesses nine electrons; therefore, one of them is unpaired. It is a highly reactive free radical and can diffuse a short distance to reach a critical target in a cell. For example, it is thought that free radicals can diffuse to DNA from within a cylinder with a diameter about twice that of the DNA double helix. It is estimated that about two thirds of the x-ray damage to DNA in mammalian cells is caused by the hydroxyl radical. The best evidence for this estimate comes from experiments using free-radical scavengers, which can reduce the biologic effect of sparsely ionizing radiations, such as x-rays, by a factor of close to 3. This is discussed further in Chapter 9. Indirect action is illustrated in Figure 1.8. This component of radiation damage is most easily modified by chemical means—either protectors or sensitizers—unlike direct action.

For the indirect action of x-rays, the chain of events, from the absorption of the incident photon to the final observed biologic change, may be described as follows:

Incident x-ray photon
↓
Fast electron (e^-)
↓
Ion radical
↓
Free radical
↓
Chemical changes from the breakage of bonds
↓
Biologic effects

There are vast differences in the time scale involved in these various events. The physics of the process, the initial ionization, may take only 10^{-15} second. The primary radicals produced by the ejection of an electron generally have a lifetime of 10^{-10} second. The OH· radical has a lifetime of about 10^{-9} second in cells, and the DNA radicals formed either by direct ionization or by reaction with OH· radicals have a lifetime of perhaps 10^{-5} second (in the presence of air). The period between the breakage of chemical bonds and the expression of the biologic effect may be hours, days, months, years, or generations, depending on the consequences involved (Fig. 1.9). If cell killing is the result, the biologic effect may be expressed hours to days later, when the damaged cell attempts to divide. If the radiation damage is oncogenic, its expression as an overt cancer may be delayed 40 years. If the damage is a mutation in a germ cell leading to hereditary changes, it may not be expressed for many generations.

ABSORPTION OF NEUTRONS

Neutrons are uncharged particles. For this reason, they are highly penetrating compared with charged particles of the same mass and energy. They are indirectly ionizing and are absorbed by elastic or inelastic scattering.

Fast neutrons differ basically from x-rays in the mode of their interaction with tissue. *X-ray photons* interact with the *orbital electrons* of atoms of the absorbing material by the Compton or photoelectric process and set in motion fast electrons. *Neutrons*, on the other hand, interact with the *nuclei* of

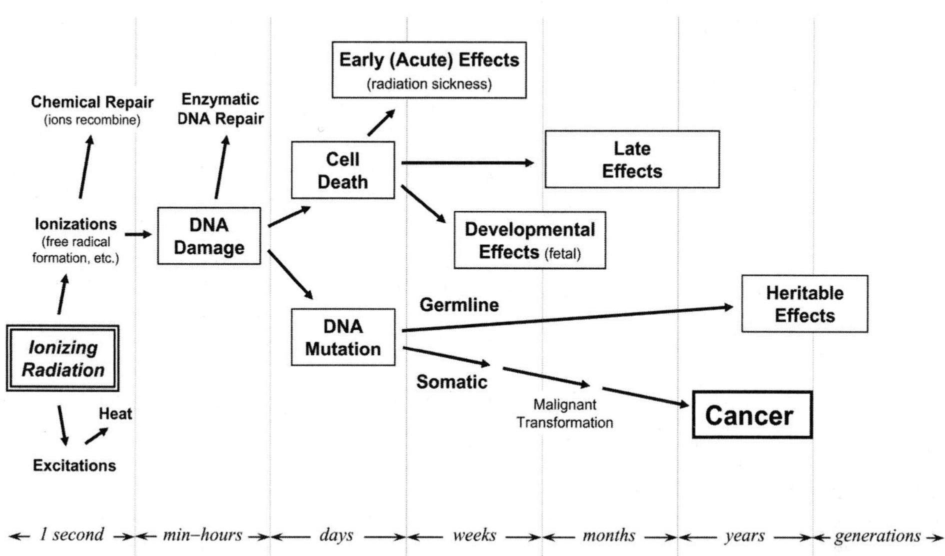

FIGURE 1.9 ● Illustration of the generally accepted sequence of events from the absorption of radiation to the expression of the various forms of biological damage. (Developed in collaboration with Dr. Noelle Metting, U.S. Department of Energy.)

atoms of the absorbing material and set in motion *fast recoil protons*, *α-particles*, and *heavier nuclear fragments*.

In the case of intermediate fast neutrons, **elastic scattering** is the dominant process. The incident neutron collides with the nucleus of an atom of the absorber; part of its kinetic energy is transferred to the nucleus and part is retained by the deflected neutron, which may go on to make further collisions.

In soft tissues, the interaction between incident neutrons and hydrogen nuclei—which are, of course, single protons—is the dominant process of energy transfer. There are several reasons for this. First, a large proportion of energy is transferred if a neutron interacts with a proton because the particles are of similar mass. Second, hydrogen is the most abundant atom in tissue. Third, the collision cross section for hydrogen is large. This process is illustrated in Figure 1.10. The recoil protons that are set in motion lose energy by excitation and ionization as they pass through the biologic material. These recoil protons deposit much of their energy at an LET of less than 30 keV/μm, and the maximum LET associated with protons as they come to rest is about 100 keV/μm. (See Chapter 7 for a discussion of LET.) Elastic collisions of neutrons with heavier elements in tissue make a small contribution to the dose, although the energy is deposited at a high LET.

At energies above about 6 MeV, **inelastic scattering** begins to take place, and it assumes increasing importance as the neutron energy rises.

The neutron may interact with a carbon nucleus to produce three α-particles or with an oxygen nucleus to produce four α-particles (Fig. 1.11). These are known as **spallation products**, which become very important at higher energies. The α-particles

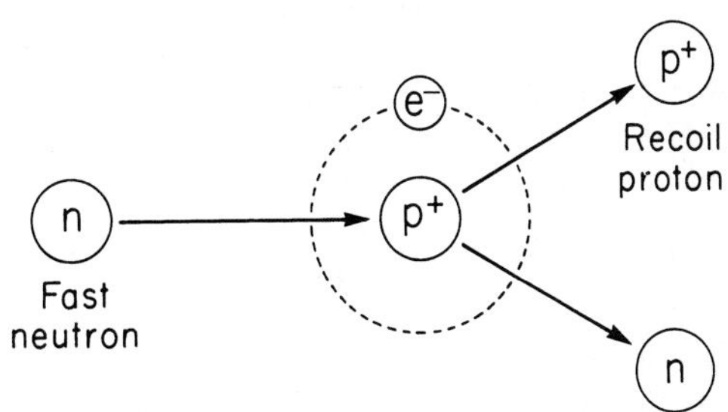

FIGURE 1.10 ● Interaction of a fast neutron with the nucleus of a hydrogen atom of the absorbing material. Part of the energy of the neutron is given to the proton as kinetic energy. The neutron, deflected from its original direction, proceeds with reduced energy.

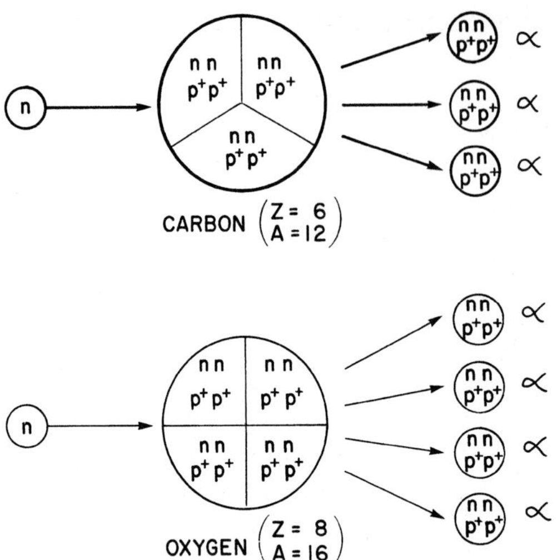

FIGURE 1.11 • The production of spallation products. As the neutron energy rises, the probability increases of a neutron interacting with a carbon or oxygen nucleus to produce three or four α-particles, respectively. Z, atomic number; A, mass number.

produced in this way represent a relatively modest proportion of the total absorbed dose, but they are densely ionizing and have an important effect on the biologic characteristics of the radiation.

CONTRAST BETWEEN NEUTRONS AND PHOTONS

X- and γ-rays are indirectly ionizing and give rise to fast-moving secondary electrons. *Fast neutrons* are also indirectly ionizing but give rise to recoil protons, α-particles, and heavier nuclear fragments.

The electrons that are set in motion if x-rays are absorbed are very light, negatively charged particles. By contrast, the particles set in motion if neutrons are absorbed are heavy and densely ionizing. They also, for the most part, carry a positive charge, but this difference appears to be relatively trivial biologically. What is important is that they are heavy compared with the electron. A proton, for example, has a mass almost 2,000 times greater than an electron; an α-particle has a mass four times larger still; and nuclear fragments may occur that are an order of magnitude larger again in mass. The pattern of ionizations and excitations along the tracks of these various charged particles is very different; in particular, the density of ionization is greater for neutrons, pions, and heavy ions than is the case for x- or γ-rays, and this accounts for the dramatic differences in the biologic effects observed. This is discussed further in Chapter 7.

For heavy particles, as for x-rays, the mechanism of biologic effect may be direct or indirect action, but there is a shift in the balance between the two modes of action (Fig. 1.12). For x-rays, indirect action is dominant; for the heavy particles set in motion by neutrons, direct action assumes a greater importance, which increases with the density of ionization. As the density of ionization increases, the probability of a direct interaction between the particle track and the target molecule increases.

It is important to note at this stage that the indirect effect involving free radicals is most easily modified by chemical means. Radioprotective compounds have been developed that work by scavenging free radicals. Such compounds, therefore, are quite effective for x- and γ-rays but of little use for neutrons or α-particles.

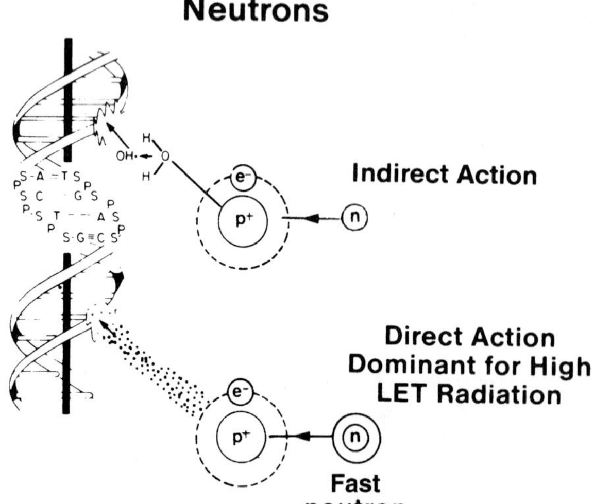

FIGURE 1.12 • Direct action dominates for more densely ionizing radiations, such as neutrons, because the secondary charged particles produced (protons, α-particles, and heavier nuclear fragments) result in a dense column of ionizations more likely to interact with the DNA. The local density of DNA radicals produced by direct ionization of DNA is so high that the additional contribution of DNA radicals produced by OH· radical attack does not add substantially to the severity of the lesion.

Summary of Pertinent Conclusions

- X- and γ-rays are indirectly ionizing; the first step in their absorption is the production of fast recoil electrons.
- Neutrons are also indirectly ionizing; the first step in their absorption is the production of fast recoil protons, α-particles, and heavier nuclear fragments.
- Biologic effects of x-rays may be caused by direct action (the recoil electron directly ionizes the target molecule) or indirect action (the recoil electron interacts with water to produce a hydroxyl radical, which diffuses to the target molecule).
- About two thirds of the biologic damage by x-rays is caused by indirect action.
- DNA radicals produced by both the direct and indirect action of radiation are modifiable with sensitizers or protectors.
- DNA lesions produced by high-LET radiations involve large numbers of DNA radicals. Chemical sensitizers and protectors are ineffective in modifying such lesions.
- The physics of the absorption process is over in 10^{-15} second; the chemistry takes longer because the lifetime of the DNA radicals is about 10^{-5} second; the biology takes hours, days, or months for cell killing, years for carcinogenesis, and generations for hereditary damage.

BIBLIOGRAPHY

Goodwin PN, Quimby EH, Morgan RH: *Physical Foundations of Radiology*. New York, Harper & Row, 1970

Johns HE, Cunningham JR: *The Physics of Radiology*. Springfield, IL, Charles C Thomas, 1969

Rossi HH: Neutron and heavy particle dosimetry. In Reed GW (ed): *Radiation Dosimetry: Proceedings of the International School of Physics*, pp. 98–107. New York, Academic Press, 1964

Smith VP (ed): *Radiation Particle Therapy*. Philadelphia, American College of Radiology, 1976

CHAPTER 2

DNA Strand Breaks and Chromosomal Aberrations

DNA STRAND BREAKS

There is strong circumstantial evidence (described in Chapter 3) that DNA is the principal target for the biologic effects of radiation, including cell killing, carcinogenesis, and mutation. A consideration of the biologic effects of radiation therefore begins logically with a description of the breaks in DNA caused by charged-particle tracks and by the chemical species produced.

Deoxyribonucleic acid (**DNA**) is a large molecule with a well-known double helix structure. It consists of two strands, held together by hydrogen bonds between the bases. The "backbone" of each strand consists of alternating sugar and phosphate groups. The sugar involved is deoxyribose. Attached to this backbone are four bases, the sequence of which specifies the genetic code. Two of the bases are single-ring groups (pyrimidines); these are thymine and cytosine. Two of the bases are double-ring groups (purines); these are adenine and guanine. The structure of a single strand of DNA is illustrated in Figure 2.1. The bases on opposite strands must be complementary; adenine pairs with thymine, and guanine pairs with cytosine. This is illustrated in the simplified model of DNA in Figure 2.2**A**.

If cells are irradiated with a modest dose of x-rays, many breaks of a single strand occur. These can be observed and scored as a function of dose if the DNA is denatured and the supporting structure stripped away. In intact DNA, however, **single-strand breaks** (**SSBs**) are of little biologic consequence as far as cell killing is concerned because they are repaired readily using the opposite strand as a template (Fig. 2.2**B**). If the repair is incorrect (misrepair), it may result in a mutation. If both strands of the DNA are broken and the breaks are well separated (Fig. 2.2**C**), repair again occurs readily, because the two breaks are handled separately.

By contrast, if the breaks in the two strands are opposite one another or separated by only a few base pairs (Fig. 2.2**D**), this may lead to a **double-strand break** (**DSB**); that is, the piece of chromatin snaps into two pieces. Double-strand breaks are believed to be the most important lesions produced in chromosomes by radiation; as described in the next section, the interaction of two double-strand breaks may result in cell killing, carcinogenesis, or mutation. The repair of DNA double-strand breaks at the molecular level will be discussed in Chapter 5.

There are many kinds of double-strand breaks, varying in the distance between the breaks on the two DNA strands and the kinds of end groups formed. Their yield in irradiated cells is about 0.04 times that of single-strand breaks, and they are induced linearly with dose, indicating that they are formed by single tracks of ionizing radiation.

Both free radicals and direct ionizations may be involved in the formation of the type of strand break

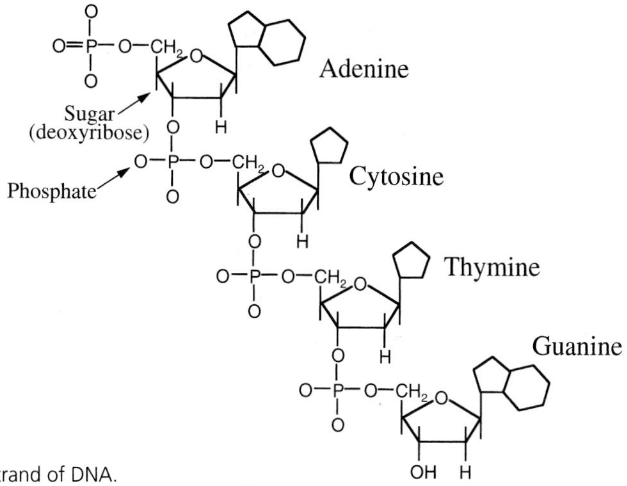

FIGURE 2.1 • The structure of a single strand of DNA.

illustrated in Figure 2.2**D**. As described in Chapter 1, the energy from ionizing radiations is not deposited uniformly in the absorbing medium but is located along the tracks of the charged particles set in motion—electrons in the case of x- or γ-rays, protons and α-particles in the case of neutrons. Radiation chemists speak in terms of "spurs," "blobs," and "short tracks." There is, of course, a full spectrum of energy event sizes, and it is quite arbitrary to divide them into just three categories, but it turns out to be instructive. A spur contains up to 100 eV of energy and involves, on average, three ion pairs. In the case of x- or γ-rays, 95% of the energy deposition events are spurs, which have a diameter of about 4 nm, which is about twice the diameter of the DNA double helix (Fig. 2.3). Blobs are much less frequent for x- or γ-rays; they have a diameter of about 7 nm and contain on average about 12 ion pairs with an energy range of 100–500 eV (Fig. 2.3). Because spurs and blobs have dimensions similar to the DNA double helix, multiple radical attack occurs if they overlap the DNA helix. There is likely to be a wide variety of complex lesions, including base damage as well as double-strand breaks. The term

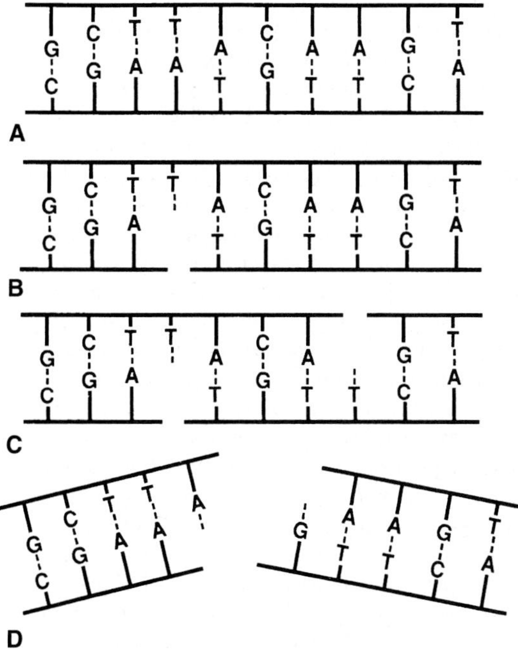

FIGURE 2.2 • Diagrams of single- and double-strand DNA breaks caused by radiation. **A:** Two-dimensional representation of the normal DNA helix. The base pairs carrying the genetic code are complementary (i.e., adenine pairs with thymine, guanine pairs with cytosine). **B:** A break in one strand is of little significance because it is repaired readily, using the opposite strand as a template. **C:** Breaks in both strands, if well separated, are repaired as independent breaks. **D:** If breaks occur in both strands and are directly opposite or separated by only a few base pairs, this may lead to a double-strand break in which the chromatin snaps into two pieces. (Courtesy of Dr. John Ward.)

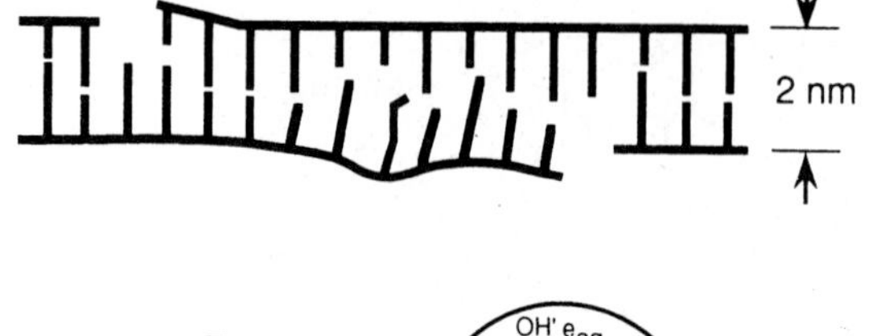

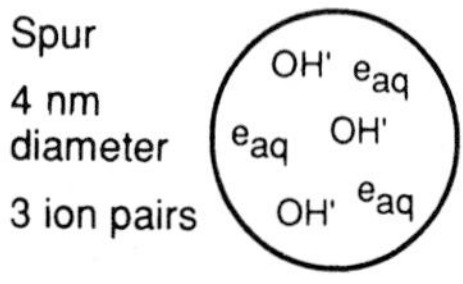

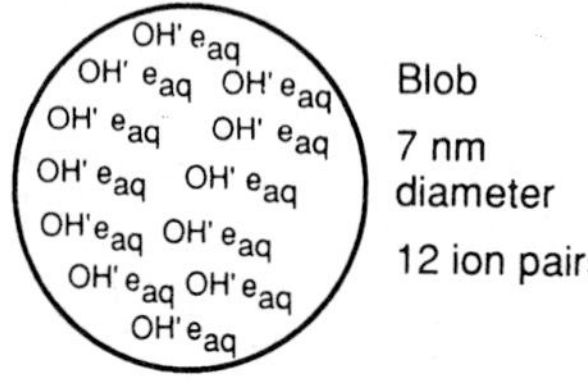

FIGURE 2.3 • Illustration of a locally multiply damaged site. Energy from x-rays is not absorbed uniformly but tends to be localized along the tracks of charged particles. Radiation chemists speak in terms of spurs and blobs, which contain a number of ion pairs and which have dimensions comparable to the DNA double helix. A double-strand break is likely to be accompanied by extensive base damage. John Ward coined the term *locally multiply damaged site* to describe this phenomenon.

locally multiply damaged site has been coined by John Ward to describe this phenomenon. Given the size of a spur and the diffusion distance of hydroxyl free radicals, the multiple damage could be spread out up to 20 base pairs. This is illustrated in Figure 2.3, in which a double-strand break is accompanied by base damage and the loss of genetic information.

In the case of densely ionizing radiations, such as neutrons or α-particles, a greater proportion of blobs is produced. The damage produced, therefore, is qualitatively different from that produced by x- or γ-rays and much more difficult for the cell to repair.

MEASURING DNA STRAND BREAKS

Both single-strand and double-strand DNA breaks can be measured readily by isolating the DNA from irradiated cells and causing the pieces to pass through a porous substrate, such as a gel or filter. The DNA pieces move under the influence of either flow through the filter or electrical field in the gel (using the fact that DNA is negatively charged). Smaller pieces move faster and farther than larger pieces of DNA and thus can be separated and counted. The larger the dose of radiation, the more the DNA is broken up. DNA is denatured and lysed by a strong alkaline preparation so that single-strand breaks are measured. Double-strand breaks are measured in a neutral preparation.

Over the years, a variety of techniques have been used to measure DNA strand breaks, including sucrose gradient sedimentation, alkaline and neutral filter elution, nucleoid sedimentation, pulsed-field gel electrophoresis, and single-cell gel electrophoresis (also known as the comet assay). Of these techniques, pulsed-field gel electrophoresis and single-cell electrophoresis are still commonly used to measure DNA strand breaks.

Pulsed-field gel electrophoresis (PFGE) is the method most widely used to detect the induction and repair of double-strand breaks. It is based on the electrophoretic elution of DNA from agarose plugs within which irradiated cells have been embedded and lysed. Pulsed-field gel electrophoresis allows separation of DNA fragments according to size in the mega-base-pair range, with the assumption that DNA double-strand breaks are induced randomly. The fraction of DNA released from the agarose plug is directly proportional to dose (Fig. 2.4**A**). The kinetics of DNA double-strand break rejoining exhibit a fast initial rate, which then decreases with repair time. The most widely accepted description of this kinetic behavior uses two first-order components (fast and slow) plus some fraction of residual DSBs. Studies have supported the finding that rejoining of incorrect DNA ends originates solely from slowly rejoining DSBs, and this subset of radiation-induced double-strand breaks is what is manifested as chromosomal damage (i.e., chromosome translocations and exchanges).

Single-cell electrophoresis (comet assay) has the advantage of detecting differences in DNA damage and repair at the single-cell level. This is particularly advantageous for biopsy specimens from tumors in which a relatively small number of cells can be assayed to determine DNA damage and repair. Similar to PFGE (described above), cells are exposed to ionizing radiation, embedded in agarose, and lysed under neutral buffer conditions to quantitate induction and repair of DNA double-strand breaks. To assess DNA single-strand breaks and alkaline-sensitive sites, lysis is performed with an alkaline buffer. If the cells are undamaged, the DNA remains compact and does not migrate. If the cell has incurred DNA double-strand breaks, the amount of damage is directly proportional to the migration of DNA in the agarose. As a result of the lysis and electrophoresis conditions, the fragmented DNA

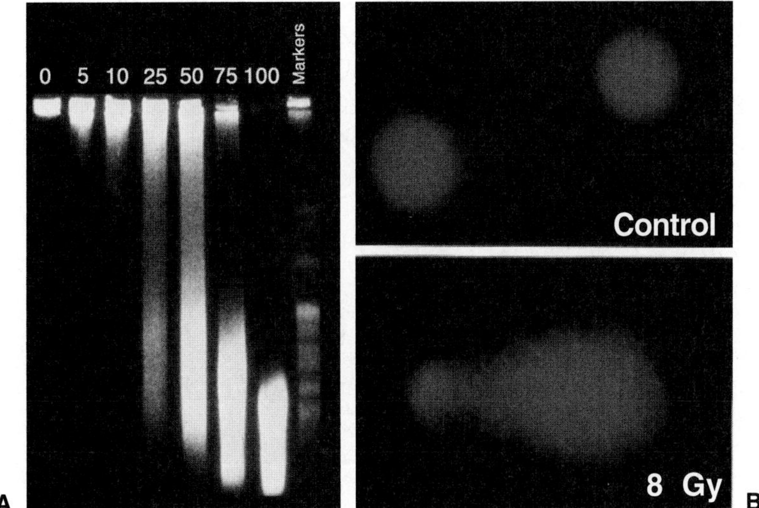

FIGURE 2.4 • **A:** The effect of ionizing radiation on DNA strand break induction as measured by pulsed-field gel electrophoresis. As the dose of ionizing radiation increases from 5 to 100 Gy, the size of the DNA fragments as detected by ethidium brodime staining decreases. Thus, more DNA enters the gel with increasing dose of ionizing radiation. In these experiments, cells were embedded in agarose and irradiated on ice to eliminate the effects of repair. The number above each lane refers to the dose in Gy to which each group of cells was exposed. (Courtesy of Dr. Nicholas Denko.) **B:** Photomicrograph of control and 8-Gy irradiated cells as detected by the comet assay. Unirradiated cells possess a near-spherical appearance, whereas the fragmented DNA in irradiated cells gives the appearance of a comet when stained with ethidium bromide. (Courtesy of Drs. Ester Hammond and Mary Jo Dorie.)

that migrates takes the appearance of a comet's tail (Fig. 2.4**B**). This assay has high sensitivity and specificity for single-strand breaks and alkaline sensitive sites and to a lesser degree DNA double-strand breaks. By changing the lysis conditions from an alkaline to a neutral pH, the comet technique can be used to measure DNA double-strand break repair.

Both of these assays are cell based, where DNA in cells is much more resistant to damage by radiation than would be expected from studies on free DNA. There are two reasons for this: the presence in cells of low-molecular-weight scavengers that mop up some of the free radicals produced and the physical protection afforded the DNA by packaging. Certain regions of DNA, particularly actively translating genes, appear to be more sensitive to radiation, and there is some evidence also of sequence-specific sensitivity.

Radiation induces a large number of lesions in DNA, most of which are repaired successfully by the cell. A dose of radiation that induces an average of one lethal event per cell leaves 37% still viable; this is called the D_0 dose and is discussed further in Chapter 3. For mammalian cells, the x-ray D_0 usually lies between 1 and 2 Gy (between 100 and 200 rad). The number of DNA lesions per cell detected immediately after such a dose is approximately:

Base damage, >1,000
Single-strand breaks, 1,000
Double-strand breaks, 40

Cell killing does not correlate at all with single-strand breaks but relates better to double-strand breaks. Agents (such as hydrogen peroxide) that produce single-strand breaks efficiently but very few double-strand breaks also kill very few cells. On the basis of evidence such as this, it is concluded that double-strand breaks are the most relevant lesions leading to most biologic insults from radiation, including cell killing. The reason for this is that double-strand breaks can lead to chromosomal aberrations, which are discussed in the next section.

CHROMOSOMES AND CELL DIVISION

The backbone of DNA is made of molecules of sugar and phosphates, which serve as a framework to hold the bases that carry the genetic code.

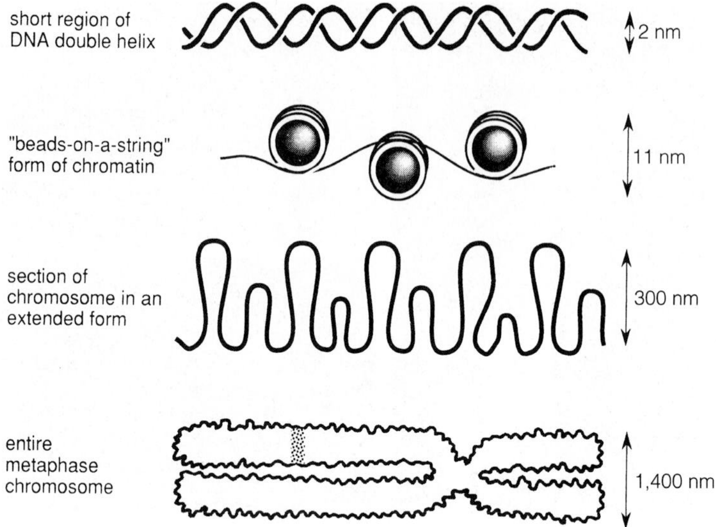

FIGURE 2.5 • Illustration of the relative sizes of the DNA helix, the various stages of folding and packing of the DNA, and an entire chromosome condensed at metaphase.

Attached to each sugar molecule is a base: thymine, adenine, guanine, or cytosine. This whole configuration is coiled tightly in a double helix.

Figure 2.5 is a highly schematized illustration of the way an organized folding of the long DNA helix might be achieved as a closely packed series of looped domains wound in a tight helix. The degree of packing also is illustrated by the relative dimensions of the DNA helix and the condensed metaphase chromosome.

The largest part of the life of any somatic cell is spent in interphase, during which the nucleus, in a stained preparation, appears as a lacework of fine, lightly stained material in a translucent, colorless material surrounded by a membrane. In the interphase nucleus in most cells, one or more bodies of various sizes and shapes, called **nucleoli,** are seen. In most cells, little more than this can be identified with a conventional light microscope. In fact, a great deal is happening during this time: The quantity of DNA in the nucleus doubles as each chromosome lays down an exact replica of itself next to itself. When the chromosomes become visible at mitosis, they are each present in duplicate. Even during interphase, there is good evidence that the chromosomes are not free to move about within the nucleus but are restricted to "domains."

The various events that occur during **mitosis** are divided into several phases. The first phase of division is called **prophase**. The beginning of this phase is marked by a thickening of the chromatin and an increase in its stainability as the chromosomes condense into light coils. By the end of prophase, each chromosome has a lightly staining constriction known as a **centromere**; extending from the centromere are the arms of the chromosome. Prophase ends when the chromosomes reach maximal condensation and the nuclear membrane disappears, as do any nucleoli.

With the disappearance of the nuclear membrane, the nuclear plasm and the cytoplasm mix. **Metaphase** then follows, in which two events occur simultaneously. The chromosomes move to the center of the cell (i.e., to the cell's equator), and the spindle forms. The spindle is composed of fibers that cross the cell, linking its poles. Once the chromosomes are stabilized at the equator of the cell, their centromeres divide, and metaphase is complete.

The phase that follows, **anaphase**, is characterized by a movement of the chromosomes on the spindle to the poles. The chromosomes appear to be pulled toward the poles of the cell by fibers attached to the centromeres. The arms, particularly the long arms, tend to trail behind.

Anaphase is followed by the last phase of mitosis, **telophase**. In this phase, the chromosomes, congregated at the poles of the cell, begin to uncoil. The nuclear membrane reappears, as do the nucleoli; and as the phase progresses, the chromosome coils unwind until the nucleus regains the appearance characteristic of interphase.

THE ROLE OF TELOMERES

Telomeres cap and protect the terminal ends of chromosomes. The name *telomere* literally means "end part." Mammalian telomeres consist of long arrays of TTAGGG repeats that range in total length anywhere from 1.5 to 150 kilobases. Each time a normal somatic cell divides, telomeric DNA is lost from the lagging strand, because DNA polymerase cannot synthesize new DNA in the absence of an RNA primer. Successive divisions lead to progressive shortening, and after 40 to 60 divisions, the telomeres in human cells are shortened dramatically, so that vital DNA sequences begin to be lost. At this point, the cell cannot divide further and undergoes senescence. Telomere length has been described as the "molecular clock" or generational clock, because it shortens with age in somatic tissue cells during adult life. Stem cells in self-renewing tissues, and cancer cells in particular, avoid this problem of aging by activating the enzyme telomerase. Telomerase is a reverse transcriptase that includes the complementary sequence to the TTAGGG repeats and so continually rebuilds the chromosome ends to offset the degradation that occurs with each division. In this way, the cell becomes immortal.

In tissue culture, immortalization of cells—that is, the process whereby cells pass through a "crisis" and continue to be able to divide beyond the normal limit— is associated with telomere stabilization and telomerase activity.

Virtually all human tumor cell lines and approximately 90% of human cancer biopsy specimens exhibit telomerase activity. By contrast, normal human somatic tissues, other than stem cells, do not possess detectable levels of this enzyme. It is an attractive hypothesis that both immortalization and carcinogenesis are associated with telomerase expression.

RADIATION-INDUCED CHROMOSOME ABERRATIONS

In the traditional study of chromosome aberrations, the effects of ionizing radiations are described in terms of their appearance when a preparation is made at the first metaphase after exposure to radiation. This is the time when the structure of the chromosomes can be discerned.

The study of radiation damage in mammalian cell chromosomes is hampered by the large number of mammalian chromosomes per cell and by their small size. Most mammalian cells currently available for experimental purposes have a diploid complement of 40 or more chromosomes. There are exceptions, such as the Chinese hamster, with 22 chromosomes, and various marsupials, such as the rat kangaroo and woolly opossum, which have chromosome complements of 12 and 14, respectively. Many plant cells, however, contain fewer and generally much larger chromosomes; consequently, until recently, information on chromosomal radiation damage accrued principally from studies with plant cells.

If cells are irradiated with x-rays, double-strand breaks are produced in the chromosomes. The broken ends appear to be "sticky" because of unpaired bases and can rejoin with any other sticky end. It would appear, however, that a broken end cannot join with a normal, unbroken chromosome, although this is controversial. Once breaks are produced, different fragments may behave in a variety of ways:

1. The breaks may restitute, that is, rejoin in their original configuration. In this case, of course, nothing amiss is visible at the next mitosis.
2. The breaks may fail to rejoin and give rise to an aberration, which is scored as a deletion at the next mitosis.
3. Broken ends may reassort and rejoin other broken ends to give rise to chromosomes that appear to be grossly distorted if viewed at the following mitosis.

The aberrations seen at metaphase are of two classes: *chromosome* aberrations and *chromatid* aberrations. **Chromosome aberrations** result if a cell is irradiated early in interphase, before the chromosome material has been duplicated. In this case, the radiation-induced break is in a single strand of chromatin; during the DNA synthetic phase that follows, this strand of chromatin lays down an identical strand next to itself and replicates the break that has been produced by the radiation. This leads to a chromosome aberration visible at the next mitosis, because there is an identical break in the corresponding points of a pair of chromatin strands. If, on the other hand, the dose of radiation is given later in interphase, after the DNA material has doubled and the chromosomes consist of two strands of chromatin, then the aberrations produced are called **chromatid aberrations**. In regions removed from the centromere, chromatid arms may be fairly well separated, and it is reasonable to suppose that the radiation might break one chromatid without breaking its sister chromatid, or at least not in the same place. A break that occurs in a single chromatid arm after chromosome replication and leaves the opposite arm of the same chromosome undamaged leads to chromatid aberrations.

EXAMPLES OF RADIATION-INDUCED ABERRATIONS

Many types of chromosomal aberrations and rearrangements are possible, but an exhaustive analysis is beyond the scope of this book. Three types of aberrations that are *lethal* to the cell are described, followed by two common rearrangements that are consistent with cell viability but are frequently involved in carcinogenesis. The three lethal aberrations are the dicentric and the ring, which are chromosome aberrations, and the anaphase bridge, which is a chromatid aberration. All three represent gross distortions and are clearly visible. Many other aberrations are possible but are not described here.

The formation of a **dicentric** is illustrated in diagrammatic form in Figure 2.6**A**. This aberration involves an interchange between two separate chromosomes. If a break is produced in each one early in interphase and the sticky ends are close to one another, they may rejoin as shown. This bizarre interchange is replicated during the DNA synthetic phase, and the result is a grossly distorted chromosome with two centromeres (hence, dicentric). There also are two fragments that have no centromere (acentric fragment), which will therefore be lost at a subsequent mitosis. The appearance at metaphase is shown in the bottom panel of Figure 2.6**A**. An example of a dicentric and fragment in a metaphase human cell is shown in Figure 2.7**B**; Figure 2.7**A** shows a normal metaphase for comparison.

The formation of a **ring** is illustrated in diagrammatic form in Figure 2.6**B**. A break is induced by radiation in each arm of a single chromatid early in the cell cycle. The sticky ends may rejoin to form a ring and a fragment. Later in the cycle, during the DNA synthetic phase, the chromosome replicates. The ultimate appearance at metaphase is shown in the lower panel of Figure 2.6**B**. The fragments have no centromere and probably will be lost at mitosis because they will not be pulled to either pole of the cell. An example of a ring chromosome in a human cell at metaphase is illustrated in Figure 2.7**C**.

An **anaphase bridge** may be produced in a variety of ways. As illustrated in Figure 2.6**C** and Figure 2.8, it results from breaks that occur late in the cell cycle (in G_2), after the chromosomes have replicated. Breaks may occur in both chromatids of the same chromosome, and the sticky ends may rejoin incorrectly to form a sister union. At anaphase, when the two sets of chromosomes move to opposite poles, the section of chromatin between the two centromeres is stretched across the cell between the poles, hindering the separation into two new progeny cells, as illustrated in Figure 26**C** and Figure 2.8**B**. The two fragments may join as shown, but because there is no centromere, the joined fragments will probably be lost at the first mitosis. This type of aberration occurs in human cells and is essentially always lethal. It is hard to demonstrate because preparations of human chromosomes usually are made by accumulating cells at metaphase, and the bridge is only evident at anaphase. Figure 2.8 is an anaphase preparation of *Tradescantia paludosa*, a plant used extensively for cytogenetic studies because of the small number of large chromosomes. The anaphase bridge is seen clearly as the replicate sets of chromosomes move to opposite poles of the cell.

Gross chromosome changes of the types discussed previously inevitably lead to the reproductive death of the cell.

Two important types of chromosomal changes that are not lethal to the cell are symmetric translocations and small deletions. The formation of a **symmetric translocation** is illustrated in Figure 2.9**A**. It involves a break in two prereplication (G_1) chromosomes, with the broken ends being exchanged between the two chromosomes as illustrated. An aberration of this type is difficult to see in a conventional preparation but is easy to observe with the technique of fluorescent *in situ* hybridization (FISH), or *chromosome painting*, as it commonly is called. Probes are available for every human chromosome that make them fluorescent in a bright color. Exchange of material between two different chromosomes then is readily observable. Translocations are associated with several human malignancies caused by the activation of an oncogene; Burkitt's lymphoma and certain types of leukemia are examples.

The other type of nonlethal chromosomal change is a **small interstitial deletion**. This is illustrated in Figure 2.9**B** and may result from two breaks in the same arm of the same chromosome, leading to the loss of the genetic information between the two breaks. The actual sequence of events in the formation of a deletion is easier to understand from Figure 2.10, which shows an interphase chromosome. It is a simple matter to imagine how two breaks may isolate a loop of DNA—an acentric ring—which is lost at a subsequent mitosis. Deletions may be associated with carcinogenesis if the lost genetic material includes a tumor suppressor gene. This is discussed further in Chapter 10 on radiation carcinogenesis.

The interaction between breaks in different chromosomes is by no means random. There is great heterogeneity in the sites at which deletions and exchanges between different chromosomes occur; for example, chromosome 8 is particularly sensitive to exchanges. As mentioned previously, each chromosome is restricted to a domain, and most interactions occur at the edges of domains, which probably

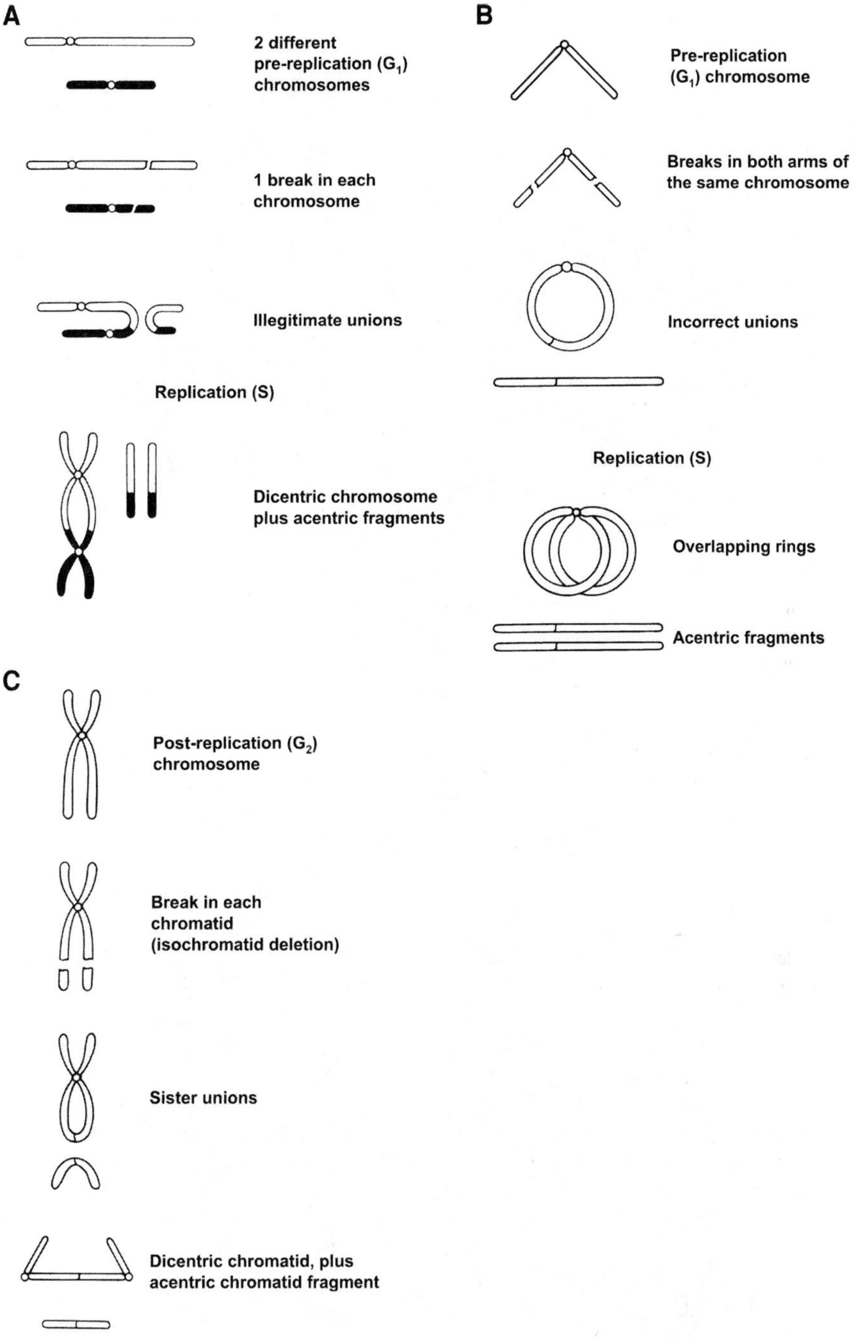

FIGURE 2.6 ● **A:** The steps in the formation of a dicentric by irradiation of prereplication (i.e., G_1) chromosomes. A break is produced in each of two separate chromosomes. The "sticky" ends may join incorrectly to form an interchange between the two chromosomes. Replication then occurs in the DNA synthetic period. One chromosome has two centromeres: a dicentric. The acentric fragment will also replicate and both will be lost at a subsequent mitosis because, lacking a centromere, they will not go to either pole at anaphase. **B:** The steps in the formation of a ring by irradiation of a prereplication (i.e., G_1) chromosome. A break occurs in each arm of the same chromosome. The sticky ends rejoin incorrectly to form a ring and an acentric fragment. Replication then occurs. **C:** The steps in the formation of an anaphase bridge by irradiation of a postreplication (i.e., G_2) chromosome. Breaks occur in each chromatid of the same chromosome. Incorrect rejoining of the sticky ends then occurs in a sister union. At the next anaphase, the acentric fragment will be lost, one centromere of the dicentric will go to each pole, and the chromatid will be stretched between the poles. Separation of the progeny cells is not possible; this aberration is likely to be lethal. (Courtesy of Dr. Charles Geard.)

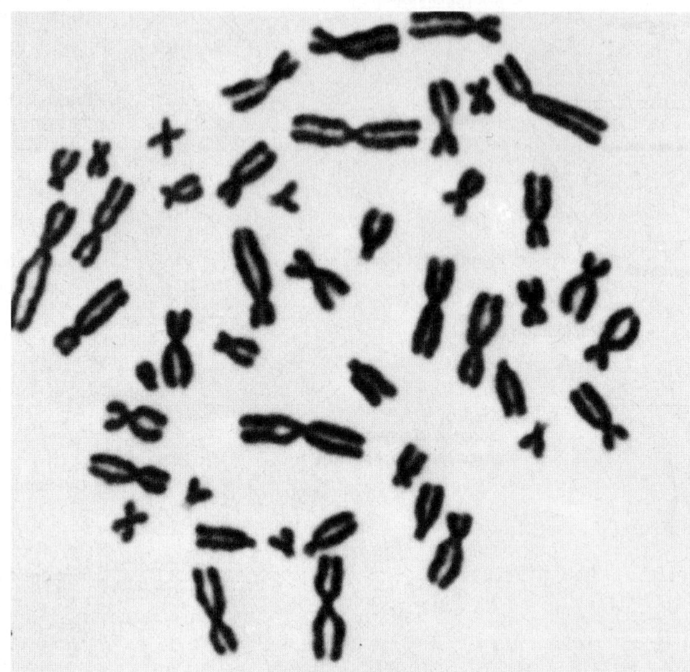

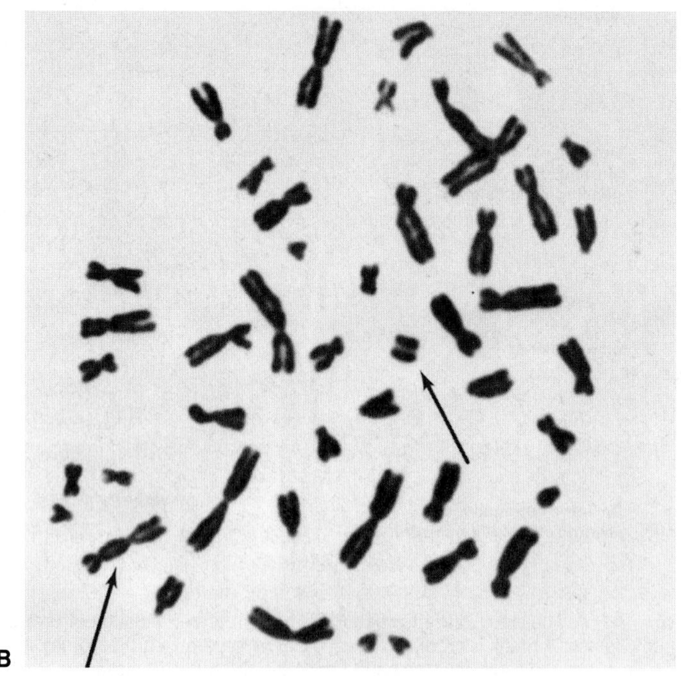

FIGURE 2.7 ● Radiation-induced chromosome aberrations in human leukocytes viewed at metaphase. **A:** Normal metaphase. **B:** Dicentric and fragment (arrows). *(Continued)*

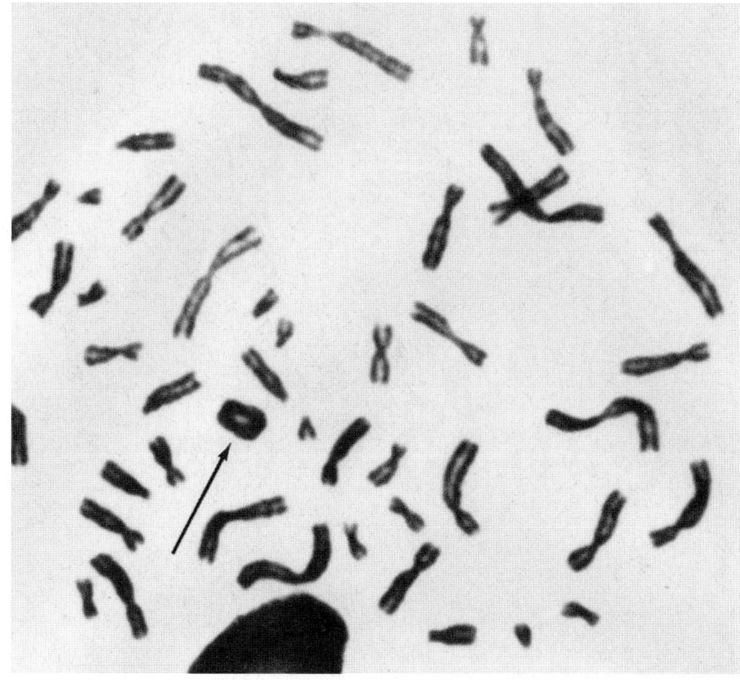

FIGURE 2.7 *(Continued)* • **C:** Ring (arrow). (Courtesy of Drs. Brewen, Luippold, and Preston.)

involves the nuclear matrix. Active chromosomes are therefore those with the biggest surface area to their domains.

CHROMOSOME ABERRATIONS IN HUMAN LYMPHOCYTES

Chromosomal aberrations in peripheral lymphocytes have been used widely as biomarkers of radiation exposure. In blood samples obtained for cytogenetic evaluation within a few days to a few weeks after total-body irradiation, the frequency of asymmetric aberrations (dicentrics and rings) in the lymphocytes reflects the dose received. Lymphocytes in the blood sample are stimulated to divide with a mitogen such as phytohemagglutinin and are arrested at metaphase, and the incidence of rings and dicentrics is scored. The dose can be estimated by comparison with *in vitro* cultures exposed to known doses. Figure 2.11 shows a dose–response curve for aberrations in human lymphocytes produced by γ-rays. The data are fitted by a linear-quadratic relationship, as would be expected, because rings and dicentrics result from the interaction of two chromosome breaks, as previously described. The linear component is a consequence of the two breaks resulting from a single charged particle. If the two breaks result from different charged particles, the probability of an interaction is a quadratic function of dose. This also is illustrated for the formation of a dicentric in Figure 2.11.

If a sufficient number of metaphases are scored, cytogenetic evaluations in cultured lymphocytes readily can detect a recent total-body exposure of as low as 0.25 Gy (25 rad) in the exposed person. Such studies are useful in distinguishing between "real" and "suspected" exposures, particularly in those instances involving "black film badges" or in potential accidents in which it is not certain whether individuals who were at risk for exposure actually received radiation doses.

Mature T lymphocytes have a finite life span of about 1,500 days and are eliminated slowly from the peripheral lymphocyte pool. Consequently, the yield of dicentrics observed in peripheral lymphocytes declines in the months and years after a radiation exposure.

During *in vivo* exposures to ionizing radiation, chromosome aberrations are induced not only in mature lymphocytes but also in lymphocyte progenitors in marrow, nodes, or other organs. The stem cells that sustain asymmetric aberrations (such as dicentrics) die in attempting a subsequent mitosis,

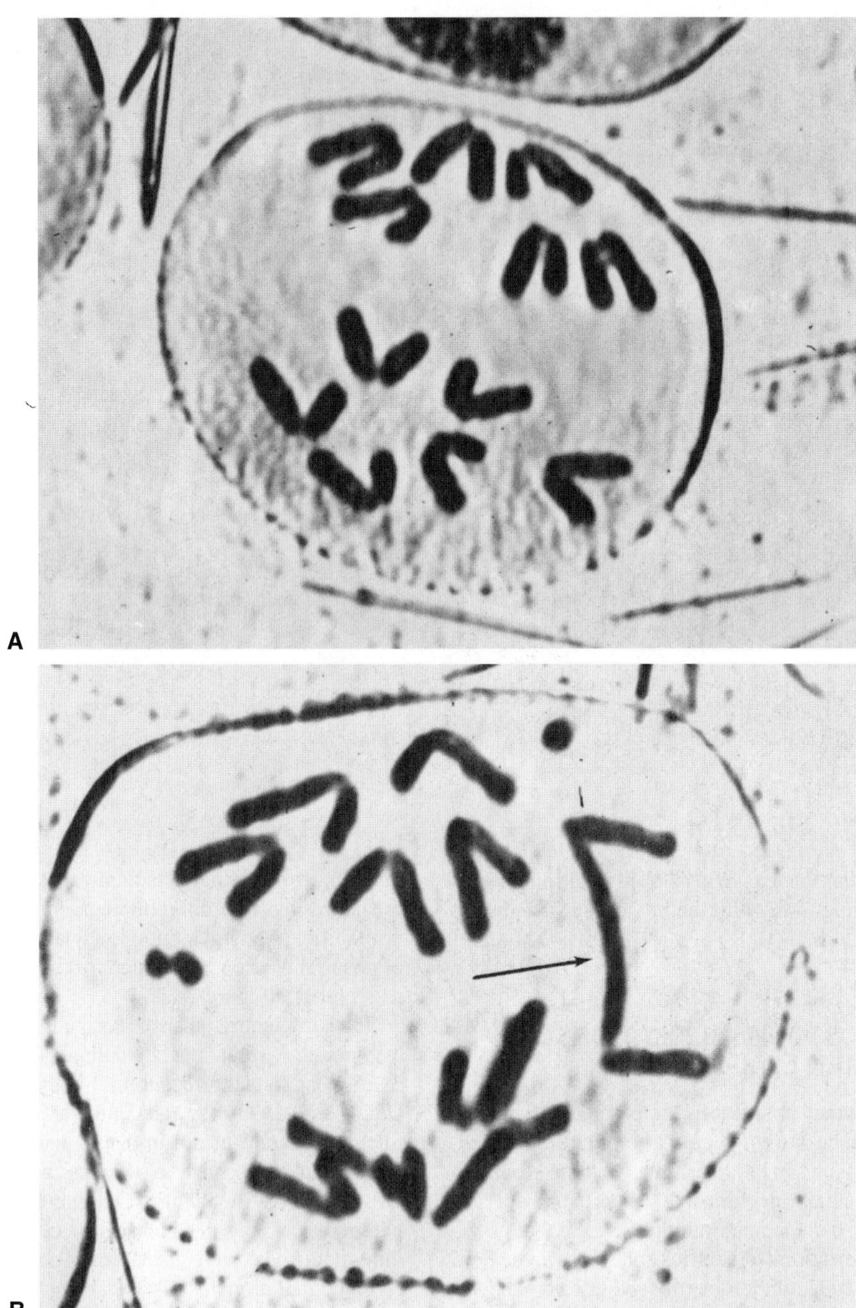

FIGURE 2.8 ● Anaphase chromosome preparation of *Tradescantia paludosa*. **A:** Normal anaphase. **B:** Bridge and fragment resulting from radiation (arrow). (Courtesy of Drs. Brewen, Luippold, and Preston.)

but those that sustain a symmetric nonlethal aberration (such as a translocation) survive and pass on the aberration to their progeny. Consequently, dicentrics are referred to as "unstable" aberrations, because their number declines with time after irradiation. Symmetric translocations, by contrast, are referred to as "stable" aberrations, because they persist for many years. Either type of aberration can be used to estimate dose soon after irradiation, but if many years have elapsed, scoring dicentrics

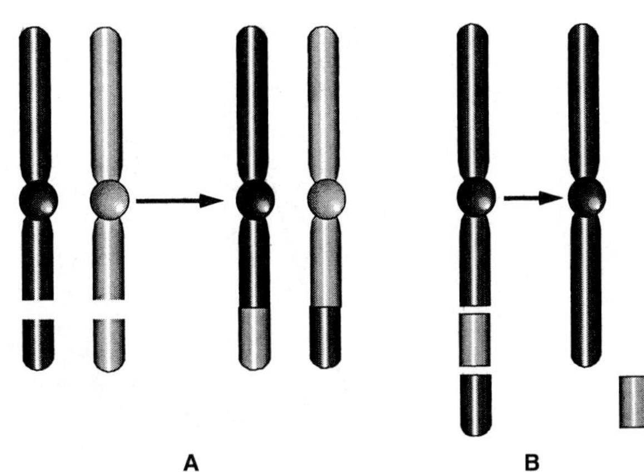

FIGURE 2.9 ● **A:** Formation of a symmetric translocation. Radiation produces breaks in two different prereplication chromosomes. The broken pieces are exchanged between the two chromosomes, and the "sticky" ends rejoin. This aberration is not necessarily lethal to the cell. There are examples in which an exchange aberration of this type leads to the activation of an oncogene. See Chapter 10 on radiation carcinogenesis. **B:** Diagram of a deletion. Radiation produces two breaks in the same arm of the same chromosome. What actually happens is illustrated more clearly in Figure 2.10.

underestimates the dose, and only stable aberrations such as translocations give an accurate picture. Until recently, translocations were much more difficult to observe than dicentrics, but now the technique of fluorescent *in situ* hybridization makes the scoring of such symmetric aberrations a relatively simple matter. The frequency of translocations assessed in this way correlates with total-body dose in exposed individuals even after more than 50 years, as was shown in a study of the survivors of the atomic-bomb attacks on Hiroshima and Nagasaki.

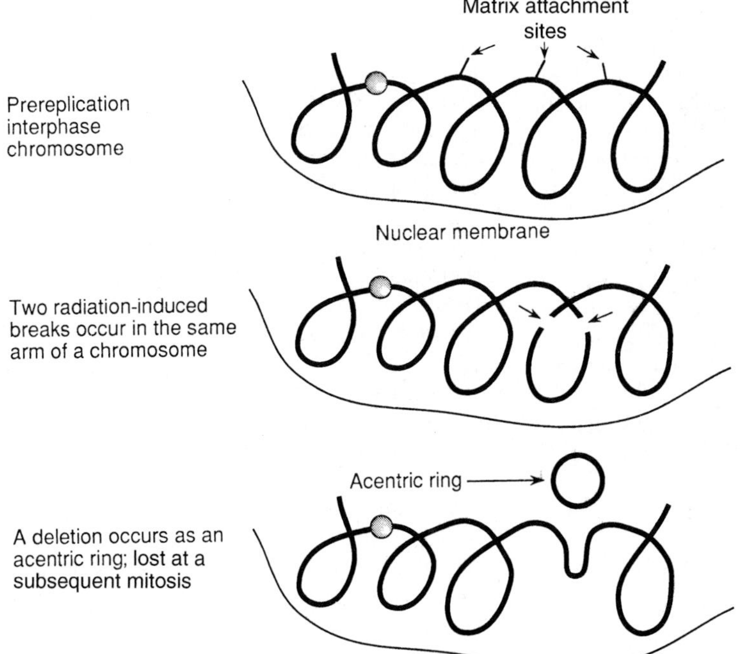

FIGURE 2.10 ● Formation of a deletion by ionizing radiation in an interphase chromosome. It is easy to imagine how two breaks may occur (by a single or two different charged particles) in such a way as to isolate a loop of DNA. The "sticky" ends rejoin, and the deletion is lost at a subsequent mitosis because it has no centromere. This loss of DNA may include the loss of a suppressor gene and lead to a malignant change. See Chapter 10 on radiation carcinogenesis.

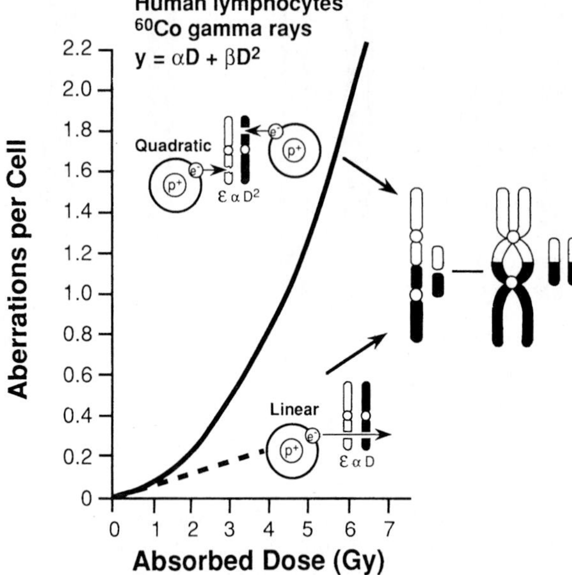

FIGURE 2.11 • The frequency of chromosomal aberrations (dicentrics and rings) is a linear-quadratic function of dose because the aberrations are the consequence of the interaction of two separate breaks. At low doses, both breaks may be caused by the same electron; the probability of an exchange aberration is proportional to dose (D). At higher doses, the two breaks are more likely to be caused by separate electrons. The probability of an exchange aberration is proportional to the square of the dose (D^2).

Summary of Pertinent Conclusions

- Many single-strand breaks are produced in DNA by radiation but are repaired readily using the opposite DNA strand as a template.
- Breaks in both strands, if well separated, also are repaired readily because they are handled individually.
- Breaks in both strands that are opposite or separated by only a few base pairs may lead to a double-strand break.
- Energy from x-rays is deposited unevenly in "spurs" and "blobs." This may lead to locally multiply damaged sites, that is, combinations of double-strand breaks and base damage.
- A variety of techniques have been used to measure DNA double-strand breaks, including sucrose gradient sedimentation, alkaline and neutral filter elution, nucleoid sedimentation, pulsed-field gel electrophoresis, and single-cell gel electrophoresis (the comet assay).
- There is good reason to believe that double-strand breaks rather than single-strand breaks lead to important biologic end points, including cell death, carcinogenesis, and mutation.
- Radiation-induced breakage and incorrect rejoining in prereplication (G_1) chromosomes may lead to chromosome aberrations.
- Radiation-induced breakage and incorrect rejoining in postreplication (late S or G_2) chromosomes may lead to chromatid aberrations.
- Lethal aberrations include dicentrics, rings, and anaphase bridges. Symmetric translocations and small deletions are nonlethal.
- There is a good correlation between cells killed and cells with asymmetric exchange aberrations (i.e., dicentrics or rings).
- The incidence of most radiation-induced aberrations is a linear-quadratic function of dose.
- Scoring aberrations in lymphocytes from peripheral blood may be used to estimate total-body doses in humans accidentally irradiated. The lowest single dose that can be detected readily is 0.25 Gy (25 rad).
- Dicentrics are "unstable" aberrations; they are lethal to the cell and are not passed on to progeny. Consequently, the incidence of dicentrics declines slowly with time after exposure.
- Translocations are "stable" aberrations; they persist for many years because they are not lethal to the cell and are passed on to the progeny.

BIBLIOGRAPHY

Alper T, Fowler JF, Morgan RL, Vonberg DD, Ellis F, Oliver R: The characterization of the "type C" survival curve. *Br J Radiol* 35:722–723, 1962

Andrews JR, Berry RJ: Fast neutron irradiation and the relationship of radiation dose and mammalian cell reproductive capacity. *Radiat Res* 16:76–81, 1962

Barendsen GW, Beusker TLJ, Vergroesen AJ, Budke L: Effects of different ionizing radiations on human cells in tissue culture: II. Biological experiments. *Radiat Res* 13:841–849, 1960

Bender M: Induced aberrations in human chromosomes. *Am J Pathol* 43:26a, 1963

Blackburn EH: Telomeres. *Annu Rev Biochem* 61:113–129, 1992

Carrano AV: Chromosome aberrations and radiation-induced cell death: II. Predicted and observed cell survival. *Mutat Res* 17:355–366, 1973

Cornforth MN, Bedford JS: A quantitative comparison of potentially lethal damage repair and the rejoining of interphase chromosome breaks in low passage normal human fibroblasts. *Radiat Res* 111:385–405, 1987

Cornforth MN, Bedford JS: X-ray-induced breakage and rejoining of human interphase chromosomes. *Science* 222:1141–1143, 1983

Cremer C, Munkel C, Granzow M, et al.: Nuclear architecture and the induction of chromosomal aberrations. *Mutat Res* 366(2):97–116, 1996

Elkind MM, Sutton H: Radiation response of mammalian cells grown in culture: I. Repair of x-ray damage in surviving Chinese hamster cells. *Radiat Res* 13:556–593, 1960

Evans HJ: Chromosome aberrations induced by ionizing radiation. *Int Rev Cytol* 13:221–321, 1962

Frankenberg D, Frankenberg-Schwager M, Harbich R: Split-dose recovery is due to the repair of DNA double-strand breaks. *Int J Radiat Biol* 46:541–553, 1984

Gasser SM, Laemmli UK: A glimpse at chromosomal order. *Trends Genet* 3:16–22, 1987

Geard CR: Effects of radiation on chromosomes. In Pizzarello D (ed): *Radiation Biology*, pp. 83–110. Boca Raton, FL, CRC Press, 1982

Georgiev GP, Nedospasov SA, Bakayev VV: Supranucleosomal levels of chromatin organization. In Busch H (ed): *The Cell Nucleus*, vol 6, pp. 3–34. New York, Academic Press, 1978

Gilson E, Laroche T, Gasser SM: Telomeres and the functional architecture of the nucleus. *Trends Cell Biol* 3:128–134, 1993

Grell RF: The chromosome. *J Tenn Acad Sci* 37:43–53, 1962

Ishihara T, Sasaki MS (eds): *Radiation-Induced Chromosome Damage in Man*. New York, Alan R Liss, 1983

Lea DEA: *Actions of Radiations on Living Cells*, 2nd ed. Cambridge, UK, Cambridge University Press, 1956

Littlefield LG, Lushbaugh CC: Cytogenetic dosimetry for radiation accidents: "The good, the bad, and the ugly." In Ricks RC, Fry SA (eds): *The Medical Basis for Radiation Accident Preparedness*, vol 2, *Clinical Experience and Follow-up Since 1979*, pp. 461–478. New York, Elsevier, 1990

Littlefield LG, Kleinerman RA, Sayer AM, Tarone R, Boice JD Jr: Chromosome aberrations in lymphocytes-biomonitors of radiation exposure. In Barton L, Gledhill I, Francesco M (eds): *New Horizons in Biological Dosimetry*, pp. 387–397. New York, Wiley Liss, 1991

Marsden M, Laemmli UK: Metaphase chromosome structure: Evidence for a radial loop model. *Cell* 17:849–858, 1979

Moorhead PS, Nowell PC, Mellman WJ, Battips DM, Hungerford DA: Chromosome preparation of leukocytes cultured from human peripheral blood. *Exp Cell Res* 20:613–616, 1960

Muller HJ: The remaking of chromosomes. In *Studies in Genetics: The Selected Papers of HJ Muller*, pp. 384–408. Bloomington, Indiana University Press,1962

Munro TR: The relative radiosensitivity of the nucleus and cytoplasm of the Chinese hamster fibroblasts. *Radiat Res* 42:451–470, 1970

Puck TT, Markus PI: Action of x-rays on mammalian cells. *J Exp Med* 103:653–666, 1956

Revell SH: Relationship between chromosome damage and cell death. In Ishihara T, Sasaki MS (eds): *Radiation-Induced Chromosome Damage in Man*, pp. 215–233. New York, Alan R Liss, 1983

Ris H: Chromosome structure. In McElroy WD, Glass B (eds): *Chemical Basis of Heredity*. Baltimore, Johns Hopkins University Press, 1957

Spear FG: On some biological effects of radiation. *Br J Radiol* 31:114–124, 1958

Ward JF: DNA damage produced by ionizing radiation in mammalian cells: identities, mechanisms of formation and repairability. *Prog Nucleic Acid Res Mol Biol* 35:95–125, 1988

Ward JF: Some biochemical consequences of the spatial distribution of ionizing radiation produced free radicals. *Radiat Res* 86:185–195, 1981

CHAPTER 3

Cell Survival Curves

REPRODUCTIVE INTEGRITY

A **cell survival curve** describes the relationship between the radiation dose and the proportion of cells that survive. What is meant by "survival"? Cell survival, or its converse, cell death, may mean different things in different contexts; therefore, a precise definition is essential. For differentiated cells that do not proliferate, such as nerve, muscle, or secretory cells, death can be defined as the loss of a specific function. For proliferating cells, such as stem cells in the hematopoietic system or the intestinal epithelium, loss of the capacity for sustained proliferation—that is, loss of *reproductive integrity*—is an appropriate definition. This is sometimes called **reproductive death**. This is certainly the end point measured with cells cultured *in vitro*.

This definition reflects a narrow view of radiobiology. A cell still may be physically present and apparently intact, may be able to make proteins or synthesize DNA, and may even be able to struggle through one or two mitoses; but if it has lost the capacity to divide indefinitely and produce a large number of progeny, it is by definition dead; it has not survived. A survivor that has retained its reproductive integrity and is able to proliferate indefinitely to produce a large clone or colony is said to be *clonogenic*.

This definition is generally relevant to the radiobiology of whole animals and plants and their tissues. It has particular relevance to the radiotherapy of tumors. For a tumor to be eradicated, it is only necessary that cells be "killed" in the sense that they are rendered unable to divide and cause further growth and spread of the malignancy. Cells may die by different mechanisms, as is described here subsequently. For most cells, death while attempting to divide, that is, **mitotic death**, is the dominant mechanism following irradiation. For some cells, programmed cell death, or **apoptosis**, is important.

Whatever the mechanism, the outcome is the same: The cell loses its ability to proliferate indefinitely, that is, its reproductive integrity.

In general, a dose of 100 Gy (10,000 rad) is necessary to destroy cell function in nonproliferating systems. By contrast, the mean lethal dose for loss of proliferative capacity is usually less than 2 Gy (200 rad).

THE *IN VITRO* SURVIVAL CURVE

The capability of a single cell to grow into a large colony that can be seen easily with the naked eye is a convenient proof that it has retained its reproductive integrity. The loss of this ability as a function of radiation dose is described by the dose–survival curve.

With modern techniques of tissue culture, it is possible to take a specimen from a tumor or from many normal regenerative tissues, chop it into small pieces, and prepare a single-cell suspension by the use of the enzyme trypsin, which dissolves and loosens the cell membrane. If these cells are seeded into a culture dish, covered with an appropriate complex growth medium, and maintained at 37°C under aseptic conditions, they attach to the surface, grow, and divide.

In practice, most fresh explants grow well for a few weeks but subsequently peter out and die. A few pass through a crisis and continue to grow for many years. Every few days, the culture must be "farmed": The cells are removed from the surface with trypsin, most of the cells are discarded, and the culture flask is reseeded with a small number of cells, which quickly repopulate the culture flask. These are called **established cell lines**; they have been used extensively in experimental cellular radiobiology.

Survival curves are so basic to an understanding of much of radiobiology that it is worth going through the steps involved in a typical experiment using an established cell line in culture.

Cells from an actively growing stock culture are prepared into a suspension by the use of trypsin, which causes the cells to round up and detach from the surface of the culture vessel. The number of cells per unit volume of this suspension is counted in a hemocytometer or with an electronic counter. In this way, for example, 100 individual cells may be seeded into a dish; if this dish is incubated for 1 to 2 weeks, each single cell divides many times and forms a colony that is easily visible with the naked eye, especially if it is fixed and stained (Fig. 3.1). All cells making up each colony are the progeny of a single ancestor. For a nominal 100 cells seeded into the dish, the number of colonies counted may be expected to be in the range of 50 to 90. Ideally, it should be 100, but it seldom is for a variety of reasons, including suboptimal growth medium, errors and uncertainties in counting the cell suspension, and the trauma of trypsinization and handling. The term **plating efficiency** indicates the percentage of cells seeded that grow into colonies. The plating

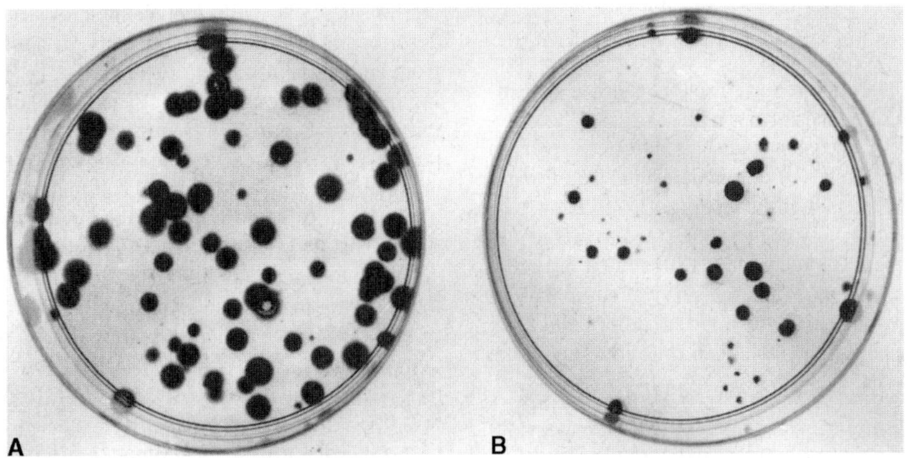

FIGURE 3.1 ● Colonies obtained with Chinese hamster cells cultured *in vitro*. **A:** In this unirradiated control dish, 100 cells were seeded and allowed to grow for 7 days before being stained. There are 70 colonies; therefore, the plating efficiency is 70/100, or 70%. **B:** Two thousand cells were seeded and then exposed to 8 Gy (800 rad) of x-rays. There are 32 colonies on the dish. Thus:

$$\begin{aligned}\text{Surviving fraction} &= \text{Colonies counted}/[\text{Cells seeded} \times (\text{PE}/100)] \\ &= 32/(2{,}000 \times 0.7) \\ &= 0.023\end{aligned}$$

efficiency is given by the formula

$$PE = \frac{\text{Number of colonies counted}}{\text{Number of cells seeded}} \times 100$$

There are 70 colonies on the control dish in Figure 3.1**A**; therefore the plating efficiency is 70%. If a parallel dish is seeded with cells, exposed to a dose of 8 Gy (800 rad) of x-rays, and incubated for 1 to 2 weeks before being fixed and stained, then the following may be observed: (1) Some of the seeded single cells are still single and have not divided, and in some instances the cells show evidence of nuclear deterioration as they die an apoptotic death; (2) some cells have managed to complete one or two divisions to form a tiny abortive colony; and (3) some cells have grown into large colonies that differ little from the unirradiated controls, although they may vary more in size. These cells are said to have survived, because they have retained their reproductive integrity.

In the example shown in Figure 3.1**B**, 2,000 cells had been seeded into the dish exposed to 8 Gy (800 rad). Because the plating efficiency is 70%, 1,400 of the 2,000 cells plated would have grown into colonies if the dish had not been irradiated. In fact, there are only 32 colonies on the dish; the fraction of cells surviving the dose of x-rays is thus

$$\frac{32}{1{,}400} = 0.023$$

In general, the surviving fraction is given by

$$\text{Surviving fraction} = \frac{\text{Colonies counted}}{\text{Cells seeded} \times (\text{PE}/100)}$$

This process is repeated so that estimates of survival are obtained for a range of doses. The number of cells seeded per dish is adjusted so that a countable number of colonies results: Too few reduces statistical significance; too many cannot be counted accurately because they tend to merge into one another. The technique is illustrated in Figure 3.2. This technique, and the survival curve that results, does not distinguish the mode of cell death, that is, whether the cells died mitotic or apoptotic deaths.

THE SHAPE OF THE SURVIVAL CURVE

Survival curves for mammalian cells usually are presented in the form shown in Figure 3.3, with dose plotted on a linear scale and surviving fraction on a logarithmic scale. Qualitatively, the shape of the survival curve can be described in relatively simple terms. At "low doses" for sparsely ionizing (low linear energy transfer) radiations, such as x-rays, the survival curve starts out straight on the log-linear plot with a finite initial slope; that is, the surviving fraction is an exponential function of dose. At higher doses, the curve bends. This bending or curving region extends over a dose range of a few gray (a few hundred rad). At very high doses, the survival curve often tends to straighten again; the surviving fraction returns to being an exponential function of dose. In general, this does not occur until doses in excess of those used as daily fractions in radiotherapy have been reached.

By contrast, for densely ionizing (high linear energy transfer) radiations, such as α-particles or low-energy neutrons, the cell survival curve is a straight line from the origin; that is, survival approximates to an exponential function of dose (see Fig. 3.3).

Although it is a simple matter to qualitatively describe the shape of the cell survival curve, finding an explanation of the biologic observations in terms of biophysical events is another matter. Many biophysical models and theories have been proposed to account for the shape of the mammalian cell survival curve. Almost all can be used to deduce a curve shape that is consistent with experimental data, but it is never possible to choose among different models or theories on the basis of goodness of fit to experimental data. The biologic data are not sufficiently precise, nor are the predictive theoretic curves sufficiently different, for this to be possible.

Two descriptions of the shape of survival curves are discussed briefly, with a minimum of mathematics (see Fig. 3.3). First, the **multitarget model** that was widely used for many years still has some merit (Fig. 3.3**B**). In this model, the survival curve is described in terms of an *initial slope*, D_1, resulting from single-event killing; a *final slope*, D_0, resulting from multiple-event killing; and some quantity (either n or D_q) to represent the size or width of the shoulder of the curve. The quantities D_1 and D_0 are the reciprocals of the initial and final slopes. In each case, it is the dose required to reduce the fraction of surviving cells to 37% of its previous value. As illustrated in Figure 3.3**B**, D_1, the initial slope, is the dose required to reduce the fraction of surviving cells to 0.37 on the initial straight portion of the survival curve. The final slope, D_0, is the dose required to reduce survival from 0.1 to 0.037, or from 0.01 to 0.0037, and so on. Because the surviving fraction is on a logarithmic scale and the survival curve becomes straight at higher doses, the dose required to reduce the cell population by a given factor (to 0.37) is the same at all survival levels. It is, on average, the dose required to deliver one inactivating event per cell.

The **extrapolation number**, n, is a measure of the width of the shoulder. If n is large (e.g., 10 or 12), the survival curve has a broad shoulder. If n is

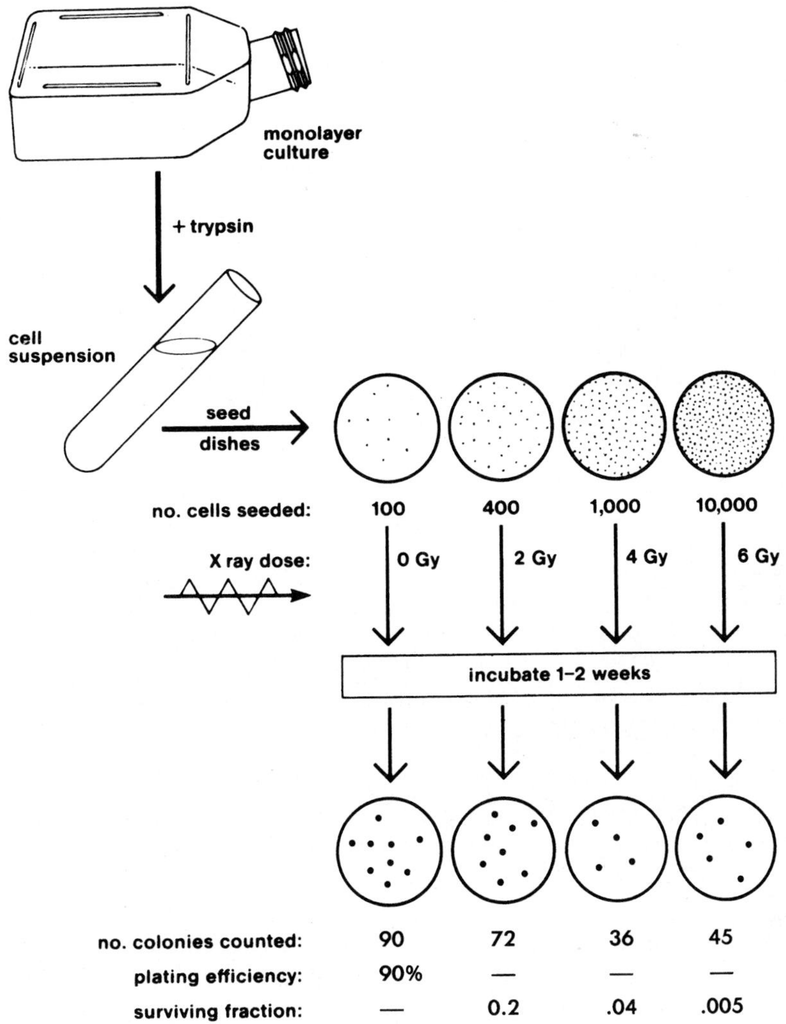

FIGURE 3.2 ● The cell culture technique used to generate a cell survival curve. Cells from a stock culture are prepared into a single-cell suspension by trypsinization, and the cell concentration is counted. Known numbers of cells are inoculated into petri dishes and irradiated. They then are allowed to grow until the surviving cells produce macroscopic colonies that can be counted readily. The number of cells per dish initially inoculated varies with the dose so that the number of colonies surviving is in the range that can be counted conveniently. Surviving fraction is the ratio of colonies produced to cells plated, with a correction necessary for plating efficiency (i.e., for the fact that not all cells plated grow into colonies, even in the absence of radiation).

small (e.g., 1.5 to 2), the shoulder of the curve is narrow. Another measure of shoulder width is the **quasithreshold dose**, shown as D_q in Figure 3.3. This sounds like a term invented by a committee, which in a sense it is. An easy way to remember its meaning is to think of the hunchback of Notre Dame. When the priest was handed the badly deformed infant who was to grow up to be the hunchback, he cradled him in his arms and said, "We will call him Quasimodo—he is almost a person!" Similarly, the quasithreshold dose is almost a threshold dose. It is defined as the dose at which the straight portion of the survival curve, extrapolated backward, cuts the dose axis drawn through a survival fraction of unity. A threshold dose is the dose below which there is no effect. There is no dose below which radiation produces no effect, so there can be no true threshold dose; D_q, the quasithreshold dose, is the closest thing.

At first sight this might appear to be an awkward parameter, but in practice it has certain merits that become apparent in subsequent discussion. The

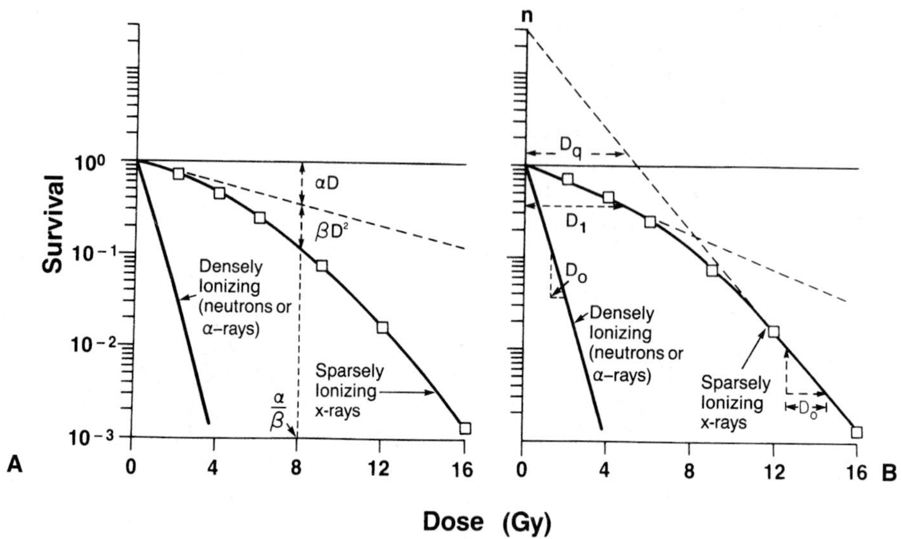

FIGURE 3.3 ● Shape of survival curve for mammalian cells exposed to radiation. The fraction of cells surviving is plotted on a logarithmic scale against dose on a linear scale. For α-particles or low-energy neutrons (said to be densely ionizing), the dose–response curve is a straight line from the origin (i.e., survival is an exponential function of dose). The survival curve can be described by just one parameter, the slope. For x- or γ-rays (said to be sparsely ionizing), the dose–response curve has an initial linear slope, followed by a shoulder; at higher doses, the curve tends to become straight again. **A:** The linear quadratic model. The experimental data are fitted to a linear-quadratic function. There are two components of cell killing: One is proportional to dose (αD); the other is proportional to the square of the dose (βD^2). The dose at which the linear and quadratic components are equal is the ratio α/β. The linear-quadratic curve bends continuously but is a good fit to experimental data for the first few decades of survival. **B:** The multitarget model. The curve is described by the initial slope (D_1), the final slope (D_0), and a parameter that represents the width of the shoulder, either n or D_q.

three parameters, n, D_0, and D_q, are related by the expression

$$\log_e n = D_q/D_0$$

The linear-quadratic model has taken over as the model of choice to describe survival curves. It is a direct development of the relation used to describe exchange-type chromosome aberrations that are clearly the result of an interaction between two separate breaks. This is discussed in some detail in Chapter 2.

The **linear-quadratic model**, illustrated in Figure 3.3**A**, assumes that there are two components to cell killing by radiation, one that is proportional to dose and one that is proportional to the square of the dose. The notion of a component of cell inactivation that varies with the square of the dose introduces the concept of dual-radiation action. This idea goes back to the early work with chromosomes in which many chromosome aberrations are clearly the result of two separate breaks. (Examples discussed in Chapter 2 are dicentrics, rings, and anaphase bridges, all of which are likely to be lethal to the cell.)

By this model, the expression for the cell survival curve is

$$S = e^{-\alpha D - \beta D^2}$$

in which S is the fraction of cells surviving a dose D, and α and β are constants. The components of cell killing that are proportional to dose and to the square of the dose are equal if

$$\alpha D = \beta D^2$$

or

$$D = \alpha/\beta$$

This is an important point that bears repeating: The linear and quadratic contributions to cell killing are equal at a dose that is equal to the ratio of α to β.

A characteristic of the linear-quadratic formulation is that the resultant cell survival curve is continuously bending; there is no final straight portion. This does not coincide with what is observed experimentally if survival curves are determined down to seven or more decades of cell killing, in which case the dose–response relationship closely approximates to a straight line in a log-linear plot; that is, cell killing is an exponential function of dose. In the first decade or so of cell killing and up to any doses used as daily fractions in clinical radiotherapy, however, the linear-quadratic model is an adequate representation of the data. It has the distinct advantage of having only two adjustable parameters, α and β.

MECHANISMS OF CELL KILLING

DNA as the Target

Abundant evidence shows that the principal sensitive sites for radiation-induced cell lethality are located in the nucleus as opposed to the cytoplasm.

Early experiments with nonmammalian systems, such as frog eggs, amoebae, and algae, were designed so that either the cell nucleus or the cytoplasm could be irradiated selectively with a microbeam. The results indicated that the nucleus was much more radiosensitive than the cytoplasm.

Evidence for chromosomal DNA as the principal target for cell killing is circumstantial but overwhelming. There is evidence that the nuclear membrane may also be involved. Indeed, the one does not exclude the other, because some portion of the DNA may be intimately involved with the membrane during some portions of the cell cycle.

The evidence implicating the chromosomes, specifically the DNA, as the primary target for radiation-induced lethality may be summarized as follows:

1. Cells are killed by radioactive tritiated thymidine incorporated into the DNA. The radiation dose results from short-range α-particles and is therefore very localized.
2. Certain structural analogues of thymidine, particularly the halogenated pyrimidines, are incorporated selectively into DNA in place of thymidine if substituted in cell culture growth medium. This substitution dramatically increases the radiosensitivity of the mammalian cells to a degree that increases as a function of the amount of the incorporation. Substituted deoxyuridines, which are not incorporated into DNA, have no such effect on cellular radiosensitivity.
3. Factors that modify cell lethality, such as variation in the type of radiation, oxygen concentration, and dose rate, also affect the production of chromosome damage in a fashion qualitatively and quantitatively similar. This is at least prima facie evidence to indicate that damage to the chromosomes is implicated in cell lethality.
4. Early work showed a relationship between virus size and radiosensitivity; later work showed a better correlation with nucleic acid volume. The radiosensitivity of a wide range of plants has been correlated with the mean interphase chromosome volume, which is defined as the ratio of nuclear volume to chromosome number. The larger the mean chromosome volume, the greater the radiosensitivity.

The Bystander Effect

Generations of students in radiation biology have been taught that hereditary biologic effects require direct damage to DNA, however, experiments in the last decade have demonstrated the existence of a "bystander effect," defined as the induction of biologic effects in cells that are not directly traversed by a charged particle, but are in close proximity to cells that are. Interest in this effect was sparked by the 1992 report of Nagasawa and Little that following a low dose of α-particles, a larger proportion of cells showed biologic damage than was estimated to have been hit by an α-particle; specifically, 30% of the cells showed an increase in sister chromatid exchanges even though less than 1% were calculated to have undergone a nuclear traversal. The number of cells hit was arrived at by a calculation based on the fluence of α-particles and the cross-sectional area of the cell nucleus. The conclusion was thus of a statistical nature, since it was not possible to know on an individual basis which cells were hit and which were not.

This observation has been extended by the use of sophisticated single-particle microbeams, which make it possible to deliver a known number of particles through the nucleus of specific cells whereas biologic effects can be studied in unirradiated close neighbors. Most microbeam studies have utilized α-particles because it is easier to focus them accurately, but a bystander effect has also been shown for protons and soft x-rays. Using single-particle microbeams, a bystander effect has been demonstrated for chromosomal aberrations, cell killing, mutation, oncogenic transformation, and alteration of gene expression. The effect is most pronounced when the bystander cells are in gap-junction communication with the irradiated cells. For example, up to 30% of bystander cells can be killed in this situation. The bystander effect is much smaller when cell monolayers are sparsely seeded so that cells are separated by several hundred micrometers. In this situation, 5 to 10% of bystander cells are killed, the effect being due, presumably, to cytotoxic molecules released into the medium. The existence of the bystander effect indicates that the target for radiation damage is larger than the nucleus and indeed larger than the cell itself. Its importance is primarily at low doses, where not all cells are "hit," and it may have important implications in risk estimation.

In addition to the experiments described above involving sophisticated single-particle microbeams, there is a body of data involving the transfer of medium from irradiated cells, which results in a biologic effect (cell killing) when added to unirradiated cells. These studies, which also evoke the term *bystander effect*, suggest that irradiated cells secrete a molecule into the medium, that is capable of killing cells when that medium is transferred onto unirradiated cells. The majority of bystander experiments involving medium transfer have utilized low-LET x- or γ-rays.

Apoptotic and Mitotic Death

Apoptosis was first described by Kerr and colleagues as a particular set of changes at the microscopic level associated with cell death. The word *apoptosis* is derived from the Greek word meaning "falling off," as in petals from flowers or leaves from trees. Apoptosis, or programmed cell death, is common in embryonic development, in which some tissues become obsolete. It is the mechanism, for example, by which tadpoles lose their tails.

This form of cell death is characterized by a stereotyped sequence of morphologic events. One of the earliest steps a cell takes if it is committed to die in a tissue is to cease communicating with its neighbors. This is evident as the dying cell rounds up and detaches from its neighbors. Condensation of the chromatin at the nuclear membrane and fragmentation of the nucleus are then evident. The cell shrinks because of cytoplasmic condensation, resulting from cross-linking of proteins and loss of water. Eventually, the cell separates into a number of membrane-bound fragments of differing sizes termed *apoptotic bodies*, which may contain cytoplasm only or nuclear fragments. The morphologic hallmark of apoptosis is the condensation of the nuclear chromatin in either crescents around the periphery of the nucleus or a group of spheric fragments.

Double-strand breaks occur in the linker regions between nucleosomes, producing DNA fragments that are multiples of approximately 185 base pairs. These fragments result in the characteristic ladders seen in gels. In contrast, necrosis causes a diffuse "smear" of DNA in gels. Apoptosis occurs in normal tissues, as described previously, and also can be induced in some normal tissues and in some tumors by radiation.

As a mode of radiation-induced cell death, apoptosis is highly cell-type dependent. Hemopoietic and lymphoid cells are particularly prone to rapid radiation-induced cell death by the apoptotic pathway. In most tumor cells, mitotic cell death is at least as important as apoptosis, and in some cases it is the only mode of cell death. A number of genes appear to be involved. First, apoptosis after radiation seems commonly to be a *p53*-dependent process; *bcl-2* is a suppressor of apoptosis.

The most common form of cell death from radiation is mitotic death: Cells die attempting to divide because of damaged chromosomes. Death may occur in the first or a subsequent division following irradiation. Many authors have reported a close quantitative relationship between cell killing and the induction of specific chromosomal aberrations. The results of one of the most elegant studies, by Cornforth and Bedford, are shown in Figure 3.4. It should be noted that these experiments were carried out in a cell line where apoptosis is not observed. The log of the surviving fraction is plotted against the average number of putative "lethal" aberrations per cell, that is, asymmetric exchange-type aberrations such as rings and dicentrics. There is virtually a one-to-one correlation. In addition, there is an excellent correlation between the fraction of cells surviving and the fraction of cells without visible aberrations.

Data such as these provide strong circumstantial evidence to support the notion that asymmetric exchange-type aberrations represent the principle mechanism for radiation-induced mitotic death in mammalian cells.

Figure 3.5 illustrates, in a much oversimplified way, the relationship between chromosome aberrations and cell killing. As explained in Chapter 2, cells in which there is an asymmetric exchange-type aberration (such as a dicentric or a ring) lose their reproductive integrity. Exchange-type aberrations require *two* chromosome breaks. At low doses, the two breaks may result from the passage of a single electron set in motion by the absorption of a photon of x- or γ-rays. The probability of an interaction between the two breaks to form a lethal exchange-type aberration is proportional to dose. Consequently, the survival curve is linear at low doses. At higher doses, the two chromosome breaks may result from two *separate* electrons. The probability of an interaction between the two breaks is then proportional to the square of the dose. If this quadratic component dominates, the survival curve bends over and becomes curved. Thus, the

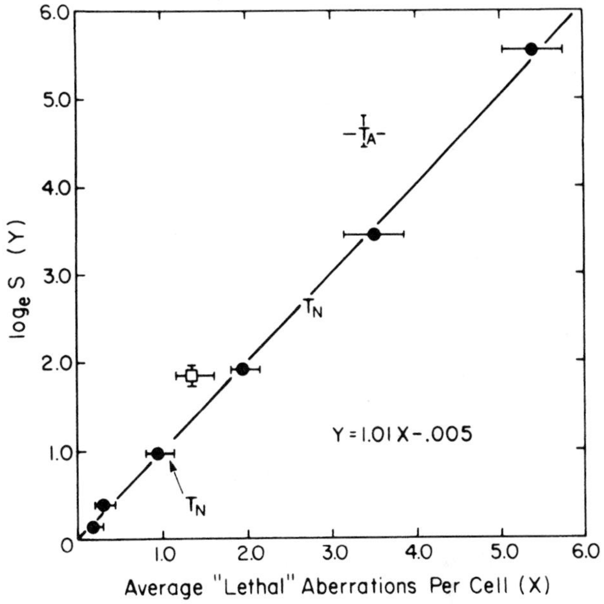

FIGURE 3.4 ● Relationship between the average number of "lethal" aberrations per cell (i.e., asymmetric exchange-type aberrations such as dicentrics and rings) and the log of the surviving fraction in AC 1522 normal human fibroblasts exposed to x-rays. There is virtually a one-to-one correlation. (From Cornforth MN, Bedford JS: A quantitative comparison of potentially lethal damage repair and the rejoining of interphase chromosome breaks in low passage normal human fibroblasts. *Radiat Res* 111:385–405, 1987, with permission.)

linear-quadratic relationship characteristic of the induction of chromosome aberrations is carried over to the cell survival curve.

SURVIVAL CURVES FOR VARIOUS MAMMALIAN CELLS IN CULTURE

Survival curves have been measured for many established cell lines grown in culture. These cell lines have been derived from the tissues of humans or other mammals, such as small rodents. In some cases, the parent tissue has been neoplastic; in other cases, it has been normal. The first *in vitro* survival curve for mammalian cells irradiated with x-rays is shown in Figure 3.6. All mammalian cells studied to date, normal or malignant, regardless of their species of origin, exhibit x-ray survival curves similar to those in Figure 3.6; there is an initial shoulder followed by a portion that tends to become straight on a log-linear plot. The size of the initial shoulder is extremely variable. For some cell lines, the survival curve appears to bend continuously, so that the linear-quadratic relationship is a better fit and n has no meaning. The D_0 of the x-ray survival curves for most cells cultured *in vitro* fall in the range of 1 to 2 Gy (100–200 rad). The exceptions are cells from patients with cancer-prone syndromes, such as ataxia telangiectasia (AT); these cells are much more sensitive to ionizing radiations, with a D_0 for x-rays of about 0.5 Gy (50 rad). This *in vitro* sensitivity

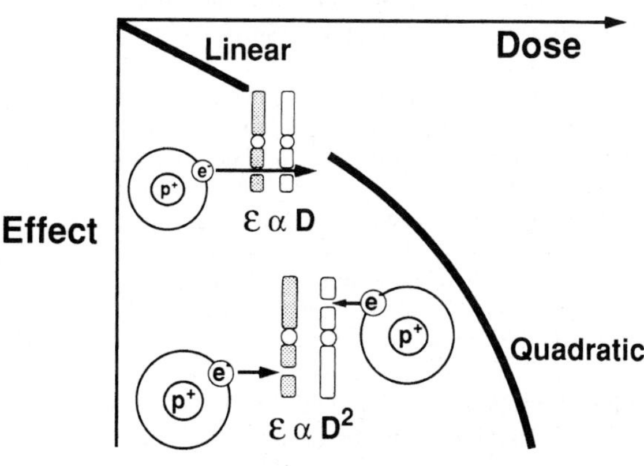

FIGURE 3.5 ● Relationship between chromosome aberrations and cell survival. Cells that suffer exchange-type chromosome aberrations (such as dicentrics) are unable to survive and continue to divide indefinitely. At low doses, the two chromosome breaks are the consequence of a single electron set in motion by the absorption of x- or γ-rays. The probability of an interaction between the breaks is proportional to dose; this is the linear portion of the survival curve. At higher doses, the two chromosome breaks may result also from two separate electrons. The probability of an interaction is then proportional to the square of the dose. The survival curve bends if the quadratic component dominates.

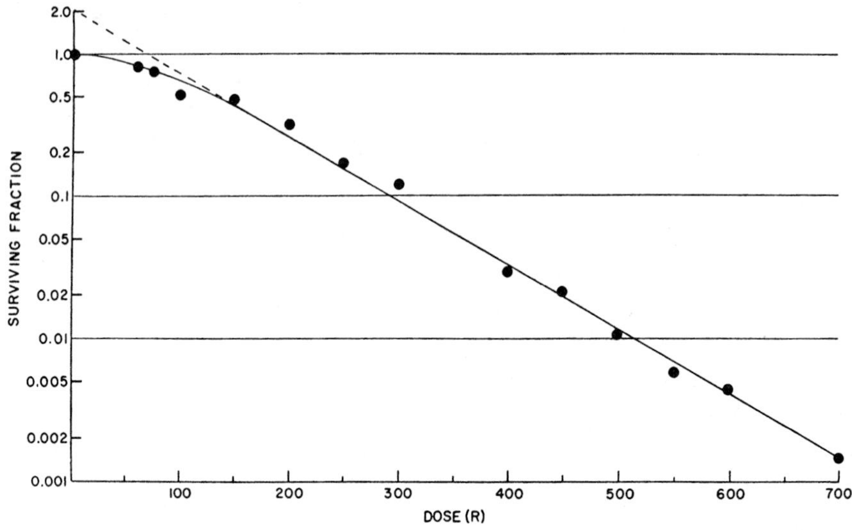

FIGURE 3.6 • Survival curve for HeLa cells in culture exposed to x-rays. Characteristically, this cell line has a small initial shoulder. (From Puck TT, Markus PI: Action of x-rays on mammalian cells. *J Exp Med* 103:653–666, 1956, with permission.)

correlates with a hypersensitivity to radiotherapy found in these patients.

The first *in vitro* survival curve was reported in 1956 and generated great excitement in the field of radiobiology. It was thought that at last, with a quantitative system available to relate absorbed dose with surviving fraction of cells, great strides would be made in understanding the effect of ionizing radiation on biologic materials. In particular, it was anticipated that significant contributions would be made toward understanding radiotherapeutic practice. This enthusiasm was not shared by everyone. Some researchers were skeptical that these *in vitro* techniques, which involved growing cells in petri dishes in very artificial conditions, would ever benefit clinical radiotherapy. The fears of these skeptics were eloquently voiced by F. G. Spear in the MacKenzie Davidson Memorial Lecture given to the British Institute of Radiology in 1957:

> An isolated cell *in vitro* does not necessarily behave as it would have done if left *in vivo* in normal association with cells of other types. Its reactions to various stimuli, including radiations, however interesting and important in themselves, may indeed be no more typical of its behavior in the parent tissue than Robinson Crusoe on his desert island was representative of social life in York in the mid-seventeenth century.

The appropriate answer to this charge was given by David Gould, then professor of radiology at the University of Colorado. He pointed out that the *in vitro* culture technique measured the reproductive integrity of cells and that there was no reason to suppose that Robinson Crusoe's reproductive integrity was any different on his desert island from what it would have been had he remained in York; all that Robinson Crusoe lacked was the opportunity. The opportunity to reproduce to the limit of their capability is afforded to cells cultured *in vitro* if they find themselves in the petri dish, with temperature and humidity controlled and with an abundant supply of nutrients.

At the time, it required a certain amount of faith and optimism to believe that survival curves determined with the *in vitro* technique could be applied to the complex *in vivo* situation. Such faith and optimism were completely vindicated, however, by subsequent events. When techniques became available to measure cell survival *in vivo*, the parameters of the dose–response relationships were shown to be similar to those *in vitro*.

In more recent years, extensive studies have been made of the radiosensitivity of cells of human origin, both normal and malignant, grown and irradiated in culture. In general, cells from a given normal tissue show a narrow range of radiosensitivities if many hundreds of people are studied (Fig. 3.7). By contrast, cells from human tumors show a very broad range of D_0 values; some cells, such as those from squamous carcinomas, tend to be more radioresistant, and sarcomas are somewhat

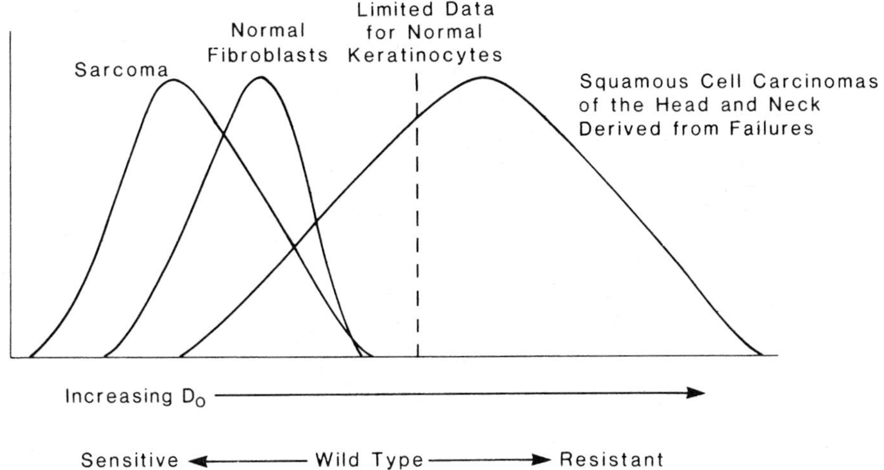

FIGURE 3.7 • Summary of D_0 values for cells of human origin grown and irradiated *in vitro*. Cells from human tumors tend to have a wide range of radiosensitivities, which brackets the radiosensitivity of normal human fibroblasts. In general, squamous cell carcinoma cells are more resistant than sarcoma cells, but the spectra of radiosensitivities are broad and overlap. (Courtesy of Dr. Ralph Wechselbaum.)

more radiosensitive. Each tumor type, however, has a broad spectrum of radiosensitivities that tend to overlap. Tumor cells bracket the radiosensitivity of cells from normal tissues; that is, some are more sensitive, and others are more resistant.

SURVIVAL CURVE SHAPE AND MECHANISMS OF CELL DEATH

Mammalian cells cultured *in vitro* vary considerably in their sensitivity to killing by radiation. This is illustrated in Figure 3.8**A**, which includes survival curves for asynchronous cultures of mouse tumor cells (EMT6) as well as for six cell lines derived from human tumors.

Asynchronous EMT6 cells are the most radioresistant, followed closely by glioblastoma cells of human origin; thereafter radiosensitivity increases, with two neuroblastoma cell lines being the most sensitive. Although asynchronous cells show this wide range of sensitivities to radiation, it is a remarkable finding that mitotic cells from all of these cell lines have essentially the same radiosensitivity. The implication of this is that if the chromosomes are condensed during mitosis, all cell lines have the same radiosensitivity governed simply by DNA content; but in interphase, the radiosensitivity differs because of different conformations of the DNA. Another interesting observation comes from a comparison of the survival curves in Figure 3.8**A** with the DNA laddering in Figure 3.8**B**.

Characteristic laddering is indicative of programmed cell death, or apoptosis, during which the DNA breaks up into discrete lengths as previously described. Comparing Figure 3.8**A** and **B**, it is evident that there is a close and impressive correlation between radiosensitivity and the importance of apoptosis. The most radioresistant cell lines, which have broad shoulders to their survival curves, show no evidence of apoptosis; the most radiosensitive, for which survival is an exponential function of dose, show clear DNA laddering as an indication of apoptosis. The increased clarity of the laddering correlates with increasing radiosensitivity together with a smaller and smaller shoulder to the survival curve. Many of the established cell lines that have been cultured *in vitro* for many years, and with which many of the basic principles of radiation biology were demonstrated, show no apoptotic death and have an abrogated *p53* function. Continued culture *in vitro* appears often to select for cells with this characteristic.

Mitotic death results (principally) from exchange-type chromosomal aberrations; the associated cell survival curve therefore is curved in a log-linear plot, with a broad initial shoulder. As is shown subsequently here, it also is characterized by a substantial dose-rate effect. Apoptotic death results from mechanisms that are not yet clearly understood, but the associated cell survival curve appears to be a straight line on a log-linear plot—that is, survival is an exponential function of dose.

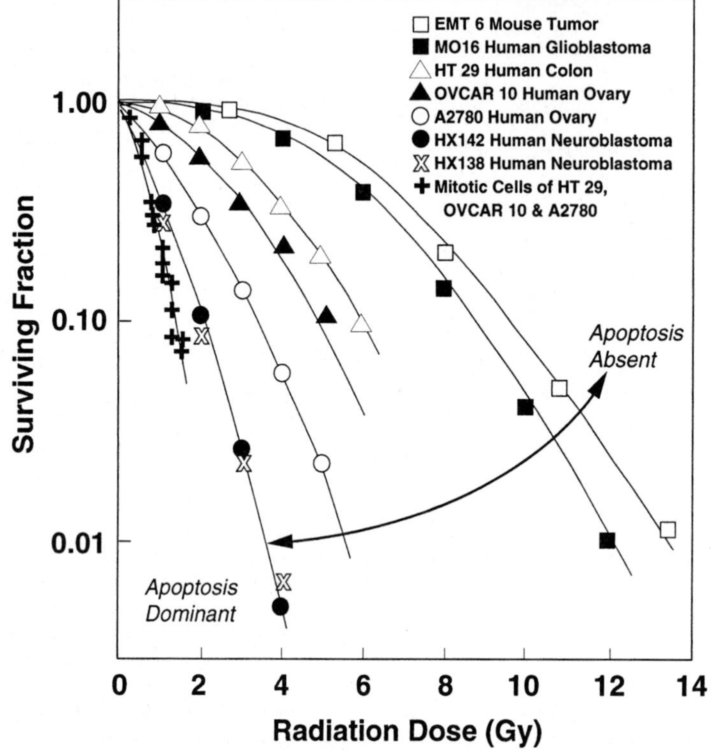

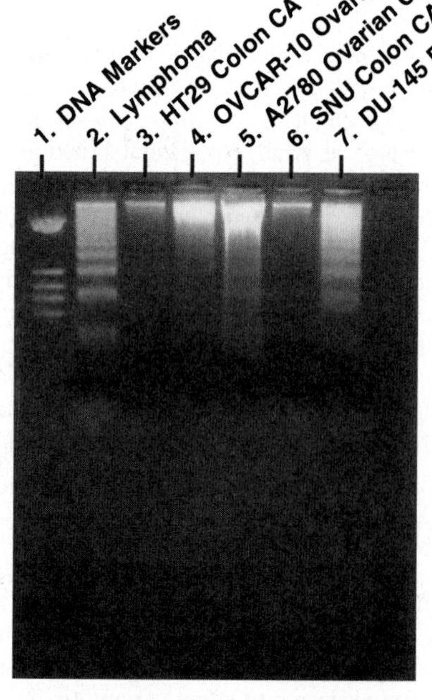

FIGURE 3.8 • **A:** Compilation of survival curves for asynchronous cultures of a number of cell lines of human and rodent origin. Note the wide range of radiosensitivity (most notably the size of the shoulder) between mouse EMT6 cells, the most resistant, and two neuroblastoma cell lines of human origin (the most sensitive). The cell survival curve for mitotic cells is very steep, and there is little difference in radiosensitivity for cell lines that are very different in asynchronous culture. (Data compiled by Dr. J.D. Chapman, Fox Chase Cancer Center, Philadelphia.) **B:** DNA purified from various cell lines (survival curves shown in Fig. 3.8**A**) 18 hours after irradiation with 10 Gy (1,000 rad) and electrophoresed for 90 minutes at 6 V/cm. Note the broad variation in the amount of "laddering"—which is characteristic of an apoptotic death. In this form of death, double-strand breaks occur in the linker regions between nucleosomes, producing DNA fragments that are multiples of about 185 base pairs. Note that cell lines that show prominent laddering are radiosensitive. (Gel prepared by Drs. S. Biade and J.D. Chapman, Fox Chase Cancer Center, Philadelphia.)

In addition, there appears to be little or no dose-rate effect, though data are sparse on this point.

Although there are some cell lines in which mitotic death dominates and others in which apoptosis is the rule, most cell lines fall somewhere in between, with contributions from both mitotic and apoptotic death following a radiation exposure, in varying proportions. It has been proposed that the dose–response relationship be described by the following relation:

$$S = e^{-(\alpha_M + \alpha_A)D - \beta_M D^2}$$

in which S is the fraction of cells surviving a dose D, α_M and α_A describe the contributions to cell killing from mitotic and apoptotic death that are linear functions of dose, and β_M describes the contribution to mitotic death that varies with the square of the dose.

ONCOGENES AND RADIORESISTANCE

Numerous reports have appeared in the literature that transfection of activated oncogenes into cells cultured *in vitro* increases their radioresistance, as defined by clonogenic survival. Reports include the transfection of activated N-*ras*, *raf*, or *ras* + *myc*, a combination that is particularly effective in transforming primary explants of rodent embryo cells to a malignant state. Results, however, are equivocal and variable. The change of radiosensitivity did not correlate with cell-cycle distribution or double-strand DNA breaks or their repair; the best correlation was with the length of the G_2 phase delay induced by radiation. It is by no means clear that oncogene expression is directly involved in the induction of radioresistance, and it is far less clear that oncogenes play any major role in radioresistance in human tumors.

GENETIC CONTROL OF RADIOSENSITIVITY

The molecular biology of repair processes in lower organisms, such as yeast and bacteria, has been studied extensively. In a number of instances, a dramatically radiosensitive mutant can result from a mutation in a single gene that functions as a repair or checkpoint gene. In mammalian cells, the situation is much more complicated, and it would appear that a large number of genes may be involved in determining radiosensitivity. Many radiosensitive mutants have been isolated from cell lines maintained in the laboratory, especially rodent cell systems. In many but not all cases, their sensitivity to cell killing by radiation has been related to their greatly reduced ability to repair double-strand DNA breaks (DSBs). Examples of these genes are *XRCC5 Ku 80, XRCC6 Ku 70*, and *XRCC7*. The first of these two genes are involved in DNA-dependent kinase activity that binds to the free ends at the site of a double-strand break, so that if they are defective, repair of double-strand breaks is prejudiced. The third gene codes for a protein that is defective in mice with the "severe combined immune deficiency syndrome" that are sensitive to radiation.

TABLE 3.1

Inherited Human Syndromes Associated with Sensitivity to X-Rays

Ataxia telangiectasia (AT)
Basal cell nevoid syndrome
Cockayne's syndrome
Down's syndrome
Fanconi's anemia
Gardner's syndrome
Nijmegan breakage syndrome
Usher's syndrome

Some patients who show an abnormally severe normal tissue reaction to radiation therapy exhibit the traits of specific inherited syndromes. These are listed in Table 3.1. The most striking example is AT. Fibroblasts taken from patients suffering from this syndrome are two or three times as radiosensitive as normal, and patients with AT receiving radiation therapy show considerable normal tissue damage unless the doses are reduced appropriately. They also have an elevated incidence of spontaneous cancer. Cells from AT heterozygotes are slightly more radiosensitive than normal, and there is some controversy as to whether AT heterozygotes are predisposed to cancer.

The gene associated with AT has been identified and sequenced and called the *ATM* (AT-mutated) gene. The *ATM* protein appears to be part of signal transduction pathways involved in many physiologic processes, though the exact mechanism by which the genetic defect in AT cells leads to radiosensitivity is not altogether clear.

INTRINSIC RADIOSENSITIVITY AND PREDICTIVE ASSAYS

Predictive assays of individual tumor radiosensitivity require cells to be grown from fresh explants of human tumor biopsies. These do not grow well as attached cells in regular clonogenic assays. Better results have been obtained with the Courtenay assay, in which cells grow in a semisolid agar gel supplemented with growth factors. In addition, a number of nonclonogenic assays have been developed based on cell growth in a multiwell plate. Growth is assessed in terms of the ability of cells to reduce a compound that can be visualized by staining or is based on total DNA or RNA content of the well. These end points are surrogates for clonogenicity or reproductive integrity. See Chapter 23 for a discussion of predictive assays.

EFFECTIVE SURVIVAL CURVE FOR A MULTIFRACTION REGIMEN

Because multifraction regimens are used most often in clinical radiotherapy, it is frequently useful to think in terms of an effective survival curve.

If a radiation dose is delivered in a series of equal fractions, separated by sufficient time for repair of sublethal damage to occur between doses, the *effective dose–survival curve* becomes an exponential function of dose. The shoulder of the survival curve is repeated many times, so that the effective survival curve is a straight line from the origin through a point on the single-dose survival curve corresponding to the daily dose fraction. This is illustrated in Figure 3.9. The effective survival curve is an exponential function of dose whether the single-dose survival curve has a constant terminal slope (as shown) or is continuously bending, as implied by the linear-quadratic relation. The D_0 of the effective survival curve (i.e., the reciprocal of the slope), defined to be the dose required to reduce the fraction of cells surviving to 37%, has a value close to 3 Gy (300 rad) for cells of human origin. This is an average value and can differ significantly for different tumor types.

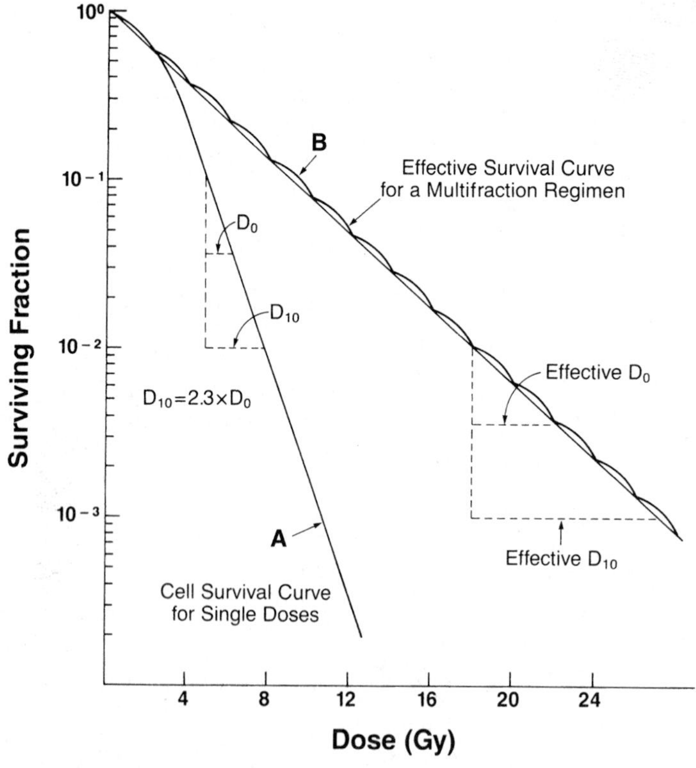

FIGURE 3.9 • The concept of an "effective" survival curve for a multifraction regimen is illustrated. If the radiation dose is delivered in a series of equal fractions separated by time intervals sufficiently long for the repair of sublethal damage to be complete between fractions, the shoulder of the survival curve is repeated many times. The effective dose–survival curve is an exponential function of dose, that is, a straight line from the origin through a point on the single-dose survival curve corresponding to the daily dose fraction (e.g., 2 Gy, or 200 rad). The dose resulting in one decade of cell killing (D_{10}) is related to the D_0 by the expression $D_{10} = 2.3 \times D_0$.

For calculation purposes, it is often useful to use the D_{10}, the dose required to kill 90% of the population. For example:

$$D_{10} = 2.3 \times D_0$$

in which 2.3 is the natural logarithm of 10.

CALCULATIONS OF TUMOR CELL KILL

The concept outlined previously of an effective survival curve for a multifraction radiation treatment may be used to perform simple calculations of tumor cell kill after radiotherapy. Although such calculations are greatly oversimplified, they are nevertheless instructive. Four examples are given here.

Problem 1

A tumor consists of 109 clonogenic cells. The effective dose–response curve, given in daily dose fractions of 2 Gy, has no shoulder and a D_0 of 3 Gy. What total dose is required to give a 90% chance of tumor cure?

Answer

To give a 90% probability of tumor control in a tumor containing 109 cells requires a cellular depopulation of 10^{-10}. The dose resulting in one decade of cell killing (D_{10}) is given by

$$D_{10} = 2.3 \times D_0 = 2.3 \times 3 = 6.9 \text{ Gy}$$

Total dose for 10 decades of cell killing, therefore, is $10 \times 6.9 = 69$ Gy.

Problem 2

Suppose that, in the previous example, the clonogenic cells underwent three cell doublings during treatment. About what total dose would be required to achieve the same probability of tumor control?

Answer

Three cell doublings would increase the cell number by

$$2 \times 2 \times 2 = 8$$

Consequently, about one extra decade of cell killing would be required, corresponding to an additional dose of 6.9 Gy. Total dose is $69 + 6.9 = 75.9$ Gy.

Problem 3

During the course of radiotherapy, a tumor containing 10^9 cells receives 40 Gy. If the D_0 is 2.2 Gy, how many tumor cells will be left?

Answer

If the D_0 is 2.2 Gy, the D_{10} is given by

$$\begin{aligned} D_{10} &= 2.3 \times D_0 \\ &= 2.3 \times 2.2 = 5 \text{ Gy} \end{aligned}$$

Because the total dose is 40 Gy, the number of decades of cell killing is $40/5 = 8$.

Number of cells remaining is $10^9 \times 10^{-8} = 10$.

Problem 4

If 10^7 cells were irradiated according to single-hit kinetics so that the average number of hits per cell is one, how many cells would survive?

Answer

A dose that gives an average of one hit per cell is the D_0, that is, the dose that on the exponential region of the survival curve reduces the number of survivors to 37%. The number of surviving cells is therefore

$$10^7 \times \frac{37}{100} = 3.7 \times 10^6$$

THE RADIOSENSITIVITY OF MAMMALIAN CELLS COMPARED WITH MICROORGANISMS

The final illustration in this chapter (Fig. 3.10) is a compilation from the literature of survival data for many types of cells. The steepest dose–response relationship (curve A) is an average curve for mammalian cells; it is evident that they are exquisitely radiosensitive compared with microorganisms. The bacterium *Escherichia coli* is more resistant, yeast is more resistant still, and the most resistant is *Micrococcus radiodurans*, which shows no significant cell killing even after a dose of 1,000 Gy (10^5 rad). There are several important points to be made from this:

1. The dominant factor that accounts for this huge range of radiosensitivities is the DNA content. Mammalian cells are sensitive because they have a large DNA content, which represents a large target for radiation damage.
2. DNA content is not the whole story, however. *E. coli* and *E. coli* B/r have the same DNA content but differ in radiosensitivity because B/r has a mutant and more efficient DNA repair system.

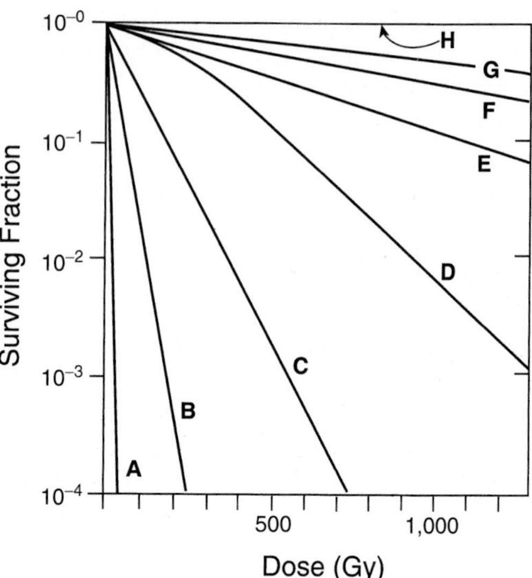

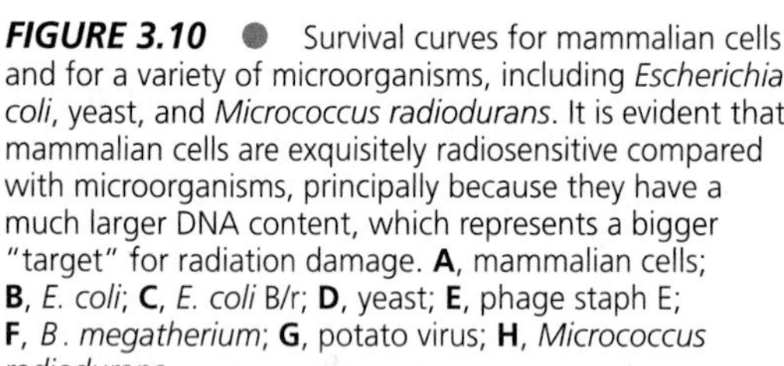
FIGURE 3.10 ● Survival curves for mammalian cells and for a variety of microorganisms, including *Escherichia coli*, yeast, and *Micrococcus radiodurans*. It is evident that mammalian cells are exquisitely radiosensitive compared with microorganisms, principally because they have a much larger DNA content, which represents a bigger "target" for radiation damage. **A**, mammalian cells; **B**, *E. coli*; **C**, *E. coli* B/r; **D**, yeast; **E**, phage staph E; **F**, *B. megatherium*; **G**, potato virus; **H**, *Micrococcus radiodurans*.

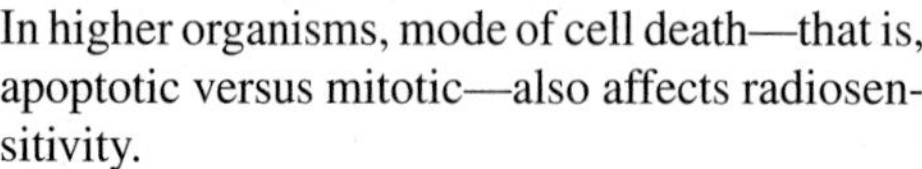
In higher organisms, mode of cell death—that is, apoptotic versus mitotic—also affects radiosensitivity.

3. Figure 3.10 explains why, if radiation is used as a method of sterilization, doses of the order of 20,000 Gy (2 million rad) are necessary. Even if objects are socially clean, such huge doses are necessary to reduce the population of contaminating microorganisms because of their extreme radioresistance.

Summary of Pertinent Conclusions

- Cells from tumors and many normal regenerative tissues grow and form colonies *in vitro*.
- Fresh explants of normal tissues often grow well in culture for a few weeks before they peter out and die. A few pass through a "crisis" and become immortal; these are the established cell lines.
- A cell is said to have retained its reproductive integrity if it is capable of sustained proliferation, that is, if it can grow into a macroscopic colony.
- A survivor that has retained its reproductive integrity is said to be *clonogenic*.
- The percentage of untreated cells seeded that grow into macroscopic colonies is known as the plating efficiency. Thus:

$$PE = \frac{\text{Number of colonies counted}}{\text{Number of cells seeded}} \times 100$$

- The plating efficiency may be close to 100% for some established cell lines but 1% or less for fresh explants of human cells.
- The fraction of cells surviving a given dose is determined by counting the number of macroscopic colonies as a fraction of the number of cells seeded. Allowance must be made for the plating efficiency. Thus:

$$SF = \frac{\text{Number of colonies counted}}{\text{Number of cells seeded} \times (PE/100)}$$

- A cell survival curve is the relationship between the fraction of cells retaining their reproductive integrity and the absorbed dose.
- Conventionally, surviving fraction on a logarithmic scale is plotted on the ordinate against dose on the abscissa. The shape of the survival curve is important.
- The cell survival curve for α-particles and low-energy neutrons (densely ionizing radiations) is a straight line on a log-linear plot; that is, survival approximates to an exponential function of dose.
- The cell survival curve for x- or γ-rays (sparsely ionizing radiations) has an initial slope, followed by a bending region or shoulder, after which it tends to straighten again at higher doses.
- Survival data are adequately fitted by many models and theories. The data are never sufficiently precise, nor are the models sufficiently different for experimental results to discriminate among models.

(continued)

Summary of Pertinent Conclusions (Continued)

- For the first one or two decades of survival and up to doses used in single fractions in radiotherapy, survival data are adequately represented by the linear-quadratic relationship

$$S = e^{-\alpha D - \beta D^2}$$

  in which S is the fraction of cells surviving a dose D and α and β are constants representing the linear and quadratic components of cell killing.
- The initial slope of the cell survival curve is determined by α; the quadratic component of cell killing (β) causes the curve to bend at higher doses.
- The ratio α/β is the dose at which linear and quadratic components of cell killing are equal.
- There is good evidence that the nucleus, specifically the DNA, is the principal target for radiation-induced cell lethality. Membrane damage also may be a factor.
- Following exposure to radiation, cells may die attempting the next or a subsequent mitosis (mitotic death), or they may die programmed cell deaths (apoptotic death).
- In cells that die a mitotic death, there is a one-to-one correlation between cell survival and the average number of putative "lethal" chromosomal aberrations per cell, that is, asymmetric exchange-type aberrations such as dicentrics and rings.
- Cells that die apoptotic deaths follow a stereotyped sequence of morphologic events, culminating in the breaking up of the DNA into fragments that are multiples of 185 base pairs; this leads to the characteristic DNA laddering seen in gels.
- In some cell types (such as lymphoid cells), apoptotic death is dominant following irradiation. Survival is then an exponential function of dose; that is, the survival curve is straight and shoulderless on the usual log-linear plot. There is also no dose-rate effect.
- In some cell types (such as CHO or V79 cells in culture), mitotic death is dominant following irradiation. Survival is then a linear-quadratic function of dose; that is, the survival curve has a shoulder on the usual log-linear plot. There is usually a large dose-rate effect.
- Many cell populations die both mitotic and apoptotic deaths. There is, in general, a correlation between the importance of apoptosis and radiosensitivity. If apoptosis is dominant, cells are radiosensitive; if apoptosis is absent, cells are radioresistant.
- Cells cultured from different tumors in humans show a broad range of radiosensitivities that bracket the sensitivity of normal cells from different people.
- There is some evidence in cells cultured *in vitro* that transfection of activated oncogenes in cells increases their radioresistance. It is not clear that oncogenes play a role in the radioresistance of human tumors *in vivo*.
- A number of genes that influence the radiosensitivity of mammalian cells have been identified.
- If these genes are defective, the repair of double-strand breaks is often prejudiced.
- A number of human syndromes have been found to be associated with radiosensitivity; AT is the best example.
- There is often a link between sensitivity to killing by radiation and predisposition to cancer.
- Predictive assays for intrinsic radiosensitivity of tumor cells from individual patients require special assays. This is discussed in Chapter 23.
- The effective survival curve for a multifraction regimen is an exponential function of dose: a straight line from the origin through a point on the single-dose survival curve corresponding to the daily dose fraction.
- The average value of the effective D_0 for the multifraction survival curve for human cells is about 3 Gy (300 rad).
- The D_{10}, the dose resulting in one decade of cell killing, is related to the D_0 by the expression:

$$D_{10} = 2.3 \times D_0$$

- Calculations of tumor cell kill can be performed for fractionated clinical radiotherapy regimens using the concept of effective survival curve.
- Mammalian cells are exquisitely radiosensitive compared with microorganisms such as bacteria and yeast, principally because of their larger DNA content, which represents a bigger "target" for radiation damage.

BIBLIOGRAPHY

Alper T, Fowler JF, Morgan RL, Vonberg DD, Ellis F, Oliver R: The characterization of the "type C" survival curve. *Br J Radiol* 35:722–723, 1962

Andrews JR, Berry RJ: Fast neutron irradiation and the relationship of radiation dose and mammalian cell reproductive capacity. *Radiat Res* 16:76–81, 1962

Barendsen GW, Beusker TLJ, Vergroesen AJ, Budke L: Effects of different ionizing radiations on human cells in tissue culture: II. Biological experiments. *Radiat Res* 13:841–849, 1960

Bender M: Induced aberrations in human chromosomes. *Am J Pathol* 43:26a, 1963

Carrano AV: Chromosome aberrations and radiation induced cell death: II. Predicted and observed cell survival. *Mutat Res* 17:355–366, 1973

Cornforth MN, Bedford JS: A quantitative comparison of potentially lethal damage repair and the rejoining of interphase chromosome breaks in low passage normal human fibroblasts. *Radiat Res* 111:385–405, 1987

Cornforth MN, Bedford JS: X-ray-induced breakage and rejoining of human interphase chromosomes. *Science* 222:1141–1143, 1983

Elkind MM, Sutton H: Radiation response of mammalian cells grown in culture: I. Repair of x-ray damage in surviving Chinese hamster cells. *Radiat Res* 13:556–593, 1960

Evans HJ: Chromosome aberrations induced by ionizing radiation. *Int Rev Cytol* 13:221–321, 1962

Frankenberg D, Frankenberg-Schwager M, Harbich R: Split-dose recovery is due to the repair of DNA double strand breaks. *Int J Radiat Biol* 46:541–553, 1984

Gatti RA, Berkel L, Boder E, et al.: Localisation of an ataxia telangiectasia gene to chromosome 11q22-23. *Nature* 336:577–580, 1988

Geard CR: Effects of radiation on chromosomes. In Pizzarello D (ed): *Radiation Biology*, pp 83–110. Boca Raton, FL, CRC Press, 1982

Grell RF: The chromosome. *J Tenn Acad Sci* 37:43–53, 1962

Ishihara T, Sasaki MS (eds): *Radiation-Induced Chromosome Damage in Man*. New York, Alan R Liss, 1983

Jackson SP, Jeggo PA: DNA double-strand break repair and V(D)J recombination: involvement of DNA-PK. *TIBS* 20:412–415, 1995

Jeggo PA, Holliday R: Azacytidine-induced reactivation of a DNA repair gene in Chinese hamster ovary cells. *Mol Cell Biol* 6:2944–2949, 1986

Jeggo PA, Kemp LM: X-ray sensitive mutants of Chinese hamster ovary cell line. Isolation and cross sensitivity to other DNA-damaging agents. *Mutat Res* 112:313–327, 1983

Kerr JFR, Wyllie AH, Currie AR: Apoptosis: a basic biological phenomenon with wide ranging implications in tissue kinetics. *Br J Cancer* 26:239–257, 1972

Kuerbitz SJ, Plunkett BS, Walsh WV, Kastan MB: Wild-type p53 is a cell cycle check point determinant following irradiation. *Proc Natl Acad Sci* 89:7491–7495, 1992

Lea DEA: Actions of Radiations on Living Cells, 2nd ed. Cambridge, UK, Cambridge University Press, 1956

Lowe SW, Schmitt EM, Smith SW, Osborne BA, Jacks T: p53 is required for radiation-induced apoptosis in mouse thymocytes. *Nature* 362:847–849, 1993

McKenna WG, Iliakis G, Muschel RJ: Mechanism of radioresistance in oncogene transfected cell lines. In Dewey WC, Eddington M, Fry RJM, Hall EJ, and Whitmore GF (eds): *Radiation Research: A Twentieth Century Perspective*, pp 392–397. San Diego, Academic Press, 1992

Moorhead PS, Nowell PC, Mellman WJ, Battips DM, Hungerford DA: Chromosome preparation of leukocytes cultured from human peripheral blood. *Exp Cell Res* 20:613–616, 1960

Munro TR: The relative radiosensitivity of the nucleus and cytoplasm of the Chinese hamster fibroblasts. Radiat Res 42:451–470, 1970

Puck TT, Markus Pl: Action of x-rays on mammalian cells. *J Exp Med* 103:653–666, 1956

Ris H: Chromosome structure. In McElroy WD, Glass B (eds): *Chemical Basis of Heredity*. Baltimore, Johns Hopkins University Press, 1957

Savitsky K, Bar-Shira A, Gilad S, et al.: A single ataxia telangiectasia gene with a product similar to PI-3 kinase. *Science* 268:1749–1753, 1995

Spear FG: On some biological effects of radiation. *Br J Radiol* 31:114–124, 1958

Swift M: Ionizing radiation, breast cancer and ataxia-telangiectasia. *J Natl Cancer Inst* 21:1571–1572, 1994

Taccioli CE, Gottlieb TM, Blunt T, et al.: Ku80: product of the XRCC5 gene and its role in DNA repair and V(D)J recombination. *Science* 265:1442–1445, 1994

CHAPTER 4

Radiosensitivity and Cell Age in the Mitotic Cycle

THE CELL CYCLE

Mammalian cells propagate and proliferate by mitosis. When a cell divides, two progeny cells are produced, each of which carries a chromosome complement identical to that of the parent cell. After an interval of time has elapsed, each of the progeny may undergo a further division. The time between successive divisions is known as the **mitotic-cycle time**, or, as it is commonly called, the **cell-cycle time** (T_C).

If a population of dividing cells is observed with a conventional light microscope, the only event in the entire cell cycle that can be identified and distinguished is mitosis, or division itself. Just before the cell divides to form two progeny, the chromosomes (which are diffuse and scattered in the nucleus in the period between mitoses) condense into clearly distinguishable forms. In addition, in monolayer cultures of cells, just before mitosis, the cells round up and become loosely attached to the surface of the culture vessel. This whole process of mitosis—in preparation for which the cell rounds up, the chromosome material condenses, and the cell divides into two and then stretches out again and attaches to the surface of the culture vessel—lasts only about 1 hour. The remainder of the cell cycle, the interphase, occupies all of the intermitotic period. No events of interest can be identified with a conventional microscope during this time.

Because cell division is a cyclic phenomenon, repeated in each generation of the cells, it is usual to represent it as a circle, as shown in Figure 4.1. The circumference of the circle represents the full mitotic-cycle time for the cells (T_C); the period of mitosis is represented by M. The remainder of the cell cycle can be further subdivided by using some marker of DNA synthesis. The original technique was autoradiography, introduced by Howard and Pelc in 1953.

The basis of the technique, illustrated in Figure 4.2, is to feed the cells thymidine, a basic building block used for making DNA, which has been labeled with radioactive tritium (^{3}H-TdR). Cells that are actively synthesizing new DNA as part of the process of replicating their chromosome complements incorporate the radioactive thymidine.

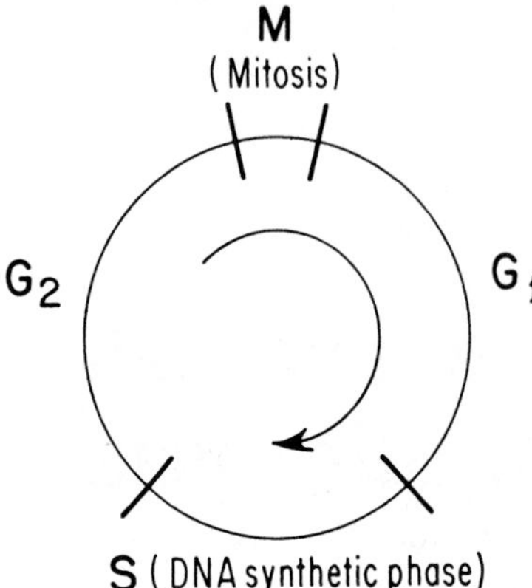

FIGURE 4.1 • The stages of the mitotic cycle for actively growing mammalian cells. M, mitosis; S, DNA synthetic phase; G_1 and G_2, "gaps," or periods of apparent inactivity between the major discernible events in the cycle.

Then the surplus radioactive thymidine is flushed from the system, the cells are fixed and stained so that they may be viewed easily, and the preparation of cells is coated with a very thin layer of nuclear (photographic) emulsion.

β-Particles from cells that have incorporated radioactive thymidine pass through the nuclear emulsion and produce a latent image. When the emulsion subsequently is developed and fixed, the area through which a β-particle has passed appears as a black spot. It is then a comparatively simple matter to view the preparation of cells and to observe that some of the cells have black spots or "grains" over them, which indicates that they were actively synthesizing DNA at the time radioactive thymidine was made available. Other cells do not have any grains over their nuclei; this is interpreted to mean that the cells were not actively making DNA when

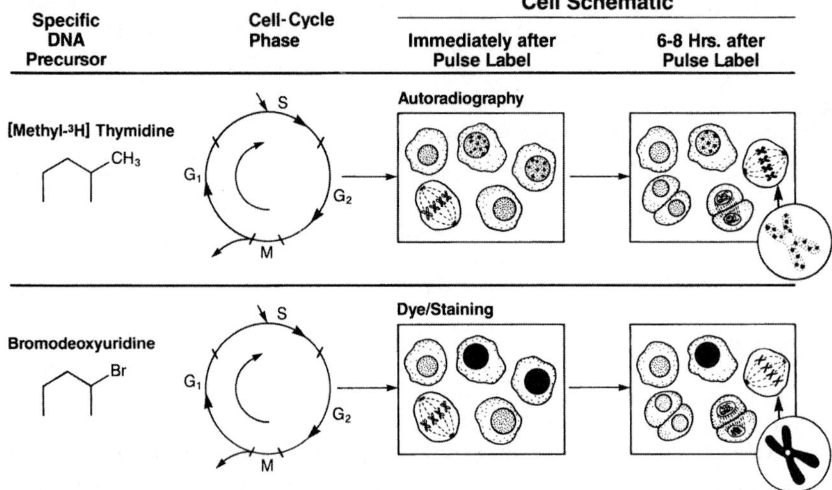

FIGURE 4.2 • Cell-labeling techniques. **Top panels:** The principle of autoradiography, which may be applied to cells in culture growing as a monolayer on a glass microscope slide or to thin sections cut from a tumor or normal tissue. Cells in the DNA synthetic phase (S) take up tritiated thymidine. After the cells are fixed and stained so that they are visible by light microscopy, they are covered with a layer of nuclear (photographic) emulsion and left for several weeks in a cool refrigerator. As β-particles from the tritiated thymidine pass through the emulsion, they form latent images that appear as black grains when the emulsion is subsequently developed and fixed. If cells are stained and autoradiographed immediately after incorporation of the tritiated thymidine, cells that are labeled are in S phase (**top middle panel**). If staining and autoradiography are delayed for 6 to 8 hours after the pulse label, some cells may move from S to M, and labeled mitotic cells are observed (**top right panel**). The lengths of the various phases of the cycle can be determined in this way. **Bottom panels:** The principle of cell-cycle analysis using 5-bromodeoxyuridine as the DNA precursor instead of radioactively labeled thymidine. The bromodeoxyuridine is incorporated into cells in S. It can be recognized by the use of a Giemsa stain (which is purple) or a monoclonal antibody to bromodeoxyuridine-substituted DNA. The antibody is tagged with a fluorescing dye (e.g., fluorescein), which shows up bright green under a fluorescence microscope. If cells are stained immediately after labeling with bromodeoxyuridine, those staining darkly are in S phase (**bottom middle panel**). If staining is delayed for 6 to 8 hours, cells incorporating bromodeoxyuridine may move from S to M, and a darkly staining mitotic cell is seen (**bottom right panel**). (Courtesy of Dr. Charles Geard.)

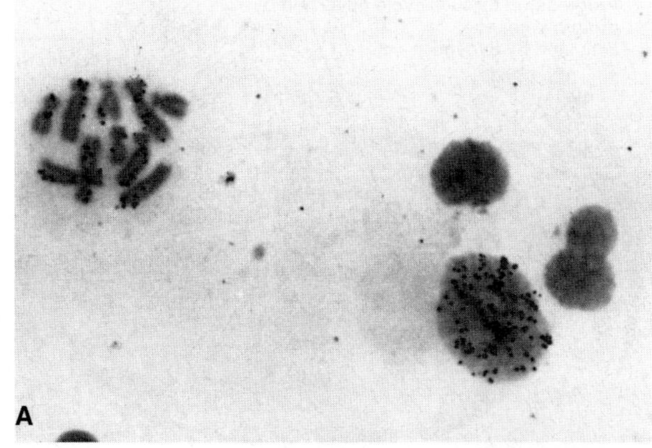

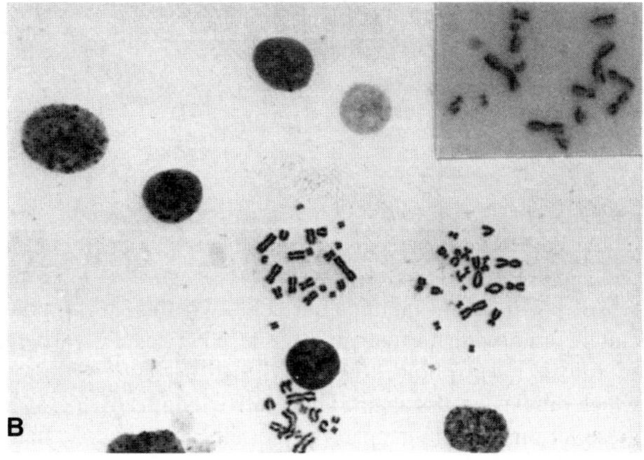

FIGURE 4.3 • **A:** Autoradiograph of Chinese hamster cells in culture flash-labeled with tritiated thymidine. The black grains over some cells indicate that they were synthesizing DNA when they were labeled. Also shown is a labeled mitotic cell. This cell was in S phase when the culture was flash-labeled but moved to M phase before it was stained and autoradiographed. **B:** Photomicrograph showing cells labeled and unlabeled with bromodeoxyuridine. Cells were grown in the presence of bromodeoxyuridine and then fixed and stained 20 hours later. Incorporated bromodeoxyuridine stains purple, which shows up dark in this black-and-white print; the rest of the cell is light blue. The stained interphase cell indicates that it was in S phase during the time the bromodeoxyuridine was available. Also shown is a first-generation mitotic cell, which had been in S phase at the time the bromodeoxyuridine was available and had moved to M phase by the time it was fixed and stained. It can be identified as first-generation because both chromatids of each chromosome are stained uniformly. **Inset:** A second-generation mitotic cell, which passed through two S phases during bromodeoxyuridine availability. One chromatid of each chromosome is darker because both strands of the DNA double helix have incorporated bromodeoxyuridine. One chromatid is lighter because only one strand of the DNA has incorporated bromodeoxyuridine. (Courtesy of Dr. Charles Geard.)

the radioactive label was made available to them. Examples of labeled cells are shown in Figure 4.3. If the cells are allowed to grow for some time after labeling with tritiated thymidine, so that they move into mitosis before being fixed, stained, and autoradiographed, then a labeled mitotic cell may be observed (Fig. 4.3**A**).

The use of tritiated thymidine to identify cells in the DNA synthetic phase (S) has been replaced largely with the use of 5-bromodeoxyuridine, which differs from thymidine only by the substitution of a bromine atom for a methyl group. If this halogenated pyrimidine is fed to the cells, it is incorporated into DNA in place of thymidine, and its presence can be detected by using an appropriate stain (see Fig. 4.2 bottom panel). In a black-and-white print, cells incorporating bromodeoxyuridine appear darkly stained. In practice they are easier to recognize because the stain is brightly colored. To identify cells that are in S phase and have incorporated bromodeoxyuridine even more readily, one can use an antibody against bromodeoxyuridine-substituted DNA which fluoresces brightly under a fluorescence microscope. Examples of stained and unstained cells are shown in Figure 4.3**B**. If time is allowed between labeling with bromodeoxyuridine and staining, then a cell may move from S to M phase, and a stained mitotic cell is observed (Fig. 4.3**B**). If the cell is in the first mitosis after bromodeoxyuridine incorporation, both chromatids of each chromosome are equally stained, as shown in the figure, but by the second mitosis, one chromatid is stained darker than the other (illustrated in the inset to Fig. 4.3**B**).

The use of bromodeoxyuridine has two advantages over conventional autoradiography using tritiated thymidine. First, it does not involve radioactive material. Second, it greatly shortens the time to produce a result, because if cells are coated with emulsion to produce an autoradiograph, they must be stored in a refrigerator for about a month to allow β-particles from the incorporated tritium to produce a latent image in the emulsion.

By using either of these techniques, it can be shown that cells synthesize DNA only during a discrete well-defined fraction of the cycle, the S phase. There is an interval between mitosis and DNA synthesis in which no label is incorporated. This first "gap" in activity was named G_1 by Howard and Pelc, and the nomenclature is used today. After

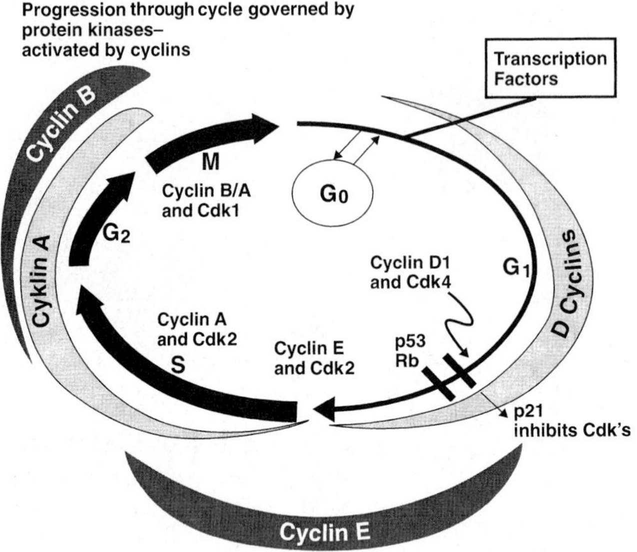

FIGURE 4.4 • Update of the phases of the cell cycle, showing how they are regulated by the periodic activation of different members of the cyclin-dependent kinase family. Various cyclin-dependent kinase–cyclin complexes are required to phosphorylate a number of protein substrates, which drive key events, including the initiation of DNA replication and the onset of mitosis.

DNA synthesis has been completed, there is a second gap before mitosis, G_2.

All proliferating mammalian cells, whether in culture or growing normally in a tissue, have a cycle of mitosis (M), followed by G_1, S, and G_2, after which mitosis occurs again. The relative lengths of these various constituent parts of the cell cycle vary according to the particular cells studied. If cells stop progressing through the cycle (i.e., are arrested), they are said to be in G_0 (see Fig. 4.4).

The characteristics of two cell lines commonly used for *in vitro* culture are summarized in Table 4.1. HeLa cells have a total cell-cycle time of about 24 hours, which is more than double that of the Chinese hamster cell, which has a cell-cycle time of about 11 hours. Mitosis lasts only a relatively short time, about 1 hour, and is not very different for those two cell lines or for most others. The S phase is 8 hours for HeLa cells and 6 hours for hamster cells; in all cell lines studied in culture or growing *in vivo,* the S phase never exceeds about 15 hours. The G_2 period is very similar in HeLa and hamster cells; in fact, the difference in the total cell-cycle time between these two cell lines is accounted for almost entirely by the difference in the length of the G_1 period.

This is an important point: The difference among mammalian cell-cycle times in different circumstances, varying from about 10 hours for a hamster cell grown in culture to hundreds of hours for stem cells in some self-renewal tissues, is the result of a dramatic variation in the length of the G_1 period. The remaining components of the cell cycle, M, S, and G_2, vary comparatively little among different cells in different circumstances.

The description of the principal phases of the cell cycle (M, G_1, S, G_2) dates from Howard and Pelc in 1953, as previously discussed. During a complete cell cycle, the cell must accurately replicate the DNA once during S phase and distribute an identical set of chromosomes equally to two progeny cells during M phase. In recent years, we have learned much more about the mechanisms by which the cycle is regulated in eukaryotic cells. Regulation occurs by the periodic activation of different members of the cyclin-dependent kinase (Cdk) family. In its active form, each Cdk is complexed with a particular cyclin. Different Cdk–cyclin complexes are required to phosphorylate a number of protein substrates that drive such cell-cycle events as the

TABLE 4.1

Phases of the Cell Cycle for Two Commonly Used Cell Lines Cultured *in Vitro*

	Hamster Cells, h	HeLa Cells, h
T_C	11	24
T_M	1	1
T_S	6	8
T_{G1}	1	11
T_{G2}	3	4

initiation of DNA replication or the onset of mitosis. Cdk–cyclin complexes are also vital in preventing the initiation of a cell-cycle event at the wrong time.

Extensive regulation of Cdk–cyclin activity by a number of transcriptional and posttranscriptional mechanisms ensures perfect timing and coordination of cell-cycle events. The Cdk catalytic subunit by itself is inactive, requiring association with a cyclin subunit and phosphorylation of a key threonine residue to become fully active. The Cdk–cyclin complex is reversibly inactivated either by phosphorylation on a tyrosine residue located in the adenosine triphosphate–binding domain, or by association with Cdk inhibitory proteins. After the completion of the cell-cycle transition, the complex is inactivated irreversibly by ubiquitin-mediated degradation of the cyclin subunit.

Entry into S phase is controlled by Cdks that are sequentially regulated by cyclins D, E, and A. D-type cyclins act as growth-factor sensors, with their expression depending more on the extracellular cues than on the cell's position in the cycle. Mitogenic stimulation governs both their synthesis and complex formation with Cdk4 and Cdk6, and catalytic activity of the assembled complexes persists through the cycle as long as mitogenic stimulation continues. Cyclin E expression in proliferating cells is normally periodic and maximal at the G_1/S transition, and throughout this interval it enters into active complexes with its catalytic partner, Cdk2. Figure 4.4 illustrates this view of the cell cycle and its regulation. This is in essence an update of Figure 4.1 and is discussed in more detail in Chapter 17.

SYNCHRONOUSLY DIVIDING CELL CULTURES

In the discussion of survival curves in Chapter 3, the assumption was implicit that the population of irradiated cells was asynchronous; that is, it consisted of cells distributed throughout all phases of the cell cycle. Study of the variation of radiosensitivity with the position or age of the cell in the cell cycle was made possible only by the development of techniques to produce synchronously dividing cell cultures—populations of cells in which all of the cells occupy the same phase of the cell cycle at a given time.

There are essentially two techniques that have been used to produce a synchronously dividing cell population. The first is the **mitotic harvest** technique, first described by Terasima and Tolmach. This technique can be used only for cultures that grow in monolayers attached to the surface of the growth vessel. It exploits the fact that if such cells are close to mitosis, they round up and become loosely attached to the surface. If at this stage the growth medium over the cells is subjected to gentle motion (by shaking), the mitotic cells become detached from the surface and float in the medium. If this medium is then removed from the culture vessel and plated out into new petri dishes, the population consists almost entirely of mitotic cells. Incubation of these cell cultures at 37°C then causes the cells to move together synchronously in step through their mitotic cycles. By delivering a dose of radiation at various times after the initial harvesting of mitotic cells, one can irradiate cells at various phases of the cell cycle.

An alternative method for synchronizing cells, which is applicable to cells in a tissue as well as cells grown in culture, involves the use of a drug. A number of different substances may be used. One of the most widely applicable is hydroxyurea. If this drug is added to a population of dividing cells, it has two effects on the cell population. First, all cells that are synthesizing DNA (S phase) take up the drug and are killed. Second, the drug imposes a block at the end of the G_1 period; cells that occupy the G_2, M, and G_1 compartments when the drug is added progress through the cell cycle and accumulate at this block.

The dynamics of the action of hydroxyurea are illustrated in Figure 4.5. The drug is left in position for a period equal to the combined lengths of G_2, M, and G_1 for that particular cell line. By the end

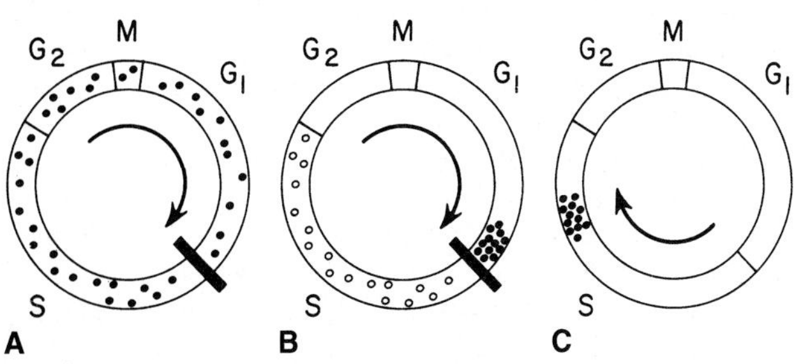

FIGURE 4.5 • Mode of action of hydroxyurea as an agent to induce synchrony. This drug kills cells in S phase and imposes a "block" at the end of the G_1 phase. Cells in G_2, M, and G_1 accumulate at this block when the drug is added. If the block is removed, the synchronized cohort of cells moves on through the cycle.

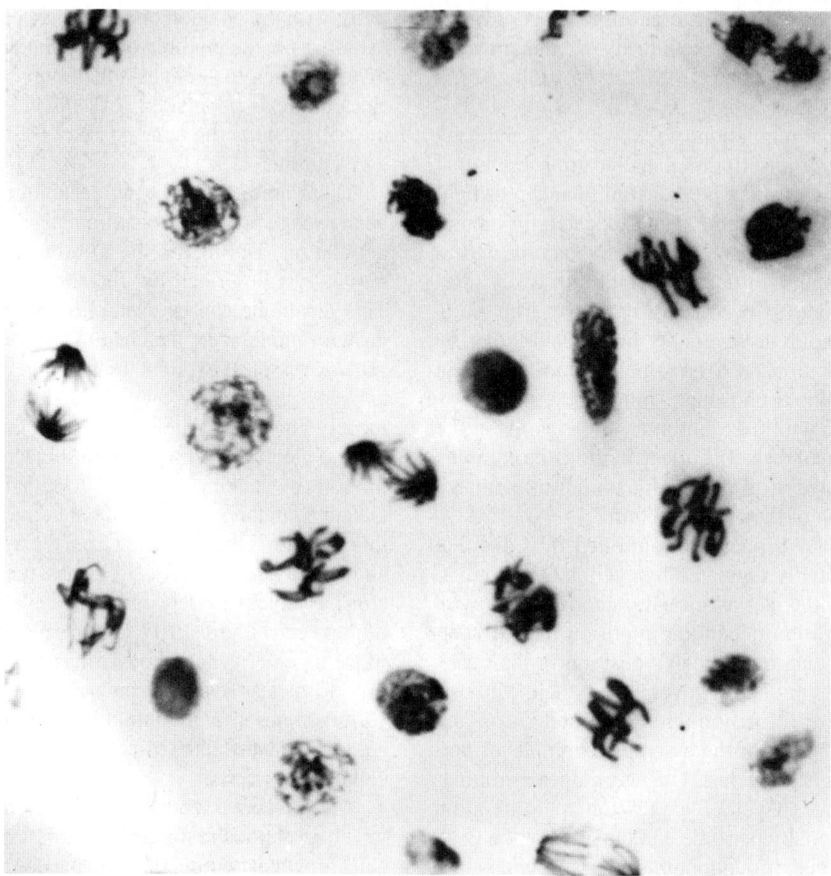

FIGURE 4.6 ● Photomicrograph of a squash preparation of the root tip of a *Vicia* seedling 11 hours after synchrony was induced with hydroxyurea. Note the large proportion of cells in mitosis. (From Hall EJ, Brown JM, Cavanagh J: Radiosensitivity and the oxygen effect measured at different phases of the mitotic cycle using synchronously dividing cells of the root meristem of *Vicia faba*. *Radiat Res* 35:622–634, 1968, with permission.)

of the treatment period, all of the viable cells left in the population are situated in a narrow "window" at the end of G_1, poised and ready to enter S. If the drug is then removed from the system, this synchronized cohort of cells proceeds through the cell cycle. For example, in hamster cells, 5 hours after the removal of the drug, the cohort of synchronized cells occupies a position late in the S phase. Some 9 hours after the removal of the drug, the cohort of cells is at, or close to, mitosis.

Techniques involving one or another of a wide range of drugs have been used to produce synchronously dividing cell populations in culture, in organized tissues (in a limited number of cases), and even in the whole animal. Figure 4.6 is a photomicrograph of a squash preparation of the root tip of a *Vicia* faba plant seedling 11 hours after synchrony was induced with hydroxyurea. A very large proportion of the cells is in mitosis.

THE EFFECT OF X-RAYS ON SYNCHRONOUSLY DIVIDING CELL CULTURES

Figure 4.7 shows results of an experiment in which mammalian cells, harvested at mitosis, were irradiated with a single dose of 6.6 Gy (660 rad) at various times afterward, corresponding to different phases of the cell cycle. The data (from Sinclair) were obtained using Chinese hamster cells in culture. As can be seen from the figure, 1 hour after the mitotic cells are seeded into the petri dishes, when the cells are in G_1, a dose of 6.6 Gy (660 rad) results in a surviving fraction of about 13%.

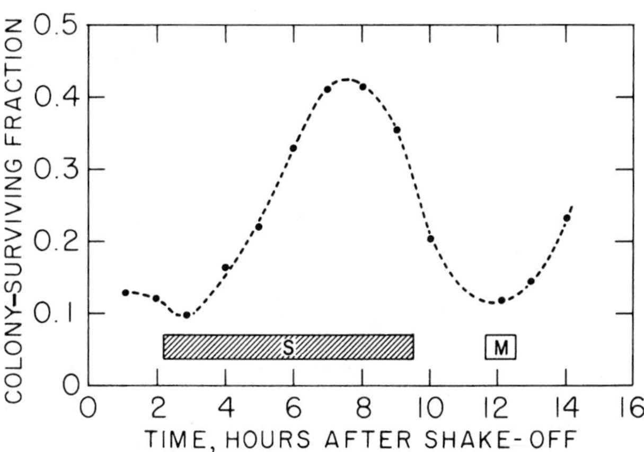

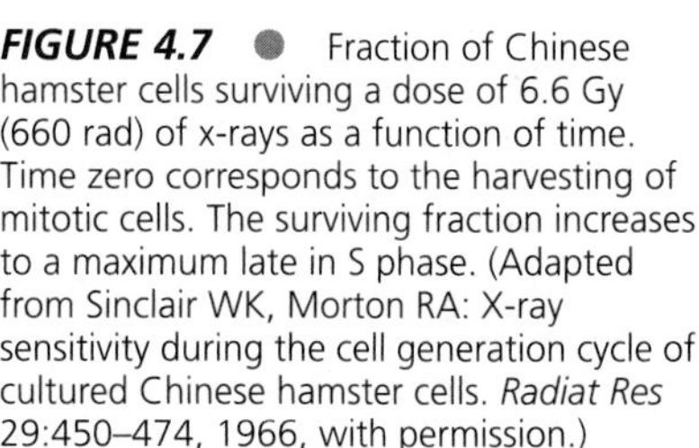

FIGURE 4.7 • Fraction of Chinese hamster cells surviving a dose of 6.6 Gy (660 rad) of x-rays as a function of time. Time zero corresponds to the harvesting of mitotic cells. The surviving fraction increases to a maximum late in S phase. (Adapted from Sinclair WK, Morton RA: X-ray sensitivity during the cell generation cycle of cultured Chinese hamster cells. *Radiat Res* 29:450–474, 1966, with permission.)

The proportion of cells that survive the dose increases rapidly with time as the cells move into S phase; by the time the cells near the end of S phase, 42% of the cells survive this same dose. When the cells move out of S into G_2 and subsequently to a second mitosis, the proportion of surviving cells falls again. This pattern of response is characteristic for most lines of Chinese hamster cells and has been reported by a number of independent investigators.

Complete survival curves at a number of discrete points during the cell cycle were measured by Sinclair. The results are shown in Figure 4.8. Survival curves are shown for mitotic cells, for cells in G_1 and G_2, and for cells in early and late S phase. It is at once evident that the most sensitive cells are those in M and G_2, which are characterized by a survival curve that is steep and has no shoulder. At the other extreme, cells in the latter part of S phase exhibit a survival curve that is less steep, but the essential difference is that the survival curve has a very broad shoulder. The other phases of the cycle, such as G_1 and early S, are intermediate in sensitivity between the two extremes.

The broken line in Figure 4.8 is the calculated survival curve that would be expected to apply for mitotic cells under conditions of hypoxia; that is, the slope is 2.5 times shallower than the solid line for

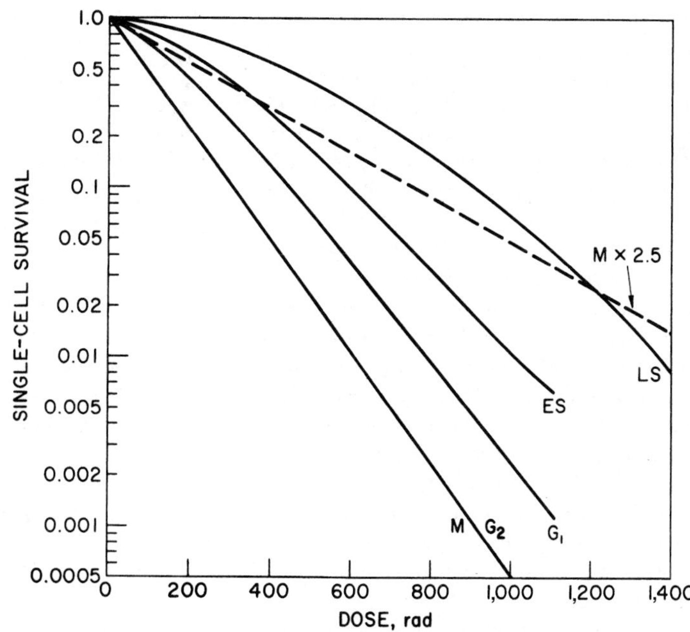

FIGURE 4.8 • Cell survival curves for Chinese hamster cells at various stages of the cell cycle. The survival curve for cells in mitosis is steep and has no shoulder. The curve for cells late in S phase is shallower and has a large initial shoulder. G_1 and early S phases are intermediate in sensitivity. The *broken line* is a calculated curve expected to apply to mitotic cells under hypoxia. (From Sinclair WK: Cyclic x-ray responses in mammalian cells *in vitro*. *Radiat Res* 33:620–643, 1968, with permission.)

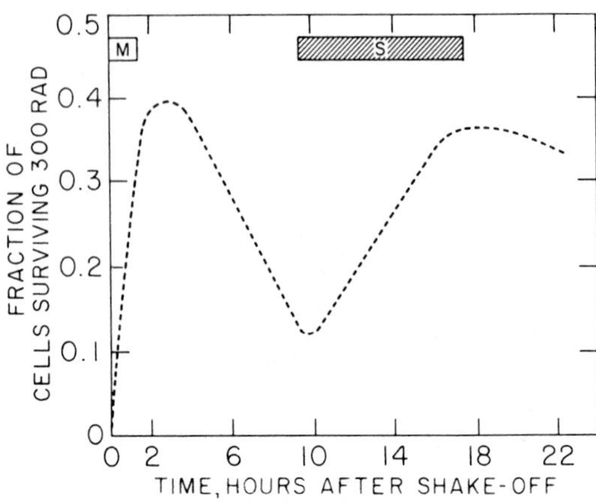

FIGURE 4.9 • Fraction of HeLa cells surviving a dose of 3 Gy (300 rad) of x-rays administered at different times in the division cycle. Time zero represents mitosis. (Adapted from Terasima T, Tolmach LJ: Variations in several responses of HeLa cells to x-irradiation during the division cycle. *Biophys J* 3:11–33, 1963, with permission.)

mitotic cells, which applies to the aerated condition. This line is included in the figure to show that the range of sensitivity between the most sensitive cells (mitotic) and the most resistant cells (late S) is of the same order of magnitude as the oxygen effect (the oxygen effect is discussed in Chapter 6).

The experiments of Terasima and Tolmach with HeLa cells, in which a dose of 3 Gy (300 rad) was delivered to cultures at various intervals after mitotic harvesting of the cells, are shown in Figure 4.9. From the beginning of S phase onward, the pattern of sensitivity is very similar to that of hamster cells; the cells become progressively more resistant as they proceed toward the latter part of S, and after the cells move from S into G_2, their sensitivity increases rapidly as they approach mitosis. The important difference between HeLa and hamster cells is the length of the G_1 phase. The G_1 of HeLa cells is appreciably long, and there appears to be a fine structure in the age–response function during this period. At the beginning of G_1 there is a peak of resistance, followed by a sensitive trough toward the end of G_1. This pattern cannot be distinguished in the hamster cell because G_1 is too short.

Figure 4.10 compares the age–response curves for cells with short G_1, represented by V79 hamster cells, and cells with a long G_1, represented by HeLa cells. If the time scales are adjusted so that S phase has a comparable length for both cell lines, it is evident that the general pattern of cyclic variation is very similar, the only important difference being the extra structure during G_1 in the HeLa cells. In later experiments, other sublines of hamster cells were investigated for which G_1 had an appreciable length; an extra peak of resistance was noted for hamster cells that was similar to the one observed for HeLa cells.

The sensitivity of cells in different parts of G_2 is difficult to determine if synchrony is produced by mitotic selection because of synchrony decay during the passage of the starting population of mitotic cells through their first G_1 and S phases and because G_2 transit times are relatively short (about 1 to 2 hours). A modification of the technique, however, allows a much greater resolution for studying G_2 sensitivity. This is sometimes called "retroactive synchronization": Cells first are irradiated, and then, as a function of time, cells arriving in mitosis are harvested by mitotic shake-off and plated for survival. In this way, it was shown that early G_2 cells are as radioresistant as late S cells, and late G_2 cells are nearly as sensitive as mitotic cells; that is, a sharp transition in radiosensitivity occurs around the so-called x-ray transition point (now often called a "checkpoint") for G_2 cell-cycle delay.

The following is a summary of the main characteristics of the variation of radiosensitivity with cell age in the mitotic cycle:

1. Cells are most sensitive at or close to mitosis.
2. Resistance is usually greatest in the latter part of S phase. The increased resistance is thought to be due to homologous recombination repair between sister chromatids that is more likely to occur after the DNA has replicated (see Chapter 2).
3. If G_1 phase has an appreciable length, a resistant period is evident early in G_1, followed by a sensitive period toward the end of G_1.
4. G_2 phase is usually sensitive, perhaps as sensitive as M phase.

A number of cells lines other than HeLa and hamster have been investigated, some of which tend to agree with these results and some of which are contradictory. The summary points listed here are widely applicable, but exceptions to every one of these generalizations have been noted for one cell line or another.

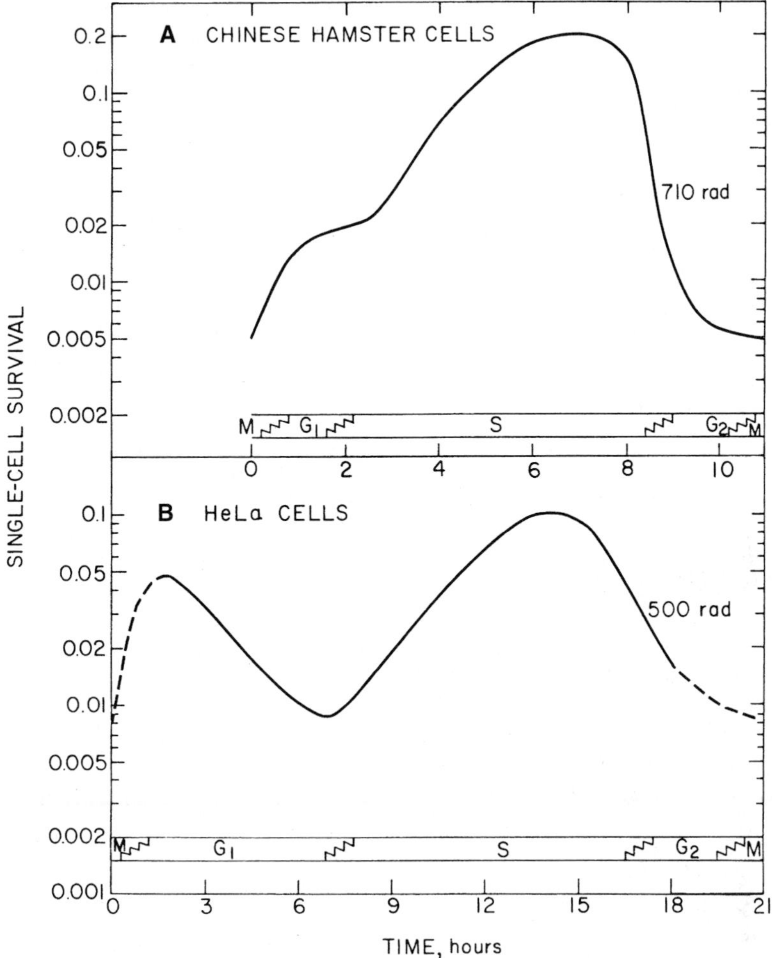

FIGURE 4.10 ● Age–response curves for cells with short G_1 phase, represented by hamster cells (**A**), and cells with long G_1 phase, represented by HeLa cells (**B**). The time scales have been adjusted so that S phase has a comparable length on the figure for both cell lines. (From Sinclair WK: Dependence of radiosensitivity upon cell age. In *Proceedings of the Carmel Conference on Time and Dose Relationships in Radiation Biology as Applied to Radiotherapy*, pp 97–107. BNL Report 50203 (C-57). Upton, NY, 1969, with permission.)

MOLECULAR CHECKPOINT GENES

Cell-cycle progression is controlled by a family of genes known as **molecular checkpoint genes**. It has been known for many years that mammalian cells exposed to a small dose of radiation tend to experience a block in the G_2 phase of the cell cycle. For example, the inverse dose-rate effect has been reported for cells of human origin, whereby over a limited range of dose rates around 0.30 to 0.40 Gy/h (30–40 rad/h) cells become more sensitive to radiation-induced cell killing as the dose rate is reduced, resulting in their accumulation in G_2, which is a radiosensitive phase of the cell cycle. This is described in Chapter 5. The mechanisms for this observation in human cells are not understood in detail, but the molecular genetics in yeast have been worked out, and the search is on for homologous pathways in mammalian cells.

In several strains of yeast, mutants have been isolated that are more sensitive than the wild type to both ionizing radiation and ultraviolet light by a factor between 10 and 100. The mutant gene has been cloned and sequenced and found to be a "G_2 molecular checkpoint gene."

In the most general terms, the function of checkpoint genes is to ensure the correct order of cell-cycle events, that is, to ensure that the initiation of later events is dependent on the completion of

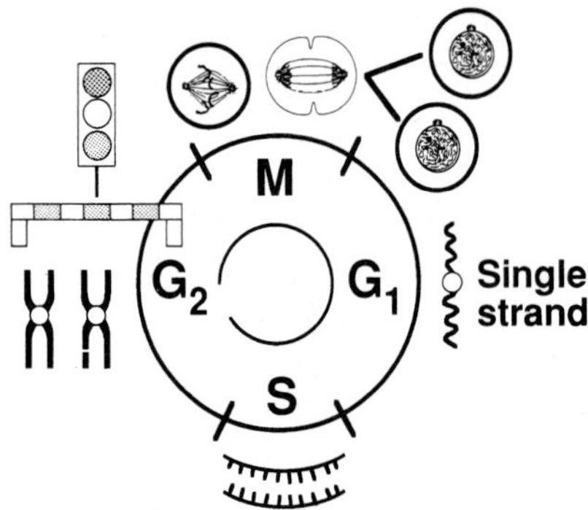

FIGURE 4.11 • Diagram illustrating the site of action and function of the molecular checkpoint gene. Cells exposed to any DNA-damaging agent, including ionizing radiation, are arrested in G_2 phase. The function of the pause in cell-cycle progression is to allow a check of chromosome integrity before the complex task of mitosis is attempted. Cells in which the checkpoint gene is inactivated are much more sensitive to killing by γ-rays or ultraviolet light. The mutant gene isolated from a sensitive strain of yeast functions as a checkpoint gene.

earlier events. The particular genes involved in radiation effects halt cells in G_2, so that an inventory of chromosome damage can be taken, and repair initiated and completed, before the complex task of mitosis is attempted (Fig. 4.11). Mutant cells that lose this G_2 checkpoint gene function move directly into mitosis with damaged chromosomes and are therefore at a higher risk of dying—hence their greater sensitivity to radiation or, for that matter, to any DNA-damaging agent.

It has been proposed that a checkpoint control monitors spindle function during mitosis. If the spindle is disrupted by a microtubular poison, progression through mitosis is blocked. The checkpoint control is involved in this dependency of mitosis on spindle function. It is thought that the mechanism of action of G_2 checkpoint genes involves Cdk1 (p34 protein kinase), levels of which control passage through mitosis. It is likely that mammalian cells that lack checkpoint genes would be sensitive not only to radiation-induced cell killing but also to carcinogenesis. Cells with damaged chromosomes that survive mitosis are likely to give rise to errors in chromosome segregation at mitosis, and this is one of the hallmarks of cancer.

THE EFFECT OF OXYGEN AT VARIOUS PHASES OF THE CELL CYCLE

By combining the most sophisticated techniques of flow cytometry to separate cells in different phases of the cycle with the most sensitive assays for cell survival, it has been shown that the **oxygen enhancement ratio (OER)** varies significantly through the cycle, at least if measured for fast-growing proliferating cells cultured *in vitro*. The OER was measured at 2.3 to 2.4 for G_2 phase cells, compared with 2.8 to 2.9 for S phase, with G_1 phase cells showing an intermediate value. This is discussed in more detail in Chapter 6.

For any given phase of the cell cycle, oxygen was purely dose modifying; that is, the value of the OER was the same for all dose levels. For an asynchronous population of cells, however, the OER does vary slightly with dose or survival level. This is illustrated in Figure 6.1. The OER appears to be smaller at high levels of survival, at which the survival curve is dominated by the killing of the most sensitive moieties of the population; the OER appears to be larger at higher doses and lower levels of survival, at which the response of the most resistant (S phase) cells, which also happen to exhibit the largest OER, dominates.

This is an interesting radiobiologic observation, but the small change of OER is of little or no clinical significance in radiation therapy.

THE AGE–RESPONSE FUNCTION FOR A TISSUE *IN VIVO*

Most studies of the variation in radiosensitivity with phase of the mitotic cycle have been done with mammalian cells cultured *in vitro* because of the ease with which they can be made to divide synchronously. The mitotic harvest technique is clearly only applicable to monolayer cultures, but techniques that involve a drug, such as hydroxyurea, to produce a synchronously dividing population can be applied to some organized tissues.

The epithelial lining of the mouse jejunum represents a classic self-renewal tissue. (The technique used to obtain a survival curve for the crypt cells is described in Chapter 18.) The rapidly dividing crypt cells can be synchronized by giving each mouse five intraperitoneal injections of hydroxyurea every hour. The rationale for this regimen is that all S cells are killed by the drug, and cells in other phases of the cycle are accumulated at the G_1/S boundary for at least 4 hours (the overall time of the five injections).

Figure 4.12, from Withers and his colleagues, shows the response of the jejunal crypt cells to a single dose of 11 Gy (1,100 rad) of γ-rays (uppermost curve) delivered at various times after the synchronizing action of the five injections of hydroxyurea. The number of crypt cells per circumference of the sectioned jejunum varies by a factor of 100, according to the phase in the cycle at which the radiation is delivered, ranging from about 2 survivors

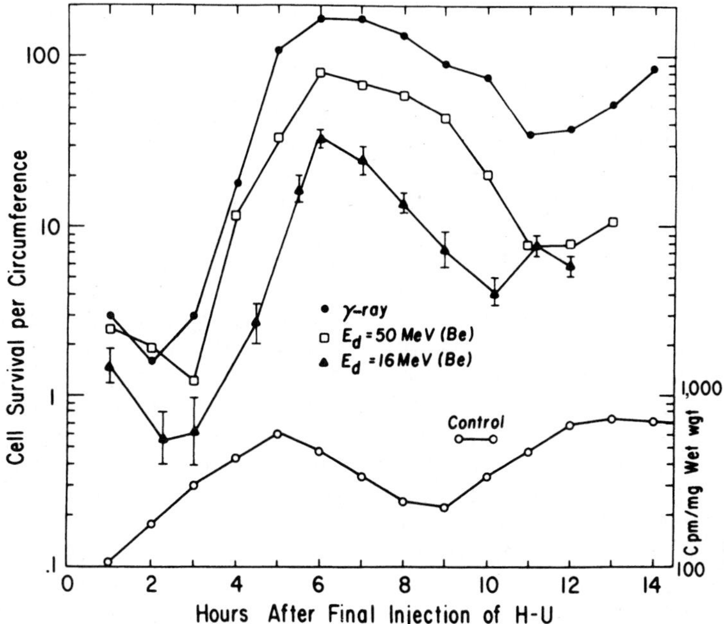

FIGURE 4.12 ● The upper three curves represent fluctuations in the survival of jejunal crypt cells exposed to γ-rays or neutrons as they pass through the cell cycle after synchronization with hydroxyurea (H-U). The doses were 11 Gy (1,100 rad) of γ-rays; 7 Gy (700 rad) of neutrons generated by 50 MeV $d^+ \rightarrow$ Be; and 6 Gy (600 rad) of neutrons generated by 16 MeV $d^+ \rightarrow$ Be. The lower curve represents the uptake of tritiated thymidine (expressed as counts per minute) per wet weight of jejunum as a function of time after the last injection of hydroxyurea. The first wave indicates crypt stem cells passing through S phase after synchronization at G_1–S phase by hydroxyurea. (From Withers HR, Mason K, Reid BO, et al.: Response of mouse intestine to neutrons and gamma rays in relation to dose fractionation and division cycle. *Cancer* 34:39–47, 1974, with permission.)

per circumference for irradiation 2 hours after the last injection of hydroxyurea to about 200 survivors per circumference by 6 hours. The DNA synthetic activity of the synchronized jejunal mucosa was monitored by injecting groups of mice with tritiated thymidine at hourly intervals after the last injection of hydroxyurea and subsequently removing a sample of the jejunum and assaying the radioactive content. The bottom curve of Figure 4.12 shows the variation of thymidine uptake with time. The first wave of the thymidine uptake represents the period of DNA synthesis of the synchronized crypt cells. The peak coincides closely with the period of maximum resistance to x-rays (about 5 hours after the last injection of hydroxyurea).

These data indicate clearly that the radiosensitivity of crypt cells in the mouse jejunum varies substantially with the phase of the cell cycle at which the radiation is delivered. Further, the pattern of response in this organized normal tissue, with a sensitive period between G_1 and S and maximum radioresistance late in S, is very similar to that characteristic of many cell lines cultured *in vitro*.

VARIATION OF SENSITIVITY WITH CELL AGE FOR HIGH-LET RADIATIONS

Figure 4.12 compares the fluctuations in survival of jejunal crypt cells in the mouse after irradiation with γ-rays or neutrons. The variation in radiosensitivity as a function of cell age is qualitatively similar for neutrons and x-rays; that is, with both types of radiation, maximum sensitivity is noted at or close to mitosis, and maximum resistance is evident late in S phase. There is, however, a quantitative difference in that the range of radiosensitivity between the most resistant and the most sensitive phases of the cell cycle is much less for fast neutrons than for x-rays. As LET increases, the variation in radiosensitivity through the cell cycle decreases, so that at very high LET, the age–response function is almost flat—that is, radiosensitivity varies little with the phase of the cell cycle.

MECHANISMS FOR THE AGE–RESPONSE FUNCTION

The reasons for the sensitivity changes through the cell cycle are not at all understood. Several correlations have been proposed, of which two are mentioned here. First, if DNA is the primary target for radiation-induced cell lethality, as commonly is supposed, then changes in the amount or form of the DNA might be expected to result in variations in sensitivity. During S phase, the DNA content doubles as the genome is replicated; just before mitosis, the chromosome material appears to condense into discrete entities. These two events coincide with the periods of minimum and maximum radiosensitivity. The nature of any cause-and-effect relationship is not clear; all that is observed really is a correlation. Second, there is also a correlation between changing radiosensitivity through the cell cycle and varying levels of naturally occurring sulfhydryl compounds in the cell. As noted in Chapter 9, these compounds are powerful radioprotectors.

Either or both of these factors may be at the root of the important and substantial changes in radiosensitivity that cells exhibit as they progress through their generation cycle. In addition, the efficiencies of different repair processes in different phases of the cell cycle can also impact radiosensitivity.

THE POSSIBLE IMPLICATIONS OF THE AGE–RESPONSE FUNCTION IN RADIOTHERAPY

If a single dose of radiation is delivered to a population of cells that are asynchronous—that is, distributed throughout the cell cycle—the effect is different on cells occupying different phases of the cell cycle at the time of the radiation exposure. A greater proportion of cells is killed in the sensitive portions of the cell cycle, such as those at or close to mitosis; a smaller proportion of those in the DNA synthetic phase is killed. The overall effect is that a dose of radiation, to some extent, tends to synchronize the cell population, leaving the majority of cells in a resistant phase of the cycle. Between dose fractions, movement of cells through the cycle into more sensitive phases may be an important factor in "sensitizing" a cycling population of tumor cells to later doses in fractionated regimen. This is considered sensitization resulting from reassortment. It results in a therapeutic gain, because sensitization by this mechanism occurs only in rapidly dividing cells and not in late-responding normal tissues.

Summary of Pertinent Conclusions

- The cell cycle for mammalian cells can be divided into four phases: mitosis (M), followed by G_1, followed by the DNA synthetic phase (S), then G_2, and into mitosis again.
- The phases of the cycle are regulated by the periodic activation of different members of the cyclin-dependent kinase family.
- The fastest-cycling mammalian cells in culture, as well as crypt cells in the intestinal epithelium, have cycle times as short as 9 to 10 hours. Stem cells in resting mouse skin may have cycle times of more than 200 hours. Most of this difference results from the varying length of G_1, the most variable phase of the cycle. The M, S, and G_2 phases do not vary much.
- In general, cells are most radiosensitive in the M and G_2 phases and most resistant in late S phase.
- For cells with longer cell-cycle times and significantly long G_1 phases, there is a second peak of resistance early in G_1.
- Molecular checkpoint genes stop cells from cycling if exposed to x-rays or any other DNA-damaging agent, allowing the chromosomes to be checked for integrity before the complex task of mitosis is attempted.
- The oxygen enhancement ratio (OER) varies little with phase of the cell cycle but may be slightly lower for cells in G_1 than for cells in S.
- The age–response function for crypt cells in the mouse jejunum is similar to that for cells in culture. This is the only tissue in which this has been studied.
- The age–response function for neutrons is qualitatively similar to that for x-rays, but the magnitude of changes through the cycle is smaller.
- The pattern of resistance and sensitivity correlates with the level of sulfhydryl compounds in the cell. Sulfhydryls are natural radioprotectors and tend to be at their highest levels in S phase and at their lowest near mitosis.
- Variations in sensitivity through the cell cycle may be important in radiation therapy because they lead to "sensitization resulting from reassortment" in a fractionated regimen.

BIBLIOGRAPHY

Dewey WC, Highfield DP: G_2 block in Chinese hamster cells induced by x-irradiation, hyperthermia, cycloheximide, or actinomycin-D. *Radiat Res* 65:511–528, 1976

Dolbeare F, Beisker W, Pallavicini M, Vanderlaan M, Gray JW: Cytochemistry for BrdUrd/DNA analysis: Stoichiometry and sensitivity. *Cytometry* 6:521–530, 1985

Dolbeare F, Gratzner H, Pallavicini M, Gray JW: Flow cytometric measurement of total DNA content and incorporated bromodeoxyuridine. *Proc Natl Acad Sci USA* 80:5573–5577, 1983

Freyer JP, Jarrett K, Carpenter S, Raju MR: Oxygen enhancement ratio as a function of dose and cell cycle phase for radiation-resistant and sensitive CHO cells. *Radiat Res* 127:297–307, 1991

Gray JW: Quantitative cytokinetics: Cellular response to cell cycle specific agents. *Pharmacol Ther* 22:163–197, 1983

Gray JW, Dolbeare F, Pallavicini MG, Beisker W, Waldman F: Cell cycle analysis using flow cytometry. *Int J Radiat Biol* 49:237–255, 1986

Griffith TD, Tolmach LJ: Lethal response of HeLa cells to S-irradiation in the latter part of the generation cycle. *Biophys J* 16:303–318, 1976

Hall EJ: Radiobiological measurements with 14-MeV neutrons. *Br J Radiol* 42:805–813, 1969

Hall EJ, Brown JM, Cavanagh J: Radiosensitivity and the oxygen effect measured at different phases of the mitotic cycle using synchronously dividing cells of the root meristem of *Vicia faba*. *Radiat Res* 35:622–634, 1968

Hartwell LH, Weiner TA: Checkpoints: Controls that ensure the order of cell cycle events. *Science* 246:629–634, 1989

Hoshino T, Yagashima T, Morovic J, Livin E, Livin V: Cell kinetic studies of *in situ* human brain tumors with bromodeoxyuridine. *Cytometry* 6:627–632, 1985

Howard A, Pelc SR: Synthesis of deoxyribonucleic acid in normal and irradiated cells and its relation to chromosome breakage. *Heredity* 6(suppl):261–273, 1953

Hoyt MA, Totis L, Roberts BT: *S. cerevisiae* genes required for cell cycle arrest in response to loss of microtubule function. *Cell* 66:507–517, 1991

Legrys GA, Hall EJ: The oxygen effect and x-ray sensitivity in synchronously dividing cultures of Chinese hamster cells. *Radiat Res* 37:161–172, 1969

Li R, Murray AW: Feedback control of mitosis in budding yeast. *Cell* 66:519–531, 1991

Lieberman HB, Hopkins KM, Laverty M, Chu HM: Molecular cloning and analysis of *Schizosaccharomyces pombe rad 9*, a gene involved in DNA repair and mutagenesis. *Mol Gen Genet* 232:367–376, 1992

Morstyn G, Hsu MS-M, Kinsella T, Gratzner H, Russo A, Mitchell J: Bromodeoxyuridine in tumors and chromosomes detected with a monoclonal antibody. *J Clin Invest* 72:1844–1850, 1983

Schneiderman MH, Dewey WC, Leeper DB, Nagasawa H: Use of the mitotic selection procedure for cell cycle analysis: Comparison between the x-ray and G_2 markers. *Exp Cell Res* 74:430–438, 1972

Sinclair WK: Cyclic x-ray responses in mammalian cells *in vitro*. *Radiat Res* 33:620–643, 1968

Sinclair WK: Dependence of radiosensitivity upon cell age. In *Proceedings of the Carmel Conference on Time and Dose Relationships in Radiation Biology as Applied to Radiotherapy*, pp 97–107. BNL Report 50203 (C-57). Upton, NY, 1969

Sinclair WK: Radiation survival in synchronous and asynchronous Chinese hamster cells *in vitro*. *In Biophysical Aspects of Radiation Quality: Proceedings of the Second IAEA Panel*, pp 39–54. Vienna, IAEA, 1968

Sinclair WK, Morton RA: X-ray sensitivity during the cell generation cycle of cultured Chinese hamster cells. *Radiat Res* 29:450–474, 1966

Steel G, Hanes S: The technique labelled mitoses: Analysis by automatic curve fitting. *Cell Tissue Kinet* 4:93–105, 1971

Terasima T, Tolmach LJ: Variations in several responses of HeLa cells to x-irradiation during the division cycle. *Biophys* J 3:11–33, 1963

Terasima R, Tolmach LJ: X-ray sensitivity and DNA synthesis in synchronous populations of HeLa cells. *Science* 140:490–492, 1963

Withers HR, Mason K, Reid BO, et al.: Response of mouse intestine to neutrons and gamma rays in relation to dose fractionation and division cycle. *Cancer* 34:39–47, 1974

CHAPTER 5

Repair of Radiation Damage and the Dose-Rate Effect

GENERAL OVERVIEW OF DNA REPAIR PATHWAYS

Mammalian cells on average experience over 100,000 DNA lesions per day as a result of replication errors, chemical decay of their bases, attack by reactive oxygen species, or exposure to ionizing radiation. However, the mutation rate in mammalian cells is quite low owing to the development of DNA repair pathways that handle each type of damage. As described in Chapter 2, ionizing radiation can induce base damage, single-strand breaks, double-strand breaks, sugar damage and DNA-DNA and DNA-protein cross-links. Mammalian cells have developed specialized pathways to sense, respond to, and repair these different types of damage. Research from yeast to mammalian cells has demonstrated that the mechanisms used to repair ionizing radiation-induced base damage are different from the mechanisms used to repair DNA double-strand breaks. As discussed below, different repair pathways are used to repair DNA damage, depending on the stage of the cell cycle. In fact, we know little about how DNA repair and cell-cycle regulation are coordinately regulated at the molecular level. For example, an ionizing radiation-induced double-strand break in an S phase cell would benefit from the cell inhibiting DNA replication until the break is repaired.

Much of our knowledge of DNA repair is the result of studying how mutations in individual genes result in radiation hypersensitivity. Recently, the

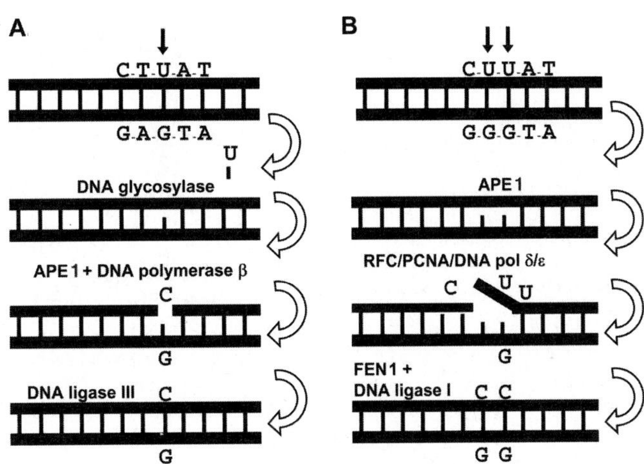

FIGURE 5.1 ● Base Excision Repair pathways. **A:** Base excision repair of a single nucleotide. Bases on opposite strands must be complementary; adenine (A) pairs with thymine (T), and guanine (G) pairs with cytosine (C). U represents a putative mutation that is first removed through a DNA glycosylase–mediated incision step. **B:** Base excision repair of multiple nucleotides. In this case, the double UU represents a putative mutation that is first removed through apurinic endonuclease 1 (APE1). See text for details.

creation of systematic deletions in all the genes of the budding yeast *Saccharomyces cerevisiae* has resulted in the identification of all nonessential yeast genes whose loss results in hypersensitivity to x-rays. The advantage of this approach is that the entire yeast genome can be tested in one experiment, and more importantly, the identity of individual radiation-sensitive mutants is known from a molecular bar tag (see Chapter 16 for more details). Radiation-sensitive mutants identified from screening both yeast and mammalian cells appear either to be involved directly in the repair process or to function as molecular checkpoint–controlling elements. This chapter focuses on DNA damage repair pathways that are involved in the cellular response to ionizing radiation.

Base Excision Repair (BER)

Base damage is repaired through the base excision repair (BER) pathway illustrated in Figure 5.1. As discussed in Chapter 2, bases on opposite strands must be complementary; adenine (A) pairs with thymine (T), and guanine (G) pairs with cytosine (C). U therefore represents a putative single-base mutation that is first removed by a glycosylase/DNA lyase (Fig. 5.1**A**). This is followed by the removal of the sugar residue by an AP endonuclease, then replacement with the correct nucleotide by DNA polymerase β, and completed by DNA ligase III–*XRCC1*–mediated ligation. If more than one nucleotide is to be replaced (illustrated by the putative mutation UU in Figure 5.1**B**), then the complex of RFC/PCNA/DNA polymerase δ/ϵ performs the repair synthesis, the overhanging flap structure is removed by the FEN1 endonuclease, and DNA strands are sealed by ligase I (Fig. 5.1**B**). Whereas ionizing radiation–induced base damage is efficiently repaired, defects in base excision repair may lead to an increased mutation rate, but usually do not result in cellular radiosensitivity. One exception to this is the mutation of the *XRCC1* gene (x-ray cross complementing factor 1), which confers about a 1.7-fold increase in radiation sensitivity. However, the radiation sensitivity of *XRCC1*-deficient cells may come from *XRCC1*'s involvement in other repair processes, such as single-strand breaks.

Nucleotide Excision Repair (NER)

Nucleotide excision repair (NER) removes bulky adducts in the DNA, such as pyrimidine dimers. The essential steps in this pathway are (1) damage recognition, (2) DNA incisions that bracket the lesion, usually between 24 and 32 nucleotides in length, (3) removal of the region containing the adducts, (4) repair synthesis to fill in the gap region, and (5) DNA ligation. Mutation in nucleotide excision repair genes does not lead to ionizing radiation sensitivity. However, defective nucleotide excision repair increases sensitivity to UV-induced DNA damage and anticancer agents such as alkylating agents that induce bulky adducts. Germline mutations in nucleotide excision repair genes lead to human DNA repair deficiency disorders such as xeroderma pigmentosum, in which patients are hypersensitive to ultraviolet light.

DNA Double-Strand Break Repair

As discussed in Chapter 2, there are multiple lines of evidence to support the importance of DNA double-strand breaks as the critical lesion induced by ionizing radiation. In eukaryotic cells, DNA double-strand breaks can be repaired by two basic processes: homologous recombination repair

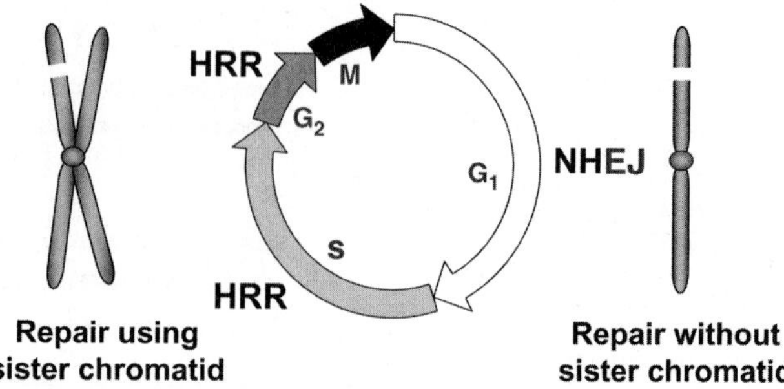

FIGURE 5.2 • Illustration showing that nonhomologous recombination occurs in the G_1 phase of the cell cycle, at which stage there is no sister chromatid to use as a template for repair. In contrast, homologous recombination occurs in the S and G_2 phases of the cell cycle, when there is a sister chromatid to use as a template in repair.

(HRR), requiring an undamaged DNA strand as a participant in the repair as a template, and nonhomologous end joining (NHEJ), which mediates end-to-end joining. In lower eukaryotes such as yeast, homologous recombination repair is the predominant pathway used for repairing DNA double-strand breaks. Double-strand break repair by homologous recombination is an error-free process because repair is performed by copying information from the undamaged homologous chromatid/chromosome. In mammalian cells, the choice of repair is biased by the phase of the cell cycle and by the abundance of repetitive DNA (Fig. 5.2). HRR occurs primarily in the late S/G_2 phase of the cell cycle, when an undamaged sister chromatid is available to act as a template, and NHEJ occurs in the G_1 phase of the cell cycle, when no such template exists. NHEJ is error prone and probably accounts for many of the premutagenic lesions induced in the DNA of human cells by ionizing radiation. However, it is important to keep in mind that NHEJ and HRR are not mutually exclusive, and both have been found to be active in the late S/G_2 phase of the cell cycle, indicating that other as yet unidentified factors in addition to cell-cycle phase are important in determining what repair program is used.

Nonhomologous End Joining (NHEJ)

The ligation of DNA double-strand breaks does not require sequence homology and is therefore termed nonhomologous end joining (NHEJ). However, the damaged ends of DNA double-strand breaks cannot simply be ligated together; they must first be modified before they can be rejoined by a ligation reaction. NHEJ can be divided into four steps: (1) end recognition, (2) end processing, (3) fill-in synthesis, or end bridging, and (4) ligation (Fig. 5.3**A**).

End recognition occurs when the Ku heterodimer, composed of 70-kDa and 83-kDa subunits, and the DNA-dependent protein kinase catalytic subunit (DNA-PKcs) bind to the ends of the DNA double-strand break. Although the Ku/DNA-PKcs complex is thought to bind ends first, it is still unknown what holds the two DNA double-strand break ends together. Although microhomology between one to four nucleotides can aid in end alignment, there is no absolute requirement for microhomology for NHEJ. In fact, Ku does not only recruit DNA-PKcs to the DNA ends, but an additional protein, Artemis, forms a physical complex with DNA-PKcs. DNA-PKcs that is bound can phosphorylate Artemis and activate its endonuclease activity to deal with 5′ and 3′ overhangs as well as hairpins. End processing is followed by fill-in synthesis of gaps formed by the Artemis endonuclease activity. This aspect of NHEJ may not necessarily be essential, for example, in the ligation of blunt ends or ends with compatible termini. It is unclear what the signal is for a fill-in reaction to proceed after endonuclease processing and what polymerase is used in this step. DNA polymerase μ has been found to be associated with the Ku/DNA/XRCC4/DNA ligase IV complex and serves as a strong candidate polymerase for the fill-in reaction. In the final step of NHEJ, ligation of nicked DNA ends that have been processed is mediated by an XRCC4/DNA ligase IV complex that is probably recruited by the Ku heterodimer. NHEJ is error prone and plays an important physiologic role in generating antibodies through V(D)J rejoining. The error-prone nature of NHEJ is essential for generating antibody diversity and often goes undetected in mammalian cells, as errors in the noncoding DNA that composes the majority of the human genome has little consequence. Nonhomologous end joining is primarily found in the G_1 phase of the cell cycle, where there is no sister chromatid.

Homologous Recombination Repair (HRR)

Homologous recombination repair (HRR) provides the mammalian genome a high-fidelity mechanism of repairing DNA double-strand breaks (Fig. 5.3**B**). In particular, the increased activity of this

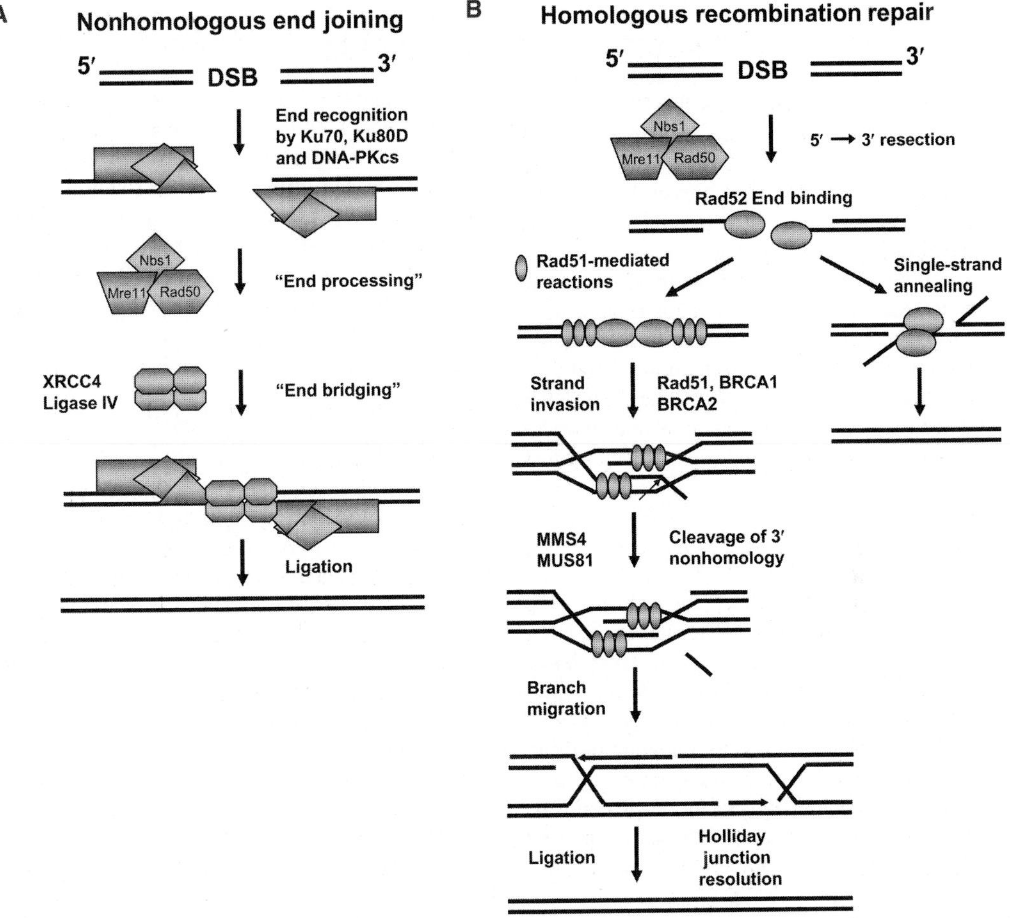

FIGURE 5.3 • DNA double-strand break repair via homologous and nonhomologous recombination. **A:** A double-strand break with no template to guide gap filling. Consequently, errors are more likely to occur in this process, which is called nonhomologous end joining. See text for details. **B:** A double-strand break that has occurred after replication (in S or G_2 phase of the cell cycle), so that identical sister chromatids are available. In homologous recombination (also termed single-strand annealing), the exposed 3′ end invades the homologous duplex, so that the complementary strand acts as a template for gap filling.

recombination pathway in late S/G_2 suggests that its primary function is to repair and restore the functionality of replication forks with DNA double-strand breaks. Compared to NHEJ, which requires no sequence homology to rejoin broken ends, HRR requires physical contact with an undamaged chromatid or chromosome (to serve as a template) for repair to occur.

The immediate response of a cell to a DNA double-strand break is the activation of a group of sensors that serve both to promote DNA repair and to prevent the cell from proceeding in the cell cycle until the break is faithfully repaired. These sensors, ATM (ataxia-telangiectasia mutated) and ATR (ataxia-telangiectasia and Rad3 related), are protein kinases that belong to the phosphatidylinositol-3-kinase-related kinase (PIKK) family and are recruited to the sites of DNA strand breaks induced by ionizing radiation. It is hypothesized that ATM and ATR phosphorylate H2AX, which then recruits the breast cancer tumor suppressor protein BRCA1 to the site of the break to regulate the activity of the NBS/MRE11/Rad50s protein complex (Fig. 5.3**B**). MRE11 and as yet unidentified endonucleases resect the DNA, resulting in a 3′ single-strand DNA that serves as a binding site for Rad51. BRCA2, which is attracted to the double-strand break by BRCA1, facilitates the loading of Rad51 onto RPA-coated single-strand overhangs produced by endonuclease resection. Rad51 protein is a homologue of the *E. coli* recombinase RecA and possesses the ability to form nucleofilaments and catalyze strand exchange with the complementary strand in the undamaged chromosome. Five additional paralogues of Rad51 also bind to the RPA-coated single-stranded region and recruit Rad52, which protects against exonucleoyltic degradation. To facilitate repair, Rad54 uses its ATPase activity to unwind the double-stranded molecule. The two invading ends serve as primers for DNA synthesis, and the so-called Holliday junctions (MMS4 and MUS81) are resolved by MMS4 and MUS81 by non-crossing over, in which case the Holliday junctions disengage and DNA strands pair followed by gap filling, or by crossing over of the Holliday junctions and gap filling. The identities of the polymerase and ligase involved in these latter steps are unknown. Because inactivation of HRR genes results in radiosensitivity and genomic instability, these genes provide a critical link between HRR and chromosome stability. Dysregulated homologous recombination can also lead to cancer by loss of heterozygosity (LOH).

Single-Strand Annealing (SSA)

Single-strand annealing (SSA) plays a transitional role between HRR and NHEJ. The ends of the DNA double-strand break are digested by an exonuclease, most probably by the NBS/MRE11/Rad50 complex, until regions of homology are exposed on both ends of the breaks. The nonhomologous tails are removed so that the two ends can be ligated. Therefore, while SSA shares parts of the HRR pathway, it results in loss of genetic information owing to the exonuclease degradation of the DNA ends.

Cross-Link Repair

The number of DNA-DNA and DNA-protein cross-links induced by ionizing radiation has not been extensively studied to arrive at a quantitative estimate. The genes and pathways used for DNA-DNA or DNA-protein cross-link repair are still under investigation. The current thinking is that a combination of nucleotide excision repair and recombinational repair pathways is needed to repair DNA cross-links. Chromatin that contains actively transcribed genes is more susceptible to DNA-protein cross-links, and the cross-linked proteins are usually nuclear matrix proteins.

Mismatch Repair

The mismatch repair pathway removes base-base and small insertion mismatches that occur during replication. In addition, the mismatch repair pathway removes base-base mismatches in homologous recombination intermediates. Mutations in any of the mismatch *MSH, MLH*, and *PSM* families of repair genes lead to microsatellite instability (small base insertions or deletions) and cancer, especially hereditary nonpolyposis colon cancer (HNPCC).

HEREDITARY SYNDROMES THAT AFFECT RADIOSENSITIVITY

The DNA damage response in mammalian cells is comprised of multiprotein complexes that sense, signal, and respond to DNA strand breaks. Disruption of the function of these multiprotein complexes by mutation of a single gene leads to cancer-prone syndromes that are characterized by hypersensitivity to DNA damage and genomic instability. Syndromes that exhibit hypersensitivity to ionizing radiation are discussed here.

Ataxia-Telangiectasia (AT)

Ataxia-telangiectasia (AT) is a rare autosomal recessive disease in which afflicted individuals present with progressive cerebellar ataxia due to increased loss of Purkinje cells in the cerebellum as well as oculocutaneous telangiectasia. AT patients are immune deficient and have a high incidence of cancer, especially of the reticular endothelial system. Individuals with AT exhibit a hypersensitive skin reaction to ionizing radiation and DNA breaking agents, but not to ultraviolet light. Both lymphocytes and fibroblasts derived from these individuals are also hypersensitive to killing by ionizing radiation.

The genetic defect responsible for the AT phenotype is the result of mutations in the *ATM* (ataxia-telangiectasia mutated) gene. The *ATM* gene encodes for a kinase that phosphorylates a serine or threonine that is followed by a glutamine motif (S/T-Q) in target proteins. ATM is involved in the rapid response of cells to DNA double-strand breaks (it signals to the DNA repair machinery) as well as the activation of cell-cycle checkpoints. However, it is important to recognize that while the ATM kinase is activated by DNA damage and chromatin alterations throughout the cell cycle, it uses different downstream effectors to mediate a checkpoint response in each of the different phases of the cell cycle. For example, the activation of a G_1 checkpoint is in large part mediated by ATM signaling to p53, which results in the transcriptional induction of the p21 cell-cycle inhibitor. Perhaps the most distinctive hallmark of AT cells is their failure to arrest in S phase in response to DNA damage. This phenomenon has been termed radioresistant DNA synthesis, and at least two pathways regulated by ATM control the passage of cells through S phase.

Much is known about the way in which ATM and its family members control cell-cycle checkpoints, but the mechanism by which loss of ATM leads to increased radiosensitivity is still under investigation. It may involve both *direct* mechanisms, such as direct phosphorylation of the cohesin family member SMC or NBS (Nijmegen breakage syndrome) protein, and *indirect* mechanisms, such as dysregulated homologous recombination. Lymphoid cells in ATM homozygotes often exhibit increased chromosomal instability, and the lymphomas that develop demonstrate the importance of DNA repair and chromosome maintenance in tumor suppression.

In mammalian cells, ATM belongs to the phosphatidylinositol 3-kinase-related kinase (PIKK) family and shares homology with two other family members—ATR (ataxia-telangiectasia and Rad3 related) and DNA-PKcs (DNA-dependent protein kinase catalytic subunit)—that are also activated by DNA strand breaks. At the molecular level, ATR and DNA-PKcs-like ATM regulate DNA repair and cell-cycle regulatory proteins. Interestingly, while *ATM* is not an essential gene, *ATR* is essential. Some individuals afflicted with Seckel's syndrome, a rare autosomal recessive disorder characterized by microcephaly and abnormal development, can possess an alteration in the *ATR* gene that reduces its absolute quantity but does not eliminate its activity. Seckel's syndrome patients do not appear to be radiosensitive, as they possess some ATR activity. The third member of this family, DNA-PKcs, is an essential component of nonhomologous recombination and is the defect in murine SCID (severe combined immunodeficiency) syndrome. However, human SCID patients do not possess DNA-PKcs mutations, but instead possess mutations in Artemis, a target of DNA-PKcs. Artemis-deficient human SCID cells are radiosensitive, and fibroblasts from afflicted individuals exhibit increased chromosomal instability.

Ataxia-Telangiectasia-Like Disorder (ATLD)

Ataxia-telangiectasia-like disorder (ATLD) is an autosomal recessive disease caused by mutations in the gene *MRE11* that forms a complex with Rad50 and NBS in irradiated cells. Cells derived from ATLD patients are radiosensitive but repair their DNA double-strand breaks similar to wild-type levels, leaving the mechanism for their radiosensitivity in question. ATLD1 cells are also defective in their checkpoint response following DNA damage.

Nijmegen Breakage Syndrome (NBS)

Nijmegen breakage syndrome (NBS) is a direct phosphorylation target of ATM and forms a complex with Rad50 and *MRE11*. This complex possesses nuclease activity that is necessary for DNA double-strand break repair. The relationship between NBS and ATM is complex, as ATM phosphorylates NBS in response to DNA damage, but NBS may also be required for activation of some ATM checkpoint responses. Thus, the mechanism of AT, ATLD1, and NBS sensitivity to ionizing radiation is probably the same.

Fanconi Anemia (FA)

Eight different proteins give rise to the autosomal recessive disorder Fanconi anemia (FA), which is characterized by spontaneous chromosomal instability, sensitivity to interstrand DNA cross-links, and in some cases sensitivity to ionizing radiation. The *FANCD2* gene is thought to be a key player in the FA pathway because it is the only *FANC* gene conserved through evolution, and most of the other *FANC* proteins form a complex that results in the monoubiquitination of *FANCD2* that results in its localization to foci that contain the breast cancer tumor suppressor genes *BRCA* and *BRCA2* (also known as *FANCD1*). The identification of *BRCA2* as an FA gene, together with its localization in foci with *FANCD2*, suggests an important role for *FANC* genes in homologous recombination. In addition, *FANCD2* has been implicated in the DNA damage checkpoint response and is phosphorylated by the ATM kinase on serine 222. The roles of *FANCD2* in the radiation response and cross-link response are separable, because inhibition of phosphorylation on serine 222 inhibits the FA-mediated radiation response, and inhibition of ubiquitination of lysine 561 results in hypersensitivity to cross-linking agents.

Clinical reports have suggested that tumors derived from patients with FA are hypersensitive to radiotherapy. However, fibroblasts derived from individuals that possess mutated forms of each of the eight different FA proteins were not always found to exhibit radiosensitivity, and never to the same level as AT cells. Therefore, the clinical response of FA patients to radiotherapy does not always correlate with intrinsic radiosensitivity of fibroblasts derived from the same patients, suggesting that additional genetic alterations in tumor cells from patients with FA may be responsible for the enhanced radiosensitivity that has been observed.

OPERATIONAL CLASSIFICATIONS OF RADIATION DAMAGE

Radiation damage to mammalian cells can operationally be divided into three categories: (1) **lethal damage**, which is irreversible and irreparable and, by definition, leads irrevocably to cell death; (2) **potentially lethal damage (PLD)**, the component of radiation damage that can be modified by postirradiation environmental conditions; and (3) **sublethal damage (SLD)**, which under normal circumstances can be repaired in hours unless additional sublethal damage is added (e.g., from a second dose of radiation) with which it can interact to form lethal damage (sublethal damage repair, therefore, is manifest by the increase in survival observed if a dose of radiation is split into two fractions separated by a time interval).

Potentially Lethal Damage (PLD) Repair

Varying environmental conditions after exposure to x-rays can influence the proportion of cells that survive a given dose because of the expression or repair of PLD. This damage is potentially lethal because under ordinary circumstances it causes cell death, but if survival is increased as a result of the manipulation of the postirradiation environment, PLD is considered to have been repaired. PLD is repaired if cells are incubated in a balanced salt solution instead of full growth medium for several hours after irradiation. This is a drastic treatment, however, and does not mimic a physiologic condition that is ever likely to occur. Little and his colleagues chose to study PLD repair in density-inhibited stationary-phase cell cultures, which are considered a better *in vitro* model for tumor cells *in vivo* (Fig. 5.4). Cell survival was enhanced considerably if the cells were allowed to remain in the density-inhibited state for 6 or 12 hours after irradiation before being subcultured and assayed for colony-forming ability.

The relevance of PLD to radiotherapy became much more obvious when it was shown that repair,

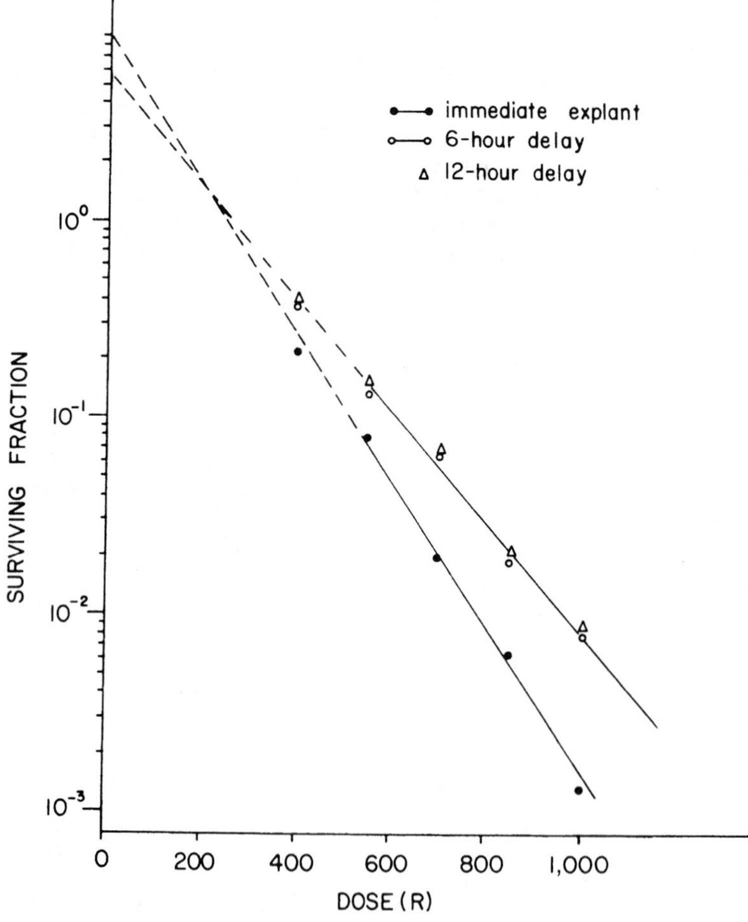

FIGURE 5.4 • X-ray survival curves for density-inhibited stationary-phase cells, subcultured (trypsinized and plated) either immediately or 6 or 12 hours after irradiation. Cell survival is enhanced if cells are left in the stationary phase after irradiation, allowing time for the repair of potentially lethal damage. (From Little JB, Hahn GM, Frindel E, Tubiana M: Repair of potentially lethal radiation damage *in vitro* and *in vivo*. *Radiology* 106:689–694, 1973, with permission.)

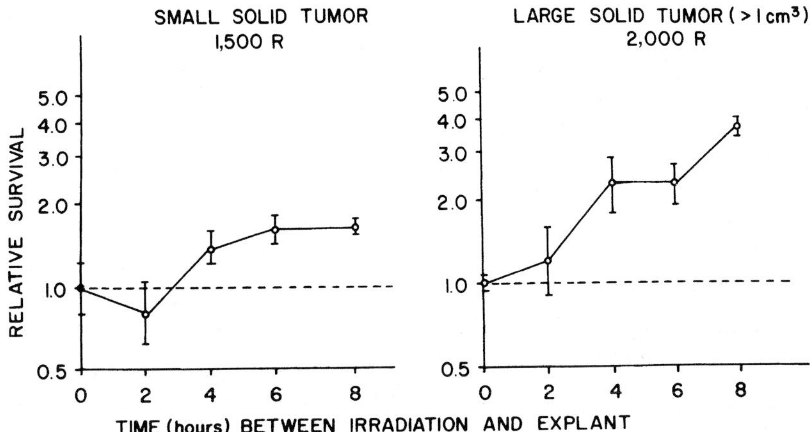

FIGURE 5.5 • Repair of potentially lethal damage in mouse fibrosarcomas. The tumors were irradiated *in situ* and then removed and prepared into single-cell suspensions. The number of survivors was determined by their ability to form colonies *in vitro*. The fraction of cells surviving a given dose increases if a time interval is allowed between irradiation and removal of the tumor, because during this interval, potentially lethal damage is repaired. (From Little JB, Hahn GM, Frindel E, Tubiana M: Repair of potentially lethal radiation damage *in vitro* and *in vivo*. *Radiology* 106:689–694, 1973, with permission.)

comparable in magnitude and kinetics to that found *in vitro*, also occurred *in vivo* in experimental tumors. In this case, repair took the form of significantly enhanced cell survival if several hours were allowed to elapse between irradiation of the tumor *in situ* and removal of the cells from the host to assess their reproductive integrity (Fig. 5.5).

To summarize the available experimental data, there is general agreement that PLD is repaired and the fraction of cells surviving a given dose of x-rays enhanced if postirradiation conditions are suboptimal for growth, so that cells do not have to attempt the complex process of mitosis while their chromosomes are damaged. If mitosis is delayed by suboptimal growth conditions, DNA damage can be repaired.

The importance of PLD repair to clinical radiotherapy is a matter of debate. That it occurs in transplantable animal tumors has been documented beyond question, and there is no reason to suppose that it does not occur in human tumors. It has been suggested that the radioresistance of certain types of human tumors is linked to their ability to repair PLD; that is, radiosensitive tumors repair PLD inefficiently, but radioresistant tumors have efficient mechanisms to repair PLD. This is an attractive hypothesis, but it has never been proven.

Sublethal Damage (SLD) Repair

Sublethal damage repair is the operational term for the increase in cell survival that is observed if a given radiation dose is split into two fractions separated by a time interval.

Figure 5.6 shows data obtained in a split-dose experiment with cultured Chinese hamster cells. A single dose of 15.58 Gy (1,558 rad) leads to a

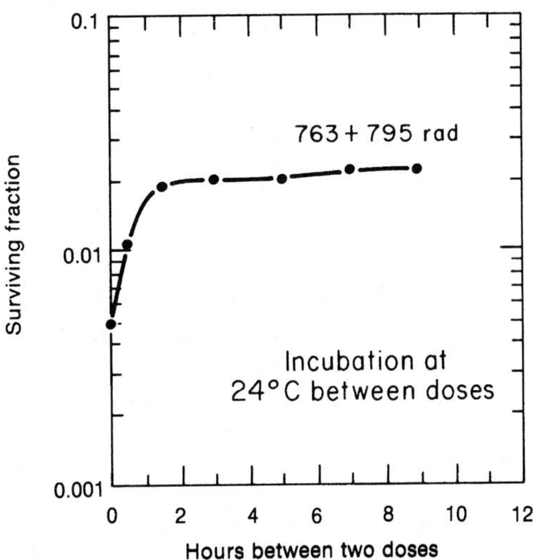

FIGURE 5.6 • Survival of Chinese hamster cells exposed to two fractions of x-rays and incubated at room temperature for various time intervals between the two exposures. (From Elkind MM, Sutton-Gilbert H, Moses WB, Alescio T, Swain RB: Radiation response of mammalian cells in culture: V. Temperature dependence of the repair of x-ray damage in surviving cells [aerobic and hypoxic]. *Radiat Res* 25:359–376, 1965, with permission.)

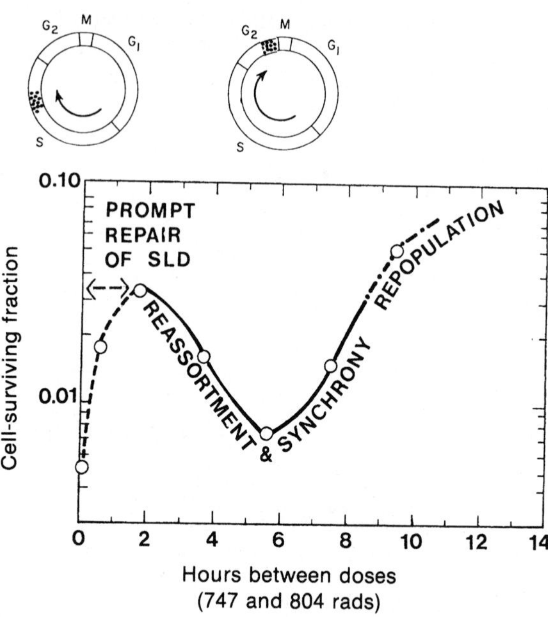

FIGURE 5.7 ● Survival of Chinese hamster cells exposed to two fractions of x-rays and incubated at 37°C for various time intervals between the two doses. The survivors of the first dose are predominantly in a resistant phase of the cycle (late S). If the interval between doses is about 6 hours, these resistant cells have moved to the G_2/M phase, which is sensitive. (Adapted from Elkind MM, Sutton-Gilbert H, Moses WB, Alescio T, Swain RB: Radiation response of mammalian cells in culture: V. Temperature dependence of the repair of x-ray damage in surviving cells [aerobic and hypoxic]. *Radiat Res* 25:359–376, 1965, with permission.)

surviving fraction of 0.005. If the dose is divided into two approximately equal fractions separated by 30 minutes, the surviving fraction is already appreciably higher than for a single dose. As the time interval is extended, the surviving fraction increases until a plateau is reached at about 2 hours, corresponding to a surviving fraction of 0.02. This represents about four times as many surviving cells as for the dose given in a single exposure. A further increase in the time interval between the dose fractions is not accompanied by any significant additional increment in survival. The increase in survival in a split-dose experiment results from the repair of sublethal radiation damage.

The data shown in Figure 5.6 were obtained with cultured mammalian cells maintained at room temperature (24°C) between the dose fractions to prevent the cells from moving through the cell cycle during this interval. This rather special experiment is described first because it illustrates repair of sublethal radiation damage uncomplicated by the movement of cells through the cell cycle.

Figure 5.7 shows the results of a parallel experiment in which cells were exposed to split doses and maintained at their normal growing temperature of 37°C. The pattern of repair seen in this case differs from that observed for cells kept at room temperature. In the first few hours, prompt repair of sublethal damage is again evident, but at longer intervals between the two split doses, the surviving fraction of cells decreases, reaching a minimum with about a 5-hour separation.

An understanding of this phenomenon is based on the age–response function described in Chapter 4. If an asynchronous population of cells is exposed to a large dose of radiation, more cells are killed in the sensitive than in the resistant phases of the cell cycle. The surviving population of cells, therefore, tends to be partly synchronized.

In Chinese hamster cells, most of the survivors from a first dose are located in the S phase of the cell cycle. If about 6 hours are allowed to elapse before a second dose of radiation is given, this cohort of cells progresses around the cell cycle and is in G_2/M, a sensitive period of the cell cycle, at the time of the second dose. If the increase in radiosensitivity in moving from late S to the G_2/M period exceeds the effect of repair of sublethal damage, the surviving fraction falls.

The pattern of repair shown in Figure 5.7 is therefore a combination of three processes occurring simultaneously. First, there is the prompt repair of sublethal radiation damage. Second, there is progression of cells through the cell cycle during the interval between the split doses, which has been termed **reassortment**. Third, there is an increase of surviving fraction resulting from cell division, or **repopulation**, if the interval between the split doses is 10 to 12 hours, because this exceeds the length of the cell cycle of these rapidly growing cells.

This simple experiment, performed *in vitro*, illustrates three of the "four Rs" of radiobiology: **repair**, **reassortment**, and **repopulation**. The fourth "R," **reoxygenation**, is discussed in Chapter 6. It should be emphasized that the dramatic dip in the split-dose curve at 6 hours, caused by reassortment, and the increase in survival by 12 hours, because of repopulation, are seen only for rapidly

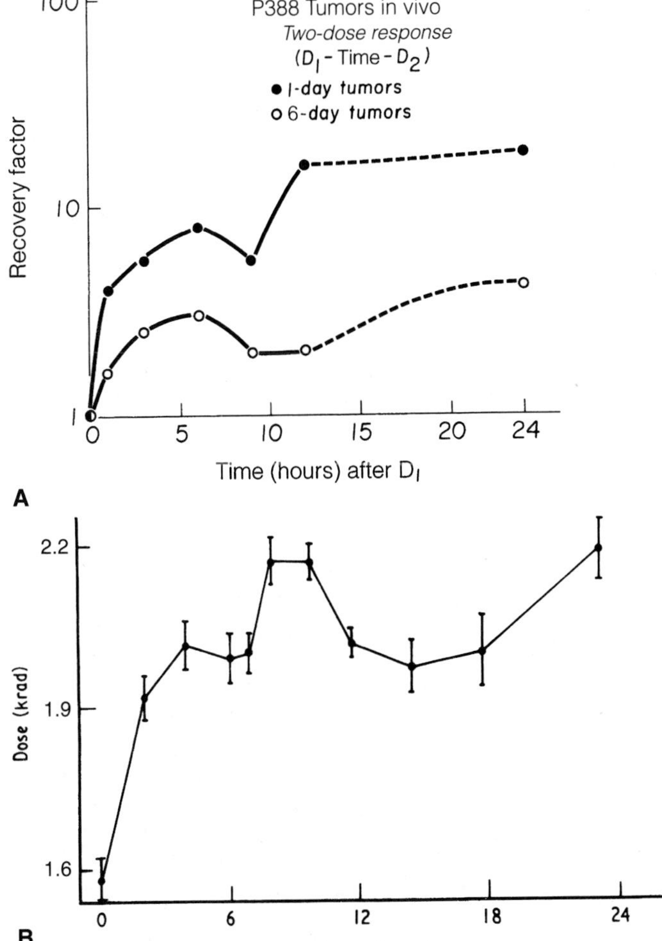

FIGURE 5.8 ● Repair of sublethal damage in two *in vivo* mammalian cell systems. **A:** Split-dose experiments with P388 lymphocytic leukemia cells in the mouse. The recovery factor is the ratio of the surviving fraction resulting from two-dose fractionation to the survival from a single equivalent dose. One-day-old tumors are composed predominantly of oxygenated cells; the cells in 6-day-old tumors are hypoxic. (From Belli JA, Dicus GJ, Bonte FJ: Radiation response of mammalian tumor cells: 1. Repair of sublethal damage *in vivo*. *J Natl Cancer Inst* 38:673–682, 1967, with permission.) **B:** Split-dose experiments with skin epithelial cells in the mouse. The total x-ray dose, given as two fractions, required to result in one surviving epithelial cell per square millimeter is plotted against the time interval between the two doses. (From Emery EW, Denekamp J, Ball MM: Survival of mouse skin epithelial cells following single and divided doses of x-rays. *Radiat Res* 41:450–466, 1970, with permission.)

growing cells. Hamster cells in culture have a cycle time of only 9 or 10 hours. The time sequence of these events would be longer in more slowly proliferating normal tissues *in vivo*.

Repair of sublethal radiation damage has been demonstrated in just about every biologic test system for which a quantitative end point is available. Figure 5.8 illustrates the pattern for repair of sublethal radiation damage in two *in vivo* systems in mice, P388 lymphocytic leukemia and skin cells. In neither case is there a dramatic dip in the curve at 6 hours resulting from movement of cells through the cycle, because the cell cycle is long. In resting skin, for example, the cell cycle of stem cells may be as long as 10 days rather than the 9 hours of the rapidly growing cells in Figure 5.7. The mouse tumor data show more repair in small 1-day tumors than in large hypoxic 6-day tumors; this important point illustrates that repair is an active process requiring oxygen and nutrients.

The various factors involved in the repair of sublethal damage are summarized in Figure 5.9. Figure 5.9**A** shows that if a dose is split into two fractions separated by a time interval, more cells survive than for the same total dose given in a single fraction, because the shoulder of the curve must be repeated with each fraction. In general, there is a good correlation between the extent of repair of sublethal damage and the size of the shoulder of the survival curve. This is not surprising, because both are manifestations of the same basic phenomenon: the accumulation and repair of sublethal damage. Some mammalian cells are characterized by a survival curve with a broad shoulder, and split-dose experiments then indicate a substantial amount of sublethal damage repair. Other types of cells show a survival curve with a minimal shoulder, and this is reflected in more limited repair of sublethal damage. In the terminology of the linear-quadratic (α/β) description of the survival curve, it

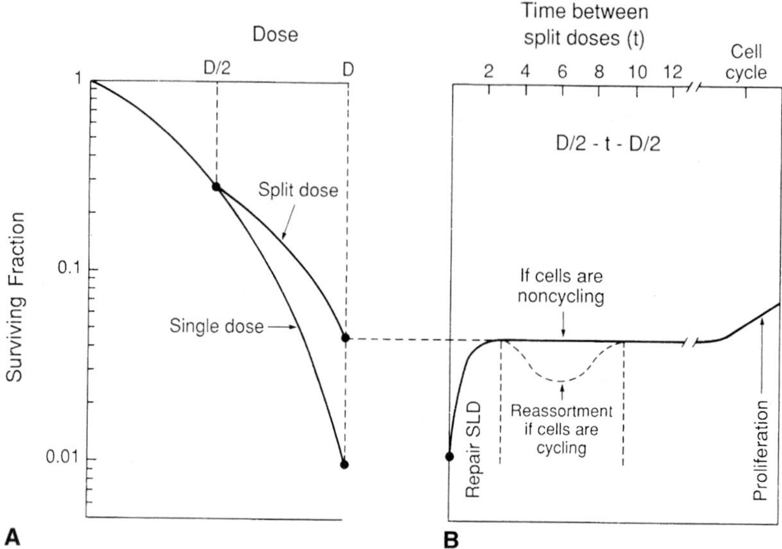

FIGURE 5.9 • Summary of the repair of sublethal damage as evidenced by a split-dose experiment. **A:** If the dose is delivered in two fractions separated by a time interval, there is an increase in cell survival because the shoulder of the curve must be expressed each time. **B:** The fraction of cells surviving a split dose increases as the time interval between the two dose fractions increases. As the time interval increases from 0 to 2 hours, the increase in survival results from the repair of sublethal damage. In cells with a long cell cycle or that are out of cycle, there is no further increase in cell survival by separating the dose by more than 2 or 3 hours. In a rapidly dividing cell population, there is a dip in cell survival caused by reassortment. However, as shown in Figure 5.7, if the time interval between the split doses exceeds the cell cycle, there is an increase in cell survival owing to proliferation or repopulation between the doses.

is the quadratic component (β) that causes the curve to bend and that results in the sparing effect of a split dose. A large shoulder corresponds to a small α/β ratio.

The time course of the increase in cell survival that results from the repair of sublethal damage is charted in Figure 5.9**B**. As the time interval between the two dose fractions is increased, there is a rapid increase in the fraction of cells surviving owing to the prompt repair of sublethal damage. This repair is complete by 1 or 2 hours for cells in culture but may take longer for late-responding tissues *in vivo* (Chapter 22). As the time interval between the two dose fractions is increased, there is a dip in the curve owing to the movement of surviving cells through the cell cycle, as explained in Figure 5.7. This occurs only in a population of fast-cycling cells. In cells that are noncycling, there can be no dip. If the time interval between the two dose fractions exceeds the cell cycle, there is an increase in the number of cells surviving because of cell proliferation; that is, cells can double in number between the dose fractions.

MECHANISM OF SUBLETHAL DAMAGE REPAIR

In Chapter 3, evidence was summarized of the correlation between cell killing and the production of asymmetric chromosomal aberrations, such as dicentrics and rings. This, in turn, is a consequence of an interaction between two (or more) double-strand breaks in the DNA. Based on this interpretation, the repair of sublethal damage is simply the repair of double-strand breaks. If a dose is split into two parts separated by a time interval, some of the double-strand breaks produced by the first dose are rejoined and repaired before the second dose. The breaks in two chromosomes that must interact to form a lethal lesion such as a dicentric may be formed by (1) a single track breaking both chromosomes (i.e., single-track damage) or (2) separate tracks breaking the two chromosomes (i.e., multiple-track damage).

The component of cell killing that results from single-track damage is the same whether the dose is given in a single exposure or fractionated. The same is not true of multiple-track damage. If the dose is given in a single exposure (i.e., two fractions with t = 0 between them), all breaks produced by separate electrons can interact to form dicentrics. But, if the two dose fractions, D/2, are separated by (for example) 3 hours, breaks produced by the first dose may be repaired before the second dose is given. Consequently, there are fewer interactions between broken chromosomes to form dicentrics, and more cells survive. Based on this simple interpretation, the repair of sublethal damage reflects the repair and rejoining of double-strand breaks before they can interact to form lethal lesions. This may not be the whole story, but it is a useful picture to keep in mind.

REPAIR AND RADIATION QUALITY

For a given biologic test system, the shoulder on the acute survival curve and therefore the amount of sublethal damage repair indicated by a split-dose experiment vary with the type of radiation used. The effect of dose fractionation with x-rays and neutrons is compared in Figure 5.10. For x-rays, dividing the total dose into two equal fractions, separated by 1 to 4 hours, results in a marked increase in cell survival because of the prompt repair of sublethal damage. By contrast, dividing the dose into two fractions has little effect on cell survival if neutrons are used, indicating little repair of sublethal damage.

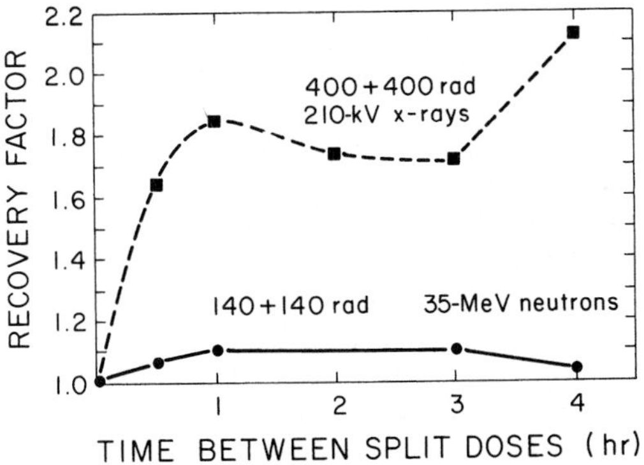

FIGURE 5.10 • Split-dose experiments with Chinese hamster cells. For 210-kV x-rays, two 4-Gy (400-rad) doses, separated by a variable interval, were compared with a single dose of 8 Gy (800 rad). For neutrons (35-MeV $d^+ \rightarrow$ Be), two 1.4-Gy (140-rad) doses were compared with a single exposure of 2.8 Gy (280 rad). The data are plotted in terms of the recovery factor, defined as the ratio of surviving fractions for a given dose delivered as two fractions compared with a single exposure. It is evident that repair of sublethal damage during the interval between split doses is virtually nonexistent for neutrons but is a significant factor for x-rays. (From Hall EJ, Roizin-Towie L, Theus RB, August LS: Radiobiological properties of high energy cyclotron produced neutrons used for radiotherapy. *Radiology* 117:173–178, 1975, with permission.)

THE DOSE-RATE EFFECT

For x- or γ-rays, dose rate is one of the principal factors that determine the biologic consequences of a given absorbed dose. As the dose rate is lowered and the exposure time extended, the biologic effect of a given dose generally is reduced.

The classic dose-rate effect, which is very important in radiotherapy, results from the repair of sublethal damage that occurs during a long radiation exposure. To illustrate this principle, Figure 5.11 shows an idealized experiment in which each dose (D_2, D_3, D_4, and so on) is delivered in a number of equal fractions of size D, with a time interval between fractions that is sufficient for repair of sublethal damage. The shoulder of the survival curve is repeated with each fraction. The broken line, F, shows the overall survival curve that would be observed if only single points were determined, corresponding to equal-dose increments. This survival curve has no shoulder. Because continuous low-dose-rate irradiation may be considered to be an infinite number of infinitely small fractions, the survival curve under these conditions also would be expected to have no shoulder and to be shallower than for single acute exposures.

EXAMPLES OF THE DOSE-RATE EFFECT *IN VITRO* AND *IN VIVO*

Survival curves for HeLa cells cultured *in vitro* over a wide range of dose rates, from 7.3 Gy/min to 0.535 cGy/min (from 730 to 0.535 rad/min), are summarized in Figure 5.12. As the dose rate is reduced, the survival curve becomes shallower and the shoulder tends to disappear (i.e., the survival curve becomes an exponential function of dose). The dose-rate effect caused by repair of sublethal damage is most dramatic between 0.01 and 1 Gy/min (between 1 and 100 rad/min). Above and below this dose-rate range, the survival curve changes little, if at all, with dose rate.

The magnitude of the dose-rate effect from the repair of sublethal damage varies enormously among different types of cells. HeLa cells are characterized by a survival curve for acute exposures that has a small initial shoulder, which goes hand in hand with a modest dose-rate effect. This is to be expected, because both are expressions of the cell's capacity to accumulate and repair sublethal radiation damage. By contrast, Chinese hamster cells have a broad shoulder to their acute x-ray survival curve and show a correspondingly large dose-rate effect. This is evident in Figure 5.13; there is a clear-cut difference in biologic effect, at least at high doses, between dose rates of 1.07, 0.30, and 0.16 Gy/min

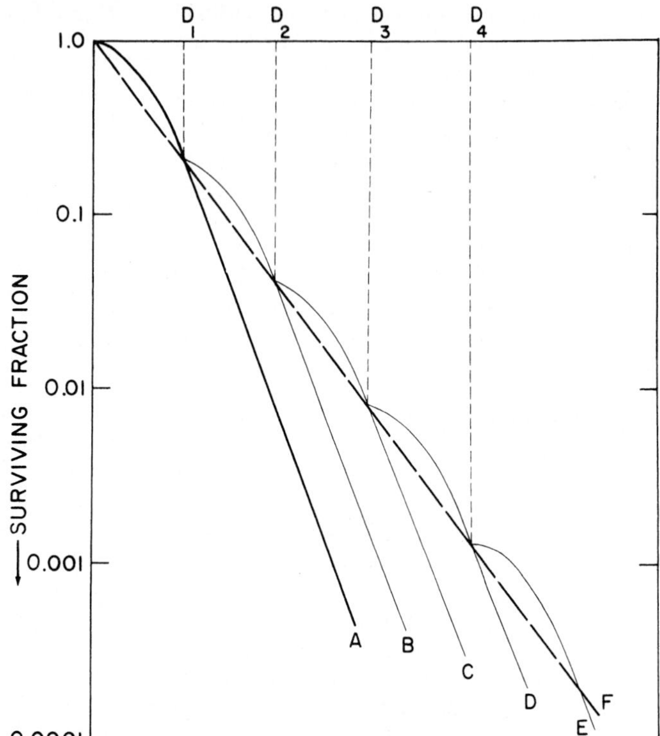

FIGURE 5.11 ● Idealized fractionation experiment. Curve A is the survival curve for single acute exposures of x-rays. Curve F is obtained if each dose is given as a series of small fractions of size D_1 with an interval between fractions sufficient for repair of sublethal damage. Multiple small fractions approximate to a continuous exposure to a low dose rate. (From Elkind MM, Whitmore GF: *Radiobiology of Cultured Mammalian Cells*. New York, Gordon and Breach, 1967, with permission.)

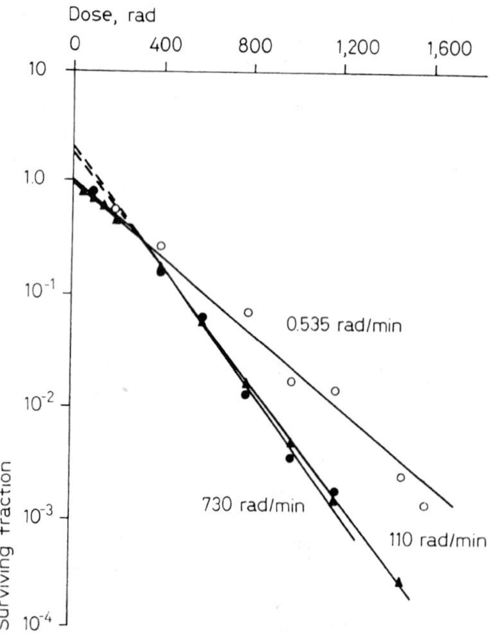

FIGURE 5.12 ● Survival curves for HeLa cells cultured *in vitro* and exposed to γ-rays at high and low dose rates.

(107, 30, and 16 rad/min). The differences between HeLa and hamster cells in the size of the shoulder to the acute survival curve and the magnitude of the dose-rate effect reflect differences in the importance of apoptosis. In the case of HeLa cells, apoptosis is an important form of cell death following radiation, whereas for hamster cells, apoptotic death is rarely seen.

Figure 5.14 shows survival curves for 40 different cell lines of human origin, cultured *in vitro* and irradiated at high dose rates and low dose rates. At low dose rates, the survival curves "fan out" and show a greater variation in slope because, in addition to the variation of inherent radiosensitivity evident at a high dose rate, there is a range of repair times of sublethal damage. Some cell lines repair sublethal damage rapidly, some more slowly, and this is reflected in the different survival curves at low dose rates.

Survival curves for crypt cells in the mouse jejunum irradiated with γ-rays at various dose rates are shown in Figure 5.15. There is a dramatic dose-rate effect owing to the repair of sublethal radiation damage from an acute exposure at 2.74 Gy/min (274 rad/min) to a protracted exposure at 0.92 cGy/min (0.92 rad/min). As the dose rate is lowered further, cell division begins to dominate the picture, because the exposure time is longer than the cell cycle. At 0.54 cGy/min (0.54 rad/min), there is little

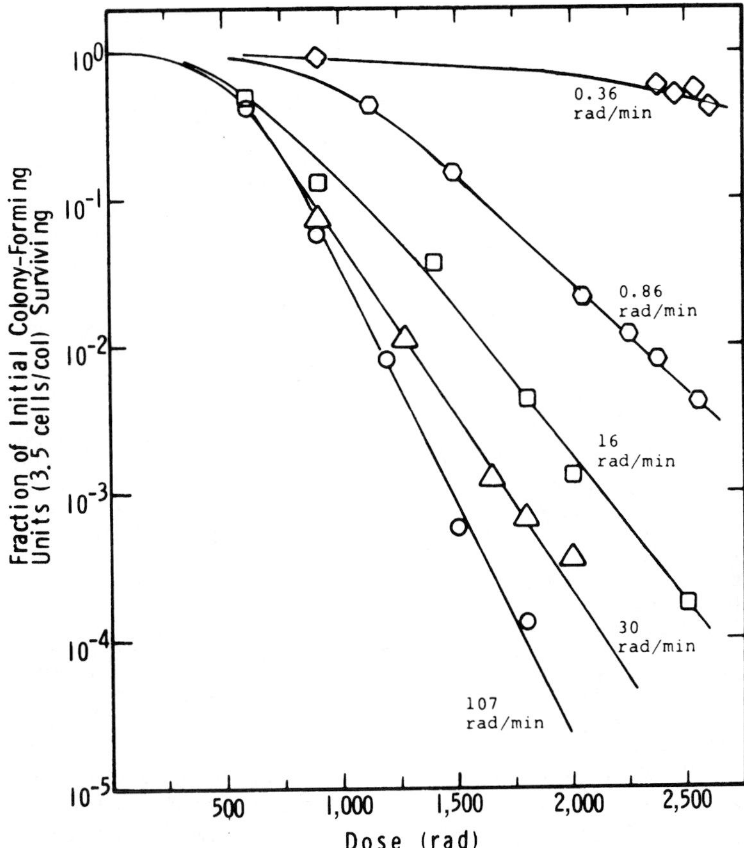

FIGURE 5.13 • Dose–response curves for Chinese hamster cells (CHL-F line) grown *in vitro* and exposed to cobalt-60 γ-rays at various dose rates. At high doses, a substantial dose-rate effect is evident even when comparing dose rates of 1.07, 0.30, and 0.16 Gy/min (107, 30, and 16 rad/min). The decrease in cell killing becomes even more dramatic as the dose rate is reduced further. (From Bedford JS, Mitchell JB: Dose-rate effects in synchronous mammalian cells in culture. *Radiat Res* 54:316–327, 1973, with permission.)

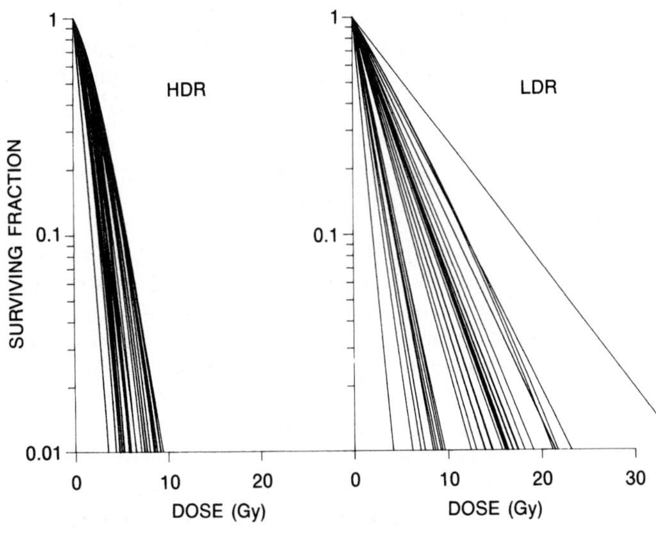

FIGURE 5.14 • Dose–survival curves at high dose rates (HDR) and low dose rates (LDR) for a large number of cell lines of human origin cultured *in vitro*. Note that the survival curves fan out at low dose rates because in addition to a range of inherent radiosensitivities (evident at HDR), there is also a range of repair times of sublethal damage.

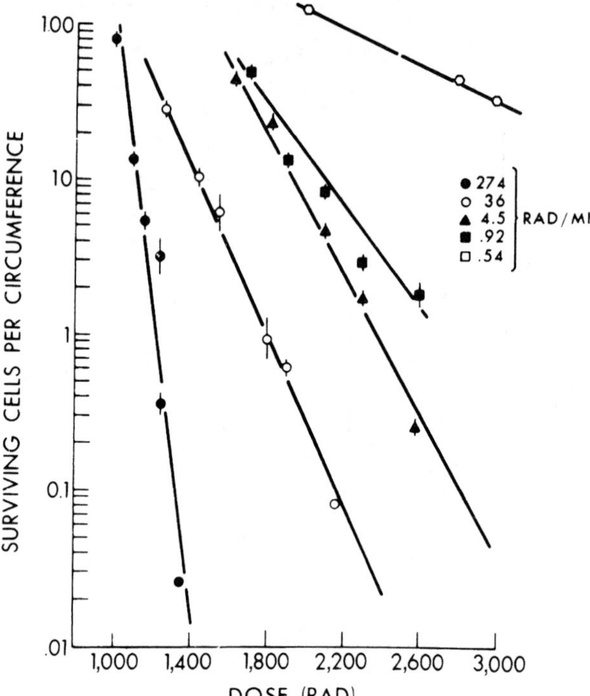

FIGURE 5.15 ● Response of mouse jejunal crypt cells irradiated with γ-rays from cesium-137 over a wide range of dose rates. The mice were given total-body irradiation, and the proportion of surviving crypt cells was determined by the appearance of regenerating microcolonies in the crypts 3 days later. Note the large dose-rate effect. (From Fu KK, Phillips TL, Kane LJ, Smith V: Tumor and normal tissue response to irradiation *in vivo*: variation with decreasing dose rates. *Radiology* 114:709–716, 1975, with permission.)

reduction in the number of surviving crypts, even for very large doses, because cellular proliferation occurs during the long exposure and makes up for cell killing by the radiation.

THE INVERSE DOSE-RATE EFFECT

There is at least one example of an inverse dose-rate effect, in which decreasing the dose rate results in increased cell killing. This is illustrated in Figure 5.16. Decreasing the dose rate for this HeLa cell line from 1.54 to 0.37 Gy/h (from 154 to 37 rad/h) increases the efficiency of cell killing such that this low dose rate is almost as damaging as an acute exposure. The explanation is illustrated in Figure 5.17. At about 0.37 Gy/h (37 rad/h), cells tend to progress through the cycle and become arrested in G_2, a radiosensitive phase of the cycle. At higher dose rates, they are "frozen" in the phase of the cycle they are in at the start of the irradiation; at lower dose rates, they continue to cycle during irradiation.

THE DOSE-RATE EFFECT SUMMARIZED

Figure 5.18 summarizes the entire dose-rate effect. For acute exposures at high dose rates, the survival curve has a significant initial shoulder. As the dose rate is lowered and the treatment time protracted, more and more sublethal damage can be repaired during the exposure. Consequently, the survival curve becomes progressively more shallow (D_0 increases), and the shoulder tends to disappear. A point is reached at which all sublethal damage is repaired, resulting in a limiting slope. In at least some cell lines, a further lowering of the dose rate allows cells to progress through the cycle and accumulate in G_2. This is a radiosensitive phase, and so the survival curve becomes steeper again. This is the inverse dose-rate effect. A further reduction in dose rate allows cells to pass through the G_2 block and divide. Proliferation then may occur during the radiation exposure if the dose rate is low enough and the exposure time is long compared with the length of the mitotic cycle. This may lead to a further reduction in biologic effect as the dose rate is progressively lowered, because cell birth tends to offset cell death.

BRACHYTHERAPY OR ENDOCURIETHERAPY

Implanting radioactive sources directly into a tumor was a strategy first suggested by Alexander Graham Bell in 1901. Over the years, various groups in different countries coined various names for this type of therapy, using the prefix *brachy-*, from the Greek for "short range," or *endo-*, from the Greek for "within." There are two distinct forms of **brachytherapy**, also called **endocurietherapy**: (1) *intracavitary* irradiation, using radioactive sources placed in body cavities in close proximity to the tumor, and (2) *interstitial* brachytherapy, using

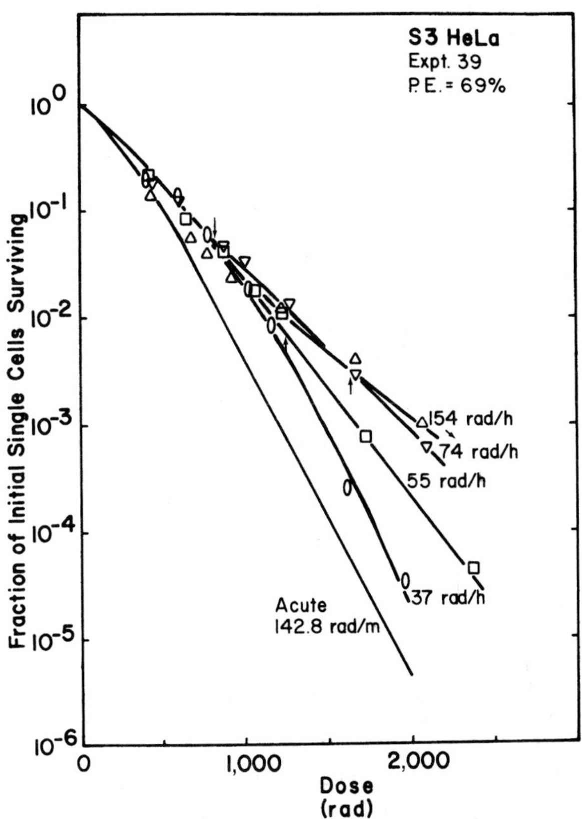

FIGURE 5.16 • The inverse dose-rate effect. A range of dose rates can be found for HeLa cells such that lowering the dose rate leads to more cell killing. At 1.54 Gy/h (154 rad/h), cells are "frozen" in the various phases of the cycle and do not progress. As the dose rate is dropped to 0.37 Gy/h (37 rad/h), cells progress to a block in G_2, a radiosensitive phase of the cycle. (From Mitchell JB, Bedford JS, Bailey SM: Dose-rate effects on the cell cycle and survival of S3 HeLa and V79 cells. *Radiat Res* 79:520–536, 1979, with permission.)

radioactive wires or "seeds" implanted directly into the tumor volume.

Both intracavitary and interstitial techniques were developed to an advanced stage at an early date because the technology was readily available. Radium in sufficient quantities was extracted and purified in the early 1900s, whereas radioactive sources of sufficient activity for **teletherapy** (or external-bean radiotherapy) sources of adequate dose rate only came as a spin-off of World War II nuclear technology.

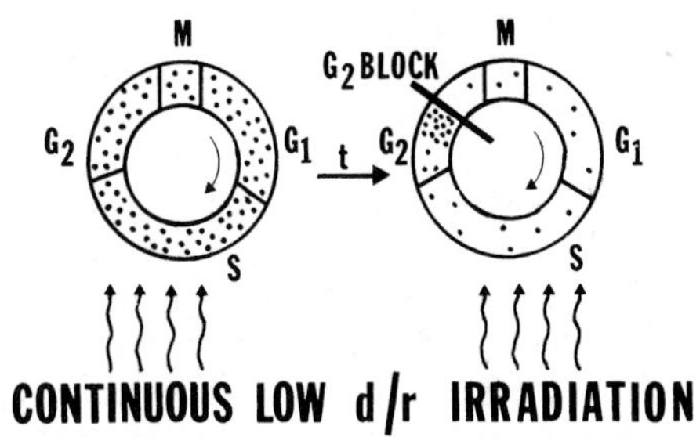

FIGURE 5.17 • The inverse dose-rate effect. A range of dose rates can be found, at least for HeLa cells, that allows cells to progress through the cycle to a block in late G_2. Under continuous low-dose-rate irradiation, an asynchronous population becomes a population of radiosensitive G_2 cells. (From Hall EJ: The biological basis of endocurietherapy: The Henschke Memorial Lecture 1984. *Endocurie Hypertherm Oncol* 1:141–151, 1985, with permission.)

Intracavitary Brachytherapy

Intracavitary brachytherapy at a low dose rate is always temporary and usually takes 1 to 4 days (with a dose rate of about 50 cGy/h, or 50 rad/h). It can be used for a number of anatomic sites, but by far the most common is the uterine cervix. There has been a continual evolution in the radionuclide used; in the early days, radium was used, but this went out of favor because of the safety concern of using an encapsulated source that can leak radioactivity. As an interim measure, cesium-137 was introduced, but today most treatment centers use iridium-192; its shorter half-life and lower γ-ray energy make for ease of radiation protection, especially in conjunction with a remote afterloader.

To an increasing extent, low-dose-rate intracavitary brachytherapy is being replaced by high-dose-rate intracavitary therapy, delivered in 3 to 12 dose fractions. Replacing continuous low-dose-rate therapy with a few large-dose fractions gives up much of the radiobiologic advantage and the sparing of late-responding normal tissues, as described in Chapter 22. It is only possible because

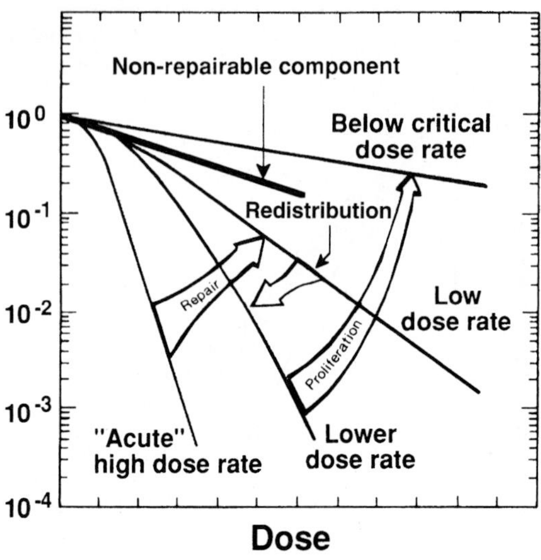

FIGURE 5.18 • The dose-rate effect resulting from repair of sublethal damage, redistribution in the cycle, and cell proliferation. The dose–response curve for acute exposures is characterized by a broad initial shoulder. As the dose rate is reduced, the survival curve becomes progressively more shallow as more and more sublethal damage is repaired, but cells are "frozen" in their positions in the cycle and do not progress. As the dose rate is lowered further and for a limited range of dose rates, the survival curve steepens again because cells can progress through the cycle to pile up at a block in G_2, a radiosensitive phase, but still cannot divide. A further lowering of dose rate below this critical dose rate allows cells to escape the G_2 block and divide; cell proliferation then may occur during the protracted exposure, and survival curves become shallower as cell birth from mitosis offsets cell killing from the irradiation. (Based on the ideas of Dr. Joel Bedford.)

the treatment of carcinoma of the cervix is a special case in which the dose-limiting normal tissues (e.g., bladder, rectum) receive a lower dose than the prescribed dose to the tumor (or to point A). For high-dose-rate treatments lasting a few minutes, it is possible to use retractors that result in even lower doses to the critical normal tissues than are possible with an insertion that lasts 24 hours or more. These physical advantages offset the radiobiologic disadvantages, so that the general principle, that administration of a few large fractions at a high dose rate gives poorer results than at a low dose rate, does not apply to this special case.

Interstitial Brachytherapy

Interstitial brachytherapy can be either temporary or permanent. Temporary implants in earlier times utilized radium, but the most widely used radionuclide at the present time is iridium-192. Implants at low dose rates are considered by many radiotherapists to be the treatment of choice for the 5% or so of human cancers that are accessible to such techniques.

The dose-rate range used in these treatments is in the region of the dose-rate spectrum in which the biologic effect varies rapidly with dose rate. The maximum dose that can be delivered without unacceptable damage to the surrounding normal tissue depends on the volume of tissue irradiated and on the dose rate, which is in turn a function of the number of radioactive sources used and their geometric distribution. To achieve a consistent biologic response, the total dose used should be varied according to the dose rate employed.

Paterson and Ellis independently published curves to relate total dose to result in normal-tissue tolerance to dose rate (Fig. 5.19); there is remarkable agreement between the two sets of data based on clinical judgment.

Quoting Paterson:

> The graph for radium implants is an attempt to set out the doses in five to ten days which are equivalent to any desired seven-day dose. In its original form it perhaps owed more to inspiration than to science but it has gradually been corrected to match actual experience.

Both Paterson and Ellis regarded a dose of 60 Gy (6,000 rad) in 7 days as the standard treatment for interstitial therapy, corresponding to a dose rate of 0.357 Gy/h (35.7 rad/h). If the sources are of higher activity and the treatment dose rate is higher, then a lower total dose should be used. For example, a dose rate of 0.64 Gy/h (64 rad/h) would produce an equivalent biologic effect with a total dose of only 46 Gy (4,600 rad) in a treatment time of 3 days.

Also shown in Figure 5.19 are isoeffect curves, matched to 60 Gy in 7 days, based on radiobiologic data for early- and late-responding tissues. The variation of total dose with dose rate is much larger for late- than for early-responding tissues because of the lower α/β characteristic of such tissues. It is interesting to note that the curve for late-responding tissues calculated from radiobiologic data agrees closely with the clinical estimates of Paterson and of Ellis, as it should, because their judgment was stated unequivocally to be based on late equalizing effects.

In the 1990s, Mazeron and his colleagues in Paris published two papers that show clearly that a dose-rate effect is important in interstitial implants. They have, perhaps, the most experience in the world with the use of iridium-192 wire implants. Their first report describes the analysis of

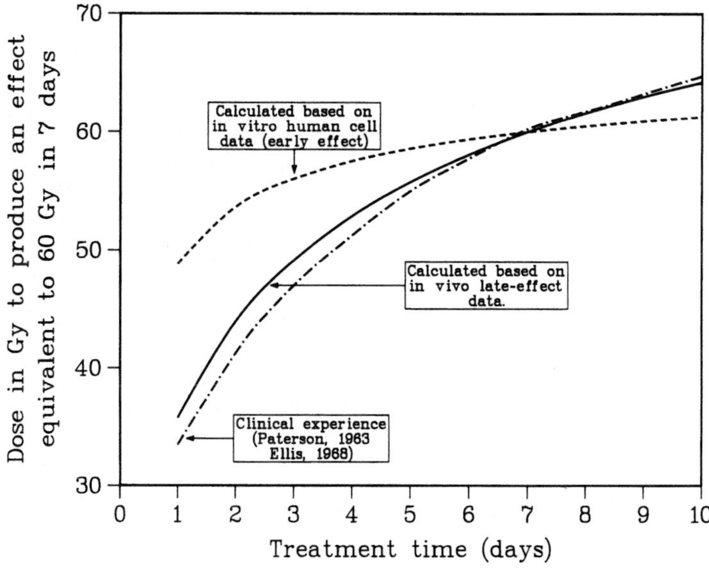

FIGURE 5.19 ● Dose equivalent to 60 Gy (6,000 rad) in 7 days as proposed by Paterson (in 1963) and by Ellis (in 1968) based on clinical observation of normal-tissue tolerance or calculated from radiobiologic principles. The α/β ratios and the half-time of repair of sublethal damage were chosen for early- or late-responding tissues (Chapter 22).

local tumor control and the incidence of necrosis in a large cohort of patients with T1-2 squamous cell carcinoma of the mobile tongue and the floor of the mouth who were treated with interstitial iridium-192. The data are shown in Figure 5.20. Patients were grouped according to dose rate, either more or less than 0.5 Gy/h (50 rad/h). It is evident that there was a substantially higher incidence of necrosis in patients treated at the higher dose rates. By contrast, dose rate makes little or no difference to local control provided the total dose is high enough, 65 to 70 Gy (6,500–7,000 rad), but there is a clear separation at lower doses (60 Gy, or 6,000 rad), with the lower dose rate being less effective. These results are in good accord with the radiobiologic predictions.

Their second report analyzes data from a large group of patients with carcinoma of the breast who received iridium-192 implants as a boost to external-beam radiotherapy. These results allow an assessment of the effect of dose rate on tumor control, but provide no information on the effect of dose rate on late effects, because there was only one case that involved necrosis. The interstitial implant was only part of the radiotherapy, and a fixed standard dose was used, so only limited conclusions can be drawn from these data. The results (Fig. 5.21), however, show a correlation between the proportion of recurrent tumors and the dose rate. For a given total dose, there were markedly fewer recurrences if the radiation was delivered at a higher dose rate rather than a lower dose rate.

The relatively short half-life of iridium-192 (70 days) means that a range of dose rates is inevitable, because the activity of the sources decays during the months that they are in use. It is important,

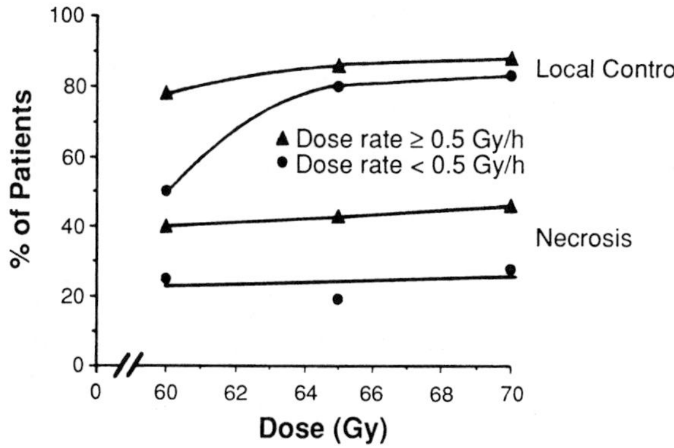

FIGURE 5.20 ● Local tumor control and necrosis rate at 5 years as a function of dose in patients with T1-2 squamous-cell carcinomas of the mobile tongue and the floor of the mouth who were treated with interstitial iridium-192 implants. The patients were grouped according to whether the implant was characterized by a high dose rate (equal to or above 0.5 Gy/h, or 50 rad/h) or low dose rate (below 0.5 Gy/h, or 50 rad/h). The necrosis rate was higher for the higher-dose-rate group at all dose levels. Local tumor control did not depend on dose rate, provided the total dose was sufficiently large. (Data from Mazeron JJ, Simon JM, Le Pechoux C, et al.: Effect of dose rate on local control and complications in definitive irradiation of T1-2 squamous cell carcinomas of mobile tongue and floor of mouth with interstitial iridium-192. *Radiother Oncol* 21:39–47, 1991.)

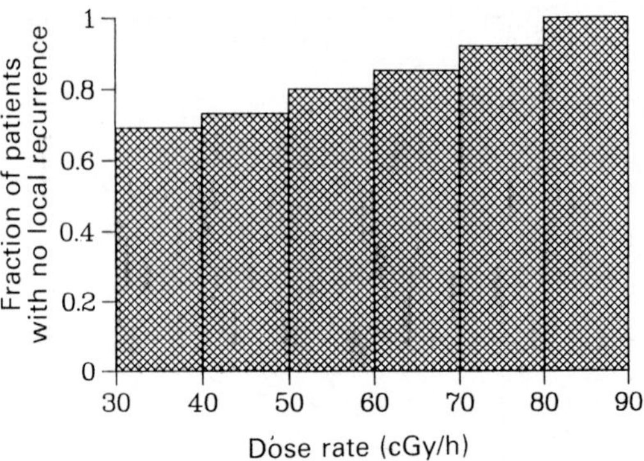

FIGURE 5.21 • Percentage of patients who showed no local recurrence as a function of dose rate in treatment for breast carcinoma by a combination of external-beam irradiation plus iridium-192 interstitial implant. The implant was used to deliver a total dose of 37 Gy (3,700 rad); the dose rate varied by a factor of 3 (30–90 cGy/hr), owing to different linear activities of the iridium-192 wire and different volumes implanted. (Data from Mazeron JJ, Simon JM, Crook J, et al.: Influence of dose rate on local control of breast carcinoma treated by external beam irradiation plus iridium-192 implant. *Int J Radiat Oncol Biol Phys* 21:1173–1177, 1991.)

therefore, to correct the total dose for the dose rate because of the experience of Mazeron and his colleagues described previously. Iridium-192 has two advantages: (1) The source size can be small, and (2) its lower photon energy makes radiation protection easier than with radium or cesium-137. Sources of this radionuclide are ideal for use with computer-controlled remote afterloaders introduced in the 1990s (Fig. 5.22). Catheters can be implanted into the patient while inactive and then the sources transferred from the safe by remote control after the patient has returned to his own room. The sources can be returned to the safe if the patient needs nursing care.

Permanent Interstitial Implants

Encapsulated sources with relatively short half-lives can be left in place permanently. There are two advantages for the patient: (1) An operation to remove the implant is not needed, and (2) the patient can go home with the implant in place. On the other hand, this does involve additional expense, because the sources are not reused. The initial dose rate is

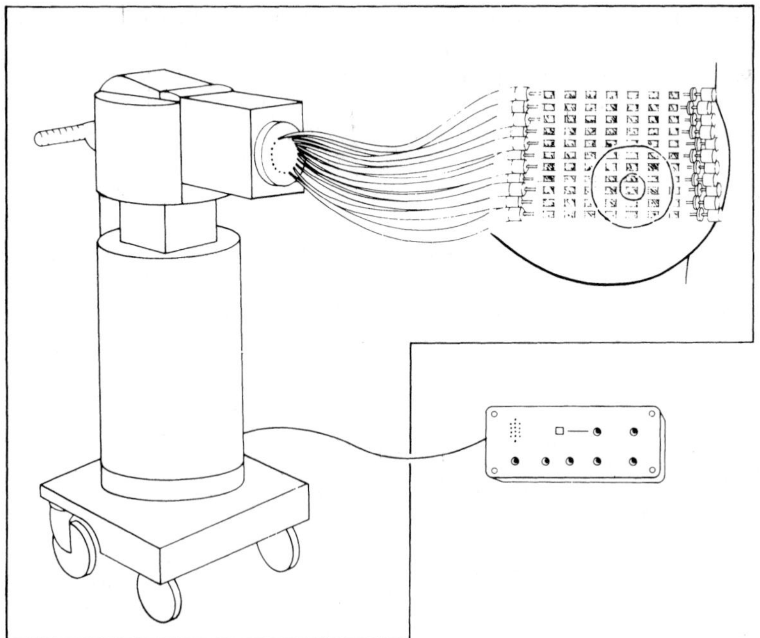

FIGURE 5.22 • Diagram illustrating the use of a computer-controlled remote afterloader to minimize radiation exposure of personnel during brachytherapy. Catheters are implanted into the tumor, and radiographs are made to check the validity of the implant using "dummy" nonradioactive sources. The catheters then are connected to a shielded safe containing the radioactive (iridium-192) sources, which are transferred by remote control to the implant in the patient. The control panel is located outside a lightly shielded room. The sources can be retracted temporarily to the safe so that personnel can care for the patient, thus effectively eliminating radiation exposure to personnel.

TABLE 5.1

Characteristics of Radionuclides for Intracavitary or Interstitial Brachytherapy

	Photon Energy, keV			
Radionuclide	Average	Range	Half-Life	HVL[a], mm Lead
Conventional				
Cesium-137	662	—	30 y	5.5
Iridium-192	380	136–1060	74.2 d	2.5
New				
Iodine-125	28	3–35	60.2 d	0.025
Gold-198	412	—	2.7 d	2.5
Americium-241	60	—	432 y	0.125
Palladium-103	21	20–23	17 d	0.008
Samarium-145	41	38–61	340 d	0.06
Ytterbium 169	100	10–308	32 d	0.1

Data computed by Dr. Ravinder Nath, Yale University.
[a] HVL = Half Valve Layer, the thickness required to reduce the incident radiation by 50%.

high and falls off as the implanted sources decay. Iodine-125 has been used most widely to date for permanent implants. The total prescribed dose is usually about 160 Gy (16,000 rad) at the periphery of the implanted volume, with 80 Gy (8,000 rad) delivered in the first half-life of 60 days. The soft emission from iodine has a relative biologic effectiveness (explained in Chapter 7) of about 1.5; this corresponds to 80 × 1.5 or 120 Gy (12,000 rad) of high-energy α-rays. This is a big dose, even at a low dose rate, and corresponds to a good level of cell kill. It is, however, spread over 60 days; consequently, the success of the implant in sterilizing the tumor depends critically on the cell cycle of the clonogenic cells. In a rapidly growing tumor, cell birth by mitosis compensates for cell killing by the radiation during the prolonged exposure time. This is much less of a problem with slowly growing tumors, such as carcinoma of the prostate, and it is in such sites that permanent implants with iodine-125 have found a place.

A major advantage of a radionuclide such as iodine-125 is the low energy of the photons emitted (about 30 keV). This makes little difference to the dose distribution in an implanted tumor but greatly simplifies radiation protection problems, because medical and nursing staff are easily shielded. In addition, the dose falls off rapidly outside the treatment volume, so that doses to parts of the patient's body remote from the implant are greatly reduced.

A number of other new radionuclides are under consideration as sources for brachytherapy that share with iodine-125 the properties of a relatively short half-life and a low-energy photon emission to reduce problems of radiation protection. By contrast, americium-241 emits a low-energy photon but has a long half-life of hundreds of years. Table 5.1 summarizes some of the physical characteristics of the newly developed sources and contrasts them with the characteristics of radionuclides more commonly used for brachytherapy.

RADIOLABELED IMMUNOGLOBULIN THERAPY FOR HUMAN CANCER

Radiolabeled immunoglobulin therapy is radiotherapy for cancer using an antibody to deliver a radioactive isotope to the tumor. Much of the pioneering work in this field was done by Stanley Order and his colleagues in the 1980s, with the primary focus on antiferritin labeled with radioactive iodine or yttrium.

Ferritin is an iron-storage protein that is synthesized and secreted by a broad range of malignancies, including hepatoma, lung cancer, neuroblastoma, acute myelogenous leukemia, cancer of the breast and pancreas, and Hodgkin's disease. It is not known why ferritin is produced preferentially in tumors. It has been suggested that messenger RNA for ferritin may resemble that for many viruses. This suggestion is highly speculative but consistent with the observation that ferritin is present in tumors that are suspected of having a viral cause. This connection is strongly suspected for hepatomas, which have been associated with the hepatitis B virus, and probably exists for Hodgkin's disease, too.

Although ferritin is also present in normal tissues, selective tumor targeting has been demonstrated in animal models and in clinical scanning, historically performed first for Hodgkin's disease. This differential is the basis of the potential therapeutic gain and thus the clinical usefulness of radiolabeled immunoglobulin therapy.

In the early years of radiolabeled immunoglobulin therapy, radiolabeled polyclonal antibodies were used. These were replaced with murine monoclonal antibodies carrying iodine-131, which could be used for both diagnosis and therapy. More recently, chimeric mouse–human antibodies, which are human antibodies derived by tissue culture or produced in genetically altered mice, and synthetically derived antibodies have become available. These developments have progressively reduced the possibility of inducing an immune response, lengthened the effective half-life, and hence increased the tumor dose.

Radionuclides

Early studies utilized iodine-131, which is easily linked to antibodies. The disadvantage of using iodine-131 is that it requires large amounts of radioactivity (about 30 mCi); as a consequence of this, patients must be hospitalized, self-care is needed, and pediatric patients are excluded. In addition, the dose and dose rate to the tumor are limited by the relatively weak β-emission (0.3 MeV) and by the total-body dose resulting from the γ-emission, which causes systemic hematopoietic toxicity.

In more recent developments, iodine-131 has been replaced by yttrium-90, which is characterized by a pure β-emission of relatively high energy (0.9 MeV). This allows a higher tumor dose and dose rate and enables the applications to be administered on an outpatient basis. More recently, rhenium-188, rhenium-186, and phosphorus-32 have been used. New chemical linkages, including a variety of chelates, have also been used, all seeking to bind the isotope firmly to the antibody.

Tumor Target Visualization

When iodine-131 was used, the γ-ray emission allowed tumor localization as well as providing the bulk of the therapeutic dose. When pure β-emitters such as yttrium-90 were first introduced, it was necessary to add a γ-emitter such as indium-111 to allow visualization. Today, it is no longer acceptable to scan with a conventional γ-camera because single-photon emission computed tomography provides a clearer picture. The bremsstrahlung from β-emitters can be scanned by this means, so that radionuclides such as yttrium-90 can be used without the need to add a γ-emitter for visualization.

Targeting

The ability to target tumors with antiferritin mirrors the vascularity of the tumor nodules. In general, tumors with a high degree of vascularity are better targeted with antiferritin than less vascularized tumors. The presence of ferritin per se is not enough to ensure targeting. The need for neovasculature means that uptake tends to be greater in smaller tumors. Uptake also can be affected by radiation or hyperthermia. A dose of external radiation can act as an initiator. This first was observed empirically but now is used routinely to enhance the targeting of the radiolabeled antiferritin. This is probably a consequence of damage to tumor vasculature, which allows antiferritin to leak out of vessels and into tumor cells. The targeting ratio of a tumor to the average for normal tissue is about 2.9 for antiferritin labeled with iodine-131; the corresponding ratios are 1.2 for bone and gastrointestinal tract and 0.8 for lung.

Clinical Results

The most promising results have been in the treatment of unresectable primary hepatoma, for which 48% partial remission and 7% complete remission rates have been reported by the Johns Hopkins group for patients receiving iodine-131–labeled antiferritin in combination with low doses of doxorubicin (Adriamycin) and 5-fluorouracil. Some success also has been reported by other groups using similar techniques in the treatment of metastatic neuroblastoma, relapsed grade IV gliomas after radiotherapy and chemotherapy, metastatic ovarian cancer resistant to prior radiotherapy, and malignant pleural and pericardial effusions of diverse causes.

Iodine-131–labeled antiferritin led to partial remissions in patients with Hodgkin's disease, but yttrium-90 antiferritin produced complete remissions, indicating the increased effectiveness of the larger doses possible with radionuclides emitting pure β-rays. Radiolabeled immunoglobulin therapy has been used with varying degrees of success for a wide range of other malignancies, including hepatomas, ovarian cancer, gliomas, and leukemia. Although a variety of radiolabeled antibodies have been shown to achieve remissions in lymphoma, the question of the effect of the total-body exposure versus tumor targeting is still open.

Dosimetry

For iodine-131–labeled antiferritin treatment of unresectable primary hepatoma, 30 mCi is administered on day 1, followed by 20 mCi on day 5.

Escalation of dose beyond these levels is not helpful, because the deposition of labeled antiferritin becomes saturated. This translates into a peak dose rate of 45 to 50 mGy/h (4.5–5 rad/h) on days 1 and 5 and a total accumulated dose of 10 to 12 Gy (1,000–1,200 rad) by about 15 days. The corresponding dose rate to normal liver is 10 mGy/h (1 rad/h), and the total-body dose is 2 to 3 mGy/h (0.2–0.3 rad/h), which results limits hematologic toxicity. It is remarkable that such a small dose at such a low dose rate can produce remissions in patients with tumors of 1 kg or more. This response is difficult to explain on the basis of conventional radiobiologic data, but the clinical results are exciting.

For yttrium-90–labeled antiferritin treatment, a single application of 20 mCi results in a peak dose rate of about 0.16 Gy/h (16 rad/h), which decays with a tumor-effective half-life of 2 days and results in a total accumulated dose of about 20 to 35 Gy (2,000–3,500 rad).

Summary of Pertinent Conclusions

DNA Repair Pathways

- Ionizing radiation induces base damage, single-strand breaks, double-strand breaks, and DNA protein cross-links.
- The cell has evolved an intricate series of sensors and pathways to respond to each type of radiation-induced damage.
- DNA double-strand breaks, the most lethal form of ionizing radiation–induced damage, is repaired by nonhomologous recombination in the G_1 phase of the cell cycle and homologous recombination (mainly) in the S/G_2 phase of the cell cycle.
- Defective nonhomologous recombination leads to chromosome aberrations, immune deficiency, and ionizing radiation sensitivity.
- Defective homologous recombination leads to chromatid and chromosome aberrations, decreased proliferation, and ionizing radiation sensitivity.

Hereditary Syndromes that Affect Radiosensitivity

- AT (ataxia-telangiectasia) is an autosomal recessive disorder that is due to a defect in the ATM kinase. AT cells fail to activate checkpoints in response to DNA damage, exhibit increased genomic instability at the chromosome level, and have an increased risk of lymphomas. AT cells and individuals are hypersensitive to ionizing radiation.
- The *ATR* gene expression (AT and Rad3 related) is decreased in patients with Seckel's syndrome. Although it belongs to the same PIKK family as ATM, it is an essential gene at the cellular level. It has an important role in responding to DNA breaks in S phase.
- SCID (severe combined immunodeficiency syndrome) mice are immune deficient and radiosensitive due to a mutation in the DNA-PKcs gene. Cells defective in DNA-PKcs are defective in nonhomologous recombination and are extremely radiosensitive.
- SCID humans are also immune deficient and radiosensitive owing to a mutation in Artemis. Cells defective in Artemis are defective in nonohomologous recombination and are radiosensitive.
- NBS (Nijmegen Breakage Syndrome) is a very rare disorder that results in increased cancer incidence. Cells defective in NBS lack an S phase checkpoint and are radiosensitive.
- ATLD (AT-Like Disorder) patients are clinically similar to AT patients except that their defect lies in the *MRE11* gene. Cells from these patients are also sensitive to ionizing radiation.
- FA (Fanconi Anemia) patients are characterized by their hypersensitivity to cross-linking agents. Although fibroblasts derived from these patients are not sensitive to ionizing radiation, tumors arising in these patients are hypersensitive. The reasons for this are currently unknown.

Potentially Lethal Damage Repair

- The component of radiation damage that can be modified by manipulation of the postirradiation conditions is known as potentially lethal damage.
- Potentially lethal damage repair can occur if cells are prevented from dividing for 6 hours or more after irradiation; this is manifest as an increase in survival. This repair can be demonstrated *in vitro* by keeping cells in saline or plateau phase for 6 hours after irradiation and *in vivo* by delayed removal and assay of animal tumors or cells of normal tissues.

(continued)

Summary of Pertinent Conclusions (Continued)

- Potentially lethal damage repair is significant for x-rays but does not occur after neutron irradiation.
- It has been suggested that resistant human tumors (e.g., melanoma) owe their resistance to large amounts of potentially lethal damage repair. This is still controversial.

Sublethal Damage Repair

- Sublethal damage repair is an operational term that describes the increase in survival if a dose of radiation is split into two fractions separated in time.
- The half-time of sublethal damage repair in mammalian cells is about 1 hour, but it may be longer in late-responding normal tissues *in vivo*.
- Sublethal damage repair occurs in tumors and normal tissues *in vivo* as well as in cells cultured *in vitro*.
- The repair of sublethal damage reflects the repair of DNA breaks before they can interact to form lethal chromosomal aberrations.
- Sublethal damage repair is significant for x-rays but almost nonexistent for neutrons.

Dose-Rate Effect

- If the radiation dose rate is reduced from about 1 Gy/min to 0.3 Gy/h (from 100 rad/min to 30 rad/h), there is a reduction in the cell killing from a given dose, because sublethal damage repair occurs during the protracted exposure.
- As the dose rate is reduced, the slope of the survival curve becomes shallower (D_0 increases), and the shoulder tends to disappear.
- In some cell lines, an inverse dose-rate effect is evident (i.e., reducing the dose rate increases the proportion of cells killed) owing to the accumulation of cells in G_2, which is a sensitive phase of the cycle.

Brachytherapy

- Implanting sources into or close to a tumor is known as brachytherapy (from the Greek *brachy-*, meaning "short") or endocurietherapy (from *endo-*, meaning "within").
- Intracavitary radiotherapy involves placing radioactive sources into a body cavity close to a tumor. The most common example is the treatment of carcinoma of the uterine cervix.
- Interstitial therapy involves implanting radioactive sources directly into the tumor and adjacent normal tissue.
- Temporary implants, which formerly utilized radium needles, now are performed most often with iridium-192 wires or seeds.
- If the implant is used as a sole treatment, a commonly used dose is 50 to 70 Gy (5,000–7,000 rad) in 5 to 9 days. Total dose should be adjusted for dose rate. Clinical studies show that both tumor control and late effects vary with dose rate for a given total dose. Often the implant is used as a boost to external-beam therapy, and only half the treatment is given with the implant.
- Because of their small size and low photon energy, iridium-192 seeds are suitable for use with computer-controlled remote afterloaders.
- Permanent implants can be used with radionuclides (such as iodine-125 or palladium-103) that have relatively short half-lives.
- A number of novel radionuclides are being considered as sources for brachytherapy. Most emit low-energy photons, which simplifies the problems of radiation protection.

Radiolabeled Immunoglobulin Therapy

- In the early days of radiolabeled immunoglobulin therapy, radiolabeled polyclonal antibodies were used. These were replaced with murine monoclonal antibodies. More recently, chimeric mouse–human antibodies, which are human antibodies derived by tissue culture or produced in genetically altered mice, have become available. Finally, synthetically derived antibodies have been produced.
- Iodine-131 largely has been replaced by pure β-ray emitters such as yttrium-90, resulting in an increased tumor dose and decreased total-body toxicity.
- Single-photon emission computed tomography can now be used to visualize the tumor, using the bremsstrahlung from the β-rays, so it is no longer necessary to add a γ-emitter when using yttrium-90.
- Radiolabeled immunoglobulin therapy has produced promising results in unresectable primary hepatoma and in patients with Hodgkin's lymphoma. It has been used with varying degrees of success for a wide range of other malignancies.

BIBLIOGRAPHY

Ang KK, Thames HD, van der Vogel AG, et al.: Is the rate of repair of radiation induced sublethal damage in rat spinal cord dependent on the size of dose per fraction? *Int J Radiat Oncol Biol Phys* 13:557–562, 1987

Bakkenist CJ, Kastan MB: Initiating cellular stress responses. *Cell* 118:9–17, 2004

Bedford JS, Hall EJ: Survival of HeLa cells cultured *in vitro* and exposed to protracted gamma irradiation. *Int J Radiat Biol* 7:377–383, 1963

Bedford JS, Mitchell JB: Dose-rate effects in synchronous mammalian cells in culture. *Radiat Res* 54:316–327, 1973

Bell AC: The uses of radium. *Am Med* 6:261, 1903

Belli JA, Bonte FJ, Rose MS: Radiation recovery response of mammalian tumor cells *in vivo*. *Nature* 211:662–663, 1966

Belli JA, Dicus GJ, Bonte FJ: Radiation response of mammalian tumor cells: 1. Repair of sublethal damage *in vivo*. *J Natl Cancer Inst* 38:673–682, 1967

Belli JA, Shelton M: Potentially lethal radiation damage: Repair by mammalian cells in culture. *Science* 165:490–492, 1969

Berry RJ, Cohen AB: Some observations on the reproductive capacity of mammalian tumor cells exposed *in vivo* to gamma radiation at low dose rates. *Br J Radiol* 35:489–491, 1962

Bryant PE: Survival after fractionated doses of radiation: Modification by anoxia of the response of Chlamydomonas. *Nature* 219:75–77, 1968

Cromie GA, Connelly JC, Leach DRF: Recombination at double-strand breaks and DNA ends: Conserved mechanisms from phage to humans. *Mol Cell* 8:1163–1174, 2001

Dale RG: The use of small fraction numbers in high dose-rate gynaecological afterloading: Some radiobiological considerations. *Br J Radiol* 63:290–294, 1990

De la Torre C, Pincheira J, López-Sáez: Human syndromes with genomic instability and multiprotein machines that repair DNA double-strand breaks. *Histol Histopathol* 18:225–243, 2003

Denekamp J, Fowler JF: Further investigations of the response of irradiated mouse skin. *Int J Radiat Biol* 10:435–441, 1966

Elkind MM, Sutton H: Radiation response of mammalian cells grown in culture: 1. Repair of x-ray damage in surviving Chinese hamster Cells. *Radiat Res* 13:556–593, 1960

Elkind MM, Sutton-Gilbert H, Moses WB, Alescio T, Swain RB: Radiation response of mammalian cells in culture: V. Temperature dependence of the repair of x-ray damage in surviving cells (aerobic and hypoxic). *Radiat Res* 25:359–376, 1965

Elkind MM, Whitmore GF: *Radiobiology of Cultured Mammalian Cells*. New York, Gordon and Breach, 1967

Ellis F: Dose time and fractionation in radiotherapy. In Elbert M, Howard A (eds): *Current Topics in Radiation Research*, vol 4, pp 359–397. Amsterdam, North-Holland Publishing Co., 1968

Emery EW, Denekamp J, Ball MM: Survival of mouse skin epithelial cells following single and divided doses of x-rays. *Radiat Res* 41:450–466, 1970

Fu KK, Phillips TL, Kane LJ, Smith V: Tumor and normal tissue response to irradiation *in vivo:* Variation with decreasing dose rates. *Radiology* 114:709–716, 1975

Hahn GM, Bagshaw MA, Evans RG, Gordon LF: Repair of potentially lethal lesions in x-irradiated, density-inhibited Chinese hamster cells: Metabolic effects and hypoxia. *Radiat Res* 55:280–290, 1973

Hahn GM, Little JB: Plateau-phase cultures of mammalian cells: An *in vitro* model for human cancer. *Curr Top Radiat Res* 8:39–43, 1972

Hall EJ: The biological basis of endocurietherapy: The Henschke Memorial Lecture 1984. *Endocurie Hypertherm Oncol* 1:141–151, 1985

Hall EJ: Radiation dose rate: A factor of importance in radiobiology and radiotherapy. *Br J Radiol* 45:81–97, 1972

Hall EJ, Bedford JS: Dose rate: Its effect on the survival of HeLa cells irradiated with gamma rays. *Radiat Res* 22:305–315, 1964

Hall EJ, Brenner DJ: The dose-rate effect revisited: Radiobiological considerations of importance in radiotherapy. *Int J Radiat Oncol Biol Phys* 21:1403–1414, 1991

Hall EJ, Brenner DJ: The 1991 George Edelstyn Memorial Lecture: Needles, wires and chips—advances in brachytherapy. *Clin Oncol* 4:249–256, 1992

Hall EJ, Cavanagh J: The effect of hypoxia on the recovery of sublethal radiation damage in *Vicia* seedlings. *Br J Radiol* 42:270–277, 1969

Hall EJ, Fairchild RG: Radiobiological measures with californium-252. *Br J Radiol* 42:263–266, 1970

Hall EJ, Kraljevic U: Repair of potentially lethal radiation damage: Comparison of neutron and x-ray RBE and implications for radiation therapy. *Radiology* 121:731–735, 1976

Hall EJ, Roizin-Towie L, Theus RB, August LS: Radiobiological properties of high energy cyclotron produced neutrons used for radiotherapy. *Radiology* 117:173–178, 1975

Hall EJ, Rossi HH, Roizin LA: Low dose-rate irradiation of mammalian cells with radium and californium-252: A comparison of effects on an actively proliferating cell population. *Radiology* 99:445–451, 1971

Henschke UK, Hilaris BS, Mahan GD: Afterloading in interstitial and intracavitary radiation therapy. *Am J Roentgenol Radium Ther Nucl Med* 90:386–395, 1963

Hornsey S: The radiosensitivity of melanoma cells in culture. *Br J Radiol* 45:158, 1972

Hornsey S: The recovery process in organized tissue. In Silini G (ed): *Radiation Research*, pp 587–603. Amsterdam, North-Holland Publishing Co., 1967

Howard A: The role of oxygen in the repair process. In Bond VP (ed): *Proceedings of the Carmel Conference on Time and Dose Relationships in Radiation Biology as Applied to Radiotherapy*, pp 70–81. Upton, NY, BNL Report 50203 (C-57), 1969

Jackson SP: Sensing and repairing DNA double-strand breaks. *Carcinogenesis* 23:687–696, 2002

Jeggo PA, Hafezparast M, Thompson AF, et al.: Localization of a DNA repair gene (XRCC5) involved in double-strand-break rejoining to human chromosome 2. *Proc Natl Acad Sci USA* 89:6423–6427, 1992

Joslin CAF: High-activity source afterloading in gynecological cancer and its future prospects. *Endocurie Hypertherm Oncol* 5:69–81, 1989

Joslin CAF, Liversage WE, Ramsay NW: High dose-rate treatment moulds by afterloading techniques. *Br J Radiol* 42:108–112, 1969

Joslin CAF, Smith CW: The use of high activity cobalt-60 sources for intracavitary and surface mould therapy. *Proc R Soc Med* 63:1029–1034, 1970

Khanna K, Gatti R, Concannon P, Weemaes CMR, Hoekstra MF, Lavin M, D'Andrea A: Cellular responses to DNA damage and human chromosome instability syndromes. In Nickoloff JA Hoekstra MF (eds): *DNA Damage and Repair*, vol 2: *DNA Repair in Higher Eukaryotes*, pp 395–442. Totowa, NJ, Humana Press, 1998

Lajtha LG, Oliver R: Some radiobiological considerations in radiotherapy. *Br J Radiol* 34:252–257, 1961

Lamerton LF: Cell proliferation under continuous irradiation. *Radiat Res* 27:119–139, 1966

Lamerton LF, Courtenay VD: The steady state under continuous irradiation. In Brown DG, Cragle RG, Noonan JR (eds): *Dose Rate in Mammalian Radiation Biology*, pp 3-1–3-12. Conference 680410. Washington, DC, United States Atomic Energy Commission, Division of Technical Information, 1968

Lenhard RE Jr, Order SE, Spunberg JJ, Asbell SO, Leibel SA: Isotopic immunoglobulin: A new systemic therapy for advanced Hodgkin's disease. *J Clin Oncol* 3:1296–1300, 1985

Lieberman HB, Hopkins KM: A single nucleotide base-pair change is responsible for the radiosensitivity exhibited by S pombe cells containing the mutant allele RAD-192 (abstr). In Chapman JD, Devey WC, Whitmore GF (eds): *Radiation Research: A Twentieth Century Perspective,* vol 1, p 333. San Diego, Academic Press, 1991

Lieberman HB, Hopkins KM, Chu HM, Laverty M: Molecular cloning and analysis of *Schizosaccharomyces pombe rad 9*, a gene involved in DNA repair and mutagenesis. *Mol Gen Genet* 232:367–376, 1992

Little JB, Hahn GM, Frindel E, Tubiana M: Repair of potentially lethal radiation damage *in vitro* and *in vivo*. *Radiology* 106:689–694, 1973

Mazeron JJ, Simon JM, Crook J, et al.: Influence of dose rate on local control of breast carcinoma treated by external beam irradiation plus iridium-192 implant. *Int J Radiat Oncol Biol Phys* 21:1173–1177, 1991

Mazeron JJ, Simon JM, Le Pechoux C, et al.: Effect of dose rate on local control and complications in definitive irradiation of T1-2 squamous cell carcinomas of mobile tongue and floor of mouth with interstitial iridium-192. *Radiother Oncol* 21:39–47, 1991

Mitchell JB, Bedford JS, Bailey SM: Dose-rate effects on the cell cycle and survival of S3 HeLa and V79 cells. *Radiat Res* 79:520–536, 1979

Order SE: Monoclonal antibodies: Potential in radiation therapy and oncology. *Int J Radiat Oncol Biol Phys* 8:1193–1201, 1982

Order SE, Klein JL, Ettinger D, et al.: Use of isotopic immunoglobulin in therapy. *Cancer Res* 40:3001–3007, 1980

Order SE, Porter M, Hellman S: Hodgkin's disease: Evidence for a tumor-associated antigen. *N Engl J Med* 285:471–474, 1971

Order SE, Stillwagon GB, Klein JL, et al.: Iodine-131 antiferritin: A new treatment modality in hepatoma: A Radiation Therapy Oncology Group study. *J Clin Oncol* 3:1573–1582, 1985

Orton CG: What minimum number of fractions is required with high dose-rate afterloading? *Br J Radiol* 60:300–302, 1987

Paterson R: *Treatment of Malignant Disease by Radiotherapy*. Baltimore, Williams & Wilkins, 1963

Petrini JHJ, Bressan DA, Yao MS: The rad52 epistasis group in mammalian double strand break repair. *Semin Immunol* 9:181–188, 1997

Phillips RA, Tolmach LJ: Repair of potentially lethal damage in x-irradiated HeLa cells. *Radiat Res* 29:413–432, 1966

Phillips TL, Ainsworth EJ: Altered split-dose recovery in mice irradiated under hypoxic conditions. *Radiat Res* 39:317–331, 1969

Phillips TL, Hanks GE: Apparent absence of recovery in endogenous colony-forming cells after irradiation under hypoxic conditions. *Radiat Res* 33:517–532, 1968

Pierquin B: L'effet differential de l'irradiation continué (ou semi-continué) a faible debit des carcinoms épidermoides. *J Radiol Electrol* 51:533–536, 1970

Pierquin B, Chassagne D, Baillet F, Paine CH: Clinical observations on the time factor in interstitial radiotherapy using iridium-192. *Clin Radiol* 24:506–509, 1973

Sancar A, Lindsey-Boltz LA, Ünsal-Kaçmaz K, Linn S: Molecular mechanisms of mammalian DNA repair and the DNA damage checkpoints. *Annu Rev Biochem* 73:39–85, 2004

Shipley WU, Stanley JA, Courtenay VC, Field SB: Repair of radiation damage in Lewis lung carcinoma cells following in situ treatment with fast neutrons and gamma rays. *Cancer Res* 35:932–938, 1975

Shuttleworth E, Fowler JF: Nomograms for radiobiologically equivalent fractionated x-ray doses. *Br J Radiol* 39:154–155, 1966

Stout R, Hunter RD: Clinical trials of changing dose rate in intracavitary low dose-rate therapy. In Mould RF (ed): *Brachytherapy*. Amsterdam, Nucletron, 1985

Suit H, Urano M: Repair of sublethal radiation injury in hypoxic cells of a C3H mouse mammary carcinoma. *Radiat Res* 37:423–434, 1969

Thacker J, Zdzienicka MZ: The mammalian *XRCC* genes: Their roles in DNA repair and genetic stability. *DNA Repair* 2:655–672, 2003

Thompson LH, Brookman KW, Jones NJ, Allen A, Carrano V: Molecular cloning of the human *XRCC1* gene, which corrects defective DNA strand break repair and sister chromatid exchange. *Mol Cell Biol* 20:6160–6271, 1990

Travis EJ, Thames HD, Watkins TL, et al.: The kinetics of repair in mouse lung after fractionated irradiation. *Int J Radiat Biol* 52:903–919, 1987

Tubiana N, Malaise E: Growth rate and cell kinetics in human tumors: Some prognostic and therapeutic implications. In Symington T, Carter RL (eds): *Scientific Foundations of Oncology*, pp 126–136. Chicago, Year Book Medical Publishers, 1976

Turesson I, Thames HD: Repair capacity and kinetics of human skin during fractionated radiotherapy: Erythema, desquamation, and telangiectasia after 3 and 5 years' follow-up. *Radiother Oncol* 15:169–188, 1989

Van't Hooft E: The selection HDR: Philosophy and design. In: Mould RF: *Selectron Brachytherapy Journal*. Amsterdam, Nucletron, 1985

Weichselbaum RR, Little JB, Nove J: Response of human osteosarcoma *in vitro* to irradiation: Evidence for unusual cellular repair activity. *Int J Radiat Biol* 31:295–299, 1977

Weichselbaum RR, Nove J, Little JB: Deficient recovery from potentially lethal radiation damage in ataxia-telangiectasia and xeroderma pigmentosum. *Nature* 271:261–262, 1978

Weichselbaum RR, Schmitt A, Little JB: Cellular repair factors influencing radiocurability of human malignant tumors. *Br J Cancer* 45:10–16, 1982

Weichselbaum RR, Withers HR, Tomkinson K, Little JB: Potentially lethal damage repair (PLDR) in x-irradiated cultures of a normal human diploid fibroblast cell strain. *Int J Radiat Biol* 43:313–319, 1983

Wells RL, Bedford JS: Dose-rate effects in mammalian cells: IV. Repairable and non-repairable damage in noncycling C3H 10T1/2 cells. *Radiat Res* 94:105–134, 1983

Whitmore GF, Gulyas S: Studies on recovery processes in mouse L cells. *Natl Cancer Inst Monogr* 24:141–156, 1967

Winans LF, Dewey WC, Dettor CM: Repair of sublethal and potentially lethal x-ray damage in synchronous Chinese hamster cells. *Radiat Res* 52:333–351, 1972

Withers HR: Capacity for repair in cells of normal and malignant tissues. In Bond VP (ed): *Proceedings of the Carmel Conference on Time and Dose Relationships in Radiation Biology as Applied to Radiotherapy*, pp 54–69. BNL Report 50203 (C-57). Upton, NY, 1969

CHAPTER 6

Oxygen Effect and Reoxygenation

A host of chemical and pharmacologic agents that modify the biological effect of ionizing radiations have been discovered. None is simpler than oxygen, none produces such a dramatic effect, and, as it turns out, no other agent has such obvious practical implications.

The oxygen effect was observed as early as 1912 in Germany by Swartz, who noted that the skin reaction produced on his forearm by a radium applicator was reduced if the applicator was pressed hard onto the skin. He attributed this to the interruption in blood flow. By 1921, it had been noted by Holthusen that *Ascaris* eggs were relatively resistant to radiation in the absence of oxygen, a result wrongly attributed to the absence of cell division under these conditions. The correlation between radiosensitivity and the presence of oxygen was made by Petry in 1923 from a study of the effects of radiation on vegetable seeds. All of these results were published in the German literature but were apparently little known in the English-speaking world.

In England in the 1930s, Mottram explored the question of oxygen in detail, basing his investigations on work of Crabtree and Cramer on the survival of tumor slices irradiated in the presence or absence of oxygen. He also discussed the importance of these findings to radiotherapy. Mottram began a series of experiments that culminated in a quantitative measurement of the oxygen effect by his colleagues Gray and Read, using as a biologic test system the growth inhibition of the primary root of the broad bean *Vicia faba*.

THE NATURE OF THE OXYGEN EFFECT

Survival curves for mammalian cells exposed to x-rays in the presence and absence of oxygen are illustrated in Figure 6.1. The ratio of doses administered under hypoxic to aerated conditions needed

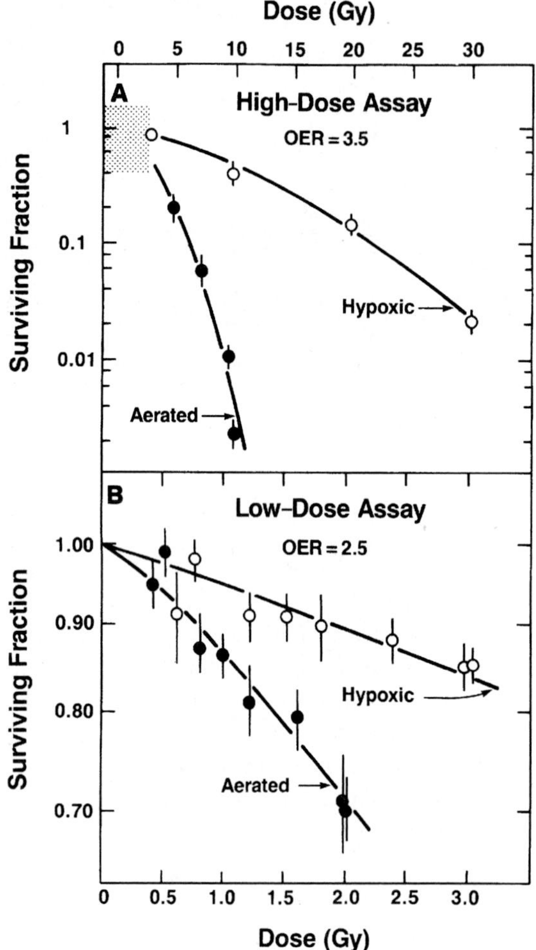

FIGURE 6.1 • Cells are much more sensitive to x-rays in the presence of molecular oxygen than in its absence (i.e., under hypoxia). The ratio of doses under hypoxic to aerated conditions necessary to produce the same level of cell killing is called the oxygen enhancement ratio (OER). It has a value close to 3.5 at high doses (**A**), but may have a lower value of about 2.5 at x-ray doses below about 2 to 3 Gy (200–300 rad) (**B**). (Adapted from Palcic B, Skarsgard LD: Reduced oxygen enhancement ratio at low doses of ionizing radiation. *Radiat Res* 100:328–339, 1984, with permission.)

to achieve the same biological effect is called the **oxygen enhancement ratio (OER)**. For sparsely ionizing radiations, such as x- and γ-rays, the OER at high doses has a value of between 2.5 and 3.5. The OER has been determined for a wide variety of chemical and biologic systems with different endpoints, and its value for x-rays and γ-rays always tends to fall in this range. There is some evidence that for rapidly growing cells cultured *in vitro*, the OER has a smaller value of about 2.5 at lower doses, on the order of the daily dose per fraction generally used in radiotherapy. This is believed to result from the variation of OER with the phase of the cell cycle: Cells in G_1 phase have a lower OER than those in S, and because G_1 cells are more radiosensitive, they dominate the low-dose region of the survival curve. For this reason, the OER of an asynchronous population is slightly smaller at low doses than at high doses. This result has been demonstrated for fast-growing cells cultured *in vitro*, for which precise survival measurements are possible, but would be difficult to show in a tissue. There is some evidence also that for cells in culture, the survival curve has a complex shape for doses below 1 Gy (100 rad). What effect, if any, this has on the OER is not yet clear.

Figure 6.2 illustrates the oxygen effect for other types of ionizing radiations. For a densely ionizing radiation, such as low-energy α-particles, the survival curve does not have an initial shoulder. In this case, survival estimates made in the presence or absence of oxygen fall along a common line; the OER is unity—in other words, there is no oxygen effect. For radiations of intermediate ionizing density, such as neutrons, the survival curves have a much reduced shoulder. In this case, the oxygen effect is apparent, but it is much smaller than is the

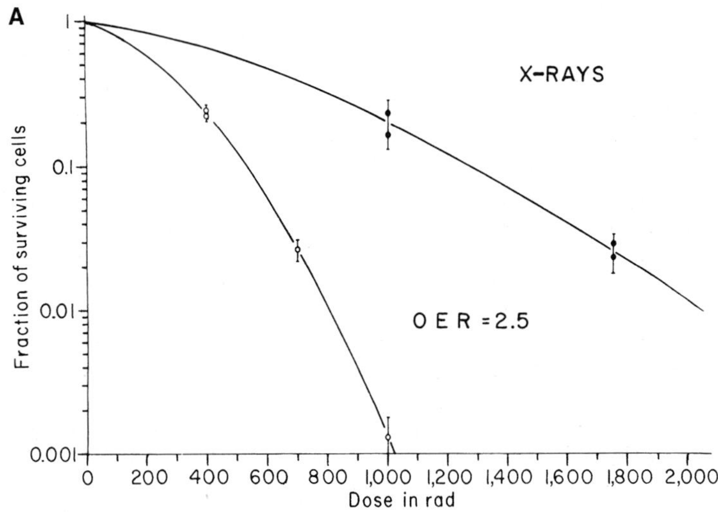

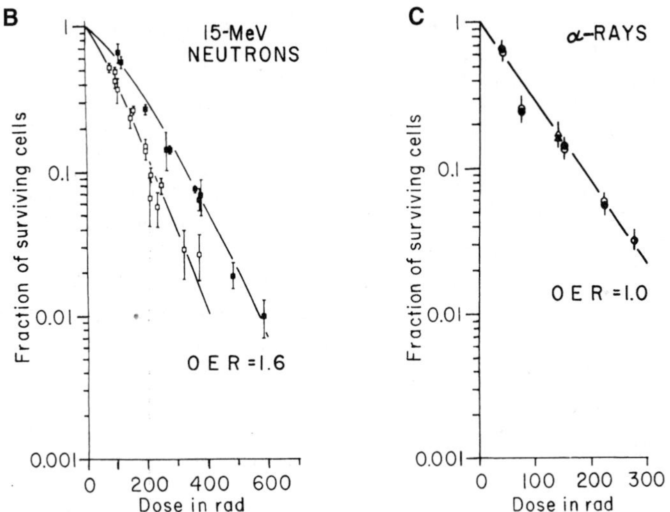

FIGURE 6.2 • The oxygen enhancement ratio (OER) for various types of radiation. The OER for low-energy α-particles is unity (**C**). X-rays exhibit a larger OER of 2.5 (**A**). Neutrons (15-MeV $d^+ \rightarrow T$) are between these extremes, with an OER of 1.6 (**B**). (Adapted from Barendsen GW, Koot CJ, van Kersen GR, Bewley DK, Field SB, Parnell CJ: The effect of oxygen on impairment of the proliferative capacity of human cells in culture by ionizing radiations of different LET. *Int J Radiat Biol Relat Stud Phys Chem Med* 10:317–327, 1966; and Broerse JJ, Barendsen GW, van Kersen GR: Survival of cultured human cells after irradiation with fast neutrons of different energies in hypoxic and oxygenated conditions. *Int J Radiat Biol Relat Stud Phys Chem Med* 13:559–572, 1968, with permission.)

case for x-rays. In the example shown in Figure 6.2, the OER for neutrons is about 1.6.

In summary, the oxygen effect is large and important in the case of sparsely ionizing radiations, such as x-rays; is absent for densely ionizing radiations, such as α-particles; and has an intermediate value for fast neutrons.

THE TIME AT WHICH OXYGEN ACTS AND THE MECHANISM OF THE OXYGEN EFFECT

For the oxygen effect to be observed, oxygen must be present during the radiation exposure or, to be precise, *during or within microseconds after* the radiation exposure. Sophisticated experiments have been performed in which oxygen, contained in a chamber at high pressure, was allowed to "explode" onto a single layer of bacteria (and later mammalian cells) at various times before or after irradiation with a 2-μs electron pulse from a linear accelerator. It was found that oxygen need not be present during the irradiation to sensitize but could be added *afterward*, provided the delay was not too long. Some sensitization occurred with oxygen added as late as 5 ms after irradiation.

Experiments such as these shed some light on the mechanism of the oxygen effect. There is general agreement that oxygen acts at the level of the free radicals. The chain of events from the absorption of radiation to the final expression of biologic damage has been summarized as follows: The absorption of radiation leads to the production of fast charged particles. The charged particles, in passing through the biologic material, produce a number of ion pairs. These ion pairs have very short life spans (about 10^{-10} second) and produce free radicals, which are highly reactive molecules because they have an unpaired valence electron. The free radicals are important because although their life spans are only about 10^{-5} second, that is appreciably longer than that of the ion pairs. To a large extent, it is these free radicals that break chemical bonds, produce chemical changes, and initiate the chain of events that results in the final expression of biologic damage; however, it has been observed that the extent of the damage depends on the presence or absence of oxygen.

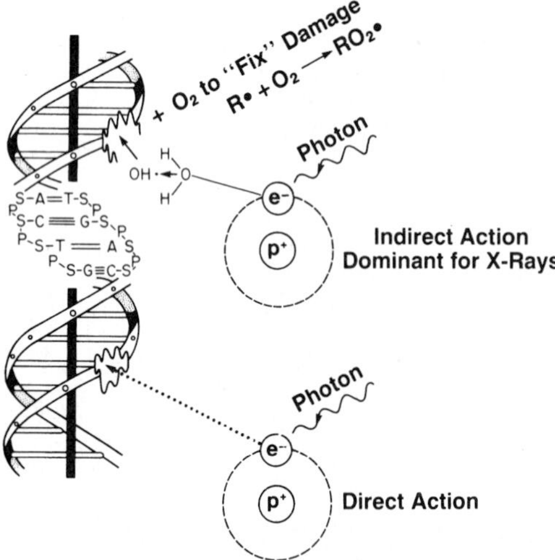

FIGURE 6.3 • The oxygen fixation hypothesis. About two thirds of the biologic damage produced by x-rays is by indirect action mediated by free radicals. The damage produced by free radicals in DNA can be repaired under hypoxia but may be "fixed" (made permanent and irreparable) if molecular oxygen is available.

If molecular oxygen is present, DNA reacts with the free radicals (R·). The DNA radical can be chemically restored to its reduced form through reaction with an SH group. However, the formation of $RO_2\cdot$, an organic peroxide, represents a non-restorable form of the target material; that is, the reaction results in a change in the chemical composition of the material exposed to the radiation. This reaction cannot take place in the absence of oxygen, since then many of the ionized target molecules are able to repair themselves and recover the ability to function normally. In a sense, then, oxygen may be said to "fix" or make permanent the radiation lesion. This is known as the *oxygen fixation hypothesis*. The process is illustrated in Figure 6.3.

THE CONCENTRATION OF OXYGEN REQUIRED

A question of obvious importance is the concentration of oxygen required to potentiate the effect of radiation. Is the amount required small or large? Many investigations have been performed using bacteria, plants, yeast, and mammalian cells, and the similarities between them are striking.

The simple way to visualize the effect of oxygen is by considering the change of slope of the mammalian cell survival curve. Figure 6.4 is a dramatic representation of what happens to the survival curve in the presence of various concentrations of oxygen. Curve A is characteristic of the response under conditions of equilibration with air. Curve B is a survival curve for irradiation in as low a level of hypoxia as usually can be obtained under experimental conditions (10 ppm of oxygen in the gas phase). The introduction of a very small quantity of oxygen, 100 ppm, is readily noticeable in a change in the slope of the survival curve. A concentration of 2,200 ppm, which is about 0.22% oxygen, moves the survival curve about halfway toward the fully aerated condition.

Other experiments have shown that generally by the time a concentration of oxygen corresponding to 2% has been reached, the survival curve is virtually indistinguishable from that obtained under conditions of normal aeration. Furthermore, increasing the amount of oxygen present from that characteristic of air to 100% oxygen does not further affect the slope of the curve. This has led to the more usual "textbook representation" of the variation of radiosensitivity with oxygen concentration as shown in Figure 6.5. The term used here

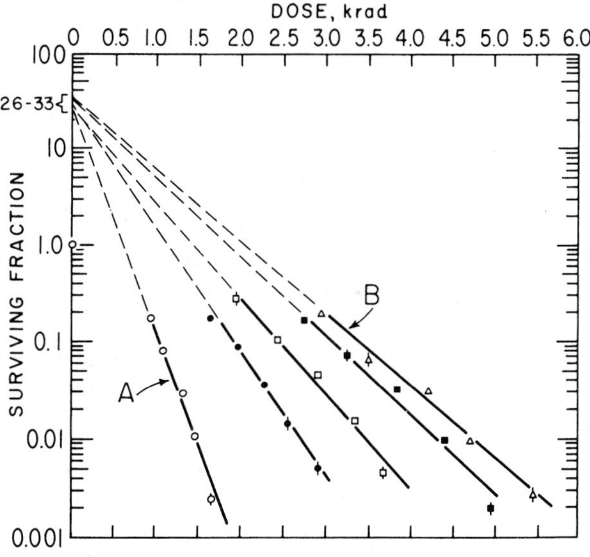

FIGURE 6.4 • Survival curves for Chinese hamster cells exposed to x-rays in the presence of various oxygen concentrations. Open circles, air (**A**); closed circles, 2,200 ppm of oxygen or pO_2 of 1.7 mm Hg; open squares, 355 ppm of oxygen or pO_2 of 0.25 mm Hg; closed squares, 100 ppm of oxygen or pO_2 of 0.075 mm Hg; open triangles, 10 ppm of oxygen or pO_2 of 0.0075 mm Hg (**B**), which corresponded to the lowest level of hypoxia that could usually be obtained under experimental conditions. (From Elkind MM, Swain RW, Alescio T, Sutton H, Moses WB: Oxygen, nitrogen, recovery and radiation therapy. In *Cellular Radiation Biology*, pp 442–461. Baltimore, Williams & Wilkins, 1965, with permission.)

to represent radiosensitivity is proportional to the reciprocal of the D_0 of the survival curve. It is arbitrarily assigned a value of unity for anoxic conditions. As the oxygen concentration increases, the biologic material becomes progressively more sensitive to radiation, until, in the presence of 100% oxygen, it is about three times as sensitive as under complete anoxia. Note that the rapid change of radiosensitivity occurs as the partial pressure of oxygen is increased from zero to about 30 mm Hg (5% oxygen). A further increase in oxygen tension to an atmosphere of pure oxygen has little, if any, further effect. An oxygen concentration of 0.5% (or about 3 mm Hg) results in a radiosensitivity halfway between the characteristic of hypoxia and that of fully oxygenated conditions.

It is evident, then, that very small amounts of oxygen are necessary to produce the dramatic and important oxygen effect observed with x-rays. Although it is usually assumed that the oxygen tension of most normal tissues is similar to that of venous blood or lymph (20–40 mm Hg), in fact, oxygen probe measurements indicate that the oxygen tension between different tissues may vary over a wide range from 1 to 100 mm Hg. Many tissues are therefore borderline hypoxic and contain a small proportion of cells that are radiobiologically hypoxic. This is particularly true of, for example, the liver and skeletal muscles. Even mouse skin has a small proportion of hypoxic cells that shows up as a change of slope if the survival curve is pushed to low survival levels.

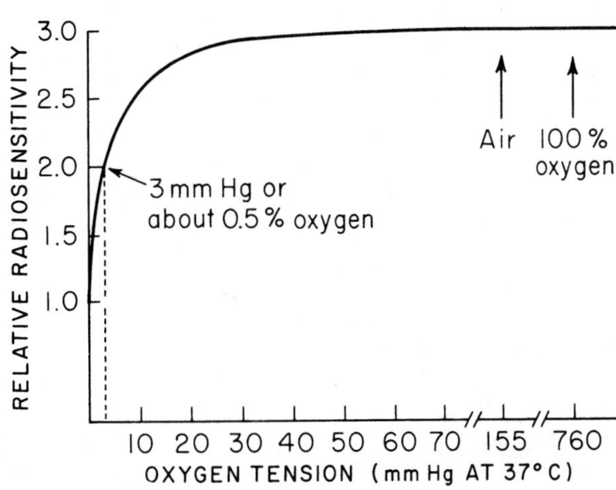

FIGURE 6.5 • An idealized representation of the dependence of radiosensitivity on oxygen concentration. If the radiosensitivity under extremely anoxic conditions is arbitrarily assigned a value of unity, the relative radiosensitivity is about 3 under well-oxygenated conditions. Most of this change of sensitivity occurs as the oxygen tension increases from 0 to 30 mm Hg. A further increase of oxygen content to that characteristic of air or even pure oxygen at high pressure has little further effect. A relative radiosensitivity halfway between anoxia and full oxygenation occurs for a pO_2 of about 3 mm Hg, which corresponds to a concentration of about 0.5% oxygen. This illustration is idealized and does not represent any specific experimental data. Experiments have been performed with yeast, bacteria, and mammalian cells in culture; the results conform to the general conclusions summarized here.

CHRONIC AND ACUTE HYPOXIA

It is important to recognize that hypoxia in tumors can result from two quite different mechanisms. *Chronic* hypoxia results from the limited diffusion distance of oxygen through tissue that is respiring. The distance to which oxygen can diffuse is largely limited by the rapid rate at which it is metabolized by respiring tumor cells. Many tumor cells may remain hypoxic for long periods of time. In contrast to chronic hypoxia, *acute* hypoxia is the result of the temporary closing of a tumor blood vessel owing to the malformed vasculature of the tumor, which lacks smooth muscle and often has an incomplete endothelial lining and basement membrane. Tumor cells are exposed to a continuum of oxygen concentrations, ranging from the highest in cells surrounding the capillaries to almost anoxic conditions in cells more distant from the capillaries. This is significant because both chronic and acute hypoxia have been shown to drive malignant progression.

Chronic Hypoxia

As already mentioned, radiotherapists began to suspect that oxygen influences the radiosensitivity of tumors in the 1930s. It was, however, a paper by Thomlinson and Gray in 1955 that triggered the tremendous interest in oxygen as a factor in radiotherapy; they described the phenomenon of chronic hypoxia that they observed in their histologic study of fresh specimens of bronchial carcinoma. Cells of the stratified squamous epithelium, normal or malignant, generally remain in contact with one another; the vascular stroma on which their nutrition depends lies in contact with the epithelium, but capillaries do not penetrate between the cells. Tumors that arise in this type of tissue often grow in solid cords that, seen in section, appear to be circular areas surrounded by stroma. The centers of large tumor areas are necrotic and are surrounded by intact tumor cells, which consequently appear as rings. Figure 6.6**A**, reproduced from Thomlinson and Gray, shows a transverse section of a tumor cord and is typical of areas of a tumor in which necrosis is not far advanced. Figure 6.6**B** shows large areas of necrosis separated from stroma by a narrow band of tumor cells about 100 μm wide.

By viewing a large number of these samples of human bronchial carcinomas, Thomlinson and Gray recognized that as the tumor cord grows larger, the necrotic center also enlarges, so that the thickness of the sheath of viable tumor cells remains essentially constant. This is illustrated in Figure 6.7.

The obvious conclusion was that tumor cells could proliferate and grow actively only if they were close to a supply of oxygen or nutrients from the stroma. Thomlinson and Gray then went on to calculate the distance to which oxygen could diffuse in respiring tissue and came up with a distance of about 150 μm. This was close enough to the thickness of viable tumor cords on their histologic sections for them to conclude that oxygen depletion was the principal factor leading to the development of necrotic areas in tumors. Using more appropriate values of oxygen diffusion coefficients and consumption values, a better estimate of the distance oxygen can diffuse in respiring tissue is about 70 μm. This, of course, varies from the arterial to the venous end of a capillary, as illustrated in Figure 6.8.

By histologic examination of sections, it is possible to distinguish only two classes of cells: (1) those that appear to be proliferating well and (2) those that are dead or dying. Between these two extremes, and assuming a steadily decreasing oxygen concentration, one would expect a region in which cells would be at an oxygen tension high enough for cells to be clonogenic but low enough to render the cells protected from the effect of ionizing radiation. Cells in this region would be relatively protected from a treatment with x-rays because of their low oxygen tension and could provide a focus for the subsequent regrowth of the tumor (Fig. 6.8). On the basis of these ideas, it was postulated that the presence of a relatively small proportion of hypoxic cells in tumors could limit the success of radiotherapy in some clinical situations.

These ideas about the role of oxygen in cell killing dominated the thinking of radiobiologists and radiotherapists in the late 1950s and early 1960s. A great deal of thought and effort was directed toward solving this problem. The solutions proposed included the use of high-pressure oxygen chambers and the development of novel radiation modalities, such as neutrons, negative π-mesons, and heavy charged ions.

Acute Hypoxia

Regions of acute hypoxia develop in tumors as a result of the temporary closing or blockage of a particular blood vessel. If this blockage were permanent, the cells downstream, of course, would eventually die and be of no further consequence. There is, however, good evidence that tumor blood vessels open and close in a random fashion, so that different regions of the tumor become hypoxic intermittently. In fact, acute hypoxia results from transient fluctuations in blood flow due to the malformed vasculature. At the moment when a dose of radiation is delivered, a proportion of tumor cells may be hypoxic, but if the radiation is delayed until a later time, a different group of cells may be hypoxic. The

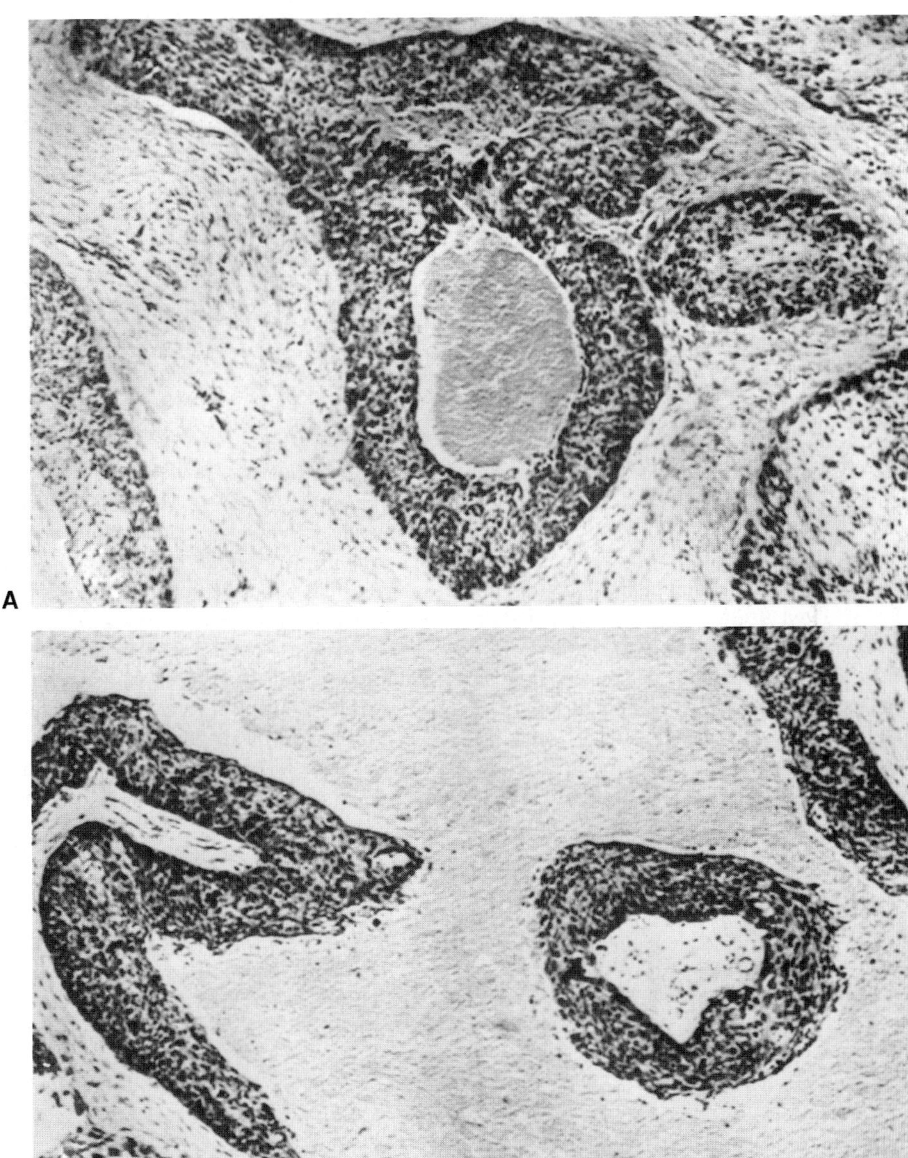

FIGURE 6.6 • Transverse sections of tumor cords surrounded by stroma from human carcinoma of the bronchus. **A:** A typical tumor area in which necrosis is not far advanced. **B:** Large areas of necrosis separated from the stroma by a band of tumor cells about 100 μm wide. (From Thomlinson RH, Gray LH: The histological structure of some human lung cancers and the possible implications for radiotherapy. *Br J Cancer* 9:539–549, 1955, with permission.)

occurrence of acute hypoxia was postulated in the early 1980s by Martin Brown and was later demonstrated unequivocally in rodent tumors by Chaplin and his colleagues. Figure 6.9, which illustrates how acute hypoxia is caused by fluctuating blood flow, also depicts the difference between acute and chronic hypoxia. In contrast to acutely hypoxic cells, chronically hypoxic cells are less likely to become reoxygenated and will die unless they are able to access a blood supply.

THE FIRST EXPERIMENTAL DEMONSTRATION OF HYPOXIC CELLS IN A TUMOR

The dilution assay technique, described in Chapter 20, was used by Powers and Tolmach to investigate the radiation response of a solid subcutaneous lymphosarcoma in the mouse. Survival estimates were made for doses from 2 to 25 Gy (200 to 2,500 rad). The results are shown in Figure 6.10, in

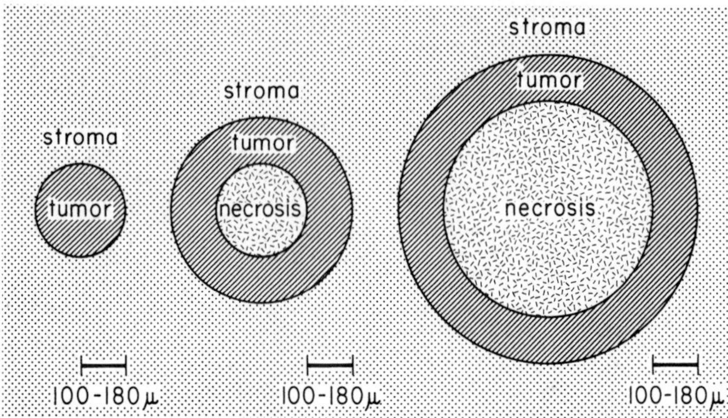

FIGURE 6.7 ● The conclusions reached by Thomlinson and Gray from a study of histologic sections of human bronchial carcinoma. No necrosis was seen in small tumor cords with a radius of less than about 160 μm. No tumor cord with a radius exceeding 200 μm was without a necrotic center. As the diameter of the necrotic area increased, the thickness of the sheath of viable tumor cells remained essentially constant at 100 to 180 μm.

which the dose on a linear scale is plotted against the fraction of surviving cells on a logarithmic scale.

The survival curve for this solid tumor clearly consists of two separate components. The first, up to a dose of about 9 Gy (900 rad), has a D_0 of 1.1 Gy (110 rad). The second has a shallower D_0 of 2.6 Gy (260 rad). This biphasic survival curve has a final slope about 2.5 times shallower than the initial portion, which strongly suggests that the tumor consists of two separate groups of cells, one oxygenated and the other hypoxic. If the shallow component of the curve is extrapolated backward to cut the surviving-fraction axis, it does so at a survival level of about 1%. From this it may be inferred that about 1% of the clonogenic cells in the tumor were deficient in oxygen.

The response of this tumor to single doses of radiation of various sizes is explained readily on this basis. If 99% of the cells are well oxygenated and 1% are hypoxic, the response to lower doses is dominated by the killing of the well-oxygenated cells.

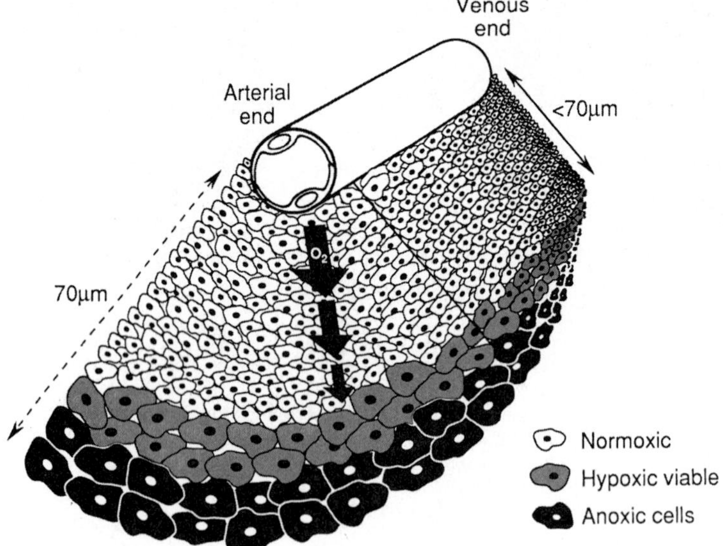

FIGURE 6.8 ● The diffusion of oxygen from a capillary through tumor tissue. The distance to which oxygen can diffuse is limited largely by the rapid rate at which it is metabolized by respiring tumor cells. For some distance from a capillary, tumor cells are well oxygenated (white). At greater distances, oxygen is depleted, and tumor cells become necrotic (black). Hypoxic tumor cells form a layer, perhaps one or two cells thick, in between (gray). In this region, the oxygen concentration is high enough for the cells to be viable but low enough for them to be relatively protected from the effects of x-rays. These cells may limit the radiocurability of the tumor. The distance to which oxygen can diffuse is about 70 μm at the arterial end of a capillary and less at the venous end.

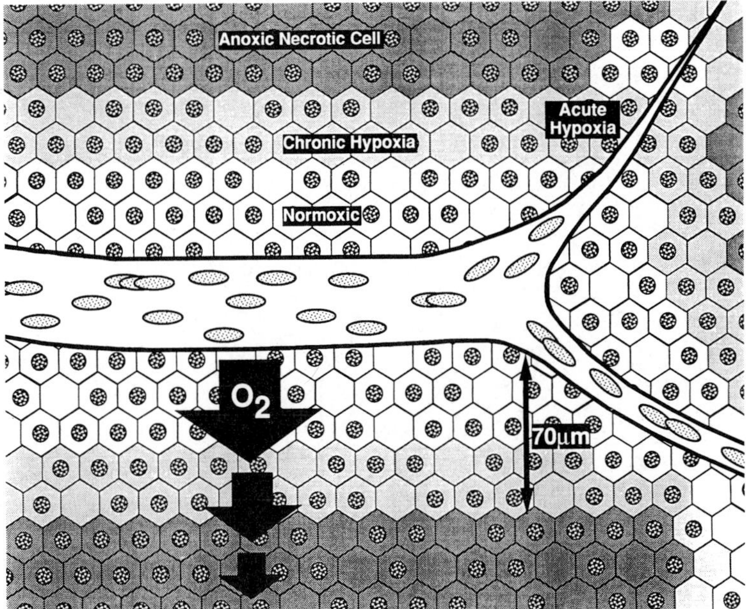

FIGURE 6.9 ● Diagram illustrating the difference between chronic and acute hypoxia. Chronic hypoxia results from the limited diffusion distance of oxygen in respiring tissue that is actively metabolizing oxygen. Cells that become hypoxic in this way remain hypoxic for long periods of time until they die and become necrotic. Acute hypoxia results from the temporary closing of tumor blood vessels. The cells are intermittently hypoxic because normoxia is restored each time the blood vessel opens up again. (Adapted from Brown JM: Tumor hypoxia, drug resistance, and metastases. *JNCI* 82:338–339 1990, with permission.)

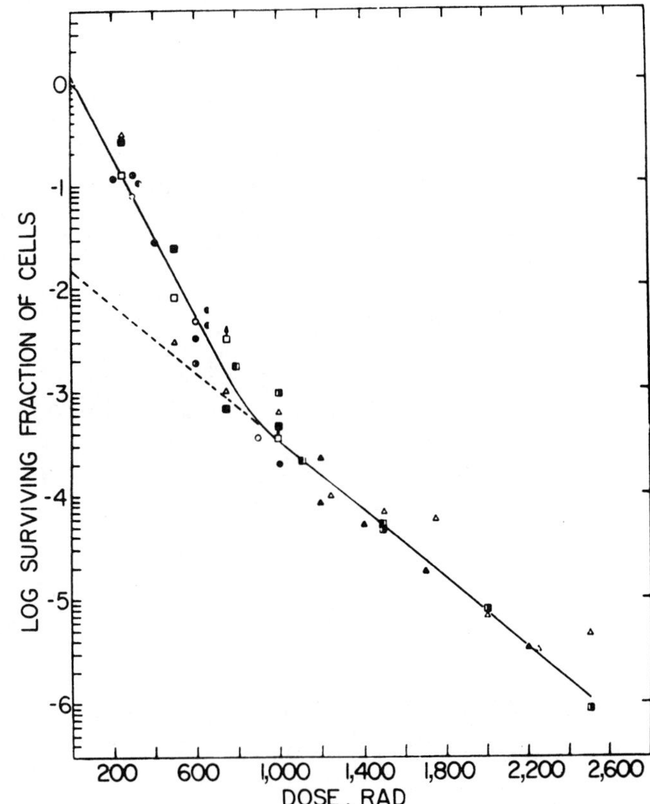

FIGURE 6.10 ● Fraction of surviving cells as a function of dose for a solid subcutaneous lymphosarcoma in the mouse irradiated *in vivo*. The first part of the curve has a slope D_0 of 1.1 Gy (110 rad); the second component of the curve has a shallower slope D_0 of 2.6 Gy (260 rad), indicating that these cells are hypoxic. (From Powers WE, Tolmach LJ: A multicomponent x-ray survival curve for mouse lymphosarcoma cells irradiated *in vivo*. *Nature* 197:710–711, 1963, with permission.)

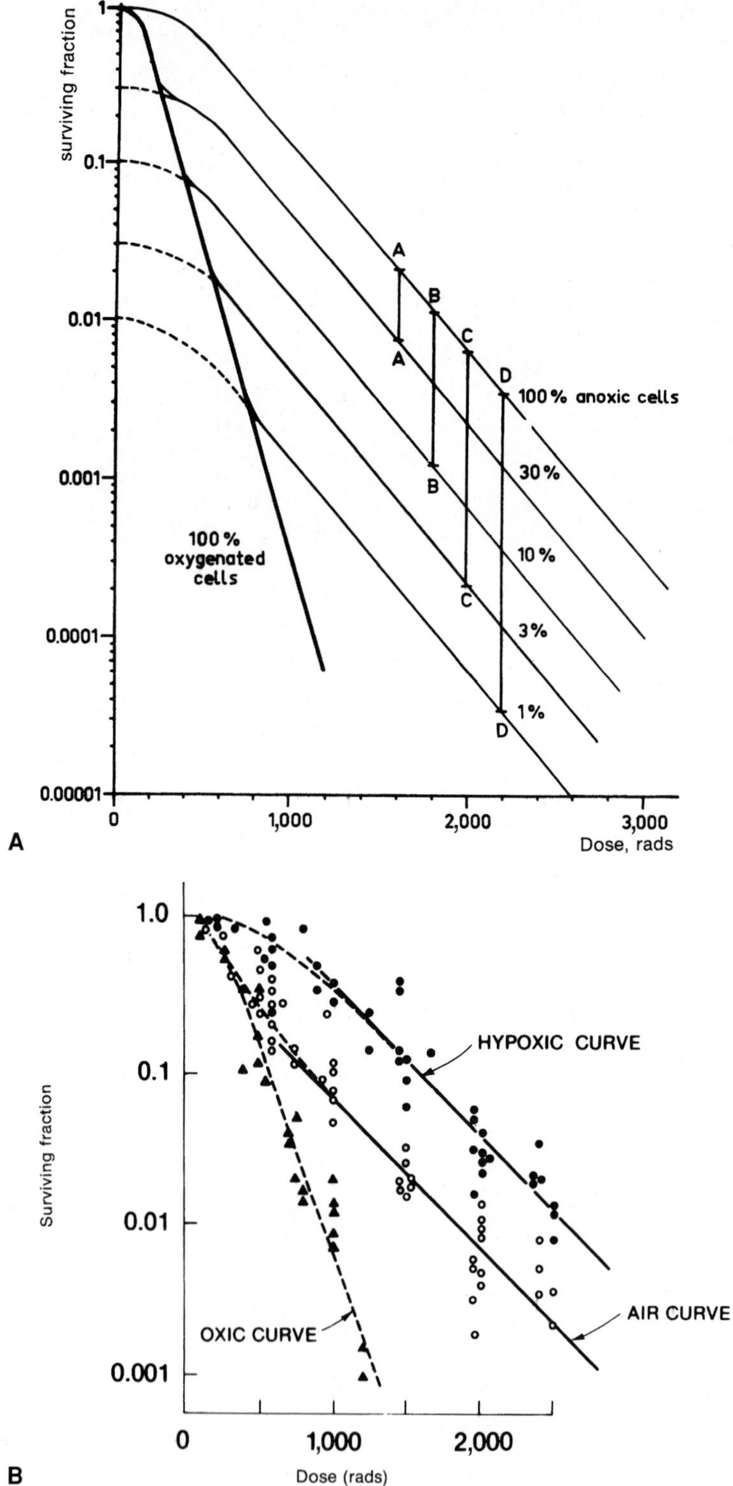

FIGURE 6.11 ● **A:** Theoretic survival curves for cell populations containing different fractions of hypoxic cells. The fraction of hypoxic cells in each population determines the distance between its survival curve and the curve for the completely hypoxic population. From the relative radiosensitivity at any dose level at which the

For these doses, the hypoxic cells are depopulated to a negligibly small extent. Once a dose of about 9 Gy (900 rad) is exceeded, however, the oxygenated compartment of the tumor is depopulated severely, and the response of the tumor is characteristic of the response of hypoxic cells. This biphasic survival curve was the first unequivocal demonstration that a solid tumor could contain cells sufficiently hypoxic to be protected from cell killing by x-rays but still clonogenic and capable of providing a focus for tumor regrowth.

PROPORTION OF HYPOXIC CELLS IN VARIOUS ANIMAL TUMORS

Over the years, many investigators have determined the fraction of hypoxic cells in a wide variety of tumors in experimental animals. The most satisfactory and most widely used method is to obtain paired survival curves (Fig. 6.11**A**). The steepest curve relates to a fully oxygenated population of cells; the uppermost curve, to a population made up entirely of hypoxic cells. The intermediate curves refer to mixed populations of hypoxic and oxygenated cells. At low doses, the survival curve for a mixed population closely follows that for the oxygenated population. At higher doses, the number of surviving oxygenated cells is negligible compared with the number of anoxic cells, and consequently the curve representing the mixed population is parallel to (i.e., has the same slope as) the curve for the hypoxic population. The fraction of hypoxic cells in the tumor determines the distance between the parallel terminal slopes of the dose–response curves, as shown in Figure 6.11**A**. This fraction is identical to the ratio of the surviving cells from the partially hypoxic tumor to those from the entirely hypoxic tumor.

In practice, the procedure is as follows: Survival measurements are made at several dose levels under two different conditions:

1. The animal (e.g., a mouse) is asphyxiated several minutes before irradiation by breathing nitrogen. Under these conditions, all of the tumor cells are hypoxic, and the data points obtained define a line comparable to the upper curve in Figure 6.11**A**.
2. The animal is alive and breathing air when irradiated, so that the proportion of hypoxic cells in the tumor is at its normal level. The data points obtained define a lower line typical of a mixed population of hypoxic and oxygenated cells. The vertical separation between the two lines gives the proportion of hypoxic cells characteristic of that particular type of tumor.

An example of experimental data for a determination of the hypoxic fraction in a mouse tumor is shown in Figure 6.11**B**. Hypoxic fractions also can be calculated from a comparison of the TCD_{50} values (i.e., the doses at which 50% of the tumors are locally controlled) for clamped and unclamped tumors or from a comparison of growth delays from tumors irradiated under these two conditions. Any of these methods involves several assumptions, notably that cells made hypoxic artificially have the same sensitivity as those that have respired to this condition in the tumor naturally and that the tumor is composed of two distinct populations, one aerated and the other hypoxic, with nothing falling in between. Consequently, measured values for hypoxic fractions can serve only as a guide and must not be taken too seriously.

Moulder and Rockwell published a survey of all published data on hypoxic fractions and reported that of 42 tumor types studied, 37 were found to contain hypoxic cells in at least one study. Hypoxic fractions range from 0 to 50%, with a tendency for many results to average about 15%. Comparable measurements cannot be made in human tumors, of course, to determine precisely the proportion of hypoxic cells.

EVIDENCE FOR HYPOXIA IN HUMAN TUMORS

Over the last decade, a variety of techniques have been used to determine the oxygenation of human tumors, including measuring the distance between

FIGURE 6.11 • *(Continued)* survival curves are approximated by parallel lines, the fraction of hypoxic cells can be determined from the ratio of survival of the completely and partially hypoxic populations, as indicated by the vertical lines A-A, B-B, and so on. This illustration is based on the model proposed by Hewitt and Wilson. (From van Putten LM, Kallman RF: Oxygenation status of a transplantable tumor during fractionated radiotherapy. *J Natl Cancer Inst* 40:441–451, 1968, with permission.) **B:** The proportion of hypoxic cells in a mouse tumor. The biphasic curve labeled *air curve* represents data for cells from tumors irradiated in mice breathing air, which are therefore a mixture of aerated and hypoxic cells. The hypoxic curve is for cells irradiated in mice asphyxiated by nitrogen breathing or for cells irradiated *in vitro* in nitrogen, so that they are all hypoxic. The air curve is for cells irradiated *in vitro* in air. The proportion of hypoxic cells is the ratio of the air to hypoxic curves or the vertical separation between the curves, because the surviving fraction is on a logarithmic scale. (Courtesy of Dr. Sara Rockwell; based on data of Moulder and Rockwell and of Rockwell and Kallman.)

tumor cells and vessels in histologic sections, determining the oxygen saturation of hemoglobin, and monitoring changes in tumor metabolism. These techniques have been replaced by newer methods, including oxygen probes, hypoxia markers, the comet assay, and noninvasive imaging. Although each of these techniques has strengths and weaknesses, together they convincingly demonstrate that hypoxia is a common feature of human solid tumors that can influence both the malignant progression and the response of tumors to therapy. In the majority of studies, the assessment of hypoxia in human tumors has been based largely on oxygen-probe measurements. This approach has been used to group patients based on their median pO_2 values, but disregards a great deal of information that is obtained in the process, especially the heterogeneity of oxygen measurements in solid tumors. Although oxygen probes are considered the "gold standard" for measuring tumor pO_2, newer noninvasive techniques will supplant them in the future.

TECHNIQUES TO MEASURE TUMOR OXYGENATION

Oxygen Probe Measurements

Oxygen probes—that is, electrodes implanted directly into tumors to measure oxygen concentration by a polarographic technique—have a long and checkered history. The widespread use of this technique did not come about until the development of the Eppendorf probe, which has a very fast response time and can be moved quickly through a tumor under computer control to obtain large numbers of oxygen measurements along multiple tracks through the tumor. The data from polarographic oxygen electrode studies indicate that hypoxia can be used to predict treatment outcomes for a variety of tumor sites, including the cervix, prostate, and head and neck. Local control of tumors treated by radiotherapy correlates with oxygen-probe measurements, indicating that oxygen measurements may have a predictive value in radiotherapy. Oxygen electrode studies of cervical cancers and sarcomas indicated that hypoxia was also predictive of tumor aggressiveness. This is discussed subsequently in this chapter. A new fiber-optic probe has been introduced as an alternative oxygen sensor. A dye in the tip of the probe has a fluorescent lifetime that is inversely related to oxygen concentration.

2-Nitroimidazole Hypoxia Markers

The idea of using hypoxia markers originated from the development of 2-nitroimidazoles, hypoxic radiosensitizers that bind irreversibly to macromolecules in hypoxic cells. These compounds are administered systemically, but are only metabolized to form adducts under hypoxic conditions. Two examples of hypoxia markers are pimonidazole and EF5. Adduct formation in the hypoxic tumor cells is detected by tumor biopsy and immunohistochemistry (Fig. 6.12). The advantages of hypoxia markers over oxygen electrodes include (1) that they provide the relative oxygen concentrations on an individual cell basis, (2) that they make it possible to distinguish between viable and necrotic tissue, and (3) that they make it possible to distinguish between chronic and acute hypoxia.

Endogenous Hypoxia Markers

Oxygen-sensing mechanisms have been developed to maintain cell and tissue homeostasis as well as to adapt to the chronic low-oxygen conditions found in solid tumors. Immunohistochemical staining for endogenous markers of tumor hypoxia, such as carbonic anhydrase IX (CA9) and hypoxia inducible factor (HIF), has also been found to colocalize with 2-nitroimidazole binding, indicating that endogenous proteins are increased in hypoxic tumor regions. However, the expression of endogenous markers can be regulated by factors other than oxygen, complicating their use in quantifying tumor hypoxia.

Comet Assay

The comet assay measures DNA strand breaks in individual cells following irradiation. The more DNA strand breaks there are, the larger the size of the comet tail. If hypoxia is present, the same amount of DNA damage results in fewer DNA strand breaks. The major disadvantage of this technique is that it requires rapid sampling of the irradiated tumor owing to the fast repair of DNA single-strand breaks.

Noninvasive Hypoxia Imaging

Radioactively labeled 2-nitroimidazoles and other redox-sensitive compounds are currently being developed to monitor tissue hypoxia noninvasively. Although noninvasive imaging of hypoxia has a lower resolution than invasive approaches, it has the distinct advantage of monitoring changes in oxygenation of both the primary tumor and metastases. A variety of PET and SPECT imaging agents are available, including ^{18}F-miso, ^{18}F-EF5, ^{60}Cu ATSM, and ^{123}I-IAZA, and the next step will be to correlate the results of noninvasive imaging with clinical outcome. The use of these agents in combination with IMRT will allow the development of "physiologically targeted radiotherapy," in which

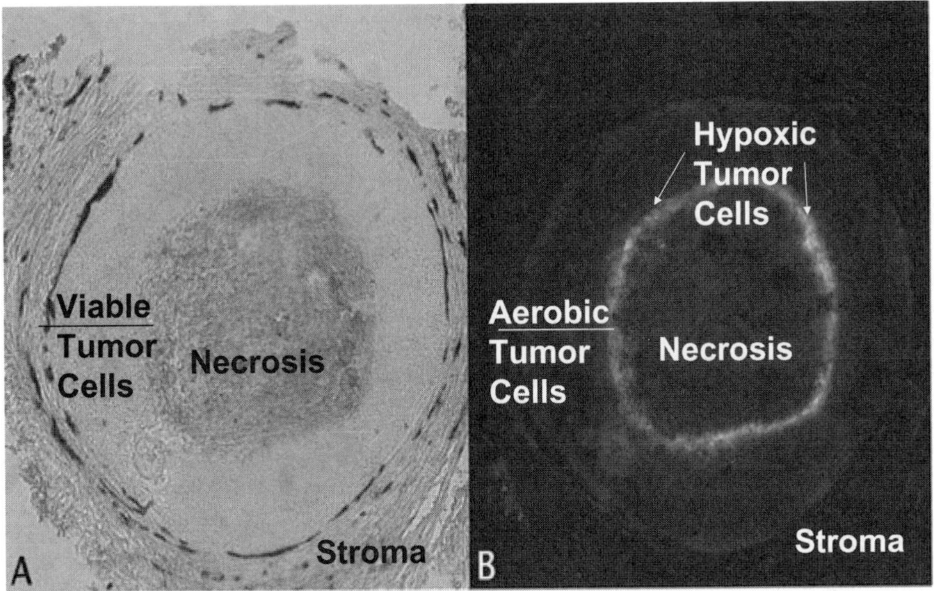

FIGURE 6.12 • These images show a section from a rodent tumor illustrating chronic hypoxic cells. The animal was treated with the 2-nitroimidazole hypoxia detection agent EF5 24 hours preceding surgical removal of the tumor. **A:** Photomicrograph of the tumor section illustrating the tumor stroma, viable tumor cells, and necrotic tumor core. **B:** The same tumor section demonstrating the presence of chronically hypoxic tumor cells that stain positive with EF5 (white rim) adjacent to the necrotic core. (Courtesy of Dr. Sydney Evans.)

different portions of the tumor can receive different radiation doses based on differences in physiology such as oxygen tension.

REOXYGENATION

Van Putten and Kallman determined the proportion of hypoxic cells in a transplantable sarcoma in the mouse. This tumor, which was of spontaneous origin, was transplanted from one generation of animals to the next by inoculating a known number of tumor cells subcutaneously. The tumor was allowed to grow for 2 weeks, by which time it had reached a size suitable for the experiment. The tumor was irradiated *in vivo* and then excised and made into a suspension of cells. The proportion of hypoxic cells was determined by the method described in Figure 6.11.

The researchers found that for this mouse sarcoma, the proportion of hypoxic cells in the untreated tumor was about 14%. The vital contribution made by van Putten and Kallman involved a determination of the proportion of hypoxic cells in this tumor after various fractionated radiation treatments. When groups of tumors were exposed to five daily doses of 1.9 Gy (190 rad), delivered Monday through Friday, the proportion of hypoxic cells was determined on the following Monday to be 18%. In another experiment, four daily fractions were given, Monday through Thursday, and the proportion of hypoxic cells measured the following day, Friday, was found to be 14%.

These experiments have far-reaching implications in radiotherapy. The fact that the proportion of hypoxic cells in the tumor is about the same at the end of a fractionated radiotherapy regimen as in the untreated tumor demonstrates that during the course of the treatment hypoxic cells become oxygenated. If this were not the case, then the *proportion* of hypoxic cells would increase during the course of the fractionated treatment, because the radiation depopulates the aerated-cell compartment more than the hypoxic-cell compartment. This phenomenon, by which hypoxic cells become oxygenated after a dose of radiation, is termed **reoxygenation**. The oxygen status of cells in a tumor is not static; it is dynamic and constantly changing.

The process of reoxygenation is illustrated in Figure 6.13. A modest dose of x-rays to a mixed population of aerated and hypoxic cells results in significant killing of aerated cells, but little killing of hypoxic cells. Consequently, the viable cell population immediately after irradiation is dominated by hypoxic cells. If sufficient time is allowed

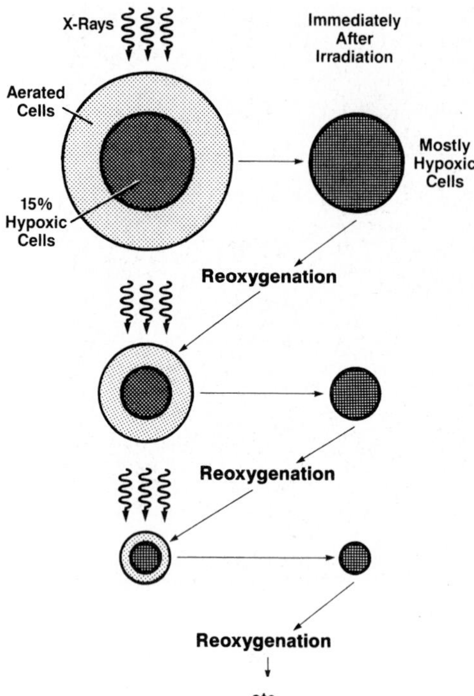

FIGURE 6.13 • The process of reoxygenation. Tumors contain a mixture of aerated and hypoxic cells. A dose of x-rays kills a greater proportion of aerated cells than hypoxic cells because aerated cells are more radiosensitive. Therefore, immediately after irradiation, most cells in the tumor are hypoxic. However, the preirradiation pattern tends to return because of reoxygenation. If the radiation is given in a series of fractions separated in time sufficient for reoxygenation to occur, the presence of hypoxic cells does not greatly influence the response of the tumor.

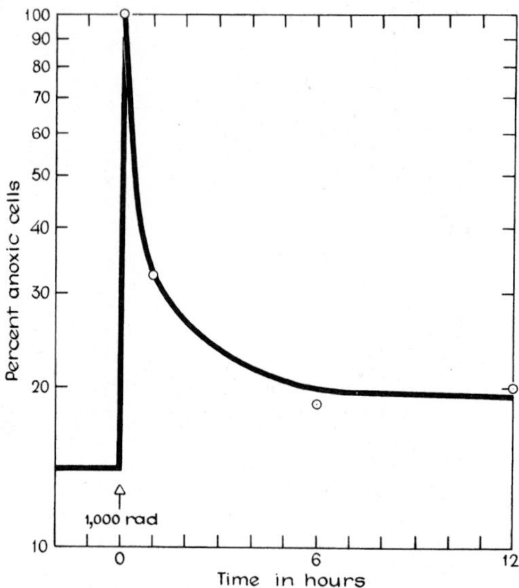

FIGURE 6.14 • Percentage of hypoxic cells in a transplantable mouse sarcoma as a function of time after a dose of 10 Gy (1,000 rad) of x-rays. Immediately after irradiation, essentially 100% of the viable cells are hypoxic, because such a dose kills a large proportion of the aerated cells. In this tumor, the process of reoxygenation is very rapid. By 6 hours after irradiation, the percentage of hypoxic cells has fallen to a value close to the preirradiation level. (From Kallman RF, Bleehen NM: Post-irradiation cyclic radiosensitivity changes in tumors and normal tissues. In Brown DG, Cragle RG, Noonan JR [eds]: *Proceedings of the Symposium on Dose Rate in Mammalian Radiobiology, Oak Ridge, TN, 1968*, pp 20.1–20.23. USAEC Report CONF-680410. Springfield, VA, Technical Information Service 1968, with permission.)

before the next radiation dose, the process of reoxygenation restores the proportion of hypoxic cells to about 15%. If this process is repeated many times, the tumor cell population is depleted, despite the intransigence to killing by x-rays of the cells deficient in oxygen. In other words, if reoxygenation is efficient between dose fractions, the presence of hypoxic cells does not have a significant effect on the outcome of a multifraction regimen.

TIME SEQUENCE OF REOXYGENATION

In the particular tumor system used by van Putten and Kallman, the proportion of hypoxic cells returned to its original pretreatment level by 24 hours after delivery of a fractionated dosage schedule. Kallman and Bleehen reported experiments in which the proportion of hypoxic cells in the same transplantable mouse sarcoma was determined at various times after delivery of a single dose of 10 Gy (1,000 rad). Their results are shown in Figure 6.14; the shape of the curve indicates that in this particular tumor, the process of reoxygenation is very rapid indeed.

Similar results subsequently have been reported by a number of researchers using a variety of tumor systems. The patterns of reoxygenation after irradiation observed in several different animal tumor systems are summarized in Figure 6.15. Four of the five animal tumors show efficient and rapid reoxygenation, with the proportion of hypoxic cells returning to or even falling below the pretreatment level in a day or two. The time sequence, however, is not the same for the five types of tumors. In particular, the mammary carcinoma investigated by Howes shows a minimum proportion of hypoxic cells that

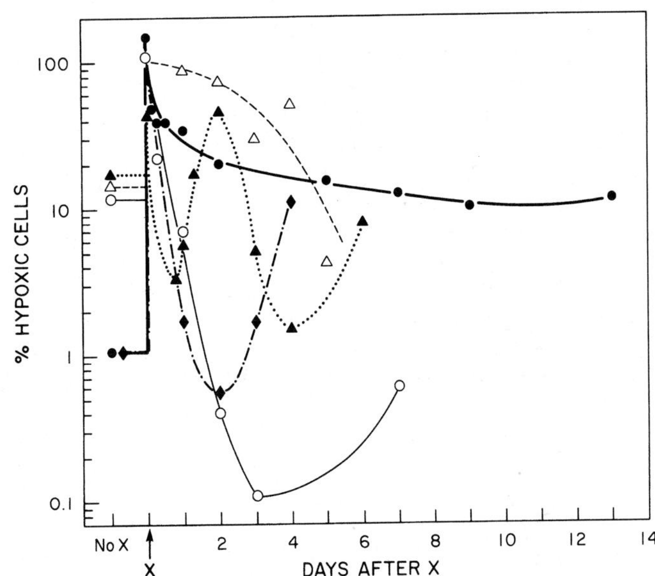

FIGURE 6.15 ● The proportion of hypoxic cells as a function of time after irradiation with a large dose of x-rays for five transplanted tumors in experimental animals. Open circles indicate mouse mammary carcinoma that reoxygenates rapidly and well (data from Howes). Closed triangles indicate rat sarcoma that shows two waves of reoxygenation (data from Thomlinson). Open triangles show mouse osteosarcoma that does not reoxygenate at all for several days and then only slowly (data from van Putten). Closed circles indicate mouse fibrosarcoma that reoxygenates quickly but not as completely as the mammary carcinoma (data from Dorie and Kallman). Closed diamonds indicate mouse fibrosarcoma that reoxygenates quickly and well (data from Kummermehr, Preuss-Bayer, and Trott). The extent and rapidity of reoxygenation are extremely variable and impossible to predict. (Courtesy of Dr. Sara Rockwell.)

is very much lower than that characteristic of the unirradiated tumor. This point is reached 3 days after the delivery of a single large dose of radiation. The only one of the five tumors that does not show any significant rapid reoxygenation is the osteosarcoma studied by van Putten, also illustrated in Figure 6.15.

MECHANISM OF REOXYGENATION

In experimental animals, some tumors take several days to reoxygenate; in others, the process appears to be complete within 1 hour or so. In a few tumors, both fast and slow components to reoxygenation are evident. The differences of time scale reflect the different types of hypoxia that are being reversed, chronic or acute. In the long term, a restructuring or a revascularization of the tumor occurs as the cells killed by the radiation are broken down and removed from the population. As the tumor shrinks in size, surviving cells that previously were beyond the range of oxygen diffusion are closer to a blood supply and so reoxygenate. This slow component of reoxygenation, taking place over a period of days as the tumor shrinks, involves reoxygenation of cells that were *chronically* hypoxic. By contrast, the first component of reoxygenation, which is complete within hours, is caused by the reoxygenation of acutely hypoxic cells. Those cells that were hypoxic at the time of irradiation because they were in regions in which a blood vessel was temporarily closed quickly reoxygenate when that vessel is reopened.

THE IMPORTANCE OF REOXYGENATION IN RADIOTHERAPY

The process of reoxygenation has important implications in practical radiotherapy. If human tumors do in fact reoxygenate as rapidly and efficiently as most of the animal tumors studied, then the use of a multifraction course of radiotherapy, extending over a long period of time, may well be all that is required to deal effectively with any hypoxic cells in human tumors.

The reoxygenation studies with mouse mammary carcinoma, included in Figure 6.15, indicate that by 2 to 3 days after a dose of radiation, the proportion of hypoxic cells is actually lower than in untreated tumors. Consequently, it was predicted that several large doses of x-rays given at 48-hour intervals would virtually eliminate the problem of hypoxic cells in this tumor. Fowler and his colleagues indeed showed that for the eradication of this tumor, the preferred x-ray schedule was five large doses in 9 days. These results suggest that x-irradiation can be an extremely effective form of therapy, but ideally requires a sharply optimal choice of fractionation pattern. Making this choice, however, demands a detailed knowledge of the time course of reoxygenation in the particular tumor to be irradiated. Unfortunately, however, this information is available for only a few animal tumors and is impossible to obtain at present for human tumors. Indeed, in humans it is not known with certainty whether any or all tumors reoxygenate, although the evidence from radiotherapy clinics that many tumors are eradicated with doses on the order of 60 Gy (6,000 rad) given in 30 treatments argues strongly in favor of reoxygenation, because the presence of a very small proportion of hypoxic cells would make "cures" unlikely at these dose levels. It is an attractive hypothesis that some of the human tumors that do not respond to conventional radiotherapy are those that do not reoxygenate quickly and efficiently.

HYPOXIA AND CHEMORESISTANCE

Hypoxia can also decrease the efficacy of some chemotherapeutic agents owing to fluctuating blood flow, drug diffusion distance, and decreased proliferation. In addition, some chemotherapeutic agents that induce DNA damage, such as doxorubicin and bleomycin, are less efficient at killing hypoxic tumor cells in part because of decreased free-radical generation. Experimental animal studies have shown that 5-FU, methotrexate, and cisplatin are less effective at killing hypoxic cells than they are at killing normoxic tumor cells. Furthermore, hypoxic tumor regions are frequently associated with a low pH that can also diminish the activity of some chemotherapy agents. (For more about chemotherapy agents and hypoxia, see Chapter 27.)

HYPOXIA AND TUMOR PROGRESSION

Evidence that low-oxygen conditions play an important role in malignant progression comes from studies of the correlation between tumor oxygenation and treatment outcome in patients, as well as from laboratory studies in cells and animals.

Patient Studies

A clinical study in Germany in the 1990s showed a correlation between local control in advanced carcinoma of the cervix, treated by radiotherapy, and oxygen-probe measurements. Specifically, patients in whom the probe measurements indicated pO_2s greater than 10 mm Hg did better than those with pO_2s less than 10 mm Hg. This suggested that the presence of hypoxic cells limited the success of radiotherapy. Later studies, however, indicated a similar improvement in outcome for patients with better oxygenated tumors if the treatment was by surgery rather than radiotherapy. This suggests that the correct interpretation is that hypoxia is a general indicator of tumor aggression in these patients, rather than the initial view that hypoxia conferred radioresistance on some cells. A Canadian study supported the concept that hypoxia drove malignant progression of cervical carcinomas in node-negative patients, as most of the failures occurred in the poorly oxygenated tumors with distant tumor spread outside the pelvis.

Studies carried out in the United States on patients receiving radiotherapy for soft-tissue sarcoma highlighted the correlation between tumor oxygenation and the frequency of distant metastases. Seventy percent of those patients with pO_2s less than 10 mm Hg developed distant metastases, versus 35% of those with pO_2s greater than 10 mm Hg. This study is particularly compelling because the primary tumor was eradicated in all patients regardless of the level of oxygenation; only the incidence of metastases varied between high and low pO_2 values. These data were subsequently confirmed in a Danish study in which 28 patients with soft-tissue sarcoma exhibited an increased risk of metastatic spread if they possessed low tumor pO_2 values. This argues strongly that the level of tumor oxygenation influences the aggressiveness of the tumor.

Laboratory Evidence

There are at least three lines of evidence from experimental studies that link hypoxia and malignant progression (Fig. 6.16). First, the combination of hypoxia and reoxygenation can induce gene amplification and genomic instability. A variety of mechanisms have been identified to explain how hypoxia induces genomic instability. It is well known that chromosome breaks at fragile sites initiate intrachromosomal amplification. Hypoxia and reoxygenation stimulate the fusion of double minute chromosomes, as well as their targeted reintegration into chromosomal fragile sites, resulting in classic homogeneously staining regions (HSRs). Gene amplification by hypoxia is associated with the expression of a small-molecular-weight DNA endonuclease that possesses an optimum pH of 6.5. This same DNA endonuclease has been found to be expressed in healing wounds that are hypoxic and in tumor samples, but not in corresponding normal tissue. In addition, recent studies have suggested

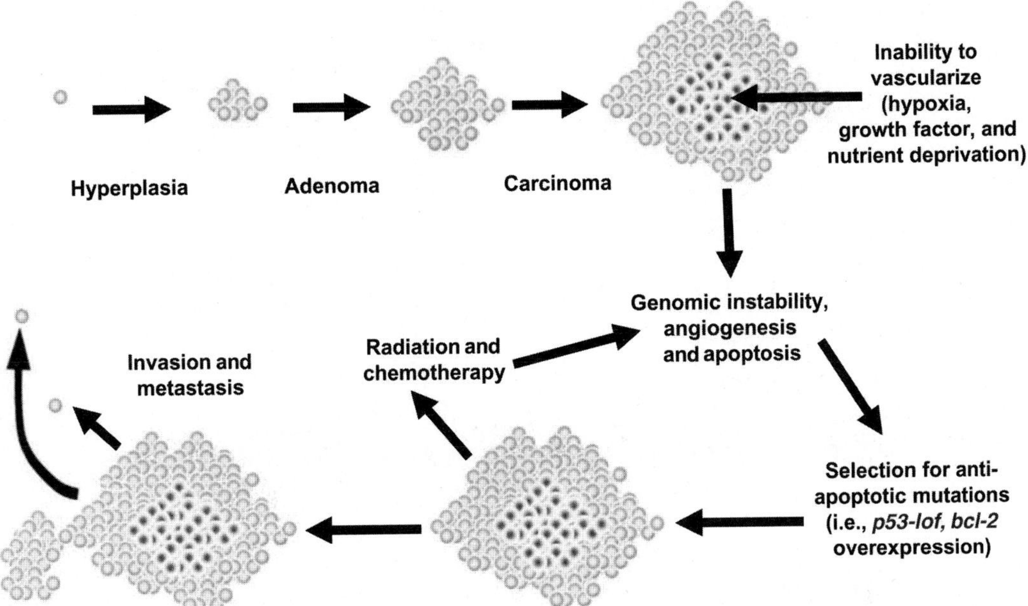

FIGURE 6.16 ● Illustration of how hypoxia may affect malignant progression of solid tumor cells by promoting genomic instability, reduced apoptotic sensitivity, and increased metastatic potential. Tumor development progresses through stages (e.g., hyperplasia, adenoma, carcinoma) that are influenced by genetic alterations and the tumor microenvironment. The interplay of these two forces is thought to drive malignant progression by increasing genomic instability through the inhibition of mismatch repair activity, stimulate angiogenesis through the induction of proangiogenic mitogens, such as vascular endothelial growth factor, and select for tumor cells with mutations that result in diminished apoptotic potential. The consequence of these events is a tumor that has its ability to die by apoptosis reduced in response to radiotherapy and chemotherapy and has an increased metastatic potential. (From Le QT, Denko NC, Giaccia AJ: Hypoxic gene expression and metastasis. *Cancer Metastasis Reviews* 23:293–310, 2004, with permission.)

that hypoxia can inhibit the expression of the mismatch repair genes *Mlh1*, *MsH2*, and *MsH6*, leading to increased dinucleotide repeat instability, and the recombinational repair gene *Rad51*, resulting in decreased levels of homologous recombination. In addition, cells with a defective apoptotic pathway, resulting from either inactivation of the p53 tumor-suppressor gene or overexpression of antiapoptotic genes such as *bcl-2*, have a survival advantage in a low-oxygen environment that increases their probability of developing genomic instability upon exposure to hypoxia and reoxygenation.

A second insight into how low-oxygen conditions may affect the aggressiveness of tumors is through hypoxia-induced proteome changes. Approximately 1% of the genome is transcriptionally regulated by hypoxic stress. A substantial portion of hypoxia-induced genes are regulated by the hypoxia-inducible transcription factor (HIF-1), which is composed of two subunits: an oxygen-sensitive HIF-1α subunit and a constitutively expressed HIF-1β subunit (also known as ARNT, the aryl hydrocarbon receptor nuclear translocator). HIF-1α protein levels in a cell are tightly regulated through protein modifications that allow it to rapidly change in response to hypoxia. Under normoxic conditions, HIF-1α is hydroxylated on two praline residues through the activity of oxygen-requiring prolyl hydroxylases. The hydroxylation of these two residues is essential for the binding of the von Hippel-Lindau (VHL) protein, an E3 ubiquitin ligase that targets HIF-1α for ubquitin-mediated degradation (Fig. 6.17). As oxygen levels decrease, prolyl hydroxylase activity decreases and HIF-1α becomes stabilized.

Although a great deal of research has focused on the HIF-1 pathway, there are several other transcriptional factors that are also activated by hypoxia. These include the cyclic-AMP response element binding (CREB) protein, the activator protein-1 (AP-1), the nuclear factor-$\kappa\beta$ (NF-$\kappa\beta$), and the early growth response-1 protein (Egr-1). Another

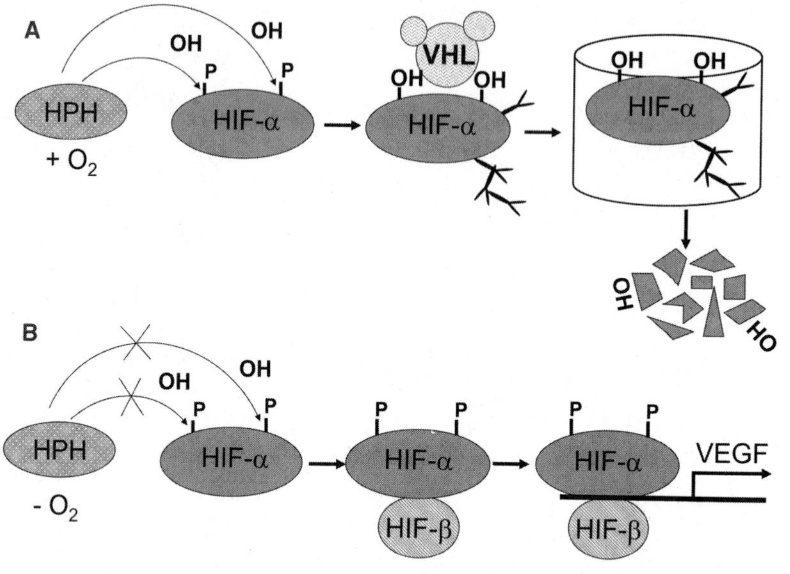

FIGURE 6.17 ● Critical steps in the regulation of the hypoxia-inducible transcription factor HIF-1α. **A:** Under normoxic conditions, a group of enzymes called prolyl hydroxylases (HPHs) add hydroxyl groups (OH) to two proline residues of HIF-1α. The hydroxylation of HIF-1α by HPH allows the VHL tumor-suppressor gene to bind and promotes the addition of ubiquitin groups. The addition of ubiquitin groups targets HIF-1α for degradation in the proteasome. **B:** Under hypoxic conditions, the HPHs cannot hydroxylate HIF-1α on proline residues owing to their requirement for molecular oxygen, and HIF-1α becomes stabilized. It then binds with the HIF-1β subunit in the nucleus and promotes transcription of at least 50 target genes that regulate angiogenesis, erythropoiesis, tissue remodeling, and glycolysis. Most of the studies to date have shown that HIF is essential for tumor growth.

important non-HIF-mediated hypoxia-signaling pathway involves the unfolded protein response and its transcriptional factors (ATF6 and XBP-1), which are critical for the induction of glucose-related proteins during chronic hypoxia exposure.

The ultimate by-products of these different signaling pathways are changes in expression of the genes and proteins that are important for cellular adaptation to a hypoxic environment. Studies indicate that there is a core set of genes involved in anaerobic metabolism, angiogenesis, tissue remodeling, proliferation, and transcriptional regulation that are induced consistently by hypoxia. Interestingly, hypoxia-induced genes can exhibit cell-type-specific induction, underscoring the importance of studying changes in gene expression in a cell-type-dependent context.

The third consequence of hypoxia is increased metastatic potential. The metastatic potential of tumor cells is influenced by both intrinsic and extrinsic factors. Intrinsic factors include the accumulation of oncogenic alterations and loss of tumor-suppressor gene function. These genetic alterations enable the tumor cell to reduce its requirements for growth factors and extracellular matrix components and increase the production of angiogenic growth factors. In addition, metastatic tumor cells develop gain-of-function activities that allow them to escape into the circulation and take up residence in a foreign location. Although a variety of genetic and epigenetic mechanisms have been proposed to explain this process, evidence is accumulating that metastasis is a rare event compared to the number of tumor cells escaping the tumor's confines at any one time. While hypoxia and reoxygenation can increase the metastatic potential of tumor cells in well-controlled experimental model systems, it is also clear that microenvironmental changes do not in themselves switch on the metastatic potential, but only enhance it. In part, the enhancement of the metastatic potential of tumor cells is due to their ability to survive a low oxygen environment and loss of attachment as well as increase their angiogenic potential.

Summary of Pertinent Conclusions

- The presence or absence of molecular oxygen dramatically influences the biologic effect of x-rays.
- The oxygen enhancement ratio (OER) is the ratio of doses under hypoxic to aerated conditions that produce the same biologic effect.
- The OER for x-rays is about 3 at high doses and is possibly lower (about 2) at doses below about 2 Gy (200 rad).
- The OER decreases as linear energy transfer increases. The OER approaches unity (i.e., no oxygen effect) for α-particles. For neutrons, the OER has an intermediate value of about 1.6.
- To produce its effect, molecular oxygen must be present during the radiation exposure or at least during the lifetime of the free radicals generated by the radiation.
- Oxygen "fixes" (i.e., makes permanent) the damage produced by free radicals. In the absence of oxygen, damage produced by the indirect action may be repaired.
- Only a small quantity of oxygen is required for radiosensitization; 0.5% oxygen (pO_2 of about 3 mm Hg) results in a sensitivity halfway between hypoxia and full oxygenation.
- There are two forms of hypoxia that are the consequence of different mechanisms: chronic hypoxia and acute hypoxia.
- Chronic hypoxia results from the limited diffusion range of oxygen through respiring tissue.
- Acute hypoxia is a result of the temporary closing of tumor blood vessels and is therefore transient.
- In either case, there may be cells present during irradiation that are at a sufficiently low oxygen tension to be intransigent to killing by x-rays but high enough to be viable.
- Most transplantable tumors in animals have been shown to contain hypoxic cells that limit curability by single doses of x-rays. Hypoxic fractions vary from 0 to 50%, with a tendency to average about 15%.
- There is strong evidence that human tumors contain hypoxic cells. This evidence includes histologic appearance, oxygen-probe measurements, the binding of nitroimidazoles, PET and SPECT studies, and pretreatment hemoglobin levels.
- Oxygen probes with fast response times, implanted in a tumor and moving quickly under computer control, may be used to obtain the oxygen profile of a tumor.
- Reoxygenation is the process by which cells that are hypoxic at the time of irradiation become oxygenated afterward.
- The extent of reoxygenation and the rapidity with which it occurs vary widely for different experimental animal tumors.
- If reoxygenation is rapid and complete, hypoxic cells have little influence on the outcome of a fractionated radiation schedule.
- The "slow" component is caused by the reoxygenation of *chronically* hypoxic cells as the tumor shrinks. The "fast" component of reoxygenation is caused by the reoxygenation of acutely hypoxic cells as tumor blood vessels open and close.
- Reoxygenation cannot be measured in human tumors, but presumably it occurs, at least in those tumors controlled by conventional fractionated radiotherapy.
- There is clinical evidence that hypoxia may play an important role in malignant progression:
  1. Clinical studies show that local control in advanced carcinoma of the cervix, treated by radiotherapy or surgery, was worse in patients with hypoxic tumors compared to patients with better oxygenated tumors.
  2. Clinical studies of patients receiving radiotherapy for soft-tissue sarcoma showed an association between low tumor pO_2 and increased risk of distant metastases.
- There is also laboratory evidence of a correlation between hypoxia and malignant progression:
  1. Hypoxia and reoxygenation induce gene amplification and genomic instability. Cells that possess diminished apoptotic programs have a survival advantage in adverse conditions and increased probability of becoming genomically unstable.
  2. Hypoxia induces changes in the proteome. The hypoxia-induced changes in the expression of genes and proteins are important for cellular adaptation to an anaerobic environment.
  3. Hypoxia increases the metastatic potential of solid tumor cells.

BIBLIOGRAPHY

Barendsen GW, Koot CJ, van Kersen GR, Bewley DK, Field SB, Parnell CJ: The effect of oxygen on impairment of the proliferative capacity of human cells in culture by ionizing radiations of different LET. *Int J Radiat Biol Relat Stud Phys Chem Med* 10:317–327, 1966

Brizel DM, Scully SP, Harrelson JM, Layfield LJ, Bean JM, Prosnitz LR, Dewhirst MW: Tumor oxygenation predicts for the likelihood of distant metastases in human soft tissue sarcoma. *Cancer Res* 56:941–943, 1996

Broerse JJ, Barendsen GW, van Kersen GR: Survival of cultured human cells after irradiation with fast neutrons of different energies in hypoxic and oxygenated conditions. *Int J Radiat Biol Relat Stud Phys Chem Med* 13:559–572, 1968

Brown JM: Evidence for acutely hypoxic cells in mouse tumours, and a possible mechanism of reoxygenation. *Br J Radiol* 52:650–656, 1979

Brown JM: Tumor hypoxia, drug resistance, and metastases. *JNCI* 82:338–339 1990

Brown JM, Graccia AJ: The unique physiology of solid tumors: Opportunities (and problems) for cancer therapy. *Cancer Res* 58:1408–1416, 1998

Chaplin DJ, Durand RE, Olive PL: Acute hypoxia in tumors: Implications for modifiers of radiation effects. *Int J Radiat Oncol Biol Phys* 12:1279–1282, 1986

Chaplin DJ, Olive PL, Durand RE: Intermittent blood flow in a murine tumor: Radiobiological effects. *Cancer Res* 47:597–601, 1987

Crabtree HG, Cramer W: The action of radium on cancer cells: I. Effects of hydrocyanic acid, iodoacetic acid, and sodium fluoride on the metabolism and transplantability of cancer cells. *Sci Rep Imp Cancer Res Fund* 11:75, 1934

Crabtree HG, Cramer W: Action of radium on cancer cells: Some factors affecting susceptibility of cancer cells to radium. *Proc R Soc Lond B Biol Sci* 113:238, 1933

Denekamp J: Cytoxicity and radiosensitization in mouse and man. *Br J Radiol* 51:636–637, 1978

Denekamp J: Discussion in session on effects of radiation on mammalian cell populations. In *Time and Dose Relationships in Radiation Biology as Applied to Radiotherapy*, NCI-AEC Carmel Conference, BNL 50203 (C-57), pp 144–145, 1970

Denekamp J, Fowler JF, Dische S: The proportion of hypoxic cells in a human tumor. *Int J Radiat Oncol Biol Phys* 2:1227–1228, 1977

Deschner EE, Gray LH: Influence of oxygen tension on x-ray-induced chromosomal damage in Ehrlich ascites tumor cells irradiated *in vitro* and *in vivo*. *Radiat Res* 11:115–146, 1959

Elkind MM, Swain RW, Alescio T, Sutton H, Moses WB: Oxygen, nitrogen, recovery and radiation therapy. In *Cellular Radiation Biology*, pp 442–461. Baltimore, Williams & Wilkins, 1965

Evans SM, Koch CJ: Prognostic significance of tumor oxygenation in humans. *Cancer Letters* 195:1–16, 2003

Fowler JF: Review of the proceedings of session V: Reoxygenation of tumour tissues. In *Time and Dose Relationships in Radiation Biology as Applied to Radiotherapy*, NCI-AEC Carmel Conference, BNL 50203 (C-57), pp 144–145, 1970

Giaccia AJ, Brown JM, Wouters B, Denko N, Kouvenis I: Cancer therapy and tumor physiology. *Science* 279:12–13, 1998

Graeber TG, Osmanian C, Jacks T, et al.: Hypoxia-mediated selection of cells with diminished apoptotic potential in solid tumors. *Nature* 379:88–91, 1996

Grau C and Overgaard J: Effect of etoposide, Carmustine, vincristine, 5-fluorouracil, or metyhotrexate on radiobiologically oxic and hypoxic cells in a C3H mouse mammary carcinoma *in situ*. *Cancer Chemother Pharmacol* 30:277–280, 1992

Gray LH, Conger AD, Ebert M, Hornsey S, Scott OC: The concentration of oxygen dissolved in tissues at the time of irradiation as a factor in radiotherapy. *Br J Radiol* 26:628–648, 1953

Groebe K, Vaupel P: Evaluation of oxygen diffusion distances in human breast cancer xenografts using tumor-specific *in vivo* data: Role of various mechanisms in the development of tumor hypoxia. *Int J Radiat Oncol Biol Phys* 15:691–697, 1988

Hill RR, Bush RS, Yeung P: The effect of anemia on the fraction of hypoxic cells in experimental tumor. *Br J Radiol* 44:299–304, 1971

Hockel M, Schlenger K, Aral B, Mitze M, Schaffer U, Vaupel P: Association between tumor hypoxia and malignant progression in advanced cancer of the uterine cervix. *Cancer Res* 56:4509–4515, 1996

Holthusen H: Beitrage zur Biologie der Strahlenwirkung. *Pflugers Arch* 187:1–24, 1921

Howard-Flanders P, Alper T: The sensitivity of microorganisms to irradiation under controlled gas conditions. *Radiat Res* 7:518–540, 1957

Howard-Flanders P, Moore D: The time interval after pulsed irradiation within which injury in bacteria can be modified by dissolved oxygen: I. A search for an effect of oxygen 0.02 second after pulsed irradiation. *Radiat Res* 9:422–437, 1958

Howes AK: An estimation of changes in the proportion and absolute numbers of hypoxic cells after irradiation of transplanted C3H mouse mammary tumors. *Br J Radiol* 42:441–447, 1969

Kallman RF: The phenomenon of reoxygenation and its implication for fractionated radiotherapy. *Radiology* 105:135–142, 1972

Kallman RF, Bleehen NM: Post-irradiation cyclic radiosensitivity changes in tumors and normal tissues. In Brown DG, Cragle RG, Noonan JR (eds): *Proceedings of the Symposium on Dose Rate in Mammalian Radiobiology, Oak Ridge, TN, 1968*, pp 20.1–20.23. USAEC Report CONF-680410. Springfield, VA, Technical Information Service 1968

Kallman RF, Jardine LJ, Johnson CW: Effects of different schedules of dose fractionation on the oxygenation status of a transplantable mouse sarcoma. *J Natl Cancer Inst* 44:369–377, 1970

Kim, CY, Tsai MH, Osmanian C, et al.: Selection of human cervical epithelial cells that possess reduced apoptotic potential to low oxygen conditions. *Cancer Res* 57:4200–4204, 1997

Le QT, Denko NC, Giaccia AJ: Hypoxic gene expression and metastasis. *Cancer Metastasis Rev* 23:293–310, 2004

Le QT, Denko NC, Giaccia AJ: Hypoxic Gene Expression and Metastasis. *Cancer Metastasis Reviews* 23:293–310, 2004

Leo C, Giaccia AJ, Denko NC: The hypoxic tumor microenvironment and gene expression. *Sem Radiat Oncol* 3:207–214, 2004

Mazure NM, Chen EY, Yeh P, Laderoute KR, Giaccia AJ: Oncogenic transformation and hypoxia synergistically act to modulate vascular endothelial growth factor expression. *Cancer Res* 56:3436–3440, 1996

Michael BD, Adams CE, Hewitt HB, Jones WBG, Watts ME: A posteffect of oxygen in irradiated bacteria: A submillisecond fast mixing study. *Radiat Res* 54:239–251, 1973

Milosevic M, Fyles A, Hedley D, Hill R: The human tumor microenvironment: Invasive (needle) measurement of oxygen and interstitial fluid pressure. *Semin Radiat Oncol* 14:249–258, 2004

Mottram JC: Factor of importance in radiosensitivity of tumours. *Br J Radiol* 9:606–614, 1936

Mottram JC: On the action of beta and gamma rays of radium on the cell in different states of nuclear division. *Rep Cancer Labs* (Middlesex Hospital, London) 30:98, 1913

Moulder JE, Rockwell S: Hypoxic fractions of solid tumors: Experimental techniques, methods of analysis and a survey of existing data. *Int J Radiat Oncol Biol Phys* 10:695–712, 1984

Palcic B, Skarsgard LD: Reduced oxygen enhancement ratio at low doses of ionizing radiation. *Radiat Res* 100:328–339, 1984

Petry E: Zur Kenntnis der Bedingungen der biologischen Wirkung der Rontgenstrahlen. *Biochem Zeitschr* 135:353, 1923

Powers WE, Tolmach LJ: A multicomponent x-ray survival curve for mouse lymphosarcoma cells irradiated *in vivo*. *Nature* 197:710–711, 1963

Read J: The effect of ionizing radiations on the broad bean root: I. The dependence of the alpha ray sensitivity on dissolved oxygen. *Br J Radiol* 25:651–661, 1952

Read J: The effect of ionizing radiations on the broad bean root: X. The dependence of the x-ray sensitivity of dissolved oxygen. *Br J Radiol* 25:89–99, 1952

Read J: Mode of action of x-ray doses given with different oxygen concentrations. *Br J Radiol* 25:336–338, 1952

Reinhold HS: The post-irradiation behaviour of transplantable solid tumors in relation to the regional oxygenation. In Turano L, Ratti A, Biagini C (eds): *Progress in Radiology*, vol 2, pp 1482–1486. Amsterdam, Excerpta Medica, 1967

Rockwell S, Moulder JE: Biological factors of importance in split-course radiotherapy. In Paliwal BR, Herbert DE, Orton CG (eds): *Optimization of Cancer Radiotherapy*, pp 171–182. New York, American Institute of Physics, 1985

Secomb TW, Hsu R, Ong ET, Gross JF, Dewhirst MW: Analysis of the effects of oxygen supply and demand on hypoxic fraction in tumors. *Acta Oncol* 34:313–316, 1995

Thomlinson RH: Changes of oxygenation in tumors in relation to irradiation. *Front Radiat Ther Oncol 3*:109–121, 1968

Thomlinson RH: Reoxygenation as a function of tumor size and histopathological type. In *Proceedings of the Carmel Conference on Time and Dose Relationships in Radiation Biology as Applied to Radiotherapy*, pp 242–254. Brookhaven National Laboratory Report 50203 (C-57). Upton, NY, BNL, 1970

Thomlinson RH, Gray LH: The histological structure of some human lung cancers and the possible implications for radiotherapy. *Br J Cancer* 9:539–549, 1955

van Putten LM: Oxygenation and cell kinetics after irradiation in a transplantable osteosarcoma. In *Effects on Cellular Proliferation and Differentiation*, pp 493–505. Vienna, IAEA, 1968

van Putten LM: Tumour reoxygenation during fractionated radiotherapy: Studies with a transplantable osteosarcoma. *Eur J Cancer* 4:173–182, 1968

van Putten LM, Kallman RF: Oxygenation status of a transplantable tumor during fractionated radiotherapy. *J Natl Cancer Inst* 40:441–451, 1968

Vaupel P, Kallinowski F, Okunieff P: Blood flow, oxygen and nutrient supply, and metabolic microenvironment of human tumors: A review. *Cancer Res* 49:6449–6465, 1989

Vaupel P, Mayer A, Hockel M: Tumor hypoxia and malignant progression. *Methods Enzymol* 381:335–354, 2004

Wright EA, Howard-Flanders P: The influence of oxygen on the radiosensitivity of mammalian tissues. *Acta Radiol* 48:26–32, 1957

CHAPTER 7

Linear Energy Transfer and Relative Biologic Effectiveness

THE DEPOSITION OF RADIANT ENERGY

If radiation is absorbed in biologic material, ionizations and excitations occur that are not distributed at random but tend to be localized along the tracks of individual charged particles in a pattern that depends on the type of radiation involved. For example, x-ray photons give rise to fast electrons, particles carrying unit electrical charge and having very small mass; neutrons, on the other hand, give rise to recoil protons, particles again carrying unit electrical charge but having mass nearly 2,000 times greater than that of the electron. α-Particles carry two electrical charges on a particle four times as heavy as a proton. The charge-to-mass ratio for α-particles therefore differs from that for electrons by a factor of about 8,000.

As a result, the spatial distribution of the ionizing events produced by different particles varies enormously. This is illustrated in Figure 7.1. The background is an electron micrograph of a human liver cell. The white dots generated by a computer simulate ionizing events. The lowest track represents a low-energy electron, such as might be set in motion by diagnostic x-rays. The primary events are well separated in space, and for this reason x-rays are said to be *sparsely ionizing*. The second track from the bottom represents an electron set in motion by cobalt-60 γ-rays, which is even more sparsely ionizing. For a given particle type, the density of ionization decreases as the energy goes up. The third track from the bottom represents a proton that might be set in motion by a fission spectrum neutron from a nuclear reactor; a dense column of ionization is produced, so the radiation is referred to as *densely ionizing*. The uppermost track refers to a 10-MeV proton, such as may be set in motion by the high-energy neutrons used for radiotherapy. The track is intermediate in ionization density.

LINEAR ENERGY TRANSFER (LET)

Linear energy transfer (LET) is the energy transferred per unit length of the track. The special unit usually used for this quantity is kiloelectron volt per micrometer (keV/μm) of unit density material. In 1962, the International Commission on Radiological Units defined this quantity as follows:

> The linear energy transfer (L) of charged particles in medium is the quotient of dE/dl, where dE is the average energy locally imparted to the medium by a charged particle of specified energy in traversing a distance of dl.

That is,

$$L = dE/dl$$

LET is an average quantity because at the microscopic level, the energy per unit length of track

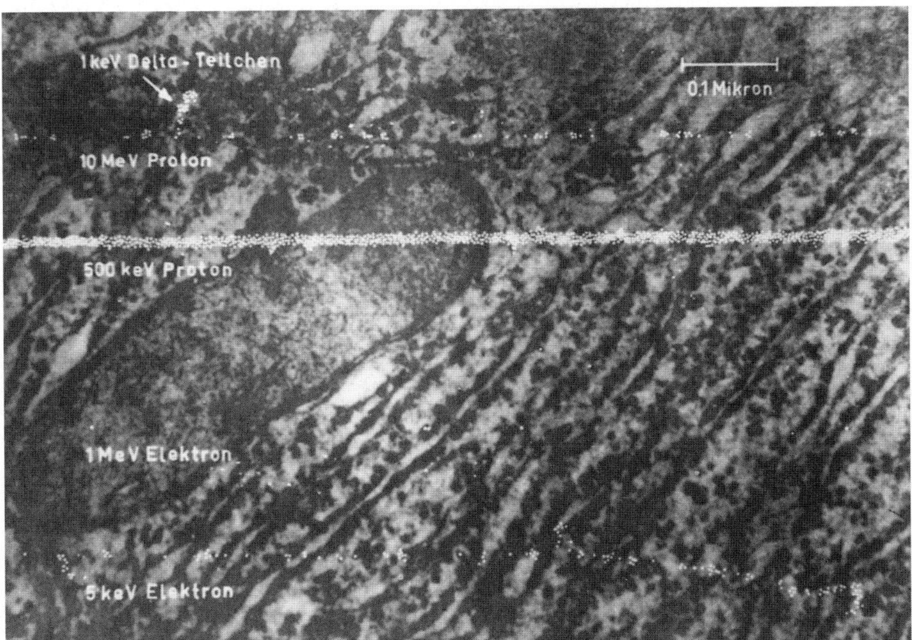

FIGURE 7.1 ● Variation of ionization density associated with different types of radiation. The background is an electron micrograph of a human cell. The white dots are a computer simulation representing ionizations. **Top to bottom:** A 10-MeV proton, typical of the recoil protons produced by high-energy neutrons used for radiotherapy. The track is intermediate in ionization density. Also shown is a secondary 1-keV δ-ray, an electron set in motion by the proton. A 500-keV proton, produced by lower-energy neutrons (e.g., from fission spectrum) or by higher-energy neutrons after multiple collisions. The ionizations form a dense column along the track of the particle. A 1-MeV electron, produced, for example, by cobalt-60 γ-rays. This particle is very sparsely ionizing. A 5-keV electron, typical of secondary electrons produced by x-rays of diagnostic quality. This particle is also sparsely ionizing but a little denser than the higher-energy electron. (Courtesy of Dr. Albrecht Kellerer.)

varies over such a wide range. Indeed, the range is so large that some believe that the concept of LET has little meaning. This can be illustrated by the story of a Martian visitor to Earth who arrives knowing that Earth is inhabited by living creatures with an average mass of 1 g. Not only is this information of very little use, but it also may be positively misleading, particularly if the first living creature that the Martian encounters is an elephant. An average quantity has little meaning if individual variation is great.

The situation for LET is further complicated by the fact that it is possible to calculate an average in many different ways. The most commonly used method is to calculate the **track average**, which is obtained by dividing the track into equal lengths, calculating the energy deposited in each length, and finding the mean. The **energy average** is obtained by dividing the track into equal energy increments and averaging the lengths of track over which these energy increments are deposited. These methods are illustrated in Figure 7.2.

In the case of either x-rays or monoenergetic charged particles, the two methods of averaging yield similar results. In the case of 14-MeV neutrons, by contrast, the track average LET is about 12 keV/μm and the energy average LET is about 100 keV/μm. The biologic properties of neutrons tend to correlate best with the energy average.

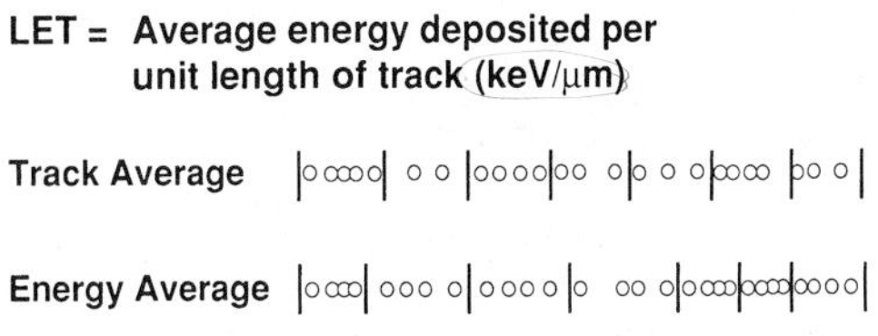

LET = Average energy deposited per unit length of track (keV/μm)

Track Average

Energy Average

FIGURE 7.2 ● Linear energy transfer (LET) is the average energy deposited per unit length of track. The track average is calculated by dividing the track into equal lengths and averaging the energy deposited in each length. The energy average is calculated by dividing the track into equal energy intervals and averaging the lengths of the track that contain this amount of energy. The method of averaging makes little difference for x-rays or for monoenergetic charged particles, but the track average and energy average are different for neutrons.

TABLE 7.1

Typical Linear Energy Transfer Values

Radiation		Linear Energy Transfer, keV/μm	
Cobalt-60 γ-rays		0.2	
250-kV x-rays		2.0	
10-MeV protons		4.7	
150-MeV proton		0.5	
	Track Avg.		Energy Avg.
14-MeV neutrons	12		100
2.5-MeV α-particles		166	
2-GeV Fe ions (space radiation)		1,000	

As a result of these considerations, LET is a quantity condemned by the purists as worse than useless, because it can in some circumstances be very misleading. It is, however, useful as a simple and naive way to indicate the quality of different types of radiation. Typical LET values for various radiations are listed in Table 7.1. Included are x- and γ-rays used for radiotherapy, protons, neutrons, and naturally occurring α-particles, as well as high-energy heavy ions encountered by astronauts in space. Note that for a given type of charged particle, the higher the energy, the lower the LET and therefore the lower its biologic effectiveness. At first sight, this may be counterintuitive. For example, γ-rays and x-rays both give rise to fast secondary electrons; therefore 1.1-MV cobalt-60 γ-rays have lower LETs than 250 kV x-rays and are less effective biologically by about 10%. By the same token, 150-MeV protons have lower LETs than 10-MeV protons and therefore are slightly less effective biologically.

RELATIVE BIOLOGIC EFFECTIVENESS (RBE)

The amount or quantity of radiation is expressed in terms of the **absorbed dose**, a physical quantity with the unit of gray or rad. Absorbed dose is a measure of the energy absorbed per unit mass of tissue. Equal doses of different types of radiation do not, however, produce equal biologic effects. For example, 1 Gy of neutrons produces a greater biologic effect than 1 Gy of x-rays. The key to the difference lies in the pattern of energy deposition at the microscopic level.

In comparing different radiations, it is customary to use x-rays as the standard. The National Bureau of Standards in 1954 defined **relative biologic effectiveness (RBE)** as follows:

> The RBE of some test radiation (r) compared with x-rays is defined by the ratio D_{250}/D_r, where D_{250} and D_r are, respectively, the doses of x-rays and the test radiation required for equal biological effect.

To measure the RBE of some test radiation, one first chooses a biologic system in which the effect of radiations may be scored quantitatively. To illustrate the process involved, we discuss a specific example. Suppose we are measuring the RBE of fast neutrons compared with 250-kV x-rays, using the lethality of plant seedlings as a test system. Groups of plants are exposed to graded doses of x-rays; parallel groups are exposed to a range of neutron doses. At the end of the period of observation, it is possible to calculate the doses of x-rays and then of neutrons that result in the death of half of the plants in a group. This quantity is known as the LD_{50}, the mean lethal dose. Suppose that for x-rays the LD_{50} turns out to be 6 Gy (600 rad) and that for neutrons the corresponding quantity is 4 Gy (400 rad). The RBE of neutrons compared with x-rays is then simply the ratio 6:4, or 1.5.

The study of RBE is relatively straightforward so long as a test system with a single, unequivocal end point is used. It becomes more complicated if, instead, a test system such as the response of mammalian cells in culture is chosen. Figure 7.3**A** shows survival curves obtained if mammalian cells in cultures are exposed to a range of doses of, on the one hand, fast neutrons and, on the other hand, 250-kV x-rays. The RBE may now be calculated from these survival curves as the ratio of doses that produce the same biologic effect. If the end point chosen for comparison is the dose required to

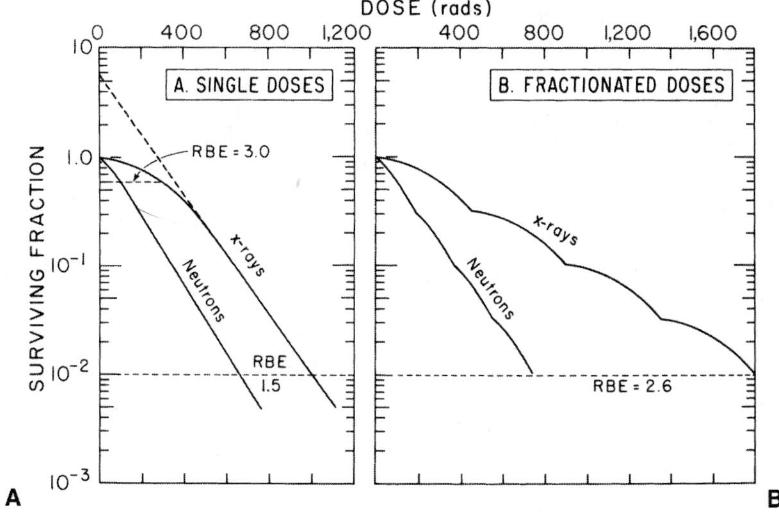

FIGURE 7.3 ● Typical survival curves for mammalian cells exposed to x-rays and fast neutrons. **A:** Single doses. The survival curve for x-rays has a large initial shoulder; for fast neutrons, the initial shoulder is smaller and the final slope steeper. Because the survival curves have different shapes, the relative biologic effectiveness (RBE) does not have a unique value but varies with dose, getting larger as the size of the dose is reduced. **B:** Fractionated doses. The effect of giving doses of x-rays or fast neutrons in four equal fractions to produce the same level of survival as in **A**. The shoulder of the survival curves is reexpressed after each dose fraction; the fact that the shoulder is larger for x-rays than for neutrons results in an enlarged RBE for fractionated treatments.

produce a surviving fraction of 0.01, then the dose of neutrons necessary is 6.6 Gy (660 rad); the corresponding dose of x-rays is 10 Gy (1,000 rad). The RBE, then, is the quotient of 10/6.6, or about 1.5. If the comparison is made at a surviving fraction of 0.6, however, the neutron dose required is only 1 Gy (100 rad), and the corresponding x-ray dose is 3 Gy (300 rad). The resultant RBE is 3:1, or 3.0. Because the x-ray and neutron survival curves have different shapes, the x-ray survival curve having an initial shoulder and the neutron curve being an exponential function of dose, the resultant RBE depends on the level of biologic damage (and therefore the dose) chosen. The RBE generally increases as the dose is decreased, reaching a limiting value that is the ratio of the initial slopes of the x-ray and neutron survival curves.

RBE AND FRACTIONATED DOSES

Because the RBE of more densely ionizing radiations, such as neutrons, varies with the dose per fraction, the RBE for a fractionated regimen with neutrons is greater than for a single exposure, because a fractionated schedule consists of a number of small doses and the RBE is large for small doses.

Figure 7.3**B** illustrates a hypothetical treatment with neutrons consisting of four fractions. For a surviving fraction of 0.01, the RBE for neutrons relative to x-rays is about 2.6. The RBE for the same radiations in Figure 7.3**A** at the same level of survival was about 1.5 because only single exposures were involved. This is a direct consequence of the larger shoulder that is characteristic of the x-ray curve, which must be repeated for each fraction. The width of the shoulder represents a part of the dose that is "wasted"; the larger the number of fractions, the greater the extent of the wastage. By contrast, the neutron survival curve has little or no shoulder, so there is correspondingly less wastage of dose from fractionation. The net result is that neutrons become progressively more efficient than x-rays as the dose per fraction is reduced and the number of fractions is increased. The same is true, of course, for exposure to continuous low-dose-rate irradiation. The neutron RBE is larger at a low dose rate than for an acute exposure, because the effectiveness of neutrons decreases with dose rate to a much smaller extent than is the case for x- or γ-rays. Indeed, for low-energy neutrons there is no loss of effectiveness.

RBE FOR DIFFERENT CELLS AND TISSUES

Even for a given total dose or dose per fraction, the RBE varies greatly according to the tissue or end

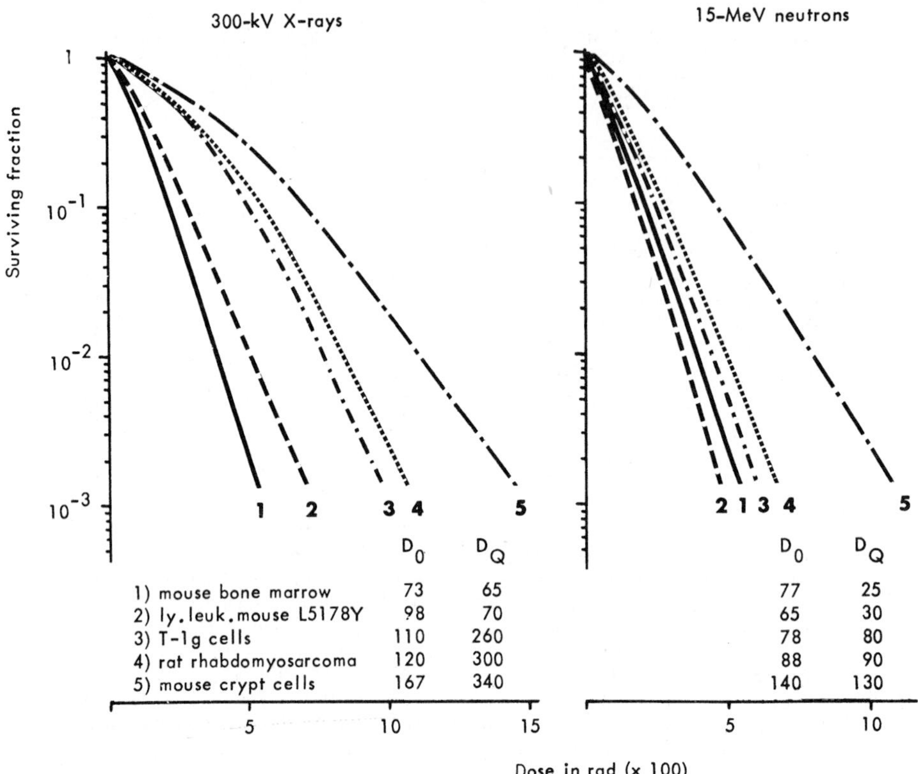

FIGURE 7.4 ● Survival curves for various types of clonogenic mammalian cells irradiated with 300-kV x-rays or 15-MeV $d^+ \rightarrow$ T neutrons: curve 1, mouse hematopoietic stem cells; curve 2, mouse lymphocytic leukemia cells L5178Y; curve 3, T1 cultured cells of human kidney origin; curve 4, rat rhabdomyosarcoma cells; curve 5, mouse intestinal crypt stem cells. Note that the variation in radiosensitivity among different cell lines is markedly less for neutrons than for x-rays. (From Broerse JJ, Barendsen GW: Relative biological effectiveness of fast neutrons for effects on normal tissues. *Curr Top Radiat Res Q* 8:305–350, 1973, with permission.)

point studied. Broerse and Barendsen and their colleagues in the Netherlands have obtained survival curves for a number of different cell lines exposed to either neutrons or x-rays. A summary of their data is shown in Figure 7.4, which illustrates the differences in intrinsic radiosensitivity among the various types of cells. In this figure, survival curves are presented for mouse bone-marrow stem cells, mouse lymphocytic leukemia cells, cultured cells of human kidney origin, rat rhabdomyosarcoma cells, and mouse intestinal crypt cells. These curves demonstrate clearly that different cells exhibit a considerable spectrum of radiosensitivities for x-rays. Of the cells tested, bone-marrow stem cells are the most sensitive; intestinal crypt cells are the most resistant.

There is still a range of radiosensitivities for irradiation with neutrons, but the differences between the various cell types is now much smaller. The principal difference is that the x-ray survival curves have large and variable initial shoulders; the shoulder region for neutrons is smaller and less variable. As a consequence, the RBE is different for each cell line. In general, cells characterized by an x-ray survival curve with a large shoulder, indicating that they can accumulate and repair a large amount of sublethal radiation damage, show larger RBEs for neutrons. Conversely, cells for which the x-ray survival curve has *little if any shoulder* exhibit smaller neutron RBE values.

In Figure 7.4, the crypt cells of the mouse jejunum have the largest shoulder to their x-ray survival curve; they also result in the highest neutron RBE. At the other end of the scale, colony-forming units in the bone marrow are characterized by a survival curve that is close to an exponential function of dose, with little if any shoulder. The RBE for neutrons is likewise smallest for this biologic system.

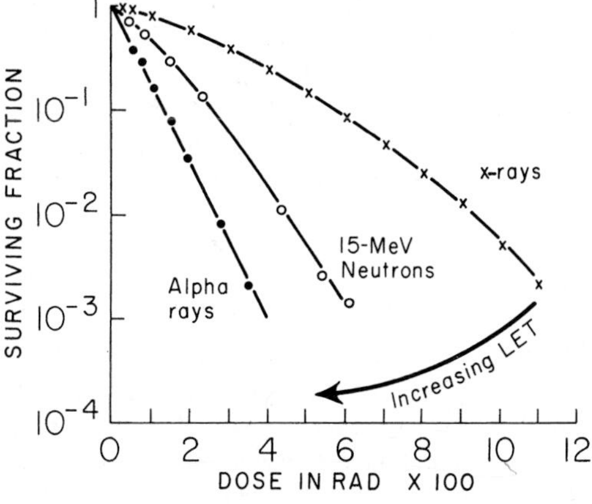

FIGURE 7.5 • Survival curves for cultured cells of human origin exposed to 250-kVp x-rays, 15-MeV neutrons, and 4-MeV α-particles. As the linear energy transfer of the radiation increases, the slope of the survival curves gets steeper and the size of the initial shoulder gets smaller. (Adapted from Broerse JJ, Barendsen GW, van Kersen GR: Survival of cultured human cells after irradiation with fast neutrons of different energies in hypoxic and oxygenated conditions. *Int J Radiat Biol Relat Stud Phys Chem Med* 13:559–572, 1968; and Barendsen GW: Responses of cultured cells, tumors, and normal tissues to radiation of different linear energy transfer. *Curr Top Radiat Res Q* 4:293–356, 1968, with permission.)

RBE AS A FUNCTION OF LET

Figure 7.5 illustrates the survival curves obtained for 250-kVp x-rays, 15-MeV neutrons, and 4-MeV α-particles. As the LET increases from about 2 keV/μm for x-rays up to 150 keV/μm for α-particles, the survival curve changes in two important respects. First, the survival curve becomes steeper. Second, the shoulder of the curve becomes progressively smaller as the LET increases. A more common way to represent these data is to plot the RBE as a function of LET (Fig. 7.6). As the LET increases, the RBE increases slowly at first and then more rapidly as the LET increases beyond 10 keV/μm. Between 10 and 100 keV/μm, the RBE increases rapidly with increasing LET and in fact reaches a maximum at about 100 keV/μm. Beyond this value for the LET, the RBE again falls to lower

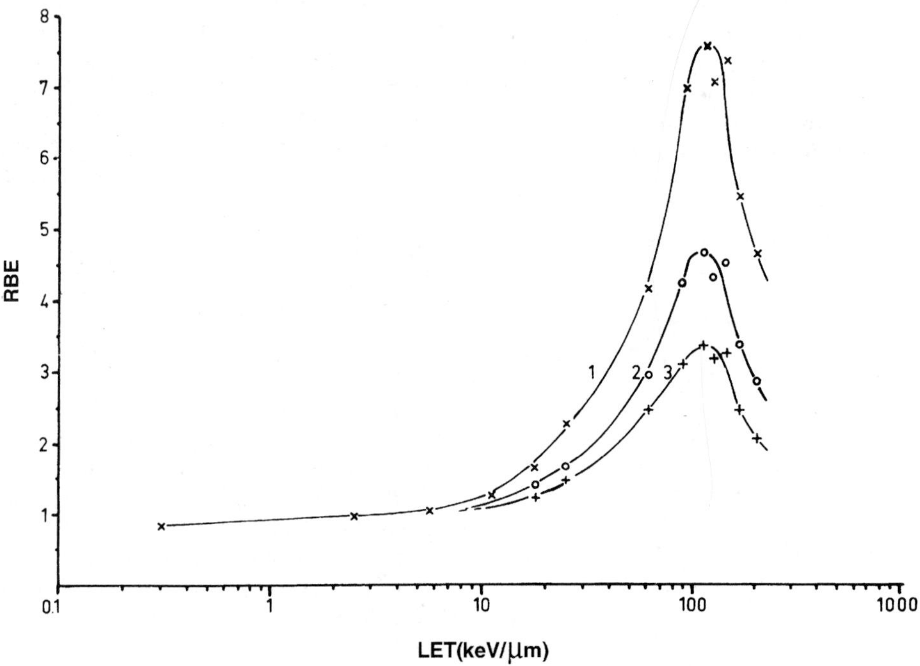

FIGURE 7.6 • Variation of relative biologic effectiveness (RBE) with linear energy transfer (LET) for survival of mammalian cells of human origin. The RBE rises to a maximum at an LET of about 100 keV/μm and subsequently falls for higher values of LET. Curves 1, 2, and 3 refer to cell survival levels of 0.8, 0.1, and 0.01, respectively, illustrating that the absolute value of the RBE is not unique but depends on the level of biologic damage and, therefore, on the dose level. (From Barendsen GW: Responses of cultured cells, tumors, and normal tissues to radiation of different linear energy transfer. *Curr Top Radiat Res Q* 4:293–356, 1968, with permission.)

values. This is an important effect and is explained in more detail in the next section.

The LET at which the RBE reaches a peak is much the same (about 100 keV/μm) for a wide range of mammalian cells, from mouse to human, and is the same for mutation as an end point as for cell killing.

THE OPTIMAL LET

It is of interest to ask why radiation with an LET of about 100 keV/μm is optimal in terms of producing a biologic effect. At this density of ionization, the average separation between ionizing events just about coincides with the diameter of the DNA double helix (20 Å, or 2 nm). Radiation with this density of ionization has the highest probability of causing a double-strand break by the passage of a single charged particle, and double-strand breaks are the basis of most biologic effects, as discussed in Chapter 2. This is illustrated in Figure 7.7. In the case of x-rays, which are more sparsely ionizing, the probability of a single track causing a double-strand break is low, and in general more than one track is required. As a consequence, x-rays have a low biologic effectiveness. At the other extreme, much more densely ionizing radiations (with an LET of 200 keV/μm, for example) readily produce double-strand breaks, but energy is "wasted" because the ionizing events are too close together. Because RBE is the ratio of doses producing equal biologic effect, this more densely ionizing radiation has a lower RBE than the optimal LET radiation. The more densely ionizing radiation is just as effective *per track*, but less effective per unit dose.

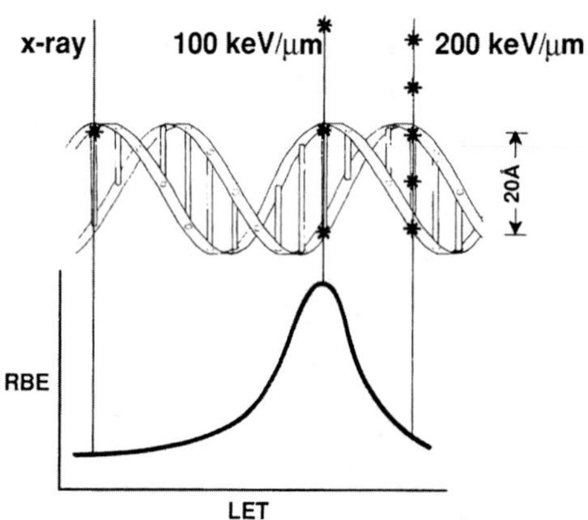

FIGURE 7.7 • Diagram illustrating why radiation with a linear energy transfer of 100 keV/μm has the greatest relative biologic effectiveness for cell killing, mutagenesis, or oncogenic transformation. For this transfer, the average separation between ionizing events coincides with the diameter of the DNA double helix (i.e., about 20 Å, or 2 nm). Radiation of this quality is most likely to produce a double-strand break from one track for a given absorbed dose.

It is possible, therefore, to understand why RBE reaches a maximum value in terms of the production of double-strand breaks, because the interaction of two double-strand breaks to form an exchange-type aberration is the basis of most biologic effects. In short, the most biologically effective LET is that at which there is a coincidence between the diameter of the DNA helix and the average separation of ionizing events. Radiations having this optimal LET include neutrons of a few hundred kiloelectron volts, as well as low-energy protons and α-particles.

FACTORS THAT DETERMINE RBE

The discussion of RBE began with a simple illustration of how this ratio may be determined for neutrons compared with x-rays using a simple biologic test system with a single, unequivocal end point, such as the LD_{50} for plant seedlings. Under these circumstances, RBE is conceptually very simple. In the years immediately after World War II, it was commonplace to see references to *the RBE* for neutrons, as if it were a single, unique quantity.

Now that more information is available from different biologic systems, many of which allow the researcher to investigate the relationship between biologic response and radiation dose rather than observing one end point at a single dose, it is apparent that RBE is a very complex quantity. RBE depends on the following:

Radiation quality (LET)
Radiation dose
Number of dose fractions
Dose rate
Biologic system or end point

Radiation quality includes the type of radiation and its energy, whether electromagnetic or particulate, and whether charged or uncharged.

RBE depends on the dose level and the number of dose fractions (or, alternatively, the dose per fraction) because in general, the shape of the dose–response relationship varies for radiations that differ substantially in their LET.

RBE can vary with the dose rate because the slope of the dose–response curve for sparsely ionizing radiations, such as x- or γ-rays, varies critically with a changing dose rate. In contrast, the biologic response to densely ionizing radiations depends little on the rate at which the radiation is delivered.

The biologic system or end point that is chosen has a marked influence on the RBE values obtained.

In general, RBE values are high for tissues that accumulate and repair a great deal of sublethal damage and low for those that do not.

THE OXYGEN EFFECT AND LET

An important relationship exists between LET and the **oxygen enhancement ratio (OER)**. Figure 7.8 shows mammalian cell survival curves for various types of radiation that have very different LETs and that exhibit very different OERs. Figure 7.8**A** refers to x-rays, which are sparsely ionizing, have a low LET, and consequently exhibit a large OER of about 2.5. Figure 7.8**B** refers to neutrons, which are intermediate in ionizing density and characteristically show an OER of 1.6. Figure 7.8**D** refers to 2.5-MeV α-particles, which have densely ionizing high-LET radiation; survival estimates, whether in the presence or absence of oxygen, fall along a common line, and so the OER is unity. Figure 7.8**C**

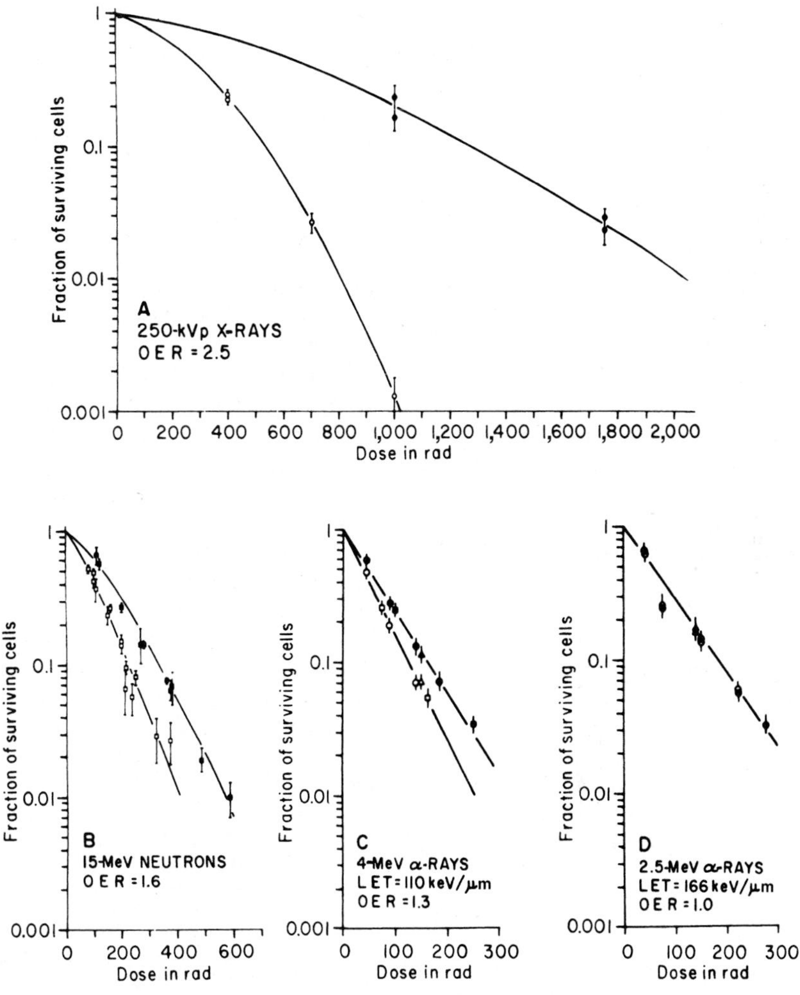

FIGURE 7.8 • Survival curves for cultured cells of human origin determined for four different types of radiation. Open circles refer to aerated conditions and closed circles to hypoxic conditions. **A:** For 250-kVp x-rays, oxygen enhancement ratio (OER) = 2.5. **B:** For 15-MeV $d^+ \rightarrow$ T neutrons, OER = 1.6. **C:** For 4-MeV α-particles, linear energy transfer (LET) = 110 keV/μm, OER = 1.3. **D:** For 2.5-MeV α-particles, LET = 166 keV/μm, OER = 1. (Adapted from Broerse JJ, Barendsen GW, van Kersen GR: Survival of cultured human cells after irradiation with fast neutrons of different energies in hypoxic and oxygenated conditions. *Int J Radiat Biol Relat Stud Phys Chem Med* 13:559–572, 1968; and Barendsen GW, Koot CJ, van Kersen GR, Bewley DK, Field SB, Parnell CJ: The effect of oxygen on impairment of the proliferative capacity of human cells in culture by ionizing radiations of different LET. *Int J Radiat Biol Relat Stud Phys Chem Med* 10:317–327, 1966, with permission.)

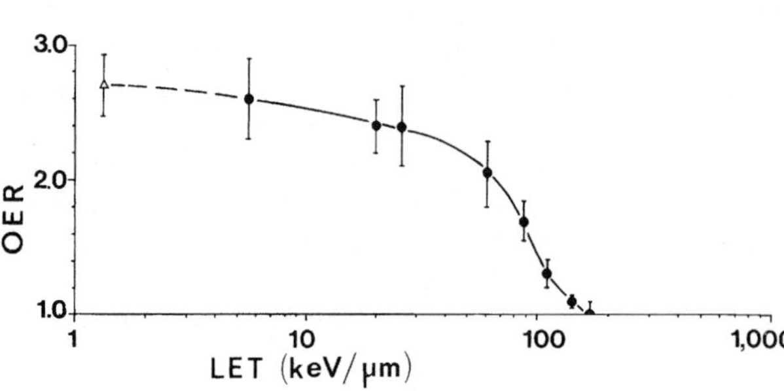

FIGURE 7.9 • Oxygen enhancement ratio as a function of linear energy transfer. Measurements were made with cultured cells of human origin. Closed circles refer to monoenergetic charged particles, the open triangle to 250-kVp x-rays with an assumed track average LET of 1.3 keV/μm. (From Barendsen GW, Koot CJ, van Kersen GR, Bewley DK, Field SB, Parnell CJ: The effect of oxygen on impairment of the proliferative capacity of human cells in culture by ionizing radiations of different LET. *Int J Radiat Biol Relat Stud Phys Chem Med* 10:317–327, 1966, with permission.)

contains data for 4-MeV α-particles, which are slightly less densely ionizing; in this case, the OER is about 1.3.

Barendsen and his colleagues have used mammalian cells cultured *in vitro* to investigate the OER for a wide range of radiation types. Their results are summarized in Figure 7.9, in which OER is plotted as a function of LET. At low LET, corresponding to x- or γ-rays, the OER is between 2.5 and 3; as the LET increases, the OER falls slowly at first, until the LET exceeds about 60 keV/μm, after which the OER falls rapidly and reaches unity by the time the LET has reached about 200 keV/μm.

Both OER and RBE are plotted as a function of LET in Figure 7.10. (The curves are taken from the more complete plots in Figures 7.6 and 7.9.) Interestingly, the two curves are virtually mirror images of each other. The optimal RBE and the rapid fall of OER occur at about the same LET value, 100 keV/μm.

RADIATION WEIGHTING FACTOR (W_R)

Radiations differ in their biologic effectiveness per unit of absorbed dose, as discussed previously. The complexities of RBE are too difficult to apply in specifying dose limits in everyday radiation protection; it is necessary to have a simpler way to consider differences in biologic effectiveness of different radiations. The term **radiation weighting factor (W_R)** has been introduced for this purpose. The quantity produced by multiplying the absorbed dose by the weighting factor is called the **equivalent dose**. When absorbed dose is expressed in gray, the equivalent dose is in sievert (Sv); if absorbed dose is in rad, the equivalent dose is in rad equivalent man (rem).

Radiation weighting factors are chosen by the International Commission on Radiological Protection (ICRP) based on a consideration of experimental RBE values, biased for biologic end points relevant to radiation protection, such as cancer at low dose and low dose rate. There is a considerable element of judgment involved. The radiation weighting factor is set at unity for all low-LET radiations (x-rays, γ-rays, and electrons), with a value of 20 for maximally effective neutrons and α-particles. Detailed values recommended by the ICRP are discussed in Chapter 15. Using this system, an absorbed dose of 0.1 Gy (10 rad) of radiation with a radiation weighting factor of 20 would result in an equivalent dose of 2 Sv (200 rem).

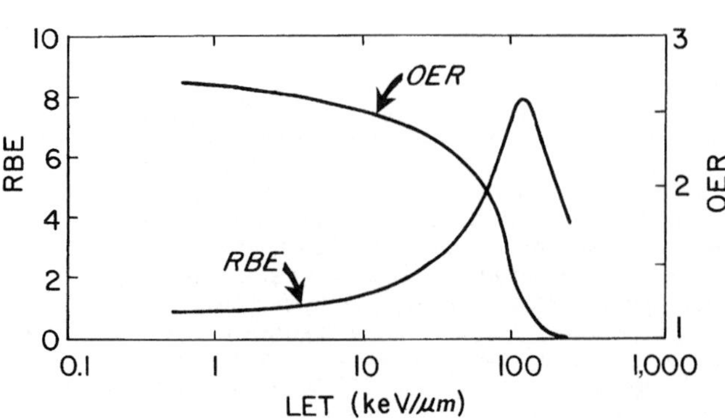

FIGURE 7.10 • Variation of the oxygen enhancement ratio and the relative biologic effectiveness as a function of the linear energy transfer of the radiation involved. The data were obtained using T1 kidney cells of human origin irradiated with various naturally occurring α-particles or with deuterons accelerated in the Hammersmith cyclotron. Note that the rapid increase in relative biologic effectiveness and the rapid fall of the oxygen enhancement ratio occur at about the same linear energy transfer, 100 keV/μm. (Redrawn from Barendsen GW: In: *Proceedings of the Conference on Particle Accelerators in Radiation Therapy*, pp 120–125. LA-5180-C. US Atomic Energy Commission, Technical Information Center, 1972, with permission.)

Summary of Pertinent Conclusions

- X- and γ-rays are said to be sparsely ionizing because along the tracks of the electrons set in motion primary ionizing events are well separated in space.
- α-Particles and neutrons are densely ionizing because the tracks consist of dense columns of ionization.
- Linear energy transfer (LET) is the energy transferred per unit length of track. Typical values are 0.2 keV/μm for cobalt-60 γ-rays, 2 keV/μm for 250-kV x-rays, and 1,000 keV/μm for heavy charged particles encountered in space.
- Relative biologic effectiveness (RBE) of some test radiation (r) is the ratio D_{250}/D_r, in which D_{250} and D_r are the doses of 250-kV x-rays and the test radiation, respectively, required to produce equal biologic effect.
- RBE increases with LET to a maximum at about 100 keV/μm, thereafter decreasing with higher LET.
- For radiation with the optimal LET of 100 keV/μm, the average separation between ionizing events is similar to the diameter of the DNA double helix (2 nm). It can most efficiently produce double-strand breaks by a single track.
- The RBE of high-LET radiations compared with that of low-LET radiations increases as the dose per fraction decreases. This is a direct consequence of the fact that the dose–response curve for low-LET radiations has a broader shoulder than for high-LET radiations.
- RBE varies according to the tissue or end point studied. In general, RBE values are high for cells or tissues that accumulate and repair a great deal of sublethal damage, so that their dose–response curves for x-rays have a broad initial shoulder.
- RBE depends on the following:

  Radiation quality (LET)
  Radiation dose
  Number of dose fractions
  Dose rate
  Biologic system or end point

- The oxygen enhancement ratio has a value of about 3 for low-LET radiations, falls when the LET rises above about 30 keV/μm, and reaches unity by an LET of about 200 keV/μm.
- The radiation weighting factor (W_R) depends on LET and is specified by the International Commission on Radiological Protection as a representative RBE at low dose and low dose rate for biologic effects relevant to radiation protection, such as cancer induction and hereditary effects. It is used in radiologic protection, to reduce radiations of different biologic effectiveness to a common scale.
- Equivalent dose is the product of absorbed dose and the radiation weighting factor. If absorbed dose is expressed in gray, equivalent dose is in sievert (Sv). If absorbed dose is in rad, equivalent dose is in rad equivalent man (rem).

BIBLIOGRAPHY

Barendsen GW: Impairment of the proliferative capacity of human cells in culture by alpha particles with differing linear energy transfer. *Int J Radiat Biol* 8:453–466, 1964

Barendsen GW: Responses of cultured cells, tumors, and normal tissues to radiation of different linear energy transfer. *Curr Top Radiat Res* Q 4:293–356, 1968

Barendsen GW: In: *Proceedings of the Conference on Particle Accelerators in Radiation Therapy*, pp 120–125. LA-5180-C. US Atomic Energy Commission, Technical Information Center, 1972

Barendsen GW, Beusker TLJ, Vergroesen AJ, Budke L: Effects of different ionizing radiations on human cells in tissue culture: II. Biological experiments. *Radiat Res* 13:841–849, 1960

Barendsen GW, Koot CJ, van Kersen GR, Bewley DK, Field SB, Parnell CJ: The effect of oxygen on impairment of the proliferative capacity of human cells in culture by ionizing radiations of different LET. *Int J Radiat Biol Relat Stud Phys Chem Med* 10:317–327, 1966

Barendsen GW, Walter HMD: Effects of different ionizing radiations on human cells in tissue culture: IV. Modification of radiation damage. *Radiat Res* 18:106–119, 1963

Berry RJ, Bewley DK, Parnell CJ: Reproductive capacity of mammalian tumor cells irradiated *in vivo* with cyclotron-produced fast neutrons. *Br J Radiol* 38:613–617, 1965

Bewley DK: Radiobiological research with fast neutrons and the implications for radiotherapy. *Radiology* 86:251–257, 1966

Bewley DK, Field SB, Morgan RL, Page BC, Parnell CJ: The response of pig skin to fractionated treatments with fast neutrons and x-rays. *Br J Radiol* 40:765–770, 1967

Broerse JJ, Barendsen GW: Relative biological effectiveness of fast neutrons for effects on normal tissues. *Curr Top Radiat Res Q* 8:305–350, 1973

Broerse JJ, Barendsen GW, van Kersen GR: Survival of cultured human cells after irradiation with fast neutrons of different energies in hypoxic and oxygenated conditions. *Int J Radiat Biol Relat Stud Phys Chem Med* 13:559–572, 1968

Field SB: The relative biological effectiveness of fast neutrons for mammalian tissues. *Radiology* 93:915–920, 1969

Field SB, Jones T, Thomlinson RH: The relative effect of fast neutrons and x-rays on tumor and normal tissue in the rat: II. Fractionation recovery and reoxygenation. *Br J Radiol* 41:597–607, 1968

Fowler JF, Morgan RL: Pretherapeutic experiments with the fast neutron beam from the Medical Research Council Cyclotron: VIII. General review. *Br J Radiol* 36:115–121, 1963

ICRP: *Recommendations of the International Commission on Radiological Protection.* International Commission on Radiological Protection Publication 26. New York, Pergamon Press, 1977

ICRP: *Recommendations of the International Commission on Radiological Protection.* Oxford, Pergamon Press, 1990

ICRP/ICRU: Report of the RBE Committee to the International Commissions on Radiological Protection and on Radiological Units and Measurements. *Health Phys* 9:357–384, 1963

ICRU: *Radiation Quantities and Units.* Report 33. Washington, DC, International Commission on Radiation Units and Measurements, 1980

International Commission on Radiation Units and Measurements: *The Quality Factor in Radiation Protection.* Report 40. Bethesda, MD, ICRU, 1986

CHAPTER 8

Acute Effects of Total-Body Irradiation

ACUTE RADIATION SYNDROME

The effect of ionizing radiation on whole organisms is discussed in this chapter. Data on the various forms of the **acute radiation syndrome (ARS)** have been drawn from many sources. Animal experiments provide the bulk of the data and result in a significant understanding of the mechanisms of death after exposure to total-body irradiation. At the human level, data have been drawn from experiences in radiation therapy and studies of the Japanese survivors of Hiroshima and Nagasaki, the Marshallese accidentally exposed to fallout in 1954, and the victims of the limited number of accidents at nuclear installations, including Chernobyl. From these various sources, the pattern of events that follows a total-body exposure to a dose of ionizing radiation has been well documented.

According to the Radiation Accident Registry maintained by the Radiation Emergency Assistance Center at Oak Ridge National Laboratory, there have been 403 radiation accidents worldwide during the period 1944 to 1999. Of these, 19 were criticalities, that is, involving nuclear reactors, but most (303) involved radiation devices, either sealed sources or x-ray machines, with the remainder (81) involving radioisotopes. These accidents have resulted in 120 deaths, including 30 in the United States, 2 in Great Britain, and 32 in the former Union of Soviet Socialist Republics.

EARLY LETHAL EFFECTS

Early radiation lethality generally is considered to be death occurring within a few weeks that can be attributed to a specific high-intensity exposure to radiation. Soon after irradiation, early symptoms appear, which last for a limited period of time; this is referred to as the **prodromal radiation syndrome**. The eventual survival time and mode of death depend on the magnitude of the dose. In most mammals, three distinct modes of death can be identified, although in actual accidental exposures, some overlap is frequently seen. At very high doses, in excess of about 100 Gy (10,000 rad), death occurs 24 to 48 hours after exposure and appears to result from neurologic and cardiovascular breakdown; this mode of death is known as the **cerebrovascular syndrome**. At intermediate dose levels, on the order of 5 to 12 Gy (500–1,200 rad), death occurs in a matter of days and is associated with extensive bloody diarrhea and destruction of the gastrointestinal mucosa; this mode of death is known as the **gastrointestinal syndrome**. At lower dose levels, on the order of 2.5 to 5 Gy (250–500 rad), death occurs several weeks to two months after exposure and is caused by effects on the blood-forming organs; this mode of death has come to be known as **bone-marrow death**, or the **hematopoietic syndrome**.

The exact cause of death in the cerebrovascular syndrome is by no means clear. In the case of both of the other modes of death—the gastrointestinal and the hematopoietic syndromes—the principal mechanisms that lead to the death of the organism are understood. Death is caused by the depletion of the stem cells of a critical self-renewal tissue: the epithelium of the gut or the circulating blood cells, respectively. The difference in the dose level at which these two forms of death occur and the difference in the time scales involved reflect variations in the population kinetics of the two cell renewal systems involved and differences in the amount of the damage that can be tolerated in these different systems before death ensues.

THE PRODROMAL RADIATION SYNDROME

The various symptoms making up the human prodromal syndrome vary with respect to time of onset, maximum severity, and duration, depending on the size of the dose. With doses of a few tens of gray (thousands of rad), all exposed individuals can be expected to show all phases of the syndrome within 5 to 15 minutes of exposure. Reaction might reach a maximum by about 30 minutes and persist for a few days, gradually diminishing in intensity until the prodromal symptoms merge with the universally fatal cerebrovascular syndrome or, after a lower dose, with the fatal gastrointestinal syndrome.

At lower doses, dose–response predictions are difficult to make because of the interplay of many different factors. A severe prodromal response usually indicates a poor clinical prognosis and portends at the least a prolonged period of acute hematologic aplasia accompanied by potentially fatal infection, anemia, and hemorrhage.

The signs and symptoms of the human prodromal syndrome can be divided into two main groups: gastrointestinal and neuromuscular. The gastrointestinal symptoms are anorexia, nausea, vomiting, diarrhea, intestinal cramps, salivation, fluid loss, dehydration, and weight loss. The neuromuscular symptoms include easy fatigability, apathy or listlessness, sweating, fever, headache, and hypotension. At doses that would be fatal to 50% of the population, the principal symptoms of the prodromal reaction are anorexia, nausea, vomiting, and easy fatigability. Immediate diarrhea, fever, and hypotension frequently are associated with supralethal exposure (Table 8.1). One of the Soviet firefighters at the Chernobyl reactor accident vividly described the onset of these symptoms as he accumulated a dose of several gray (several hundred rad) working in a high-dose-rate area.

TABLE 8.1

Symptoms of the Prodromal Syndrome

Neuromuscular	Gastrointestinal
Signs and Symptoms to be Expected at about 50% Lethal Dose	
Easy fatigability	Anorexia
	Nausea
	Vomiting
Additional Signs to be Expected after Supralethal Doses	
Fever	Immediate diarrhea
Hypotension	

The diagnosis of the acute radiation syndrome can also be based on laboratory data. During the prodromal phase, evidence of hematopoietic damage can already be observed by a drop in the lymphocyte count after an exposure as low as 0.5 Gy (50 rad). The circulating lymphocytes are one of the most radiosensitive cell lines, and a fall in the absolute lymphocyte count is the best and most useful laboratory test to determine the level of radiation exposure in the early phase of observation. Among assays for biological dosimetry, chromosomal aberration analysis from cultured circulating lymphocytes is the most widely accepted and reliable. The dose–response relationships are well established in many laboratories around the world. The lower limit of detection of a dose by using this cytogenetic method is approximately 0.2 Gy (20 rad) of γ-rays or x-rays.

THE CEREBROVASCULAR SYNDROME

A total-body dose on the order of 100 Gy (10,000 rad) of γ-rays or its equivalent of neutrons results in death in 24 to 48 hours. At these doses, all organ systems also are seriously damaged; both the gastrointestinal and hematopoietic systems are of course severely damaged and would fail if the person lived long enough, but cerebrovascular damage brings death very quickly, so that the consequences of the failure of the other systems do not have time to be expressed. The symptoms that are observed vary with the species of animal involved and also with level of radiation dose; they are summarized briefly as follows. There is the development of severe nausea and vomiting, usually within a matter of minutes. This is followed by manifestations of disorientation, loss of coordination of muscular movement, respiratory distress, diarrhea, convulsive seizures, coma, and finally death. Only a few instances of accidental human exposure have involved doses high enough to produce a cerebrovascular syndrome; two such cases are described briefly.

In 1964 a 38-year-old man working in a uranium-235 recovery plant was involved in an accidental nuclear excursion. He received a total-body dose estimated to be about 88 Gy (8,800 rad) made up of 22 Gy (2,200 rad) of neutrons and 66 Gy (6,600 rad) of γ-rays. He recalled seeing a flash and was hurled backward and stunned; he did not lose consciousness, however, and was able to run from the scene of the accident to another building 200 yards away. Almost at once he complained of abdominal cramps and headache, vomited, and was incontinent of bloody diarrheal stools. The next day the patient was comfortable but restless. On the second day, his condition deteriorated; he was restless, fatigued, apprehensive, and short of breath and had greatly impaired vision; his blood pressure could only be maintained with great difficulty. Six hours before his death, he became disoriented, and his blood pressure could not be maintained; he died 49 hours after the accident.

In a nuclear criticality accident at Los Alamos in 1958, one worker received a total-body dose of mixed neutron and γ-radiation estimated to be between 39 and 49 Gy (3,900–4,900 rad). Parts of his body may have received as much as 120 Gy (12,000 rad). This person went into a state of shock immediately and was unconscious within a few minutes. After 8 hours, no lymphocytes were found in the circulating blood, and there was virtually a complete urinary shutdown despite the administration of large amounts of fluids. The patient died 35 hours after the accident.

The exact and immediate cause of death in what is known as the cerebrovascular syndrome is not at all fully understood. Although death usually is attributed to events taking place within the central nervous system, much higher doses are required to produce death if the head alone is irradiated, rather than the entire body; this would suggest that effects on the rest of the body are by no means negligible. It has been suggested that the immediate cause of death is an increase in the fluid content of the brain owing to leakage from small vessels, resulting in a buildup of pressure within the bony confines of the skull.

THE GASTROINTESTINAL SYNDROME

A total-body exposure of more than 10 Gy (1,000 rad) of γ-rays or its equivalent of neutrons commonly leads in most mammals to symptoms characteristic of the gastrointestinal syndrome, culminating in death some days later (usually between 3 and 10 days). The characteristic symptoms are nausea, vomiting, and prolonged diarrhea. People lose their appetite, and appear sluggish and lethargic. Prolonged diarrhea, extending for several days, usually is regarded as a bad sign because it indicates that the dose received was more than 10 Gy (1,000 rad), which is inevitably fatal. The person shows signs of dehydration, loss of weight, emaciation, and complete exhaustion; death usually occurs in a few days. There is no instance on record of a human having survived a dose in excess of 10 Gy (1,000 rad).

The symptoms that appear and the death that follows are attributable principally to the depopulation of the epithelial lining of the gastrointestinal tract by the radiation. The normal lining of the intestine is a classic example of a self-renewing tissue; Figure 8.1 shows the general characteristics of such a tissue. It is composed of a stem-cell compartment, a differentiating compartment, and mature functioning cells.

The structure of the intestinal epithelium is described in some detail in Chapter 18. Dividing cells are confined to the crypts, which provide a continuous supply of new cells; these cells move up the villi, differentiate, and become the functioning cells. The cells at the top of the folds of villi are sloughed off slowly but continuously in the normal course of events, and the villi are continuously replaced by cells that originate from mitoses in the crypts.

A dose of radiation on the order of 10 Gy (1,000 rad) sterilizes a large proportion of the dividing cells in the crypts; a dose of this order of magnitude does not seriously affect the differentiated and functioning cells. As the surface of the villi is sloughed off and rubbed away by normal use, there are no replacement cells produced in the crypt. Consequently, after a few days, the villi begin to shorten and shrink, and eventually the surface lining of the intestine is completely denuded villi. The rate of cell loss and shrinkage depends on dose. It occurs faster at higher doses than at lower doses. At death the villi are very clearly flat and almost completely free of cells.

The precise time schedule of these events and the time required before the intestine is denuded of cells entirely varies with the species. In small rodents, this condition is reached between 3 and 4 days after

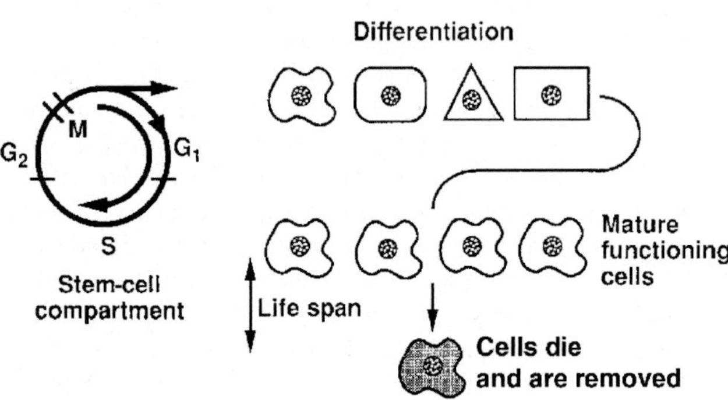

FIGURE 8.1 ● The classic self-renewal tissue. The stem-cell compartment contains the dividing cells. Of the new cells produced, some maintain the pool and some go on to differentiate and produce mature functioning cells. If the tissue is exposed to radiation, the "Achilles heel" is the stem-cell compartment. Huge doses of radiation are needed to destroy differentiated cells and prevent them from functioning, but modest doses kill some or all of the stem cells, in the sense that they lose their reproductive integrity. Irradiation does not produce an immediate effect on the tissue because it does not affect the functioning cells. The delay between the time of irradiation and the onset of the subsequent radiation syndrome is dictated by the normal life span of the mature functioning cells.

the dose of radiation is delivered. In humans it does not occur until about 10 days after irradiation. All of the individuals who received a dose large enough for the gastrointestinal syndrome to result in death have already received far more than enough radiation to result in hematopoietic death. Death from a denuding of the gut occurs, however, before the full effect of the radiation on the blood-forming organs has been expressed because of differences in the population kinetics of the stem-cell systems involved.

Before Chernobyl, there was probably only one example in the literature of a human suffering a gastrointestinal death as a result of radiation exposure. In 1946, a 32-year-old man was admitted to the hospital within 1 hour of a radiation accident in which he received a total-body dose of neutrons and γ-rays. The dosimetry is very uncertain in this early accident, and various estimates of total-body exposure range from 11 to 20 Gy (1,100–2,000 rad). In addition, the man's hands received an enormous dose, possibly as much as 300 Gy (30,000 rad). The patient vomited several times within the first few hours of the exposure. On admission, his temperature and pulse rate were slightly elevated; other than that, the results of his physical examinations were within normal limits. His general condition remained relatively good until the sixth day, at which time signs of severe paralytic ileus developed that could be relieved only by continuous gastric suction. On the seventh day, liquid stools that were guaiac-positive for occult blood were noted. The patient developed signs of circulatory collapse and died on the ninth day after irradiation. At the time of death, jaundice and spontaneous hemorrhages were observed for the first time.

At autopsy, the small intestine showed the most striking change. The mucosal surface was edematous and erythematous, and the jejunum was covered by a membranous exudate. Microscopically, there was complete erosion of the epithelium of the jejunum and ileum, as well as loss of the superficial layers of the submucosa. The duodenal epithelium was lost, except in the crypts; the colon epithelium was somewhat better preserved. The denuded surfaces were covered everywhere by a layer of exudate in which masses of bacteria were seen, and in the jejunum, the bacteria had invaded the intestinal wall. Blood cultures postmortem yielded *Escherichia coli.*

Several of the firefighters at Chernobyl, including those who received bone-marrow transplants, died between a week and 10 days after exposure, suffering from symptoms characteristic of the gastrointestinal syndrome.

THE HEMATOPOIETIC SYNDROME

At doses of 2.5 to 5 Gy (250–500 rad), death, if it occurs, is a result of radiation damage to the hematopoietic system. Mitotically active precursor cells are sterilized by the radiation, and the subsequent supply of mature red blood cells, white blood cells, and platelets is thereby diminished. The time of potential crisis, at which the number of circulating cells in the blood reaches a minimum value, is delayed for some weeks. It is only when the mature circulating cells begin to die off and the supply of new cells from the depleted precursor population is inadequate to replace them that the full effect of the radiation becomes apparent.

The concept of the 50% lethal dose (LD_{50}) as an end point for scoring radiation death from this

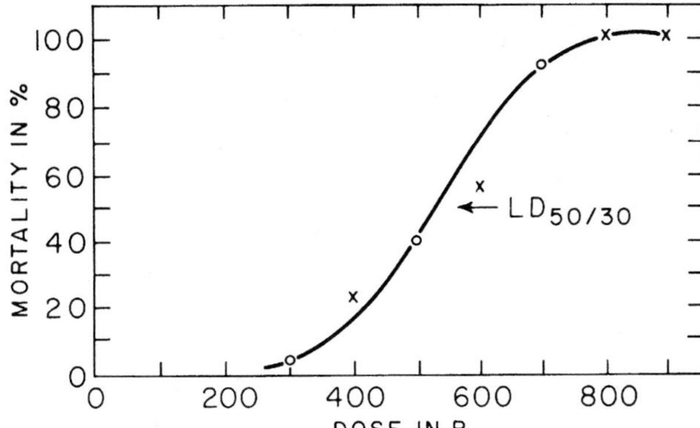

FIGURE 8.2 ● Mortality rate of rhesus monkeys at 30 days after a single total-body exposure to x-rays. (From Henschke UK, Morton JL: The mortality of rhesus monkeys after single total-body radiation. *AJR Am J Roentgenol* 77:899–909, 1957, with permission.)

cause has been borrowed from the field of pharmacology. The LD_{50} is defined as the dose of any agent or material that causes a mortality rate of 50% in an experimental group within a specified period of time.

Within a given population of humans or animals, there are many factors that influence the response of the individual to total-body irradiation. For example, the very young and the old appear to be more radiosensitive than the young adult. The female, in general, appears to have a greater degree of tolerance to radiation than does the male. Figure 8.2 shows a typical relationship between the dose of radiation and the percentage of monkeys killed by total-body irradiation. Up to a dose exceeding 2 Gy (200 rad), no animals die, whereas a dose of about 8 Gy (800 rad) kills all the animals exposed. Between these two doses, there is a very rapid increase in the percentage of animals killed as the dose increases, and it is a simple matter by visual inspection of the graph or by a more sophisticated statistical analysis to arrive at a precise estimate of the LD_{50} dose, which in this case is 5.3 Gy (530 rad).

Humans develop signs of hematologic damage and recover from it much more slowly than most other mammals. The peak incidence of human death from hematologic damage occurs at about 30 days after exposure, but deaths continue for up to 60 days. The LD_{50} estimates for hematopoietic death for humans are therefore expressed as the $LD_{50/60}$, in contrast to the $LD_{50/30}$ for mice, in which peak incidence of death occurs 10 to 15 days after exposure and is complete by 30 days.

A dose of radiation close to the LD_{50} results in the prodromal syndrome already described, the chief symptoms of which are nausea and vomiting. A symptom-free interval of time, known as the *latent period*, follows. This is, in fact, a very inappropriate name, because during this period the most important consequences of the radiation exposure, leading to its lethal effects, are in progress. About 3 weeks after the radiation exposure, there is onset of chills, fatigue, petechial hemorrhages in the skin, and ulceration of the mouth; epilation also occurs at this time. These symptoms are a manifestation of the depression of blood elements: infections and fever from granulocyte depression and impairment of immune mechanisms, bleeding, and possibly anemia caused by hemorrhage resulting from platelet depression. Anemia from red blood cell depression usually does not occur. Death occurs at this stage unless the bone marrow has begun to regenerate in time. Infection is an important cause of death, but it may be controlled to a large extent by antibiotic therapy.

As a consequence of the reactor accident at Chernobyl, 203 operating personnel, firemen, and emergency workers were hospitalized suffering from the early radiation syndrome, having received doses in excess of 1 Gy (100 rad). Of these, 35 had severe bone-marrow failure, and 13 of them died. The remainder recovered with conservative medical care.

MEAN LETHAL DOSE AND BONE-MARROW TRANSPLANTS

Studies of total-body irradiation have been performed on many species; a few LD_{50} values are listed in Table 8.2, ranging from mouse to human. Such studies were popular and important in the 1950s and 1960s, supported largely by the military. In more recent years, total-body irradiation has been of interest from the point of view of bone-marrow transplantation. This interest may stem from the treatment of radiation accidents, such as the Chernobyl disaster, or from the rescue of patients receiving cancer therapy with total-body irradiation, radiolabeled antibodies, or cytotoxic drugs.

Many attempts have been made to estimate the $LD_{50/60}$ for humans based on the experiences at Hiroshima and Nagasaki, the total-body irradiation of

TABLE 8.2

The 50% Lethal Doses for Various Species from Mouse to Human and the Relation between Body Weight and the Number of Cells that Need to be Transplanted for a Bone-Marrow "Rescue"

Species	Average Body Weight, kg	50% Lethal Total-Body Irradiation, Gy	Rescue Dose per kg $\times 10^{-8}$	Relative Hematopoietic Stem-Cell Concentration
Mouse	0.025	7	2	10
Rat	0.2	6.75	3	6.7
Rhesus monkey	2.8	5.25	7.5	7.3
Dog	12	3.7	17.5	1.1
Human	70	4	20	1

Data from Vriesendorp HM, van Bekkum DW: Susceptibility to total-body Irradiation. In Broerse JJ, MacVittle T (eds): *Response to Total-Body Irradiation in Different Species*, Amsterdam, Martinus Nijhoff, 1984.

patients with malignant disease, and the accidents that have occurred at nuclear installations. In a careful summary of all of the available data, Lushbaugh claims that the best estimate is around 3.25 Gy (325 rad) for young healthy adults without medical intervention. There does exist in the literature a surprising number of instances in which young men and women have received total-body irradiation up to a dose of around 4 Gy (400 rad) and recovered under conservative care in a modern well-equipped hospital. The LD_{50} for humans quoted in Table 8.2 is the estimate of Vriesendorp and van Bekkum, in the Netherlands. In addition to LD_{50} data for a number of species, this table also shows estimates of the bone-marrow "rescue dose" required in a bone-marrow transplant, that is, the number of transplanted bone-marrow cells that are required for a person to recover from a supralethal dose. Larger species are clearly more susceptible to hematopoietic damage than smaller species, as reflected by a lower LD_{50}. The bone-marrow transplant experience indicates that this is because of a negative correlation between body weight and hematopoietic stem-cell concentration, that is, the number of hematopoietic stem cells per body unit. The correlation between body weight and the number of bone-marrow cells needed for a rescue is illustrated in Figure 8.3 for a range of species, from mouse to human. Humans require about ten times as many bone-marrow cells per kilogram of body weight as the mouse for a successful bone-marrow rescue after supralethal total-body irradiation because of the lower concentration of hematopoietic stem cells.

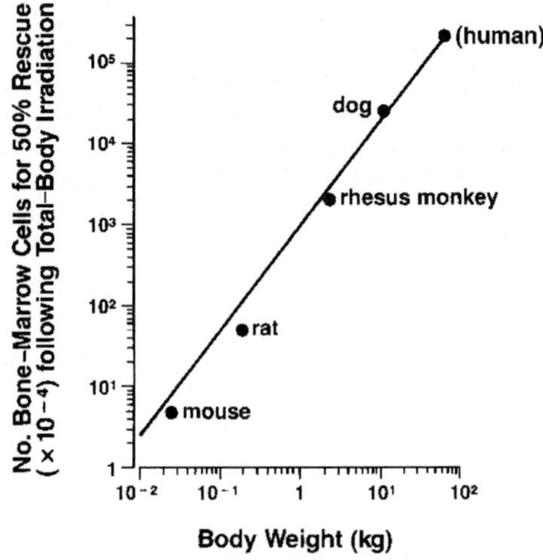

FIGURE 8.3 • Correlation between body weight and bone-marrow dose for 50% rescue (i.e., number of hematopoietic stem cells required to be transplanted) following supralethal total-body irradiation. (From Vriesendorp HM, van Bekkum DW: Role of total-body irradiation in conditioning for bone marrow transplantation. In Thierfelder S, Rodt H, Kolb HJ (eds): *Immunobiology of Bone Marrow Transplantation*, pp 349–364. Berlin, Springer Verlag, 1980, with permission.)

SYMPTOMS ASSOCIATED WITH THE ACUTE RADIATION SYNDROME

The International Atomic Energy Agency and the World Health Organization jointly sponsored a report entitled *Diagnosis and Treatment of Radiation Injuries*. Tables 8.3 and 8.4 have been adapted from

TABLE 8.3

Latent Phase (Prodromal Syndrome) of Acute Radiation Syndrome (ARS)

	Degree of ARS and Approximate Dose of Acute WBE (Gy)				
	Mild (1–2 Gy)	**Moderate (2–4 Gy)**	**Severe (4–6 Gy)**	**Very Severe (6–8 Gy)**	**Lethal (>8 Gy)**
Lymphocytes (G/L) (days 3–6)	0.8–1.5	0.5–0.8	0.3–0.5	0.1–0.3	0.0–0.1
Granulocytes (G/L)	>2.0	1.5–2.0	1.0–1.5	≤0.5	≤0.1
Diarrhea	None	None	Rare	Appears on days 6–9	Appears on days 4–5
Epilation	None	Moderate, beginning on day 15 or later	Moderate or complete on days 11–21	Complete earlier than day 11	Complete earlier than day 10
Latency period (d)	21–35	18–28	8–18	7 or less	None
Medical response	Hospitalization not necessary	Hospitalization recommended	Hospitilization necessary	Hospitalization urgently necessary	Symptomatic treatment only

Adapted from *Diagnosis and Treatment of Radiation Injuries*, International Atomic Energy Agency, Vienna, 1998.

TABLE 8.4

Critical Phase of Acute Radiation Syndrome (ARS)

	Degree of ARS and Approximate Dose of Acute WBE (Gy)				
	Mild (1–2 Gy)	**Moderate (2–4 Gy)**	**Severe (4–6 Gy)**	**Very Severe (6–8 Gy)**	**Lethal (>8 Gy)**
Onset of symptoms	>30 days	18–28 days	8–18 days	<7 days	<3 days
Lymphocytes (G/L)	0.8–1.5	0.5–0.8	0.3–0.5	0.1–0.3	0–0.1
Platelets (G/L)	60–100 10–25%	30–60 25–40%	25–35 40–80%	15–25 60–80%	<20 80–100%[a]
Clinical manifestations	Fatigue, weakness	Fever, infections, bleeding, weakness, epilation	High fever, infections, bleeding, epilation	High fever, diarrhea, vomiting, dizziness and disorientation, hypotension	High fever, diarrhea, unconsciousness
Lethality (%)	0	0–50 Onset 6–8 weeks	20–70 Onset 4–8 weeks	50–100 Onset 1–2 weeks	100 1–2 weeks
Medical response	Prophylactic	Special prophylactic treatment from days 14–20; isolation from days 10–20	Special prophylactic treatment from days 7–10; isolation from the beginning	Special treatment from day 1; isolation from the beginning	Symptomatic only

[a] In very severe cases, with a dose >50, Gy, death precedes cytopenia.

Adapted from *Diagnosis and Treatment of Radiation Injuries*, International Atomic Energy Agency, Vienna, 1998.

that report, and the expected distribution of symptoms following whole-body irradiation are summarized. Table 8.3 refers to the prodromal syndrome in the period soon after irradiation, while Table 8.4 refers to the later critical phase. These should not be taken too literally, since the information is based on a limited number of exposed individuals over the years, but they are a useful guide. They cover the dose range from 1.0 Gy (100 rad), which results in little effect, to more than 8 Gy (800 rad), which is expected to result in 100% lethality. The nature of the symptoms, their severity, and the time of onset can be a useful predictor of the eventual outcome in the absence of physical dosimetry. For example, severe immediate diarrhea indicates that a supralethal dose has been received and that any treatment is likely to be ineffective and therefore useless.

TREATMENT OF RADIATION ACCIDENT VICTIMS EXPOSED TO DOSES CLOSE TO THE $LD_{50/60}$

If the radiation exposure is known to be less than 4 to 5 Gy (400–500 rad), most experts recommend that the patient be watched carefully but only treated in response to specific symptoms, such as antibiotics for an infection, fresh platelets for local hemorrhage, and so on. Petechial hemorrhages in skin were commonly observed in the Japanese irradiated in 1945 but are not reported so commonly among individuals exposed accidentally in nuclear power installations in the United States. Blood transfusions should not be given prophylactically because they delay the regeneration of the blood-forming organs.

If the dose is known to have exceeded about 5 Gy (500 rad), then death from the hematopoietic syndrome 3 to 4 weeks later is a real possibility. In some countries, isolation and barrier nursing—that is, isolation from others so that they do not come in contact with possible infections while their blood count is low—is recommended. It has been shown in animals that the LD_{50} can be raised by a factor of about 2 by the use of antibiotics, and there is no reason to suppose that the same is not true in humans. The important things are to avoid infection, bleeding, and physical trauma during the period in which the circulating blood elements reach a nadir and to give the bone marrow a chance to regenerate.

The area of most discussion and disagreement is the use of bone-marrow transplantation. This technique was used on four Yugoslav scientists who were exposed accidentally in the 1950s to doses initially estimated to be about 7 Gy (700 rad). All of the grafts were rejected, but the exposed individuals survived anyway, probably because later estimates indicated that the dose received was much lower, in the region of 4 Gy (400 rad). In fact, many observers claim that the scientists survived in spite of the transplants, rather than because of them. Figure 8.4 shows the depression and recovery of blood elements in the Yugoslav scientists and also in victims of the famous Y-12 reactor accident at Oak Ridge, Tennessee, who received about 4 Gy (400 rad).

In more recent years, bone-marrow transplantation techniques have been greatly improved and, together with growth factors, have been used routinely to "rescue" patients given supralethal doses of radiation for the treatment of leukemia or in preparation for organ transplants. In such cases, of course, the dosimetry is accurate and the doses are just enough to suppress the immunologic response.

Of the Chernobyl accident victims, 13 received bone-marrow transplants (some matched for immune compatibility and some not). In addition, six received fetal liver transplants, but these patients all died early, some of gastrointestinal symptoms. Of the 13 who received bone-marrow transplants, only two survived, and one showed autologous bone-marrow repopulation. There was therefore only one possible successful transplant that saved a life, and even that result has been questioned.

The situation was made difficult because the doses to which individuals had been exposed were not known with any precision. After doses close to the LD_{50}, and certainly for higher doses, peripheral lymphocytes disappear before 24 hours, and then it is not possible to estimate total-body doses by counting chromosome aberrations in stimulated lymphocytes taken from peripheral blood. Because the U.S. transplant team did not arrive in Chernobyl for some time, biologic dosimetry was never possible for those exposed to higher doses. Consequently, some victims who received bone-marrow transplants already were doomed to die of the gastrointestinal syndrome, having received doses in excess of 10 Gy (1,000 rad).

In fact, the window of dose within which a bone-marrow transplant is useful is very small. Below about 8 Gy (800 rad), an exposed person is likely to survive with careful nursing and an antibiotic screen because the LD_{50} can be approximately doubled by such conservative measures. In such cases, therefore, a transplant is not necessary. Above about 10 Gy (1,000 rad) death from the gastrointestinal syndrome is inevitable, and so a bone-marrow transplant is of no use. This highlights the narrow

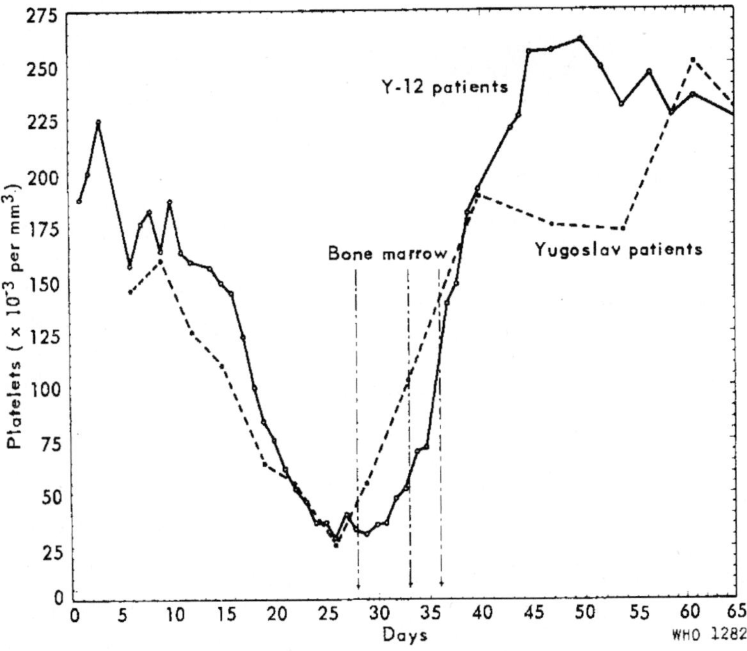

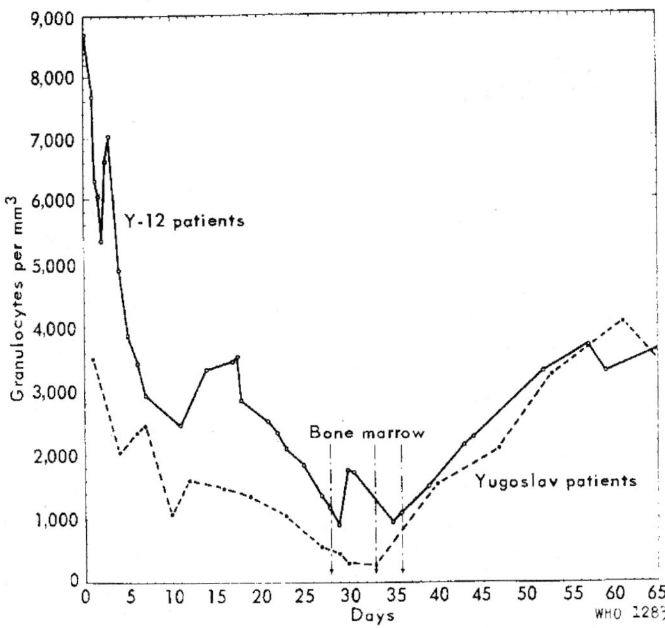

FIGURE 8.4 • Depression and recovery of circulating blood elements in victims of the Y-12 reactor accident at Oak Ridge, Tennessee, and four accidentally exposed Yugoslav scientists. (From Andrews GA, Sitterson BW, Kretchmar AL, Brucer M: *Diagnosis and Treatment of Acute Radiation Injury*, pp 27–48. Geneva, World Health Organization, 1961.)

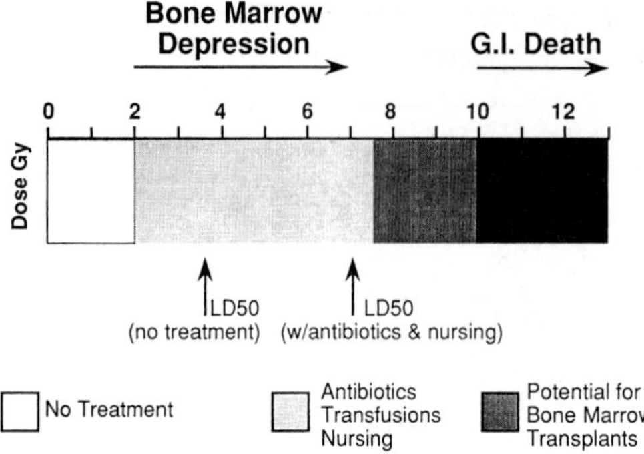

FIGURE 8.5 • Illustrating the narrow window of dose over which bone-marrow transplants might be useful following total-body irradiation. Up to about 8 Gy (800 rad), most people would survive with antibiotics and careful nursing. Above about 10 Gy (1,000 rad), most people would die as a consequence of the gastrointestinal syndrome.

"window" of dose within which a transplant can be effective (about 8–10 Gy, or 800–1,000 rad). This is illustrated in Figure 8.5. Therefore, there is an urgent need to develop better methods of *in vivo* biologic dosimetry, because chromosome aberrations in lymphocytes are not always useful in this dose range.

SURVIVORS OF SERIOUS RADIATION ACCIDENTS IN THE UNITED STATES

Over the past 50 years, there have been a number of accidents in which small numbers of people employed in the nuclear program were exposed to total-body or partial-body irradiation. Most occurred in the early days of the nuclear program and involved criticality accidents. The number involved in the United States is about 70 workers in 13 separate accidents.

The long-term survivors have been studied exhaustively over the years. The medical history of these heavily irradiated people mirrors that of any aging population. The expected high incidences of shortened lifespan, early malignancies after a short latent period, and rapidly progressing lenticular opacities have not been observed. The numbers in any group are small, but the several malignancies, cataracts, and degenerative diseases that have been seen are no more than might be expected in a similar group of unirradiated people of the same age.

The survivors of the 1958 criticality accident at the Oak Ridge Y-12 plant are a case in point. Their blood cell counts are shown in Figure 8.4. A group of eight workers, ranging in age from 25 to 56 years, received total-body doses of 0.23 to 3.65 Gy (23–365 rad); five of them received doses above 2 Gy (200 rad). Nevertheless, as of 1999, over 40 years after the accident, none had died of a classic "radiogenic" cancer. There were two cases of lung cancer in very heavy smokers, a meningioma, and prostate cancer in a 70-year-old man. In fact, the only medical finding likely to be radiation related is bilateral posterior capsular cataracts in two of these patients. Three of the workers who received the biggest doses are retired and in good health.

This highlights the problem of detecting an excess cancer incidence in any small irradiated population. For example, if a group of workers receive a total-body exposure of 3 Gy (300 rad), the biggest dose possible without suffering early death from the hematopoietic syndrome, the excess cancer incidence would be expected to be about 24%. (The cancer risk estimates of the Committee on Biological Effects of Ionizing Radiation and the United Nations Scientific Committee on the Effects of Atomic Radiation based on the Japanese atomic-bomb survivors amount to about 8% per sievert.) Thus, the biggest dose to which humans can be exposed and survive doubles the spontaneous cancer incidence. This is difficult to detect in a small group of people and is likely to be masked by other biologic factors. That is not to say that heavily irradiated individuals are not at increased risk, but an excess cancer incidence can be observed only by a careful study of a large population.

RADIATION EMERGENCY ASSISTANCE CENTER

In the context of radiation accidents, it should be noted that the Medical Sciences Division of the Oak Ridge Institute for Science and Education operates a Radiation Emergency Assistance Center/Training Site (REAC/TS). This is operated on behalf of the U.S. Department of Energy.

REAC/TS provides 24-hour direct or consultative assistance with medical and health physics problems associated with radiation accidents in local, national, and international incidents. The resources of REAC/TS consist of expertise in cytogenetics for dose assessment, calculation of doses from internally deposited radionuclides, and laboratory facilities that include total-body counting capabilities. The regular telephone number for information is (865) 576-3131, and the 24-hour emergency number is (865) 576-1005 (ask for REAC/TS). The REAC/TS website is http://www.orau.gov/reacts.

Summary of Pertinent Conclusions

- The prodromal syndrome varies in time of onset, severity, and duration.
- At doses close to the dose that would be lethal to 50% of the population (LD_{50}), the principal symptoms of the prodromal syndrome are anorexia, nausea, vomiting, and easy fatigability.
- Immediate diarrhea, fever, or hypotension indicate a supralethal exposure.
- The cerebrovascular syndrome results from a total-body exposure to about 100 Gy (10,000 rad) of γ-rays and in humans results in death in 24 to 48 hours. The cause of death may be changes in permeability of small blood vessels in the brain.
- The gastrointestinal syndrome results from a total-body exposure to about 10 Gy (1,000 rad). Death occurs in about 5 to 10 days in humans because of depopulation of the epithelial lining of the gastrointestinal tract.
- The hematopoietic syndrome results from total-body exposure to 2.5 to 5 Gy (250–500 rad). The radiation sterilizes some or all of the mitotically active precursor cells. Symptoms result from lack of circulating blood elements 3 or more weeks later.
- The LD_{50} for humans is 3 to 4 Gy (300–400 rad) for young adults without medical intervention. It may be less for the very young or the old.
- Some people who would otherwise die from the hematopoietic syndrome may be saved by antibiotics, platelet infusions, or bone-marrow transplants.
- In primates, the LD_{50} can be raised by a factor of 2 by appropriate treatment, including careful nursing and antibiotics, and the same may be assumed for humans.
- The dose window over which bone-marrow transplants may be useful is narrow, namely, 8 to 10 Gy (800–1,000 rad).
- Heavily irradiated survivors of accidents in the nuclear industry have been followed for many years; their medical history mirrors that of any aging population. An expected higher incidence of shortened lifespan, early malignancies after a short latency, and rapidly progressing cataracts has not been observed. That is not to say that heavily irradiated individuals are not at increased risk, but an excess cancer incidence can be observed only by a careful study of a large population.

BIBLIOGRAPHY

Andrews GA, Sitterson BW, Kretchmar AL, Brucer M: *Diagnosis and Treatment of Acute Radiation Injury*, pp 27–48. Geneva, World Health Organization, 1961

Bacq ZM, Alexander P: *Fundamentals of Radiobiology*, 2nd ed. New York, Pergamon Press, 1961

Bond VP, Fliedner TM, Archambeau JO: *Mammalian Radiation Lethality: A Disturbance in Cellular Kinetics.* New York, Academic Press, 1965

Fry SA, Littlefield G, Lushbaugh CC, Sipe AH, Ricks RC, Berger ME: Follow-up of survivors of serious radiation accidents in the United States. In Ricks R, Fry SA (eds): *The Medical Basis for Radiation Accident Preparedness.* New York, Elsevier Science, 1990

Hemplemann LH, Lisco H, Hoffman JG: The acute radiation syndrome: A study of nine cases and a review of the problem. *Ann Intern Med* 36:279–510, 1952

Henschke UK, Morton JL: The mortality of rhesus monkeys after single total-body radiation. *AJR Am J Roentgenol* 77:899–909, 1957

IAEA: *Diagnosis and Treatment of Radiation Injuries.* Safety Report Series No. 2, Vienna, International Atomic Energy Agency, 1998

Karas JS, Stanbury JB: Fatal radiation syndrome from an accidental nuclear excursion. *N Engl J Med* 272:755–761, 1965

Langham WH (ed): *Radiobiological Factors in Manned Space Flight: Report of the Space Radiation Study Panel of the Life Sciences Committee.* Publication No. 1487. Washington, DC, National Academy of Sciences, National Research Council, 1967

Lushbaugh CC: Reflections on some recent progress in human radiobiology. In Augenstein LC, Mason R, Zelle M (eds): *Advances in Radiation Biology*, pp 277–314. New York, Academic Press, 1969

Shipman TL, Lushbaugh CC, Peterson D, Langham WH, Harris PS, Lawrence JNP: Acute radiation death resulting from an accidental nuclear critical excursion. *J Occup Med* 3(suppl):145–192, 1961

Vriesendorp HM, van Bekkum DW: Bone marrow transplantation in the canine. In Shifrine M, Wilson FD (eds): *The Canine as a Biomedical Research Model: Immunological, Hematological and Oncological Aspects.* Washington, DC, Department of Energy, Office of Health and Environmental Research, 1980

Vriesendorp HM, van Bekkum DW: Role of total-body irradiation in conditioning for bone marrow transplantation.

In Thierfelder S, Rodt H, Kolb HJ (eds): *Immunobiology of Bone Marrow Transplantation*, pp 349–364. Berlin, Springer Verlag, 1980

Vriesendorp HM, van Bekkum DW: Susceptibility to total-body irradiation. In Broerse JJ, MacVittie T (eds): *Response to Total-Body Irradiation in Different Species*. Amsterdam, Martinus Nijhoff, 1984

Vriesendorp HM, Zurcher C: Late effects of total-body irradiation in dogs treated with bone marrow transplantation. In Fliedner TM, Grossner W, Patrick C (eds): *Proceedings of the Meeting of the European Late Effects Project Group of EURATOM*. Report EUR 8078. Luxembourg, Commission of the European Communities, 1982

CHAPTER 9

Radioprotectors

THE DISCOVERY OF RADIOPROTECTORS

Some substances, although they do not directly affect the radiosensitivity of cells, nevertheless may protect whole animals because they cause vasoconstriction or in some way upset normal processes of metabolism to such an extent that the oxygen concentration in critical organs is reduced. Because cells are less sensitive to x-rays under hypoxia, this confers a measure of protection. Examples of such protective substances are sodium cyanide, carbon monoxide, epinephrine, histamine, and serotonin. Such compounds are not really radioprotectors per se and are not discussed further here.

The most remarkable group of true radioprotectors is the sulfhydryl compounds. The simplest is **cysteine**, a sulfhydryl compound containing a natural amino acid, the structure of which is

$$SH{-}CH_2{-}CH\begin{matrix} \diagup NH_2 \\ \diagdown COOH \end{matrix}$$

In 1948, Patt discovered that cysteine could protect mice from the effects of total-body exposure to x-rays if the drug was injected or ingested in large amounts before the radiation exposure. At about the same time, Bacq and his colleagues in Europe independently discovered that **cysteamine** could also protect animals from total-body irradiation. This compound has a structure represented by

$$SH{-}CH_2{-}CH_2{-}NH_2$$

Animals injected with cysteamine to concentrations of about 150 mg/kg require doses of x-rays 1.8 times larger than control animals to produce the same mortality rate. This factor of 1.8 is called the *dose-reduction factor* (*DRF*), defined as

$$\text{DRF} = \frac{\begin{matrix}\text{Dose of radiation in} \\ \text{the presence of the drug}\end{matrix}}{\begin{matrix}\text{Dose of radiation in} \\ \text{the absence of the drug}\end{matrix}}$$

to produce a given level of lethality.

MECHANISM OF ACTION

Many similar sulfhydryl compounds have been tested and found to be effective as radioprotectors. The most efficient tend to have certain structural features in common: a free SH group (or potential SH group) at one end of the molecule and a strong basic function, such as amine or guanidine, at the other end, separated by a straight chain of two or three carbon atoms. Sulfhydryl compounds are efficient radioprotectors against sparsely ionizing radiations, such as x- or γ-rays.

The mechanisms most implicated in SH-mediated cytoprotection include:

1. Free-radical *scavenging* that protects against oxygen-based free-radical generation by ionizing radiations or chemotherapy agents such as alkylating agents.
2. Hydrogen atom donation to facilitate direct chemical *repair* at sites of DNA damage.

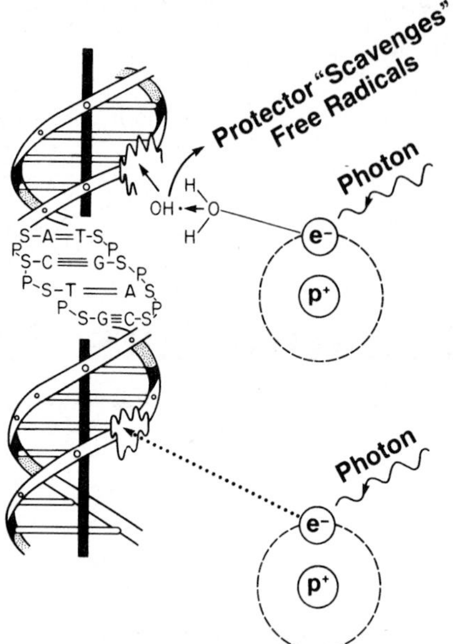

FIGURE 9.1 • Radioprotectors containing a sulfhydryl group exert their effect by scavenging free radicals and by rducing free-radical damage to DNA. They are most effective for radiations characterized by low linear energy transfer, becoming progressively less effective with increasing LET because the amount of local damage is so great.

Chapter 1 includes a discussion of the chain of events between the absorption of a photon and the eventual biologic damage, which includes the production of free radicals, which are highly reactive species. If these free radicals are scavenged before they can interact with biologic molecules, the effect of the radiation is reduced. This process is illustrated in Figure 9.1.

The protective effect of sulfhydryl compounds tends to parallel the oxygen effect, being maximal for sparsely ionizing radiations (e.g., x- or γ-rays) and minimal for densely ionizing radiations (e.g., low-energy α-particles). It might be predicted that with effective scavenging of all free radicals, the largest possible value of dose-reduction factor for sparsely ionizing radiations would equal the oxygen enhancement ratio, with a value of 2.5 to 3.0.

This simple description of the mechanism of action of sulfhydryl radioprotectors is intellectually satisfying, but it is clearly not the whole story, because radioprotectors of this class have more effect with densely ionizing radiations (such as neutrons) than would be expected based on this explanation alone. Other factors must be involved that are not fully understood.

DEVELOPMENT OF MORE EFFECTIVE COMPOUNDS

The discovery in 1948 of a compound that offered protection against radiation excited the interest of the U.S. Army because the memory of Nagasaki and Hiroshima was vivid in the years immediately after World War II. However, although cysteine is a radioprotector, it is also toxic and induces nausea and vomiting at the dose levels required for radioprotection. A development program was initiated in 1959 by the U.S. Army in studies conducted at the Walter Reed Institute of Research to identify and synthesize drugs capable of conferring protection to individuals in a radiation environment, but without the debilitating toxicity of cysteine or cysteamine. Over 4,000 compounds were synthesized and tested. At an early stage, the important discovery was made that the toxicity of the compound could be greatly reduced if the sulfhydryl group was covered by a phosphate group. This is illustrated for cysteamine, otherwise known as MEA, in Table 9.1. The 50% lethal dose of the compound in animals can be doubled and the protective effect in terms of the dose-reduction factor greatly enhanced if the SH group is covered by a phosphate. This tends to reduce systemic toxicity. Once in the cell, the phosphate group is stripped, and the SH group begins scavenging for free radicals.

TABLE 9.1

Effect of Adding a Phosphate-Covering Function on the Free Sulfhydryl of β-Mercaptoethylamine (MEA)

Drug	Formula	Mean 50% Lethal Dose (Range) in Mice	Dose-Reduction Factor
MEA	NH_2—CH—CH_2—SH	343 (323–364)	1.6 at 200 mg/kg
MEA-PO_3	NH_2—CH_2—CH—SH_2PO_3	777 (700–864)	2.1 at 500 mg/kg

TABLE 9.2

Two Radioprotectors in Practical Use

Compound	Structure	Use
WR-638	$NH_2CH_2CH_2SPO_3HNa$	Carried in field pack by Russian army (cystaphos)
WR-2721	$NH_2(CH_2)_3NHCH_2CH_2SPO_3H_2$	Protector in radiotherapy and carried by U.S. astronauts on lunar trips (amifostine)

Comparison of Gastrointestinal and Hematopoietic Dose-Reduction Factors in Mice for these Radioprotectors (the Two Compounds Listed Above)

		Dose-Reduction Factor	
Compound	Drug Dose, mg/kg	7 Days (Gastrointestinal)	30 Days (Hematopoietic)
WR-638	500	1.6	2.1
WR-2721	900	1.8	2.7

The structures of two typical compounds of the more than 4,000 synthesized in the Walter Reed series are shown in Table 9.2. The first compound, WR-638, called *cystaphos*, was said to be carried routinely in the field pack of Soviet infantry in Europe during the Cold War for use in the event of a nuclear conflict.

The second compound, WR-2721, now known as *amifostine*, is perhaps the most effective of those synthesized in the Walter Reed series. It gives good protection to the blood-forming organs, as can be seen by the dose-reduction factor for 30-day death in mice, which approaches the theoretic maximum value of 3. It was probably the compound carried by U.S. astronauts on their trips to the moon, to be used if a solar event occurred. On these missions, when the space vehicle left Earth's orbit and began coasting toward the moon, the astronauts were committed to a 14-day mission, because they did not have sufficient fuel to turn around without first orbiting the moon and using its gravitational field. If there had been a major solar event in that period, the astronauts would have been exposed to a shower of high-energy protons, resulting in an estimated dose of several gray (several hundred rad). The availability of a radioprotector with a dose-reduction factor of between 2 and 3 would have been very important in such a circumstance. As it turned out, no major solar event occurred during any manned lunar mission. The potential for this problem will be greatly magnified in future missions to Mars, which may take as long as three years.

AMIFOSTINE (WR-2721) AS A RADIOPROTECTOR IN RADIOTHERAPY

The only radioprotective drug approved by the FDA for use in radiation therapy is amifostine (WR-2721), sold under the trade name Ethyol for use in the prevention of xerostomia in patients treated for head and neck cancer. The Radiotherapy Oncology Group (RTOG) conducted a phase III randomized clinical trial, which demonstrated the efficacy of amifostine in reducing xerostomia in head and neck cancer patients receiving radiotherapy without prejudice to early tumor control. The drug was administered daily, 30 minutes before each dose fraction in a multifraction regimen. Three months posttreatment, the incidence of xerostomia was significantly reduced in those patients treated with amifostine. There was an improvement in the patients' assessments of such symptoms as dry mouth and difficulty in eating or speaking and in the need for fluids and oral comfort aids. There was no difference in locoregional tumor control between patients who received the radioprotector and those who did not. Giving the amifostine only 30 minutes before each treatment was designed to exploit the slower rate at which the drug penetrates tumors relative to normal tissues.

Amifostine is a phosphorothioate that is nonreactive and does not readily permeate cells, primarily because of its terminal phosphorothioic acid group. It is therefore a "prodrug." When dephosphorylated by the enzyme alkaline phosphatase, which is present in high concentrations in normal tissues and capillaries, it is converted to the active metabolite designated WR-1065. This metabolite readily enters normal cells by facilitated diffusion and scavenges free radicals generated by ionizing radiations or by drugs used in chemotherapy such as alkylating agents.

It might have been expected that radioprotectors would enjoy a wider use in radiation therapy, but in practice, clinical use continues to be plagued by issues relating to possible tumor protection and loss of therapeutic gain. The potential use of such protectors is based on the observation from animal studies that amifostine quickly floods normal tissues but penetrates more slowly into tumors. Consequently, if the radiation dose is given within minutes after the administration of the radioprotector, there is a differential sparing of normal tissue compared with tumor cells. Because one can never be sure that the tumor is not protected to some extent, the use of radioprotectors is not "fail safe." For this reason, radioprotectors are not widely used in radiotherapy, indeed in practice they are used only for the reduction of xerostomia.

RADIOPROTECTORS AND CHEMOTHERAPY

Although sulfhydryl compounds were developed initially as radioprotectors against ionizing radiation, they also protect against the cytotoxic effects of a number of chemotherapeutic agents. The experimental clinical use of amifostine has shown that the compound offers significant protection against nephrotoxicity, ototoxicity, and neuropathy from cisplatin and hematologic toxicity from cyclophosphamide. The same experimental studies indicated no obvious antitumor activity of the radioprotector, implying a differential uptake between normal and malignant tissues.

OTHER USES OF AMIFOSTINE

While the emphasis for the development of amifostine was to protect against cell killing, this compound also protects against radiation-induced mutagenesis and oncogenic transformation in cells in culture and against carcinogenesis in mouse model systems. Furthermore, while a dose of about 400 mg/kg is required to demonstrate optimal cytoprotection—a dose that carries with it significant side effects—its antimutagenic effect persists at a dose as low as 25 mg/km, which is nontoxic. The proposed mechanism of this effect is not explained by the antioxidant properties, since the effect occurs even when cells are exposed to amifostine up to 3 hours following irradiation. Rather, it has been proposed that the polyamine-like properties of the phosphorothioates may result in a stabilization of DNA-damaged sites, facilitating a slower and more error-free repair of damage.

Following the destruction of the World Trade Center on September 11, 2001, and the rise of a nuclear terrorism threat, there has been a revived interest in the development of novel effective and nontoxic radioprotectors for potential use in homeland defense as well as in medical applications.

Summary of Pertinent Conclusions

- Radioprotectors are chemicals that reduce the biologic effects of radiation.
- The sulfhydryl compounds cysteine and cysteamine were discovered early but are toxic. If the SH group is covered by a phosphate group, toxicity is reduced.
- The mechanism of action is the scavenging of free radicals and restitution of free-radical damage, although this is not the whole story.
- The dose-reduction factor (DRF) is the ratio of radiation doses required to produce the same biologic effect in the absence and presence of the radioprotector.
- The best available radioprotectors can attain dose-reduction factor values of 2.5 to 3.0 for bone-marrow death in mice irradiated with x-rays.
- Dose-reduction factor values close to the oxygen enhancement ratio are possible for γ-rays, but the effectiveness of radioprotectors decreases with increasing linear energy transfer.
- During the Cold War, it is said that Soviet infantry in Europe carried radioprotectors for use in a possible nuclear war. Radioprotectors were carried to the moon by U.S. astronauts to be used in the event of a solar flare.

(continued)

Summary of Pertinent Conclusions (Continued)

- More than 4,000 compounds were synthesized by the U.S. Army in studies conducted at the Walter Reed Institute of Research. Amifostine (WR-2721) appears to be the best for use in conjunction with radiotherapy.
- Amifostine, sold under the trade name Ethyol, is the only radioprotective drug approved by the FDA for use in the prevention of xerostomia in patients treated for head and neck cancer.
- An RTOG phase III trial demonstrated the efficacy of amifostine in reducing xerostomia in patients with head and neck cancer receiving radiation therapy without affecting locoregional control. The radioprotector was administered 30 minutes before radiation.
- Amifostine is a "prodrug" that is unreactive and that penetrates poorly into cells until it is dephosphorylated by the enzyme alkaline phosphatase to the active metabolite WR-1065.
- The rationale for the use of phosphorothioate radioprotectors is that they flood normal tissues rapidly after administration but penetrate tumors much more slowly. The strategy is to begin irradiation soon after administration of the drug to exploit a differential effect.
- The clinical use of radioprotectors in radiation therapy continues to be plagued by issues relating to possible tumor protection and diminution of therapeutic gain.
- Amifostine is useful as a protector for chemotherapy as well as radiotherapy. It is reported to offer protection against nephrotoxicity, ototoxicity, and neuropathy from cisplatin and hematologic toxicity from cyclophosphamide, without reduction of tumor activity.
- A dose of 400 mg/kg is required for optimal cytoprotection, which is toxic with many side effects, but its antimutagenic effect persists at a low nontoxic dose of 25 mg/kg.
- The antimutagenic effect of amifostine is not explained by its antioxidant properties, since it occurs if the drug is added 3 hours following irradiation, but is likely due to its polyamine-like properties, which may stabilize DNA-damaged sites and promote error-free repair.
- Following the destruction of the World Trade Center on September 11, 2001, and the rise of a nuclear terrorism threat, there has been a revived interest in the development of novel, effective, and nontoxic radioprotectors for potential use in homeland defense as well as in medical applications.

BIBLIOGRAPHY

Brizel DM, Overgaard J: Does amifostine have a role in chemoradiation treatment? *Lancet Oncol* 4(6):378–381, 2003

Brizel D, Sauer R, Wannenmacher M, Henke M, Eschwege F, Wasserman T: Randomized phase III trial of radiation ± amifostine in patients with head and neck cancer [abstract 1487]. *Proceedings of ASCO* 17, 1998

Bump EA, Malaker K (eds): *Radioprotectors: Chemical, Biological and Clinical Perspectives.* Boca Raton, CRC Press, 1997

Grdina DJ, Kataoka Y, Basic I, Perrin J: The radioprotector WR-2721 reduces neutron-induced mutations at the hypozanthine-guanine phosphoribosyl transferase locus in mouse splenocytes when administered prior to or following irradiation. *Carcinogenesis* 13:811–814, 1992

Grdina DJ, Kataoka Y, Murley JS: Amifostine: Mechanisms of action underlying cytoprotection and chemoprevention. *Drug Metabol Drug Inter* 16(4):237–279, 2000

Grdina DJ, Murley JS, Kataoka Y: Radioprotectants: Current status and new directions. *Oncology* 63(suppl 2):2–10, 2002

Grdina DJ, Shigematsu N, Dale P, et al.: Thiol and disulfide metabolites of the radiation protector and potential chemopreventive agent WR 2721 are linked to both its anticytotoxic and antimutagenic mechanisms of action. *Carcinogenesis* 16:767–774, 1995

Liu T, Liu Y, He S, Zhang Z, Kligerman MM: Use of radiation with or without WR-2721 in advanced rectal cancer. *Cancer* 69:2820–2825, 1992

Patt HM, Tyree B, Straube RL, Smith DE: Cysteine protection against x-irradiation. *Science* 110:213–214, 1949

Rasey JS, Nelson NJ, Mahler P, Anderson K, Krohn KA, Menard T: Radioprotection of normal tissues against gamma-rays and cyclotron neutrons with WR2721: LD50 studies and 35S-WR2721 biodistribution. *Radiat Res* 97:598–607, 1984

Sweeney TR: *A Survey of Compounds from the Antiradiations Drug Development Program of the US Army*

Medical Research and Development Command. Washington, DC, Walter Reed Army Institute of Research, 1979

Utley JF, Marlowe C, Waddell WJ: Distribution of 35S-labeled WR-2721 in normal and malignant tissues of the mouse. *Radiat Res* 68:284–291, 1976

Yuhas J: Active versus passive absorption kinetics as the basis for selective protection of normal tissues by S-2-(3-aminopropylamino)-ethyl-phosphorothioic acid. *Cancer Res* 40:1519–1524, 1980

Yuhas JM: Differential chemoprotection of normal and malignant tissues. *J Natl Cancer Inst* 42:331–335, 1969

CHAPTER 10

Radiation Carcinogenesis

DETERMINISTIC AND STOCHASTIC EFFECTS

If cellular damage occurs as a result of radiation and it is not adequately repaired, it may prevent the cell from surviving or reproducing or it may result in a viable cell that has been modified, that is, suffered a change or mutation that it retains as a legacy of the radiation exposure. The two outcomes have profoundly different implications for the person of whom the cell is a part.

Most organs or tissues of the body are unaffected by the loss of a few cells; but if the number of cells lost is sufficiently large, there is observable harm, reflecting the loss of tissue function. The probability of such harm is zero at small radiation doses, but above some level of dose, calledthe *threshold dose*, the probability increases rapidly with dose to 100%. Above the threshold, the severity of harm also increases with dose. Effects such as this are said to be *deterministic*. A deterministic effect has a threshold in dose, and the severity of the effect is dose related. Radiation-induced cataracts are an example.

The outcome is very different if the irradiated cell is viable but modified. Carcinogenesis and hereditary effects fall into this category. If somatic cells are exposed to radiation, the probability of cancer increases with dose, probably with no threshold, but the severity of the cancer is not dose related. A cancer induced by 1 Gy (100 rad) is no worse than one induced by 0.1 Gy (10 rad), but of course the probability of its induction is increased. This category of effect is called *stochastic*, a word that has been given a special meaning in radiation protection but in general just means "random." If the radiation damage occurs in germ cells, mutations may occur that could cause deleterious effects in future generations. Again, there is probably no threshold, and the severity of hereditary effects is not dose related, although the probability of it occurring is.

The belief that stochastic effects have no dose threshold is based on the molecular mechanisms involved. There is no reason to believe that even a single x-ray photon could not result in a base change leading to a mutation that could cause cancer or a hereditary defect. For this reason, it is considered prudent to assume that no dose is too small to be effective.

The two types of effects are summarized as follows:

Deterministic effect: severity increases with dose; practical threshold; probability of occurrence increases with dose; e.g., cataract.

Stochastic effect: severity independent of dose; probability of occurrance increases with dose; no threshold; e.g., cancer.

CARCINOGENESIS: THE HUMAN EXPERIENCE

Cancer induction is the most important somatic effect of low-dose ionizing radiation. In sharp contrast to the case for the hereditary effects of radiation (Chapter 11), risk estimates for leukemogenesis and carcinogenesis do not rely on animal data but can be based on experience in humans. There is a long history of a link between radiation exposure and an elevated incidence of cancer. Figure 10.1 is a beautiful photograph of Marie Curie and her daughter Irene, who are both thought to have died of leukemia as a result of the radiation exposure they received while conducting their experiments with radioactivity. Figure 10.2 is a photograph of the hand of a dentist in New York who held x-ray films in patients' mouths for many years and who suffered malignant changes as a result. Quantitative data on cancer induction by radiation come from populations irradiated for medical purposes or exposed deliberately or inadvertently to nuclear weapons. Persons exposed therapeutically received comparatively high doses, and their susceptibility to the effects of radiation might have been influenced by the medical condition for which treatment was being given. Those exposed to γ-rays and neutrons from nuclear weapons represent a wider cross section in terms of health and also include individuals exposed to lower doses. In both cases, dose rates were high and exposure times brief.

There are a few groups of exposed individuals to whom these generalizations do not apply.

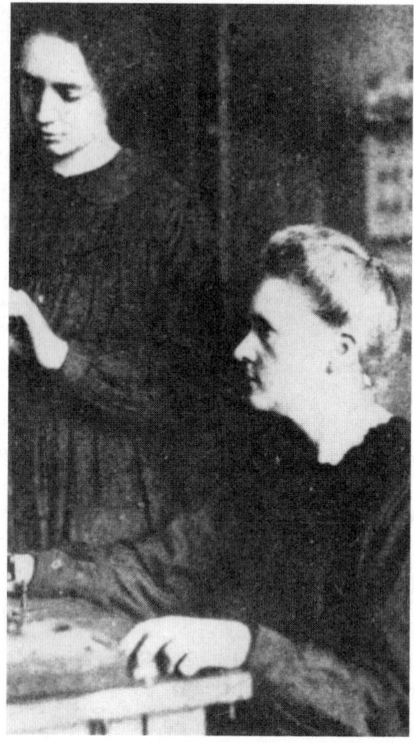

FIGURE 10.1 • Marie Curie (seated) at work with her daughter Irene. Both are thought to have died of leukemia as a consequence of the radiation exposure they received during their experiments with radioactivity. (Courtesy of the Austrian Radium Institute and the International Atomic Energy Bulletin.)

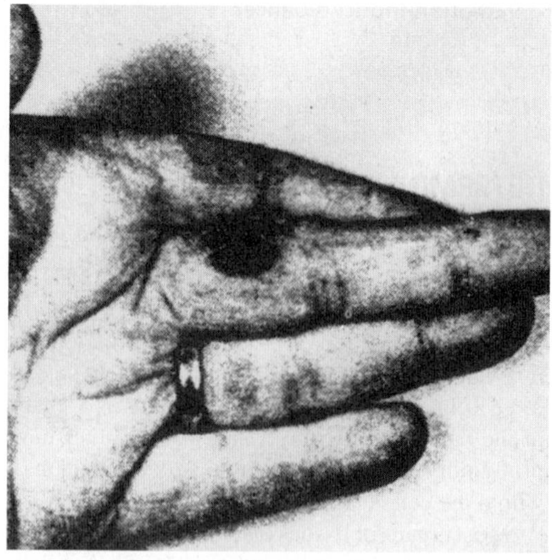

FIGURE 10.2 • Hand of a dentist who for 35 years held x-ray films in place in patients' mouths. The thumb has been partially amputated. Damaged skin on the fingers has been replaced by grafts. The lesion on the finger is a skin cancer subsequently removed. (Courtesy of Dr. Victor Bond, Brookhaven National Laboratory.)

Examples include pitchblende and uranium miners who inhaled the radioactive gas radon and its progeny products over a prolonged period of time, patients injected with radium chloride or Thorotrast for medical purposes, and individuals who ingested radionuclides while painting luminous dials on clocks and watches with paint containing radium. A large number of workers have been exposed occupationally, but the study of these workers has so far yielded few useful quantitative data on cancer risk estimates, except for miners exposed to radon.

The early human experience of radiation-induced cancer may be summarized as follows:

1. Skin cancer and leukemia were common in early x-ray workers, principally physicists and engineers who worked around accelerators before radiation safety standards were introduced.
2. Lung cancer was a frequent problem in pitchblende miners in Saxony, who dug out the ore from which radium was extracted. In the years following World War II, lung cancer also was noted in uranium miners in the central Colorado plateau. In both cases, the mines were poorly ventilated and there was a buildup of radon gas in the atmosphere of the mine; radon and its progeny were inhaled by the miners, depositing atoms of radioactive material in their lungs. The intense local α-radiation was responsible for inducing lung tumors.
3. Bone tumors were observed in the radium dial painters. The painters were mostly young women who worked in factories in which the luminous dials on clocks and watches were painted with a special paint preparation containing radium. The workers dipped their brushes into the radium paint and used their tongues to shape the brushes into sharp points to paint the small dials on watches. As a result, some radium was ingested, which, because it is in the same group of the periodic table as calcium, was deposited in the tips of the growing bones. The intense α-radiation produced bone tumors. There is also history of bone tumors in people who, in the 1920s and 1930s, received injections of radium salts for the treatment of tuberculosis or ankylosing spondylitis.
4. An excess incidence of liver tumors was reported in patients in whom the contrast material Thorotrast was used. Thorotrast contains radioactive thorium, which, when deposited in the liver, produced a small incidence of liver tumors by α-radiation.

These early examples are interesting but largely anecdotal, although they did alert scientists to the danger of radiation exposure. None of these examples involved situations that now constitute a public health hazard; these problems will never happen again, and the dosimetry in each instance is so uncertain that it is rarely possible to deduce any quantitative relationship between the dose of radiation involved and the tumor incidence.

More recent examples of the human experience with radiation-induced cancer and leukemia include the following:

1. The Japanese survivors of the atomic-bomb attacks on Hiroshima and Nagasaki are the most important single group studied because of their large number, the care with which they have been followed, and the fact that individuals of all ages and both sexes received a wide range of doses. About 120,000 people have been followed carefully, of whom about 50,000 received doses in excess of 0.005 Sv (0.5 rem). By 1990, there had been 6,000 deaths from cancer, of which about 400 were considered to be an excess mortality caused by radiation. The weapons used on the two cities were very different. The one used on Nagasaki was of a type that would be expected to emit α-rays with few neutrons and had been previously tested, so dosimetry is based partly on measurements. The weapon used at Hiroshima was of a type never tested before or since, so that dose estimates are based largely on computer simulations. The radiation from this weapon was a mixture of neutrons and γ-rays. In 1986, the dosimetry relating to the atomic bombs was revised. Computer simulations indicated that the proportion of neutrons, especially at Hiroshima, was lower than previously thought, and the γ-ray doses at greater distances were higher. The net effect was to increase cancer risk estimates substantially. The 1998 report of the United Nations Scientific Committee on Effects of Atomic Radiation (UNSCEAR) and the 1990 report of the Committee on Biologic Effects of Ionizing Radiation (BEIR V) summarized the new estimates. The numeric values are discussed later in this chapter.
2. In Britain, from 1935 through 1944, some 14,000 patients suffering from ankylosing spondylitis were given radiotherapy to various regions of their spine to relieve pain. A small risk of leukemia mortality has been reported in these individuals. Although the spondylitic series provides one of the largest bodies of data on leukemia in humans after exposure to x- or γ-radiation, and the dosimetry is quite good, it is far from ideal, because it lacks a proper control, consisting of patients with the same disease who did not receive x-ray therapy but whose

treatment was otherwise the same. A possible contribution of carcinogenic drugs to the tumor incidence also has been suggested.

3. There is also documentation of an elevated incidence of leukemia in radiologists who joined learned societies before about 1922, before the introduction of radiation safety standards. This will be discussed later in the chapter.
4. Thyroid cancer has been observed in children who received radiotherapy for what was thought to be an enlarged thymus. The thyroid was included in the treatment field, and both malignant and benign thyroid tumors have been observed. Breast cancer is also elevated in these individuals.
5. As recently as the 1950s, it was common practice to use x-rays to epilate children suffering from *tinea capitis* (ringworm of the scalp). An increased incidence of thyroid cancer from this practice was first reported by Modan and his colleagues in Israel, who treated a large number of immigrant children from North Africa in whom ringworm of the scalp reached epidemic proportions. There was also a significantly increased risk of brain tumors, salivary gland tumors, skin cancer, and leukemia mortality. A comparable group of children in New York for whom x-rays were used for epilation before treatment for tinea capitis show quite different results. There were only two malignant thyroid tumors in addition to some benign tumors. There is, however, an incidence of skin cancer around the face and scalp in those areas also subject to sunlight. The skin tumors arose only in white children, and there were no tumors in black children in the New York series.
6. Patients with tuberculosis, who were fluoroscoped many hundreds of times during artificial pneumothorax, have shown an elevated incidence of breast cancer. This was first reported in Nova Scotia, but the report was confirmed by a similar study in New England. The doses these patients received are uncertain but must have been about 0.8 to 0.9 Gy (80–90 rad), because some of the women developed skin changes in the chest wall on the side frequently fluoroscoped. Patients who received radiotherapy for postpartum mastitis were also shown to have an excess incidence of breast cancer.

THE LATENT PERIOD

The time interval between irradiation and the appearance of a malignancy is known as the **latent period**.

Leukemia has the shortest latent period. Excess cases began to appear in the survivors of Hiroshima and Nagasaki a few years after irradiation and reached a peak by 5 to 7 years; most cases occurred in the first 15 years. Solid tumors show a longer latency than the leukemias, on the order of anything from 10 to 60 years or more. For example, an excess incidence of solid tumors is still evident in Japanese survivors exposed to radiation from the atomic bombs in 1945. Indeed, for solid cancers, the excess risk is apparently more like a lifelong elevation of the natural age-specific cancer risk.

As the Japanese data have matured, the concept of a fixed time interval between irradiation and the appearance of the malignancy has been replaced by the concept of "age at expression." Regardless of the age at the time of exposure, radiation-induced solid tumors tend to be expressed later in life, at the same time as spontaneous tumors of the same type. Breast cancer in women is the most striking example. This suggests that although radiation may initiate the carcinogenic process at a young age, additional steps are required later in life, some of which may well be hormone-dependent.

ASSESSING THE RISK

To use the available human data to estimate risks as a function of dose, it is necessary to fit the data to a model. There are several reasons for this:

1. Data obtained at relatively high doses must be extrapolated to the low doses of public health concern.
2. No large human population exposed to radiation has yet been studied for its full life span, and so estimates must be projected into the future. For example, in the year 2000, about half of the Japanese survivors irradiated in 1945 were still alive.
3. The best data pertain to the Japanese irradiated by the atomic bombs, and risk estimates based on this must be transferred to other populations that have quite different characteristics, including their natural cancer incidence.

There are two types of models that are conceptually quite different: the absolute risk model and the relative risk model. The **absolute risk model** assumes that radiation induces a "crop" of cancers over and above the natural incidence and unrelated to it. The **relative risk model** assumes that the effect of radiation is to increase the natural incidence *at all ages* subsequent to exposure by a given factor. Because the natural or spontaneous cancer incidence rises significantly in old age, the relative risk model predicts a large number of radiation-induced cancers in old age.

The model favored by the BEIR committee, for the assessment of the cancer risks from the Japanese atomic-bomb survivors is the **time-dependent relative risk model**. The excess incidence of cancer was assumed to be a function of dose, the square of the dose, age at exposure, and time since exposure. For some tumors, gender must be added as a variable—for example, in the case of breast cancer.

COMMITTEES CONCERNED WITH RISK ESTIMATES AND RADIATION PROTECTION

There are two series of reports that analyze available data and come up with risk estimates for radiation-induced cancer. The first is the United Nations Scientific Committee on the Effects of Atomic Radiation (UNSCEAR) reports. This committee reports to the General Assembly at regular intervals; the most recent report appeared in 2000. The second is the committee of the U.S. National Academy of Sciences known as the Committee on the Biologic Effects of Ionizing Radiation (BEIR). Reports appear periodically, the most recent comprehensive report (BEIR V) appearing in 1990. To a large, extent, these are "scholarly" committees, inasmuch as they are under no compulsion to draw conclusions if data are not available.

On the other hand, there are committees involved with radiation protection that cannot afford to be scholarly, because they must make recommendations whether or not adequate data are available. First, there is the International Commission on Radiological Protection (ICRP). This commission originally was set up and funded by the first International Congress of Radiology. Over the years, the funding base of this commission has broadened, and it has assumed the role of an independent self-propagating committee. At a national level in the United States, there is the National Council on Radiological Protection and Measurements (NCRP). This is an independent body chartered by Congress and funded from industry, government grants, and professional societies. The NCRP formulates policies for radiation protection in the United States, often but not always following the lead of the ICRP. The recommendations of the NCRP carry no weight in law but are almost always adopted and enforced by the regulatory agencies. (See Chapter 15 on radiation protection for more regarding these committees.)

RADIATION-INDUCED CANCER IN HUMAN POPULATIONS

Under appropriate conditions, a malignancy can be induced in essentially all tissues of the body. Some of the most common are discussed below.

Leukemia

The incidence of chronic lymphocytic leukemia does not appear to be affected by radiation. Acute and chronic myeloid leukemia are the types chiefly responsible for the excess incidence observed in irradiated adults. Susceptibility to acute lymphatic, or stem-cell, leukemia seems to be highest in childhood and to decrease sharply during maturation.

Two principal population groups provide data to determine risk estimates:

1. Survivors of the atomic-bomb attacks on Hiroshima and Nagasaki.
2. Patients treated for ankylosing spondylitis.

Thyroid Cancer

The thyroid gland is an organ of high sensitivity for radiation carcinogenesis, at least in children; in adults, radiation is much less efficient in inducing thyroid cancer. The malignant tumors that have been produced, however, consistently have been of a histologically well-differentiated type, which develops slowly and often can be removed completely by surgery or treated successfully with radioactive iodine if metastasized; consequently, these tumors show a low mortality rate. It is estimated that about 5% of those with radiation-induced thyroid cancer die as a result.

Here are the principal population groups available for deriving risk estimates for thyroid cancer:

1. Survivors of the atomic-bomb attacks on Hiroshima and Nagasaki.
2. Residents of the Marshall Islands exposed to external radiation and ingested iodine-131 from fallout after the 1954 testing of a thermonuclear device, in whom there was a high incidence of nodule formation and some thyroid cancer (benign as well as malignant tumors).
3. Individuals who ingested radioactive iodine as a result of the Chernobyl accident (this experience shows how very sensitive children are and that adults are relatively resistant).
4. Children treated with x-rays for an enlarged thymus.
5. Children treated for diseases of the tonsils and nasopharynx.

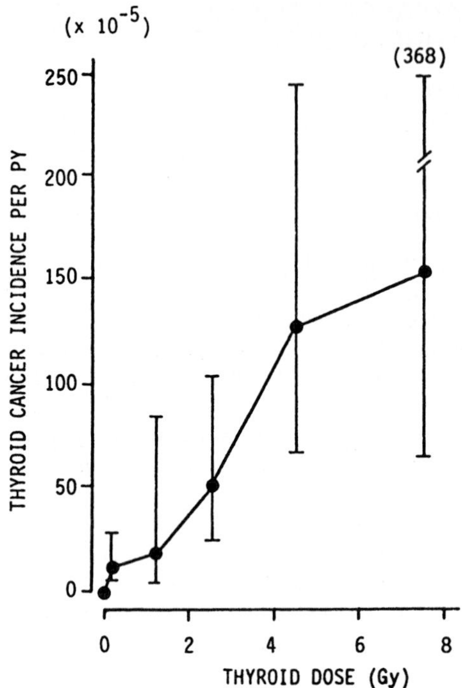

FIGURE 10.3 • Thyroid cancer incidence per person-year (PY) as a function of the radiation dose in the thyroid. Rates adjusted for gender, ethnicity, and interval after irradiation. Error bars represent 90% confidence limits. (From Shore RE, Woodard E, Hildreth N, et al.: Thyroid tumors following thymus irradiation. *JNCI* 74:1177–1184, 1985, with permission.)

6. Children epilated with x-rays for the treatment of tinea capitis.
7. Children treated for cancer.

Figure 10.3 shows the incidence of thyroid cancer per person-year as a function of thyroid dose, from the New York series of children treated for enlarged thymus.

Breast Cancer

Breast cancer may be induced with relatively high frequency by radiation. The cancer is of the type arising initially from duct cells but commonly is found to infiltrate breast tissue.

There are three principal exposed populations from which the risk of breast cancer incidence may be derived:

1. Japanese female survivors of the atomic-bomb attacks on Hiroshima and Nagasaki.
2. Female patients in a Nova Scotia sanatorium subjected to multiple fluoroscopies during artificial pneumothorax for pulmonary tuberculosis. There is doubt about the dosimetry, but the dose to breast tissue per fluoroscopy is estimated to have been 0.04 to 0.2 Gy (4–20 rad). The number of examinations commonly exceeded 100, and in some instances women received more than 500 fluoroscopies; three patients, in fact, developed radiation dermatitis. This group of exposed women probably constitutes the most convincing evidence of the production of cancer by fractionated x-rays used for diagnosis. This Canadian study also showed the importance of age at the time of exposure. The study was later confirmed by the follow-up of patients discharged from two tuberculosis sanatoria in Massachusetts. These patients were examined fluoroscopically an average of 102 times over a period of years and subsequently were found to be 80% more likely to develop breast cancer than a comparable unexposed population.
3. Females treated for postpartum mastitis and other benign conditions. Patients typically received 1 to 6 Gy (100–600 rad) and showed an excess incidence of breast cancer compared with the general female population of New York State. A legitimate objection to the use of these data for risk estimates is the uncertainty as to whether postpartum mastitis predisposes to breast cancer.

The data for excess incidence of breast cancer in these populations are shown in Figure 10.4. A number of interesting points are immediately apparent. First, the data from the New York series of postpartum mastitis patients are so poor that they do not give any clue as to the shape of the dose–response relationship. Second, there is a marked difference in the natural incidence of breast cancer in Japanese women, in whom it is low, compared with American and Canadian women, in whom it is high; nevertheless, in all cases, incidence rises with radiation dose. Third, the data for breast cancer are reasonably well fitted by a straight line.

Lung Cancer

Radiation is but one of a long list of carcinogens for lung cancer: Cigarette smoking, asbestos, chromium salts, mustard gas, hematite, and asphalt derivatives have also been implicated. Radiation risk estimates come from two principal sources:

1. Individuals exposed to external sources of radiation, including the Japanese survivors and those with the ankylosing spondylitis. An excess was found even when smoking was taken into account.

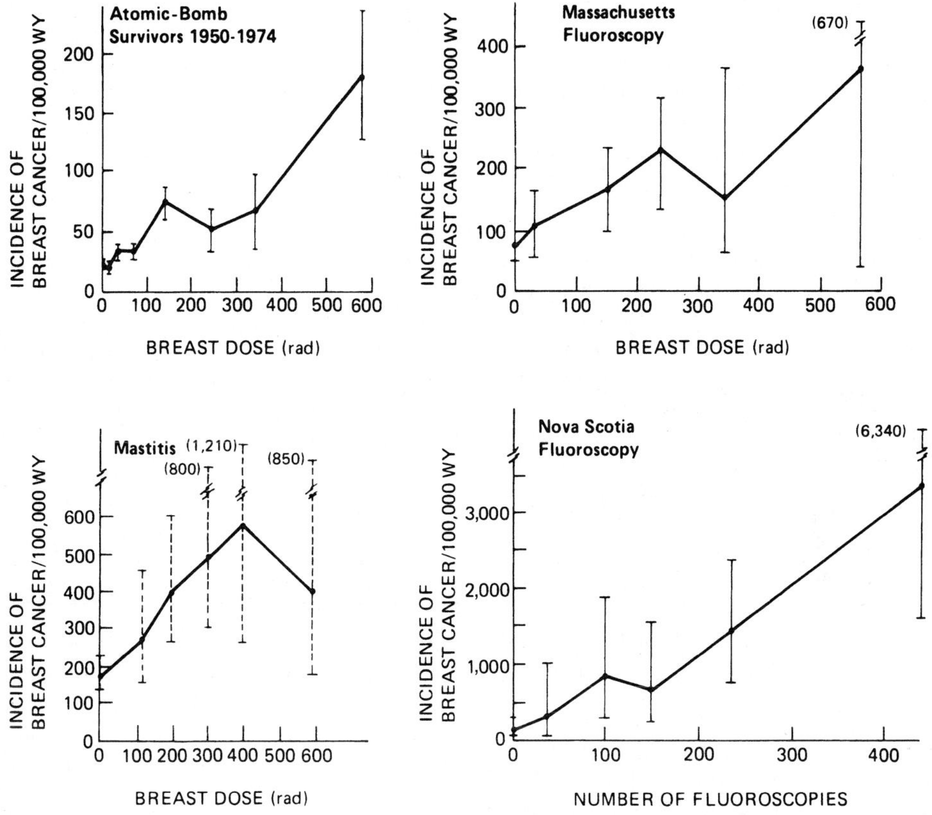

FIGURE 10.4 ● Incidence of breast cancer as a function of dose for four human populations that allow risk estimates to be made. The data are expressed in terms of the number of cases per 100,000 women-years (WY). Note that the natural incidence of breast cancer is low in Japanese women and high in American and Canadian women. (From Boice JD Jr, Land CE, Shore RE, Norman JE, Tokunaga M: Risk of breast cancer following low-dose exposure. *Radiology* 131:589–597, 1979, with permission.)

2. Underground miners exposed to radon in the mine atmosphere. The naturally occurring deposits of radioactive materials in the rocks of the earth decay through a long series of steps until they reach a stable isotope of lead. One of these steps involves radon, which, unlike the other elements in the decay series, is a gas. In the closed environment of a mine, workers inhale radon gas, and some radon atoms decay to the next member of the radioactive series, a solid, which consequently is deposited on the bronchial epithelium. Subsequent steps in the radioactive decay series take place in the lungs, causing intense α-irradiation of localized surrounding tissue.

There is a clear excess of lung cancer among workers in the uranium mines of the Colorado plateau in the United States, the uranium mines in Czechoslovakia, the nonuranium mines in Sweden, and the fluorspar mines in Newfoundland. It remains difficult to separate adequately the contributory effects of radon and cigarette smoking in causing the cancers, because there are too few nonsmoking miners to form an adequate control group. In addition, the average duration of exposure usually spans 15 to 20 years, during which standards of safety and ventilation have changed substantially. In any case, it is no easy matter to estimate the dose to the critical cells in the basal layer of the epithelium of the lung from knowledge of the radon concentration in the air that is breathed. There is also some evidence, summarized in the BEIR VI report, of an excess of lung cancer from domestic radon exposure. It is estimated that 10% of the 150,000 lung cancer deaths annually in the United States are due to radon.

Bone Cancer

There is some evidence of bone cancer induced by external x-irradiation in children epilated for the treatment of tinea capitis and in patients treated for ankylosing spondylitis. The numbers are small and the risk estimates poor. The largest body of data comes from two populations, each of which ingested isotopes of radium that emit high linear energy transfer α-particles and that follow the metabolic pathways of calcium in the body to become deposited in the bone. The populations include:

1. Young persons, mostly women, employed as dial painters, who ingested radium as a result of licking their brushes into a sharp point for application of luminous paint to watches and clocks. In this group there have been bone sarcomas and carcinomas of epithelial cells lining the paranasal sinuses and nasopharynx. None of these tumors occurred at doses below 5 Gy (500 rad); above this level, the incidence rose sharply, particularly the sarcomas. The radium in these paints consisted of the isotopes radium-226 and radium-228, with half-lives of about 1,600 years and 6 years, respectively.
2. Patients given injections of radium-224 for the treatment of tuberculosis or ankylosing spondylitis.

Three points need to be emphasized. First, the dose is made up of α-particles, which have a short range and deposit their energy close to the site at which the isotope is deposited; α-particles are also more effective than x-rays by a factor of about 20. Second, osteosarcomas arise predominantly from endosteal cells, and the relevant dose for estimating the risk of sarcoma is the dose to these cells, which lie at a distance of up to 10 μm from the bone surface, rather than the mean dose throughout the bone. Radium-224 has a short half-life (3.6 days), and its radiation therefore largely is delivered while it is still present on the bone surface. This contrasts sharply with radium-226 and radium-228, which have long half-lives and consequently become distributed throughout bone during their periods of radioactive decay. The dose to endosteal cells from radium-224 is about nine times larger than the dose averaged throughout bone, whereas it is about two thirds of the mean bone value from radium-226. Consequently, it is difficult to compare data from the two groups of people who were exposed to these very different isotopes of radium. Third, age at the time of exposure is an important factor in the development of bone cancer. For young persons, and possibly also for those exposed *in utero*, the rapid deposition of bone-seeking radioisotopes during active bone growth might confer a higher risk of cancer than in adults. There is, in general, poor agreement among the risk estimates derived from the various groups of persons showing an excess of bone cancer, so that risk estimates must be very crude. Figure 10.5 shows the incidence of bone sarcoma in female dial painters as a function of activity of radium ingested. These data imply that a linear extrapolation from high to low doses would overestimate risks at low doses. It appears that sarcomas are induced only after large doses that are sufficient to cause tissue damage and therefore to stimulate cell proliferation.

Skin Cancer

The first neoplasm attributed to x-rays was an epidermoid carcinoma on the hand of a radiologist, which was reported in 1902. In the years that

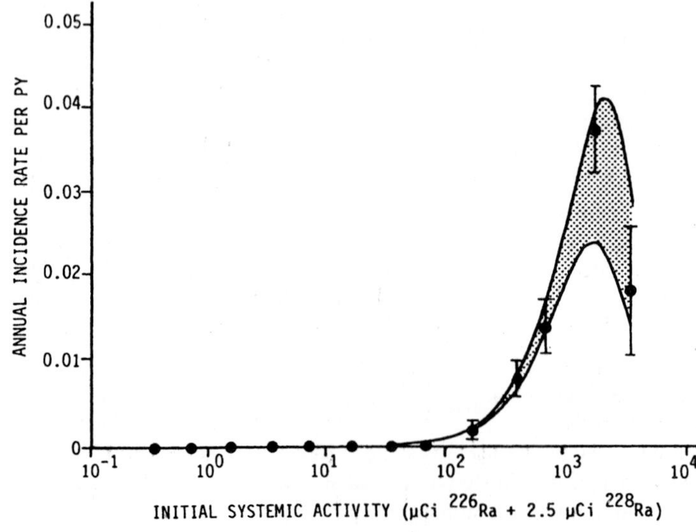

FIGURE 10.5 • A semilogarithmic plot of bone sarcoma incidence rate as a function of systemic intake for female dial painters employed before 1950, showing a dose-squared exponential fit. The shaded band indicates the range covered by the fitted function if the coefficients are allowed to vary by ±1 standard deviation. (From Rowland R, Stehner AF, Lucas HF: Dose–response relationships for radium-induced bone sarcomas. *Health Phys* 44:15–31, 1983, with permission.)

TABLE 10.1

Summary of the 1958–1994 Cancer Incidence Data in A-Bomb Survivors

Colon Dose, Sv	Number of Subjects	Solid Cancers	Estimated Excess
Beyond >3,000 m	23,493	3,230	0
<0.005 Sv within <3,000 m	10,159	1,301	1
0.005–0.1	30,524	4,119	77
0.1–0.2	4,775	739	60
0.2–0.5	5,862	982	164
0.5–1	3,048	582	177
1–2	1,570	376	165
>2	470	126	80

Based on Pierce DA, Preston DL: Radiation-related cancer risks at low doses among atomic bomb survivors. *Radiation Research* 154:178–186, 2003.

followed, several hundred such cases arose among physicians, dentists, physicists, and x-ray technicians, in an era in which safety standards were virtually nonexistent. In most cases, the onset of neoplasms followed chronic radiodermatitis and a long latent period. Squamous cell and basal cell carcinomas have been most frequently observed, and occasionally a sarcoma of the subcutaneous tissues has been seen. Since the evolution of modern safety standards, epidermoid carcinoma has ceased to be an occupational disease of radiation workers.

Radiation-induced skin cancers are diagnosed readily and treated at an early stage of development, and there is a large difference between rates of incidence and mortality. There is a small excess incidence of skin cancer in the children epilated with x-rays for the treatment of tinea capitis.

QUANTITATIVE RISK ESTIMATES FOR RADIATION-INDUCED CANCER

Despite a diverse collection of data for cancer in humans from medical sources, both the BEIR V and the latest UNSCEAR reports elected to base their risk estimates almost entirely on the data from the survivors of the atomic-bomb attacks on Hiroshima and Nagasaki.

Table 10.1 shows a summary of the data for cancer incidence in the atomic-bomb survivors for the years 1958–1994. The raw data are shown principally to emphasize the relative poverty of the data; only a few hundred excess cancer cases caused by radiation are involved, compared with many thousands of naturally occurring malignancies—and these must be allocated to different dose groups and different sites.

Figure 10.6 shows the data for cancer incidence in the A-bomb survivors for the years 1958–1994. The relative risk is a linear function of dose up to about 2 Sv (200 rem). Over the lower-dose range from 0 to 0.5 Sv (0–50 rem), there is a suggestion that the risks are slightly higher than the linear extrapolation from higher doses. There is some uncertainty in the control group, i.e., the zero-dose group, used for comparison. There are in fact two zero-dose groups; survivors beyond 3,000 m and survivors within 3,000 m who for one reason or another were not exposed (e.g., they might have been out of the city at the time). The two groups have slightly different cancer rates, which is not surprising, because one is a rural and the other an urban population. Figure 10.7 addresses the question of the lowest dose at which the A-bomb data show a significant excess cancer risk. The group of individuals exposed to an average dose of 34 mSv (3.4 rem) shows a small but statistically significant excess cancer incidence.

The BEIR V and UNSCEAR committees analyzed the data in more detail and considered a number of specific cancer sites rather than lumping together all solid cancers. Table 10.2 summarizes these data. The two committees considered slightly different groupings of cancer sites, but in general the agreement between the two is more remarkable than the differences. The risk estimates for these principal tumor types that have been shown to be radiogenic differ only by a factor of about 2 or 3. It should be noted that cancer risks in other organs or tissues are much lower or too low to be detectable.

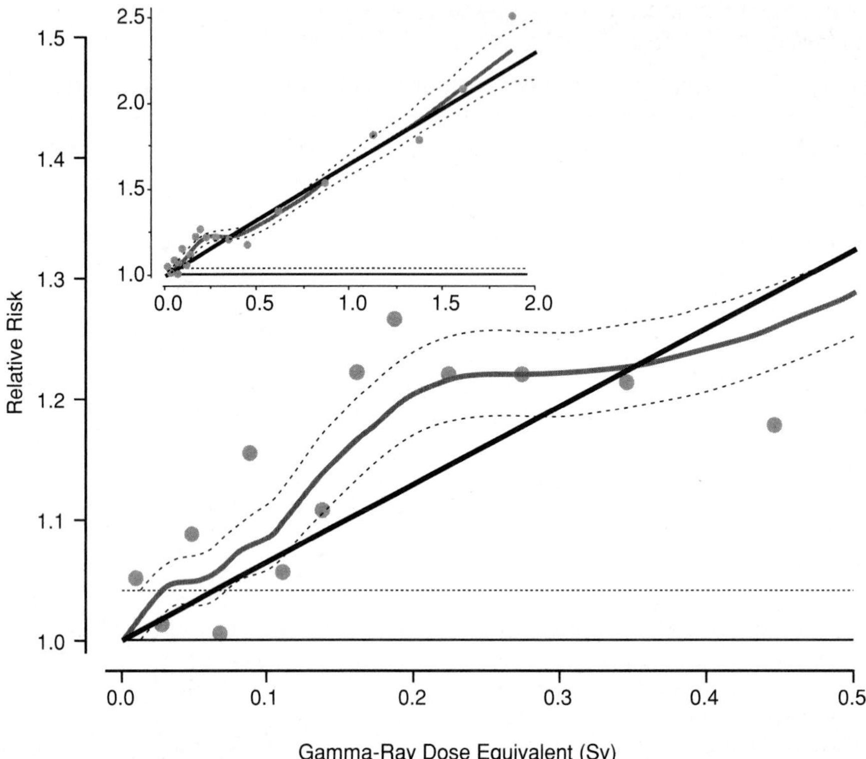

FIGURE 10.6 ● Estimated relative risks for cancer rates in the A-bomb survivors over the 1958–1994 follow-up period relative to unexposed individuals. The dashed curve represents ±1 standard error for the smoothed curve. The inset shows data over the whole dose range 0 to 2 Sv (0–200 rem), to which a straight line is fitted, i.e., relative risk is proportional to dose, with no threshold. The main figure is an expanded version of the low-dose region up to 0.5 Sv (500 rem). The straight line is taken from the inset data for the whole dose range. There is a suggestion that low-dose risks are above the line. (Redrawn from Pierce DA, Preston DL: Radiation related cancer risks at low doses among atomic bomb survivors. *Radiation Research* 154:178–186, 2000.)

As the data from Japan have matured and more detailed information has become available, it is evident that the risk of radiation-induced cancer varies considerably with age at the time of exposure. In most cases, those exposed at an early age are much more susceptible than those exposed at later times. The difference is most dramatic for thyroid cancer; children are very radiosensitive, while adults are quite resistant. It is also dramatic for breast cancer in females; females exposed before 15 years of age are most susceptible; women 50 years of age or older show little or no excess. There are exceptions to this general rule. Susceptibility to radiation-induced leukemia is relatively constant throughout life, and susceptibility to respiratory cancers increases in middle age. The overall risk, however, drops dramatically with age; children and young adults are much more susceptible to radiation-induced cancer than the middle- and old-aged. This is illustrated dramatically in Figure 10.8.

DOSE AND DOSE-RATE EFFECTIVENESS FACTOR (DDREF)

The Japanese data relate only to high doses and high dose rates because they are based on the atomic-bomb survivors. Both the UNSCEAR and BEIR committees considered that there is a dose-rate effect for low linear energy transfer radiations; that is, fewer malignancies are induced if a given dose is spread out over a period of time at low dose rate than if it is delivered in an acute exposure. The dose and dose-rate effectiveness factor (DDREF) is defined as the factor by which radiation cancer risks observed after large acute doses should be reduced when the radiation is delivered at low dose rate or in a series of small dose fractions. There are

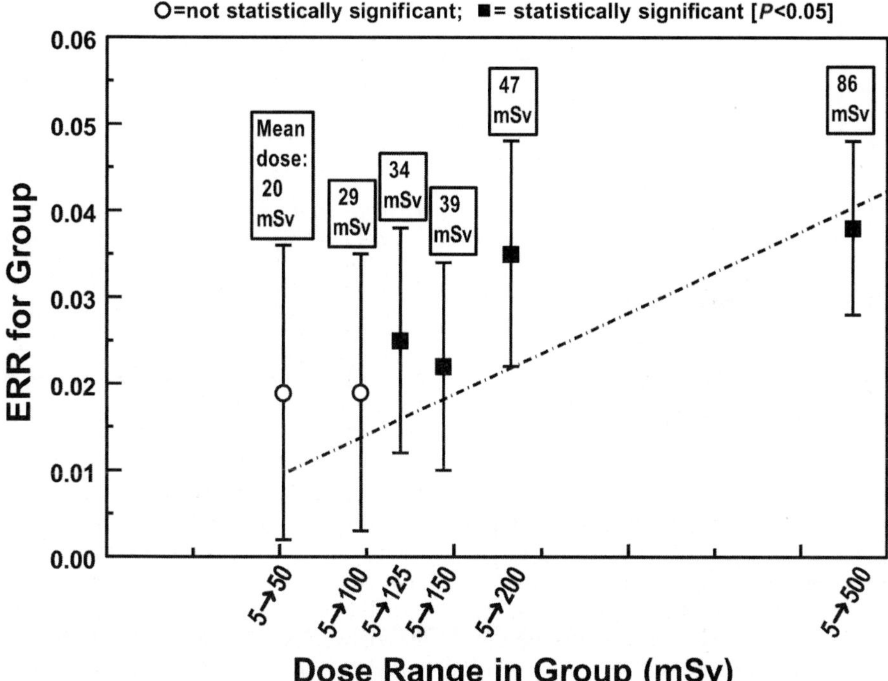

FIGURE 10.7 • Estimated excess relative risk (±1 SE) of mortality from solid cancers among groups of survivors in the life span cohort of atomic-bomb survivors who were exposed to low doses of radiation. The groups correspond to progressively larger maximum doses, with the mean doses in each group indicated above each data point. The first two data points are not statistically significant compared with the comparison population, who were exposed to <5 mSv (500 mrem), whereas the remaining four higher-dose points are statistically significant (p <0.05). The dashed straight line represents the results of a linear fit to all the data from 5 to 4,000 mSv (500 mrem–400 rem) (higher dose points are not shown). (Redrawn from Brenner DJ, Doll R, Goodhead DT, et al.: Cancer risks attributable to low doses of ionizing radiation: Assessing what we really know. *PNAS* 100:13761–13766, 2003.)

TABLE 10.2

Excess Cancer Mortality: Lifetime Risk per 100,000 at 0.1 Sv

	BEIR V (U.S. Population)		UNSCEAR 88 (Japanese Population)	
	Males	Females		
Breast	—	70	Breast	60
Respiratory	190	150	Lung	151
Digestive system	170	290	Stomach	126
			Colon	79
Other solid	300	220	Other solid	194
Leukemia	110	80	Leukemia	100
Total	770	810	Total	710

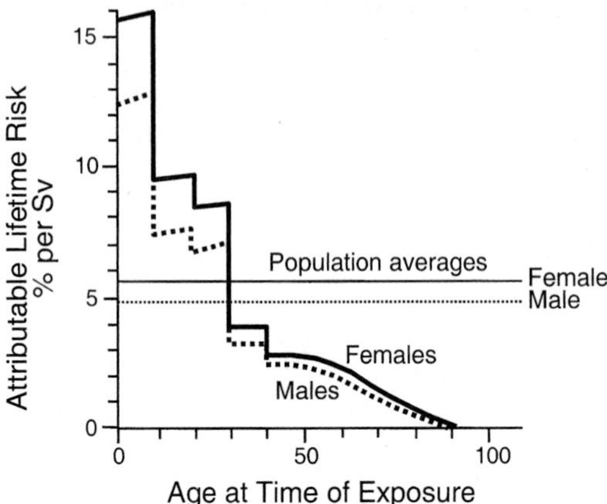

FIGURE 10.8 • The attributable lifetime risk from a single small dose of radiation at various ages at the time of exposure. Note the dramatic decrease in radiosensitivity with age. The higher risk for the younger age-groups is not expressed until late in life. These estimates are based on a relative risk model and on a dose and dose-rate effectiveness factor (DDREF) of 2. (Adapted from ICRP: Recommendations. *Annals of the ICRP Publication 60*, Oxford, England, Pergamon Press, 1990.)

insufficient data, however, in the human to be certain of a quantitative value for the magnitude of the dose-rate effect; consequently, a range of 2 to 10 was proposed, based on animal data. For purposes of radiation protection, the ICRP recommends a DDREF of 2 for doses below 0.2 Gy (20 rad) at any dose rate and higher doses if the dose rate is less than 0.1 Gy/h (10 rad/h). Choosing the lower value for the DDREF follows their policy of being conservative.

SUMMARY OF RISK ESTIMATES

In summarizing all of these risk estimates for the practical purposes of radiation protection, the ICRP recommends the following figures, listed in Table 10.3. For a working population composed of both sexes, the lifetime risk of fatality from cancer is 8×10^{-2} per sievert for high dose and dose rate and 4×10^{-2} per sievert for low dose and low dose rate.

TABLE 10.3

International Commission on Radiological Protection Summary of Risks of Cancer Lethality by Radiation

	High Dose High Dose Rate	Low Dose Low Dose Rate
Working population	8×10^{-2} per Sv	4×10^{-2} per Sv
Whole population	10×10^{-2} per Sv	5×10^{-2} per Sv

International Commission on Radiological Protection: Recommendations. *Annals of the ICRP Publication 60*, Oxford, England, Pergamon Press, 1990, with permission.

The comparable values for the whole population are a little higher because of the sensitivity of the young: 10×10^{-2} per sievert for high dose and dose rate and 5×10^{-2} per sievert for low dose and dose rate. Based on all of the assumptions inherent in the relative risk projection model, the ICRP has estimated that, on average, 13 to 15 years of life are lost for each radiation-induced cancer, but that, again on average, death occurs at 68 to 70 years of age.

SECOND MALIGNANCIES IN RADIOTHERAPY PATIENTS

The risk of second malignancies after radiotherapy is a subject not without controversy. One of the reasons for the uncertainty is that patients undergoing radiotherapy are often at high risk of a second cancer because of their lifestyles, and this factor is more dominant than the radiation risk.

There are many single-institution studies in the literature involving radiotherapy for a variety of sites that conclude that there is no increase in second malignancies, although a more accurate assessment would have been that the studies had limited statistical power to detect a relatively small increased incidence of second malignancies induced by the treatment.

Whenever large studies have been performed, radiotherapy has been shown to be associated with a statistically significant, though very small, enhancement in the risk of second malignancies, particularly in long-term survivors. The three requirements for a study to be credible are:

1. A sufficiently large number of patients.
2. A suitable comparison group, that is, patients with the same cancer treated by some means other than radiation.
3. A sufficiently long follow-up for radiation-induced solid tumors to become manifest.

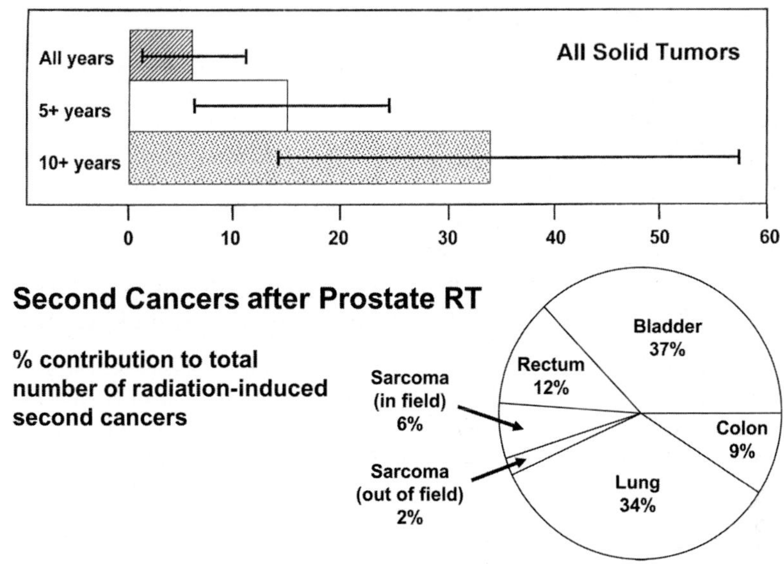

FIGURE 10.9 • **Top panel:** Percentage increase in relative risk for all solid tumors (except prostate cancer) for individuals who received radiotherapy for prostate cancer relative to the risk for individuals who underwent surgery for prostate cancer. **Bottom panel:** Distribution of radiation-induced second cancer at 5+ years post radiotherapy. (Illustration prepared by Dr. David Brenner based on the data from Brenner DJ, Curtis RE, Hall EJ, Ron E: Second cancers after radiotherapy for prostate cancer. *Cancer* 88:398–406, 2000.)

Only a few studies satisfy these criteria; these will be discussed in some detail.

Second Cancers after Radiotherapy for Prostate Cancer

Brenner and colleagues described a study using data from the National Cancer Institute's Surveillance, Epidemiology and End Results (SEER) program. The SEER program is a set of geographically defined, population-based tumor registries, covering approximately 10% of the U.S. population. The database contained information on 51,584 men with prostate cancer treated by radiotherapy and 70,539 who underwent surgery. There was no evidence of a difference in the risk of leukemia for radiotherapy versus surgery patients, but the risk of a second solid tumor at any time postdiagnosis was significantly greater after radiotherapy than after surgery, by about 6%. The relative risk increased with time posttreatment and reached 34% after 10 years or more. The most dramatic increases were for the bladder (77%) and the rectum (105%) for 10 years or more following diagnosis. The relative risks are shown in Figure 10.9, together with the distribution of second cancers; note that even sites remote from the treatment area (e.g., lung) show an increased incidence. Figure 10.10 shows the relative risk of sarcomas in the heavily irradiated tissues in or near the treatment field. It can be seen that the relative

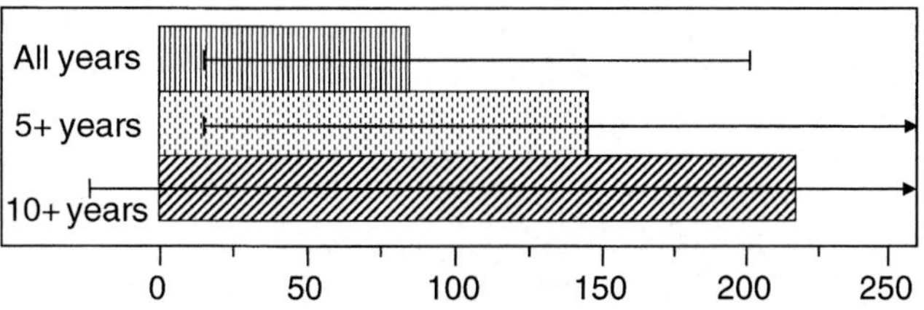

FIGURE 10.10 • Percentage increase in relative risk for sarcomas in or near the treatment field for individuals who received radiotherapy for prostate cancer relative to individuals who underwent surgery. Although the number of tumors involved is much smaller than for all solid tumors (shown in Figure 10.9), the relative risks are extremely high. (Adapted from Brenner DJ, Curtis RE, Hall EJ, Ron E: Second cancers after radiotherapy for prostate cancer. *Cancer* 88:398–406, 2000, with permission.)

risk increases to more than 200% at 10 years or more, compared with the surgical patients.

It is interesting to note that the increase in relative risk for carcinoma of the lung, which was exposed to a relatively low dose (about 0.5 Gy, or 50 rad), is of the same order as that for carcinomas of the bladder, rectum, and colon, all of which were subject to much higher doses (typically more than 5 Gy, or 500 rad). This pattern may reflect the fact that carcinomas, originating in actively dividing cells or cells under hormonal control, can be efficiently induced by relatively low doses of radiation, as evidenced by the atomic-bomb survivors, but the cancer risk at high doses decreases because of the effects of cell killing. In contrast to this pattern for radiation-induced carcinomas, radiation-induced sarcomas appear only in heavily irradiated sites, close to the treatment volume, because large radiation doses are needed to produce sufficient tissue damage to stimulate cellular renewal in mostly dormant cells. The sarcoma data in this study appear to follow this pattern, with significant radiation-related risks being exhibited for sites in and close to the treatment volume, but no significant increases being shown for more distant sites.

Radiation Therapy for Carcinoma of the Cervix

In the largest study of its kind, Boice and colleagues studied the risk of second malignancies in a wide range of organs and tissues as a consequence of the treatment by radiation of carcinoma of the uterine cervix. This huge international study was a *tour de force*. The paper had 42 authors from 38 institutions representing both sides of the Atlantic. Such a collaboration allowed the accumulation of data from 150,000 patients to be studied. This study is strengthened enormously by the fact that an ideal control group is available for comparison. This malignancy is equally well treated by radiation or surgery. The results can be summarized as follows:

1. Very high doses, on the order of several hundred gray (several tens of thousands of rad), were found to increase the risk of cancer of the bladder, rectum, and vagina and possibly bone, uterine corpus, and cecum as well as non-Hodgkin's lymphoma. The risk ratios vary from a high of 4.0 for the bladder to a low of 1.3 for bone. For all female genital cancers combined, a steep dose–response curve was observed, with a 5-fold excess at doses of more than 150 Gy (15,000 rad).
2. Doses of several gray (several hundred rad) increased the risk of stomach cancer and leukemia.
3. Perhaps surprisingly, radiation was found not to increase the overall risk of cancers of the small intestine, colon, ovary, vulva, connective tissue, or breast or of Hodgkin's disease, multiple myeloma, or chronic lymphocytic leukemia.

The overall conclusion of this study was that excess cancers certainly were associated with radiotherapy, as opposed to surgery, and that the risks were highest among long-term survivors and concentrated among women irradiated at relatively young ages.

Second Cancers among Long-Term Survivors from Hodgkin's Disease

Second cancer represents the leading cause of death in long-term survivors of Hodgkin's disease, with exceptionally high risks of breast cancer among women treated at a young age. A number of studies have been reported. Bhatia and colleagues reported that 17 of 483 girls in whom Hodgkin's disease was diagnosed before the age of 16 years subsequently developed breast cancer, with radiotherapy implicated in the majority of cases. The ratio of observed to expected cases is 75.3. Another study (by Sankila and colleagues) involved 1,641 patients treated for Hodgkin's disease as children in five Nordic countries and reported a relative risk that was 17 times higher than the general population, based on 16 cases of breast cancer. Travis and colleagues evaluated 3,869 women in population-based registries participating in the SEER program. All these women received radiotherapy as an initial treatment for Hodgkin's disease. Breast cancer developed in a total of 55 patients, which represents a ratio of observed to expected cases of 2.24. The risk of breast cancer, however, was 60.57% in women treated before the age of 16 years, with most tumors appearing 10 or more years later. This agrees with previous studies that have shown the female breast to be very radiosensitive to carcinogenesis at young ages. The risk of breast cancer decreased with increasing age at the time of therapy and was only slightly elevated in women who were 30 years old or older when treated. In a later study, Travis and colleagues followed 3,817 female survivors of Hodgkin's disease, diagnosed at age 30 years or younger, over a long period of time. A radiation dose of 4 Gy (400 rad) or more delivered to the breast was associated with a 3.2-fold increase in risk. Risk increased 8-fold with a dose of more than 40 Gy (4,000 rad). Hormonal stimulation appears to be important for the development of radiation-induced breast cancer, as evidenced by the reduced risk in patients who received alkylating agents, as well as radiation, which caused ovarian damage.

These studies clearly show that if an adequate cohort can be studied, there is a clear excess of

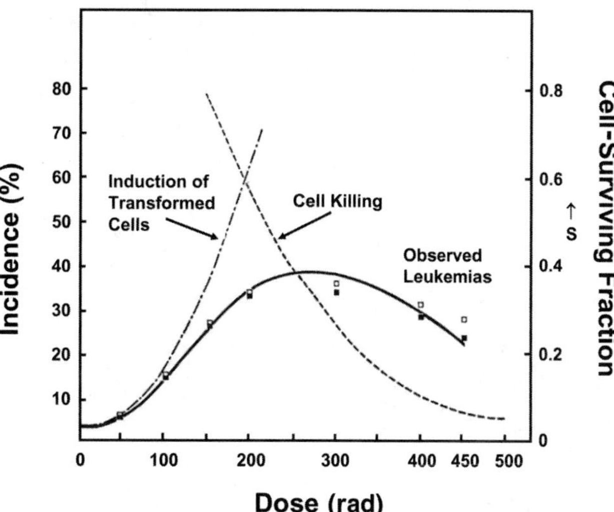

FIGURE 10.11 • Illustrating the concept, introduced by Gray, that the incidence of radiation-induced leukemia in mice follows a "bell" shape because of the balance between the induction of transformed cells and cell killing. (Adapted from Gray LH: Radiation biology and cancer. In: *Cellular Radiation Biology: A Symposium Considering Radiation Effects in the Cell and Possible Implications for Cancer Therapy; A Collection of Papers*. Published for the University of Texas MD Anderson Hospital and Tumor Institute by William & Wilkins, Baltimore, pp 8–25, 1965.)

second cancers induced by radiotherapy. The data confirm previous studies that show that in the young, the breast is especially sensitive to the carcinogenic effects of radiation. In addition, excess cancers develop with a latency of 10 years or more and persist for decades after exposure.

DOSE–RESPONSE RELATIONSHIP FOR RADIATION CARCINOGENESIS AT HIGH DOSES

In the 1960s, Gray proposed that the dose–response relationship for radiation-induced malignancies would be bell shaped, as illustrated in Figure 10.11—that is, the incidence would rise at low doses but fall at high doses. He explained this shape by the concurrent presence of two phenomena: (1) a "dose-related" *increase* in the proportion of normal cells that are transformed to a malignant state and (2) a dose-related *decrease* in the probability that transformed cells may survive the radiation exposure. Gray argued that whatever sequence of changes has taken place in the course of cell transformation, the changes must have been such as to leave the cell capable of indefinite proliferation—that is, with full reproductive integrity. The balance between transformation and cell killing leads to the overall shape, with cell killing becoming dominant at increasingly high doses. With Figure 10.11, Gray was specifically attempting to explain the shape of the dose–response relationship for the induction of leukemia in mice exposed to total body irradiation, which is why the dose goes up only to 500 rad (5 Gy); but it has been tacitly assumed ever since that this bell-shaped curve applies to radiation-induced carcinogenesis in general. However, several recent studies challenge the validity of this assumption by examining whether the linear dose response for radiation-induced cancer, evident in the A-bomb survivors at doses up to 2 Sv (200 rem), extends to the higher-dose ranges used for radiotherapy. Two studies involved the incidence of breast cancer in women treated for Hodgkin's disease with a mantle field, which results in a large dose gradient across the breast (3–42 Gy, or 300–4,200 rad). There was an increasing risk of breast cancer over this entire dose range, with an 8-fold risk for the highest dose category (42 Gy) compared to the lowest (less than 3 Gy).

Another study from St. Jude Children's Research Hospital evaluated 1,612 patients with acute lymphoblastic leukemia, whose primary treatment was chemotherapy, but who also received prophylactic cranial irradiation because many chemotherapy agents do not effectively cross the blood–brain barrier. An excess of high-grade gliomas and meningiomas were evident during the first decade of follow-up, while an increased risk of low-grade brain tumors was observed at later follow-up intervals. The risk of brain tumors increased significantly with increasing radiation dose, as shown in Figure 10.12, but there is no sign of the cancer incidence falling at high doses. There is some indication of a plateau, but no fall as would be predicted as cell killing takes over. As a consequence of these studies, prophylactic cranial radiotherapy has been largely replaced by intrathecal methotrexate.

These examples are further evidence that the incidence of radiation-induced solid cancers does not fall at the high doses typically used therapeutically and accords with the clinical observation that secondary cancers often occur in or near the treatment field in high-dose areas, as well as in more remote locations.

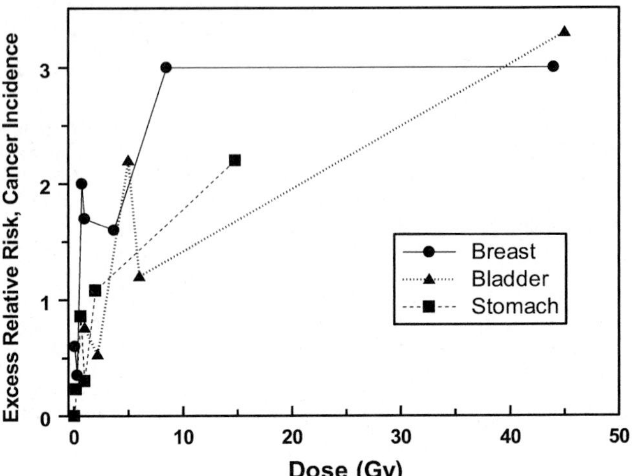

FIGURE 10.12 • Excess relative risk as a function of dose for three types of radiation-induced human solid cancers. The low-dose data (up to 2 Gy) came from the A-Bomb survivors, while the high-dose data refer to radiotherapy patients. (Data compiled by Dr. Elaine Ron.)

CANCER RISKS IN NUCLEAR-INDUSTRY WORKERS

The International Agency for Research on Cancer carried out a huge study involving over 95,000 nuclear-industry workers in the United States, the United Kingdom, and Canada. For all solid cancers combined, there was no evidence of an increased risk associated with radiation in any of the three countries. There was a small statistically significant excess of leukemia in U.K. workers. In U.S. workers, there was a deficit in leukemia, the familiar "healthy worker" syndrome noted in previous studies in the U.S. because in the past, radiation workers tended to belong to higher socioeconomic groups and also needed to pass a medical examination to be hired. The excess disappears if the data for all three countries are pooled. Figure 10.13 shows the excess relative risks for leukemia and solid cancers in this study, which have sufficiently

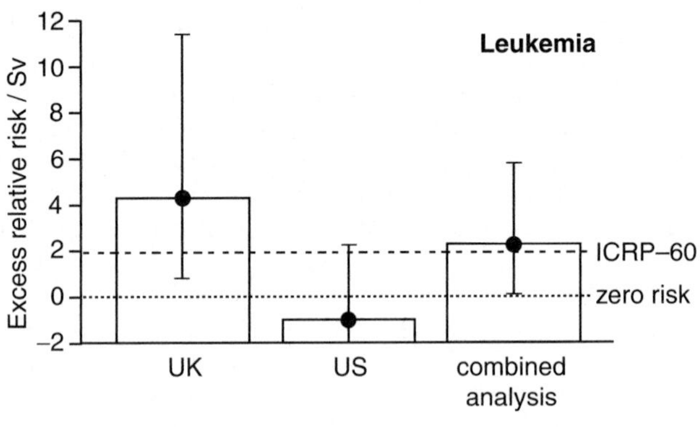

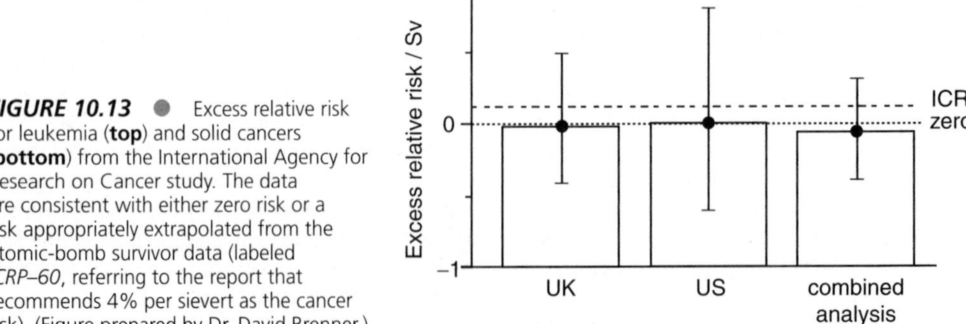

FIGURE 10.13 • Excess relative risk for leukemia (**top**) and solid cancers (**bottom**) from the International Agency for Research on Cancer study. The data are consistent with either zero risk or a risk appropriately extrapolated from the atomic-bomb survivor data (labeled *ICRP–60*, referring to the report that recommends 4% per sievert as the cancer risk). (Figure prepared by Dr. David Brenner.)

large standard errors that they are equally consistent with zero risk or with the risk estimated by ICRP based on the Japanese atomic-bomb survivors (4% per sievert). The study illustrates the futility of trying to detect the possible slight excess of cancer in radiation workers against the high natural background, even if 95,000 are studied. On the other hand, significant excesses of cancer have been detected in nuclear workers from the former Soviet Union, where much higher doses were involved.

MORTALITY PATTERNS IN RADIOLOGISTS

An extensive and interesting report was published by Sir Richard Doll and colleagues in 2003 that assessed 100 years of observations in terms of mortality from cancer and other causes. Relative to all male physicians, male British radiologists who entered the field between 1897 and 1979 showed a small but significant overall increase in cancer mortality (standardized mortality ratio, or SMR = 1.16) and a small but significant decrease in noncancer mortality (SMR = 0.86). The increased cancer risk is not surprising in that estimated annual doses to early radiologists were typically in the range of 1 Gy (100 rad) per year.

When British radiologists were stratified by time of entry into the profession, the most recent cohort (1955–1970) showed a decrease in cancer mortality compared with the control group (SMR = 0.71), though this difference in cancer mortality was not statistically significant. However, there was also a decrease in noncancer mortality (SMR = 0.64), which is statistically significant. These decreases in risk relative to all physicians have attracted much interest, leading to speculation by some that low doses of radiation may be beneficial and may actually lead to a longer life!

The corresponding, but much larger, study of male U.S. radiologists has, surprisingly, received much less attention. Some comparisons between the two studies, both of which are retrospective cohort studies, are given in Table 10.4, in which only radiologists who entered the profession after 1920 are considered, when at least minimal radiation protection practices were in place. There are advantages and disadvantages to both studies; the British study has a longer follow-up and included radiologists who entered the field more recently, while the U.S. study has the advantage of considerably larger numbers and a more direct analysis of the "all physicians" control groups (in the British, studies, the control mortality rates for "all male medical practitioners" were estimated indirectly from census data).

If only radiologists who entered the field after 1920 are analyzed, the U.S. study shows good evidence of significantly increased standardized mortality ratios, relative to all physicians, both for cancer and noncancer mortality. The British study

TABLE 10.4

Comparison between Two Retrospective Cohort Studies of Mortality among Radiologists

	British study[a]	U.S. study
Number of radiologists in study	2,629	6,510
Control physicians	Rates estimated from census data	23,215
Year of entry into profession	1920–1979	1920–1969
Last year of follow-up	1996	1974
Number of radiologists deceased	837 (35%)	1,871 (29%)
SMR for all cancer mortality[b]	1.04 (n.s.)	1.31 (s.s.)
SMR for noncancer mortality[b]	0.86 (s.s.)	1.18 (s.s.)
SMR for all cancer mortality for most recent entry cohort[b]	0.71 (n.s.) (profession entry 1955–1979)	1.15 (n.s.) (profession entry 1940–1969)

Abbreviations: SMR, standardized mortality ratio; n.s., not statistically significant ($p > 0.05$); s.s., statistically significant ($p < 0.05$)

[a] Restricted to radiologists who entered the profession after 1920.

[b] SMRs relative to all physicians (this is the most appropriate comparison group, as death rates in 25 to 74-year-old British physicians are about half those of the general public).

Based on Brenner DJ, Hall EJ: Mortality patterns in British and US radiologists: What can we really conclude? *Br J Radiol* 76:1–2, 2003.

shows no evidence for a different SMR between the radiologists and all physicians for cancer mortality and a significant decrease in SMR for noncancer mortality.

How are we to interpret this apparent difference in risk between British and U.S. radiologists, since year by year the doses to the two cohorts are quite similar, decreasing with time? An appraisal of the SMR data in Table 10.4 would suggest that if the U.S. and British studies were appropriately combined, (1) the SMR for all radiologists entering the field after 1920 compared with all physicians would be significantly greater than unity for cancer mortality, but would be close to unity for noncancer mortality, and (2) for the more recent lower-dose cohorts, the estimated SMR for cancer mortality compared with all physicians would not be significantly different from unity.

In short, in the early "preshielding" era, radiation risks to radiologists were large and easily demonstrable. In the current era, where annual doses are more than a thousandfold lower, the radiation effects may be below the limit of detectability for a retrospective cohort study and arguably for any current epidemiological method. Thus, it is entirely to be expected that some studies will produce null results, some will produce slightly positive results, and others will produce slightly negative results, which is the case for the British and U.S. studies discussed here. With regard to the proposition that low doses of radiation may be beneficial and prolong life, one has to pick and choose the data to reach such a conclusion. When all of the studies are considered, the weight of evidence does not support the suggestion.

CHILDHOOD CANCER AFTER RADIATION EXPOSURE *IN UTERO*

In several widely publicized British studies in the 1950s and 1960s, Stewart and her colleagues reported an excess of leukemia and childhood cancer in children irradiated *in utero* as a consequence of diagnostic x-ray examinations involving the pelvis of the mother. An association between leukemia and x-rays *in utero* was confirmed in the United States by MacMahon.

This has been a highly controversial topic. It is discussed in more detail in Chapter 12. In a 1997 paper, Doll and Wakeford summarized all of the available data and came to the conclusion that radiation was the causative agent. They concluded that:

- Low-dose irradiation of the fetus *in utero*, particularly in the last trimester, causes an increased risk of childhood malignancies.
- An obstetric x-ray examination, even though the dose is only about 10 mGy (1 rad), increases the risk of childhood cancer by 40%.
- The excess absolute risk is about 6% per gray.

The relative risk of 40% is very high because, of course, cancer is relatively rare in children. The absolute risk works out to be about 6% per gray, which is not very different from the cancer risk calculated for the atomic-bomb survivors following adult exposure.

Summary of Pertinent Conclusions

- A deterministic effect has a threshold in dose, and the severity of the effect is dose related. Radiation-induced cataracts are an example of a deterministic effect.
- Radiation carcinogenesis is a stochastic effect; that is, the probability of an effect increases with dose, with no dose threshold, but the severity of the effect is not dose related. Hereditary effects are also stochastic.
- The human experience of radiation-induced carcinogenesis includes the survivors of the atomic-bomb attacks on Hiroshima and Nagasaki, patients exposed to medical irradiation, and early workers exposed occupationally. Some examples include:
  1. Leukemia and solid tumors in Japanese survivors of the atomic bomb
  2. Leukemia in patients irradiated for ankylosing spondylitis
  3. Thyroid cancer in children irradiated for benign conditions of the head and neck, such as enlarged thymus or tonsils, and children epilated for tinea capitis
  4. Breast cancer in patients treated with x-rays for postpartum mastitis and patients fluoroscoped repeatedly during the management of tuberculosis
  5. Lung cancer in uranium miners
  6. Bone cancer in dial painters who ingested radium and patients who had injections of radium for tuberculosis or ankylosing spondylitis
- Latency refers to the time interval between irradiation and the appearance of the malignancy.

(continued)

Summary of Pertinent Conclusions (Continued)

- The shortest latency is for leukemia, with a peak at 5 to 7 years. For solid tumors, the latency may extend for 60 years or more.
- Regardless of the age at exposure, radiation-induced malignancies tend to appear at the same age as spontaneous malignancies of the same type. Indeed, for solid cancers, the excess risk is apparently more like a lifelong elevation of the natural age-specific cancer risk.
- To determine risk estimates for radiation-induced cancer from observed data (the Japanese atomic-bomb survivors), a model must be assumed because:
  1. Data must be extrapolated from relatively high doses to the low doses of public health concern.
  2. Data must be projected out to a full lifespan, because no exposed population has yet lived out its lifespan.
  3. Risks must be "transferred" from the Japanese population to (for example) a Western population with different natural cancer rates.
- There are two principal risk models. The absolute risk model assumes that radiation produces a discrete "crop" of cancers, over and above the spontaneous level and unrelated to the spontaneous level. The relative risk model assumes that radiation increases the spontaneous incidence by a factor. Because the natural cancer incidence increases with age, this model predicts a large number of excess cancers appearing late in life after irradiation.
- The reassessment of radiation-induced cancer risks by the BEIR V committee was based on a time-related relative risk model. Excess cancer deaths were assumed to depend on dose, square of the dose, age at exposure, time since exposure, and, for some cancers, gender.
- For solid tumors, the excess cancer incidence was found to be a linear function of dose up to about 2 Sv (200 rem).
- Leukemia data were best fitted by a linear-quadratic function of dose.
- The Japanese atomic-bomb data refer to acute exposure at a high dose rate. A dose and dose-rate effectiveness factor (DDREF) is needed to convert risk estimates to the low dose and low dose rates encountered in radiation protection. From animal studies, this is anywhere from 2 to 10. The ICRP conservatively assumes a value of 2.
- Based on reports of the UNSCEAR and BEIR V committees, the ICRP suggests a risk estimate of excess cancer mortality in a working population of 8×10^{-2} per sievert for high doses and high dose rates and 4×10^{-2} per sievert for low doses and low dose rates.
- For the general population, slightly higher risks apply because of the increased susceptibility of the young. The ICRP estimates are 10×10^{-2} per sievert for high doses and dose rates and 5×10^{-2} per sievert for low doses and dose rates.
- The ICRP estimates that, on average, 13 to 15 years of life are lost for each radiation-induced cancer and that death occurs at age 68 to 70 years.
- There is a clear excess of second cancers induced by radiation therapy, both in heavily irradiated tissue and in more remote organs. This is evident if a sufficiently large number of patients and an adequate control group are available for study and if there is a sufficiently long follow-up for solid tumors to become manifest.
- Large studies show a clear excess of second cancers after radiotherapy for prostate cancer, carcinoma of the cervix, and Hodgkin's lymphoma. An excess has also been shown following radiation therapy for breast cancer, carcinoma of the testes, and various childhood malignancies.
- The International Agency for Research on Cancer studied 95,000 workers in the nuclear industry in the United States, United Kingdom, and Canada. It was not possible to distinguish between zero risk and the ICRP risk of 4% per sievert extrapolated to the doses received by the workers.
- Early radiologists who practiced prior to the 1920s showed an excess of malignancies. No excess is evident in radiologists in recent years. The report that British radiologists live longer is not confirmed in other studies.
- Irradiation *in utero* by diagnostic x-rays appears to increase the spontaneous incidence of leukemia and childhood cancers by a factor of about 1.4. This is a high relative risk because malignancies in children are rare, but the absolute risk is about 6% per gray—not very different from the risk estimate calculated for the A-bomb survivors following adult exposure.

BIBLIOGRAPHY

Andersson M, Carstensen B, Storm HH: Mortality and cancer incidence after cerebral arteriography with or without Thorotrast. *Radiat Res* 142:305–320, 1995

Berrington A, Darby SC, Weiss HA, Doll R: 100 years of observation on British radiologists: Mortality from cancer and other causes 1897–1997. *Br J Radiol* 74:507–519, 2001

Bhatia S, Robison LL, Oberlin O, et al.: Breast cancer and other second neoplasms after childhood Hodgkin's disease. *N Engl J Med* 334:745–751, 1996

Boice JD Jr, Engholm G, Kleinman RA, et al.: Radiation dose and second cancer risk in patients treated for cancer of the cervix. *Radiat Res* 116:3–55, 1988

Boice JD, Hutchison GB: Leukemia in women following radiotherapy for cervical cancer: Ten-year follow-up of an international study. *J Natl Cancer Inst* 65:115–129, 1980

Boice JD Jr, Land CE, Shore RE, Norman JE, Tokunaga M: Risk of breast cancer following low-dose exposure. *Radiology* 131:589–597, 1979

Boice JD Jr., Preston D, David FG, Monson RR: Frequent chest x-ray fluoroscopy and breast cancer incidence among tuberculosis patients in Massachusetts. *Radiat Res* 125:214–222, 1991

Brenner DJ, Curtis RE, Hall EJ, Ron E: Second malignancies in prostate patients after radiotherapy compared with surgery. *Cancer* 88:398–406, 2000

Brenner DJ, Doll R, Goodhead DT, et al.: Cancer risks attributable to low doses of ionizing radiation: Assessing what we really know. *PNAS* 100:13761–13766, 2003

Brenner DJ, Hall EJ: Mortality patterns in British and US radiologists: What can we really conclude? *Br J Radiol* 76:1–2, 2003

Cardis E, Gilbert ES, Carpenter L, et al.: Effects of low doses and low dose rates of external ionizing radiation: Cancer mortality among nuclear industry workers in three countries. *Radiat Res* 142:117–132, 1995

Carpenter LM, Swerdlow AJ, Fear NT: Mortality of doctors in different specialties: Findings from a cohort of 20,000 NHS hospital consultants. *Occup Environ Med* 54:388–395, 1997

Coleman CN: Second malignancy after treatment of Hodgkin's disease: An evolving picture. *J Clin Oncol* 4:821–824, 1986

Committee on the Biological Effects of Ionizing Radiation: *The Effects on Populations of Exposure to Low Levels of Ionizing Radiations*. Washington, DC, National Academy of Sciences, National Research Council, 1972

Committee on the Biological Effects of Ionizing Radiation: *The Effects on Populations of Exposure to Low Levels of Ionizing Radiations*. Washington, DC, National Academy of Sciences, National Research Council, 1980

Committee on the Biological Effects of Ionizing Radiation: *Health Effects of Exposure of Low Levels of Ionizing Radiations*. Washington, DC, National Academy of Sciences, National Research Council, 1990

Czesnin K, Wronkowski Z: Second malignancies of the irradiated area in patients treated for uterine cervix cancer. *Gynecol Oncol* 6:309–315, 1978

Darby SC, Reeves G, Key T, Doll R, Stovall M: Mortality in a cohort of women given x-ray therapy for metropathia haemorrhagica. *Int J Cancer* 56:793–801, 1994

Delobngchamp RR, Mabuchi K, Yoshimoto Y, Preston DL: Cancer mortality among atomic bomb survivors exposed *in utero* or as young children, October 1950–May 1992. *Radiat Res* 147:385–395, 1997

Doll R, Wakeford R: Risk of childhood cancer from fetal irradiation. *Br J Radiol* 70:130–139, 1997

Fry SA: Studies of US radium dial workers: An epidemiological classic. *Radiat Res* 150:S21–S29, 1998

Giles D, Hewitt D, Stewart A, Webb J: Malignant disease in childhood and diagnostic irradiation *in utero*. *Lancet* ii:447, 1956

Gray LH: Radiation biology and cancer. In: *Cellular Radiation Biology: A Symposium Considering Radiation Effects in the Cell and Possible Implications for Cancer Therapy; A Collection of Papers*. Published for the University of Texas MD Anderson Hospital and Tumor Institute, by William & Wilkins, Baltimore, pp 8–25, 1965

Hildreth NG, Shore RE, Hempelmann LH, Rosenstein M: Risk of extrathyroid tumors following radiation treatments in infancy for thymic enlargement. *Radiat Res* 2: 378–392, 1985

Howe GR, McLaughlin J: Breast cancer mortality between 1950 and 1987 after exposure to fractionated moderate-dose-rate ionizing radiation in the Canadian Fluoroscopy cohort study and a comparison with breast cancer mortality in the atomic bomb survivors study. *Radiat Res* 145:694–707, 1996

IARC Study Group on Cancer Risk Among Nuclear Industry Workers: Direct estimates of cancer mortality due to low doses of ionizing radiation: An international study. *Lancet* 344:1039–1043, 1994

International Commission on Radiological Protection: Recommendations of the ICRP. *ICRP Publication 60*. Oxford, England, Pergamon Press, 1990

International Commission on Radiation Units and Measurements: *Radiation Quantities and Units*. Report 33. Washington, DC, ICRU, 1967

Kapp DS, Fisher D, Grady KJ, Schwartz PE: Subsequent malignancies associated with carcinoma of uterine cervix, including an analysis of the effects of patient and treatment parameters on incidence and site metachronous malignancies. *Int J Radiat Oncol Biol Phys* 8:192–205, 1982

Kleinerman RA, Boice JD Jr, Storm HH, et al.: Second primary cancer after treatment for cervical cancer. An international registries study. *Cancer* 76:442–452, 1995

Land CE: Studies of cancer and radiation dose among atomic bomb survivors. The example of breast cancer. *JAMA* 274:402–407, 1995

Land H, Parada LF, Weinberg RA: Tumorigenic conversion of primary embryo fibroblasts requires at least two cooperating oncogenes. *Nature* 304:596–602, 1983

Lee JY, Perez CA, Ettinger N, et al.: The risk of second primaries subsequent to irradiation for cervix cancer. *Int J Radiat Oncol Biol Phys* 8:207–211, 1982

MacMahon B: Prenatal x-ray exposure and childhood cancer. *JNCI* 28:1173–1191, 1962

Matanoski GM: Risk of cancer associated with occupational exposure in radiologists and other radiation workers. In Burchenal JH, Oettgen HF (eds): *Cancer—Achievements, Challenges and Prospects for the 1980s*. New York, Grune and Stratton, pp 241–254, 1981

Matanoski GM, Sternberg A, Elliott EA: Does radiation exposure produce a protective effect among radiologists? *Health Phys* 52:637–643, 1987

Modan B, Baidatz D, Mart H, Steinitz R, Levin SG: Radiation-induced head and neck tumors. *Lancet* 1:277–279, 1974

Mole RH: Endosteal sensitivity to tumor induction by radiation in different species: A partial answer to an unsolved question? In Mays C, Jee W, Lloyd R, Stover B, Dougherty J, Taylor G (eds): *Delayed Effects of Bone-Seeking Radionuclides*, pp 249–258. Salt Lake City, University of Utah Press, 1969

Nekolla EA, Kellerer AM, Kuse-Isingschulte M, Eder E, Spiess H: Malignancies in patients treated with high doses of radium-224. *Radiat Res* 152:S3–S7, 1999

Nyandoto P, Muhonen T, Joensuu H: Second cancers among long-term survivors from Hodgkin's disease. *Int J Radiat Oncol Biol Phys* 42:373–378, 1998

Pederson BJ, Larson SD: Incidence of acute nonlymphocytic leukemia, preleukemia and acute myeloproliferative syndrome up to 10 years after treatment of Hodgkin's disease. *N Engl J Med* 307:965–975, 1982

Pierce DA, Preston DL: Radiation-related cancer risks at low doses among atomic bomb survivors. *Radiation Research* 154:178–186, 2003

Pierce DA, Shimizu Y, Preston DL, Vaeth M, Mabuchi K: Studies of the mortality of atomic bomb survivors: Report 12, Part I. Cancer: 1950–1990. *Radiat Res* 146:1–27, 1996

Preston DL, Pierce DA: The effect of changes in dosimetry on cancer mortality risk estimates in the atomic bomb survivors. *Radiat Res* 114:437–466, 1988

Preston DL, Kumusumi S, Tomonaga M, et al.: Cancer incidence in atomic bomb survivors. Part III: Leukemia lymphoma and multiple myeloma, 1950–1987. *Radiat Res* 137:S68–S97, 1994

Rowland RE, Stehney AF, Lucas HF: Dose-response relationships for radium-induced bone sarcomas. *Health Phys* 44:15–31, 1983

Ron E, Lubin JH, Shore RE, et al.: Thyroid cancer after exposure to external radiation: A pooled analysis of seven studies. *Radiat Res* 141:259–277, 1995

Rotblat J, Lindop P: Long-term effects of a single whole-body exposure of mice to ionizing radiations: II. Causes of death. *Proc R Soc Lond B Biol Sci* 154:350–368, 1961

Saenger EL, Thoma BE, Tompkins EA: Leukemia after treatment of hyperthyroidism. *JAMA* 205:855–862, 1968

Sankila R, Garwicz S, Olsen JH, et al.: Risk of subsequent malignant neoplasms among 1,641 Hodgkin's disease patients diagnosed in childhood and adolescence: A population-based cohort study in the five Nordic countries. *J Clin Oncol* 14:1442–1446, 1996

Shore RE, Hildreth N, Woodard E, Dvoretsky P, Hempelmann L, Pasternack B: Breast cancer among women given x-ray therapy for acute postpartum mastitis. *J Natl Cancer Inst* 77:689–696, 1986

Shore RE, Woodard E, Hildreth N, Dvoretsky P, Hempelmann L, Pasternack B: Thyroid tumors following thymus irradiation. *J Natl Cancer Inst* 74:1177–1184, 1985

Stewart A, Kneale GW: Changes in the cancer risk associated with obstetric radiography. *Lancet* 1:104–107, 1968

Stewart A, Webb J, Hewitt D: A survey of childhood malignancies. *Br Med J* 1:1495–1508, 1958

Tatsuo A, Takashi N, Fukushia K, et al.: Second cancer after radiation therapy for cancer of the uterine cervix. *Cancer* 67:398–405, 1991

Thompson DE, Mabucghi K, Ron E, et al.: Cancer incidence in atomic bomb survivors. Part II: Solid tumors, 1958–1987. *Radiat Res* 138:209–223, 1994

Tokunaga M, Land CE, Tokuoka S, Nishimori I, Soda M, Akiba S: Incidence of female breast cancer among atomic bomb survivors, 1950–1985. *Radiat Res* 138:209–223, 1994

Travis LB, Curtis RE, Boice JD Jr: Late effects of treatment for childhood Hodgkin's disease. *N Engl J Med* 335:352–353, 1996

Travis LB, Hill DA, Dores GM, et al.: Breast cancer following radiotherapy and chemotherapy among young women with Hodgkin's disease. *JAMA* 290:465–475, 2003. Erratum in: *JAMA* 290:1318, 2003

United Nations Scientific Committee on the Effects of Atomic Radiation: *Sources and Effects of Ionizing Radiation*. New York, UNSCEAR, 1988

United Nations Scientific Committee on the Effects of Atomic Radiation: *Sources and Effects of Atomic Radiation: UNSCEAR 1994 Report to the General Assembly, with Scientific Annexes*. E 94 IXII. New York, United Nations, 1994

Upton AC: The dose-response relation in radiation-induced cancer. *Cancer Res* 21:717–729, 1961

van Kaick G, Dahlmeimer A, Hornik S, et al.: The German Thorotrast study: Recent results and assessment of risks. *Radiat Res* 152: S64–S71, 1999

van Leeuwen FE, Klokman WJ, Stovall M, et al.: Roles of radiation dose, chemotherapy and hormonal factors in breast cancer following Hodgkin's disease. *J Natl Cancer Inst.* 95:971–980, 2003

Walter AW, Hancock ML, Pui CH, et al.: Secondary brain tumors in children treated for acute lymphoblastic leukemia at St Jude Children's Research Hospital. *J Clin Oncol.* 16:3761–3767, 1998

Wall PL, Clausen KP: Carcinoma of urinary bladder in patients receiving cyclophosphamide. *N Engl J Med* 293:271–273, 1975

Weiss HA, Darby SC, Doll R: Cancer mortality following x-ray treatment for ankylosing spondylitis. *Int J Cancer* 59:327–338, 1994

Yamamoto T, Kopecky KJ, Fujikura T, Tokuoka S, Monzen T, Nishimori I, Nakashima E, Kato H: Lung cancer incidence among Japanese A-bomb survivors, 1950–1980. *J Radiat Res* 28:156–171, 1987

CHAPTER 11

Hereditary Effects of Radiation

GERM-CELL PRODUCTION AND RADIATION EFFECTS ON FERTILITY

In the male mammal, spermatozoa arise from the germinal epithelium in the seminiferous tubules of the testes, and their production is continuous from puberty to death. The spermatogonial (stem) cells consist of several different populations that vary in their sensitivity to radiation. The postspermatogonial cells pass through several stages of development: primary spermatocytes, secondary spermatocytes, spermatids, and finally spermatozoa. The division of a spermatogonium to the development of mature sperm involves a period of 6 weeks in the mouse and 10 weeks in the human. The effect of radiation on fertility is not apparent immediately, because the postspermatogonial cells are relatively resistant compared with the sensitive stem cells. After exposure to a moderate dose of radiation, the individual remains fertile as long as mature sperm cells are available, but decreased fertility or even temporary sterility follows if these are used up. The period of sterility lasts until the spermatogonia are able to repopulate by division.

Radiation doses as low as 0.15 Gy (15 rad) result in oligospermia (diminished sperm count) after a latent period of about 6 weeks. Doses above 0.5 Gy (50 rad) result in azoospermia (absence of living spermatozoa) and therefore temporary sterility. The duration of azoospermia is dose dependent; recovery can begin within 1 year after doses of less than 1 Gy (100 rad) but requires 2 to 3½ years after a dose of 2 Gy (200 rad). The original single-dose data came from the irradiation of prisoners, which showed that a dose in excess of 6 Gy (600 rad) is needed to result in permanent sterility. In contrast to most organ systems, where fractionation of dose results in sparing, fractionated courses cause more gonadal damage than a single dose. Studies of patients receiving radiation therapy indicate that permanent sterility can result from 2.5 to 3 Gy (250–300 rad) in a fractionated regime over 2 to 4 weeks. The induction of sterility by radiation in human males does not produce significant changes in hormone balance, libido, or physical capability.

Gonadal kinetics in women are opposite to those in men, as the germ cells are nonproliferative. All cells in the oogonial stages progress to the oocyte stage in the embryo. By 3 days after birth, in the mouse or human, all of the oocytes are in a resting phase and there is no cell division. Consequently, in the adult there are no stem (oogonial) cells, but there

TABLE 11.1

Radiation Sterility—Comparing Male and Female

Male	Female
Self-renewal system: Spermatogonia → spermatocytes → spermatids → spermatozoa	Gonadal kinetics opposite of males: by 3 days after birth, all cells progressed to oocyte stage; no further cell division
Latent period between irradiation and sterility Oligospermia and reduced fertility: 0.15 Gy Azoospermia and temporary sterility: 0.5 Gy Recovery is dose dependant (1 yr after 2 Gy)	Neither latent period nor temporary sterility in females
Permanent sterility: 6 Gy, single dose 2.5–3 Gy, fractionated, 2–4 wks	Radiation can induce permanent ovarian failure; marked age dependence Permanent sterility: 12 Gy, prepuberty 2 Gy, premenopausal
Induction of sterility does not affect hormone balance, libido, or physical capability	Radiation sterility produces hormonal changes like those seen in natural menopause

are three types of follicles: immature, nearly mature, and mature. At birth, a woman has about 1 million oocytes, which are reduced to about 300,000 at puberty.

In women, radiation is highly effective at inducing permanent ovarian failure, but there is a marked age dependence in sensitivity. The dose required to induce permanent sterility varies from 12 Gy (1,200 rad) prepubertal to 2 Gy (200 rad) premenopausal. Pronounced hormonal changes, comparable to those associated with the natural menopause, accompany radiation-induced sterilization in females.

Overall, radiation sterility is very different between men and women, and these differences are compared and contrasted in Table 11.1.

REVIEW OF BASIC GENETICS

The study of the inheritance of observable characteristics includes molecular as well as morphologic and some behavioral traits. The **chromosomes** carry, in code form, all of the information that specifies a particular human, with all of his or her individual characteristics. The chromosomes are long threadlike structures, the essential ingredient of which is DNA, itself a long complex molecule with a sugar-phosphate backbone. Attached to each sugar molecule is an organic base; these come in four varieties: thymine, adenine, guanine, and cytosine. This whole configuration is tightly coiled in a double helix, rather like a miniature spiral staircase, with chains of sugar molecules linked by phosphates forming the rails on either side, bridged at regular intervals by pairs of bases, which form the steps. The order, or sequence, of the bases contains the genetic information in code form.

A **gene** is a finite segment of DNA specified by an exact sequence of bases. Genes occur along chromosomes in linear order like beads on a string, and the position of a gene is referred to as its **locus.**

The human chromosome complement consists of 22 pairs of autosomes present in both sexes, plus a pair of sex chromosomes, the X and Y. Males have 22 pairs of autosomes plus an X and a Y. Females have 22 pairs of autosomes plus a pair of Xs. One chromosome of each pair is derived from each parent.

The human **genome** is composed of the DNA of chromosomes and, to a minute extent, the DNA of mitochondria. The 46 chromosomes contain about 6×10^9 base pairs of DNA, with each chromosomal arm including a single supercoiled molecule of DNA associated with chromosomal proteins. The total number of genes is in the range of 50,000 to 100,000 per haploid set of chromosomes. The average gene would therefore contain 30 to 60 kilobases of DNA if no DNA were unrelated to genes. The study of individual genes hardly has begun, but it is apparent that some genes are smaller than this and at least one, whose mutation can cause Duchenne-type muscular dystrophy, has been reported to contain more than 103 kilobases of DNA. Because most protein products of genes are less than 300 kDa, the translated portions of genes are seldom larger than 10 kilobases, so a major part of the genome appears to be untranslated. Some of this DNA appears to be transcribed but not translated. Much of the untranslated DNA consists of **introns** that reside between translated **exons**. In addition, much of the DNA outside the exons is involved in gene function through regulation and RNA polymerase attachment.

Not only does this genome recombine in each generation, but it also may undergo **mutation**, a term used here to denote any change in chromosomes, their genes, and their DNA. Thus, alterations in chromosome number and structure would be included along with changes not visible microscopically. These latter changes include an array of changes in DNA, such as deletion, rearrangement, breakage in the sugar-phosphate backbone, and base alterations. Gene function can be disturbed not only by loss or modification of translated exons but also through alteration of nonexonic sites that regulate transcription and translation. Mutation occurs in both germ cells and somatic cells, although it is much less apparent in the latter unless it occurs under conditions of clonal proliferation, as happens with cancer. On the other hand, many mutations in the germline are lethal during embryonic development.

In humans, every normal cell has 46 chromosomes, 23 derived from the mother and 23 from the father. The two members of a pair of chromosomes normally have the same genes for given characteristics lined up in the same sequence. In this case, the two chromosomes are said to be **homologous**. The pair of chromosomes that determine sex are XX in the female and XY in the male; in the case of the male, therefore, the two chromosomes of this pair are **heterologous**; they do not contain parallel genes. If the two members of a pair of genes are alike, the person is said to be **homozygous** for that pair of genes; if they are different, the person is said to be **heterozygous**.

The fact that pairs of chromosomes contain corresponding sets of genes introduces the idea of dominant and recessive genes. A dominant gene, by definition, expresses itself if its corresponding gene is recessive, the recessive gene in this case being either ineffective or suppressed. A completely recessive gene is expressed only if both corresponding genes of a pair of chromosomes are recessive (i.e., the person must be homozygous for the recessive gene) or if the recessive gene is on the X chromosome in a male. Eye color is the simplest example. The gene for blue eyes is recessive; that for brown eyes is dominant. A child will have blue eyes only if he or she receives the gene for blue eyes from both parents. If both or only one of the genes that determine eye color is for brown eyes, then the child will have brown eyes, because this gene is dominant. It should be pointed out that not all genes are completely dominant; some permit expression of the recessive counterpart to a varying extent, depending on the particular characteristics involved.

The Y sex chromosome in humans has genes that determine maleness but appears to have few other genes. The X chromosome, on the other hand, has many genes. If a mother carries a recessive mutant gene on the single X chromosome that she donates to her son, there is no matching gene from the father, and consequently the recessive gene is expressed. If the offspring is a daughter, there may well be a dominant gene on the X chromosome supplied by the father, which would suppress the expression of the recessive mutant. The daughter, however, could transmit the mutant gene to her sons, in whom it would be expressed. Characteristics that result from recessive genes on the X chromosome, so that they are expressed almost exclusively in male children, are said to be sex-linked. The most common examples are color blindness and hemophilia.

An elementary discussion of genetics, such as presented here, may give the impression that each characteristic of a person is determined by a single pair of genes. On the contrary, this is the exception rather than the rule, because most characteristics are the result of an interplay in the expression of many genes.

MUTATIONS

Exposure of a population to radiation can cause adverse health effects in the descendants as a consequence of mutations induced in the germ cells. **Hereditary diseases**, also known as **genetic diseases,*** may result when mutations occurring in the germ cells of parents are transmitted to progeny; in contrast, most cancers result from mutations in somatic cells. Because the human genome includes between 50,000 and 100,000 genes, the potential number of mutations, and thus hereditary diseases, is staggering.

It is a commonly held view that radiation produces bizarre mutants and monsters, as illustrated in Figure 11.1. This view is absolutely false. Radiation does not result in hereditary effects that are new or unique but rather increases the frequencies of the same mutations that already occur spontaneously or naturally in that species.

**Such diseases were formerly called* genetic *diseases, but the term* hereditary *is more descriptive, reflecting the transfer from one generation to the next, to distinguish them from cancer, which is also, in essence, genetic.*

My father was a radiologist and he assured me that radiation is NOT hazardous.

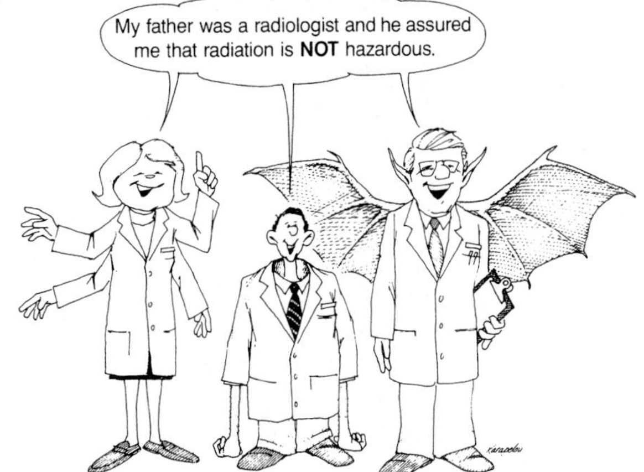

FIGURE 11.1 • It is a commonly held view that radiation produces bizarre mutations or monsters that may be recognized readily. This is not true. Radiation increases the incidence of the same mutations that occur spontaneously in a given population. The study of radiation-induced hereditary effects is difficult because the mutations produced by the radiation must be identified on a statistical basis in the presence of a high natural incidence of the same mutations.

Hereditary diseases are classified into three principal categories: **Mendelian chromosomal**, and **multifactorial** (Table 11.2). The baseline frequencies of these different classes of hereditary diseases in the human population have been estimated by the UNSCEAR 2001 committee and are summarized in Table 11.3.

Mendelian

Mendelian diseases are those caused by mutations in single genes located on either the autosomes or the sex chromosomes. The mutation may be a change in the structure of DNA, which may involve either the base composition, the sequence, or both. An alteration so small that it involves the substitution, gain, or loss of a single base can be the cause of significant hereditary changes. A striking example is sickle-cell anemia, which results from the substitution of only one base. The important point with respect to Mendelian diseases is that the relationship between mutation and disease is simple and predictable.

These diseases are subdivided into autosomal dominant, autosomal recessive, and X-linked conditions, depending on which chromosome the

TABLE 11.2

Hereditary Effects of Radiation

Hereditary Effect	Example
Gene mutations*	
Single dominant 736 (753)	Ploydactyly, Huntington's chorea
Recessive 521 (596)	Sickle-cell anemia, Tay–Sachs disease, cystic fibrosis, retinoblastoma
Sex-linked 80 (60)	Color blindness, hemophilia
Chromosomal changes	
Too many or too few	Down's syndrome (extra chromosome 21), mostly embryonic death
Chromosome aberrations, physical abnormalities	Embryonic death or mental retardation
Robertsonian translocation	
Multifactorial	
Congenital abnormalities present at birth	Neural tube defects, cleft lip, cleft plalate
Chroinc diseases of adult onset	Diabetes, essential hypertension, coronary heart disease

* The numbers following types of gene mutations refer to the number of human diseases known to be caused by such a mutation. The numbers in parentheses refer to additional possible diseases.

TABLE 11.3

Baseline Frequencies of Genetic Diseases in Human Populations (from UNSCEAR 2001)

Disease Class	Frequency per Million[a]	
Mendelian diseases		24,000
Autosomal dominant diseases	15,000	
X-linked diseases	1,500	
Autosomal recessive diseases	7,500	
Chromosomal diseases		4,000
Multifactorial diseases		710,000
Chronic diseases	650,000	
Congenital abnormalities	60,000	
Total		738,000

[a] For Mendelian and chromosomal diseases and for congenital abnormalities, the frequencies are per million live births; for chronic multifactorial diseases, the frequency is per million of the population.

From United Nations Scientific Committee on the Effects of Atomic Radiation: *Hereditary Effects of Radiation: The UNSCEAR 2001 Report to the General Assembly with Scientific Annex.* New York, United Nations, 2001.

mutant genes are located on and the pattern of transmission. In the case of dominant diseases, one mutant gene received from either one of the parents is sufficient to cause disease, although the copy of the gene from the other parent is normal.

A **dominant** gene mutation is expressed in the first generation after its occurrence. More than 700 such conditions have been identified with certainty, and an additional 700 or more are less well established. Some examples are polydactyly, achondroplasia, and Huntington's chorea.

By contrast, **recessive** mutations, unless sex-linked, require that the gene be present in duplicate to produce the trait, which means that the mutant gene must be inherited from each parent; consequently, many generations may pass before it is expressed. If one copy of the gene is mutant and the other is normal, the individual is not affected. More than 500 recessive diseases are known, and another 600 are suspected. Some examples are sickle-cell anemia, cystic fibrosis, and Tay–Sachs disease.

X-linked recessive diseases are caused by mutations in genes located on the X-chromosome. The Y chromosome contains far fewer genes than the X. Because males have only one X chromosome, all males having a mutation in the X chromosome show the effect of mutation; like dominant mutations, they are expressed soon after the mutation occurs. Since females have two X chromosomes, they need two mutant genes to show the effect of an X-linked recessive mutation. The best known examples of sex-linked disorders are hemophilia, color blindness, and a severe form of muscular dystrophy, but altogether there are more than 80 well-established and another 60 probable conditions of this sort.

In the case of Mendelian diseases, about 67% are caused predominantly by point mutations (base-pair changes in the DNA), 22% by both point mutations and DNA deletions within genes (i.e., they are intragenic), and 13% by intragenic deletions and large multilocus deletions. In some genes, the mutational sites of mutations are distributed throughout the gene; in a large proportion, however, these are nonrandomly distributed—that is, restricted to specific sites along the gene (specificities). Likewise, the break points of deletions are also nonrandomly distributed, showing specificities.

Some dominant and some recessive mutant genes cause traits that are regarded by society as normal or acceptable, such as different eye colors or blood groups. The majority, however, cause diseases ranging from mild to severe in their impact on the person.

The three types of Mendelian diseases are summarized as follows:

Autosomal dominant: The disease is due to a mutation in a single gene on one chromosome.
Autosomal recessive: The disease is due to a defective copy of the same gene from each parent.
Sex-linked: Males have one X chromosome, so one mutation can cause the disease; females have two

Xs, so two mutant genes are needed to cause the disease.

Chromosomal Changes

Chromosomal diseases are caused by gross abnormalities either in the structure of the chromosomes or in the number of chromosomes (too many or too few). With a few important exceptions, gross chromosome changes that can be seen under the microscope are not compatible with viability in the fertilized egg. Down's syndrome is the best-known example: It results from an extra chromosome 23. It is estimated that at least 40% of the spontaneous abortions that occur from the 5th through the 28th week of gestation and about 6% of stillbirths are associated with chromosomal anomalies. This kind of chromosome error is not believed to be influenced strongly by radiation, particularly at low doses. Chromosome breakage is less frequent than aberrations among spontaneous instances of severe human anomalies, but radiation is much more effective at breaking chromosomes than in causing errors in chromosome distribution. Chromosomes that are broken may rejoin in various ways (Chapter 2). A translocation, for example, involves the reciprocal exchange of parts between two or more chromosomes and is not necessarily harmful as long as both rearranged chromosomes are present and contain the full gene complement. Children of a person with a translocation often receive only one of the rearranged chromosomes, and their cells are therefore genetically unbalanced. The nature and extent of the abnormality varies enormously, and the harm to the person ranges from rather mild to very severe. Chromosome imbalance, if it does not cause the death of the embryo, typically leads to physical abnormalities, usually accompanied by mental deficiency.

Robertsonian translocations are the most common type found in normal humans. These are fusions of two chromosomes, each having a spindle attachment at the end of the chromosome, to produce a single chromosome with the spindle attachment in the center. The children of a person with this type of translocation are usually normal, because they inherit either the translocated pair or a pair of normal chromosomes. Radiation does not appear to be a major cause of Robertsonian translocations but rather tends to induce those of the reciprocal-exchange type.

Multifactorial

The term *multifactorial* is a general designation assigned to a disease known to have a genetic component but whose transmission patterns cannot be described as simple Mendelian. The common congenital abnormalities that are present at birth (e.g., neural tube defects, cleft lip with or without cleft palate) and many chronic diseases of adult onset, such as diabetes, essential hypertension, and coronary heart disease, are examples of multifactorial diseases. These diseases result from a number of causes, both genetic and environmental, the nature of which can vary among individuals, families, and populations. For these diseases, there is no simple relationship between mutation and disease, but the fact that genetic factors are involved is evident from observations of familial clustering; that is, these diseases run in families, but the recurrence risk to first-degree relatives is in the range of 5 to 10%, depending on the multifactorial disease, but never close to the 25 to 50% characteristic of Mendelian diseases. The potential role of some of the environmental factors has been delineated for only a few of these diseases; for example, excess caloric intake rich in saturated fat is an environmental risk factor for coronary heart disease, as are environmental allergens for asthma. Mendelian and chromosomal diseases are rare and account for only a very small proportion of hereditary diseases in the population; the major load is from multifactorial diseases.

Characteristics of multifactorial diseases include the following:

- Known to have a genetic component
- Transmission pattern not simple Mendelian
- Congenital abnormalities: cleft lip with or without cleft palate; neural tube defects
- Adult onset: diabetes, essential hypertension, coronary heart disease
- Interaction with environmental factors

RADIATION-INDUCED HEREDITARY EFFECTS IN FRUIT FLIES

As early as 1927, Müller reported that exposure to x-rays could cause readily observable mutations in the fruit fly, *Drosophila melanogaster*. These included a change of eye color from red to white, the ebony mutant with its jet-black color, the "vestigial wing" mutant, and the easiest of all to observe, the recessive lethal mutation. The fact that mutants produced by radiation cannot be identified as different compared with those that occur spontaneously makes their study particularly difficult. Sample sizes must be sufficiently large to detect the small excess by radiation, which made *Drosophila* an attractive and economical biologic test system, since huge numbers can be accommodated in a small space (compared, for example, with mice). Indeed, it was hereditary data from the fruit fly that led to the recommendation of a 5 R maximum permissible annual dose for radiation workers in the 1950s. The units have changed from R to rem to mSv, and the justification has also changed, but the quantity remains to this day. In the 1950s, hereditary changes were considered the principal hazard of exposure to ionizing radiation. There were three reasons for this:

1. A low **doubling dose** (5–150 R) for mutations was estimated from fruit fly experiments. (The doubling dose is the dose required to double the spontaneous mutation rate.)
2. Based again in the fruit fly, it was thought that hereditary effects were cumulative; that is, a little radiation now, some next week, and some next year all added up and contributed to the genetic load carried by the human race.
3. In the 1950s, little was known of the carcinogenic potential of low doses of radiation. An excess incidence of leukemia was evident in the Japanese survivors of the A-bomb attacks, but the much larger number of solid cancers did not appear until many years later.

Over the past 50 years, the hereditary risks from radiation have been progressively reduced, replaced by a concern over carcinogenesis as the data from the A-bomb survivors have matured.

RADIATION-INDUCED HEREDITARY EFFECTS IN MICE

The most common way to estimate the hereditary risks of radiation is to compare radiation-induced mutations with those that occur spontaneously and to express the results in terms of the doubling dose—the amount of radiation required to produce as many mutations as occur spontaneously in a generation. The idea is based on the assumption that "if nature can do it, radiation can do it, too." This is the **relative mutation risk**.

In the years following World War II, the husband-and-wife team of Russell and Russell, working at Oak Ridge National Laboratory, mounted an experiment of heroic proportions to determine specific locus mutation rates in the mouse under a variety of irradiation conditions. This experiment often is referred to as the "megamouse project" because of the enormous number of animals involved. Before the study ended, 7 million mice had been used.

An inbred mouse strain was chosen in which seven specific locus mutations occur, six involving a change of coat color and one expressed as a stunted ear. Figure 11.2 shows three coat-color variations: a piebald, a light honey, and a darker brown. These mutations occur spontaneously, and their incidence is increased by radiation.

These extensive studies included the irradiation of both male and female mice with a range of doses, dose rates, and fractionation patterns. Five major conclusions are pertinent to the radiologist:

1. The radiosensitivity of different mutations varies by a significant factor of about 35, so that it is only possible to speak in terms of average mutation rates. We now know that this is due simply to a size difference between the various genes involved.
2. In the mouse, there is a substantial dose-rate effect, so that spreading the radiation dose over a period of time results in fewer mutations for a given dose than in an acute exposure. This is in complete contrast to the data on *Drosophila*, where fractionated doses are cumulative. The big dose-rate effect discovered in the mouse, between 90 and 0.8 R/min (between about 90 and 0.8 cGy/min), was attributed to a repair process. The data are shown in Figure 11.3.
3. Essentially all of the radiation-induced hereditary data come from experiments with male mice. In the mouse, the oocytes are exquisitely radiosensitive and are readily killed by even low doses of radiation. For this reason, the mouse was an unfortunate choice as an experimental animal.
4. The hereditary consequences of a given dose can be reduced greatly if a time interval is allowed between irradiation and conception. This was first noticed in the male and a correlation was found to exist with the stage of spermatogenesis at which the radiation was delivered. If animals were irradiated and used immediately for mating in genetic experiments, so that the sperm used for fertilization had been irradiated in a mature state, then a relatively large number of mutations were produced. In contrast, if animals were irradiated and mating delayed for a number of weeks, so that the sperm used for fertilization had been irradiated in a primitive state, then fewer mutations were produced. It is inferred that this decrease in mutation rate with time after irradiation is the consequence of some repair process. Whatever the explanation, it is an important empirical observation that the hereditary consequences of a given dose of radiation can be reduced if a time interval is allowed between irradiation and conception.

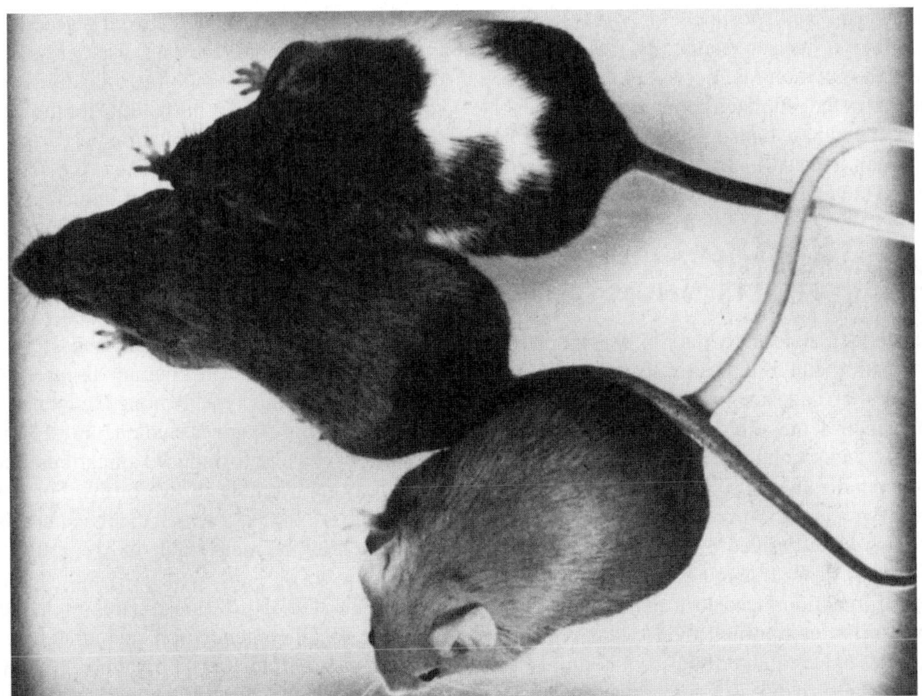

FIGURE 11.2 • In the megamouse project, seven specific locus mutations were used to study radiation-induced hereditary effects. This photo shows three of the mutations, which involve changes of coat color. (Courtesy of Dr. William L. Russell, Oak Ridge National Laboratory.)

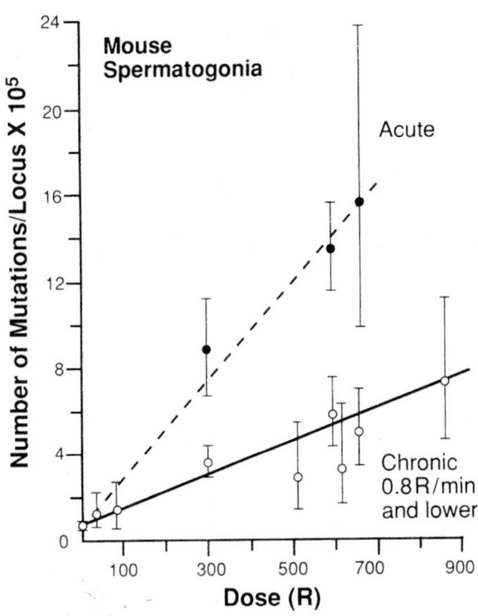

FIGURE 11.3 • Mutations in mice as a function of dose, delivered at high and low dose rates. (Courtesy of Dr. William L. Russell, Oak Ridge National Laboratory.)

This information is already used in genetic counseling given to people who have received radiation. In the mouse, a time interval between irradiation and insemination of 2 months in the male and rather longer in the female is sufficient to produce a maximum reduction in the effect of radiation. Although data are not available for humans, by analogy a period of 6 months usually is recommended. Consequently, if people are exposed to significant doses of radiation, either accidentally or as a result of their occupation, it is recommended that 6 months be allowed to elapse between the exposure to the radiation and a planned conception, to minimize the genetic consequence. This would be good advice to a person accidentally exposed to, say 0.1 Gy (10 rad), to young patients with Hodgkin's disease receiving radiotherapy, or even to patients subjected to diagnostic x-ray procedures involving the lumbar spine or the lower gastrointestinal tract in which a large exposure is used and the gonads must be included within the radiation field.

5. The estimate of the doubling dose favored by the Committee on the Biological Effects of Ionizing Radiation (BEIR V) and the United Nations Scientific Committee on the Effects of Atomic Radiation (UNSCEAR 88) is 1 Gy (100 rad) based

on low dose-rate exposure. This is a calculated rather than a measured quantity, based on the measured mutation rate per locus in the mouse adjusted for the estimated comparable number of loci in the human. It also allows for the fact that the human is usually exposed at low dose-rate, whereas the mouse data reflect acute exposures.

RADIATION-INDUCED HEREDITARY EFFECTS IN HUMANS

To estimate the risk of hereditary effects in the human population due to exposure to radiation, two basic pieces of data are needed: first, the baseline spontaneous mutation rate, which is known for humans, and second, the doubling dose, which can only come from mouse experiments (1 Gy, or 100 rad). Two correction factors must then be applied, which were derived by a task force of the ICRP in 2000. The first must allow for the fact that not all mutations lead to a disease. This so-called **mutation component (MC)** varies for different classes of hereditary diseases; it is simple for autosomal recessive diseases and very complex for multifactorial diseases. For the first generation following radiation exposure, the MC is about 0.3 for autosomal dominant and X-linked diseases, close to zero for autosomal recessive diseases, and about 0.01 to 0.02 for chronic multifactorial diseases. The second correction factor must allow for the fact that the seven specific locus mutations used to assess the doubling dose in the megamouse project are not representative of the spectrum of inducible hereditary diseases in humans. The success of experimental radiation mutagenesis studies in the mouse is mainly due to the fortunate choice of genes that are nonessential for survival of the animal or the cell and also happen to be located in nonessential regions of the genome. Most human disease-causing genes are not of this type. Among the human autosomal and X-linked genes studied, only 15 to 30% may be responsive to induced mutations that are potentially recoverable in live births. For chronic multifactorial diseases, which involve a number of genes, the fraction recoverable in live births would be even lower.

The UNSCEAR 2001 estimates of hereditary risks for the first generation and first two generations of an irradiated population are listed in Table 11.4. The risk of autosomal dominant and X-linked diseases for the first generation after irradiation is on the order of 750 to 1,500 cases

TABLE 11.4

Current Estimates of Genetic Risks from Continuing Exposure to Low-LET, Low-Dose, or Chronic Irradiation (from UNSCEAR 2001) (Assumed Doubling Dose: 1 Gy)

Disease Class	Based Frequency per 10^6 Live Births	Risk per Gy per 10^6 Progeny	
		First Generation	Up to Second Generation
Mendelian			
Autosomal dominant and X-linked	16,500	~750–1,500	~1,300–2,500
Autosomal recessive	7,500	0	0
Chromosomal	4,000	[a]	[a]
Multifactorial			
Chronic	650,000	~250–1,200	~250–1,200
Congenital abnormalities	60,000	~2,000	~2,400–3,000
Total	738,000	~3,000–4,700	~3,950–6,700
Total risk per Gy expressed as percent of baseline		~0.41–0.64	~0.53–0.91

[a]Assumed to be subsumed in part under the risk of autosomal dominant and X-linked diseases and in part under congenital abnormalities.

From United Nations Scientific Committee on the Effects of Atomic Radiation: *Hereditary Effects of Radiation: The UNSCEAR 2001 Report to the General Assembly with Scientific Annex.* New York, United Nations, 2001.

per million progeny per gray of chronic low-LET radiation (compared to the baseline of 16,500 cases per million). The risk of autosomal recessive diseases is essentially zero (compared to the baseline of 7,500 per million). The risk of chronic diseases is on the order of 250 to 1,200 cases per million (compared to the baseline of 650,000 per million). The risk of multisystem developmental or congenital abnormalities may be of the order of about 2,000 cases per million. Note that the total risk per gray is only about 0.41 to 0.64% of the baseline risk of 738,000 per million live births—that is, a relatively small proportion.

ICRP ESTIMATES OF HEREDITARY RISKS

The strategy of ICRP to estimate hereditary risks is based on the data for the first two generations calculated by UNSCEAR 2001, shown in Table 11.4. These data refer to a "reproductive" population and apply when the radiation doses received by all individuals in the population are genetically significant. However, when the *total* population of all ages is considered, the genetically significant dose will be markedly lower than the total dose received over a lifetime. Genetic damage sustained by germ cells of individuals who are beyond the reproductive period or who are not procreating for any reason poses no hereditary risks. Assuming an average life expectancy of 75 years, with mean reproductive age stopping at 30 years, the risk coefficients for a total population of all ages will be 30/75, that is, 40% of that for a reproductive population. This rounds out at 0.2%/Sv. For a *working* population, the relevant age range is only from 18 to 30 years, since no one is allowed to be a radiation worker before 18 years and the reproductive cycle is assumed to end at 30 years; consequently, the risk coefficients will be 12/75, or, 16% of that for a reproductive population, which rounds out at 0.1%/Sv.

MUTATIONS IN THE CHILDREN OF THE A-BOMB SURVIVORS

The survivors of the atomic-bomb attacks on Hiroshima and Nagasaki constitute the largest irradiated human population studied carefully for hereditary effects. Over the years, a cohort of 31,150 children born to parents receiving significant amounts of radiation (within 2 km of the bomb's hypocenter) and a somewhat larger control cohort (41,066) have been studied with respect to a variety of indicators: first, in the early years, for congenital defects, gender of child, physical development, and survival; then, in the middle years, for cytogenetic abnormality; and, more recently, for the occurrence of malignant disease and for electrophoretic or functional defects in a battery of some 30 serum proteins or erythrocyte enzymes. None of these indicators was related significantly to parental radiation exposure, but the net regression was slightly positive.

TABLE 11.5

Doubling Dose (Gametic) in the Offspring of Survivors of the Atomic-Bomb Attacks on Hiroshima and Nagasaki

Genetic Indicator	Doubling Dose, Sv
Untoward pregnancy outcome	0.69
Childhood mortality	1.47
Sex chromosome aneuploidy	2.52
Simple average	1.56

Adapted from Schull WJ, Otake M, Neal JV: Genetic effects of the atomic bomb: A reappraisal. *Science* 213:1220–1227, 1981, with permission.

For these various measures of hereditary effects, the differences between the children of proximally and distally exposed survivors is in the direction expected if a hereditary effect did result from the radiation, but in fact none of the findings are statistically significant. Nevertheless, the differences between these groups of children were used to calculate doubling doses.

Only three of these indicators lend themselves to an estimate of doubling dose, and the results are shown in Table 11.5, taken from a study in the early 1980s. The simple average of the three estimates is 1.56 Sv (156 rem). In a more recent review paper, Neel estimated the doubling dose for the human to be about 2 Sv; this is subject to considerable uncertainties, with a lower limit of 1 Sv and an upper limit that is indeterminate. This, of course, refers to an acute radiation dose, because it depends on the Japanese survivors.

The sparse human data support the current impression that the doubling dose derived from the mouse specific locus experiments is too low. The lack of a statistically significant excess of hereditary effects in the children of the A-bomb survivors is consistent with the numeric risk estimates developed by ICRP. The number of children involved and the range of doses to which their parents were exposed are too small for a statistically significant hereditary effect to be expected.

Summary of Pertinent Conclusions

- In the male, doses as low a 0.15 Gy (15 rad) result in oligospermia (diminished sperm count) after a latent period of about 6 weeks. Doses above 0.5 Gy (50 rad) result in azoospermia (absence of living spermatozoa) and therefore temporary sterility. Recovery time depends on dose.
- Permanent sterility in the male requires a single dose in excess of 6 Gy (600 rad).
- In the male, fractionated doses cause *more* gonadal damage than a single dose. Permanent sterility can result from a dose of 2.5 to 3 Gy (250–300 rad) in a fractionated regime over 2 to 4 weeks.
- In the female, radiation is highly effective in inducing permanent ovarian failure, with a marked age dependence on the dose required.
- The dose required for permanent sterility in the female varies from 12 Gy (1,200 rad) prepubertal to 2 Gy (200 rad) premenopausal.
- The induction of sterility in males does not produce significant changes in hormone balance, libido, or physical capability, but in the female leads to pronounced hormonal changes comparable to natural menopause.
- Exposure of a population can cause adverse health effects in the descendants as a consequence of mutations induced in germ cells. These used to be called "genetic" effects but are now more often called "hereditary" effects.
- Hereditary diseases are classified into three principal categories: Mendelian, chromosomal, and multifactorial.
- Radiation does not produce new, unique mutations but increases the incidence of the same mutations that occur spontaneously.
- Information on the hereditary effects of radiation comes almost entirely from animal experiments.
- The earlier mutation experiments were carried out with the fruit fly *Drosophila melanogaster*.
- Relative mutation rates have been measured in the megamouse project by observing seven specific locus mutations. This leads to an estimate of the "doubling dose."
- The doubling dose is the dose required to double the spontaneous mutation incidence; put another way, it is the dose required to produce an incidence of mutations equal to the spontaneous rate. Based on the mouse data, the doubling dose for low dose-rate exposure is estimated to be 1 Gy (100 rad).
- Not more than 1 to 6% of spontaneous mutations in humans may be ascribed to background radiation.
- To estimate the risk of radiation-induced hereditary diseases in the human, two quantities are required: (1) the baseline mutation rate for humans, which is estimated to be 738,000 per million, and (2) the doubling dose from the mouse data, which is about 1 Gy (100 rad).
- Two correction factors are needed: (1) to allow that not all mutations lead to a disease—this is the mutation component (MC), which varies for different classes of hereditary diseases; (2) to allow for the fact that the seven specific locus mutations used in the mouse experiments are not representative of inducible hereditary diseases in the human because they are all nonessential for the survival of the animal or cell.
- The International Commission on Radiological Protection (ICRP) estimates that the hereditary risk of radiation is about 0.2%/Sv for the general population and about 0.1%/Sv for a working population.
- In terms of detriment, expressed in years of life lost or impaired, congenital anomalies (i.e., resulting from effects on the developing embryo and fetus) are much more important than hereditary disorders.
- Children of the atomic-bomb survivors have been studied for a number of indicators, including congenital defects, gender ratio, physical development, survival, cytogenetic abnormalities, malignant disease and electrophoretic variants of blood proteins. A recent paper estimated the doubling dose to be about 2 Sv (200 rem), with a lower limit of 1 Sv (100 rem) and an upper limit that is indeterminate because the increase in mutations is not statistically significant.

BIBLIOGRAPHY

Bacq ZM, Alexander P: *Fundamentals of Radiobiology*, 2nd ed, pp 436–450. New York, Pergamon Press, 1961

Committee on the Biological Effects of Ionizing Radiation: *The Effects on Populations of Exposure to Low Levels of Ionizing Radiation.* Washington, DC, National Academy of Sciences, National Research Council, 1972

Committee on the Biological Effects of Ionizing Radiation: *The Effects on Populations of Exposure to Low Levels of Ionizing Radiation.* Washington, DC, National Academy of Sciences, National Research Council, 1980

Committee on the Biological Effects of Ionizing Radiation: *The Effects on Populations of Exposure to Low Levels of Ionizing Radiation.* Washington, DC, National Academy of Sciences, National Research Council, 1990

International Commission on Radiological Protection and International Commission on Radiation Units and Measurements: Exposure of man to ionizing radiation arising from medical procedures. *Phys Med Biol* 2:107–151, 1957

International Commission on Radiological Protection: *Report of the Task Group on Risk Estimation for Multifactorial Diseases*, ICRP Publication 83, Annals of the ICRP 29(3-4), Oxford, Pergamon Press, 1999

McKusick VAP: *Human Genetics.* Englewood Cliffs, NJ, Prentice Hall, 1969

Müller HJ: Advances in radiation mutagenesis through studies on *Drosophila.* In Bugher JC (ed): *Progress in Nuclear Energy* Series VI, pp 146–160. New York, Pergamon Press, 1959

Müller HJ: Artificial transmutation of the gene. *Science* 66:84–87, 1927

National Academy of Science: *The Effects on Populations of Exposure to Low Levels of Ionizing Radiation.* Washington, DC, National Academy of Sciences, National Research Council, 1972

Neel JV, Schull WJ, Awa AA, et al.: The children of parents exposed to atomic bombs: Estimates of genetic doubling dose of radiation for humans. *Am J Hum Genet* 46:1053–1072, 1990

Neel JV: Reappraisal of studies concerning the genetic effects of the radiation of human, mice and *Drosophila. Environ Mol Mutagen* 31:4–10, 1998

Pochin EE: Sizewell 13 inquiry: The biological basis of the assumption made by NRPB in the calculation of health effects and proof of evidence. NRPB/P/2 (Rev). Chilton, Oxon, UK, National Radiological Protection Board, 1983

Russell LB, Russell WL: The sensitivity of different stages in oogenesis to the radiation induction of dominant lethals and other changes in the mouse. In Mitchell JS, Holmes BE, Smith CL (eds): *Progress in Radiobiology*, pp 187–192. Edinburgh, Oliver & Boys, 1956

Russell WL: Effect of the interval between irradiation and conception on mutation frequency in female mice. *Proc Natl Acad Sci* USA 54:1552–1557, 1965

Russell WL: Genetic hazards of radiation. *Proc Am Phil Soc* 107:11–17, 1963

Russell WL: Studies in mammalian radiation genetics. *Nucleonics* 23:53–56, 1965

Russell WL: The effect of radiation dose rate and fractionation on mutation in mice. In Sobels FH (ed): *Repair of Genetic Radiation Damage*, pp 205–217, New York, Pergamon Press, 1963

Sankaranarayanan K, Chakraborty R: Ionizing radiation and genetic risks. XIII. Summary and synthesis of papers VI to XII and estimates of genetic risks in the year 2000. *Mutat Res* 453:183–197, 2000

Sankaranarayanan K, Chakraborty R: Ionizing radiation and genetic risks. XI. The doubling dose estimates from the mid-1950s to the present and the conceptual change to the use of human data for spontaneous mutation rates and mouse data for induced rates for doubling dose calculations. *Mutat Res* 453:107–127, 2000

Sankaranarayanan K, Chakraborty R: Ionizing radiation and genetic risks. XII. The concept of potential recoverability correction factor (PRCF) and its use for predicting the risk of radiation-inducible genetic diseases in human live births. *Mutat Res* 453:129–179, 2000

Sankaranarayanan K, Chakraborty R: Ionizing radiation and genetic risks. X. The potential "disease phenotypes" of radiation-induced genetic damage in humans: perspectives from human molecular biology and radiation genetics. *Mutat Res* 429:45–83, 1999

Sankaranarayanan K: Ionizing radiation and genetic risks. IX. Estimates of the frequencies of Mendelian diseases and spontaneous mutation rates in human populations. *Mutat Res* 411:129–179, 1998

Schull WL, Otake M, Neal JV: Genetic effects of the atomic bomb: A reappraisal. *Science* 213:1220–1227, 1981

Searle GH, Phillips RJS: Genetic effect of high LET radiation in mice. *Space Radiol Biol Radiat Res* 7(suppl):294–303, 1967

Selby PB, Selby PR: Gamma-ray-induced dominant mutations that cause skeletal abnormalities in mice: I. Plan, summary of results, and discussion. *Mutat Res* 43:357–375, 1977

Selby PB: Induced skeletal mutations. *Genetics* 92(suppl):127–133, 1979

Selby PB: Radiation-induced dominant skeletal mutations in mice: Mutation rate, characteristics, and usefulness in estimating genetic hazard to human from radiation. In Okada S, Imamura M, Terasima T, Yamaguchi M (eds): *Radiation Research: Proceedings of the Sixth International Congress of Radiation Research*, pp 537–544. Tokyo, Toppan Printing, 1979

Selby PB: The doubling dose for radiation, or for any other mutagen, is actually several times larger than has been previously thought if it is based on specific-locus mutation frequencies in mice. *Environ Mol Mutagen* 27(suppl 27):61, 1996

Spencer WP, Stern C: Experiments to test the validity of the linear R-dose mutation frequency relation in *Drosophila* at low dosage. *Genetics* 33:43–74, 1948

United Nations Scientific Committee on the Effects of Atomic Radiation: *Genetic Effect of Radiation.* New York, United Nations, 1977

United Nations Scientific Committee on the Effects of Atomic Radiation: *Ionizing Radiation Sources and Biological Effects.* New York, United Nations, 1982

United Nations Scientific Committee on the Effects of Atomic Radiation: *Ionizing Radiation Sources and Biological Effects.* New York, United Nations, 1988

United Nations Scientific Committee on the Effects of Atomic Radiation: *Hereditary Effects of Radiation: The UNSCEAR 2001 Report to the General Assembly with Scientific Annex.* New York, United Nations, 2001

United Nations Scientific Committee on the Effects of Atomic Radiation: *The 1993 Report to the General Assembly, with Annexes.* New York, United Nations, 1993

CHAPTER 12

Effects of Radiation on the Embryo and Fetus

HISTORICAL PERSPECTIVE

In the early years of the 20th century, case reports began to appear in the medical literature that described mental retardation in children with small head size, as well as other gross malformations, born to mothers who had received pelvic radiotherapy before realizing that they were pregnant. As early as 1929, Goldstein and Murphy reviewed 38 such cases. Interestingly enough, they concluded that large doses were needed to produce such effects and did not consider diagnostic pelvic irradiation of the mother to be a hazard.

We now have a great deal of information concerning the effects of radiation on the developing embryo and fetus from both animal experiments and the human experience.

OVERVIEW OF RADIATION EFFECTS ON THE EMBRYO AND FETUS

Among the somatic effects of radiation other than cancer, developmental effects on the unborn child are of greatest concern. The classic effects are listed here:

1. *Lethal effects* are induced by radiation before or immediately after implantation of the embryo into the uterine wall or are induced after increasingly higher doses during all stages of intrauterine development, to be expressed either before birth (prenatal death) or at about the time of birth (neonatal death).
2. *Malformations* are characteristic of the period of major organogenesis, in which the main body structures are formed, and especially of the most active phase of cell multiplication in the relevant structures.
3. *Growth disturbances without malformations* are induced at all stages of development but particularly in the latter part of pregnancy.

The principal factors of importance are the *dose* and the *stage of gestation at which it is delivered. Dose rate* is also of significance because many pathologic effects on the embryo are reduced significantly by reducing the dose rate.

It should be recognized that congenital anomalies arise in all animal species, even in the absence of any radiation beyond that received from natural sources. The incidence depends to a large extent on the time at which the anomalies are scored. In humans, the average incidence of malformed infants at birth is about 6%. Some malformations

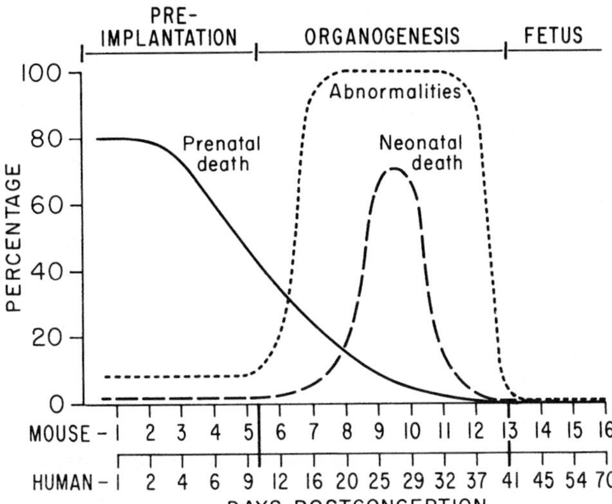

FIGURE 12.1 • Incidence of abnormalities and of prenatal and neonatal death in mice given a dose of 200 R of x-rays at various times after fertilization. The lower scale consists of Rugh's estimates of the equivalent stages for the human embryo. (Data from Russell LB, Russell WL: An analysis of the changing radiation response of the developing mouse embryo. *J Cell Physiol* 43[suppl 1]:130–149, 1954.)

disappear after birth, but more become evident later that are not scored at birth. The global incidence roughly doubles to 12% if grown children rather than infants are examined. Any assessment of the effectiveness of radiation in inducing damage *in utero* must be viewed against this natural level of inborn defects and its variable expression.

DATA FROM MICE AND RATS

Most experimental data on the effect of radiation on the developing embryo or fetus have been obtained with the mouse or rat, animals that reproduce in quantity with relatively short gestation periods. Russell and Russell divided the total developmental period *in utero* into three stages: (1) **preimplantation**, which extends from fertilization to the time at which the embryo attaches to the wall of the uterus; (2) **organogenesis**, the period during which the major organs are developed; and (3) the **fetal period**, during which growth of the structures already formed takes place. There is a very large variability in the relative duration of these periods among animal species, as well as in the total duration of intrauterine life. Also, at any given stage of development, the state of differentiation or maturation of any one structure, with respect to all the others, varies considerably in different species.

In the mouse, preimplantation corresponds to days 0 through 5; organogenesis, days 5 through 13; and the fetal period, day 13 through full term, which is about 20 days. The effect of about 2 Gy (200 rad) of x-rays delivered at various times after conception is illustrated in Figure 12.1. The lower scale contains Rugh's estimates of the equivalent ages for human embryos, based solely on comparable stages of organ development. It is a nonlinear match, because preimplantation, organogenesis, and the fetal period in the mouse are about equal in length, whereas the fetal period in the human is proportionately much longer.

Figure 12.2 is taken from the work of Brent and Ghorson, who performed an extensive series of experiments with rats. It shows the various periods during gestation in which the principal effects of radiation are most evident. The horizontal scale refers to the times of the major events during gestation for the rat and gives an estimate of the comparable stages for the human. The following discussion of the principal effects of radiation delivered during preimplantation, organogenesis, and the fetal stages represents a consensus view, combining conclusions from various experiments with either rats or mice.

Preimplantation

Preimplantation is the most sensitive stage to the lethal effects of radiation. This high incidence of prenatal death may be expressed in a decrease in litter size. Growth retardation is not observed after irradiation at this stage; if the embryo survives, it grows normally *in utero* and afterward. Few if any abnormalities are produced by irradiation at this stage. Rugh has shown that in mice, an x-ray dose of 0.05 to 0.15 Gy (5–15 rad) can kill the fertilized egg.

Thus, the irradiated preimplanted embryo that survives grows normally in the prepartum and postpartum periods; that is, there is an "all-or-nothing" effect of radiation because if the number of cells in the conceptus is small and their nature is not yet specialized, the effect of damage to these cells is most likely to take the form of a failure to implant or an undetected death of the conceptus. This is

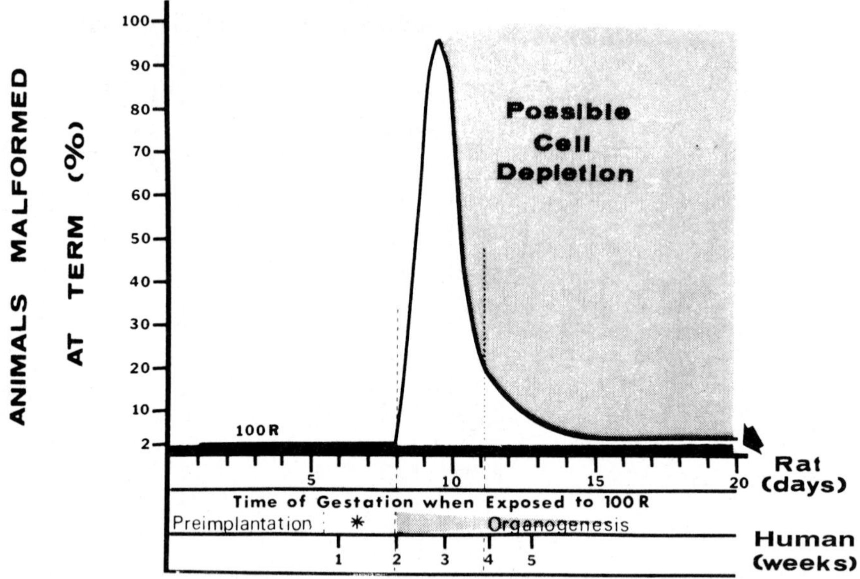

FIGURE 12.2 • Relative incidence of congenital malformations in the rat after an x-ray exposure of 100 R, delivered at various stages during gestation. The control incidence in this species is about 2%, indicated by the arrow on the right. The incidence of malformation after irradiation before the 8th day is not detectably different from controls. A large incidence, approaching 100%, occurs if the radiation is delivered during early organogenesis, corresponding to the 2nd through 4th week of a human pregnancy. The number of malformations produced falls off rapidly as organogenesis diminishes, though some organogenesis of the central nervous system continues to term. During the fetal stage, a dose of 100 R causes an irreversible loss of cells that is expressed as growth retardation persisting to adulthood. The asterisk shows the stage of implantation at which radiation causes growth retardation that is expressed as a decrease in weight at term. (From Brent RL, Ghorson RO: Radiation exposure in pregnancy. *Curr Probl Radiol* 2:1–48, 1972, with permission.)

illustrated in the remarkable pictures produced by Pedersen and reproduced in Figure 12.3. If too many cells are killed by irradiation, the embryo dies and is resorbed. If only a few cells are killed, one or two cell divisions can make good the damage.

Organogenesis

During organogenesis, the principal effect of radiation in small rodents is the production of a variety of congenital anomalies of a structural nature. As seen in Figure 12.1, a dose of about 2 Gy (200 rad) of x-rays to the mouse embryo during the period of maximum sensitivity can result in a 100% incidence of malformations at birth. A similar result is seen in Figure 12.2 for rats exposed to about 1 Gy (100 rad). During organogenesis, most of the embryonic cells are in their blastula, or differentiating, stage and are particularly sensitive. This corresponds to the period in the human at which the tranquilizer thalidomide produced such disastrous effects (i.e., at about 35 days after conception), and it is also the time of maximum risk of deleterious effects from the rubella virus.

Examples of gross anomalies resulting from irradiation during the period of organogenesis are shown in Figures 12.4 and 12.5. It is characteristic of mice and rats that a wide variety of structural malformations are seen. The production of a specific defect is associated with a definite time during this period of organogenesis, usually the time of the first morphologic evidence of differentiation in the organ or portion of the organ involved.

Embryos exposed during early organogenesis also exhibit the greatest intrauterine growth retardation. This is expressed as a weight reduction at term and is a phenomenon resulting from cell depletion. Animals show a remarkable ability to recover from the growth retardation produced by irradiation during organogenesis, and although they may be smaller than usual at birth, they may achieve a normal weight as adults. There is an association between growth retardation and teratogenesis: Irradiated embryos that show major congenital anomalies also suffer an overall reduction of growth. In animals, a dose of about 1 Gy (100 rad) of x-rays produces growth retardation if delivered at any stage of gestation (except during preimplantation); 0.25 Gy (25 rad) does not produce an observable effect, even at the most sensitive stage.

If death occurs as a result of irradiation in organogenesis, it is likely to be neonatal

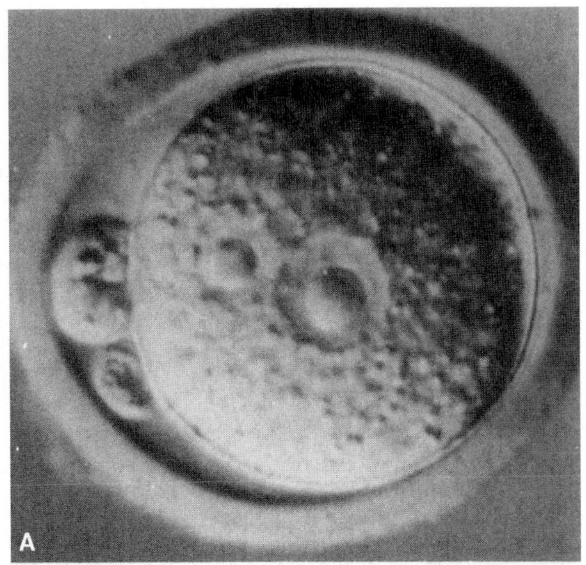

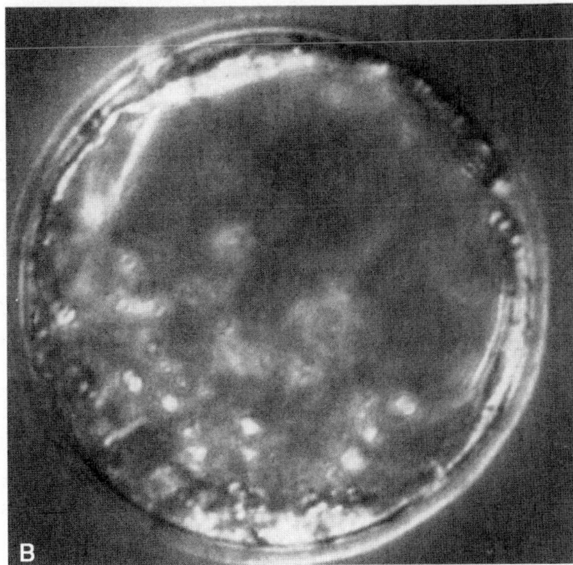

FIGURE 12.3 • During preimplantation, the embryo consists of a limited number of cells. **A:** Newly fertilized mouse egg. **B:** By the 3rd day, the mouse embryo consists of only 16 cells. About 5 days after conception in the mouse, which corresponds to about 9 or 10 days in the human, the embryo becomes embedded in the wall of the uterus, and at about this time, cells begin to differentiate to form specific tissues and organs. (Courtesy of Dr. Pedersen, University of California at San Francisco.)

death—occurring at or about the time of birth. The transition from prenatal death from irradiation mainly during preimplantation to neonatal death resulting from irradiation mainly in organogenesis is very clear from Figure 12.1. The neonatal deaths peak at 70% for mice receiving about 2 Gy (200 rad) on about the 10th day.

The Fetal Period

The remainder of pregnancy, the fetal period, extends from about day 13 onward in the mouse; this corresponds to about 6 weeks onward in the human. A variety of effects have been documented in the experimental animal after irradiation during the fetal stages, including effects on the hematopoietic system, liver, and kidney, all occurring, however, after relatively high radiation doses. The effects on the developing gonads have been documented particularly well, both morphologically and functionally. There appears at present to be little correspondence between the cellular and functional damage as a function of dose, but doses of a few tenths of a gray as a minimum are necessary to produce fertility changes in various animal species.

Much higher doses of radiation are required to cause lethality during this period than at earlier stages of development, although the irradiated early fetus exhibits the largest degree of permanent growth retardation, in contrast to the embryo in

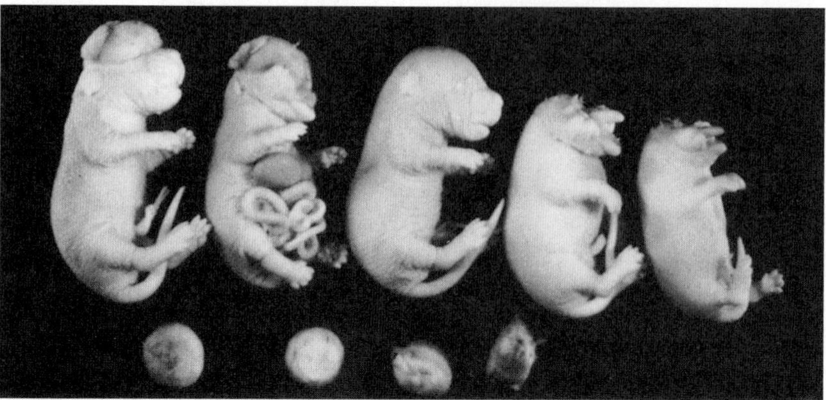

FIGURE 12.4 ● Litter from a female mouse irradiated with x-rays during organogenesis and sacrificed at 19 days. A number of anomalies are demonstrated in this litter. There are four resorbed embryos (bottom) and five fetuses that would have been born alive (top). From left to right, the first shows exencephaly; the second, exencephaly and evisceration; the third is apparently normal; and the remaining two are anencephalics with stunting. (Photograph by Dr. Roberts Rugh.)

early organogenesis, which exhibits the most temporary growth retardation, which is evident at term but from which the animal is able to recover later.

EXPERIENCE IN HUMANS

Information on the irradiation of human concepti comes from two major sources: studies of atomic-bomb survivors in Japan and medical exposures (particularly therapeutic irradiations), especially during the early part of the century, when hazards were not yet fully appreciated. These will be discussed in turn.

Survivors of the A-Bomb Attacks on Hiroshima and Nagasaki Irradiated *in Utero*

The growth to maturity of children exposed *in utero* at Hiroshima and Nagasaki has been studied carefully. There are difficulties associated with the dosimetry, but the conclusions have far-reaching implications.

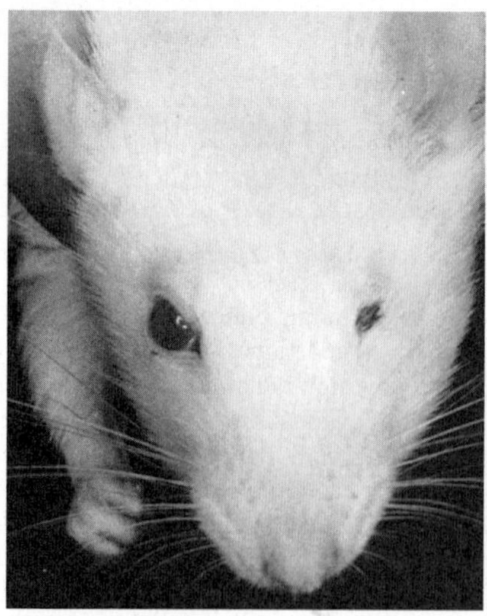

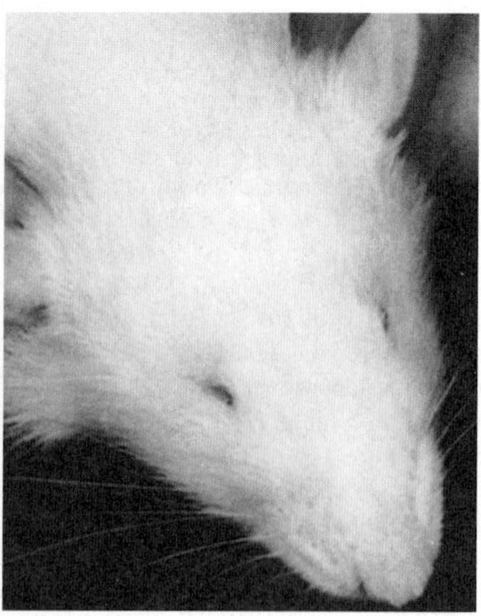

FIGURE 12.5 ● Two rats from the same litter exposed to a dose of 100 R of x-rays 9.5 days after conception. The rat on the left has a normal right eye and microphthalmus of the left. The rat on the right shows anophthalmia of both eyes. (From Rugh R, Caveness WF, Duhamel L, Schwarz GS: Structural and functional [electroencephalographic] changes in the post-natal mammalian brain resulting from x-irradiation of the embryo. *Mil Med* 128:392–408, 1963, with permission.)

TABLE 12.1

Growth Retardation at Hiroshima from *in Utero* Irradiation:[a] Comparison of Those Exposed within 1,500 m[b] of the Hypocenter with Those More than 3,000 m from the Hypocenter

Height	2.25 cm shorter
Weight	3 kg lighter
Head diameter	1.1 cm smaller

[a] 80% of 1,613 children exposed *in utero* followed to age 17 years.
[b] Average kerma, 25 rad (0.25 Gy), but doses are subject to modification.
Data from Committee on the Biological Effects of Ionizing Radiations: *The Effects on Populations of Exposure to Low Levels of Ionizing Radiation.* Washington, DC, National Academy of Sciences, 1980.

Data on the children exposed *in utero* in Hiroshima and Nagasaki show too few individuals who were younger than 4 weeks of gestational age at the time the bomb was dropped. This deficiency presumably results from increased fetal loss or infant mortality rate. This stage of development is so early that damage to a single cell or group of cells is likely to impair the function of all the progeny cells and lead to death of the embryo. In accord with this reasoning is the observation that no birth defects were found as a result of irradiation before 15 days of gestational age. This is in accord with the experimental data for rats and mice in which exposure during preimplantation had an all-or-nothing effect: death of the embryo or normal development.

Exposure to radiation resulted in growth retardation (Table 12.1). Children exposed as embryos closer than 1,500 m to the hypocenter of the atomic explosion were shorter, weighed less, and had head diameters significantly smaller than children who were more than 3,000 m from the hypocenter and received negligibly small doses. It is of interest to note that there was no catch-up growth, because the smallness in head size was maintained into adulthood.

The principal effects of irradiation *in utero* of the Japanese at Hiroshima and Nagasaki are small head size (microcephaly) and mental retardation. Figure 12.6 is one of the few photographs available of young Japanese adults, exposed *in utero* to radiation from the atomic bomb, whose head circumference is evidently smaller than normal. The prevalence of small head diameter and mental retardation has been evaluated in individuals exposed *in utero* to the A-bombs in Japan. The study involved about 1,600 exposed children, of whom about 62 had small heads, and 30 showed clinically severe mental retardation.

1. *Microcephaly.* A significant effect of radiation on the frequency of small heads is observed only in the periods 0 to 7 and 8 to 15 weeks postovulation. No significant excess was seen among individuals exposed at 16 weeks or more. The proportion of exposed individuals with microcephaly increases with dose, and there is little evidence for a threshold in dose (Fig. 12.7). As pointed out earlier, radiation-related small head size is related to a generalized growth retardation, including reduced height and weight.
2. *Mental retardation.* A child was deemed to be severely retarded if he or she was "unable to perform simple calculations, to make simple conversation, to care for himself or herself, or if he or she was completely unmanageable or has been institutionalized." Most of these children never were enrolled in public schools, but among the few who were, the highest IQ was 68. In all, 30 children were judged to be severely mentally retarded; in 5 of these children, causes other than radiation were considered likely, including Down's syndrome, neonatal jaundice, encephalitis, or birth trauma. Nevertheless, the remaining number represents an incidence far higher than normal. Severe mental retardation

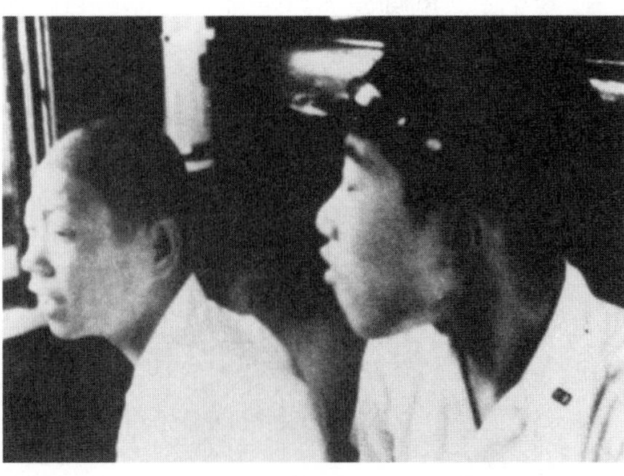

FIGURE 12.6 ● One of the few photographs available of Japanese youths with reduced head circumference as a result of radiation exposure *in utero* from the atomic bombs. (From Committee for the Compilation of Materials on Damage Caused by the Atomic Bomb in Hiroshima and Nagasaki: *Hiroshima and Nagasaki: The Physical, Medical and Social Effects of the Atomic Bombings.* New York, Basic Books, 1981, with permission.)

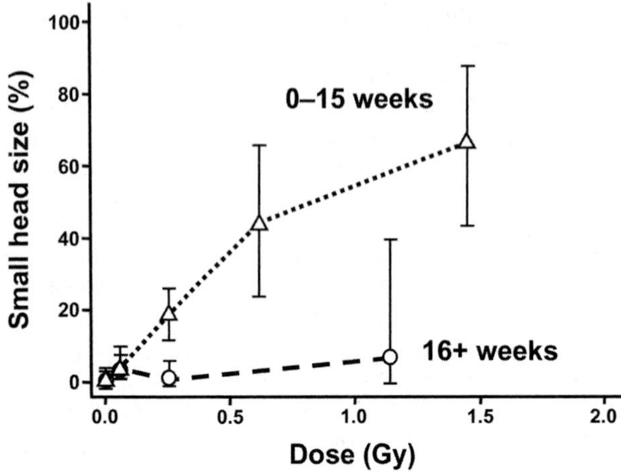

FIGURE 12.7 • Proportion of exposed individuals with small head sizes as a function of dose and gestational age. (Redrawn from the data of Otake M, Schull WJ: Radiation-related small head size among prenatally exposed A-bomb survivors. *Int J of Radiat Biol* 63:255–270, 1993.)

was not observed to be induced by radiation before 8 weeks after conception or after 25 weeks. The most sensitive period is 8 to 15 weeks after conception; for exposure during weeks 16 to 25, the risk is four times smaller. Figure 12.8 shows the relation between the incidence of mental retardation and absorbed dose for this most sensitive period. The relationship appears to be linear, and the data are consistent with a probability of occurrence of mental retardation of 40% at a dose of 1 Gy (100 rad). The possibility of a dose threshold cannot be excluded. By using the most recent dosimetry and discarding two cases of mental retardation for which *in utero* irradiation was unlikely to be the cause, the dose–response relationship is consistent with a threshold of 0.12 to 0.2 Gy (12–20 rad). A linear, nonthreshold response is unlikely in view of the presumed deterministic nature of mental retardation that would require the killing of a minimum number of cells to be manifest.

Microcephaly and mental retardation differ somewhat in the gestational ages at which they occur. Both occur in the 8–15 week period, but in the earlier period (0–7 weeks), microcephaly appears without mental retardation, while in the later period (16–25 weeks), mental retardation is observed in the absence of microcephaly. The highest risk of mental retardation occurs at a gestational age at which the relevant tissue, that is, the brain cortex, is being formed. It is thought to be associated with impaired proliferation, differentiation, and, most of all, migration of cells from their place of birth to their site of function. Cells killed before 8 weeks of gestation can cause small head size without mental retardation because the neurons that lead to the formation of the cerebrum are at a stage not yet sensitive to impairment by radiation. Glial cells that provide structural support for the brain are, however, susceptible to depletion. Magnetic resonance images of individuals irradiated *in utero* at 3 to 15 weeks of gestation show evidence of massive impairment of

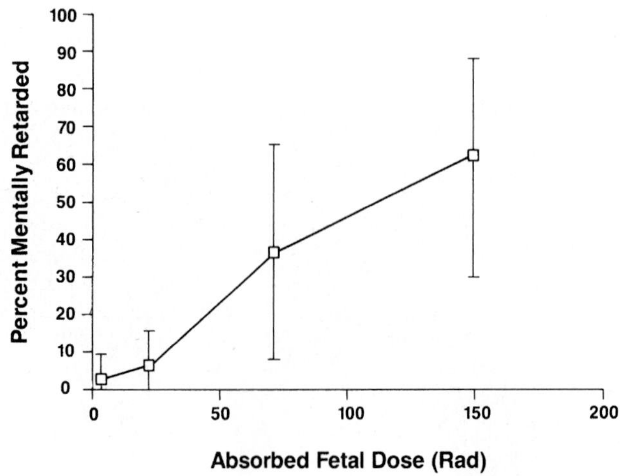

FIGURE 12.8 • The frequency of mental retardation as a function of dose among those exposed *in utero* to atomic-bomb radiation. The data are pooled from Hiroshima and Nagasaki for those exposed at 8 to 15 weeks gestational age. The vertical bars represent the 90% confidence intervals. There was no risk at 0 to 8 weeks after conception, and for exposure at later periods during gestation (16+ weeks), the excess is barely significant, even at the higher doses. (Adapted from Otake M, Schull WJ: *In utero* exposure to A-bomb radiation and mental retardation: A reassessment. *Br J Radiol* 57:409–414, 1984, with permission.)

cells to migrate from proliferative zones. A typical distribution of gray matter is often seen in patients with spontaneous mental retardation, but it is usually *unilateral*; that caused by radiation exposure is *bilateral*.

Although severe mental retardation requiring the children to be institutionalized has been known for some time in those exposed *in utero* at Hiroshima, more recent studies have shown mental impairment of less severity, indicated by IQ test scores. For irradiation during the sensitive period of 8 to 15 weeks after conception, the observed shift in intelligence test scores corresponds to about 30 IQ points per gray (100 rad). Extrapolating these data to situations in which a fetus is knowingly or unwillingly exposed to diagnostic radiology, resulting in doses of perhaps 0.05 Gy (5 rad), the loss of IQ, using a linear model, would be too small to be detected.

Exposure to Medical Radiation

A relationship between microcephaly and x-irradiation during intrauterine life has been recognized since Goldstein and Murphy first focused attention on the subject in 1929. The numbers are small and the doses are not known with any certainty, though most were in the therapeutic range. Microcephaly was reported as well as mental retardation and a variety of defects, including spina bifida, bilateral clubfoot, ossification defects of the cranial bones, deformities of the upper extremities, hydrocephaly, alopecia of the scalp, divergent squint, and blindness at birth.

Dekaban surveyed the literature for instances of pelvic x-irradiation in pregnant women. On the basis of the available data, the following generalizations were proposed:

1. Large doses of radiation (2.5 Gy, or 250 rad) delivered to the human embryo before 2 to 3 weeks of gestation are not likely to produce severe abnormalities in most children born, although a considerable number of the embryos may be resorbed or aborted.
2. Irradiation between 4 and 11 weeks of gestation would lead to severe abnormalities of many organs in most children.
3. Irradiation between 11 and 16 weeks of gestation may produce a few eye, skeletal, and genital organ abnormalities; stunted growth, microcephaly, and mental retardation are frequently present.
4. Irradiation of the fetus between 16 and 25 weeks of gestation may lead to a mild degree of microcephaly, mental retardation, and stunting of growth.
5. Irradiation after 30 weeks of gestation is not likely to produce gross structural abnormalities leading to a serious handicap in early life but could cause functional disabilities.

COMPARISON OF HUMAN AND ANIMAL DATA

Figure 12.9 is an attempt to summarize the data for the effects of radiation on the developing embryo and fetus, comparing the information from animals and human A-bomb survivors.

Exposure to radiation during preimplantation leads to a high incidence of embryonic death, but embryos that survive develop normally. This has been shown clearly in experiments with both rats and mice and is consistent with the data from Japan. In animals, irradiation during organogenesis leads to neonatal death, temporary growth retardation, and, above all, a wide range of malformations affecting many different limbs and organs. By contrast, the principal effect in the Japanese survivors of the atomic-bomb attacks is microcephaly with or without mental retardation, and this begins in the 8th week, that is, after the period classically described as organogenesis. The wide array of congenital malformations found in rats and mice irradiated during organogenesis (and in humans in medical exposures) was not reported in the Japanese survivors. Much has been made of this difference. On the one hand, it has been suggested that the gross structural deformities in Japan simply were not recorded in the chaos that followed the dropping of the atomic bombs. On the other hand, it is argued that humans differ from rats and mice in that the period of susceptibility to a wide array of congenital malformations (i.e., during organogenesis) is short compared with the period during which mental retardation can be induced. Because the number of children involved is quite small, it might be expected that effects on the central nervous system, which is developing over a larger period of time, would dominate. The situation is different in laboratory animals: Their susceptibility to radiation-induced small head size is of similar duration to that for the induction of other deformities. The data from patients exposed to therapeutic doses of medical radiation show a range of congenital malformations that more closely mirrors the animal results, although the numbers are small and the doses high. To be on the safe side, it must be assumed that the entire period of gestation from about 10 days to 25 weeks is sensitive to the induction of malformations by radiation.

Table 12.2 summarizes the lowest doses at which effects on the embryo and fetus have been observed.

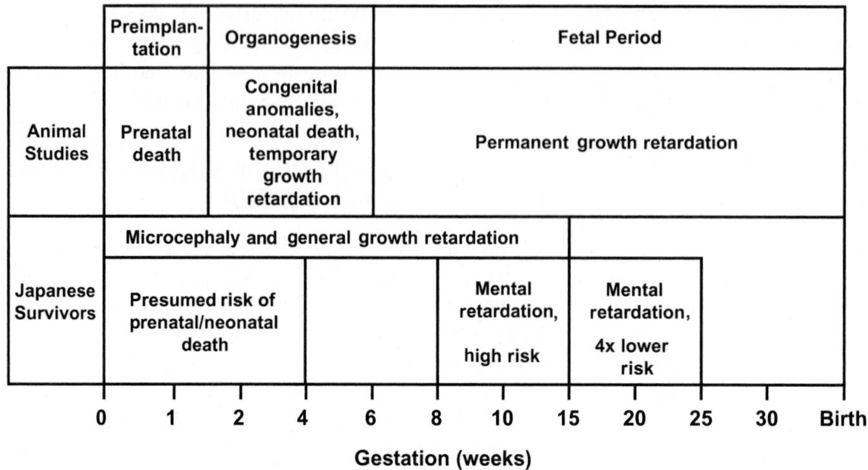

FIGURE 12.9 • Chart illustrating the similarities and differences between data from small laboratory animals and data from the Japanese survivors of the atomic-bomb attacks. The gestation weeks are for the human; the equivalent gestation periods have been matched for animal studies. Both sets of data indicate that irradiation early in gestation may result in the death of the embryo but that malformations do not occur. The animal data show a high incidence of a wide spectrum of malformations during organogenesis. The principal finding in the Japanese is microcephaly, which occurred up to 15 weeks, and mental retardation, which occurred most frequently following irradiation at 8 to 15 weeks of gestation and, to a lesser extent, at 16 to 25 weeks.

This table summarizes the conclusions of the third report of the Committee on the Biological Effects of Ionizing Radiation (BEIR III). Readily measurable damage can be observed at doses below 0.1 Gy (10 rad) delivered at sensitive stages of gestation. The principal abnormalities produced by radiation are almost certainly the consequence of damage to many cells (i.e., *deterministic* effects) and therefore would be consistent with a threshold in dose. There is also some indication of this in the data for mental retardation.

CANCER IN CHILDHOOD AFTER IRRADIATION *IN UTERO*

The Oxford Survey of Childhood Cancers, published by Stewart and Kneale in the 1950s, suggested an association between the risk of cancer, principally leukemia, up to 15 years of age and exposure *in utero* to diagnostic x-rays. This was a retrospective case-controlled study and is summarized in Table 12.3. Of 7,649 children who died of leukemia or childhood cancers, 1,141 had been

TABLE 12.2

Minimum Doses at Which Effects on the Embryo and Fetus Have Been Observed

Animal data	
Oocyte killing (primates)	50% lethal dose at 5 rad (0.5 Gy)
Central nervous system damage (mouse)	Threshold at 10 rad (0.1 Gy)
Brain damage and behavioral damage (rat)	Threshold at 6 rad (0.06 Gy)
Human data	
Small head circumference	Air kerma 10–19 rad (0.1–0.19 Gy)
Summary	Fetal dose 6 rad (0.06 Gy)
Readily measurable damage caused by doses below 10 rad (0.1 Gy) (acute exposure) delivered at sensitive stages	

Summarized from Committee on the Biological Effects of Ionizing Radiation: *The Effects on Populations of Exposure to Low Levels of Ionizing Radiation*. BEIR III Washington, DC, National Academy of Sciences, 1980.

TABLE 12.3

Childhood Cancer and Irradiation *in Utero*

Number of children with leukemia or cancer before age 10 years	7,649
Number x-rayed *in utero*	1,141
Number of matched controls	7,649
Number of controls irradiated *in utero*	774
Number of films	1 to 5
Fetal dose per film	0.46–0.2 rad (4.6–2 mGy)
Relative cancer risk estimate assuming radiation to be the causative agent	1.52

Based on Stewart A. Kneale GW: Radiation dose effects in relation to obstetric x-rays and childhood cancer. *Lancet* 1:1185–1188, 1970.

x-rayed *in utero*. Of an equal number of controls who did not develop childhood cancer, only 774 had been irradiated prenatally. The irradiated children received one to five films, with a fetal dose per film of 0.46 to 0.2 rad (4.6–2 mGy); however, the estimated doses are uncertain and probably varied over the period of the study. A subsequent study in New England by MacMahon also reported an association between prenatal x-rays and childhood leukemia.

This subject has been the source of great controversy for many years. No one seriously doubts the *association* between *in utero* irradiation and childhood cancer; the debate is whether the radiation is *causative* or whether it involves the selection of a particular group of children prone to cancer.

In a careful paper in 1997, Doll and Wakeford summarized all of the studies of *in utero* exposure and came to the following conclusions:

- Low-dose irradiation of the fetus *in utero* causes an increased risk of childhood malignancies. Most of the data refer to exposure in the third trimester.
- An obstetric x-ray examination results in a 40% increase in the risk of childhood cancer over the spontaneous level.
- Radiation doses of around 10 mGy (1 rad) increase the risk.
- The excess absolute risk is about 6% per gray (100 rad).
- These risk estimates are highly uncertain except to say that they are not zero.

In a later (2003) paper, Wakeford and Little compared the risk of childhood cancer per unit dose of radiation received *in utero* for the obstetric x-ray examinations and the Japanese A-bomb survivors. They concluded that once all sources of uncertainty are taken into account, the risks are not inconsistent, which supports a causal explanation for the cancers seen in the Oxford survey.

OCCUPATIONAL EXPOSURE OF WOMEN

The National Council on Radiological Protection and Measurements in this (NCRP Report 116) recommends a monthly limit of 0.5 mSv (0.05 rem) to the embryo or fetus once pregnancy is declared. This recommendation is designed to limit the risk of mental retardation, congenital malformations, and carcinogenesis. NCRP no longer recommends specific controls for occupationally exposed women *until* a pregnancy is declared. Once a pregnancy is declared, the radiation worker should be interviewed by the radiation safety officer or the chair of the radiation safety committee to discuss the advisability of changing or curtailing duties to limit exposure.

THE PREGNANT OR POTENTIALLY PREGNANT PATIENT

Most practicing radiologists at some time in their careers are faced with a patient who has discovered in retrospect that she was pregnant at a time when extensive x-ray procedures were performed involving the pelvis or lower abdomen.

The only completely satisfactory solution to this problem is to ensure that the situation never occurs in the first place. Patients should always be asked if they are, or may be, pregnant, and in the case of procedures involving larger doses of radiation to the pelvis, a pregnancy test may be in order.

Despite the best-laid plans and the most careful precautions, there still are occasional instances in which, because of clinical urgency or unusual accident, an early developing embryo is exposed to a substantial dose of radiation amounting to several centigray (rad) or more. The first step in evaluating whether or not damage may have been done to the embryo is to estimate the dose involved. It is sometimes useful to solicit the help of an experienced medical physicist to make measurements in a phantom after carefully reconstructing the setup that was used. No dose level can be regarded as completely safe. Congenital abnormalities occur in 5 to 10% of the human population anyway, so it is impossible in retrospect to attribute a given anomaly to a small dose of radiation received by an embryo or fetus. All that can be said is that radiation increases the probability of an anomaly and that this increase is a function of dose.

The figure of 0.1 Gy (10 rad) often is mentioned as the dose to a developing embryo or fetus at a

TABLE 12.4

Major Events in Understanding Effects of Radiation on the Developing Embryo and Fetus

Investigators	Year	Observations
Goldstein and Murphy	1929	Various abnormalities, including mental retardation and small head diameter in children born to mothers who received pelvic radiation therapy during pregnancy
Job et al.	1935	Recognition that different periods of gestation differ in radiosensitivity
Russell	1950	Nature of developmental abnormality determined by gestational age at exposure
Russell and Russell	1952	Clinical Implications of irradiation in pregnancy
Plummer	1952	Mental retardation and microcephaly observed in children of atomic-bomb survivors
Stewart and Kneale	1952	Leukemia and childhood cancer in children irradiated *in utero* with diagnostic x-rays
Otake and Schull	1984	Mental retardation caused by irradiation at 8–15 weeks of pregnancy in Japanese survivors

gestational age sensitive to the induction of congenital malformations, including reduced head diameter and mental retardation, above which a therapeutic abortion should be considered. As noted above, this period extends from about 10 days to 25 weeks of gestation. The basis of this recommendation is as follows: The data from Japan for severe mental retardation could be interpreted as having a threshold, and the mechanism of the radiation effect is consistent with this conclusion. At the same time, the loss of IQ measured at 1 Gy (100 rad) would be undetectable if extrapolated linearly to 0.1 Gy (10 rad).

Not everyone would agree with this view, and the cutoff point is clearly not sharp. If a dose approaching this value has been given during the sensitive period, however, it is prudent to consider the relative merits of terminating the pregnancy in consultation with the referring physician as well as with the patient and her family.

There are a number of factors to consider in conjunction with the dose. These include the hazard of the pregnancy to the expectant mother, the probability of future pregnancies, the extent to which the prospective parents want the unborn infant, their mental outlook on the possibility of a deformed child, and the ethnic and religious background of the family. The exact dose level at which it is justifiable to terminate the pregnancy may be flexible within broad limits around the guideline figure, depending on a combination of these other circumstances.

There are special problems involved in the use of nuclear-medicine procedures in pregnant or potentially pregnant females. This is particularly true in the case of radionuclides that are able to cross the placenta. This topic is discussed in Chapter 14.

Table 12.4 is a historical summary of events in our gradual understanding of radiation effects on the developing embryo and fetus.

Summary of Pertinent Conclusions

- Moderate doses of radiation can produce catastrophic effects on the developing embryo and fetus.
- The effects depend on the stage of gestation, the dose, and also the dose rate.
- Gestation is divided into preimplantation, organogenesis, and the fetal period. In humans, these periods correspond to about 0 through 9 days, 10 days through 6 weeks, and 6 weeks through term, respectively.
- The principal effects of radiation on the developing embryo and fetus, aside from cancer, are embryonic, fetal, or neonatal death; congenital malformations; growth retardation; and functional impairment, such as mental retardation.
- Irradiation during preimplantation leads to potential death of the embryo. Growth retardation or malformations are not seen in animals from irradiation at this time. The human data are consistent with this conclusion.
- In animals, embryos exposed to radiation in early organogenesis exhibit the most severe

(continued)

Summary of Pertinent Conclusions (Continued)

intrauterine growth retardation, from which they can recover later (i.e., temporary growth retardation). Irradiation in the fetal period leads to the greatest degree of permanent growth retardation.

- In animals, lethality from irradiation varies with stage of development. The embryonic 50% lethal dose is lowest during early preimplantation; at this stage, embryos killed by radiation suffer a prenatal death and are resorbed. In organogenesis, prenatal death is replaced by neonatal death—death at or about the time of birth. During the fetal stage, the 50% lethal dose approaches that of the adult.
- In animals, the peak incidence of teratogenesis, or gross malformations, occurs if the fetus is irradiated in organogenesis.
- In contrast to what is observed in experimental animals, radiation-induced malformations of body structures other than the central nervous system are uncommon in the Japanese survivors irradiated *in utero*, although they have been reported in patients exposed to therapeutic doses of medical radiation.
- In the Japanese survivors, irradiation *in utero* resulted in small head size (microcephaly) and mental retardation.
- Mental retardation from irradiation occurred primarily at 8 to 15 weeks of gestational age, with a smaller excess at 16 to 25 weeks. It is thought to be caused by radiation effects on cell migration within the brain.
- The incidence of severe mental retardation as a function of dose is apparently linear without threshold at 8 to 15 weeks, with a risk coefficient of 0.4 per Gy (0.4 per 100 rad). The incidence is about four times lower at 16 to 25 weeks. The data are also consistent with a dose threshold of 0.12 to 0.2 Gy (12–20 rad).
- Small head circumference was more common than mental retardation.
- Data on atomic-bomb survivors indicate that microcephaly can result from exposure at 0 to 7 and 8 to 15 weeks postovulation, but not at later times. There is little evidence for a threshold in dose.
- A variety of effects have been documented in experimental animals after irradiation during fetal stages, including effects on the hematopoietic system, liver, and kidney, all occurring, however, after quite high radiation doses.
- There is an association between exposure to diagnostic x-rays *in utero* and the subsequent development of childhood malignancies.
- The original study of diagnostic x-ray exposure *in utero* and subsequent malignancies, principally leukemia, was done by Stewart and Kneale at Oxford University, but the same association was observed in the United States by MacMahon. If x-rays are the causative agent, these studies imply that radiation at low doses *in utero* increases the spontaneous cancer incidence in the first 10 to 15 years of life by 50%—that is, by a factor of 1.5 to 2.
- It has been argued for years whether radiation is the causative agent or whether there are other factors involved, such as the selection of a particular group of children prone to cancer.
- Doll and Wakeford in 1997 summarized all of the evidence for and against and concluded that an obstetric x-ray examination, particularly in the third trimester, increased the risk of childhood cancer by 40%. The risk is increased by a dose of only 10 mGy (1 rad). The excess absolute risk is about 6% per gray (100 rad), which is not very different from the risk estimates from the atomic-bomb survivors for adult exposure.
- Until a pregnancy is declared, no special limits apply to women other than those applicable to any radiation worker. Once a pregnancy is declared, the maximum permissible dose to the fetus is 0.5 mSv (0.05 rem) per month.
- Once a pregnancy is declared, the duties of a radiation worker should be reviewed to ensure that this limit is not exceeded.
- A dose of 0.1 Gy (10 rad) to the embryo during the sensitive period of gestation (10 days to 25 weeks) often is regarded as the cutoff point above which a therapeutic abortion should be considered to avoid the possibility of an anomalous child. The decision to terminate a pregnancy should be flexible and must depend on many factors in addition to dose.

BIBLIOGRAPHY

Adelstein SJ: Administered radionuclides in pregnancy. *Teratology* 59:236–239, 1999

Antypas C, Sandilos P, Kouvaris J, Balafouta E, Karinou E, Kollaros N, Vlahos L: Fetal dose evaluation during breast cancer radiotherapy. *Int J Radiat Oncol Biol Phys* 40: 995–999, 1998

Balakier H, Pedersen RA: Allocation of cells to inner cell mass and trophectoderm lineages in preimplantation mouse embryos. *Dev Biol* 90:352–362, 1982

Bithel JF, Stiller CA: A new calculation of the carcinogenic risk of obstetric x-raying. *Stat Med* 7:857–864, 1988

Boice JD, Jr., Miller RW: Childhood and adult cancer after intrauterine exposure to ionizing radiation. *Teratology* 59:227–233, 1999

Brent RL, Ghorson RO: Radiation exposure in pregnancy. *Curr Probl Radiol* 2:1–48, 1972

Committee for the Compilation of Materials on Damage Caused by the Atomic Bomb in Hiroshima and Nagasaki: *Hiroshima and Nagasaki: The Physical, Medical and Social Effects of the Atomic Bombings.* New York, Basic Books, 1981

Committee on the Biological Effects of Ionizing Radiation: *Health Effects of Exposure to Low Levels of Ionizing Radiations.* Washington, DC, National Academy of Sciences/National Research Council, 1990

Committee on the Biological Effects of Ionizing Radiations: *The Effects on Populations of Exposure to Low Levels of Ionizing Radiation.* Washington, DC, National Academy of Sciences, 1980

Dekaban AS: Abnormalities in children exposed to x-radiation during various stages of gestation: Tentative timetable of radiation to the human fetus. *Int J Nucl Med* 9:471–477, 1968

Delongchamp RR, Mabuchi K, Yoshimoto Y, Preston DL: Cancer mortality among atomic bomb survivors exposed *in utero* or as young children, October 1950–May 1992. *Radiat Res* 147:385–395, 1997

Doll R, Wakeford R: Risk of childhood cancer from fetal irradiation. *Br J Radiol* 70:130–139, 1997

Goldstein L, Murphy DP: Microcephalic idiocy following radium therapy for uterine cancer during pregnancy. *Am J Obstet Gynecol* 18:189–195, 281–282, 1929

Hammer-Jacobsen E: Therapeutic abortion on account of x-ray examination during pregnancy. *Dan Med Bull* 6:113–121, 1959

Harvey EB, Boice JD, Honeyman M, Fannery JT: Prenatal x-ray exposure and childhood cancer in twins. *N Engl J Med* 312:541–545, 1985

Little MP, Charles MW, Wakeford R: A review of the risks of leukemia in relation to parental preconception exposure to radiation. *Health Phys* 68:299–310, 1995

Mayr NA, Wen BC, Saw CB: Radiation therapy during pregnancy. *Obstet Gynecol Clin North Am* 25:301–321, 1998

MacMahon B: Prenatal x-ray exposure and childhood cancer. *JNCI* 28:1173–1191, 1962

Meinert R, Kaletsch U, Kaatsch P, Schuz J, Michaelis J: Associations between childhood cancer and ionizing radiation: Results of a population-based case-control study in Germany. *Cancer Epidemiol Biomarkers Prev* 8:793–799, 1999

Miller RW, Mulvihill JJ: Small head size after atomic irradiation. In Sever JL, Brent RL (eds): *Teratogen Update: Environmentally Induced Birth Defect Risks,* pp 141–143. New York, Alan R Liss, 1986

Mole RH: Childhood cancer after prenatal exposure to diagnostic x-ray examinations in Britain. *Br J Cancer* 62:152–168, 1990

Mole RH: The biology and radiobiology of *in utero* development in relation to radiological protection. *Br J Radiol* 66:1095–1102, 1993

National Council on Radiation Protection and Measurements: *Limitation of Exposure to Ionizing Radiation.* NCRP Report No. 116. Bethesda, NCRP, 1993

Otake M, Schull WJ: In utero exposure to A-bomb radiation and mental retardation: A reassessment. *Br J Radiol* 57:409–414, 1984

Otake M, Schull WJ: Radiation-related brain damage and growth retardation among the prenatally exposed atomic bomb survivors. *Int J Radiat Biol* 74:159–171, 1998

Otake M, Schull WJ: Radiation-related small head size among prenatally exposed A-bomb survivors. *Int J of Radiat Biol* 63:255–270, 1993

Otake M, Schull WJ, Lee S: Threshold for radiation-related severe mental retardation in prenatally exposed A-bomb survivors: A re-analysis. *Int J Radiat Biol* 70:755–763, 1996

Rodvall Y, Pershagen G, Hrubec Z, Ahlbom A, Pederson NL, Boice JD: Prenatal x-ray exposure and childhood cancer in Swedish twins. *Int J Cancer* 46:362–365, 1990

Rugh R: The impact of ionizing radiation on the embryo and fetus. *AJR* 89:182–190, 1963

Rugh R, Caveness WF, Duhamel L, Schwarz GS: Structural and functional (electroencephalographic) changes in the post-natal mammalian brain resulting from x-irradiation of the embryo. *Mil Med* 128:392–408, 1963

Russell LB, Montgomery CS: Radiation sensitivity differences within cell-division cycles during mouse cleavage. *Int J Radiat Biol* 10:151–164, 1966

Russell LB, Russell WL: An analysis of the changing radiation response of the developing mouse embryo. *J Cell Physiol* 43(Suppl 1):130–149, 1954

Russell WL: Effect of the interval between irradiation and conception on mutational frequency in female mice. *Proc Natl Acad Sci USA* 54:1552–1557, 1965

Schull WJ, Otake M: Cognitive function and prenatal exposure to ionizing radiation. *Teratology* 59:222–226, 1999

Seigel DG: Frequency of live births among survivors of Hiroshima and Nagasaki atomic bombs. *Radiat Res* 28:278–288, 1966

Stabin MG: Health concerns related to radiation exposure of the female nuclear medicine patient. *Environ Health Perspect* 105 (Suppl 6):1403–1409, 1997

Stewart A, Kneale GW: Radiation dose effects in relation to obstetric x-rays and childhood cancers. *Lancet* 1:1185–1188, 1970

United Nations Scientific Committee on the Effects of Atomic Radiation: *Sources and Effects of Ionizing Radiation.* New York, UNSCEAR, 1986

Wakeford R, Little MP: Risk coefficients for childhood cancer after intrauterine irradiation: A review. *Int J Radiat Biol* 79:293–309, 2003

CHAPTER 13

Radiation Cataractogenesis

CATARACTS OF THE OCULAR LENS

The word **cataract** is used to describe any detectable change in the normally transparent lens of the eye. The effect may vary from tiny flecks in the lens to complete opacification, resulting in total blindness. Cataracts are usually associated with old age or, less commonly, with some abnormal metabolic disorder, chronic ocular infection, or trauma. It is also well known that sufficient exposure to ionizing radiations (such as x- or γ-rays, charged particles, or neutrons) may cause a cataract.

The ocular lens is enclosed in a capsule (Fig. 13.1); the lens itself consists largely of fiber cells and is covered with an epithelium anteriorly. The lens has no blood supply. Dividing cells are limited to the preequatorial region of the epithelium. The progeny of these mitotic cells differentiate into lens fibers and accrete at the equator.

Because cell division continues throughout life, the lens may be regarded as a self-renewal tissue. It is, however, a most curious cellular system in that there appears to be no mechanism for cell removal. If dividing cells are injured by radiation, the resulting abnormal fibers are not removed from the lens but migrate toward the posterior pole; because they are not translucent, they constitute the beginning of a cataract.

LENS OPACIFICATION IN EXPERIMENTAL ANIMALS

Some species of animals, especially the mouse, are very sensitive to radiation as far as lens opacification is concerned. A large proportion of a mouse population naturally develop opacifications as they become older. A dose of a few centigray of x-rays or a fraction of a centigray of fast neutrons produces readily discernible changes in the lens. As the dose is increased, the *latent period*, the time that elapses before an opacity of given severity is evident, becomes shorter. Put another way, radiation advances in time a process that occurs normally.

Neutrons and other densely ionizing radiations are very effective at inducing cataracts, as evidenced by the number of physicists and engineers who developed cataracts as a result of working around high-energy accelerators in the early days before safety procedures were introduced. The relative biologic effectiveness (RBE) of fast neutrons is a strong function of dose, with a value of about 10 pertaining to high dose levels on the order of several gray (several hundred rad), relative to x-rays, but rising to 50 or more for small doses of a fraction of a centigray (rad). Worgul and his associates have reported similar RBEs for lens damage in rat eyes exposed to accelerated heavy ions. The increase in

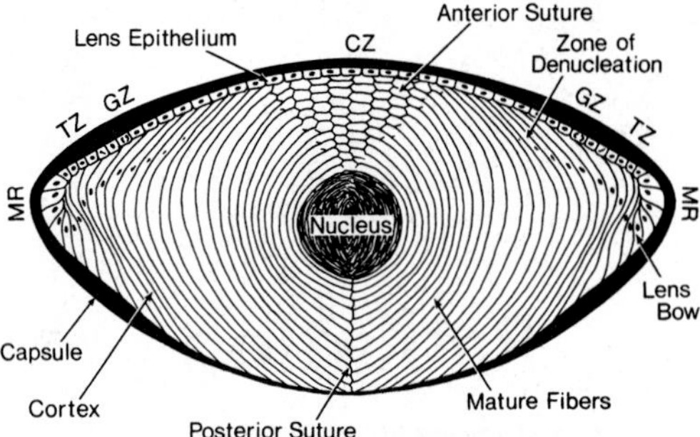

FIGURE 13.1 • Diagram of a sagittal section of a human lens, illustrating the various cellular relationships. Cells are produced by mitosis in the germination zone (GZ) of the epithelium. They begin to differentiate into lens fibers at the meridional rows (MR) and accumulate at the equator. Cells in the central zone (CZ) do not normally divide. (From Merriam GR, Worgul BV: Experimental radiation cataract: Its clinical relevance. *Bull NY Acad Med* 59:372–392, 1983, with permission.)

RBE at low doses is caused largely by the sharply declining effectiveness of x-rays with decreasing dose, rather than an increase in effect per unit dose of neutrons or charged particles.

CATARACTS IN HUMANS

Radiologists have known for many years that the lens of the eye may be damaged by radiation. A study of patients treated with x- or γ-rays, in which a proportion of the dose reached the eye, has provided some insight into radiation cataractogenesis in humans. Figure 13.2 shows a typical cataract in a patient on radiotherapy. An early radiation cataract viewed through an ophthalmoscope may appear as a dot, usually situated at the posterior pole. As it enlarges, small granules and vacuoles appear around it. With further enlargement, to the point at which the opacity is several millimeters in diameter, it may develop with a relatively clear center, so that it is shaped like a doughnut. At the same time, granular opacities and vacuoles may appear in the anterior subcapsular region, usually in the pupillary area. This sequence of events is not unique to radiation, but its appearance in an individual with a radiation history strongly suggests radiation as the causative agent. By the same token, an absence of this sequence of events would exclude radiation as a cause. In other words, while it is never possible to state unequivocally that a given cataract is radiation induced, it is possible to say with some certainty that some cataracts—for example, nuclear cataracts—do not have a radiation etiology. Depending on dose, the cataract frequently remains stationary at this stage, confined to the posterior subcapsular region. If it continues to progress, it becomes nonspecific and cannot be distinguished from other types of cataracts.

THE DEGREE OF OPACITY

At low doses, the opacity may become stationary at a level that involves little or no impairment of vision. At higher doses, the opacity may progress until it results in a significant loss of vision. Of patients on radiotherapy who received low dose levels to the eye (2.2–6.5 Gy, or 220–650 rad), only about

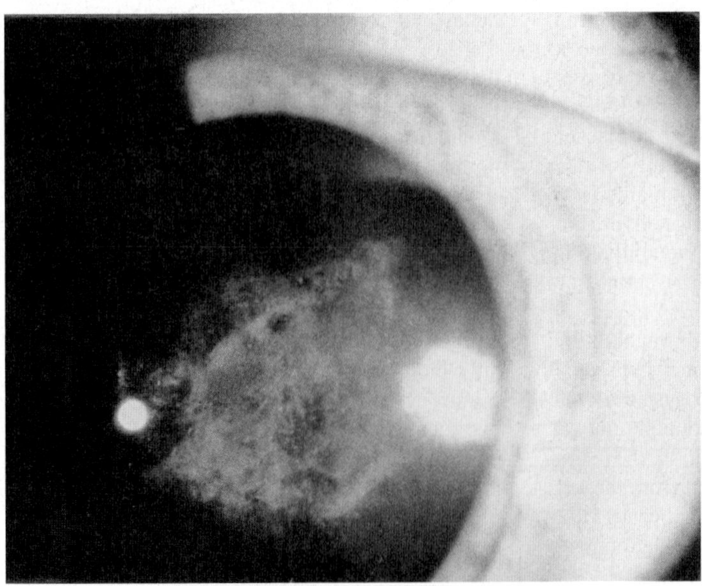

FIGURE 13.2 • Cataract in the posterior subcapsular region 4 years after a dose of 24 Gy (2,400 rad) of x-rays to a patient on radiotherapy. (From Merriam GR, Worgul BV: Experimental radiation cataract: Its clinical relevance. *Bull NY Acad Med* 59:372–392, 1983, with permission.)

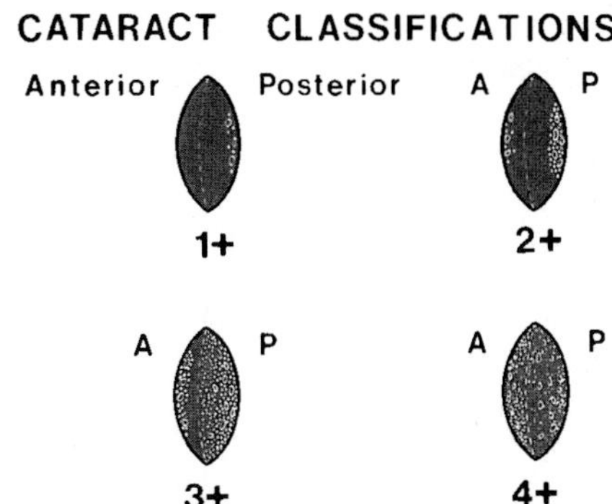

FIGURE 13.3 • The system of cataract classification devised by Merriam and Focht, illustrating the arbitrary numeric scores assigned to progressive severities of cataracts. (Courtesy of Dr. Basil Worgul.)

12% developed *progressive* opacities. Conversely, in higher-dose groups (6.5–11.5 Gy, or 650–1,150 rad), only 12% had *stationary* opacities.

Figure 13.3 shows the system of cataract classification devised in the 1950s by Merriam and Focht. The accumulation of some opaque fibers at the posterior pole is labeled a 1+ cataract; as the severity of this opacity increases and some impaired fibers show up in the anterior part of the lens, the score edges up progressively to 4+.

The severity of the cataract can be assessed quantitatively and objectively by using the Scheimpflug imaging system. This device provides a distortion-free digitized image for densitometric analysis of the cataract. Figure 13.4 shows a cross section of the lens of one of the "liquidators" who worked on the roof of the reactor at Chernobyl and accumulated a significant dose. The degree of opacity, measured with the Scheimpflug system, is shown in the lower panel.

Figure 13.5, deduced from accumulated clinical experience, represents a time–dose relationship for the production of cataracts. A combination of a dose and a treatment time that falls *below* the shaded band *does not* produce injury to the lens. A combination of dose and overall time that falls *above* the shaded area *would* be expected to produce a progressive opacity with impairment of vision. Within the shaded zone, a cataract may or may not be produced. The probability of a progressive cataract increases with increasing dose. It is clear

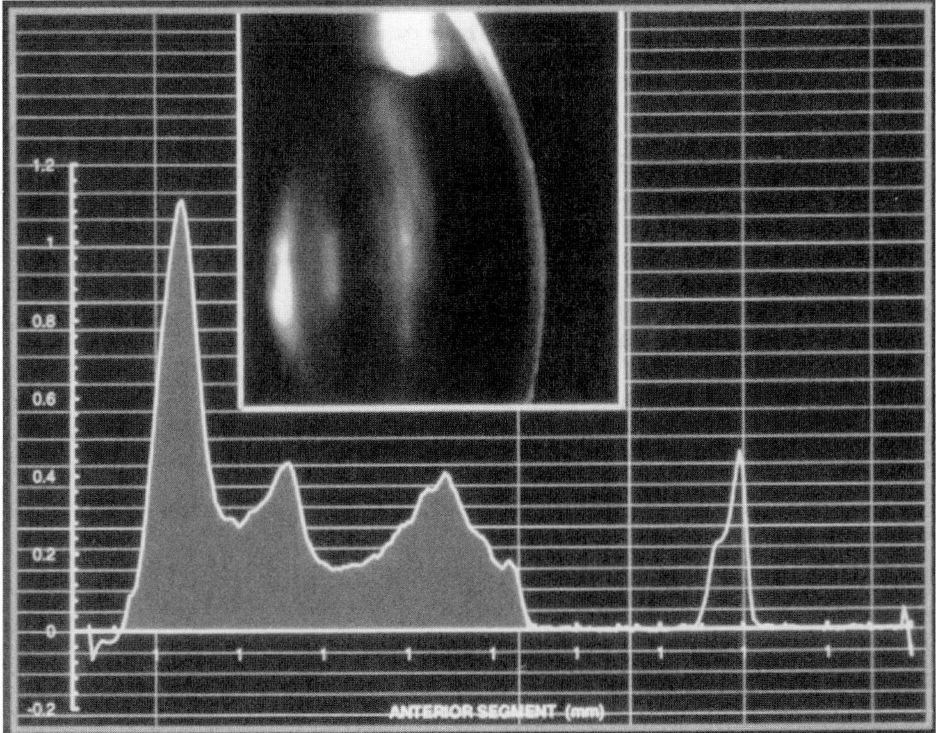

FIGURE 13.4 • **Top:** Photograph of the lens of a "liquidator" who worked on top of the reactor at Chernobyl and accumulated a substantial radiation dose. **Bottom:** Degree of opacity through the lens measured with the Scheimpflug imaging system. This equipment gives a quantitative and objective assessment of the severity of the cataract. The area under the curve represents a densitometric reading of the lens. The region of greatest opacification is under the posterior capsule. (Courtesy of Dr. Basil Worgul.)

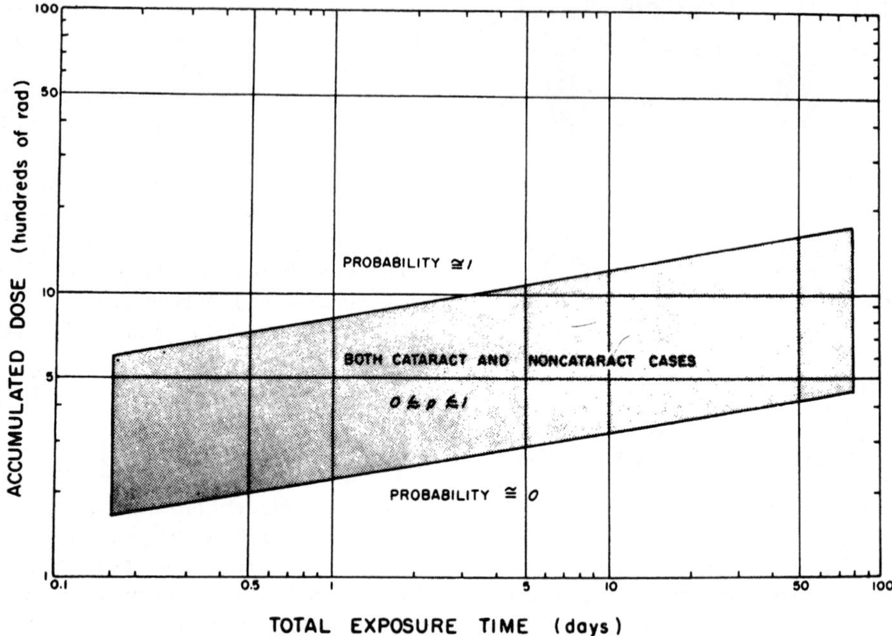

FIGURE 13.5 ● Time–dose relationship indicating radiation dosage for cataract production in humans with a probability between 0 and 1. A combination of a total dose and overall treatment time that falls above the shaded area would produce a progressive vision-impairing opacity. A dose and treatment time falling below the shaded area would not be expected to produce injury to the lens. Within the shaded area, a cataract may or may not be produced; the probability increases with increasing dose. (From Merriam GR, Szechter A, Focht EF: The effects of ionizing radiations on the eye. *Front Radiat Ther Oncol* 6:346–385, 1972, with permission.)

that the lens is able to tolerate a higher dose with increased fractionation and overall treatment time.

Table 13.1 shows estimates of the minimum cataractogenic and maximum noncataractogenic doses for a single acute exposure, a protracted exposure of 3 weeks to 3 months, and an even more protracted exposure. A vision-impairing ocular cataract is considered a deterministic effect (Chapter 15). The minimum dose required to produce a progressive cataract is about 2 Gy (200 rad) in a single exposure; larger doses are necessary in a fractionated or protracted exposure.

THE LATENT PERIOD

The time period between irradiation and the appearance of lens opacities in humans has been reported in the literature variously to be from 6 months to 35 years. In patients who had received 2.5 to 6.5 Gy (250–650 rad), the average latent period was about 8 years. At higher doses of between 6.51 to 11.5 Gy (651–1,150 rad), the average latent period was reduced to about 4 years. This and other evidence indicate that the latent period becomes shorter as dose is increased.

TABLE 13.1

Relation between Overall Exposure Time and the Radiation Dose Needed to Produce a Cataract

Duration of Treatment	Minimum Cataractogenic Dose, Gy	Maximum Noncataractogenic Dose, Gy
Single	2.0	2.0
3 weeks–3 months	4.0	10.0
Over 3 months	5.5	10.5

DOSE–RESPONSE RELATIONSHIP FOR CATARACTS IN HUMANS

Merriam, Szechter, and Focht carefully reviewed the case histories of 233 patients on radiotherapy who received radiation to the lens of the eye and for whom dose estimates were available. Of these, 128 developed cataracts, 105 did not.

Britten and his colleagues reported 14 cases of radiation-induced cataracts in 38 patients treated with radon gold seed implants for tumors of the eyelid; in 6, visual acuity was seriously affected. These cataracts were thought to be progressive between 6 and 11 years after treatment. Doses were calculated to the center of the lens, and it appeared that 4,000 R (about 40 Gy) produced a cataract in all cases, whereas 2,000 R (about 20 Gy) resulted in no cataracts at all. In a parallel series treated by superficial x-rays, only one case of radiation cataract was observed in 57 patients treated; this was in the contralateral eye, which received a dose of 9.5 Gy (950 rad) in a single exposure, which presumably was transmitted through the nose to the opposite eye. The lens dose on the treated side that was shielded with lead was only 0.16 Gy (16 rad).

Observations of the survivors of Hiroshima and Nagasaki have been consistent with the data from patients on radiotherapy. Large doses of radiation are required to produce vision-impairing cataracts. Physicists exposed to neutrons during the operation of cyclotron accelerators and survivors of reactor accidents also have developed cataracts, but the numbers are too small and the doses are not known with sufficient certainty to allow a meaningful construction of a dose–response relationship.

The available information appears to indicate the existence of a threshold for the induction of detectable lens opacification in humans. This does not exclude the possibility that the smallest doses do produce some damage; but in practical terms, a dose of several gray (several hundred rad) is required to result in a demonstrable effect, and even larger doses are needed to produce a cataract that impairs vision. Great care should be exercised in the use of neutrons and indeed all forms of high linear energy transfer radiations, because animal experiments indicate that they have a high RBE for lens opacification. There is evidence of early cataracts in some of the 300 or so astronauts who have flown in space, particularly in those who flew in the lunar missions or in shuttle missions of high inclination—that is, close to the poles, where the dose from high-energy heavy ions is greatest.

Radiation-induced cataracts are considered a deterministic late effect, because there is a practical threshold dose below which they do not occur, and above the threshold the severity of the biologic response is dose related.

Summary of Pertinent Conclusions

- A cataract is an opacification of the normally transparent lens of the eye.
- Dividing cells are limited to the preequatorial region of the epithelium. Progeny of these mitotic cells differentiate into lens fibers and accrete at the equator. It is the failure of these cells to differentiate correctly that leads to a cataract, whether spontaneous or radiation induced.
- A unique feature of the lens is that there is no mechanism for the removal of dead or damaged cells.
- The minimum dose required to produce a progressive cataract is about 2 Gy (200 rad) in a single exposure; larger doses are necessary in a fractionated or protracted exposure. The minimum dose increases to 4 Gy (400 rad) spread over 3 weeks to 3 months and 5.5 Gy (550 rad) for more than 3 months.
- The latent period between irradiation and the appearance of a lens opacity is dose related. The latency is about 8 years after exposure to a dose in the range of 2.5 to 6.5 Gy (250–650 rad).
- It is never possible to state unequivocally that a given cataract is radiation induced; however, the appearance of a cataract at the posterior pole of the lens in an individual with a radiation history strongly suggests radiation as the causative agent. On the other hand, it is possible to say with some certainty that some cataracts—for example, nuclear cataracts—do not have a radiation etiology.
- The RBE of neutrons or heavy ions is about 10 at high doses but rises to 50 or more for small doses.
- There is evidence of early cataracts in astronauts exposed to high-energy heavy ions.
- A radiation-induced cataract is a deterministic late effect. There is a practical threshold dose below which cataracts are not produced, and above this threshold the severity of the biologic response is dose related.

BIBLIOGRAPHY

Bateman JL, Bond VP: Lens opacification in mice exposed to fast neutrons. *Radiat Res* 7(suppl):239–249, 1967

Britten MJA, Halnan KE, Meredith WJ: Radiation cataract: New evidence on radiation dosage to the lens. *Br J Radiol* 39:612–617, 1966

Cucinotta FA, Manuel FK, Jones J, Iszard G, Murrey J, Djojonegro B, Wear M: Space radiation and cataracts in astronauts. *Radiat Res* 156:460–466, 2001

Langham WH (ed): *Radiobiological Factors in Manned Space Flight.* Publication No. 1487. Washington, DC, National Academy of Sciences, National Research Council, 1967

Merriam CR, Focht EF: Clinical study of radiation cataracts and the relationship to dose. *AJR Am J Roentgenol* 77:759–785, 1957

Merriam GR, Focht EF: Radiation dose to the lens in treatment of tumors of the eye and adjacent structures: Possibilities of cataract formation. *Radiology* 71:357–369, 1958

Merriam GR, Szechter A, Focht EF: The effects of ionizing radiations on the eye. *Front Radiat Ther Oncol* 6:346–385, 1972

Merriam GR, Worgul BV: Experimental radiation cataract: Its clinical relevance. *Bull NY Acad Med* 59:372–292, 1983

Worgul BV, Merriam GR, Medvedovsky C: Accelerated heavy particles and the lens: II. Cytopathological changes. *Invest Ophthalmol Vis Sci* 27:108–114, 1985

CHAPTER 14

Doses and Risks in Diagnostic Radiology, Interventional Radiology and Cardiology, and Nuclear Medicine

The purpose of this chapter is to review the doses involved, and to estimate the associated risks, in radiology, cardiology, and nuclear medicine. The bulk of radiation exposure is received by patients as part of their diagnosis or treatment, so there is a tangible medical benefit to balance against the risk; but medical radiation exposure is also conducted for medicolegal reasons, and on volunteers (patients or healthy persons) for research purposes, and here the risk–benefit equation is quite different. However, to put things in perspective, we first summarize the radiation doses from natural background sources. This usually is regarded as an important benchmark, because life on earth has evolved in the presence of this continuous background radiation.

DOSES FROM NATURAL BACKGROUND RADIATION

Natural sources of radiation include cosmic rays from outer space, terrestrial radiation from natural radioactive materials in the ground, and radiation from radionuclides naturally present in the body, inhaled, or ingested. The sources of natural background radiation are illustrated in Figure 14.1.

Enhanced natural sources are sources that are natural in origin but to which exposure is increased as a result of human activity (inadvertent or otherwise). Examples include air travel at high altitude, which increases cosmic-ray levels, and movement of radionuclides on the ground in phosphate mining, which can increase the terrestrial component

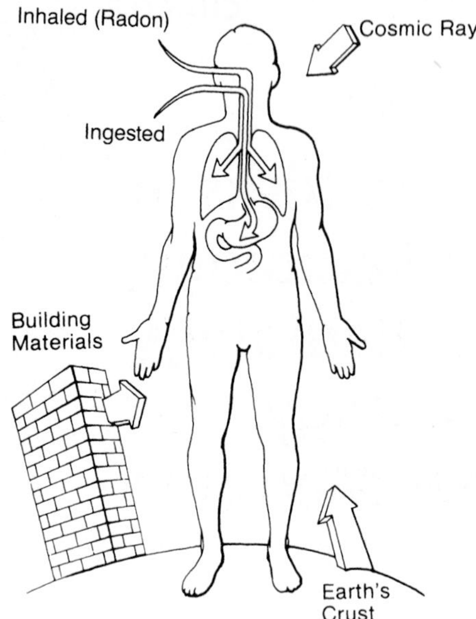

FIGURE 14.1 ● Three principal components of natural background radiation: (1) cosmic rays from solar flares in the sun or from outer space; (2) ingested radioactivity, principally potassium-40 in food, and inhaled radioactivity, principally radon; and (3) radiation from the earth's crust, which in practice means radiation emanating from building materials, because most people spend much of their lives indoors.

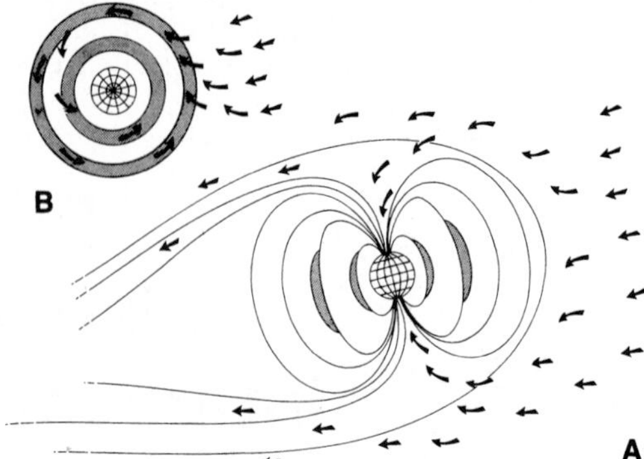

FIGURE 14.2 ● **A:** The earth behaves like a giant magnet. Showers of charged particles from solar events on the surface of the sun are deflected away from the equator by the earth's magnetic field; most miss the earth altogether; others are funneled into the polar regions. This explains why cosmic-ray dose is low near the equator and high in the polar regions. It is also the basis of the aurora borealis, or northern lights, caused by intense showers of cosmic-ray particles that spiral down the lines of magnetic field into the poles. **B:** Viewed from above the poles, the earth is ringed with lines of magnetic field that form regions of high radiation dose known as the *Van Allen belts*. Humans could not live for long in the dose rates characteristic of these belts. On lunar missions, spaceships pass quickly through the Van Allen belts; the space shuttle orbits well below them.

to persons living in houses built on waste landfills. Radon exposure indoors might be considered in some instances an enhanced natural source, inasmuch as it is not natural to live in an insulated house. In a sense, also, all operations associated with the nuclear fuel cycle, starting with mining, involve natural radionuclides, but these are more generally classified as a consequence of human activity.

Cosmic Radiation

Cosmic rays are made up of radiations originating from outside the solar system and from charged particles (largely protons) emanating from the surface of the sun. The intensity of cosmic rays arriving at the earth's surface varies with both latitude and altitude above sea level. The variation with latitude is a consequence of the magnetic properties of the earth: Cosmic rays are charged particles that tend to be deflected away from the equator and funneled into the poles. This is illustrated in Figure 14.2. The aurora borealis, or northern lights, results from charged particles spiraling down the lines of magnetic field in the polar regions. Consequently, cosmic-ray intensity is least in equatorial regions and rises toward the poles. There is an even larger variation in cosmic-ray intensity with altitude, because at high elevations above sea level, there is less atmosphere to absorb the cosmic rays, so their intensity is greater. For example, the cosmic-ray annual equivalent dose in the United States is about 0.26 mSv (26 mrem) at sea level. This essentially doubles for each 2,000-m increase in altitude in the lower atmosphere, so that in Denver, Colorado, the annual effective dose* from cosmic radiation is about 0.5 mSv (50 mrem). Long flights at high altitudes involve some increased dose too. For example, the extra dose from cosmic rays received by a passenger on a commercial flight flying from the United States to Europe is about 0.05 mSv (5 mrem). Flight crews on northerly routes accumulate larger doses than most radiology staff in hospitals; in fact, airline crews are already classified as radiation workers in Europe, but that is not yet the case in the United States.

**Readers unfamiliar with terms such as* effective dose *or any other quantities or units of dose should read the definitions in Chapter 15.*

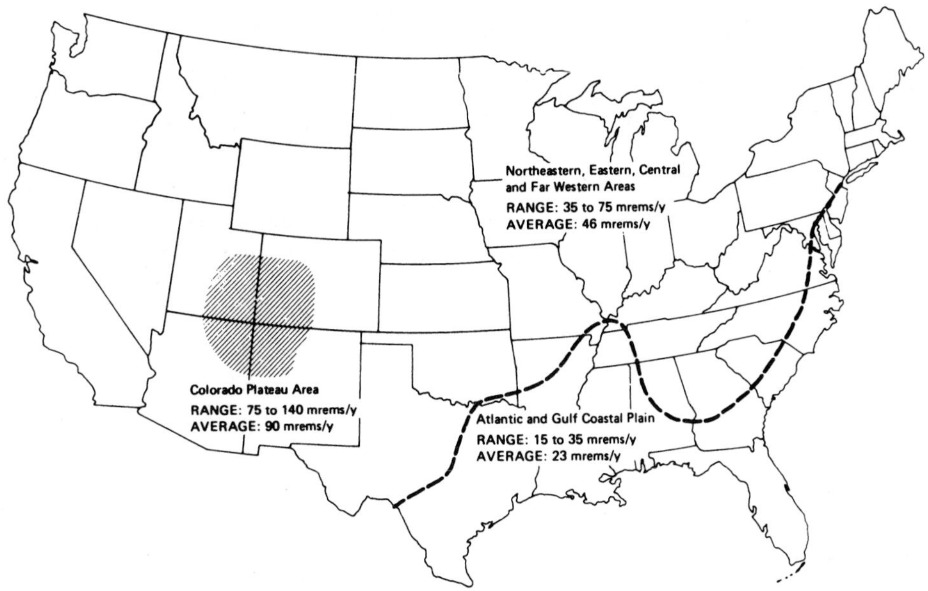

FIGURE 14.3 • The variation of the component of natural background radiation originating from the earth's crust. (Committee on the Biological Effects on Ionizing Radiations: *The Effects on Populations of Exposure to Low Levels of Ionizing Radiation.* BEIR III Washington, DC, National Academy Press, National Research Council, 1980.)

Natural Radioactivity in the Earth's Crust

Naturally occurring radioactive materials are widely distributed throughout the earth's crust, and humans are exposed to the γ-rays from them. In the United States, there is a big variation between the Colorado plateau area, where the rocks and soil contain relatively more radioactive thorium and uranium (75–140 mrem/y), and the Atlantic seaboard, where radioactivity is low (15–35 mrem/y). This is shown in Figure 14.3.

Internal Exposure

Small traces of radioactive materials are normally present in the human body, ingested from the tiny quantities present in food or inhaled as airborne particles. Radioactive thorium, radium, and lead can be detected in most persons, but the amounts are small and variable, and the figure usually quoted for the average dose rate resulting from these deposits is less than 10 μSv/y (1 mrem/y). Only radioactive potassium-40 makes an appreciable contribution to human exposure from ingestion. The dose rate is about 0.2 mSv/y (20 mrem/y), which cannot be ignored as a source of mutations in humans.

The biggest source of natural background radiation is radon gas, which seeps into the basements of houses from rocks underground. Radon, a decay product in the uranium series, is a noble gas that does little harm, but in the confined space of an underground mine or the basement of a house, it decays with a 3-day half-life to form solid progeny that stick to dust particles and, if inhaled, become lodged on the surface of the bronchus or lung. Radon progeny emit α-particles that, it is believed, are responsible for lung cancer. Radon levels in houses vary enormously, but the average concentration in the United States appears to be about 37 Bq/m^3 (1 pCi/L) in aboveground living areas and much, much more in basements. It is a sobering thought that in an average home, in every cubic meter of air, 37 atoms of radon decay each second, producing radioactive progeny. Only the bronchi and lungs are irradiated by this source, but α-particles are highly effective and have a radiation weighting factor of 20 (radiation weighting factor is explained in Chapters 7 and 15). This translates into an annual average effective dose of about 2 mSv (200 mrem) (Table 14.1). There is no question that radon is by far the largest component of natural background radiation. The Environmental Protection Agency action level for radon is 148 Bq/m^3 (4 pCi/L); remedial action is suggested for houses above this level. The Committee on the Biological Effects of Ionizing Radiation of the National Academy of Sciences

TABLE 14.1

Annual Effective Dose in the U.S. Population Circa 1980–1982

Source	Thousands of Persons Exposed	Average Annual Effective Dose in Exposed Population, mSv[a]	Annual Collective Effective Dose, person-Sv[b]	Average Annual Effective Dose in U.S. Population mSv[a]
Natural sources				
Radon	230,000	2.0	460,000	2.0
Other	230,000	1.0	230,000	1.0
Occupational	930[c]	2.3	2,000	0.009
Nuclear fuel cycle	—	—	136	0.0005
Consumer products				
Tobacco[d]	50,000	—	—	—
Other	120,000	0.05–0.3	12,000–29,000	0.05–0.13
Miscellaneous environmental sources	~25,000	0.006	160	0.0006
Medical				
Diagnostic x-rays	—[e]	—	91,000	0.39
Nuclear medicine	—[f]	—	32,000	0.14
Rounded total	230,000	—	835,000	3.6

[a] 1 mSv = 100 mrem.
[b] 1 person-Sv = 100 man-rem.
[c] Those nominally exposed total 1.68×10^6.
[d] Effective dose equivalent difficult to determine; dose to a segment of bronchial epithelium estimated to be 0.16 Sv/y (16 rem/y).
[e] Number of persons exposed is not known. Number of examinations was 180 million and effective dose per examination 500 μSv.
[f] Number of persons exposed is not known. Number of examinations was 7.4 million and effective dose per examination 4,300 μSv.
Data from National Council on Radiation Protection and Measurements: *Exposure of the Population in the United States to Ionizing Radiation*. Report 93. Bethesda, MD, NCRP, 1987.

(BEIR IV report, 1998) estimates that radon may be responsible for between 15,400 and 21,800 lung cancer deaths per year in the United States (i.e., about 10% of the total lung cancer deaths).

Areas of High Natural Background

There are several inhabited areas of the world in which background radiation is considerably elevated because of radioactivity in rocks or soil or in building materials from which houses are made. These areas are in Brazil, France, India, Niue Island (in the South Pacific), and Egypt.

In Brazil, some 30,000 people who live in coastal areas are exposed to dose rates of 5 mSv/y (500 mrem/y). About one sixth of the population of France live in areas, largely in the Burgundy wine-growing district, in which the rocks are principally granite, and they receive 1.8 to 3.5 mSv/y (180–350 mrem/y) from background radiation. Undoubtedly, the highest natural background radiation is in Kerala, India, where more than 100,000 people receive an average annual dose of about 13 mSv (1,300 mrem), reaching a high in certain locations on the coast of 70 mSv (7,000 mrem).

Many studies have been made of these human populations who have lived for many generations in areas of high natural background radiation. So far, no excess incidence of cancer or hereditary anomalies has been observed that can reasonably be attributed to the radiation. Such studies, of course, are beset with difficulties. Nevertheless, in spite of the obvious problems involved in making comparisons, it is an important and significant fact that human populations who have lived for generations at levels of background radiation that differ by an order of magnitude do not show noticeable differences in the incidence of cancer or genetic disorders. This is

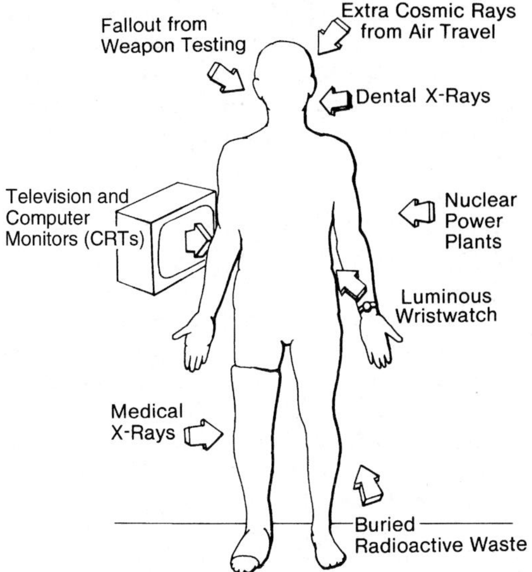

FIGURE 14.4 • The various sources of radiation resulting from human activity to which the human population is exposed. In developed countries, the effective dose is dominated by medical radiation.

the basis for believing that as long as human-made radiation does not exceed the average background value, it is unlikely to produce any detectable deleterious effects on the world's population.

COMPARISON OF RADIATION DOSES FROM NATURAL SOURCES AND HUMAN ACTIVITIES

In addition to natural background radiation, the human population is exposed to a variety of sources of radiation resulting from human activity, as illustrated in Figure 14.4.

Radiation doses to the U.S. population from all sources are summarized in Figure 14.5 and in somewhat more detail in Table 14.1. The average annual effective dose from all sources amounts to 3.6 mSv (360 mrem). There is a large extra dose to the bronchial epithelium in smokers from naturally occurring radionuclides in tobacco products, primarily polonium-120, but it is difficult to estimate with any precision.

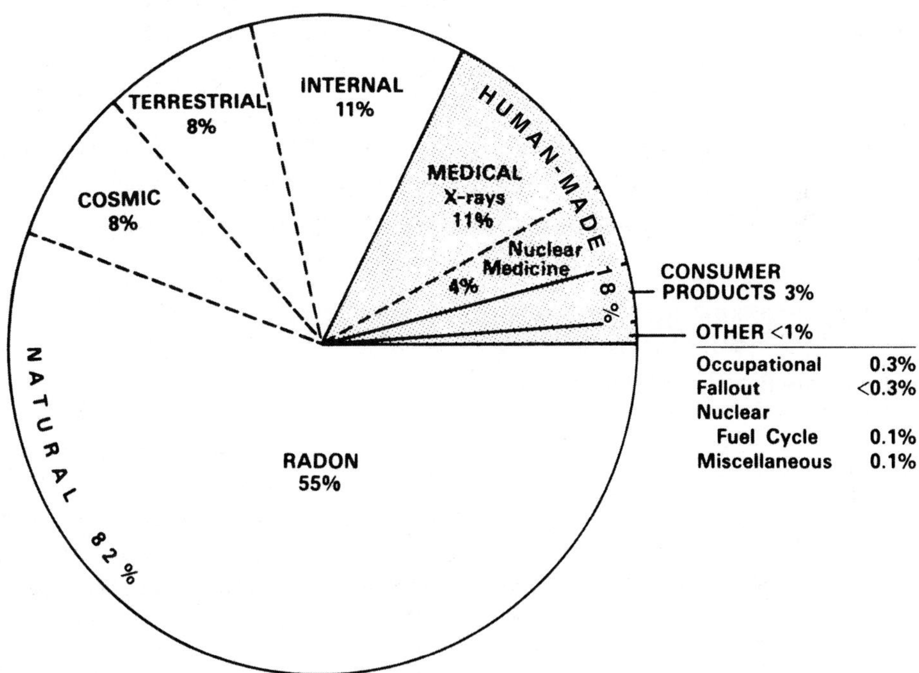

FIGURE 14.5 • This pie diagram, which appeared in 1987, is from a study that showed for the first time that the average effective dose to the population of the United States is dominated by indoor radon progeny products. The effective dose, of course, is the dose in gray (or rad) multiplied by the radiation weighting factor, which is 20 for the α-particles emitted by radon progeny products, and multiplied by the tissue weighting factor, which is about 0.12 Sv (12 rem) for the lungs. The total annual effective dose to the U.S. population is about 3.6 mSv (360 mrem). More than one half of this is a result of radon, and altogether 82% comes from natural sources. Medical x-rays contribute only 11% and nuclear medicine 4%. (From National Council on Radiation Protection and Measurements: *Ionizing Radiation Exposure of the Population of the United States.* Report 93. Bethesda, MD, NCRP, 1987.)

There are several obvious conclusions to be drawn from this summary of doses from various sources. First, radon represents the largest source of radiation to the U.S. population. Second, medical diagnostic x-rays represent by far the largest source of radiation resulting from human activities. Third, the overall effective dose from medical radiation is about equal to that from natural background, excluding radon, and only about a quarter of the total effective dose to which the U.S. population is exposed if radon is included.

DIAGNOSTIC RADIOLOGY

The use of x-rays for diagnosis in medicine varies significantly between countries, depending on the standard of health care. Table 14.2, based on UNSCEAR 2000, summarizes the availability of radiologists and the number of specialized units such as **Computed Tomography (CT)** scanners and mammography units in the United States, the United Kingdom, and several other industrialized countries. The UNSCEAR reports from 1977 on are available free of charge at the website www.unscear.org.

The radiation doses involved in radiology other than interventional procedures are seldom sufficiently large to result in *deterministic effects*. By definition, a deterministic effect has a practical threshold in dose, the severity of the effect increases with dose, and it results from damage to many cells. The one exception is inadvertent exposure of the developing embryo or fetus, with a possible consequence of reduced head diameter (microcephaly) and mental retardation. The threshold for radiation-induced mental retardation is thought to be 0.1 to 0.2 Gy (10–20 rad), so few procedures are likely to cause this effect.

Apart from this important exception, the potential deleterious consequences of diagnostic radiology involve *stochastic effects*, that is, carcinogenesis and hereditary effects. The characteristic of stochastic effects is that there is no threshold in dose; that is, there is no dose below which the effect does not occur, though the probability of carcinogenesis or hereditary effects increases with dose. A stochastic effect may result from irradiation of one or a few cells, and the severity of the response is not dose related. As a consequence, *absorbed dose* to a limited portion of an individual's body does not by itself provide the overall perspective on risk associated with a given procedure.

Effective dose is a more relevant quantity; it takes into account the tissues and organs irradiated, as well as the dose involved. This is important, because some tissues and organs are more susceptible than others to radiation. (Effective dose is discussed in detail in Chapter 15.) The technical definition of effective dose is the sum of the equivalent doses to each tissue and organ exposed multiplied by the appropriate tissue weighting factors. What this amounts to in simpler terms is that effective dose

TABLE 14.2

Overview of the Practice of Radiology

	Population $\times 10^6$	Mammography Units/10^6 Population	CT Scanners—Total (per 10^6 Population)	Medical X-Rays—Number of Annual Radiation Exams and Treatments $\times 10^6$ (per 10^6 Population)	Physicians Conducting Radiology (per 10^6 Population)
Canada	27.9	20.2	223 (8.0)	24.9 (0.89)	74
France	57.7	42.2	561 (9.7)	92.0 (1.59)	119
Germany	81.5	43.6	1,400 (17.2)	102.2 (1.25)	405
Japan	125.0	11.7	7,959 (63.7)	184.7 (1.48)	94
Sweden	8.8	19.3	115 (13.1)	5.0 (0.57)	125
United Kingdom	58.2	4.4	350 (6.0)	28.9 (0.50)	41
United States	260.0	38.6	6,800 (26.2)	250.0 (0.96)	92

Based on UNSCEAR 2000, which in turn is based on UNSCEAR surveys 1991–1996.

is the whole-body dose of x-rays that would have to be delivered to produce the same stochastic risk as the partial-body dose that actually was delivered. This quantity provides an easy assessment of overall risk and makes comparison of risks much simpler; for example, risk from a diagnostic examination is more readily compared with that from background radiation if effective dose is quoted. If absorbed dose is in gray, the effective dose is in sievert; if absorbed dose is in rad, effective dose is in rem. Many recent reports in the literature use effective dose in discussing the potential consequences of diagnostic radiology.

Last but not least, the overall population impact of diagnostic radiology can be assessed in terms of the *collective effective dose*, the product of effective dose and the number of individuals exposed.

These three quantities—dose, effective dose, and collective effective dose—are discussed in turn. (In general, whenever the term *dose* is used alone, it refers to the absorbed dose.)

Dose

Table 14.3 is a summary of entrance skin exposures, as well as absorbed doses to various organs, characteristic of a representative sample of standard diagnostic procedures. The data do not contain any big surprises. As would be expected, radiographs of the lumbar spine, barium enema series, and upper gastrointestinal series involve substantial doses of radiation because of the need to penetrate these thick and dense regions of the body. These are the procedures, too, that inevitably lead to large gonadal doses.

The Nationwide Evaluation of X-ray Trends (NEXT) series of reports give doses for a number of common examinations:

- The 1992 report summarized mammography x-ray data. It was shown that over the years, the mean glandular dose per examination has fallen and is now about 2 mGy while the image quality has improved. This is illustrated in Figure 14.6.
- The 1994 report summarized data for adult chest x-rays. The average entrance air kerma was 0.14 mGy at an average clinical kVp of 101, with an average exposure time of 31 ms.
- The 1995 report referred to abdomen and lumbosacral spine x-ray data, which are shown in Table 14.4.
- The 1998 report focused on pediatric chest x-ray data. In contrast to the adult chest x-ray data of 1994, the average entrance air kerma was 0.05 mGy at an average kVp of 71, with an average exposure time of 12 ms.
- Dental x-ray data were the subject of the 1999 survey. The average entrance air kerma was 1.6 mGy with an average clinical kVp of 71.

Some of the largest doses in diagnostic radiology are associated with fluoroscopy. In this case, the dose rate is greatest at the skin, where the x-ray beam first enters the patient. Dose rates from fluoroscopy from the NEXT 1996 Upper G.I. Fluoroscopy Survey is shown in Table 14.5. Although dose rates in the literature are now reported in the new SI unit of milligray per minute, existing regulations still specify limits in terms of an exposure rate (röntgen per minute). The entrance exposure limit for standard operation of a fluoroscope is 10 R/min. Some fluoroscopes are equipped with a high-output or "boost" mode, and the limit for operation in this mode on state-of-the-art equipment is 20 R/min. There is no limit on entrance exposure rate during any type of recorded fluoroscopy, such as cinefluorography or digital acquisitions.

A typical fluoroscopic entrance exposure rate for a man of medium build is approximately 3 R/min. Much higher dose rates may be encountered during recorded interventional and cardiac catheterization studies, such as those that involve a series of multiple, still-frame image acquisitions.

The number of CT scanners in clinical use has risen steadily over the years, reaching a global total in 1997 of about 20,000 units, with an associated annual total of some 67 million CT procedures. The distribution of scanners throughout the world is far from uniform, as shown by Table 14.6. By far the largest number of scanners per million population is found in the United States, and this is reflected in the highest number of annual procedures per thousand population. The figures in Table 14.6 are from the mid-1990s but are already out of date because the use of CT continues to grow rapidly. At the time of this writing, the NEXT report for 2000 was not yet available in final form, but the estimate is that 57 million scans were performed in the United States alone—almost as many as in the whole world in 1995!

Several surveys have been completed of the doses of radiation resulting from CT scans of the head. The 1990 NEXT survey evaluated some 252 CT scanning systems and found that the average central dose from a series of contiguous slices through the head was 34 to 55 mGy (3.4–5.5 rad). A similar survey of 14 CT scanners in Australia, evaluating doses from a series of 10 contiguous 10-mm slices, essentially all of the head, found an average dose of 45.8 mGy (4.58 rad). Both surveys emphasized wide variations in dose with different

TABLE 14.3

Entrance Skin Exposure and Absorbed Doses to Various Organs from Radiographic Studies in Adults[a]

Examination and View	Free-in-Air Exposure at Skin Entrance, mR	Dose, mGy (mrad)					
		Active Bone Marrow	Thyroid	Breast	Lungs	Ovaries	Testes
Chest							
PA	20	0.02 (2)	0.01 (1)	0.01 (1)	0.07 (7)	N	N
Lateral	65	0.02 (2)	0.07 (7)	0.15 (15)	0.12 (12)	N	N
Series	—	0.04 (4)	0.07 (7)	0.16 (16)	0.19 (19)	N	N
Skull							
AP	330	0.08 (8)	0.06 (6)	—	N	N	N
Lateral	190	0.05 (5)	0.21 (21)	—	N	N	N
Series	—	0.24 (24)	0.34 (34)	—	0.01 (1)	N	N
Cervical spine							
AP	150	0.02 (2)	1.00 (100)	—	0.02 (2)	N	N
Lateral	100	0.02 (2)	0.06 (6)	—	0.02 (2)	N	N
Series	—	0.09 (9)	2.60 (260)	—	0.11 (11)	N	N
Thoracic spine							
AP	280	0.05 (5)	0.25 (25)	0.95 (95)	0.35 (35)	N	N
Lateral	630	0.12 (12)	0.05 (5)	0.05 (5)	0.75 (75)	N	N
Series	—	0.17 (17)	0.30 (30)	1.00 (100)	1.10 (110)	N	N
Lumbar spine							
AP	640	0.18 (18)	N	—	0.40 (40)	1.10 (110)	0.02 (2)
Lateral	2,300	0.44 (44)	N	—	0.30 (30)	0.90 (90)	0.02 (2)
Series	—	1.10 (110)	N	—	1.70 (170)	3.70 (370)	0.06 (6)
Urography							
KUB (AP)	600	0.20 (20)	N	—	0.07 (7)	1.30 (130)	0.10 (10)
Series	—	0.90 (90)	N	—	0.27 (27)	5.50 (550)	0.40 (40)
Series + 4 tomograms	—	1.70 (170)	N	—	0.54 (54)	6.50 (650)	0.50 (50)
Mammography[b]	—	—	—	2.40 (240)	—	—	—
Upper gastrointestinal series	—	3.00 (300)	0.03 (3)	0.50 (50)	1.00 (100)	12.00 (1,200)	0.80 (80)
Barium enemia series	—	5.20 (520)	N	—	—	—	—

[a]Values given are exposures and doses received by some patients at some facilities. Values can be much higher or lower depending on patient size, the technology employed, and the examination protocols established by the radiologist. Key: —, no estimate is made; N, negligible dose (<0.01 mGy [<1 mrad]).

[b]Two-view screening with film-screen grid.

Adapted from Wagner LK: *Radiation Bioeffects and Management Test and Syllabus*. Reston, VA, American College of Radiology, 1991, with permission.

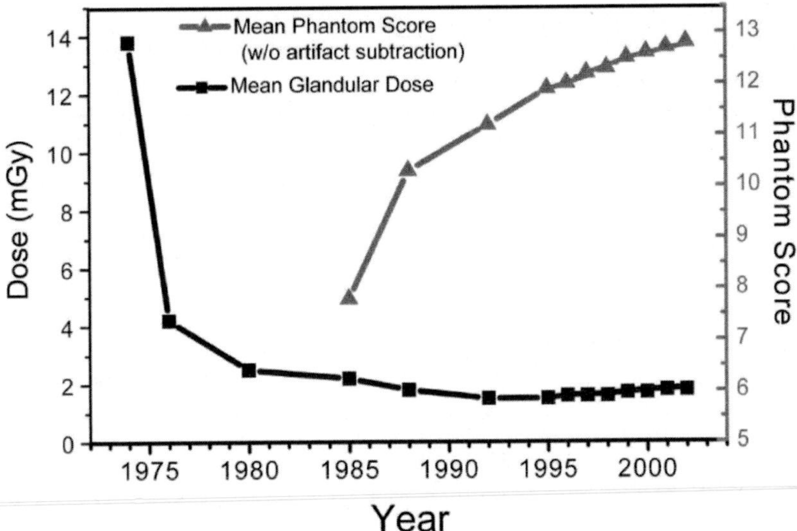

FIGURE 14.6 • Graph showing how the mean glandular dose for mammography fell dramatically between 1970 and 1990 and is now about 1.4 mGy (14 rad). Meanwhile the image quality improved. Image quality is measured in terms of phantom score; a phantom contains fiber specks and spheres of different sizes, and the score indicates how many can be seen. (From "Twenty five years of NEXT" Feb. 2003.)

model scanners and different techniques. In general, the multiple-scan average dose ranges are 40 to 60 mGy (4–6 rad) for head scans and 10 to 40 mGy (1–4 rad) for body scans.

Effective Dose

Many recent surveys of doses in diagnostic radiology emphasize the effective dose because this is related to the risk of stochastic effects, such as the induction of cancer or hereditary effects.

Table 14.7 shows the results of a study conducted in the United States by the FDA, listing the entrance skin exposure and the corresponding effective dose resulting from a representative sample of diagnostic procedures. Comparable data for both dose and effective dose from the United Kingdom are shown in Table 14.8.

It is not difficult to understand why CT scans involve relatively larger effective doses, because larger volumes of tissue are exposed to higher doses than with plain x-rays.

Table 14.9 summarizes effective doses from CT around the world in the 1990s, taken from an UNSCEAR survey. The comparable data for the United States is shown in Table 14.10, taken from

TABLE 14.4

Abdomen and Lumbosacral Spine (NEXT 1995)

	1995 Abdomen	1995 LS Spine
Entrance air kerma (mGy)	2.8	3.2
Clinical kVp	76	78
Exposure time (ms)	145	247
Percent using grids	97	96
Phantom film optical density	1.74	1.32

From the NEXT 1995 Abdomen and LS Spine X-Ray Data Survey.

TABLE 14.5

Dose Rates from Fluoroscopy (NEXT 1996)

	1996 Upper GI	1996 Cardiac Cath Labs	1996 C-Arm Units
Entrance air kerma (mGy/min)[a]	45	38	22
Clinical kVp	99	82	78
Fluoroscope tube current (mA)	2.3	5.1	3.0
Air kerma rate w/contrast[b] (mGy/min)[a]	67	71	41
Maximum air kerma rate[a]	70	74	44

[a] Determined at 1 cm of the table top and does not include contributions from over-table units.
[b] Copper is used to simulate the presence of barium contrast medium.
From the NEXT 1996 Upper G.I. Fluoroscopy Survey.

the NEXT survey in 2000. A comprehensive survey of data from CT scans in the United Kingdom was published in 1999 and is shown in Table 14.11.

Pediatric CT scans are a special case. If the same parameters (kV and mAs) are used for babies and small children as for adults, much larger doses and effective doses are received by the pediatric cases. This was common practice until 2001, when it was pointed out that children are at least ten times as sensitive as adults to radiation-induced cancer. As a consequence, a major effort has been made by pediatric radiologists to tailor the appropriate parameters to the size of the individual being scanned. This has led to a substantial dose reduction in children receiving CT scans.

The next two tables address special and very different circumstances. Table 14.12 compares the effective dose from cerebral angiography, which at about 10.6 mSv (1,060 mrem) is similar to that from an alternative nuclear-medicine study, but much more than a CT scan and nearly two orders of magnitude more than from a plain skull x-ray. Bone mineral densitometry is the subject of Table 14.13. There are wide variations for different techniques, but note that the effective doses are very small, in the microsievert range.

TABLE 14.6

Global Activity in Computed Tomography for 1995

Region	Scanners per Million Population	Annual Procedures per Thousand Population
World	3.5	11
United States	26.4	91
European Union	10.1	33
France	7.7	33
Germany	16.6	53
Italy	9.6	30
Spain	5.7	15
United Kingdom	6.2	21

Adapted from Bahador B: *Trends in Diagnostic Imaging to 2000*. London, FT Pharmaceutical and Health Care Publishing, 1996, with permission.

TABLE 14.7

Effective Doses for Common Diagnostic Procedures (United States)

	ESAK, mGy	Entrance Skin Exposure, mR	Effective Dose, mSv (mrem)	
			Male	Female
Chest (PA)	0.18	20	0.03 (3)	0.03 (3)
Chest (lateral)	0.57	65	0.05 (5)	0.08 (8)
Skull (AP)	2.9	330	0.04 (4)	0.04 (4)
Skull (lateral)	1.5	166	0.02 (2)	0.02 (2)
C-spine (AP)	1.3	150	0.05 (5)	0.05 (5)
C-spine (lateral)	0.88	100	0.02 (2)	0.02 (2)
T-spine (AP)	2.5	280	0.27 (27)	0.54 (54)
T-spine (lateral)	6.0	680	0.25 (25)	0.27 (27)
L-spine (AP)	5.6	640	0.40 (40)	0.78 (78)
L-spine (lateral)	20	2300	0.53 (53)	0.84 (84)
Abdomen (AP)	5.3	600	0.37 (37)	0.73 (73)

Entrance skin exposure values taken from Wagner LK: *Radiation Bioeffects and Management Test and Syllabus*. Reston, VA, American College of Radiology, 1991.

Effective doses calculated by Dr. Beth A. Schueler using Rosenstein M: *Handbook of Selected Tissue Doses for Projections, Common in Diagnostic Radiology.* Rockville, MD, US Department of Health and Human Services, Public Health Service, Food and Drug Administration Publication 89-8031, 1988 for organ doses and ICRP weighting factors.

TABLE 14.8

Mean Values of Patient Dose and Effective Dose from Computed Tomographic Examinations in the United Kingdom for 1989

	Organ Dose, mGy[a]				
Examination	Eyes	Uterus	Ovaries	Testes	Effective Dose, mSv[a]
Routine head	50	—	0	0	1.8
Posterior fossa	53	—	—	0	0.72
Pituitary	60	—	—	0	0.57
Internal auditory meatus	2.6	—	0	0	0.35
Orbits	50	—	—	0	0.64
Facial bones	9.0	—	—	0	0.68
Cervical spine	0.62	—	—	0	2.6
Thoracic spine	0.04	0.02	0.02	—	4.9
Routine chest	0.14	0.06	0.08	—	7.8
Mediastinum	0.11	0.03	0.04	—	7.6
Routine abdomen	—	8.0	8.0	0.70	7.6
Liver	—	1.0	1.2	0.03	7.2
Pancreas	—	0.35	0.41	0.01	4.8
Kidneys	—	1.1	1.3	0.03	6.3
Adrenals	—	0.10	0.12	—	3.4
Lumbar spine	—	2.4	2.7	0.06	3.3
Routine pelvis	—	26	23	1.7	7.1

[a] Multiply by 100 to convert mGy to mrad and mSv to mrem.

Adapted from Shrimpton PC: Protection of the patient in x-ray computed tomography, in documents of the NRPB, Vol. 3, No. 4, London, HMSO, 1992.

TABLE 14.9

Effective Doses to Patients from Computed Tomography, 1991–1995

	Mean Effective Dose per Procedure, mSv						
Country/Area	**Head**	**Chest**	**Abdomen**	**Liver**	**Kidneys**	**Pelvis**	**Lumbar Spine**
Australia	2.6	10.4	16.7	12.7	—	11.0	5.2
Finland	1.3	5.1	11.6	—	—	—	5.0
Germany	2.6	20.5	27.4	—	—	—	9
Japan	—	4.6–10.8	6.7–13.3	—	—	—	—
Netherlands	0.8–5.0	6–18	6–24	—	—	—	2–12
New Zealand	1.8	8.9	9.7	6.5	7.6	6.9	4.7
Norway	2.0	11.5	12.8	11.9	9.9	9.8	4.5
Sweden	2.1	10	10	10	10	10	6
United Kingdom (Wales)	1.6	9.7	12	10.3	9.1	9.8	3.3

Based on the United Nations Scientific Committee on the Effects of Atomic Radiation: *Annex C Medical Radiation Exposures*. New York, UNSCEAR, 2000.

Collective Effective Dose

Next to be considered is the effect of diagnostic radiology on the population as a whole, rather than on the individual. The relevant quantity here is the *collective effective dose*, which is the product of the effective dose and the number of individuals exposed. It can give a very rough indication of the harm or detriment to an exposed population in terms of the number of radiation-induced cancers or hereditary effects that may be expected to be produced.

There are two values of the collective effective dose that are of interest in diagnostic radiology, that to patients and that to health-care workers.

First we consider the patients. Table 14.14 shows the collective effective dose from all diagnostic x-ray procedures performed in both doctors' offices and hospitals in the United States in 1980. The total amounts to 92,000 person-Sv (9.2 million man-rem). This estimate is out of date and may be much too low for the present time because of the greatly increased use of CT scans in the past 2 decades. On the other hand, it may be too high, because the population receiving diagnostic x-rays is substantially skewed with regard to age distribution compared with the working population, for which the concept of effective dose initially was developed. Over one half are older than 45 years of age, and a quarter are older than 64 years. It also has been claimed that half of all x-ray diagnostic procedures are performed on patients during a terminal illness within 18 months of their death; clearly, radiation-induced cancer and hereditary effects are irrelevant to this segment of the population.

Although the collective effective doses in Table 14.14 may be too low or too high for various reasons, they nevertheless represent the best data available and may be considered as providing "ballpark figures." Based on the International Commission on Radiological Protection (ICRP) estimates of 5% per sievert for fatal cancer induction, 0.9% per sievert for nonfatal cancer, and 0.2% per sievert for severe hereditary effects, it can be concluded that one year's practice of diagnostic radiology in the United States results in the induction of about 4,600 cancer deaths in the individuals exposed, 828 cases of nonfatal cancer, and 184 severe hereditary defects in future generations. This detriment must be balanced against the diagnostic benefit to over

TABLE 14.10

Effective Doses Characteristic of CT Scans in the United States in the Year 2000

	Head	**Chest**	**Abdomen**	**Pelvis**
mAs	355	—	—	—
kVp	127	—	—	—
MSAD, mGy	50.3	—	—	—
Effective dose, mSv	2	7	7	6

Based on the NEXT 2000 Computed Tomography Protocol Survey.

TABLE 14.11

Effective Doses from Computed Tomography in the United Kingdom

Examination	Mean Effective Dose, mSv[a]	
	United Kingdom, 1989	Wales, 1994
Routine head	1.8	1.6
Posterior fossa	0.7	1.2
Pituitary	0.6	0.9
Internal auditory meatus	0.4	1.0
Facial bones	0.7	0.3
Orbits	0.6	0.8
Cervical spine	2.6	1.5
Thoracic spine	4.9	2.4
Lumbar spine	3.3	3.3
Chest	7.8	9.7
High-resolution lung	—	1.9
Abdomen	7.6	12.0
Liver	7.2	10.3
Pancreas	4.8	7.4
Kidneys	6.3	9.1
Pelvis	7.1	9.8

[a] Multiply by 100 to convert mSv to mrem.
Adapted from Shrimpton PC, Wall BF, Hart D: Diagnostic medical exposures in the UK. *Appl Radiat Isot* 50:261–269, 1999, with permission.

100 million individuals receiving the various procedures. Put another way, less than 0.004% of the examined population is potentially at risk, according to these estimates.

TABLE 14.12

Effective Doses from Cerebral Angiography

Procedure	Effective Dose, mSv
Cerebral angiography	10.6
Nuclear medicine: brain imaging	About 10
Computed tomography	2
Skull x-ray	0.15

Adapted from Feygelman VM, Huda W, Peters K: Effective dose equivalents to patients undergoing cerebral angiography. *AJNR* 13:845–849, 1992, with permission.

More recent data are available from the United Kingdom concerning CT scanning. A CT scanner with a full workload may result in an annual effective dose of about 22.5 person-Sv (2,250 man-rem). This may vary by a factor of up to 3 between different models from various manufacturers because of design differences. On the broad basis of such scanner workloads, however, it has been estimated that in the late 1990s, CT scanning may have contributed around 40% of the collective effective dose to the population from radiologic procedures, although it represents only about 4% of the total number of procedures. By the year 2000, it is estimated that CT scans accounted for 11% of all radiologic procedures in the United States, but represented two thirds of the collective effective dose. This is a sobering thought.

In 1989, the NCRP published an extensive report on collective effective doses to radiation workers, including medical staff. Table 14.15 shows the estimated collective effective dose. Table 14.16 shows the breakdown for the various environments in which x-rays are used for medical purposes; the

TABLE 14.13

Representative Effective Doses from Bone Mineral Densitometry

Type of Measurement	Effective Dose, μSv	Comments
Dual-energy x-ray absorptiometry	~2.5	Representative value for single PA scan
Single-energy quantitative CT[a]	~300	SPR + 3 CT slices @ 80 kVp
Dual-energy quantitative CT	~1,000	SPR + 3 CT slices @ 80 kVp + 3 CT slices @120 kVp
Radiographs	~100	Single (collimated) view (AP or lateral)

[a]CT, computed tomography.
Adapted from Huda W, Morin RL: Patient doses in bone mineral densitometry. *Brit J Radiol* 69:422–425, 1996, with permission.

bulk of the collective dose is about equally divided between hospitals and private practice. If this total collective dose of 410 person-Sv (41,000 man-rem) for medical workers is multiplied by the ICRP risk estimate for radiation-induced fatal cancer at a low dose rate of 4% per sievert, it leads to the conclusion that about 16 individuals in the U.S. health-care industry will develop a fatal cancer as a consequence of each year's use of medical radiation.

Estimating Risks at Low Doses

In this chapter, ICRP risk estimates for radiation-induced cancer and hereditary effects, combined with values of the collective effective dose, have been used to estimate the detriment caused by diagnostic radiology to patients and medical staff. It is important to note that there is no direct evidence that small doses of radiation, similar to those used

TABLE 14.14

Collective Effective Dose from Diagnostic Medical X-Rays: United States, 1980

Examination Type	Effective Dose, mSv[a]	Thousands of Examinations	Collective Effective Dose, person-Sv[b]
Computed tomography (head and body)	1.11	3,300	3,660
Chest	0.08	64,000	5,120
Skull	0.22	8,200	1,800
Cervical spine	0.20	5,100	1,020
Biliary	1.89	3,400	6,430
Lumbar spine	1.27	12,900	16,400
Upper gastrointestinal	2.44	7,600	18,500
Abdomen (kidneys, ureters, bladder)	0.56	7,900	4,420
Barium enema	4.06	4,900	19,900
Intravenous pyelogram	1.58	4,200	6,640
Pelvis	0.44 } 0.64		
Hip	0.83 }	4,700	3,010
Extremities	0.01	45,000	450
Other	0.50	(8,400)	4,200
Rounded total			92,000

[a] 1 mSv = 100 mrem.
[b] 1 person-Sv = 100 man-rem.
Adapted from National Council on Radiation Protection and Measurements: *Exposure of the US Population from Diagnostic Medical Radiation*. Report 100. Bethesda, MD, NCRP, 1989, with permission.

TABLE 14.15

Collective Effective Doses to Radiation Workers

Occupational Category	Annual Collective Effective Dose, person-Sv[a]
Industrial personnel (other than nuclear fuel cycle)	390
Nuclear power plant personnel	551
Department of Energy personnel	224
Uranium miners	112
Uranium mill and fuel fabrication personnel	6
Well loggers	30
U.S. Public Health Service personnel	0.3
U.S. Navy	51
Flight crews and attendants	165
Medical staff (non-Federal)	410
Government	120
Other workers	145
Education and transportation personnel	50
Rounded total	2,200

[a] 1 person-Sv = 100 man-rem.
Adapted from National Council on Radiation Protection and Measurements: *Exposures of the US Population from Occupational Radiation.* Report 101. Bethesda, MD, NCRP, 1989, with permission.

in diagnostic radiology, cause harmful effects in the persons who are exposed. Discussions in this chapter involve inferences and estimates of the biologic effects that might occur if a large number of people are exposed to small doses of radiation, based on extrapolation from the known deleterious effects observed if a smaller number of people (or animals) are exposed to much larger doses of radiation. All that can be done in the case of low doses of radiation is to make estimates based on plausible

TABLE 14.16

Summary of Mean Collective Equivalent Doses to Monitored Medical Workers

Sources of Occupational Exposures	Thousands of Workers	Collective Equivalent Dose,[a] person-Sv
Dentistry	259	60
Private medical practice	155	160
Hospital	126	170
Other[b]	44	20
Total	584	410

[a]Collective equivalent doses are reported in the source of these data, but because the data were obtained from personnel monitors worn at waist level, the readings are assumed to represent total-body exposures; hence, collective equivalent dose is identical to collective effective dose.
[b]"Other" includes chiropractic medicine with 15,000, podiatry with 8,000, and veterinary medicine with 21,000 potentially exposed workers.
Adapted from National Council on Radiation Protection and Measurements: *Exposures of the US Population from Occupational Radiation.* Report 101. Bethesda, MD, NCRP, 1989, with permission.

assumptions, but these are estimates for which there is no direct evidence. They are not measurements or observations.

INTERVENTIONAL RADIOLOGY AND CARDIOLOGY

The past two decades have witnessed a major increase in high-dose fluoroscopically guided interventional procedures in medicine. These procedures include cardiac radiofrequency ablation, coronary artery angioplasty and stent placement, neuroembolization, and transjugular intrahepatic portosystemic shunt placement. Such procedures tend to be lengthy and involve fluoroscopy of a single area of anatomy for a prolonged period of time—frequently for longer than 30 minutes and occasionally for over 1 hour. In addition, the need for multiple sequential treatment sessions can occur. Because of the high skin doses that can be generated in the course of these interventions, some procedures have resulted in early or late skin reactions, including necrosis in some cases. In all cases of skin reactions, the doses are thought to have been high, and the severity of some reactions has required skin grafts or myocutaneous flaps for treatment. Procedures have evolved to include increasingly complex curative interventions that are associated with higher radiation exposures to both patients and health-care workers.

Angiography consists of inserting a catheter into a patient, guiding it along with the aid of fluoroscopy, and injecting contrast material into the vascular system. Stenosis, or blockage of one or more of these vessels, can lead to a myocardial infarction, but it can be visualized and treated with surgery or coronary angioplasty. Coronary angiography is a procedure that uses cineangiography in angulated projections, which can expose the operator to higher doses than when the x-ray equipment is used in the standard posteroanterior position.

Percutaneous transluminal coronary angioplasty is a therapeutic procedure to open blocked arteries by either inflating a small balloon inside the artery, compressing and fracturing the obstruction, or using rotating blades to cut and remove the obstruction. It often requires the deployment of stents, as well, to maintain vessel patency. During conventional coronary angioplasty, prolonged fluoroscopy in severely angulated positions increases the dose to the operator and the patient. For coronary angioplasty, the overall potential radiation exposure to the operators is medium to high. The usual arterial accesses are the femoral artery in the groin and the brachial artery in the shoulder. Large doses also are involved in the placement of transjugular intrahepatic portosystemic shunts.

The clinical application of electrophysiology in cardiology is to study the electrical conduction pathways of the heart. In the cardiac catheterization laboratory, fluoroscopic control is used to position catheters in the heart to measure electrical activity and to map electrical conduction pathways. This technique is being used increasingly because abnormal conduction pathways, which may lead to life-threatening cardiac arrhythmias, can be controlled by ablation, now being performed using catheter-directed methods. Either a direct current or radiofrequency generator is used to produce a voltage of 20 or 30 V, which heats tissue to approximately 60°C for about 1 minute, destroying the abnormal electrical conduction pathways. These procedures usually require only posteroanterior fluoroscopy, although oblique or angulated views also are used. The successful treatment of some cardiac arrhythmias by radiofrequency ablation probably will increase the use of fluoroscopy for this type of therapy. Long fluoroscopic times and the occasional use of angulated views result in high radiation exposures to workers during these procedures.

In addition, a large number of nonvascular interventional procedures using radiation are performed, such as the drainage of a blocked kidney or ablation of liver cancer.

Patient Doses

Radiation doses received by patients from interventional radiology and cardiology are very much higher than from general diagnostic radiology, so much so that there is a risk of deterministic effects, such as early or late skin damage. This is not to say, however, that stochastic risks are absent. They are greater than for diagnostic procedures because the doses are much higher. Because the patients are, in general, older and suffering from life-threatening medical conditions, however, the possibility of a radiation-induced cancer 10, 20, or 30 years down the road is largely academic. The immediate threat of deterministic effects, however, is very real and can affect quality of life in a serious way.

There are now reports in the literature of several dozen cases of skin damage following fluoroscopically guided interventional procedures. Also frequently reported are cases showing an acute phase involving erythema and deep ulceration, followed by a late phase involving telangiectasia, and/or hyperpigmentation. Less frequent and following more than 2 hours of fluoroscopy, erythema, desquamation, and later a moist ulcer with tissue necrosis have been reported, requiring a skin graft. In view of the concerns raised by reports of adverse biologic effects, a number of attempts have been made to measure and document doses received by patients undergoing diagnostic and interventional cardiac catheterization procedures.

To put things into context, however, considering the hundreds of thousands of patients involved each year in the United States alone, problems seen in cardiac and neurologic intervention are exceedingly rare, but the potential is always there. Although the entrance exposure limit for standard operation of a fluoroscope is 100 mGy/min (10 R/min), there is no limit on entrance exposure rate during any type of recorded fluoroscopy, such as cinefluorography or digital acquisitions. Consequently, dose rates of up to 500 mGy/min (50 R/min) and higher may be encountered during recorded interventional and cardiac catheterization studies. Several authors have estimated the entrance dose to the skin of the patient's back during cardiovascular procedures. Mean entrance doses for diagnostic catheterization vary from 0.7 to 2.2 Gy (70–220 rad). Difficult cases and multiple procedures in the same patient can readily lead to much higher doses that result in erythema or more severe skin damage.

Studies have also been published on skin doses involved in patients who underwent arrhythmia ablation procedures. The average fluoroscopy time was 46 minutes, corresponding to an entrance skin dose of about 1 Gy (100 rad), but a few percent of patients recorded a skin dose in excess of 3 Gy (300 rad). It should be noted that the radiation doses involved in a given procedure vary widely owing to uncontrollable factors above and beyond the skill and experience of the operator, including the age, size, and state of health of the patient.

Table 14.17 summarizes fluoroscopy time, cine time, and area exposure product (AEP) with units of Gy cm^2 for diagnostic, interventional, and combined procedures. It is not difficult to accept the idea that above a threshold, deterministic effects such as damage to the skin depend in some way on the dose and the area exposed, but the exact form of the relationship is not obvious on radiobiologic grounds.

Table 14.18 is a much more detailed survey of the AEP values for a number of specific procedures. This survey also calculated effective doses, which are discussed in the next section. To put things into context, for a nominal irradiated area of 100 cm^2 at the skin surface, an AEP of 200 Gy cm^2 (20,000 rad cm^2) would be required for a 2-Gy (200-rad) skin exposure, which is about the threshold for early transient erythema.

Several other conclusions were drawn from this and other studies. For example, radiation exposure was increased significantly in patients with a prior history of bypass surgery because of the need for more cine runs to image the native vessels and bypass grafts, as well as more fluoroscopy time to cannulate the grafts, and in patients undergoing multivessel intervention. The entrance exposure rate may be in the region of 0.1 Gy/min (10 rad/min), and procedures may last from minutes to several hours.

TABLE 14.17

Fluoroscopy Times, Cine Times, and Area–Exposure Products for Diagnostic, Interventional, and Combined Procedures

	Diagnostic (n = 173)	Interventional (n = 225)	Combined (n = 112)
Time, min			
Fluoroscopy	6.8 ± 6.4	19.9 ± 13.6	20.4 ± 10.5
Cine	0.78 ± 0.32	0.91 ± 0.6	1.18 ± 0.55
Area–exposure product, Gy cm^2			
Fluoroscopy	39 ± 46	101 ± 76	107 ± 65
Cine	70 ± 36	62 ± 33	92 ± 38
Total	108 ± 74	163 ± 95	198 ± 87
Cine runs	95 ± 33	136 ± 58	172 ± 59
Fluoroscopy[a]	32 ± 15	58 ± 14	52 ± 12

[a] Fluoroscopy expressed as a percentage of total area–exposure product.

Adapted from Bakalyar DM, Castellani MD, Safian RD: Radiation exposure to patients undergoing diagnostic and Interventional cardiac catheterization procedures. *Cathet Cardiovasc Diagn* 42:121–125, 1997, with permission.

TABLE 14.18

Mean Fluoroscopy Screening Times, Dose–Area Product Values

Interventional Procedure	Fluoroscopy Screening Time, min	Dose–Area Product, Gy cm²			Effective Dose, mSv
		Fluoroscopy	Radiography	Total	
Diagnostic					
Cerebral angiography	12.1	28.2	45.8	74.1	7.4
Carotid angiography	10.3	22.9	26.4	49.3	4.9
Upper extremity angiography	4.6	10.5	16.8	27.3	0.3
AV fistula angiography	2.3	4.6	12.6	17.2	0.2
Thoracic angiography	22.1	49.0	36.2	85.2	11.9
Nephrostography	4.0	12.4	2.2	14.7	2.4
Renal angiography	5.1	17.7	22.1	39.8	6.4
PTC	14.6	76.9	3.3	80.2	12.8
CT arterial portography	10.0	69.0	11.6	80.6	12.9
Hepatic angiography	12.1	74.9	61.0	136	21.7
Transjugular hepatic biopsy	6.8	30.8	3.4	34.1	5.5
Abdominal angiography	8.0	46.1	72.1	118	18.9
Femoral angiography	7.2	17.2	29.6	46.7	7.5
Lower extremity angiography	7.5	28.0	51.9	79.8	0.8
Therapeutic					
Cerebral embolization	34.1	43.1	61.4	105	10.5
AV fistula angioplasty	14.6	16.4	8.7	25.1	0.3
Thoracic therapeutic procedures	14.9	59.5	56.9	116	16.3
Biliary stent insertion/removal	7.1	40.5	2.6	43.1	6.9
TIPS	48.4	400	125	524	83.9
Nephrostomy	7.0	39.8	3.2	43.0	6.9
Renal angioplasty	14.0	57.0	28.1	85.2	13.6
Other abdominal therapeutic procedures (excluding hepatic and renal)	18.4	114	54.1	168	26.9

Adapted from McPariand BJ: A study of patient radiation doses in interventional radiological procedures. *Br J Radiol* 71:175–185, 1998, with permission.

Advances in spiral or helical CT scanning have led to the development of CT fluoroscopy (CTF). CTF presently is used as an imaging aid in invasive procedures, such as accurate localization of a biopsy needle. Because the x-ray tube and detector system can rotate continually around the patient, spiral CT has made it possible to continually image the same cross section of anatomy and have the reconstructed images displayed at many frames per second, demonstrating the temporal advancement of the invasive device. To manage the radiation at an acceptable level, the tube currents for CTF are much lower than those for routine CT scanning (about 10–20% of normal). Even so, dose rates are substantive, and the potential for extremely high doses in a prolonged procedure exists. Doses to the skin of a patient after about 90 seconds of CTF range from about 0.2 to 0.5 Gy (20–50 rad). Prolonged CTF or CTF at high tube currents has the potential for serious injury to the patient. Doses to the physician performing the procedure are also substantive.

TABLE 14.19

Potential Effects of Fluoroscopic Exposures on the Reaction of the Skin

Effect	Approximate Threshold Dose, Gy	Time of Onset
Early transient erythema	2	2–24 h
Main erythema reaction	6	~1.5 wk
Temporary epilation	3	~3 wk
Permanent epilation	7	~3 wk
Dry desquamation	14	~4 wk
Moist desquamation	18	~4 wk
Secondary ulceration	24	>6 wk
Late erythema	15	8–10 wk
Ischemic dermal necrosis	18	>10 wk
Dermal atrophy (1st phase)	10	>12 wk
Dermal atrophy (2nd phase)	10	>52 wk
Telangiectasis	10	>52 wk
Delayed necrosis	12?	>52 wk (related to trauma)
Skin cancer	Not known	>15 y

Adapted from Wagner LK, Archer BR: *Minimizing Risks from Fluoroscopic X-rays*, 2nd ed. Houston, TX, Partners in Radiation Management, 1998, with permission, and modified by Hopewell (personal communication).

Because the maximum dose is to the skin, and because the skin is an external organ readily observable, it is not surprising that effects such as erythema or epilation are the most frequently reported. Radiation effects in the skin (Table 14.19) include the following:

- Early transient erythema may occur in a matter of hours following doses of more than 2 Gy (200 rad) because of changes in permeability of capillaries. The main wave of erythema peaks at 10 days to 2 weeks and requires a larger dose of about 6 Gy (600 rad).
- Epilation, or hair loss, occurs if there is sufficient reduction in the replicative capacity of germinal cells or the matrix of the hair follicles. Temporary epilation may occur after doses of about 3 Gy (300 rad), with an onset at about 3 weeks and regrowth requiring 5 weeks or more. Epilation is permanent if the dose exceeds about 7 Gy (700 rad).
- Dry desquamation, flaking sheets of corneum, much like a sunburn, may occur after single doses of more than 14 Gy (1,400 rad) because of depopulation of clonogenic cells in the epidermis. Healing requires the repopulation of basal cells from surviving clonogens.
- Moist desquamation requires higher doses exceeding 18 Gy (1,800 rad) and also results from depopulation of clonogenic cells in the epidermis. Healing is caused by repopulation of surviving clonogens or migration of clonogens from the edges of the irradiated area. These effects may cause substantial discomfort, but provided they are not too severe, they heal and clear up as the population of basal cells recovers.
- Late effects in the skin include dermal atrophy, telangiectasia, and necrosis. These effects occur months to years after higher doses of radiation (10–18 Gy, or 1,000–1,800 rad) and are caused primarily by vascular damage to the dermis. Late effects also may develop after unusually severe early effects, in which case they are referred to as "consequential" late effects.

Table 14.19 is a compilation of the approximate dose levels and relative times at which these effects are observed following a single acute radiation exposure. The doses from fluoroscopically guided interventional procedures are so large that the potential effects of immediate concern are deterministic rather than stochastic.

TABLE 14.20

Effective Doses to Patients from Radiologic and Nuclear Medicine Procedures

Procedure	Effective Dose, mSv
Arrhythmia ablation	17
Coronary angiography	12
Coronary angioplasty	22
Thallium-201 scan	21
Technetium-99 radionuclide ventriculogram	8

Adapted from Lindsay BD, Eichlin JO. Ambos HD, Cain ME: Radiation exposure to patients and medical personnel during radiofrequency catheter ablation for supraventricular tachycardia. *Am J Cardiol* 70:218–223, 1992, with permission.

Effective Dose and Cancer

Although the entrance skin dose is the most relevant to the possible induction of acute deterministic effects, the effective dose is the relevant quantity for estimating the risks of stochastic effects such as cancer. Effective dose is a function of the dose and the specific organs and tissues exposed and can be determined from mathematic models and measurements in anthropomorphic phantoms. Table 14.18 includes estimates of the effective dose for a wide range of procedures. Table 14.20 is more of a summary of mean doses, with less detail, of effective doses from arrhythmia ablation, coronary angiography, and coronary angioplasty. Quantitative estimates of the risk of cancer as a function of dose come from studies of the Japanese survivors of the atomic bombs, as described in Chapter 10, where we discuss radiation carcinogenesis. The risk of cancer death, therefore, from a typical interventional procedure can be estimated to be on the order of 1 in 1,000.

Of course, these deleterious effects of radiation must be viewed in the context of the overall clinical situation. Most patients undergoing fluoroscopically guided interventional procedures are suffering from life-threatening conditions; they are likely to die unless something is done, so the risk–benefit equation is heavily weighted by a substantial benefit balancing the undoubted risk.

Dose to Personnel

Physicians involved in cardiology, angiography, and fluoroscopically guided interventional work routinely receive radiation doses higher than any other staff in a medical facility and comparable to doses received by workers in the nuclear industry (Figure 14.7 and Table 14.21). This is principally

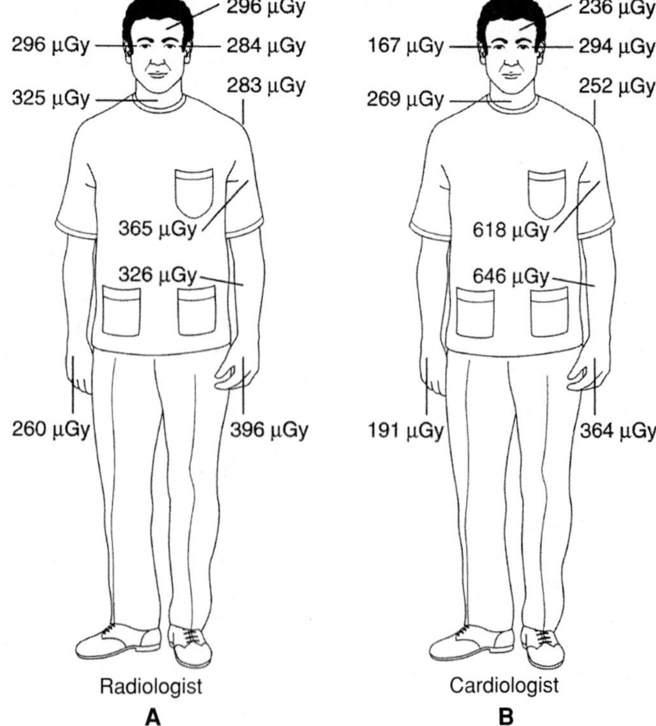

FIGURE 14.7 • Graphic representation of the mean values of doses per procedure for a radiologist (**A**) and a cardiologist (**B**) engaged in an interventional procedure. The figures are the mean of measurements taken during more than 80 procedures. (Adapted from Vano E, Gonzalez L, Guibelalde E, Fernandez JM, Ten JI: Radiation exposure to medical staff in interventional and cardiac radiology. *Br J Radiol* 71:954–960, 1998, with permission.)

TABLE 14.21

Estimated Dose to Staff during Typical Cardiac Studies

Category of Staff	One Catheterization, mSv				One Angioplasty, mSv				One Pacemaker Implant (No Cine), mSv			
	Weighted Surface Dose, No Apron	Weighted Surface Dose with Apron	Hands	Eyes	Weighted Surface Dose, No Apron	Weighted Surface Dose with Apron	Hands	Eyes	Weighted Surface Dose, No Apron	Weighted Surface Dose with Apron	Hands	Eyes
Cardiologist	1.6	0.09	2.1	0.6	3.1	0.2	4.2	1.0	0.14	0.01	0.2	0.05
Cardiologist who stands back during cine	0.3	0.01	0.3	0.2	1.5	0.1	1.9	0.7				
Technologist	0.08	<0.01	0.09	0.02	0.2	0.01	0.2	0.05	0.01	<0.01	0.01	<0.01
Technologist who stands back during cine	0.04	<0.01		0.04	0.01	0.1	0.01	0.1	0.03			
Nurse or anesthetist	0.3	0.02	0.4	0.2	0.8	0.06	0.9	0.5	0.04	<0.01	0.04	0.03

Adapted from National Council on Radiation Protection and Measurements: *Implementation of the Principle of As Low As Reasonably Achievable (ALARA) for Medical and Dental Personnel*. Report 107. Bethesda, MD, NRCP, 1990, with permission.

because of the use of fluoroscopy. CTF poses a new and additional risk.

NUCLEAR MEDICINE

Historical Perspective

The first person to suggest using radioactive isotopes to label compounds in biology and medicine was the Hungarian chemist Georg von Hevesy, whose work, beginning before World War II, earned him a Nobel Prize in 1943 (Fig. 14.8). The concept of using radioactive tracers in medicine could not be exploited until the means to produce artificial isotopes were readily available. The cyclotron was invented and developed by Ernest Lawrence in the 1930s, also leading to a Nobel Prize, and devices of this type have been used to produce short-lived isotopes and positron emitters (Fig. 14.9). Nuclear reactors were developed during World War II and are used to produce most medically used radioactive isotopes, all of which are electron or γ-ray emitters.

For these reasons, nuclear medicine was a late starter compared with radiation therapy and x-ray diagnosis. Radiopharmaceuticals of adequate quality and consistency were not available until 1946, but since then, nuclear medicine has grown into a specialty in its own right and was one of the most rapidly growing areas of medicine until slowed by the advent of CT scanning and magnetic resonance imaging. A broad array of pharmaceuticals, coupled with the development of sophisticated hardware,

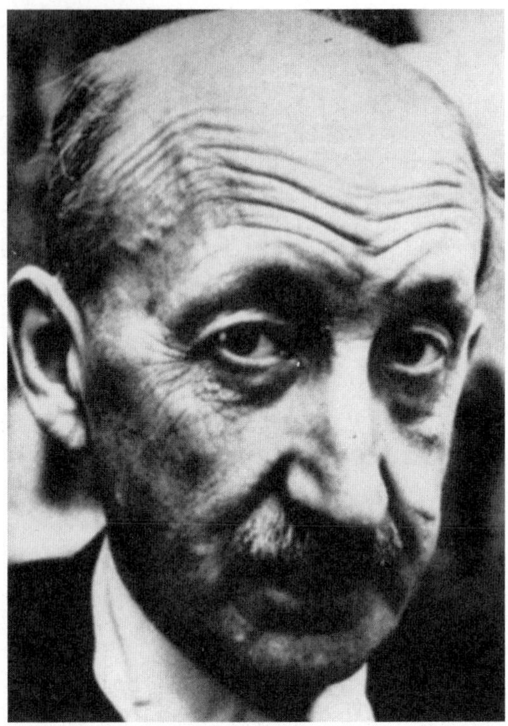

FIGURE 14.8 • The great Hungarian chemist Georg von Hevesy (1885–1966), whose work beginning before World War II earned him a Nobel Prize in 1943. He was the first to conceive of using radioactive isotopes to label compounds for biology and medicine. (Courtesy of the University of California Lawrence Berkeley Laboratory.)

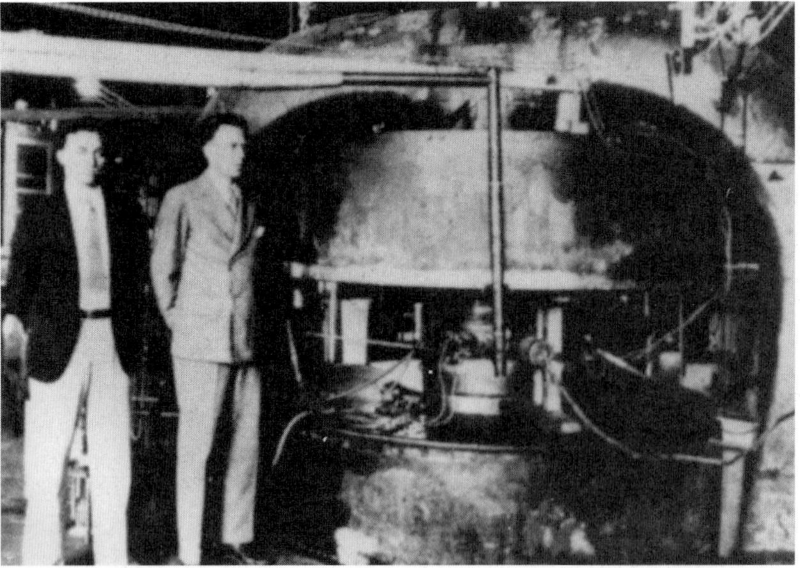

FIGURE 14.9 • The concept of using radioactive isotopes as tracers in medicine was not fully explored until the invention of the cyclotron in 1931. Its inventor, Ernest O. Lawrence, is seen here (*right*) with his second cyclotron in 1934. Many short-lived isotopes that are positron emitters are made with a device of this sort. (Courtesy of the University of California Lawrence Berkeley Laboratory.)

has made possible a widening diversity of applications. PET scanning has opened up a whole new area of rapid growth that is discussed subsequently in this chapter.

In 1989, the NCRP estimated that about 100 million procedures using radioactive materials were performed each year in the United States for diagnostic and therapeutic medical purposes. Approximately 10% of these procedures involved administration of radioactive pharmaceuticals directly to patients for diagnostic or therapeutic procedures. The remaining 90% were radioimmunoassay procedures that involved the use of small amounts of radioactivity in analysis of patient urine, blood, and so forth. It is estimated that in the year 2004, there were more than 10,000 physicians in the United States licensed to administer radiopharmaceuticals to patients for diagnostic and therapeutic purposes.

Although there are over 150 diagnostic and therapeutic nuclear-medicine procedures involving the administration of radiopharmaceuticals to patients, 10 *in vivo* diagnostic procedures comprise over 90% of all such procedures performed in a typical nuclear-medicine clinic, and only 1 therapeutic procedure constitutes the bulk of all nuclear-medicine treatments (Table 14.22 includes the typical doses

TABLE 14.22

Relative Frequency of Nuclear-Medicine Procedures (1991), Typical Activities Administered, and Typical Dose

Procedure	Relative Frequency of Procedure, %	Radiopharmaceutical	Activity Administered per Procedure, MBq	Typical Dose to Patient, mGy
Diagnostic				
Bone	20.6	^{99m}Tc medronate or oxidronate	740	1.3
Gastric emptying	4.6	^{99m}Tc sulfur colloid	40	0.2
Heart Equilibrium radiocardiography	11.8	^{99m}Tc red cells	110	4.5
Heart Myocardial perfusion	17.9	^{201}Tl thallous chloride	110	6.3
		^{99m}Tc sestamibi	1,110	5.0
		^{99m}Tc teboroxime	1,850	8.3
Hepatobiliary	2.9	^{99m}Tc disofenin	300	1.3
Kidney	9.6	^{131}I iodohippurate	15	0.4
		^{99m}Tc penetate	370	0.6
		^{99m}Tc mertiatide	370	0.7
Lung				
Perfusion	8.2	^{99m}Tc macro-aggregated albumin	110	0.5
Ventilation	7.3	^{133}Xe gas	370	0.14
		^{99m}Tc penetate aerosol	740	1.6
Thyroid (25% uptake of iodine)	5.6	^{123}I Na iodide	15	0.4
		^{131}I Na iodide	4	0.7
		^{99m}Tc pertechnetate	185	0.7
Tumor/Infection	3.8	^{67}Ga citrate	190	13.0
Other	5.7			
Therapeutic				
Hyperthyroidism	1.8	^{131}I Na iodide	740	—
Thyroid cancer	0.2	^{131}I Na iodide	3,700	—

Based on National Council on Radiation Protection and Measurements: *Sources and Magnitude of Occupational and Public Exposures from Nuclear Medicine Procedures.* Report 124. Bethesda, MD, NCRP, 1996.

involved). The distribution of studies has shifted significantly over the years, reflecting two simultaneously occurring trends. Radiologic imaging has improved significantly with the advent and application of high-contrast, high-resolution modalities (e.g., CT scanning, ultrasound, magnetic resonance imaging, and digital subtraction angiography) for anatomic definition, thereby supplanting the poorer-resolution nuclear-medicine techniques in the detection and definition of pathologic anatomy. On the other hand, pathophysiologically oriented nuclear-medicine studies have made significant progress with the availability of newer radiopharmaceuticals (e.g., myocardial perfusion agents and regional cerebral blood flow agents), instrumentation (e.g., single-photon emission CT), and computers and software (e.g., renal function evaluation).

Principles in Nuclear Medicine

A wide range of radionuclides are used in diagnostic nuclear medicine that meet the necessary requirements for effective and efficient imaging. All are produced artificially, using four principal routes of manufacture: cyclotron bombardment (producing, for example, ^{67}Ga, ^{111}In, ^{201}Tl, ^{57}Co, ^{123}I, ^{11}C, ^{15}O, ^{13}N, and ^{18}F), reactor irradiation (e.g., ^{51}Cr, ^{75}Se, ^{59}Fe, ^{58}Co, ^{125}I, and ^{131}I), fission products (e.g., ^{131}I, ^{133}Xe, and ^{90}Sr), and generators that provide secondary decay products from longer-lived parent radionuclides. The most common example of the latter is the column generator incorporating ^{99}Mo for the provision of ^{99m}Tc, which, because of its highly suitable physical characteristics for a wide range of applications, forms the basis for over 80% of the radiopharmaceuticals used in nuclear medicine. Most ^{99m}Tc generators utilize fission-produced ^{99}Mo, although techniques of neutron irradiation could provide a viable alternative source of this important parent radionuclide. Other generators include those incorporating ^{113}Sn (for the provision of ^{113m}In), ^{81}Rb (for ^{81m}Kr), and ^{68}Ge (for ^{68}Ga).

The use of radiopharmaceuticals for diagnosis or therapy is based on the accumulation or concentration of the isotope in the organ of interest, referred to as the *target organ*. A radiopharmaceutical may have an affinity for a certain organ that is not necessarily the organ of interest, in which case this organ is termed a *critical organ*. Often the dose to a critical organ limits the amount of radioisotope that may be administered. The risk to which the patient is subjected is clearly a function of the doses received in all organs and must be balanced against the expected advantages and benefits rendered by the procedure. The calculation of the dose absorbed from a radiopharmaceutical can represent a tricky problem, because it may vary with a number of factors.

In addition to conventional planar imaging, techniques have also been developed to allow emission tomography that, like x-ray CT, can demonstrate internal structures or functional information from cross-sectional slices of the patient. Two basic modalities have evolved. The most common is that of **single-photon emission computed tomography (SPECT).** This utilizes conventional γ-emitting radiopharmaceuticals and is often performed in combination with planar imaging. SPECT imaging requires a scanning system incorporating a circular array of detectors or, more often, a rotating γ-camera system with up to four detector heads. The second modality is the more specialized technique of **positron emission tomography (PET).** This is based on the simultaneous detection of the pairs of photons (511 keV) arising from positron annihilation and mostly uses the short-lived biologically active radionuclides ^{15}O, ^{11}C, ^{18}F, and ^{13}N. Dedicated PET scanners use a circular array of detectors, although PET imaging can also be performed using coincidence-adapted γ-camera systems.

The use of radionuclides in medicine is rather sharply divided into diagnostic and therapeutic procedures. There may be a thousandfold difference in the amounts of radioactive material used and therefore in the doses absorbed, depending on whether a given isotope is used to aid diagnosis or is used for therapy. Consequently, therapeutic uses are discussed under a separate heading.

In general, there are three doses of interest after the administration of a given amount of a radiopharmaceutical:

1. *Total-body dose*, because this largely determines the risk of leukemia and cancer.
2. *Gonadal dose*, because this is a measure of hereditary (genetic) effect.
3. *Dose to the critical organ*, because this may be many times larger than the total-body dose, and it is known that certain tissues are particularly susceptible to radiation-induced cancer.

The risk of cancer and hereditary effects are related to the effective dose, which must be calculated.

Dose, Effective Dose, and Collective Effective Dose

Gonadal doses characteristic of selected nuclear-medicine procedures are listed in Table 14.23. Effective doses resulting from a few common

TABLE 14.23

Administered Activity and Gonadal Doses

Examination Type	Estimated Administered Activity + Pharmaceutical per Examination[a]	Gonadal Dose for Each Radiopharmaceutical, mGy[b]		Gonadal Dose, Weighted Average, mGy[b]	
		Male	Female	Male	Female
Brain	740 MBq ^{99m}Tc DTPA (50)	2.2	4.4	1.9	4.4
	740 MBq ^{99m}Tc O_4 (50)	1.5	4.4		
Hepatobiliary	185 MBq ^{99m}Tc iminodiacetic acid (IDA) (10)	0.2	1.7	0.2	0.5
	185 MBq ^{99m}Tc sulfur colloid (90)	0.2	0.4		
Bone	740 MBq ^{99m}Tc phosphate	3.7	4.4	3.7	4.4
Respiratory				0.3	0.3
Perfusion	185 MBq ^{99m}Tc macroaggregated albumin (MAA) (66)	0.4	0.4		
Ventilation	370 MBq ^{133}Xe gas (34)	0.1	0.1		
Thyroid	185 MBq ^{99m}Tc O_4 (80)	0.4	1.1		
	3.7 MBq ^{131}I (10)	<0.1	0.1	0.3	0.9
	11,1 MBq ^{123}I (10)	<0.1	0.1		
Renal	740 MBq ^{99m}Tc DTPA (60)	2.2	4.4	1.3	2.7
	9.25 MBq ^{131}I hippuran (40)	<0.1	<0.1		
Abscess/Tumor	111 MBq ^{67}Ga citrate	7.2	8.4	7.2	8.4
Cardiovascular	740 MBq ^{99m}Tc labeled red blood cells (40)	0.2	0.8		
	111 MBq ^{201}Tl chloride (40)	45.5	11.1	18.9	5.7
	740 MBq ^{99m}Tc phosphate (20)	3.2	4.4		

[a] Number in parentheses is the estimated percent of examination type with a particular radiopharmaceutical.
[b] 1 mGy = 100 mrad.
Adapted from National Council on Radiation Protection and Measurements: *Exposure of the US Population from Diagnostic Medical Radiation.* Report 100. Bethesda, MD, NCRP, 1989, with permission.

nuclear-medicine procedures are listed in Table 14.24. Such tables have been rendered largely obsolete by the exhaustive calculations of both organ doses and effective doses for every known radionuclide and procedure by the Oak Ridge Institute for Science and Education. The doses are calculated using the MIRD (Medical Internal Radiation Dose) technique as implemented in the MIRDOSE computer code developed by the Radiation Internal Dose Information Center at the Oak Ridge Institute. Dose estimates are available for adults, for children, and for embryos or fetuses at various stages of gestation. The dose to the uterus may be used to estimate the dose to the developing embryo or fetus up to about 6 weeks of gestation.

Although the figures in Tables 14.23 and 14.24 must be regarded as purely representative, they are nevertheless instructive. For example, the effective dose for a typical nuclear-medicine procedure, such as a bone scan using technetium-99m phosphate compounds, is about 3.5 mSv (350 mrem). Using the risk estimate of 4% per sievert for radiation-induced cancer, derived in the chapter on radiation carcinogenesis (Chapter 10), this leads to a fatal cancer risk associated with a bone scan of about 1.4 in 10,000.

The other figure of interest is the collective effective dose, which is a measure of the impact of nuclear medicine on the entire U.S. population. The collective effective dose is the summed

TABLE 14.24

Maximum Usual Activity per Test Recommended in the United Kingdom and Corresponding Effective Dose for Some Common Diagnostic Nuclear-Medicine Procedures

Procedure	Radiopharmaceutical	Maximum Usual Activity per Test, MBq	Effective Dose, mSv
Bone scan	^{99m}Tc phosphate compounds	600	3.5
Renal scan	^{99m}Tc DMSA	80	0.7
Renal scan	^{99m}Tc DTPA	300	1.6
Dynamic cardiac scan	^{99m}Tc erythrocytes	800	5.3
Biliary scan	^{99m}Tc IDA	150	2.3
Brain scan	^{99m}Tc HMPAO	500	4.7
Abscess imaging	^{99m}Tc leukocytes	200	2.2
Lung perfusion scan	^{99m}Tc MAA	100	1.1
Renal scan	^{99m}Tc MAG3	100	0.7
Myocardial imaging	^{99m}Tc MIBI	400	3.4
Thyroid scan	^{99m}Tc pertechnetate	80	1.0
Tumor/Abscess imaging	^{67}Ga citrate	150	16.5
Thrombus imaging	^{111}In leukocytes	20	7.2
Thyroid scan (35% uptake)	^{123}I iodide	20	4.4
Tumor imaging	^{123}I MIBG	400	5.6
Thyroid metastase (0% uptake)	^{131}I iodide	400	24
Myocardial imaging	^{201}Tl chloride	80	18

Adapted from Shrimpton PC, Wall BF, Hart D: Diagnostic medical exposures in the UK. *Appl Radiat Isot* 50:261–269, 1999, with permission.

product of effective dose and the number of individuals exposed (see Chapter 15 for definitions). There have been no recent surveys in the United States of collective doses from nuclear medicine, but Table 14.25 is reproduced from NCRP Report 100, published in 1989. The biggest contributors to the collective effective dose are brain, bone, thyroid, and cardiovascular procedures. The age-weighted collective effective dose for nuclear medicine is reduced by an even larger factor than for diagnostic x-rays, to account for the fact that the patient population is skewed even more toward older individuals, who are less likely to be actively reproductive and who are less susceptible to cancer induction. Consequently, hereditary effects are of little importance, and even the risk of radiation-induced cancer becomes moot if the patients do not live long enough for those late effects to be manifest. The age-weighted collective dose for nuclear medicine is estimated to be about 13,500 person-Sv (Table 14.25). Based on this figure, the practice of nuclear medicine in the United States for one year may result in 675 radiation-induced fatal cancers, 121 nonfatal cancers, and 27 hereditary effects. Stated another way, less than 0.006% of those examined might be affected. This calculated possible risk must be weighted against the benefit that about 10 million patients receive from diagnosis of their medical conditions.

The UNSCEAR 2000 report includes some more recent estimates of collective effective doses for diagnostic nuclear-medicine procedures in countries of the developed world, and these are listed in Table 14.26.

Positron Emission Tomography (PET)

One exciting development in nuclear medicine in recent years involves the use of PET scanning. The important and unique feature of PET studies is

TABLE 14.25

Comparison of Collective Effective Dose versus Age-Weighted Collective Dose for U.S. Nuclear-Medicine Procedures in 1982

Examination	Effective Dose, mSv[a]	Examinations, $\times 10^3$	Collective Effective Dose, person-Sv[b]	Age-Weighted Collective Dose, person-Sv[b]
Brain	6.5	813	5,300	2,200
Hepatobiliary	3.7	180	700	300
Liver	2.4	1,424	3,400	1,300
Bone	4.4	1,811	8,000	2,900
Pulmonary	1.5	1,203	1,800	800
Thyroid	7.5	530	4,000	2,400
Renal	3.1	236	700	400
Tumor	12.2	121	1,500	600
Cardiovascular	7.1	961	6,800	2,600
Total			32,100	13,500
Per caput			140 μSv (14 mrem)	59 μSv (5.9 mrem)

[a] 1 mSv = 100 mrem.
[b] 1 person-Sv = 100 man-rem.
Adapted from National Council on Radiation Protection and Measurements: *Exposure of the US Population from Diagnostic Radiation*. Report 100. Bethesda, MD, NCRP, 1989, with permission.

TABLE 14.26

Some Reported Annual Individual and Collective Effective Doses from Diagnostic Nuclear-Medicine Procedures

Country/Area	Effective Dose, mSv: Per Examination	Effective Dose, mSv: Per Caput	Collective Effective Dose, person-Sv[a]
Australia	5.3	0.064	1,110
Canada	4	0.16	4,500
Finland	4.0	0.04	207
Germany	3	0.1	5,000
Netherlands	4.2	0.067	1,000
New Zealand	3.1	0.026	90
Romania	16.2	0.049	1,124
Russian Federation	5.4	0.075	10,000
Switzerland	4.2	0.04	300
United Kingdom	4.2	0.036	2,000
United States	4.4	0.14	35,400

[a] 1 person-Sv = 100 man-rem.
Based on the United Nations Scientific Committee on the Effects of Atomic Radiation: *Annex C Medical Radiation Exposures*. New York, UNSCEAR, 2000.

that they document physiologic abnormalities, or changes in metabolism, rather than simply alterations in anatomy.

The principle of PET imaging is that the scanner locates the tracer by detecting the collinear pairs of 0.511-MeV photons emitted if a positron annihilates after uniting with an electron. A positron is a particle with the same mass and magnitude of charge as an electron, except that the charge is positive. A positron cannot exist at rest, because if it has lost all its kinetic energy, it is electrostatically attracted to an electron with which it annihilates to produce two antiparallel 0.511-MeV photons. Radionuclides that emit positrons have excesses of protons in their nuclei and are produced by bombarding stable elements in a cyclotron. Positron emitters do not occur in nature.

Examples of radionuclides used for PET imaging include oxygen-15, carbon-11, and fluorine-18; these radionuclides have short half-lives of 2, 20, and 110 minutes, respectively, so that the PET facility is frequently close to the cyclotron.

Brain imagers showing the physiologic and functional distribution of positron tracers are currently in use at about 200 PET imaging centers around the world. The most commonly administered positron-emitting radionuclide is fluorine-18, which is used for the production of [^{18}F]-2-deoxy-2-fluoro-D-glucose, usually referred to as *FDG*. This material is used in routine clinical care. Metabolic radiopharmaceuticals are rapidly finding a place in clinical practice—for example, to map areas of tumors that are dividing rapidly, that are hypoxic, or that show a higher degree of malignancy. Many of the other positron-emitting radionuclides are used for the production of experimental compounds used in research studies. For example, oxygen-15 is used to label water for blood flow studies. The doses delivered to patients in PET studies are quite low because of the rapid decay of the radionuclides, even though the administered amounts of radioactivity are high to allow rapid and detailed imaging.

Table 14.27 shows organ doses as well as effective doses for studies with [^{18}F]FDG and for [^{15}O]H_2O. Much more detailed dosimetry is available through the Internet from the Oak Ridge Institute for Science and Education. For procedures

TABLE 14.27

Organ Doses and Effective Doses for Position Emission Tomography Compounds

	F-18 FDG		0-15 H_2O	
	mGy/MBq $\times 10^{-2}$	rad/mCi $\times 10^{-2}$	mGy/MBq $\times 10^{-3}$	rad/mCi $\times 10^{-3}$
Brain	1.9	7.0	1.3	4.9
Heart wall	6.0	22.0	2.2	8.2
Kidneys	2.0	7.4	1.9	7.2
Ovaries	1.7	6.3	0.36	1.3
Red marrow	1.3	4.8	0.90	3.3
Spleen	3.7	14.0	1.6	5.8
Testes	1.3	4.8	0.67	2.5
Thyroid	1.0	3.9	1.7	6.3
Bladder wall	19.0	70	0.22	0.81
	mSv/MBq $\times 10^{-2}$	**rem/mCi $\times 10^{-2}$**	**mSv/MBq $\times 10^{-3}$**	**rem/mCi $\times 10^{-3}$**
Effective dose	3.0	11.0	1.1	4.2

Data from the Oak Ridge Institute for Science and Education (ORISE).

TABLE 14.28

Typical Effective Doses to Patients from Diagnostic PET Imaging

Radionuclide	Chemical Form	Investigation	Administered Activity, MBq	Effective Dose, mSv	Dose to Uterus, mSv
^{11}C	L-methyl-methionine	Brain tumor imaging	400	2	1
^{11}C	L-methyl-methionine	Parathyroid imaging	400	2	1
^{13}N	Ammonia	Myocardial blood flow imaging	550	2	1
^{15}O	Water (bolus)	Cerebral blood flow imaging	2,000	2	1
^{15}O	Water (bolus)	Myocardial blood flow imaging	2,000	2	1
^{18}F	FDG	Tumor imaging	400	10	7
^{18}F	FDG	Myocardial imaging	400	10	7
^{18}F	Fluoride	Bone imaging	250	7	5

Based on UNSCEAR 2000.

using [^{18}F]FDG, the only agent used commonly in routine clinical care, the bladder wall receives the highest dose; the heart, brain, and kidney also receive relatively high absorbed doses. The ICRP, in its publication 53, estimated the effective dose from this procedure to be about 2.7×10^{-2} mSv/MBq, which is in good agreement with the Oak Ridge calculation. A typical administered activity may be 370 MBq (10 mCi), so that the effective dose would be about 11 mSv (1.1 rem). This is equal to about 4 months of natural background radiation in the United States. The associated risk of fatal radiation-induced cancer might be about 0.04%, or 4 cases per 10,000. UNSCEAR 2000 contains a more comprehensive list of effective doses from diagnostic PET procedures, as well as doses to the uterus; this is summarized in Table 14.28.

PET technologists often have higher radiation exposures than other workers in nuclear medicine. Pharmacists at cyclotron facilities have even higher exposures, especially to their hands. This is a function of two factors: (1) the relatively high energy, and therefore penetrating nature, of the photons emitted by the radionuclides used (0.511 MeV) and (2) because of the short half-lives of the commonly used positron-emitting radionuclides, the large initial activities that must be prepared so that a sufficient amount is left by the time the patient is imaged (this is especially true for oxygen-15, which has a half-life of only 2 minutes).

The Therapeutic Use of Radionuclides

Radioactive iodine-131 is widely used for the treatment of hyperthyroidism and thyroid cancer. Because this radionuclide first became generally available in 1946, there has been a gradual shift in the selection of definitive therapy for hyperthyroidism. In the late 1940s and early 1950s, iodine-131 was reserved for patients deemed to be poor surgical risks. By the 1960s, the situation had been completely reversed. Radioactive iodine had become the preferred modality, with thyroidectomy being reserved for the young and for those patients whose clinical evaluation suggested the desirability of surgery to allow an examination of the gland. As a rough estimate, 250,000 patients have now received at least one therapeutic dose of radioactive iodine. Hyperthyroidism is probably the major benign disease for which radiation is the treatment of choice.

A therapeutic treatment with iodine-131 involves an absorbed dose to the thyroid gland that varies with the person and is very nonuniform within the tissue itself but is on the order of many tens of gray (thousands of rad). In addition, there is a total-body dose of typically 70 to 150 mGy (7–15 rad), which results from the isotope circulating in the blood. Because radiation is known to be a potent carcinogen, the risk of leukemia following iodine-131 therapy has been appreciated from the outset and has been looked for carefully. There is also the risk of thyroid cancer because the isotope is concentrated in the thyroid and a large dose is delivered there. These are discussed in turn.

There is no question that thyroid cancer can be induced by external x-irradiation, though most of the data refer to children. By contrast, no excess of thyroid cancer has been observed in adults after the iodine-131 treatment of hyperthyroidism. The experience of the Chernobyl accident indicates that although children are very sensitive to the induction of thyroid cancer by radioiodine, adults are quite resistant.

Because of isolated reports of patients who developed leukemia after treatment with iodine-131 for hyperthyroidism, the Cooperative Thyrotoxicosis Therapy Follow-Up Study was initiated in 1961 under the sponsorship of the U.S. Bureau of Radiological Health. The study included 36,000 patients in 26 medical centers in the United States who were treated for hyperthyroidism either by radioiodine or surgery. The mean bone-marrow doses from the iodine-131 treatments were in the range of 70 to 150 mGy (7–15 rad). The data failed to reveal a statistically significant excess of leukemia from the radioiodine treatment per se. It is of interest to note that the age-adjusted death rate from leukemia in both treatment groups was $1\frac{1}{2}$ times higher than expected on the basis of figures for the general population, from which it was concluded that patients with hyperthyroidism have an enhanced risk of leukemia, regardless of the method by which they are treated.

Pregnancy is, of course, a contraindication to the treatment of hyperthyroidism with iodine-131. Treatment of fertile women should be preceded by the taking of a careful history and a pregnancy test. Treatment should be delayed, if possible, to eliminate the potential effects during pregnancy.

In the treatment of thyroid cancer, many hundreds of millicuries of iodine-131 may be given, which results in a total-body dose sufficient to cause severe depression of the bone marrow. For example, 3.7×10^3 MBq (100 mCi) of iodine-131 delivers 0.5 to 1 Gy (50–100 rad) to the hematopoietic tissue. The effect of such doses on the circulating blood elements is similar to the effect of total-body exposure to external radiation. Ultimately, bone-marrow depression may limit the treatment. Because the treatment of thyroid cancer involves the use of such large and repeated quantities of iodine-131, with the attendant total-body doses, it is not surprising that a few cases of myeloid leukemia have been reported in patients who have received this form of therapy. This is the risk entailed whenever therapeutic doses of radiation are involved; it is usually acceptable because of the serious and malignant character of the disease under treatment.

MEDICAL IRRADIATION OF CHILDREN AND PREGNANT WOMEN

Irradiation of Children

The hazards associated with medical radiation in children are basically the same as in adults—namely, cancer and hereditary effects (mutations)—except for the possibility that the risks associated with a given absorbed dose of radiation are higher because of an increased sensitivity in younger persons. There is good evidence for this. The Japanese survivors of the atomic-bomb attacks represent the most carefully studied human population exposed to radiation. There is a marked decrease in sensitivity to radiation-induced malignancies with increasing age. The effect is most dramatic for breast cancer, where young girls and teenagers are more radiosensitive than older adults by a factor of 10 to 15 (Chapter 10). The same appears to be true of thyroid cancer, for which the incidence per unit dose is much higher in childhood. The most reliable estimates for thyroid cancer come from children irradiated externally with x-rays for a supposedly enlarged thymus and from children irradiated in the course of treatment for tinea capitis. In both cases, the thyroid receives a dose of radiation (as little as 60 mGy (6 rad) in the children with tinea capitis), and within 20 years, an elevated incidence of thyroid cancer is evident. The overall lifetime risk for children irradiated before the age of 10 years is perhaps three times higher than for individuals irradiated as adults. The importance of age is even more obvious in the case of incorporated radioactive iodine. The Chernobyl study shows clearly that children ingesting radioactive iodine are very sensitive to the induction of both benign and malignant thyroid tumors, whereas adults appear to be relatively resistant.

Concern for possible hereditary effects induced by radiation is likewise greater in children, because they have their entire reproductive lives ahead of them. For many adult patients who are past their reproductive years, the risk of hereditary effects is clearly of no concern.

TABLE 14.29

Typical Effective Doses to Pediatric Patients from Diagnostic Nuclear Medicine Procedures

Radiopharmaceutical	Activity for Adult Patient, MBq	Effective Dose per Procedure by Patient Age[a] (mSv)				
		Adult 70 kg [1.0]	15-Year-Old 55 kg [0.9]	10-Year-Old 3.3 kg [0.69]	5-Year-Old 18 kg [0.44]	1-Year-Old 10 kg [0.27]
^{99m}Tc MAG3 (normal renal function)	100	0.7	0.8	0.7	0.6	6.0
^{99m}Tc MAG3 (abnormal renal function)	100	0.6	0.7	0.7	0.5	0.5
^{99m}Tc DTPA (normal renal function)	300	1.6	1.8	2.1	1.8	2.2
^{99m}Tc DTPA (abnormal renal function)	300	1.4	1.6	1.9	1.8	2.0
^{99m}Tc DMSA (normal renal function)	80	0.7	0.7	0.8	0.8	0.8
^{99m}Tc pertechnetate (no thyroid block)	80	1.0	1.2	1.3	1.4	1.4
^{99m}Tc IDA (normal biliary function)	150	2.3	2.4	2.9	3.0	3.7
^{99m}Tc HMPAO	500	4.7	5.0	5.9	5.7	6.5
^{99m}Tc leukocytes	200	2.2	2.7	3.0	2.9	3.4
^{99m}Tc erythrocytes	800	5.3	6.0	6.6	6.7	7.6
^{99m}Tc phosphates	600	3.6	3.7	4.1	4.2	4.9
^{99m}Tc MIBI (resting)	400	3.3	4.0	4.4	4.8	5.4
^{201}Tl chloride	80	20	30	129	95	86
^{125}I iodide (55% thyroid uptake)	20	7.2	10.2	12.1	16.3	18.8
^{125}I iodide (total thyroid block)	20	0.2	0.3	0.3	0.3	0.3
^{125}I MIBG (no impurity)	400	5.6	6.5	9.1	8.8	10.1
^{67}Ga citrate	150	15	18.9	22.8	23.1	27.9

[a] Figures in brackets are scaling factors for activity based on body weights shown. Doses are calculated using age-specific coefficients.
Based on UNSCEAR 2000.

In pediatric radiology or pediatric nuclear medicine, the general principle is that radiation exposures should be kept to the lowest practical level. In each case, the expected benefit should exceed the risk clearly. The dominant concern is the burgeoning use of CT imaging in pediatric radiology, because the doses involved are substantial and the effective doses for a given procedure are even larger in children than in adults, unless care is taken to adjust the parameters of kV and mAs to account for the smaller mass of babies and children. Physicians and patients alike are much more cautious about nuclear-medicine procedures in children than about diagnostic x-rays, even if the dose levels may be similar.

Table 14.29 compares the effective dose in children of various ages with adults for a variety of diagnostic nuclear medicine procedures. In general, effective doses are larger in young children for the same procedure, even if the administered activity is adjusted for body weight.

The implication of the review of carcinogenesis and hereditary effects on humans (Chapters 10 and 11) is that any amount of radiation, no matter how small, has a deleterious effect. This conclusion is based on the assumption of a linear, nonthreshold, dose-effect model that has been adopted by most standard-setting bodies as the most conservative basis for risk estimates. This philosophy requires that the physician have some reasonable indications that the potential gain for the patient from the use of a procedure in nuclear medicine exceeds the risks. The demand for nonessential repetitive examinations and the use of children in poorly planned "research" studies are examples of nonproductive uses of radiation.

Irradiation of Pregnant Women

The risks involved in exposure to radiation of the embryo or fetus are discussed in detail in Chapter 12. They may be summarized as follows:

1. For the first 2 weeks following conception (i.e., during preimplantation), the most significant effect of radiation may be to kill the embryo, leading to resorption. There is also a risk of carcinogenesis.
2. Between 2 and 8 weeks postconception, the risks include congenital malformation and small head size, as well as carcinogenesis.
3. Between 8 to 15 weeks, and to a lesser extent 15 to 25 weeks, the risks include mental retardation as well as small head size and carcinogenesis.
4. Beyond 25 weeks, the only risk of externally delivered diagnostic radiation is carcinogenesis, which is much reduced compared with the risk during the first trimester.

Radiation-induced carcinogenesis is considered a stochastic effect; that is, there is no threshold and the risk increases with dose. One obstetric examination involving a few films may increase the relative risk of leukemia and childhood cancer by about 40%; however, because malignancies are relatively rare in children, the absolute risk is small. The other serious effects, such as mental retardation and congenital malformations, are considered deterministic; that is, there is a threshold of about 0.1 to 0.2 Gy (10–20 rad). It is against the background of these possible risks that the irradiation of the pregnant or potentially pregnant woman must be considered.

Some radiologists instruct their technologists to ask all female patients about possible pregnancy before these women have abdominal or pelvic radiographic examinations. This would appear to be prudent and expedient. Indeed, if time permits, a pregnancy test might be desirable. If a woman requires an emergency radiologic examination, however, there should be no hesitation to do the study. The health of the woman is of primary importance, and if serious injury or illness is suspected, this takes priority in determining the need for a study. The risk to a possible conceptus must be weighed against the risks of not performing the examination.

The NCRP in 1977 recommended for pregnant women that

> if, in the best judgment of the attending physician, a diagnostic examination or nuclear medicine procedure at that time is deemed advisable to the medical well-being of the patient, it should be carried out without delay, with special efforts being made, however, to minimize the dose received by the lower abdomen (uterus).

In the case of nonemergency examinations, it sometimes may be prudent to consider delaying the proposed procedure. The physician contemplating the delay of a study on a woman early in pregnancy should consider the consequences in view of the possibility that the diagnostic examination might become necessary later in the pregnancy, when the risks are much greater. For example, during the first 2 weeks postconception, the risks are possible carcinogenesis and resorption of the embryo. If the study is delayed, however, but becomes essential during the 8th through the 15th week, the risks include small head size and carcinogenesis; in addition, this is the peak of sensitivity to mental retardation. Delay compounds the problem. Conversely, if the patient is already in this peak period of radiosensitivity when a procedure is contemplated, then a delay until after the 25th week would be an advantage, because radiation risks during this period may be at their smallest and involve only a slight risk of carcinogenesis.

The effects of radionuclides on the developing embryo or fetus have not been studied as extensively as the consequences of externally administered x-rays. The biologic effects may depend on many factors, including the chemical form of the isotope, the type and energy of the radiation emitted, whether the compounds containing the radioactivity cross the placenta, and whether they tend to be concentrated in specific target organs.

The metabolism of the radiopharmaceutical may cause high concentrations of the radionuclide in organs of a conceptus if the material crosses the placenta. This may result in dysfunctioning fetal

TABLE 14.30

Thyroidal Radioiodine Dose to the Fetus

Gestation Period	Fetal/Maternal Ratio (Thyroid Gland)	Dose to Fetal Thyroid, rad/μCi[a]
10–12 weeks	—	0.001 (precursors)
12–13 weeks	1.2	0.7
Second trimester	1.8	6
Third trimester	7.5	—
Birth imminent	—	8

[a] Rad/μCi of ^{131}I ingested by mother.
Courtesy of Dr. J. Keriakes, unpublished data.

organs. The classic example of this effect involves the uptake of iodine-131 in the thyroid of the developing embryo and fetus. Up to about 12 weeks, the fetal thyroid does not take up iodine. After this time, iodine concentrates in the fetal thyroid in amounts considerably greater than those in the maternal thyroid (Table 14.30). A number of cases from the 1950s through the 1980s have documented the induction of hypothyroidism and cretinism from doses of iodine-131 to the fetal thyroid.

Although pregnant women receive diagnostic x-rays occasionally, it is rare for them to be given radioactive isotopes. In general, physicians and patients alike are much more wary about nuclear-medicine procedures than about diagnostic x-rays, even if dose levels may be similar. Never is this truer than in the case of pregnant or potentially pregnant women. Table 14.31 includes estimates of the dose to the embryo for selected radiopharmaceuticals administered to the mother in various procedures.

TABLE 14.31

Dose Estimate to Embryo from Radiopharmaceuticals

Radiopharmaceutical	Embryo Dose, rad/mCi Administered
^{67}Ga citrate	0.25
^{5}Se methionine	3.8
^{99m}Tc DTPA	0.035
^{99m}Tc human serum albumin	0.018
^{99m}Tc lungaggregate	0.035
^{99m}Tc polyphosphate	0.036
^{99m}Tc sodium pertechnetate	0.037
^{99m}Tc stannous glucoheptonate	0.04
^{99m}Tc sulfur colloid	0.032
^{123}I sodium iodide (15% uptake)	0.032
^{131}I sodium iodide (15% uptake)	0.1
^{123}I rose bengal	0.13
^{131}I rose bengal	0.68

Courtesy of Dr. J. Kereikes, unpublished data.

Summary of Pertinent Conclusions

- Everyone is exposed to radiation from unperturbed natural sources, enhanced natural sources, and sources resulting from human activity, including medical x-rays.
- Natural background radiation comes from cosmic rays, terrestrial radiation from the earth's crust, and inhaled or ingested radioactivity.
- Cosmic-ray levels vary with altitude and latitude.
- Terrestrial radiation levels vary widely with locality.
- Radon and its progeny result in irradiation of lung tissue with α-particles; this is the largest source of natural radiation.
- Diagnostic radiology is the largest source of radiation resulting from human activities.
- More than 250 million medical and about 100 million dental x-ray examinations are performed each year in the United States.
- About 10 million doses of radiopharmaceuticals are administered each year in the United States.
- The relative importance of natural background radiation compared with radiation from human activities can be assessed from the relevant annual average total effective doses to the U.S. population (Table 14.1), which are:

Natural background, radon	2 mSv (200 mrem)
Natural background, other	1 mSv (100 mrem)
Medical diagnostic x-rays	0.39 mSv (39 mrem)
Nuclear medicine	0.14 mSv (14 mrem)
Consumer products	0.12 mSv (12 mrem)
Rounded total	3.6 mSv (360 mrem)

- The radiation doses involved in diagnostic radiology, except for interventional procedures, do not result in deterministic effects; the risks are stochastic effects (i.e., carcinogenesis and hereditary effects). The one exception is when there is inadvertent exposure to an embryo or fetus.

Computed Tomography (CT)

- The use of computed tomography has increased dramatically in the past decade.
- In 1997, there were about 20,000 CT scanners in the world, with an associated annual total of about 67 million CT procedures. In the year 2000, it is estimated that there were 57 million CT scans in the United States alone. The number of scanners per million population is much greater in the United States than elsewhere.
- The multiple-scan average dose ranges from 40 to 60 mGy (4–6 rad) for head scans to 10 to 40 mGy (1–4 rad) for body scans.
- CT scans involve relatively large effective doses because larger volumes of tissue are exposed to higher doses than occurs in common x-rays. The effective dose varies from a low of 0.35 mSv (35 mrem), when only part of the head is exposed, to a high of 7.8 mSv (780 mrem) for a routine multiple-slice chest CT.
- It is estimated in the United States that while CT comprises 11% of diagnostic procedures, it contributes 60 to 70% to the collective effective dose.
- Effective doses from CT scans are larger in small children than in adults unless care is taken to adjust the kV and mAs.

Effective Dose and Cancer

- The cancer risk to the individual is expressed in terms of the effective dose, the equivalent dose to the various organs and tissues exposed, multiplied by the appropriate tissue weighting factors (W_T).
- The collective effective dose is the product of the effective dose and the number of individuals exposed. It gives an indication of the harm or "detriment" to an exposed population.
- The annual collective effective dose to the U.S. population in 1980 from diagnostic x-rays was about 92,000 person-Sv (9.2 million man-rem). This estimate is out of date and therefore probably too low because of the increased use of CT, but it may instead be too high because the population receiving x-rays is skewed with regard to age distribution as compared with the general population. Overall, it is the best we have.
- The weighted annual collective effective dose for nuclear medicine is 13,500 person-Sv (1.35 million man-rem). An even bigger allowance is necessary to correct for the older age distribution of nuclear-medicine patients than of patients receiving diagnostic radiology.
- The "detriment" from diagnostic radiology and nuclear medicine may be calculated from the collective effective dose and the risk estimate of 5% per sievert for fatal cancer, 0.9% per sievert for nonfatal cancer, and 0.2% per sievert for serious hereditary effects.
- Detriment includes an allowance for loss of quality of life as well as for death.

(continued)

Summary of Pertinent Conclusions (Continued)

- The practice of diagnostic radiology for one year in the United States may benefit about half of the population but may result in several thousand fatal cancers, several hundred nonfatal cancers, and several hundred hereditary effects (mutations).
- The practice of nuclear medicine for one year in the United States may benefit 10 million patients but may result in several hundred fatal cancers and a very small number of nonfatal cancers and hereditary effects.

Interventional Procedures

- The 1990s have witnessed a major increase in high-dose fluoroscopically guided interventional procedures in medicine.
- Radiation doses to patients from interventional radiology and cardiology are in general much higher than from general diagnostic radiology.
- There is a risk of deterministic effects, such as early or late skin damage from interventional procedures. These include:
  1. Early transient erythema, which may occur in a matter of hours following doses of more than 2 Gy (200 rad). The main wave of erythema peaks at 10 days to 2 weeks and requires a larger dose of about 6 Gy (600 rad).
  2. Dry desquamation, which may occur after single doses of more than 10 Gy (1,000 rad) and is due to depopulation of clonogenic cells in the epidermis.
  3. Moist desquamation, which requires doses exceeding 15 Gy (1,500 rad) and is also due to depopulation of clonogenic cells in the epidermis. These effects may cause substantial discomfort, but provided they are not too severe, they will heal and clear up as the population of basal cells recovers.
  4. Temporary epilation, which may occur after doses of about 3 Gy (300 rad), with an onset at about 3 weeks and regrowth requiring 5 weeks or more. Epilation is permanent if the dose exceeds about 7 Gy (700 rad).
  5. Late effects in the skin, which include dermal atrophy, telangiectasia, and necrosis. These effects occur months to years after higher doses of radiation. Late effects may also develop after unusually severe early effects, in which case they are referred to as "consequential" late effects.
- Above a certain threshold, the risk of skin damage is a function of the AEP, the area exposure product, with units of Gy cm^2.
- To put things into context, hundreds of thousands of patients each year in the United States alone undergo interventional procedures, and yet serious problems are rare; for example, about 40 injuries were reported to the FDA in 1994.
- Because most patients undergoing interventional procedures are older and suffer from life-threatening medical conditions, the possibility of stochastic effects (such as radiation-induced cancer) 10 to 20 years in the future is largely academic.

Effects on the Embryo and Fetus

- For irradiation of the human *in utero*, the risk of severe mental retardation as a function of dose is apparently linear, with a risk coefficient as high as 40% per Sv (40% per 100 rem) at 8 to 15 weeks after conception and about four times lower at 15 to 25 weeks. The data are also consistent with a threshold of about 0.1 to 0.2 Sv (10–20 rem).
- Loss of IQ is estimated to be about 30 points per sievert (30 points per 100 rem).
- Every precaution should be taken to avoid exposure of a conceptus.
- Many x-ray exposures involve doses too small to pose a significant risk to the embryo or fetus.
- In the event of an accidental exposure of an unsuspected conceptus, the dose should be estimated carefully. Some believe that a dose exceeding 0.1 to 0.2 Sv (10–20 rem) during a sensitive period of gestation may be grounds for a therapeutic abortion. This dose is flexible and depends on many social factors, such as the religious beliefs of the parents or the number of children they already have.
- The effects of radionuclides on the developing embryo and fetus have been studied less than the effects of x-rays and are likely to be much more complex. Special care should be taken to avoid this problem.

Summary

- In the treatment of hyperthyroidism with iodine-131, the risk of death from radiation-induced leukemia or cancer is less than the risk of death from a general anesthetic used during surgery.
- The risks posed by diagnostic x-rays and nuclear-medicine procedures are small compared with other hazards in an industrialized society, such as smoking cigarettes or driving an automobile.

BIBLIOGRAPHY

Bahodar B: *Trends in Diagnostic Imaging to 2000.* London, FT Pharmaceutical and Healthcare Publishing, 1996

Bakalyar D, Castellani M, Safian R: Radiation exposure to patients undergoing diagnostic and interventional cardiac catheterization procedures. *Cathet Cardiovasc Diagn* 42:121–125, 1997

Bell MR, Berger PB, Menke KK, Holmes DR: Balloon angioplasty of chronic total coronary artery occlusions: What does it cost in radiation exposure, time and materials? *Cathet Cardiovasc Diagn* 25:10–15, 1992

Bergeron P, Carrier R, Roy D, Blais N, Raymond J: Radiation doses to patients in neurointerventional procedures. *Am J Neuroradiol* 15:1809–1812, 1994

Brenner DJ, Elliston CD, Hall EJ, Berdon WE: Estimated risks of radiation-induced fatal cancer from pediatric CT. *AJR Am J Roentgenol* 176:289–296, 2001

Broadhead DA, Chapple C-L, Faulkner K, Daview M, McCallum H: Doses received during interventional procedures. In *Proceedings of the International Congress on Radiation Protection*, pp 438–440. Vienna, IRPA (International Radiation Protection Association) 1996

Committee on the Biological Effects on Ionizing Radiations. *The Effects on Populations of Exposure to Low Levels of Ionizing Radiation.* BEIR III, Washington, DC, National Academy Press, National Research Council, 1980

Committee on the Biological Effects of Ionizing Radiations (BEIR V): *Health Effects of Exposure to Low Levels of Ionizing Radiation.* Washington, DC, National Academy Press, National Research Council, 1990

Conway BJ: *Nationwide Evaluation of X-ray Trends (NEXT) Summary of 1990 Computerized Tomography Survey and 1991 Fluoroscopy Survey.* CRCPD Publication 94-2, Conference of Radiation Control Program Directors Inc., Frankfort, Kentucky, January 1994

Conway BJ, McCrohan JL, Antonsen RG, Rueter FG, Slayton RJ, Suleiman OH: Average radiation dose in standard CT examinations of the head: Results of the 1990 NEXT survey. *Radiol* 184:135–140, 1992

Cristy M, Eckerman K: Specific absorbed fractions of energy at various ages from internal photon sources: Parts I-VII. ORNL/TM-8381/VI-V7. Oak Ridge, TN, Oak Ridge National Laboratory, 1987

Eckerman KF: Aspects of the dosimetry of radionuclides within the skeleton with particular emphasis on the active marrow. In *Proceedings: Fourth International Radiopharmaceutical Dosimetry Symposium*, pp 514–534. Oak Ridge, TN, Oak Ridge Associated Universities, 1986

Feygelman VM, Huda W, Peters K: Effective dose equivalents to patients undergoing cerebral angiography. *AJNR* 13:845–849, 1992

Hart D, Hillier MC, Wall BF: Doses to patients from medical x-ray examinations in the UK—2000 review. NRPB report, 2000

Hart D, Wall BF: Estimation of effective dose from dose-area product measurements for barium meals and barium enemas. *Br J Radiol* 67:485–489, 1994

Hart D, Wall BF: Potentially higher patient radiation doses using digital equipment for barium studies. *Br J Radiol* 68: 1112–1115, 1995

Huda W, Atherton JV, Ware DE, Cumming WA: An approach for the estimation of effective radiation dose at CT in pediatric patients. *Radiology* 203(2):417–422, 1997

Huda W, Morin RL: Patient doses in bone mineral densitometry. *Brit J Radiol* 69:422–425, 1996

International Commission on Radiological Protection: *1990 Recommendations of the International Commission on Radiological Protection.* Publication 60, Vol 21, Nos 1–3, p 24. Oxford, Pergamon Press, 1991

International Commission on Radiological Protection: *Gamma-Ray Spectrometry in the Environment.* Report 53, Bethesda, Maryland, ICRP, 1994

Jessen KA, Shrimpton PC, Geleijns J, Panzer W, Tosi G: Dosimetry for optimisation of patient protection in computed tomography. *Appl Radiat Isot.* 50(1):165–172, 1999

Jones DG, Shrimpton PC: *Normalised Organ Doses for X-ray Computed Tomography Calculated Using Monte Carlo Techniques.* NRPB-SR250. Chilton, UK, National Radiological Protection Board, 1993

Karppinen J, Parviainen T, Servoman A, Komppa T: Radiation risk and exposure of radiologists and patients during coronary angiography and percutaneous transluminal coronary angioplasty (PCTA). *Radiat Prot Dosim* 57:481–485, 1995

Knautz MA, Abele DC, Reynolds TL: Radiodermatitis after transjugular intrahepatic portosystemic shunt. *South Med J* 5:450–452, 1997

Lichtenstein DA, Klapholz L, Vardy DA, et al.: Chronic radiodermatitis following cardiac catheterization. *Arch Dermatol* 132:663–667, 1996

Lindsay BD, Eichlin JO, Ambos HD, Cain ME: Radiation exposure to patients and medical personnel during radiofrequency catheter ablation for supraventricular tachycardia. *Am J Cardiol* 70:218–223, 1992

Loevinger R, Budinger T, Watson E: *MIRD Primer for Absorbed Dose Calculations.* New York, NY, Society of Nuclear Medicine, 1991

McCrohan JL, Patterson JF, Gagne RM, Goldenstein HA: Average radiation doses in a standard head examination for 250 CT systems. *Radiology* 163:263–268, 1987

McParland BJ: A study of patient radiation doses in interventional radiological procedures. *Br J Radiol* 71:175–185, 1998

Mejia AA, Nakamura T, Masatoshi I, Hatazawa J, Masaki M, Watanuki S: Estimation of absorbed doses in humans due to intravenous administration of fluorine-19-fluorodeoxyglucose in PET studies. *J Nucl Med* 32:699–706, 1991

Mettler FA, Wiest PW, Locken JA, Kelsey CA: CT scanning: Patterns of use and dose. *J Radiol Prot* 20(4):353–9, 2000

Nahass GT: Acute radiodermatitis after radiofrequency catheter ablation. *J Am Acad Dermatol* 36:881–884, 1997

Nahass GT, Cornelius L: Fluoroscopy-induced radiodermatitis after transjugular intrahepatic portosystemic shunt. *Am J Gastroenterol* 93:1546–1549, 1998

National Center for Devices and Radiological Health. Fluoroscopically guided procedures have potential for skin injury. *Radiological Health Bulletin* 28:1–2, Rockville, MD: US Department of Health and Human Services, Public Health Services, Food and Drug Administration; 1994

National Council on Radiation Protection and Measurements: *Exposures of the Population in the United States to Ionizing Radiation.* Report 93. Bethesda, MD, NCRP, 1987

National Council on Radiation Protection and Measurements: *Exposure of the US Population from Diagnostic Medical Radiation.* Report 100. Bethesda, MD, NCRP, 1989

National Council on Radiation Protection and Measurements: *Exposures of the US Population from Occupational Radiation.* Report 101. Bethesda, MD, NCRP, 1989

National Council on Radiation Protection and Measurements: *Implementation of the Principle of As Low As Reasonably Achievable (ALARA) for Medical and Dental Personnel.* Report 107. Bethesda, MD, NCRP, 1990

National Council on Radiation Protection and Measurements: *Ionizing Radiation Exposure of the Population of the United States*. Report 93. Bethesda, MD, NCRP 1987

National Council on Radiation Protection and Measurements: *Sources and Magnitude of Occupational and Public Exposures from Nuclear Medicine Procedures*. Report 124. Bethesda, MD, NCRP, 1996

Paterson A, Frush DP, Donnelly LF: Helical CT of the body: Are settings adjusted for pediatric patients? *AJR Am J Roentgenol* 176:297–301, 2001

Pattee PL, Johns PC, Chambers RJ: Radiation risk to patients from percutaneous transluminal coronary angioplasty. *J Am Coll Cardiol* 22:1044–1051, 1993

Refetoff S, Harrison J, Karanfilski BI, Kaplan E, DeGroot LJ, Bekerman C: Continuing occurrence of thyroid carcinoma after irradiation to the neck in infancy and childhood. *N Engl J Med* 292:171–175, 1975

Robinson AE, Hill EP, Harpen MD: Radiation dose reduction in pediatric CT. *Pediatr Radiol* 16(1):53–4, 1986

Rosenstein M: *Handbook of Selected Tissue Doses for Projections Common in Diagnostic Radiology*. Publication 89-8031. Rockville, MD, US Department of Health and Human Services, Public Health Service, Food and Drug Administration, 1988

Rosenthal L, Beck TJ, Williams J, et al.: Acute radiation dermatitis following radiofrequency catheter ablation of atrioventricular nodal reentrant tachycardia. *Pacing Clin Electrophysiol* 20:1834–1839, 1997

Rowley KA: Patient exposure in cardiac catheterization and cinefluorography using the Eclair 16mm camera at speeds up to 200 frames per second. *Br J Radiol* 47:169–178, 1974

Shrimpton PC: Protection of the patient in x-ray computed tomography, in documents of the NRPB, Vol. 3, No. 4, London, HMSO, 1992

Shrimpton PC, Edyvean S: CT scanner dosimetry. *Br J Radiol.* 71(841):1–3, 1998

Shrimpton PC, Jessen KA, Geleijns J, Panzer W, Tosi G: Reference doses in computed tomography. *Radiat Prot Dos* 80:55–59, 1998

Shrimpton PC, Wall BF, Hart D: Diagnostic medical exposures in the UK. *Appl Radiat Isot* 50:261–269, 1999

Smith PG, Doll R: Mortality from cancer and all causes among British radiologists. *Br J Radiol* 54:187–194, 1981

Stern SH, Rosenstein M, Renaud L, Zankl M: *Handbook of Selected Tissue Doses for Fluoroscopic and Cineangiographic Examination of the Coronary Arteries*. Rockville, MD, Food and Drug Administration, 1995

Stern SH, Spelic DC, Kaczmarek RV: *NEXT 2000 Protocol for Survey of Computed Tomography (CT)*. Conference of Radiation Control Program Directors Inc. Frankfort, Kentucky, December 18, 2000

Stewart A, Webb J, Hewitt D: A survey of childhood malignancies. *Br Med J* 1:1495–1508, 1958

Stone MS, Robson KJ, Leboit PE: Subacute radiation dermatitis from fluoroscopy during coronary artery stenting: Evidence for cytotoxic lymphocyte mediated apoptosis. *J Am Acad Dermatol* 38:333–336, 1998

United Nations Scientific Committee on the Effects of Atomic Radiation: *Annex C Medical Radiation Exposures*. New York, UNSCEAR, 2000

United Nations Scientific Committee on the Effects of Atomic Radiation: *Sources and Effects of Ionizing Radiation*. New York, UNSCEAR, 1986

Vano E, Gonzalez L, Guibelalde E, Fernandez JM, Ten JI: Radiation exposure to medical staff in interventional and cardiac radiology. *Br J Radiol* 71:954–960, 1998

Wagner HN: F-18 FDG in oncology: Its time has come. *Appl Radiol* 26:29–31, 1997

Wagner LK: *Radiation Bioeffects and Management Test and Syllabus*. Reston, VA, American College of Radiology, 1991

Wagner LK, Archer BR: *Minimizing Risks from Fluoroscopic X-rays*, 2nd ed. Houston, TX, Partners in Radiation Management, 1998

Wagner LK, Archer BR: *Radiation Protection Management for Fluoroscopy: A Manual for Physicians*. Houston, TX, RM Partnership, 1995

Wagner LK, Eifel PJ, Geise RA: Effects of ionizing radiation. *J Vasc Interv Radiol* 6:988–989, 1995

Wagner LK, Eifel PJ, Geise RA: Potential biological effects following high x-ray dose interventional procedures. *J Vasc Interv Radiol* 5:71–84, 1994

Wagner LK, McNeese MD, Marx MV, Siegel EL: Severe skin reactions from interventional fluoroscopy: Case report and review of the literature. *Radiology* 213:773–776, 1999

Wall BF, Hart, D: Commentary: Revised radiation doses for typical x-ray examinations. *Br J Radiol* 70:437–439, 1997

Ware DE, Huda W, Mergo PJ, Litwiller AL: Radiation effective doses to patients undergoing abdominal CT examinations. *Radiology* 210:645–650, 1999

Watson RM: Radiation exposure: Clueless in the cath lab, or sayonara ALARA. *Cathet Cardiovasc Diagn* 42:126–127, 1997

Whalen JP, Balter S: *Radiation Risks in Medical Imaging*. Chicago, Yearbook Medical Publishers, 1984

Williams J: The interdependence of staff and patient doses in interventional radiology. *Br J Radiol* 70:498–503, 1997

CHAPTER 15

Radiation Protection

THE ORIGINS OF RADIATION PROTECTION

At the Second International Congress of Radiology in Stockholm in 1928, member countries were invited to send representatives to prepare x-ray protection recommendations. The British recommendations were adopted because they were most complete: guidelines on radiation protection had been set up in that country as early as 1915.

The 1928 congress set up the International X-Ray and Radium Protection Committee, which after World War II was remodeled into two commissions that survive to this day:

The International Commission on Radiological Protection (ICRP)
The International Commission on Radiation Units and Measurements (ICRU)

The U.S. representative to this 1928 congress was Dr. Lauristor Taylor, who brought back to the United States the agreed radiation protection criteria and set up a national committee, the Advisory Committee on X-Ray and Radium Protection, under the auspices of the Bureau of Standards, which was perceived to be "neutral territory" by the various radiologic societies of the day; this committee operated until World War II. In 1946, it was renamed the National Council on Radiation Protection and Measurements (NCRP), eventually receiving a charter from Congress as an independent body to provide advice and recommendations on matters pertaining to radiation protection in the United States. NCRP reports still form the basis of radiation protection policy in the United States today, though legal responsibility for the implementation of radiation safety is variously in the hands of the Nuclear Regulatory Commission, the Department of Energy, and state or city bureaus of radiation control.

ORGANIZATIONS

The organization of radiation protection and the interrelation of the various committees whose reports are quoted deserve a brief explanation.

First, there are the committees that summarize and analyze data and suggest risk estimates for radiation-induced cancer and hereditary effects. At the international level, there is the United Nations Scientific Committee on the Effects of Atomic Radiation, usually known as UNSCEAR. This committee has wide international representation, being composed of scientists from 21 member states. Comprehensive reports appeared at intervals over the years since 1958, with the latest report in 2000. The United States committee is appointed by the National Academy of Sciences and is now known as the BEIR (Biological Effects of Ionizing Radiations) Committee. The first report appeared in 1956, when it was known as the BEAR (Biological Effects of Atomic Radiations) Committee. Subsequent comprehensive reports appeared in 1972 (BEIR II), 1980 (BEIR III), and 1990 (BEIR V). BEIR VI, entitled *The Health Effects of Exposure to Indoor Radon*, appeared in 1999. The next comprehensive report on radiation effects will be BEIR VII, appeared in 2005.

These committees are "scholarly" committees in the sense that if information is not available on a particular topic, they do not feel compelled to make a recommendation. Because they do not serve an immediate pragmatic aim, they are not obliged to make a "best guess" estimate if data are uncertain. For example, both committees declined to choose a value for the dose-rate effectiveness factor for carcinogenesis in the human (for which there are no data) and simply described a range of 2 to 10 based on animal studies.

Second, there are the committees that formulate the concepts for use in radiation protection and recommend maximum permissible levels. These committees serve more pragmatic aims and therefore must make best estimates even if good data are unavailable. At the international level there is the International Commission on Radiological Protection (ICRP), which (together with the International Commission on Radiation Units and Measurements [ICRU]) was established in 1928 after a decision by the Second International Congress of Radiology (as mentioned above). In 1950, the ICRP was restructured and given its present name. The ICRP often takes the lead in formulating concepts in radiation protection and in recommending dose limits. As an international body, it has no jurisdiction over anyone and can do no more than recommend; it has established considerable credibility, however, and its views carry great weight. Its most recent comprehensive report is ICRP Publication No. 60, published in 1991, with revisions in Tables 15.2 to 15.3 from ICRP 2004. The United Kingdom, most of Europe, and Canada follow ICRP recommendations.

In the United States, there is the NCRP (also mentioned above), chartered by Congress to be an "impartial" watchdog and consisting of 100 experts from the radiation sciences—who are therefore not impartial at all. The NCRP often, but not always, follows the lead of ICRP. Their most recent comprehensive report on dose limits (NCRP Report No. 116, published in 1992) differs from ICRP in several important respects. The ICRP and NCRP suggest dose limits and safe practices, but in fact neither body has any jurisdiction to enforce their recommendations.

In the United States, the Environmental Protection Agency (EPA) has responsibility for providing guidance to federal agencies; it is the EPA that sets, for example, the action level for radon. Each state can formulate its own regulations for x-rays and radiations produced by sources other than reactors. In agreement states, the Nuclear Regulatory Commission formulates rules for by-product materials from reactors. Table 15.1 lists "agreement states" as of 2003. In other states, this responsibility falls on the U.S. Occupational Safety and Health Administration. The Department of Energy is responsible for radiation safety regulations at all of its facilities operated by contractors. Up to the present time, the various regulating bodies in the United States have accepted, endorsed, and used the reports issued by the NCRP, but they are not obligated to do so, and they are often slow to adopt the latest reports.

QUANTITIES AND UNITS

Dose

The quantity used to measure the "amount" of ionizing radiation is the **absorbed dose**, usually termed simply **dose**. This is defined as the energy absorbed per unit mass, and its unit is joules per kilogram, which is given a special name, the gray (Gy), named after the British physicist who contributed to the development of ionization chamber theory. The unit used in the past was the rad (radiation absorbed dose), defined as an energy absorption of 100 erg/g. Consequently, 1 Gy equals 100 rad.

TABLE 15.1

List of Agreement States—August 2003

State	Date of Agreement
Alabama	10/01/66
Arizona	05/15/67
Arkansas	07/01/63
California	09/01/62
Colorado	02/01/68
Florida	07/01/64
Georgia	12/15/69
Illinois	06/01/87
Iowa	01/01/86
Kansas	01/01/65
Kentucky	03/26/62
Louisiana	05/01/67
Maine	04/01/92
Maryland	01/01/71
Massachusetts	03/21/97
Mississippi	07/01/62
Nebraska	10/01/66
Nevada	07/01/72
New Hampshire	05/16/65
New Mexico	05/01/74
New York	10/15/62
North Carolina	08/01/64
North Dakota	09/01/69
Ohio	08/31/99
Oklahoma	09/29/00
Oregon	07/01/65
Rhode Island	01/01/80
South Carolina	09/15/69
Tennessee	09/01/65
Texas	03/01/63
Utah	04/01/84
Washington	12/31/66
Wisconsin	08/11/03

Radiation Weighting Factor (W_R)

The probability of a stochastic effect, such as the induction of cancer or of hereditary events, depends not only on the dose but also on the type and energy of the radiation; that is, some radiations are biologically more effective, for a given dose, than others. This is taken into account by weighting the absorbed dose by a factor related to the quality of the radiation. A **radiation weighting factor (W_R)** is a dimensionless multiplier used to place biologic effects (risks) from exposure to different types of radiation on a common scale. Radiation weighting factors are chosen by the ICRP as representative of relative biologic effectiveness (RBE), applicable to low doses and low dose rates, and for biologic end points relevant to stochastic late effects. They can be traced ultimately to experimentally determined RBE values, but a large judgmental factor is involved in their choice. The weighting factors recommended by the ICRP for different types of radiations, such as photons, electrons, protons, neutrons, and α-particles, are listed in Table 15.2.

Equivalent Dose

In radiologic protection, the **equivalent dose** is the product of the absorbed dose averaged over the tissue or organ and the radiation weighting factor selected for the type and energy of radiation involved. Thus:

$$\text{Equivalent dose} = \text{absorbed dose} \times \text{radiation weighting factor}$$

If absorbed dose is measured in gray, the equivalent dose is in sievert (Sv), named after the Swedish physicist who designed early ionization chambers. If the absorbed dose is in rad, the equivalent dose is in rem (rad equivalent man). Although 1 Gy of neutrons does not produce the same biologic effect as 1 Gy of x-rays, 1 Sv of either neutrons or x-rays does result in equal biologic effects. The ICRP has recommended a new name for this quantity: **radiation weighted dose**. The commission is also considering a new (special) name for the unit of radiation weighted dose so as to avoid the use of "sievert" for both radiation weighted dose and effective dose.

If a radiation field is made up of a mixture of radiations, the equivalent dose is the sum of the individual doses of the various types of radiations, each multiplied by the appropriate radiation weighting factor. Thus, if a tissue or organ were exposed to 0.15 Gy (15 rad) of cobalt-60 γ-rays plus 0.02 of 1-MeV neutrons, the equivalent dose would be

$$(0.15 \times 1) + (0.02 \times 20) = 0.55 \text{ Sv, or } 55 \text{ rem}$$

Effective Dose

If the body is uniformly irradiated, the probability of the occurrence of stochastic effects (cancer and hereditary effects) is assumed to be proportional to the equivalent dose, and the risk can be represented by a single value. In fact, truly uniform total-body exposures are rare, particularly if irradiation is from radionuclides deposited in tissues and organs. Sometimes, equivalent doses to various tissues differ substantially, and it is well established that different tissues vary in their sensitivities to

TABLE 15.2

Radiation Weighting Factors

Type and Energy Range	Radiation Weighting Factor, W_R
Photons	1
Electrons	1
Protons	2
α-Particles, fission fragments, heavy nuclei	20
Neutrons	A continuous curve is recommended with a maximum of 20 for the most effective neutrons of about 1 MeV

Based on International Commission on Radiological Protection: Relative biological effectiveness (RBE), quality factor (Q), and radiation weighting factor (W_R). ICRP Publication 92, Oxford, UK, Elsevier Science Ltd, 2004.

radiation-induced stochastic effects. For example, it is difficult to produce hereditary effects by irradiation of the head or hands! On the other hand, the thyroid and breast appear to be particularly susceptible to radiation-induced cancer. To deal with this situation, the ICRP introduced the concept of the **tissue weighting factor** (**W_T**), which represents the relative contribution of each tissue or organ to the total detriment resulting from uniform irradiation of the whole body. Table 15.3 lists the tissue weighting factors recommended by the ICRP.

The sum of all of the weighted equivalent doses in all the tissues or organs irradiated is called the **effective dose**, which is expressed by the formula

$$\text{Effective dose} = \Sigma \text{ absorbed dose} \times W_R \times W_T$$

for all tissues or organs exposed. Effective dose is in principle as well as in practice a nonmeasurable quantity.

Committed Equivalent Dose

In the case of external irradiation, the absorbed dose is delivered at the time of exposure; but for irradiation from internally deposited radionuclides, the total absorbed dose is distributed over time, as well as to different tissues in the body. The dose rate falls off, depending on the physical and biologic half-lives of the radionuclide.

To take into account the varying time distributions of dose delivery, the ICRP defined the **committed equivalent dose** as the integral over 50 years of the equivalent dose in a given tissue after intake of a radionuclide. This time was chosen to correspond to the working life of a person. For radionuclides with effective half-lives up to about 3 months, the committed equivalent dose is essentially equal to the annual equivalent dose in the year of intake; but for radionuclides with longer effective half-lives it

TABLE 15.3

Tissue Weighting Factors

Tissue	W_T	ΣW_T
Bone marrow, breast, colon, lung, stomach	0.12	0.60
Bladder, esophagus, gonads, liver, thyroid	0.05	0.25
Bone surface, brain, kidneys, salivary glands, skin	0.01	0.05
Remainder tissues[a]	0.10	0.10

[a] Remainder tissues (14 in total): adipose tissue, adrenals, connective tissue, extrathoracic airways, gall bladder, heart wall, lymphatic nodes, muscle, pancreas, prostate, small intestine wall, spleen, thymus, and uterus/cervix.

Based on International Commission on Radiological Protection: Relative biological effectiveness (RBE), quality factor (Q), and radiation weighting factor (W_R). ICRP Publication 92, Oxford, UK, Elsevier Science Ltd, 2004.

is greater, because it reflects the dose that will accrue over future years.

Committed Effective Dose

If the committed equivalent doses to individual organs or tissues resulting from the intake of a radionuclide are multiplied by the appropriate tissue weighting factors and then summed, the result is the **committed effective dose**.

Collective Equivalent Dose

The quantities referred to previously all relate to the exposure of an individual. They become appropriate for application to the exposure of a group or population by the addition of the term *collective*. Thus, the **collective equivalent dose** is the product of the average equivalent dose to a population and the number of persons exposed. There appears to be some confusion about the accepted name of the unit for collective equivalent dose in the new SI system of units. Some use *man-sievert*, presumably agreeing with the judgment of Sir Winston Churchill that "man embraces woman." The more liberated prefer the term *person-sievert*, which is used here. (The old unit was the man-rem.)

Collective Effective Dose

The **collective effective dose** is likewise the product of the average effective dose to a population and the number of persons exposed. The unit is again the *person-sievert* (formerly man-rem). An example is in order here. If 100 persons receive an average effective dose of 0.3 sievert (30 rem), the collective effective dose is 30 person-Sv (3,000 man-rem).

Collective Committed Effective Dose

In the case of a population ingesting or inhaling radionuclides that deposit their dose over a prolonged period of time, the integral of the effective dose over the entire population out to a period of 50 years is called the **collective committed effective dose**.

These collective quantities can be thought of as representing the total consequences of exposure of a population or group, and they can be thought of as surrogates for "harm." For example, the annual collective effective dose to the U.S. population from diagnostic radiology is about 100,000 person-Sv (10 million man-rem). Such collective quantities are much beloved by the bureaucrats because they make it possible to compare different activities or accidents, inasmuch as each can be described by a single number. The danger is that the next step is to convert the collective dose into the number of cancers or hereditary effects produced, which, of course, assumes proportionality between dose and biologic effect, which is seldom true. The quantities certainly are used widely to give a rough guide to the probability of cancer and hereditary effects in a population exposed to radiation, and in particular they can be used to compare the approximate impact of different types of radiation accidents in terms of the number of health effects that might arise in that population.

Summary of Quantities and Units

Table 15.4 is a summary of the quantities and units that have been described here, showing how they build logically on one another. If on reading this section the reader gains the impression that the bureaucrats have taken over, it is because they have—at least in the field of radiation protection. An elaborate set of definitions has been produced based on the assumption of linearity between dose and risk. The whole business needs to be taken with a generous grain of salt, because it is like a house of cards, based on somewhat shaky premises.

The concept of collective effective dose does allow a rough and quick estimate to be made of the potential health hazards to a population from, for example, an accidental release of radioactivity from a nuclear reactor. It must be emphasized again that these concepts can be used only under conditions in which it is *reasonable to assume linearity between risk and dose*—that is, that risks are directly proportional to the summation of doses from different sources. Exposures that are within the administratively allowed dose limits may cause an increased incidence of stochastic effects, such as cancer and hereditary effects, but are much below the thresholds for early deterministic effects. In the case of larger accidental releases, in which doses to some people might be high enough to exceed these thresholds to the point of causing early death, collective effective dose is an inappropriate quantity.

AIMS AND OBJECTIVES OF RADIATION PROTECTION

The fundamental aim of radiation protection has been summed up by the International Commission on Radiological Protection (ICRP) as follows:

> The primary aim of radiological protection is to provide an appropriate standard of protection for man without unduly limiting the beneficial actions giving rise to radiation exposure. This aim cannot be achieved on the basis of scientific concepts alone. All those concerned with radiological protection have to make value

TABLE 15.4

Quantities and Units Used in Radiation Protection

Quantity	Definition	Unit	
		New	Old
Absorbed dose	Energy per unit mass	Gray	Rad
For individuals			
Equivalent dose (Radiation weighted dose)	Average dose × radiation weighting factor	Sievert	Rem
Effective dose	Sum of equivalent doses to organs and tissues exposed, each multiplied by the appropriate tissue weighting factor	Sievert	Rem
Committed equivalent dose	Equivalent dose integrated over 50 years (relevant to incorporaated radionuclides)	Sievert	Rem
Committed effective dose	Effective dose integrated over 50 years (relevant to incorporated radionuclides)	Sievert	Rem
For populations			
Collective effective dose	Product of the average effective dose and the number of individuals exposed	Person-sievert	Man-rem
Collective committed effective dose	Integration of the collective dose over 50 years (relevant to incorporated radionuclides)	Person-sievert	Man-rem

judgments about the relative importance of different kinds of risk and about the balancing of risks and benefits. In this, they are no different from those working in other fields concerned with the control of hazards.

As stated by the NCRP, the objectives of radiation protection are (1) to prevent clinically significant radiation-induced deterministic effects by adhering to dose limits that are below the apparent or practical threshold, and (2) to limit the risk of stochastic effects (cancer and hereditary effects) to a reasonable level in relation to societal needs, values, and benefits gained. The difference in shape of the dose–response relationships for deterministic and stochastic effects is illustrated in Figure 15.1. The objectives of radiation protection can be achieved by reducing all exposure to as low as reasonably achievable (ALARA) and by applying dose

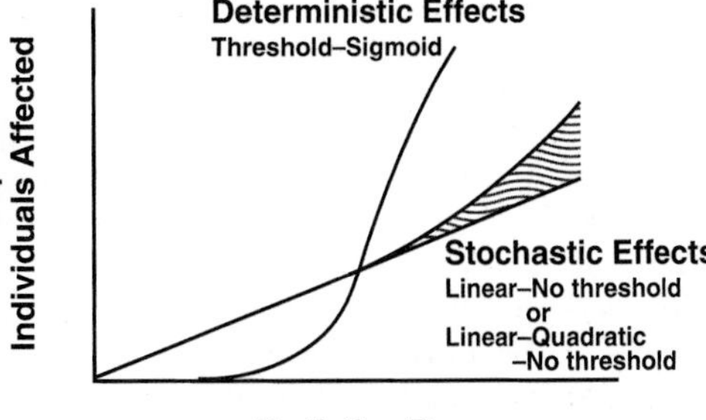

FIGURE 15.1 • The basic differences in the shape of the dose–response relationship for stochastic as opposed to deterministic effects. Deterministic effects (e.g., cataracts or mental retardation) show no threshold in dose; the severity of the effect increases with dose above this threshold, and the proportion of individuals rises rapidly with dose to 100%. The dose–response relationship is therefore sigmoid after a threshold. Stochastic effects are all-or-nothing effects (e.g., cancer and hereditary effects). The severity of the effect is not dose related, though the probability of it occurring is. The increase with dose may be linear or linear-quadratic. There is no threshold, that is, no dose below which the probability of an effect is zero. The dose–response relationship is therefore linear, or linear-quadratic, with no threshold.

limits for controlling occupational and general public exposures. For radiation protection purposes, it is assumed that *the risk of stochastic effects is strictly proportional to dose without threshold throughout the range of dose and dose rates of importance in radiation protection*. Furthermore, the probability of response (risk) is assumed to accumulate linearly with dose. This is not true at higher doses characteristic of radiation accidents, in which more complex (nonlinear) dose–risk relationships may apply.

Given these assumptions, any selected dose limit has an associated level of risk. Consequently, it is necessary to justify any use of radiation in terms of a benefit to a person or to society.

Justification of exposure is one of the basic principles of radiation protection. The concept was described in 1977 by the ICRP:

> A practice involving exposure to radiation should produce sufficient benefit to the exposed individual or to society to offset the radiation detriment it causes.

This concept is sometimes difficult to put into practice in the variety of situations in which individuals are exposed:

1. In the case of patients, the diagnostic or therapeutic benefit should outweigh the risk of detriment.
2. In the case of occupational exposure, the radiation risk must be added to and compared with other risks in the workplace.
3. The most difficult situation is exposure for the sake of research, where volunteer subjects may fall into one of three categories: patients who may benefit, patients who may receive no benefit, and healthy volunteers. In cases in which the individual receives no benefit, the benefit to society must outweigh the risks.

BASIS FOR EXPOSURE LIMITS

Exposure limits have changed over the years in step with evolving information about the biologic effects of radiation and with changes in the social philosophy within which recommended exposure limits are developed.

In the 1930s, the concept of a **tolerance dose** was used, a dose to which workers could be exposed continuously without any evident deleterious acute effects, such as erythema of the skin.

By the early 1950s, the emphasis had shifted to late effects. The **maximum permissible dose** was designed to ensure that the probability of the occurrence of injuries was so low that the risk would be readily acceptable to the average person. At about that time, based on the results of genetic studies in *Drosophila* and mice, the occupational limit was reduced substantially and a limit for exposure of the public introduced. Subsequently, the hereditary effects were found to be smaller, and cancer risks larger, than were thought at the time.

By the 1980s, the NCRP was comparing the probability of radiation-induced cancer death in radiation workers with annual accidental mortality rates in "safe" industries. Exposure standards therefore are necessarily based partly on observed effects, but with a great deal of judgment involved.

Earlier chapters described the deleterious effects of radiation in terms of hereditary effects, carcinogenesis, and effects on the developing embryo and fetus. The risk estimates derived are summarized in Table 15.5. By far the largest risk estimate is 40%/Sv for severe mental retardation for the most sensitive period of gestation and above a threshold of about 0.2 Gy (20 rad). Next comes carcinogenesis as 5%/Sv, corresponding to exposure of the general population to low doses and dose rates. Last are hereditary effects, lowered in 2004 by the ICRP to 0.2%/Sv for the general population.

TABLE 15.5

Deleterious Effects of Radiation that Highlight the Need for Protection

End Point	Risk Estimate
Severe mental retardation:	
Exposure of embryo/fetus (8–15 weeks)	40%/Sv
Carcinogenesis:	
General population (low dose, low dose rate)	5%/Sv
Hereditary effects:	
General population	0.2%/Sv

Based on ICRP, BEIR, and UNSCEAR.

LIMITS FOR OCCUPATIONAL EXPOSURE

The NCRP recommends the limits described in the following sections (and summarized in Table 15.6). These limits do not include natural background radiation or radiation for medical purposes.

Stochastic Effects

1. No occupational exposure should be permitted until the age of 18 years.

TABLE 15.6

Summary of Recommended Dose Limits

	NCRP	ICRP (If Different)
Occupational Exposure:		
Stochastic effects: effective dose limits		
Cumulative	10 mSv × age	20 mSv/y averaged over 5 years
Annual	50 mSv/y	—
Deterministic effects: dose equivalent limits for tissues and organs (annual):		
Lens of eye	150 mSv/y	—
Skin, hands, and feet	500 mSv/y	—
Embryo/Fetus Exposure:		
Effective dose limit after pregnancy declared	0.5 mSv/month	Total of 2 mSv to abdomen surface
Public Exposure (annual):		
Effective dose limit, continuous or frequent exposure	1 mSv/y	No distinction between frequent
Effective dose limit, infrequent exposure	5 mSv/y	and infrequent—1 mSv/y
Dose equivalent limits of lens of eye, skin, and extremities	50 mSv/y	—
Education and Training Exposure (annual):		
Effective dose limit	1 mSv/y	No statement
Dose equivalent limit for lens of eye	15 mSv/y	No statement
Skin and extremities	50 mSv/y	No statement
Negligible Individual Dose (annual):	0.01 mSv/y	No statement

Based on National Council on Radiation Protection and Measurements: *Recommendations on Limits for Exposure to Ionizing Radiation.* NCRP Report No. 116. Bethesda, MD, 1993; and International Commission on Radiation Protection: *Recommendations of the ICRP.* ICRP Publication 60. New York, Pergamon Press, 1991.

2. The effective dose in any year should not exceed 50 mSv (5 rem).
3. The individual worker's lifetime effective dose should not exceed age in years × 10 mSv (1 rem).

These limits apply to the sum of the effective dose from external radiation and the committed effective dose from internal exposures.

Deterministic Effects

1. 150 mSv (15 rem) per year for the lens of the eye.
2. 500 mSv (50 rem) per year for localized areas of the skin and the hands and feet.

These additional limits for deterministic effects are required because the weighting factors for, for example, the hands and the feet are so small that huge doses could be given before cancer induction became a problem. Other deterministic effects are limiting at lower doses.

AS LOW AS REASONABLY ACHIEVABLE (ALARA)

The dose limits referred to previously are all upper limits and subject to the concept of **ALARA** (as low as reasonably achievable). The recommendation that standard-setting committees would like to make for personnel protection is zero exposure. This is not feasible, however, if society is to realize the enormous benefits derived from the uses of radiations and radioactive materials.

Radiation is potentially harmful, and exposure to it should be monitored continually and controlled. No unnecessary exposure should be allowed. Equipment and facilities should be designed so that exposure of personnel and the public is kept to a minimum and not up to a standard. No exposure at all should be permitted without considering the benefits that may be derived from that exposure and the relative risks of alternative approaches.

Of course, the ultimate problem is determining what is "reasonable." There is also the question: How much expense is justified to reduce the exposure of personnel by a given amount? As a rule of thumb in the nuclear-power industry in the United States, ALARA has a cash value of about $1,000 per 10 mSv (1 rem). If the exposure of one person to 10 mSv (1 rem) can be avoided by the expenditure of this amount of money, it is considered reasonable. If the cost is more, it is considered unreasonable, and the exposure is allowed. However, the $1,000 per 10 mSv (1 rem) figure applies specifically to low dose levels. At higher dose levels, at which the accumulation of an additional exposure may threaten a worker's job by exceeding the lifetime dose limit, then the cash value of avoiding a 10 mSv (1 rem) exposure may be closer to $10,000. This sort of choice seldom has to be made in a hospital setting except, for example, in the purchase of remote afterloading equipment for brachytherapy.

PROTECTION OF THE EMBRYO/FETUS

The NCRP recommends a monthly limit of 0.5 mSv (50 mrem) to the embryo or fetus once a woman declares her pregnancy. In contrast to this, the ICRP recommends a limit of 2 mSv (200 mrem) to the surface of the woman's abdomen (lower trunk) for the remainder of the pregnancy. These recommendations are essentially similar and are designed to limit the risk of mental retardation, other congenital malformations, and carcinogenesis. The NCRP and ICRP no longer recommend specific controls for occupationally exposed women *until* the pregnancy is declared. There is a provision that a declared pregnancy can later be "undeclared" if the female worker so desires.

Internally deposited radionuclides pose special problems for protection of the embryo or fetus. Some remain in the body for long periods of time, and the doses delivered to fetal organs are not well known for all radionuclides. Consequently, particular care should be taken to limit the intake of radionuclides by pregnant women so that the equivalent dose to the embryo or fetus would not exceed the recommended limit.

EMERGENCY OCCUPATIONAL EXPOSURE

Under normal conditions, only actions involving the saving of life justify acute exposures in excess of the annual effective dose limit. The use of volunteers for exposures during emergency actions is desirable. If possible, older workers with low lifetime accumulated effective doses should be chosen from among the volunteers. Exposure during emergency actions that do not involve the saving of life should be controlled, to the extent possible, at the occupational exposure limits. If this cannot be accomplished, the NCRP and ICRP recommendation of 0.5 Sv (50 rem) should be applied.

If, for lifesaving or equivalent purposes, the exposure may approach or exceed 0.5 Sv (50 rem) to a large portion of the body, the worker not only needs to understand the potential for acute effects, but also should have an appreciation of the substantial increase in his or her lifetime risk of cancer. If the possibility of internal exposures also exists, this should also certainly be taken into account.

EXPOSURE OF PERSONS YOUNGER THAN 18 YEARS OF AGE

For educational and training purposes, it may be necessary and desirable to accept occasional exposure of persons younger than the age of 18 years, in which case an annual effective dose limit of 1 mSv (100 mrem) should be maintained (NCRP).

EXPOSURE OF MEMBERS OF THE PUBLIC (NONOCCUPATIONAL LIMITS)

The limitation of radiation exposure for members of the public from human-made sources is inevitably arbitrary because it cannot be based on direct experience. The variety of risks of accident and death regularly faced by members of the public vary greatly; the numbers range from 10^{-4} to 10^{-6} per year. Depending on their nature, these risks seem to be accepted without much thought. At the same time, everyone is exposed to natural background radiation of about 1 mSv (100 mrem) annually, excluding radon, which may result in a mortality risk of 10^{-4} to 10^{-5} annually.

Based on these considerations, the NCRP recommended limits for human-made sources other than medical are as follows: For *continuous* or *frequent* exposure, the annual effective dose should not exceed 1 mSv (100 mrem). It is clear, however, that larger exposures to more limited groups of people are not especially hazardous, provided they do not occur often to the same groups. Consequently, a maximum permissible annual effective dose equivalent of 5 mSv (500 mrem) is recommended as a limit for *infrequent* exposure. Medical exposures are excluded from these limitations because it is assumed that they confer personal benefit to the exposed person.

Because some organs and tissues are not necessarily protected against deterministic effects in the calculation of effective dose, the hands and feet, localized areas of the skin, and the lens of the eye are also subject to an annual dose limit of 50 mSv (5 rem).

The fact that the terms *frequent* and *infrequent* in the public dose limits are not defined has caused some confusion. Nevertheless, the intention of the NCRP is laudable, namely, that exceptions to the 1 mSv (100 mrem) per year for members of the public may be justified on the basis of significant benefit either to those exposed or to society as a whole. Here are three examples:

- For workers who come into contact with a coworker who is a radionuclide therapy patient, the annual effective dose limit of 1 mSv may be exceeded under carefully controlled conditions for a small number of such workers, who may receive up to 5 mSv annually.
- For adult family members exposed to a patient who has received radionuclide therapy, the annual effective dose limit is 50 mSv. Thus, adult family members under this circumstance are considered separate from other members of the public and should receive appropriate training and individual monitoring.
- Another example is the inadvertent irradiation of a stowaway in a cargo container irradiated with a pulsed fast neutron analysis system to assess the contents of the container. The NCRP has recommended that such systems be designed and operated in a manner such that the exposure of a stowaway would result in an effective dose of less than 1 mSv for that occurrence. However, an effective dose of up to 5 mSv would be permissible for such an occurrence if necessary to achieve national security objectives.

A more contentious issue is the exposure of members of the public to scattered radiation in a radiology department. For example, exposure of an individual member of the public to scattered radiation in the waiting room of a radiology facility is infrequent for a given individual. On the other hand, a secretary or receptionist may be exposed frequently or continuously, so the desk area must be protected to a lower level, which can be an expensive proposition. It might be tempting to reclassify the office personnel as "radiation workers," but to do so would offend all the basic principles of radiation protection.

EXPOSURE TO INDOOR RADON

Radon levels vary enormously with different localities, depending on the composition of the soil and the presence of cracks or fissures in the ground, which allow radon to escape to the surface. Many homes in the United States and Europe consequently contain an appreciable quantity of radon gas, which enters the living quarters through the basement. Insulating and sealing houses increased greatly as a result of the escalating cost of heating oil in the 1970s, and this has exacerbated the radon problem, because a well-sealed house allows fewer exchanges of air with the outside and consequently results in a greater concentration of radon. Radon is a noble gas and is itself relatively nonhazardous because if breathed in, it is breathed out again without being absorbed. In a confined space such as a basement, however, the decay of radon leads to the accumulation of progeny that are solids, which stick to particles of dust or moisture and tend to be deposited on the bronchial epithelium. These progeny emit α-particles and cause intense local irradiation.

An extreme example is the famous case of Stanley Watras, who wanted to work in a nuclear-power station but was turned away because the radiation monitors were set off as he entered the plant by the accumulation of radon progeny products deposited in his body and on his clothes that came from his home.

Indoor radon currently is perceived to be the most important problem involving radiation exposure of the public. In the United States and most European countries, the mean radon concentration in homes is in the range of 20 to 60 Bq/m^3 (0.5–1.6 pCi/L), with higher mean values of about 100 Bq/m^3 (2.7 pCi/L) in Finland, Norway, and Sweden. Converting radon concentrations into dose to the bronchial epithelium involves many uncertainties, because such conversion depends on the model used and the assumptions made. One widely used conversion factor equates an air concentration of 20 Bq/m^3 (0.5 pCi/L) with an effective dose to the bronchial epithelium of 1 mSv/y (100 mrem/y).

The EPA has set the "action level" at about 148 Bq/m^3 (4 pCi/L), suggesting that remedial action should be taken to reduce radon levels if they are higher than this. The action level is about four times the average radon concentration in homes, but it is estimated that about 1 in 12 homes in the United States—about 6 million in all—have radon concentrations above this action level. In the past, other countries, including Germany, Great Britain, and Canada, had much higher action levels, but these are all now under review.

The BEIR VI Committee of the National Academy of Sciences published a report on the health effects of radon in 1999. The committee's preferred central estimates, depending on which of two models is used, are that about 1 in 10 or 1 in

7 of all lung cancer deaths—amounting to 15,400 or 21,800 per year in the United States—can be attributed to radon. There are considerable uncertainties involved, and the number could be as low as 3,000 or as high as 32,000 each year. Most of the radon-related lung cancers occur among smokers because of the synergism between smoking and radon. Among those who have never smoked, the committee's best estimate is that of the 11,000 lung cancer deaths each year, 1,200 or 2,900, depending on the model used, are radon related. Of the deaths that can be attributed to radon, perhaps one third could be avoided by reducing radon in homes in which it is above the "action level" of 148 Bq/m^3 (4 pCi/L) recommended by the EPA.

DE MINIMIS DOSE AND NEGLIGIBLE INDIVIDUAL DOSE

Collective dose to a population has little meaning without the concept of ***de minimis* dose**. The idea is to define some very low threshold below which it would make no sense to make any additional effort to reduce exposure levels further. For example, suppose there is a release of radioactivity from a reactor that dissipates into the atmosphere, blows around the world, and eventually exposes many hundreds of millions of people to very low doses. The doses may be so low that the biologic effects are negligible, but because the number of persons involved is so large, the product of the dose and the number of persons would dominate the collective dose. The term *de minimis* comes from the legal saying *De minimis non curat lex*, which roughly translates to "The law does not concern itself with trifles."

Dr. Merril Eisenbud in an NCRP publication quotes this limerick of dubious origin:

There was a young lawyer named Rex
Who was very deficient in sex
When charged with exposure
He said with composure
De minimis non curat lex

The concept of *de minimis* dose has been espoused by the NCRP in the form of **negligible individual dose**, defined here to be the dose below which further efforts to reduce radiation exposure to the person are unwarranted. The NCRP considers an annual effective dose of 0.01 mSv (1 mrem) to be a negligible individual dose. This dose is associated with a risk of death between 10^{-6} and 10^{-7}, which is considered trivial compared with the risk of fatality associated with ordinary and normal societal activities and therefore can be dismissed from consideration of additional radioprotective measures.

RISKS ASSOCIATED WITH CURRENT RECOMMENDED LIMITS

Risk estimates for radiation-induced cancer and hereditary effects are discussed in Chapters 10 and 11. They are summarized in Table 15.7. The possible deleterious effects of long-term occupational exposure to radiation include the reduction of life expectancy (a combination of the probability of developing a fatal cancer and the number of years lost if it occurs), as well as the morbidity, that is, decreased quality of life, associated with nonfatal cancers and hereditary effects. The ICRP has coined the term *detriment* to cover all of these effects. The best estimate for the risk of fatal cancer in a working population exposed to a uniform total-body equivalent dose of 1 Sv (100 rem) at low dose rate is 4×10^{-2}. The contributions from nonfatal cancers and hereditary effects are more difficult to assess. The total detriment (life lost and quality of life impaired) for adult radiation workers amounts to about 4.7×10^{-2} per sievert. (See Table 15.7)

TABLE 15.7

Detriment Due to Cancer and Hereditary Effects

	Detriment 10^{-2} Sv^{-1}		
	Fatal and Non-Fatal Cancers	Hereditary Effects	Total
Adult radiation workers	4.6	0.1	4.7
Whole population	5.9	0.2	6.1

Data from International Commission on Radiation Protection: Relative biological effectiveness (RBE), quality factor (Q), and radiation weighting factor (W_R). ICRP Publication 92, Oxford, UK, Elsevier Science Ltd, 2004.

TABLE 15.8

Trends in Fatal Accident Rates (1976, 1989) for Workers in the United States

	Mean Rate 1976 $10^{-6}y^{-1}$	Mean Rate 1989 $10^{-6}y^{-1}$
All groups	142	90
Trade	64	40
Manufacture	89	60
Service	86	40
Government	111	90
Transport/public utilities	313	240
Construction	568	320
Mines and quarries	625	430
Agriculture (1973–1980)	541	400

Based on National Safety Council: Accident Facts 1976, Chicago, National Safety Council, 1977; and National Safety Council: Accident Facts 1989, Chicago, National Safety Council, 1990.

Recent surveys indicate that the average annual equivalent dose to monitored radiation workers with measurable exposures is about 2 mSv (200 mrem), which results in a total detriment per year of less than 2×10^{-4}. This is comparable to the average death rate from fatal accidents in what are considered "safe" industries, such as trade and government service (Table 15.8). For those few persons who might receive doses close to the limit over an entire working life, the total detriment is comparable to less safe industries, such as construction or working in mines or quarries.

NCRP AND ICRP COMPARED

At the present time, there is a difference in the recommendations of the national and international bodies regarding the maximum permissible effective dose for occupational exposure (stochastic effects). The differences are highlighted in Table 15.6.

Both bodies recommend a maximum of 50 mSv (5 rem) in any 1 year, but the NCRP adds a lifetime cumulative limit of the person's age × 10 mSv (1 rem), and the ICRP adds a limit of 20 mSv (2 rem) per year averaged over defined periods of 5 years.

The practical consequence of this difference is that a radiation worker starting at, for example, age 18 years can accumulate a larger dose under the NCRP recommendations in the early years up to an age in the mid 30s, but later in life could accumulate a larger dose under the ICRP recommendations. Under NCRP recommendations, a new radiation worker could receive 50 mSv (5 rem) in each of several consecutive years until the limit of age × 10 mSv (1 rem) kicks in. Under ICRP rules, the average cannot exceed 20 mSv (2 rem) per year over a 5-year period, so one or two 50-mSv (5-rem) years would have to be followed by several years at very low exposure levels. If individuals were exposed throughout their working lives to the maximum permissible dose, the excess risk of stochastic effects (cancer and hereditary effects) would be about the same under NCRP or ICRP recommendations. Under the NCRP, a person occupationally exposed from 18 to 65 years of age could receive a total dose of 650 mSv (65 rem). Under the ICRP, the same person could receive 940 mSv (94 rem), but less would be received in the early years and more at later ages.

The NCRP scheme is less restrictive for a few workers in the nuclear-power industry who tend to receive large effective doses in their early years working on nuclear reactors. Later in life, these individuals tend to occupy supervisory or administrative positions and receive little if any dose. To cope with those who do not, the NCRP has added the extra recommendation that this limit, age × 10 mSv (1 rem), can be relaxed *in individual cases after counseling* if implementation of the recommendation would mean loss of a job.

It should be emphasized that few persons exposed occupationally in a medical setting receive doses anywhere near the recommended limits. Some interventional radiologists may well receive more than 50 mSv (5 rem) per year to a monitor worn outside the lead-rubber apron or to a monitor worn at neck level or on the forearm. But the recommended maximum permissible levels refer to *effective dose*, which takes into account the parts of the body exposed.

DOSE RANGES

Doses to which individuals are exposed vary enormously by several orders of magnitude. Figure 15.2 attempts to put this into perspective by comparing the ranges of doses used in medicine with doses received occupationally and from natural sources.

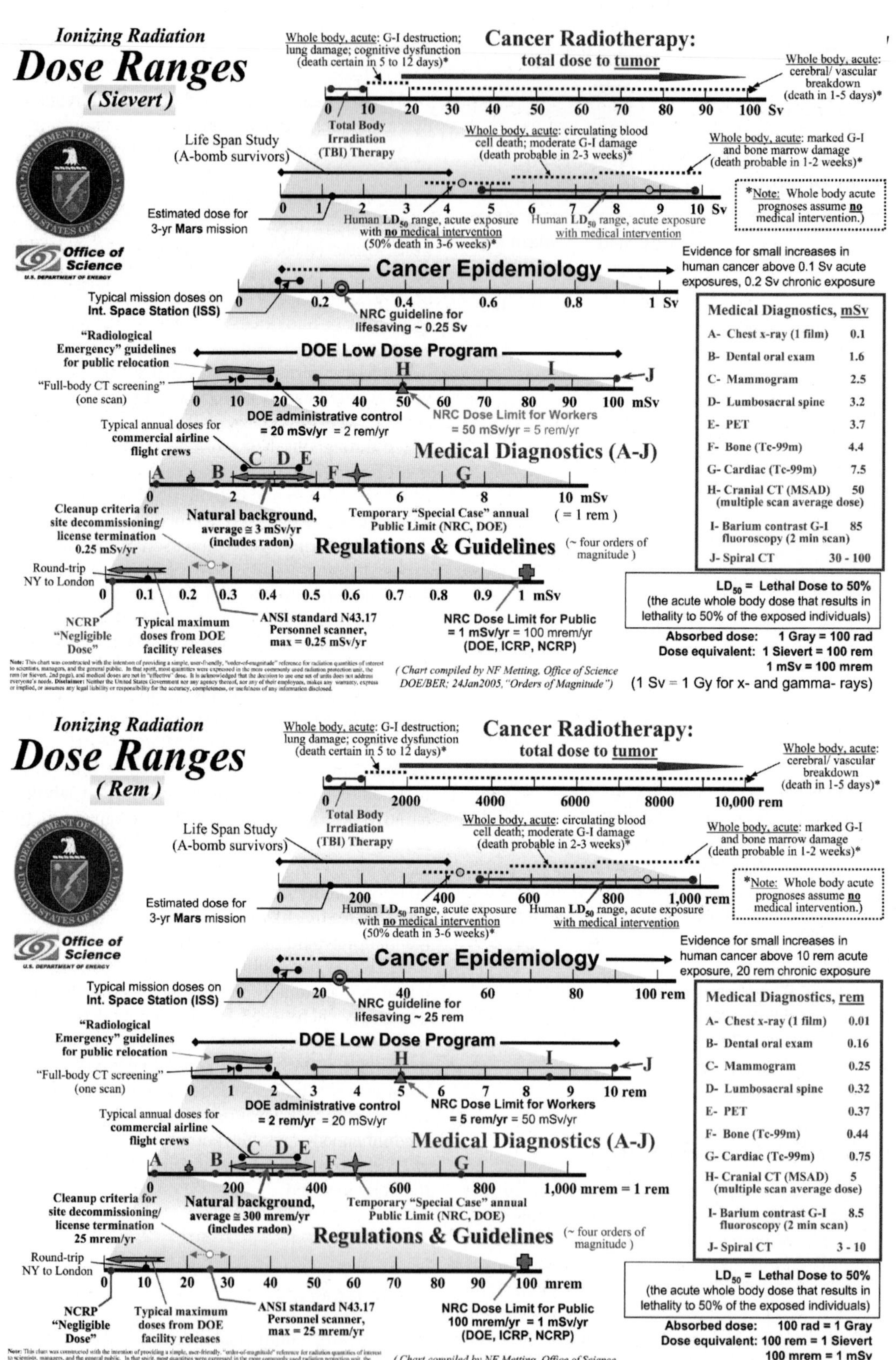

FIGURE 15.2 ● These charts, compiled by Dr. Noelle Metting, Office of Science of the U.S. Department of Energy, put into perspective the different dose ranges relevant to radiation therapy, diagnostic radiology, and background radiation. One chart uses the new SI units of gray and sievert (**top**), and the other uses the older units based on the rad and the rem (**bottom**).

Summary of Pertinent Conclusions

- The objectives of radiation protection are to prevent clinically significant deterministic effects by keeping doses below the practical threshold and to limit the risk of stochastic effects (cancer and hereditary effects) to a reasonable level in relation to societal needs, values, and benefits gained.
- Justification is one of the basic principles of radiation protection; a practice involving exposure to radiation should produce sufficient benefit to the exposed individual or to society to offset the radiation detriment it causes.
- Radiation weighting factors (W_R) are approximate values of the relative biologic effectiveness, applicable to low doses and relevant to carcinogenesis and hereditary effects. Radiation weighting factors are chosen by the ICRP based on experimental relative biologic effectiveness values with a large judgmental factor.
- Equivalent dose is the product of absorbed dose and radiation weighting factor. The units are sievert or rem for an absorbed dose in gray or rad. ICRP has recommended a new name for this quantity—radiation weighted dose—and is considering a new name for the unit.
- Tissue weighting factors (W_T) reflect the susceptibility of different organs or tissues to carcinogenesis or hereditary effects.
- Effective dose is the sum of the weighted equivalent doses for all irradiated tissues and organs multiplied by the appropriate tissue weighting factors.
- Committed equivalent dose is the integral over 50 years of the equivalent dose after the intake of a radionuclide.
- Committed effective dose is the integral over 50 years of the effective dose in the case of an incorporated radionuclide.
- Collective effective dose is a quantity for a population and is the sum of effective doses to all members of that population. The unit is person-sievert (man-rem).
- Collective committed effective dose is also a quantity for a population and is the sum of committed effective doses to all members of the population.
- All radiation exposures are governed by the ALARA (as low as reasonably achievable) principle.
- No occupational exposure should be permitted before 18 years of age.
- The effective dose in any 1 year should not exceed 50 mSv (5 rem) (NCRP).
- The individual worker's lifetime effective dose should not exceed age in years × 10 mSv (1 rem) (NCRP).
- To limit deterministic effects, the dose limit to the lens of the eye is 150 mSv (15 rem) per year, and the dose limit to localized areas of the skin, hands, and feet is 500 mSv (50 rem) per year.
- Once a pregnancy is declared, the NCRP recommends a monthly limit of 0.5 mSv (50 mrem) to the embryo or fetus.
- Specific controls for occupationally exposed women are no longer recommended until a pregnancy is declared.
- Internally deposited radionuclides pose a special problem for protection of the embryo or fetus; particular care should be taken to limit intake.
- Emergency occupational exposures normally justify doses in excess of the recommended limits only if lifesaving actions are involved. Volunteers from among older workers with low lifetime accumulated effective doses should be chosen in emergencies in which the exposure may be up to 0.5 Sv (50 rem). If the exposure may exceed 0.5 Sv (50 rem), the worker should be counseled about the short-term and long-term possible consequences.
- For educational or training purposes, it may sometimes be desirable to accept radiation exposures of persons younger than 18 years of age, in which case the annual effective dose limit of 1 mSv (100 rem) should be maintained.
- The annual effective dose limit for members of the public is 1 mSv (100 mrem), except for infrequent exposures, in which the limit may be 5 mSv (500 mrem). Medical x-rays are excluded from these limitations because they are assumed to confer personal benefit.
- For deterministic effects, the dose limits for members of the general public are 50 mSv (5 rem) to the hands and feet, to localized areas of the skin, or to the lens of the eye.
- Indoor radon is perceived to be the most important problem involving radiation exposure of the general public. Remedial action in homes is recommended by the EPA if the radon concentration exceeds 148 Bq/m^3 (4 pCi/L).

(continued)

Summary of Pertinent Conclusions (Continued)

- Negligible individual dose is the dose below which further expenditure to improve radiation protection is unwarranted. The negligible individual dose is an annual effective dose of 0.01 mSv (1 mrem), which carries a risk of between 10^{-6} and 10^{-7} of carcinogenesis or hereditary effects.
- A uniform whole-body equivalent dose of 1 Sv (100 rem) to an adult radiation worker is assumed to result in a total detriment of about 4.7×10^{-2} per sievert. This is made up of a risk of fatal and nonfatal cancer together with a risk of severe hereditary effects.
- The average annual equivalent dose to monitored radiation workers is about 2 mSv (200 mrem). This involves a total detriment of about 2×10^{-4}, which is comparable to the annual risk of a fatal accident in a "safe" industry, such as trade or government service.
- The NCRP and ICRP differ in two important recommendations:
  1. The effective dose limit for occupational exposure (stochastic effects): The NCRP recommends a lifetime cumulative limit of age × 10 mSv (1 rem), with a limit in any year of 50 mSv (5 rem). The ICRP recommends a limit of 20 mSv (2 rem) per year averaged over defined periods of 5 years, with a limit in any year of 50 mSv (5 rem).
  2. The dose limit to the developing embryo or fetus once a pregnancy is declared: The NCRP recommends a monthly limit of 0.5 mSv (50 mrem) to the embryo or fetus. The ICRP recommends a limit of 2 mSv (200 mrem) to the surface of the woman's abdomen for the remainder of pregnancy.

GLOSSARY OF TERMS

absorbed dose The energy imparted to matter by ionizing radiation per unit mass of irradiated material at the place of interest. The unit is the gray (Gy), defined as an energy absorption of 1 J/kg. The old unit was the rad, defined as an energy absorption of 100 erg/g.

ALARA As low as reasonably achievable, economic and social factors being taken into account. This is identical to the principle of optimization of protection used by the ICRP.

annual limit on intake The activity of a radionuclide taken into the body during a year that would provide a committed equivalent dose to a person, represented by a reference "man," equal to the occupational dose limit set by recommending and regulating bodies. The annual limit normally is expressed in becquerel (Bq).

becquerel (Bq) The special name for the unit of activity. 3.7×10^{10} Bq = 1 Ci.

collective committed effective dose Applies to a population ingesting or inhaling radionuclides that deposit their dose over a prolonged period of time and is the integral of the effective dose over the entire population out to a period of 50 years.

collective effective dose Applies to a group of persons and is the sum of the products of the effective dose and the number of persons receiving that effective dose.

collective equivalent dose Applies to a group of persons and is the sum of the products of the equivalent dose and the number of persons receiving that equivalent dose.

committed effective dose The sum of the committed organ or tissue equivalent doses resulting from an intake multiplied by the appropriate tissue weighting factors.

committed equivalent dose The equivalent dose averaged throughout a specified tissue in the 50 years after intake of a radionuclide into the body.

deterministic effects Effects for which the severity of the effect in affected persons varies with the dose and for which a threshold usually exists. These were formerly known as *nonstochastic effects*. An example is a cataract.

effective dose The sum over specified tissues of the products of the equivalent dose in a tissue and the appropriate tissue weighting factor for that tissue.

equivalent dose A quantity used for radiation protection purposes that takes into account the different probability of effects that occur with the same absorbed dose delivered by radiations of different quality. It is defined as the product of the averaged absorbed dose in a specified organ or tissue and the radiation weighting factor. The unit of equivalent dose is the sievert (Sv). The ICRP is now recommending that this be called the radiation weighted dose.

genetically significant dose (GSD) The dose to the gonads weighted for the age and sex distribution in those members of the population expected to have offspring. The genetically significant dose is measured in sievert (rem).

gray (Gy) The special name for the SI unit of absorbed dose, kerma, and specific energy imparted. 1 Gy = 1 J/kg. Also, 1 Gy = 100 rad.

negligible individual dose A level of effective dose that can be dismissed as insignificant and below which further efforts to improve radiation protection are not justified. The recommended negligible individual dose is 0.01 mSv/y (1 mrem/y).

nonstochastic effects Previous term for deterministic effects.

organ or tissue weighting factor (W_T) *See* tissue weighting factor.

rad The old unit for absorbed dose, kerma, and specific energy imparted. One rad is 0.01 J absorbed per kilogram of any material (also defined as 100 erg/g). The term is being replaced by the gray: 1 rad = 0.01 Gy.

radiation weighted dose New name recommended by ICRP for equivalent dose.

radiation weighting factor (W_R) A factor used for radiation protection purposes that accounts for differences in biologic effectiveness between different radiations. The radiation weighting factor is independent of the tissue weighting factor.

relative biologic effectiveness (RBE) A ratio of the absorbed dose of a reference radiation to the absorbed dose of a test radiation to produce the same level of biologic effect, other conditions being equal. It is the quantity that is measured experimentally.

rem The old unit of equivalent dose or effective dose. It is the product of the absorbed dose in rad and modifying factors and is being replaced by the sievert.

sievert (Sv) The unit of equivalent dose or effective dose in the SI system. It is the product of absorbed dose in gray and modifying factors. 1 Sv = 100 rem.

stochastic effects Effects for which the probability of their occurring, rather than their severity, is a function of radiation dose without threshold. More generally, stochastic means random in nature.

tissue weighting factor (W_T) A factor that indicates the ratio of the risk of stochastic effects attributable to irradiation of a given organ or tissue to the total risk if the whole body is uniformly irradiated. Organs that have a large tissue weighting factor are those that are susceptible to radiation-induced carcinogenesis (such as the breast or thyroid) or to hereditary effects (the gonads).

working level The amount of potential α-particle energy in a cubic meter of air that results in the emission of 2.08×10^{-5} J of energy.

working level month A cumulative exposure, equivalent to exposure to one working level for a working month (170 hours), that is, $2 \times 10^{-5}\ \text{J}\cdot\text{m}^{-3} \times 170 = 3.5 \times 10^{-3}\ \text{J}\cdot\text{h}\cdot\text{m}^{-3}$.

BIBLIOGRAPHY

Burkhart RL, Gross RE, Jans RG, McCrohen JL Jr, Rosenstein M, Reuter FA (eds): *Recommendations for Evaluation of Radiation Exposure from Diagnostic Radiology Examinations.* Health and Human Services publication No. 85-8247. Springfield, VA, Food and Drug Administration, National Technical Information Service, 1985

Committee on the Biological Effects of Ionizing Radiations: *The Effects on Populations of Exposure to Low Levels of Ionizing Radiation.* Washington, DC, National Academy Press, 1980

Committee on the Biological Effects of Ionizing Radiations: *Health Effects of Exposure to Low Levels of Ionizing Radiation.* Washington, DC, National Academy Press, 1990

International Commission on Radiation Units and Measurements: *Determination of Dose Equivalent Resulting from External Radiation Sources.* Report 39. Bethesda, MD, ICRU, 1985

International Commission on Radiation Units and Measurements: *The Quality Factor of Radiation Protection: Report of a Joint Task Group of the ICRP and ICRU to the ICRP and ICRU.* Report 40. Bethesda, MD, ICRU, 1986

International Commission on Radiological Protection: Biological Effects after Prenatal Irradiation (Embryo and Fetus). ICRP Publication 90. Oxford UK, Elsevier Science Ltd, 2004

International Commission on Radiological Protection: *Quantitative Bases for Developing a Unified Index of Harm.* ICRP Publication 45. New York, Pergamon Press, 1985

International Commission on Radiological Protection: *Recommendations of the ICRP.* ICRP Publication 26. New York, Pergamon Press, 1977

International Commission on Radiological Protection: *Recommendations of the ICRP.* ICRP Publication 60. New York, Pergamon Press, 1991

International Commission on Radiological Protection: Relative biological effectiveness (RBE), quality factor (Q), and radiation weighting factor (W_R). ICRP Publication 92. Oxford, UK, Elsevier Science Ltd, 2004

Kato H, Schull WJ: Studies of the mortality of A-bomb survivors: 7. Mortality, 1950–1978. I. Cancer mortality. *Radiat Res* 90:395–432, 1982

National Council on Radiation Protection and Measurements: *Basic Radiation Protection Criteria.* Report 39. Bethesda, MD, NCRP, 1971

National Council on Radiation Protection and Measurements: *Comparative Carcinogenicity of Ionizing Radiation and Chemicals.* Report 96. Bethesda, MD, NCRP, 1989

National Council on Radiation Protection and Measurements: *Evaluation of Occupational and Environmental Exposure to Radon and Radon Daughters in the United States.* Report 78. Bethesda, MD, NCRP, 1984

National Council on Radiation Protection and Measurements: *Implementation of the Principle of As Low As Reasonably Achievable (ALARA) for Medical and Dental Personnel.* Report 107. Bethesda, MD, NCRP, 1990

National Council on Radiation Protection and Measurements: *Radiation Protection in Educational Institutions.* Report 32. Bethesda, MD, NCRP, 1966

National Council on Radiation Protection and Measurements: *Recommendations on Limits for Exposure to Ionizing Radiation.* Report 91. Bethesda, MD, NCRP, 1987

National Council on Radiation Protection and Measurements: *Recommendations on Limits for Exposure to Ionizing Radiation.* Report 116. Bethesda, MD, NCRP, 1993

National Council on Radiation Protection and Measurements: *Review of NCRP Radiation Dose Limit for Embryo and Fetus in Occupationally-Exposed Women.* Report 53, Bethesda, MD, NCRP, 1977

National Safety Council: *Accident Facts 1976.* Chicago, National Safety Council, 1977

National Safety Council: *Accident Facts 1989.* Chicago, National Safety Council, 1990

United Nations Scientific Committee on the Effects of Atomic Radiation: *Biological Effects of Pre-Natal Irradiation.* Presented before the 35th Session of UNSCEAR. New York, UNSCEAR, 1986

United Nations Scientific Committee on the Effects of Atomic Radiation: *Ionizing Radiation: Sources and Biological Effects.* Report to the General Assembly, with Annexes, publication No. E.82.IX8. New York, UNSCEAR, 1982

United Nations Scientific Committee on the Effects of Atomic Radiation: *Sources and Effects of Ionizing Radiation.* Report to the General Assembly, with Annexes, publication No. E.77.IXI. New York, UNSCEAR, 1977

CHAPTER 16

Molecular Techniques in Radiobiology

HISTORICAL PERSPECTIVES

Recombinant DNA technology has revolutionized research in biology. It allows questions to be asked that were unthinkable just a few years ago. It is also a technology that is moving so fast that anything written in a book is likely to be out of date before it appears in print. This technology is invading every field of biologic research, and radiobiology is no exception. To keep abreast of developments in the field, it is essential to know what recombinant DNA technology is and how it works. A detailed description is beyond the scope of this book; for a more extensive account, the interested reader is referred to several excellent volumes that have appeared in recent years and are listed in the bibliography. The goal here is to provide an overview and to illustrate how recombinant techniques have been used to solve specific problems in radiobiologic research.

The birth of molecular biology could be ascribed to the one-page publication in *Nature* in 1953 by James Watson and Francis Crick describing the structure of DNA. In short order, this work led the way to breaking the genetic code and understanding the process of transcription of DNA to messenger RNA (mRNA) and the translation of mRNA into proteins. At about the same time, in the late 1940s and early 1950s, Linus Pauling realized that three-dimensional structures were formed as amino acids were folded into proteins and that function was related to structure. The whole concept emerged that the sequence of bases, which coded for a protein, ultimately determined function.

These remarkable discoveries were followed by a period of limited progress focusing mainly on simple systems such as viruses, bacteriophages, and bacteria, until new tools and techniques to work with DNA were perfected.

Recombinant DNA technology got its start with the first successful cloning experiment of Stanley Cohen, in which he joined two DNA fragments together (a plasmid containing a tetracycline resistance gene with a kanamycin resistance gene), introduced this recombinant molecule into *Escherichia coli*, and demonstrated that the bacteria now had dual antibiotic resistance.

This simple experiment was only possible because of the simultaneous development of several techniques for cutting DNA with restriction enzymes and joining the fragments with ligases and using *E. coli* as a host with the ability to take up foreign DNA through the use of plasmid vectors. This was followed quickly by the development of methods to sort pieces of DNA and RNA by size, using gel electrophoresis and blotting. The stage was set for an explosion of knowledge.

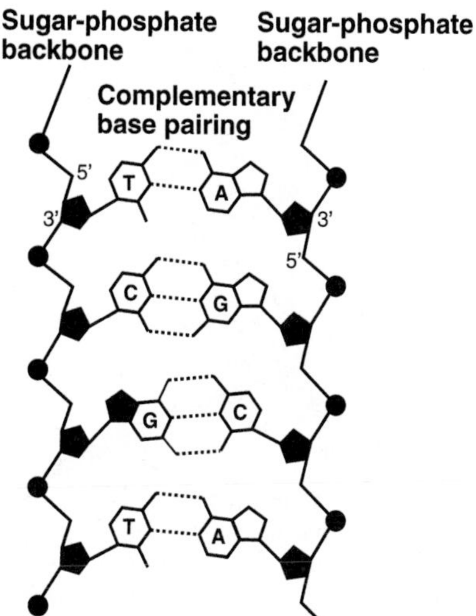

FIGURE 16.1 • The DNA double helix is held together by hydrogen bonds between base pairs. These are shown as dotted lines in the figure.

What follows is a brief and simplified description of these techniques and those that followed, together with some examples of their application to problems in radiobiology.

THE STRUCTURE OF DNA

The structure of DNA arrived at by Crick and Watson is elegant in its simplicity. The molecule is composed of two antiparallel helices, looking rather like a gently twisted ladder. The rails of the ladder, which run in opposite directions, contain units of deoxyribose sugar alternating with a phosphate. Each rung is composed of a pair of nucleotides, a base pair held together by hydrogen bonds (Fig. 16.1). There is a complementary relationship between the bases: adenine always pairs with thymine, and cytosine always pairs with guanine. Thus, the nucleotide sequence of one strand of the DNA helix determines the sequence of the other.

This structure explains how a DNA molecule replicates during cell division so that each progeny cell receives an identical set of instructions. The hydrogen bonds between the base pairs break, allowing the DNA ladder to unzip (Fig. 16.2). Each half then constitutes a template for the reconstruction of the other half. Two identical DNA molecules result, one for each progeny cell.

RNA AND DNA

Unlike DNA, which is located primarily in the nucleus, RNA is found throughout the cell. Within the nucleus, RNA is concentrated in the *nucleoli*,

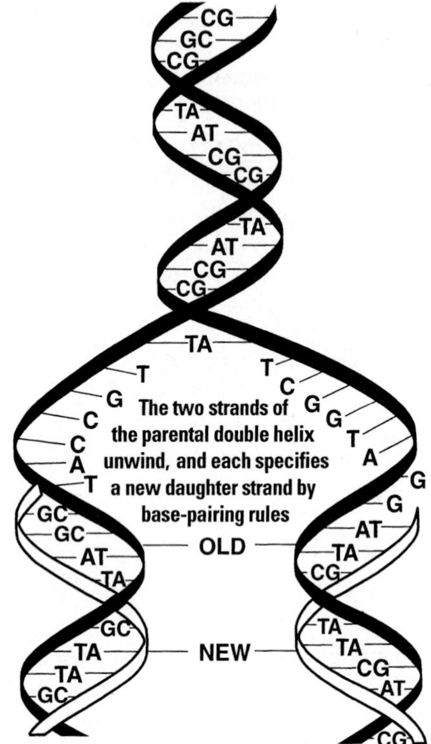

FIGURE 16.2 • The complementary nature of DNA is at the heart of its capacity for self-replication. The two strands of the parental DNA unwind and the hydrogen bonds break. Each strand then becomes a template to specify a new progeny strand obeying the base-pairing rules.

dense granules attached to chromosomes. The sugar molecule in RNA is a *ribose* (hence its name, *ribonucleic acid*), whereas in DNA the sugar molecule is a *deoxyribose* (hence *its* name, *deoxyribonucleic acid*). In both DNA and RNA, the bases are made up of two *purines* and two *pyrimidines*. The two purines, *adenine* and *guanine*, as well as the pyrimidine *cytosine,* are common to both DNA and RNA. However, although *thymine* is found only in DNA, the structurally similar pyrimidine *uracil* appears in RNA (Fig. 16.3).

TRANSCRIPTION AND TRANSLATION

The flow of genetic information from DNA to protein requires a series of steps. In the first step, the DNA code is *transcribed* in the nucleus into mRNA (Fig. 16.4). It is at once obvious from a comparison of a mature cytoplasmic mRNA transcript with its parental DNA that the mRNA sequence is not contiguous with the DNA sequence. Some blocks of DNA sequence are represented in the mRNA, others are not. DNA is transcribed into pre-mRNA. During the process of splicing, large regions called *introns* are removed and the remaining *exons* are joined together. Only the exons of the DNA are translated. Almost all genes from higher eukaryotes contain introns; genes may have only a few or as many as 100 introns. Typically, introns make up the bulk of the gene. For example, in the gene involved with muscular dystrophy, the mRNA consists of 14,000 bases, whereas the gene spans more than 2 million base pairs. The mRNA transcript associates with a ribosome, at which, with the help of ribosomal RNA and transfer RNA (tRNA), the mRNA message is translated into a protein.

THE GENETIC CODE

The genetic code was cracked by 1966. Triplet mRNA sequences specify each of the amino acids. Because there are four bases, the number of possibilities for a three-letter code is 4 × 4 × 4, or 64. There are only 20 amino acids, however; consequently, more than one triplet can code for the same amino acid—that is, there is redundancy in the code. Because nearly all proteins begin with the amino acid methionine, its codon (AUG) represents the "start" signal for protein synthesis. Three codons for which there are no naturally occurring tRNAs—UAA, UAG, and UGA—are "stop" signals that terminate translation. Only methionine and tryptophan are specified by a unique codon; all other amino acids are specified by two or more different codons. As a consequence of this redundancy, a single-base change in RNA does not necessarily change the amino acid coded for.

Given the position of the bases in a codon, it is possible from Table 16.1 to find the corresponding amino acid. For example, 5′ CAU 3′ specifies histidine, whereas AUG specifies methionine. Glycine is specified by any of four codons: GGU, GGC, GGA, or GGG.

AMINO ACIDS AND PROTEINS

The vast majority of proteins are composed of a mixture of the same 20 amino acids. Each polypeptide chain is characterized by a unique sequence of its amino acids. Chain lengths vary from 5 to more than 4,000 amino acids. Most proteins contain only one polypeptide chain, but others are formed through the aggregation of separately synthesized chains that have different sequences. Though the vast majority of proteins are enzymes (i.e., they act as catalysts, inducing chemical changes in other

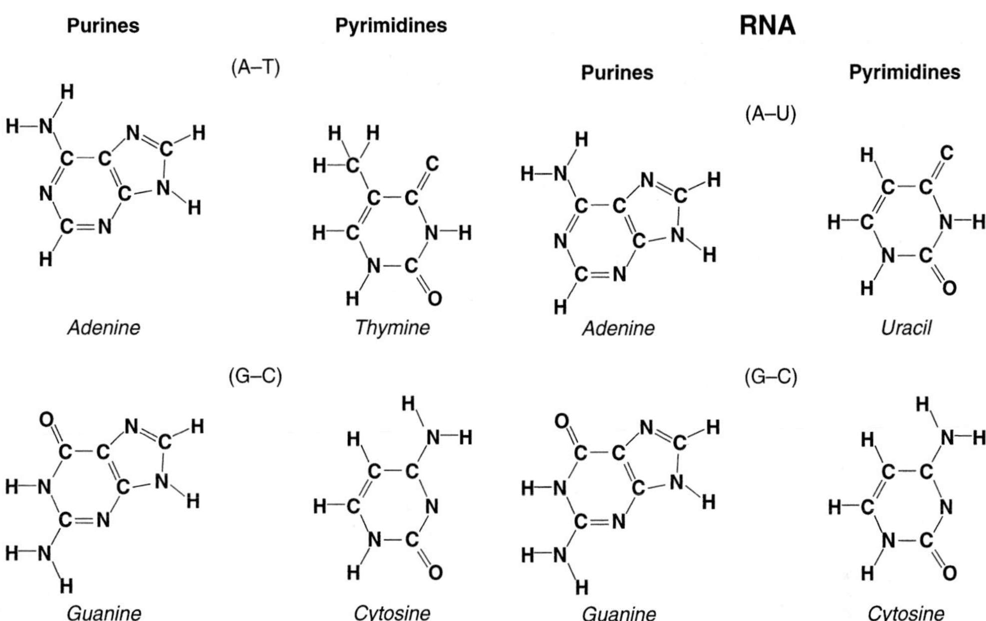

FIGURE 16.3 ● Illustrating the pairing of complementary bases in DNA and RNA. **Left:** DNA contains the purines adenine (A) and guanine (G), as well as the pyrimidines thymine (T) and cytosine (C). A purine always pairs with a pyrimidine; specifically, A pairs with T, and G pairs with C. **Right:** RNA contains uracil (U) instead of thymine. In this case, A pairs with U, and G pairs with C.

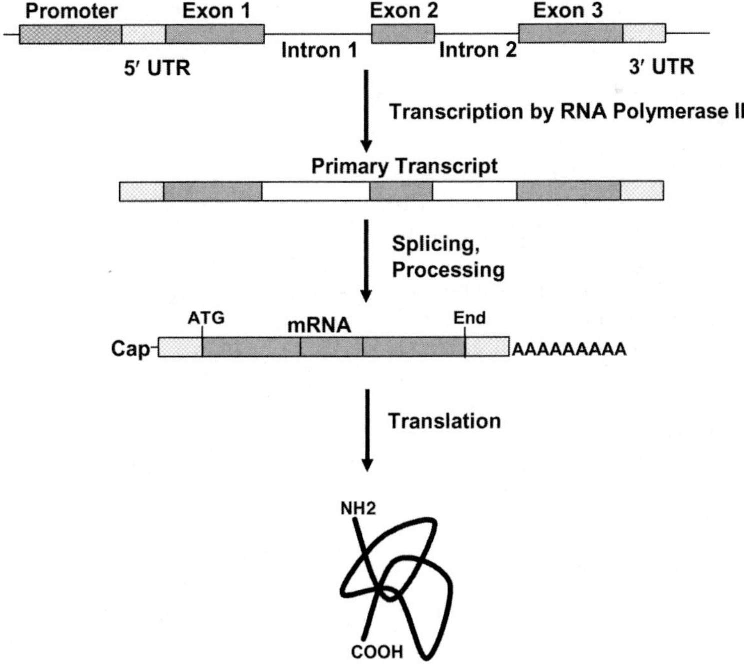

FIGURE 16.4 ● Transcription and translation. The "information" in DNA is linear, consisting of combinations of the four nucleotides, adenine, guanine, cytosine, and thymine. The information is transcribed into mRNA (messenger RNA), which in turn is a complementary version of the DNA code. The mRNA message is spliced in the nucleus to remove introns and is then transported to the cytoplasm for translation into protein. Triplet RNA codons specify each of the 20 amino acids. The sequence of amino acids determines the protein, which ultimately has three-dimensional form.

TABLE 16.1

Codes for the Amino Acids

First Position (5′ End)	Second Position U	C	A	G	Third Position (3′ End)
U	Phe	Ser	Tyr	Cys	U
	Phe	Ser	Tyr	Cys	C
	Leu	Ser	Stop	Stop	A
	Leu	Ser	Stop	Trp	G
A	Ile	Thr	Asn	Ser	U
	Ile	Thr	Asn	Ser	C
	Ile	Thr	Lys	Arg	A
	Met	Thr	Lys	Arg	G
G	Val	Ala	Asp	Gly	U
	Val	Ala	Asp	Gly	C
	Val	Ala	Glu	Gly	A
	Val	Ala	Glu	Gly	G
C	Leu	Pro	His	Arg	U
	Leu	Pro	His	Arg	C
	Leu	Pro	Gln	Arg	A
	Leu	Pro	Gln	Arg	G

substances but themselves remaining apparently unchanged), many have structural roles as well. The essential fabric of both nuclear and plasma membranes is formed of proteins.

Once a polypeptide chain is synthesized from a string of amino acids, it tends to fold up into a three-dimensional form, the shape of which is governed by the weak chemical interactions between the side groups of the amino acids. Each three-dimensional shape is unique to the amino acid sequence. The shape of a protein is the key to its function.

RESTRICTION ENDONUCLEASES

Restriction enzymes are endonucleases found in bacteria that have the property of recognizing a specific DNA sequence and cleaving at or near that site. These enzymes can be grouped into three categories, types I, II, and III. The restriction enzymes commonly used are of type II, meaning that they have endonuclease activity only (i.e., they cut the DNA without modification) at a predictable site within or adjacent to the recognition sequence. Types I and III have properties that make them impractical for use in molecular biology.

More than a thousand type II enzymes have been isolated, and more than 70 are commercially available. A few examples are shown in Table 16.2. They are named according to the following system:

1. The first letter comes from the genus of the organism from which the enzyme was isolated.
2. The second and third letters follow the organism's species name.
3. If there is a fourth letter, it refers to a particular strain of the organism.
4. The roman numerals, as often as not, refer to the order in which enzymes were discovered, although the original intent was that it would indicate the order in which enzymes of the same organism and strain are eluted from a chromatography column.

Restriction endonucleases scan the DNA molecule, stopping if they recognize a particular nucleotide sequence. The recognition sites are short, four to eight nucleotides, and usually read the same

TABLE 16.2

Examples of Type II Restriction Enzymes

Enzyme	Element of Terminology	Meaning
*Hind*III	*H*	Genus *Haemophilus*
	in	Species *influenzae*
	d	Strain Rd
	III	Third endonuclease isolated
*Eco*RI	*E*	Genus *Escherichia*
	co	Species *coli*
	R	Strain RY13
	I	First endonuclease isolated
Bam HI	*B*	Genus *Bacillus*
	am	Species *amyloliquefaciens*
	H	Strain H
	I	First endonuclease isolated

in both directions, forward and backward, which is termed a *palindromic sequence*. Some endonucleases, such as *Hind*II, for example, produce blunt-ended fragments because they cut cleanly through the DNA, cleaving both complementary strands at the same nucleotide position, most often near the middle of the recognition sequence. Other endonucleases cleave the two strands of DNA at positions two to four nucleotides apart, creating exposed ends of single-stranded sequences. The commonly used enzymes *Eco*RI, *Bam*HI, and *Hind*III, for example, leave 5′ overhangs of four nucleotides, which represent "sticky" ends, very useful for making recombinant molecules. Table 16.3 shows the recognition sequence and point of cutting of a dozen commonly used restriction enzymes. This specificity is the same, regardless of whether the DNA is from a bacterium, a plant, or a human cell.

Most restriction recognition sites have symmetry in that the sequence on one strand is the same as on the other. For example, *Eco*RI recognizes the sequence 5′ GAATTC 3′; the complementary strand is also 5′ GAATTC 3′. *Eco*RI cuts the DNA between the G and A on each strand, leaving a 5′ single-strand sequence of AATT on each strand. The strands are complementary. Therefore, all DNA fragments generated with *Eco*RI are complementary and can "base-pair" with each other. This is illustrated in Figure 16.5.

VECTORS

A vector is a self-replicating DNA molecule that has the ability to carry another foreign DNA molecule into a host cell. In the context of this chapter, the object of the exercise is usually to insert a fragment of human DNA (perhaps containing a gene of

TABLE 16.3

Specificities of Some Typical Restriction Endonucleases

Enzyme	Organism	Recognition Sequence[a]	Blunt or Sticky End
*Eco*RI	*Escherichia coli*	GAATTC	Sticky
*Bam*HI	*Bacillus amyioliquefaciens*	GGATCC	Sticky
*Bgl*fII	*Bacillus globigii*	AGATCT	Sticky
*Pvu*I	*Proteus vulgaris*	CGATCG	Sticky
*Pvu*II	*Proteus vulgaris*	CAGCTG	Blunt
*Hind*III	*Haemophilus influenzae* R_1	AAGCTT	Sticky
*Hin*tI	*Haemophilus influenzae* R_1	GANTC	Sticky
*Sau*3A	*Staphylococcus aureus*	GATC	Sticky
*Alu*I	*Arthrobacter luteus*	AGCT	Blunt
*Taq*I	*Thermus aquaticus*	TCGA	Sticky
*Hae*III	*Haemophilus aegyptius*	GGCC	Blunt
*Not*I	*Nocardia otitidis-caviarum*	GCGGCCGC	Sticky

[a] The sequence shown is that of one strand given in the 5′ to 3′ direction. Only one strand is represented.

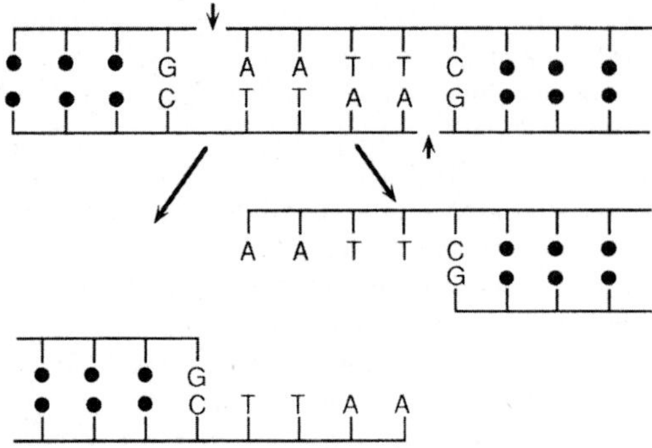

FIGURE 16.5 ● Illustration of how some endonucleases cleave each strand of the DNA off-center in the recognition site, creating fragments with exposed ends of short, single-stranded sequences. These "sticky" ends are extremely useful in making recombinant molecules because they rejoin only with complementary sequences.

interest) into a bacterium so that it can be replicated and grown into quantities suitable for study.

There are many types of vectors, including plasmids, bacteriophages (especially bacteriophage λ), bacterial artificial chromosomes (BACs), and viruses.

Plasmids

The simplest bacterial vectors are **plasmids**, which are circular DNA molecules that can exist and replicate inside a bacterium, independent of the host chromosome. A piece of foreign DNA can be inserted into a plasmid, which in turn is introduced into a bacterium. As the bacterium grows and replicates, so does the foreign DNA. The plasmid also contains a gene for resistance to an antibiotic (e.g., ampicillin), and if the bacteria are subsequently grown in a culture medium containing the antibiotic, only those bacteria that have taken up the plasmid survive and replicate. This is illustrated in Figure 16.6.

It is a relatively simple matter, subsequently, to harvest the recombinant plasmids. There are two limitations to this technique. First, plasmids are useful only for relatively small DNA inserts up to about 10,000 base pairs (bp). Second, the plasmids do not transfect into bacteria with high efficiency.

Bacteriophage λ

Bacteriophages are bacterial viruses. The bacteriophage most commonly used as a cloning vector is **bacteriophage** λ. It has two advantages compared with other vectors. As a bacteriophage particle, bacteriophage λ can infect its host at a much higher efficiency than a plasmid, and it can accommodate a larger range of DNA fragments, from a few to up to 24,000 bp, depending on the specific vector used. Many vectors have been derived from bacteriophage λ. Some have been modified to clone small DNAs, usually cDNAs, and some have been modified to clone large DNA molecules. If bacteriophage λ is used to clone large DNA molecules, the central portion of the bacteriophage DNA is deleted. This is to allow the foreign DNA to be accommodated within the bacteriophage particle, which has an upper limit of 55,000 bp. Once the bacteriophage DNA is ligated with the DNA to be cloned, the total DNA is mixed with extracts containing empty bacteriophage particles. The ligated DNA is taken up into the bacteriophage, which is then used to infect *E. coli*.

To insert itself into the *E. coli* chromosome, the phage DNA circularizes by the base pairing of the complementary single-strand tails that exist at its two ends—the **cos** sites. The resulting circular λ DNA then recombines into the *E. coli* chromosome.

If part of the wild-type DNA of the bacteriophage is removed, room can be made for a piece of human DNA to be inserted, again with a gene that

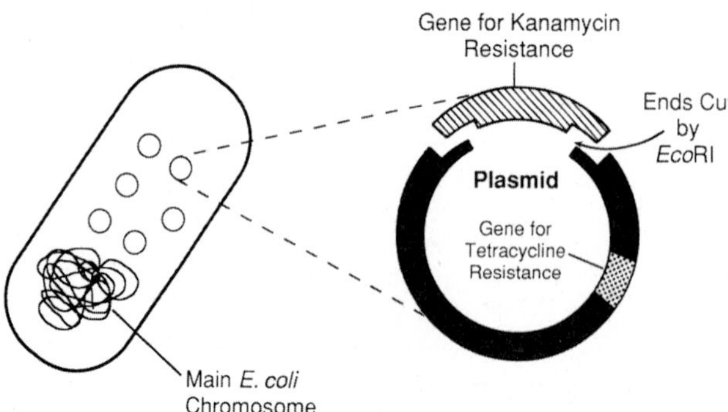

FIGURE 16.6 ● A plasmid is the simplest bacterial vector—a means of carrying foreign DNA sequences into bacteria such as *Escherichia coli*. A plasmid is a circular DNA molecule, capable of autonomous replication, that typically carries one or more genes encoding an antibiotic resistance. Foreign DNA (e.g., from a human cell) also can be incorporated into the plasmid. If inserted into a bacterium, the plasmid replicates along with the main chromosome.

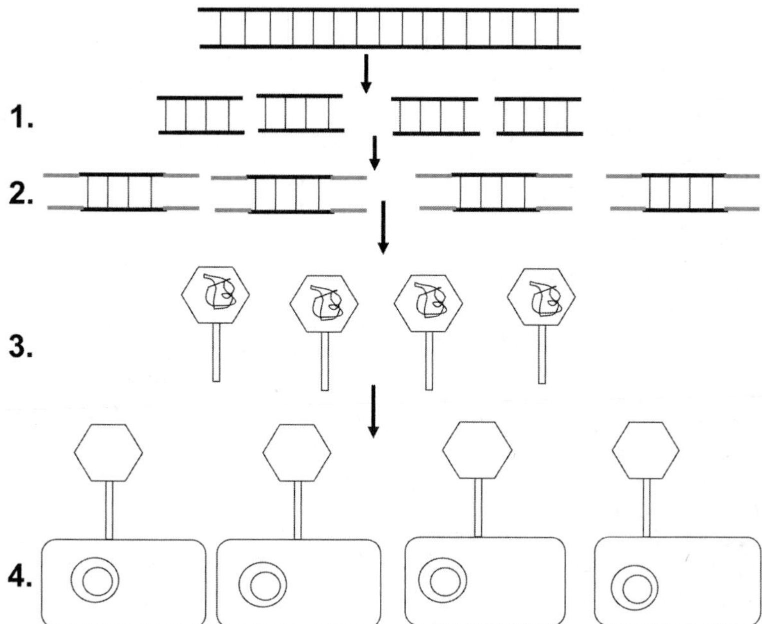

FIGURE 16.7 ● A bacteriophage is a virus that infects bacteria. It represents a much more efficient means of inserting foreign DNA into a bacterium than using a plasmid. If part of the wild-type DNA is removed, room can be made for a piece of "foreign" DNA, for example, from a human cell, as well as a gene that confers resistance to an antibiotic to allow selection. The DNA of the bacteriophage replicates along with that of the bacterium.

confers resistance to an antibiotic to allow selection. The bacteriophage can then be used to infect bacteria that multiply their own DNA as well as the integrated piece of human DNA. Bacteriophage λ accommodates DNA inserts up to about 24,000 bp (Fig. 16.7).

Bacterial Artificial Chromosomes

Sequencing large genomes requires a cloning vector capable of carrying very large fragments of DNA. **BACs (bacterial artificial chromosomes)** are vectors based on a type of plasmid with sequences encoding self-replication while maintaining a low copy number. BACs can accommodate approximately 300 kilobases (kb) of DNA, whereas plasmids are limited to approximately 10-kb insertions. BACs transform *E. coli* via electroporation more efficiently than comparable but larger constructs, compensating for the reduced amount of inserted DNA that can be accommodated. Because of the defined genetic backgrounds of their bacterial hosts, BACs are also less prone to recombination events (a common problem with large DNA vectors). BACs were the primary vector used during the genome-sequencing projects, mainly because a BAC carrying a gene of interest is easily acquired.

Viruses

Viruses are highly efficient vectors for introducing foreign genes into mammalian cells. Viral infection of mammalian cells has proved to be an effective and efficient method for delivering and stably expressing a gene of interest. The two main types of viruses used for gene transfer are retroviruses and adenoviruses. **Retroviruses** are a type of RNA virus. Unlike all other RNA viruses, the RNA genome of retroviruses is transcribed into DNA, which is then stably integrated into the host genome. Retroviruses can infect virtually every type of mammalian cell, making them very versatile. In contrast to retroviruses, **adenoviruses** are a type of DNA virus, and they can infect both proliferative and quiescent cells. Adenovirus gene expression is stable, but the genome remains epichromosomal.

LIBRARIES

Genomic Library

A **genomic library** is a compilation of DNA fragments that make up the entire genome. Making a genomic library is frequently the starting point of a gene isolation experiment. DNA is extracted from a tissue sample or from cultured cells, and a partial digest is made using *Eco*RI, for example. This enzyme has a six-nucleotide recognition sequence, so if the digest is complete, it cuts the DNA into pieces about 4,000 bp long. (The probability of cleaving a six base pair sequence is $(\frac{1}{4})^6$, or once every 4,096 bases.) By reducing the enzyme concentration and incubation time, a partial digest is obtained, so that the *Eco*RI enzyme cuts at only about one in five restriction sites, resulting in fragments of about 40,000 bp.

The genomic DNA fragments are then ligated into a suitable vector and "packaged" inside infective bacteriophage particles. The assembled bacteriophage particles are used to infect *E. coli* cells, which are spread on plates and incubated in growth medium containing the appropriate antibiotic (e.g., ampicillin), so that only bacteria that have taken up the cosmid survive and grow into colonies. Each colony contains millions of copies of a single genomic DNA insert. About 75,000 colonies encompass the entire genome. If the equivalent of several genomes worth of colonies are screened, then one or more should contain the gene of interest. The trick is to identify that particular colony out of hundreds of thousands.

cDNA Library

As an alternative to making a genomic DNA library, it is sometimes more useful to make a cDNA library. **Complementary DNA (cDNA)** is DNA that is complementary to the mRNA and therefore includes only the expressed genes of a particular cell. For eukaryotic cells, the mRNA is usually much shorter than the total size of the gene, because the coding sequences in the genome are split into exons separated by noncoding regions of DNA called introns.

cDNA libraries are made in either plasmids or bacteriophage λ. Often these vectors have been modified such that the cDNA can be transcribed into mRNA and then translated into protein. If this type of vector is used, the library can be screened using an antibody that recognizes the protein of the gene of interest, because the cells are expressing the gene. This type of cDNA library is called an **expression library**.

HOSTS

Recombinant DNA molecules can be constructed and manipulated to some extent in the test tube, but amplification and expression ideally require a host.

Escherichia Coli

E. coli is the most widely used organism in molecular biology because it is relatively simple and well understood. It contains a single chromosome consisting of about 5 million base pairs.

In addition to their main chromosomes, many bacteria, including *E. coli*, possess large numbers of tiny circular DNA molecules that may contain only a few thousand base pairs. They are called *episomes*, a subset of which are known as plasmids. Plasmids are autonomously replicating "minichromosomes." They were first identified as genetic elements separate from the main chromosome and carrying genes that conveyed resistance to antibiotics. Foreign DNA can be introduced readily into *E. coli* in the form of plasmids.

Because the DNA of all organisms is made of identical subunits, *E. coli* accepts foreign DNA from any organism. The DNA of bacteria, *Drosophila,* plants, and humans consists of the same four nucleotides: adenine, cytosine, guanine, and thymine. A foreign gene inside *E. coli* is replicated in essentially the same way as its own DNA.

Yeast

Yeast are simple eukaryotes that have many characteristics in common with mammalian cells but can be grown almost as quickly and inexpensively as bacteria.

The study of yeast has frequently provided insights into similar phenomena and functions in mammalian cells that are much more difficult to address. Yeast have been of particular value in radiobiology, because the availability of a wide array of mutants that are sensitive to ultraviolet or ionizing radiations has made the study of the genes responsible for radiosensitivity and radioresistance much simpler than if studies were conducted only in mammalian cells. Complementation of many yeast mutants with mammalian genes has proved to be a powerful screening method.

Yeast have also proved to be good systems for studying cell-cycle control. Because it appears that the cell-cycle machinery of all eukaryotes is very similar, it makes sense to concentrate on the simplest and most easily manipulated system. The availability of temperature-sensitive yeast mutants is of particular value. The yeast *Saccharomyces cerevisiae* (budding yeast, baker's yeast, or brewer's yeast) and *Schizosaccharomyces pombe* (fission yeast) have been used widely. They grow rapidly and have been well characterized genetically.

A new approach has been developed for analyzing large numbers of uniquely tagged yeast deletion

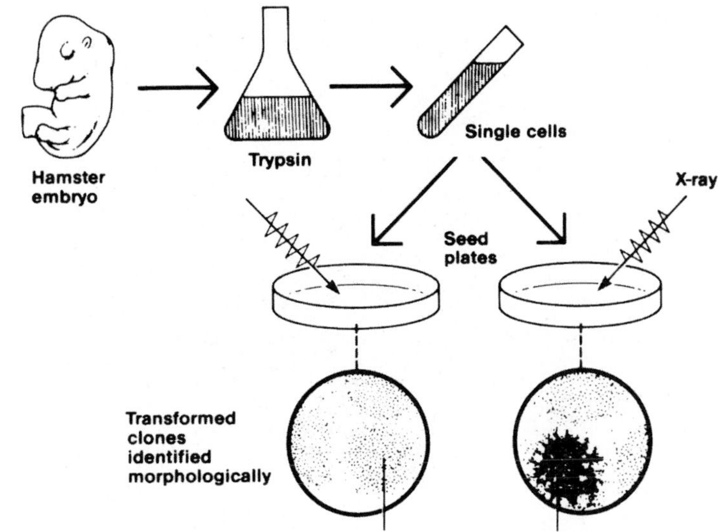

FIGURE 16.8 • Protocol for the assay of oncogenic transformation in hamster embryo cells by radiation. Midterm hamster embryos are removed, minced, enzymatically dissociated, and seeded as single cells on feeder layers. They are then treated with either radiation or chemicals, and the resultant colonies (normal and transformed) are scored after 8 to 10 days of incubation.

strains by hybridization to high-density oligonucleotide arrays. Deletion strains are generated using a PCR targeting strategy, and each deletion strain is specifically labeled with two 20-base tag sequences. (See pages 253–254 for discussion of PCR.) Each molecular tag is important, as it serves as a "bar code," allowing approximately 4,500 deletion strains to be pooled and analyzed simultaneously by hybridization to an array. The abundance of a given strain is reflective of its hybridization to its corresponding complementary sequence on a high-density oligonucleotide array. The yeast deletion strains and oligonucleotide arrays containing complementary sequences for each deletion mutant are commercially available.

Mammalian Cells

The limited number of cell systems used in radiation and chemical transformation studies can be separated broadly into two categories. The first category includes short-term explants of cells derived from rodent or human embryos with a limited life span. These include:

Hamster embryo cells
Rat embryo cells
Human skin fibroblasts
Human foreskin cells
Human embryo cells

These cell assay systems can be used to assess the expression or activity of foreign genes transfected into them, or they may be used in studies of oncogenic transformation induced by radiation or chemicals.

In practice, the bulk of the experimental work has been performed with hamster or rat embryo cells. One advantage of such systems is that they consist of diploid cells, so that parallel cytogenetic experiments can be performed. Cell survival and cell transformation can be scored simultaneously in the same dishes.

The experimental methodology is illustrated in Figure 16.8. Cells are seeded at low density into dishes or flasks and treated with radiation or chemicals. They are allowed to grow for 8 to 10 days, and the resultant colonies are fixed and stained. Transformed colonies are identifiable by dense multilayered cells, random cellular arrangement, and haphazard cell-to-cell orientation accentuated at the colony edge. Normal counterparts are flat, with an organized cell-to-cell orientation and no piling up of cells. An example of the contrast between a normal and a transformed colony is shown in Figure 16.9.

The second category of experimental systems includes established cell lines that have an unlimited lifespan. The karyotype of these cells shows various chromosomal rearrangements and heteroploidy. The two most widely used established cell lines for transformation studies are the BALB/C-3T3 cell line and the C_3H 10T1/2 cell line. Both originated from mouse embryos, are transformable by a variety of oncogenic agents, and have been used extensively in transformation studies. The advantage of these established cell lines lies in the fact that they are "immortal," so that a particular passage can be used over a long period of time and maintained

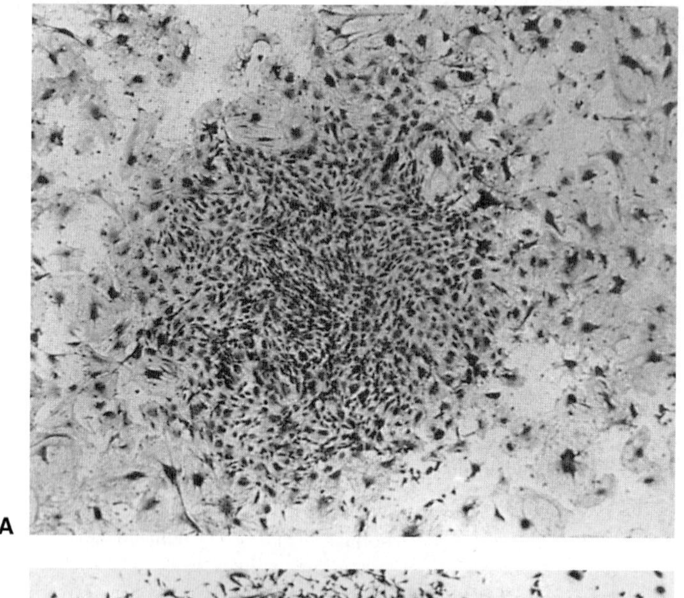

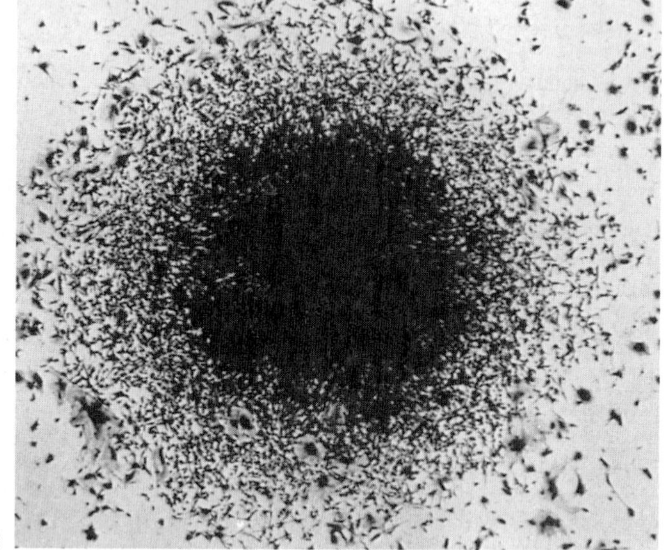

FIGURE 16.9 • **A:** A normal untransformed colony of hamster embryo cells. The cells are orderly and show contact inhibition. **B:** A colony of radiation-transformed hamster embryo cells. Note the densely stained, piled up cells and the crisscross pattern at the periphery of the colony.

in banks of frozen cells. The transformation assay is a focal assay. Cells are treated with radiation or chemicals and then allowed to grow for 6 weeks. The "normal" cells stop growing after confluence is reached, and transformed foci can be identified against a background of the contact-inhibited normal cells because they are densely stained, tend to pile up, and show a crisscross random pattern at the edge of the focus. Transformed cells, identified by their characteristic morphology, grow in soft agar, which indicates that they have lost anchorage dependence, and produce fibrosarcomas if injected into suitably prepared animals. This is illustrated in Figure 16.10.

The *in vitro* assay systems based on mammalian cells have two quite different uses in radiobiology. First, they may be used to accumulate data and information that are essentially pragmatic in nature; for example, they may be used to compare the oncogenic potential of a variety of chemical and physical agents. As such, they occupy a useful intermediate position between the bacterial mutagenesis assays, which are quick and inexpensive but score mutagenesis rather than carcinogenesis, and animal studies, which may be more relevant to humans but are quite cumbersome and inordinately expensive. Second, the assay systems can be used to study the mechanisms of carcinogenesis. In this context, transformation assays have played a vital role in unfolding the oncogene story, because transfecting DNA from human tumors into one or the other of the established cell lines used for transformation,

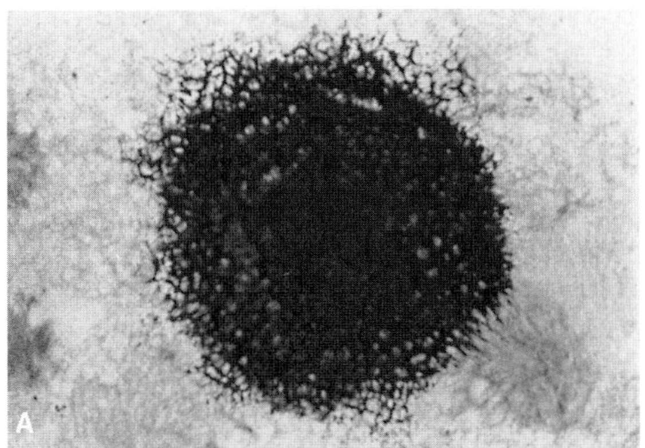

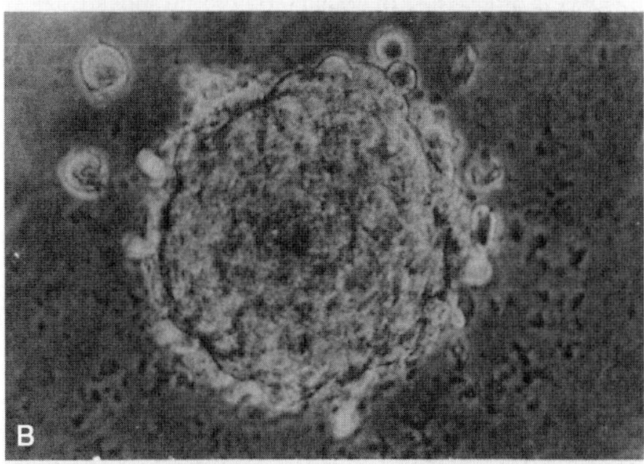

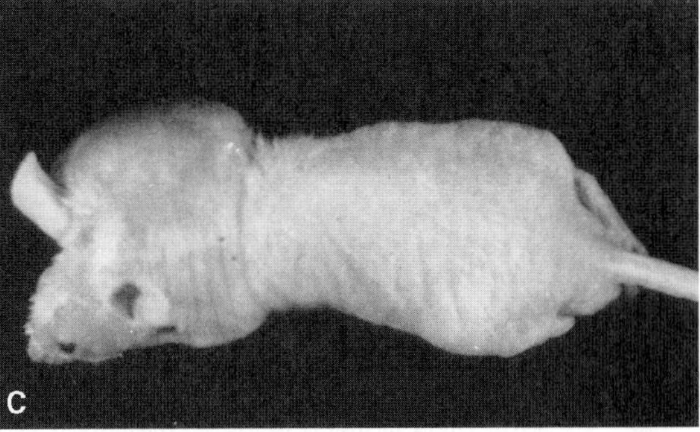

FIGURE 16.10 ● **A:** A type III transformed focus of C_3H 10TI/2 cells induced by the hypoxic cell sensitizer etanidazole (SR 2508). Note the multilayered growth and the crisscrossing of cells at the periphery of the clone over a contact-inhibited backg ̦nd of nontransformed cells. **B:** Cells from the focus shown in **A** were plucked, expanded in culture, and plated into semisolid medium; they formed colonies, indicating that they had lost anchorage dependence. This is an indication of malignancy. **C:** The ultimate test of malignancy is whether cells from a type III transformed clone injected into a suitably prepared animal produce a tumor (a fibrosarcoma) that eventually kills the animal.

most often 3T3 or rat-2 cells, and observing the induction of transformed foci is one way to detect the expression of an oncogene (see Chapter 17 for more details).

DNA-MEDIATED GENE TRANSFER

Gene transfer is now a routine tool for studying gene structure and function. Because gene transfer into mammalian cells is an inefficient process, an abundant source of starting cells is necessary to generate a workable number of transfected cells—that is, cells containing a transferred gene.

Mammalian cells do not take up foreign DNA naturally; indeed, they try to protect themselves from invading DNA. Consequently, one of several tricks must be used to bypass natural barriers:

1. **Microinjection:** This is the most direct but most difficult procedure to accomplish. DNA can be injected, cell by cell, directly into the nucleus through a fine glass needle.
2. **Calcium phosphate precipitation:** Cells take up DNA relatively efficiently in the form of a precipitate with calcium phosphate. The efficiency varies markedly from one cell line to

another. For example, NIH 3T3 cells are particularly receptive to foreign DNA introduced by this technique. High-molecular-weight DNA is mixed with insoluble calcium phosphate as a carrier and layered onto cells in petri dishes. Typically, a plasmid containing a selectable marker, such as G418 resistance, is copipetted and cotransfected into cells. In this way, cells that take up DNA can be selected. Of the cells that take up DNA, only a small percentage ultimately integrate the DNA into their genomes (are stably transfected). If a fragment of DNA containing an activated oncogene is transfected into NIH 3T3 cells, morphologic transformation of the cell occurs, leading to loss of contact inhibition, and the cells produce tumors if injected into immune-suppressed animals.

3. **Cationic lipids:** Cationic lipids offer some of the highest transfection efficiencies and expression levels to a wide variety of cells, both in suspension and attached. The protocol is very simple in that you mix lipid and DNA, vortex gently, centrifuge, and allow to sit at room temperature for 10 to 30 minutes before adding to cells. While cationic lipids produce high transfection efficiencies, some cells are sensitive to these lipids.
4. **Electroporation:** This technique is useful for cells that are resistant to transfection by calcium phosphate precipitation. Cells in solution are subjected to a brief electrical pulse that causes holes to open transiently in the membrane, allowing foreign DNA to enter.
5. **Viral vectors:** The ultimate means of transfection involves the use of a retrovirus. This is analogous to using bacteriophage to get DNA into bacteria. The genetic material of a retrovirus is RNA, and when retroviruses infect mammalian cells, their RNA genomes are converted to DNA by the viral enzyme **reverse transcriptase**. The viral DNA is incorporated efficiently into the host genome, replicating along with the host DNA at each cell cycle. If a foreign gene is incorporated into the retrovirus, it is permanently maintained in the infected mammalian cell. **Oncogenes**, genes that can cause cancer, and their counterpart, **tumor-suppressor genes**, can be studied by incorporating them into retroviral vectors.

AGAROSE GEL ELECTROPHORESIS

The purpose of agarose gel electrophoresis is to separate pieces of DNA of different size. This technique is based on the fact that DNA is negatively charged. Under the influence of an electrical field, DNA molecules move from negative to positive poles and are sorted by size in the gel. In a given time, small fragments migrate through the gel farther than large fragments.

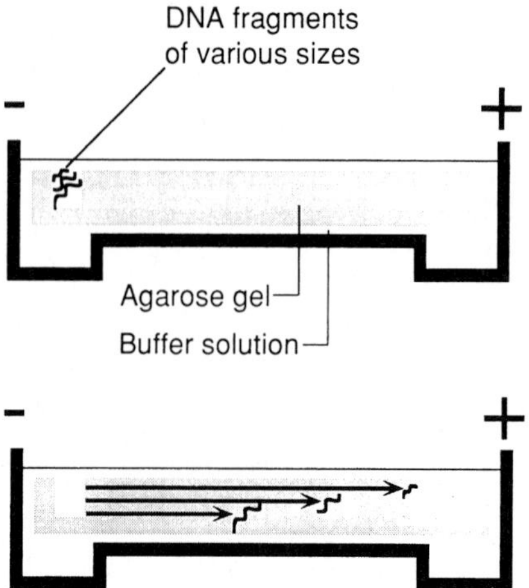

FIGURE 16.11 ● Illustration of agarose gel electrophoresis. DNA is negatively charged, so that under the influence of an electrical field, it migrates toward the anode. During electrophoresis, DNA fragments sort by size, small molecules moving farther than larger molecules. Because smaller molecules move farther than larger molecules in a given time, polyacrylamide gel electrophoresis often is employed to separate smaller DNA fragments with greater resolution than with agarose.

The technique, illustrated in Figure 16.11, is as follows: Molten agarose is poured into a tray in which a plastic comb is suspended near one end to form wells in the gel after it has solidified like gelatin. The concentration of the agarose is varied according to the size of the DNA fragment to be separated and visualized: high concentration for small fragments, lower concentration for larger fragments. The solidified gel is immersed in a tray containing an electrolyte to conduct electricity. The DNA samples, mixed with sucrose and a visible dye, are pipetted into the wells, and the electrical field is connected. Electrophoresis is monitored by observing the movement of the dye in the electrical field. After separation is complete, the gel is soaked in ethidium bromide, which intercalates into DNA and fluoresces under ultraviolet light to make the position of the DNA visible. The smaller DNA fragments migrate farther on the gel than the larger fragments, as illustrated in Figure 16.12. In fact, the distance migrated is directly related to DNA size. (Illustrations of several examples appear elsewhere in this chapter.)

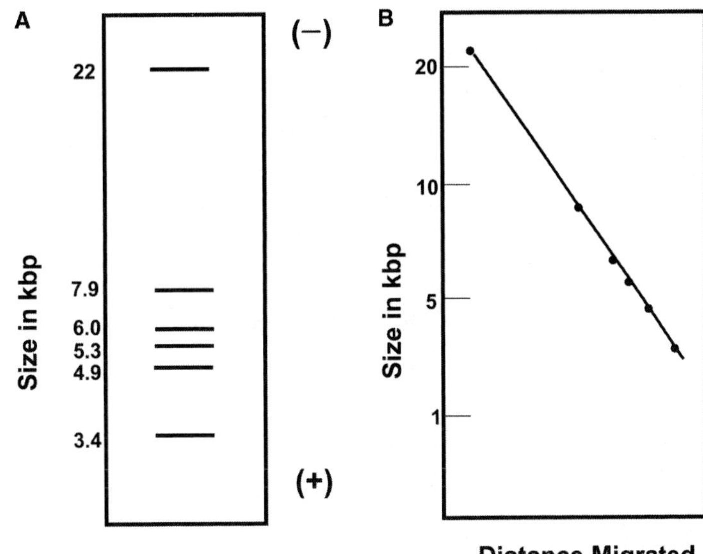

FIGURE 16.12 • **A:** Illustration of the separation of λ DNA after digestion with *Eco*RI. Agarose gels separate DNA fragments that can be quite large. By varying the percentage of agarose, the resolution of different-sized fragments can be maximized. **B:** Regardless of change in agarose concentration, the distance migrated is directly proportional to DNA size.

POLYMERASE CHAIN REACTION (PCR)

The **polymerase chain reaction (PCR)** technique uses enzymatic amplification to increase the number of copies of a DNA fragment of up to about 6,000 bp. The principle is based on primer extension by DNA polymerases, which was discovered in the 1960s. First, primers that are complementary to the 5′ end of the double-stranded DNA sequence to be amplified are synthesized. The two primers are mixed in excess with a sample of DNA that includes the fragments to be amplified, together with a heat-stable *Taq* DNA polymerase from *Thermus aquaticus*, a bacterium that inhabits hot springs. The four deoxyribonucleotide triphosphates also are provided in excess; one or more of them may be radioactively labeled. The power of the technique is that it can be used to amplify a DNA fragment from total genomic DNA. The PCR technique is illustrated in Figure 16.13.

The amount of the sequence is doubled in each cycle, which takes about 7 minutes. During each cycle, the sample is heated to about 94°C to denature the DNA strands, then cooled to about 50°C to allow the primers to anneal to the template DNA, and then heated to 72°C, the optimal temperature for *Taq* polymerase activity. In a matter of a few hours, a million copies of the DNA fragment can be obtained in an essentially automated device. PCR has found many applications in both basic research and clinical settings. For example, it has been used to detect malignant cells in patients with leukemias that are characterized by consistent translocation breakpoints. Primers that span the breakpoint are added to a bone-marrow sample and subjected to multiple cycles of PCR. Even one cell in a million with the translocation can be detected.

PCR-Mediated Site-Directed Mutagenesis

PCR-mediated site-directed mutagenesis is a technique used to create mutations such as nucleotide replacements, insertions, or deletions at a desired location in the gene or its flanking sequences to investigate the relationship between gene sequence and gene function. The starting material is usually a double-stranded DNA vector with the gene or nucleotide of interest acting as the template for PCR. In this technique, two complementary oligonucleotides containing the mutation of interest are used as the primers for PCR. The mutant strand of DNA is synthesized by denaturing the DNA template, annealing mutagenic primers to the DNA template, and extending the primers using a high-fidelity DNA polymerase such as *Pfu* polymerase to eliminate the chance of unwanted random errors being introduced during replication. Bacteria modify DNA by methylation to prevent it from being digested by restriction endonucleases. This modification of DNA is then used to eliminate the starting DNA from the PCR-amplified DNA by digestion with a methylation-specific endonuclease (*Dpn I*), leaving only the mutated DNA. This DNA is then used to transform competent bacterial cells so that it can be used for further study.

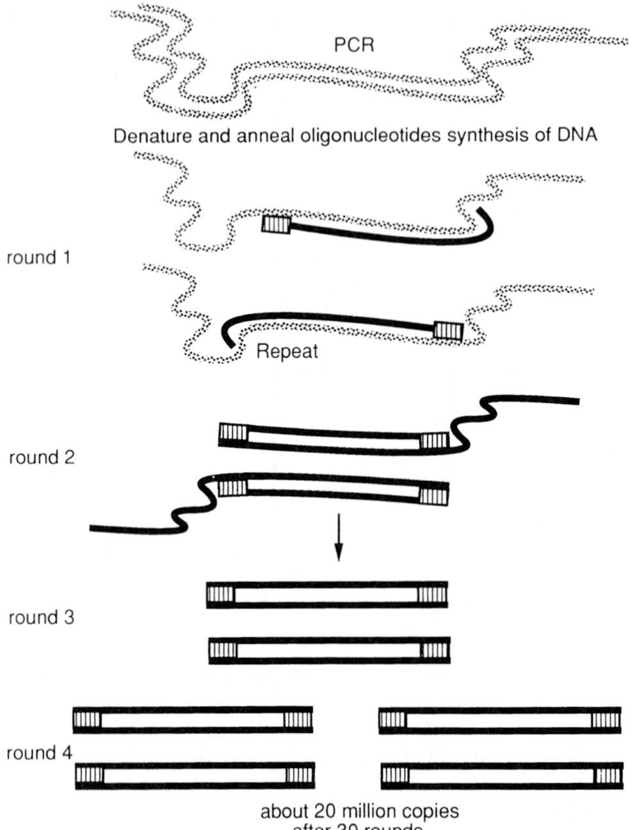

FIGURE 16.13 • The polymerase chain reaction for the amplification of DNA fragments. The number of DNA molecules is doubled in each cycle, which takes about 7 minutes, so that in a matter of several hours, millions of copies of a DNA fragment can be made. (Courtesy of Dr. Greg Freyer.)

GENE-CLONING STRATEGIES

In the most general terms, there are three steps involved in cloning a gene:

1. Choose a source of DNA, which may be genomic DNA or cDNA.
2. Construct a library, which is a collection of DNA fragments inserted into an appropriate vector.
3. Screen the library to locate the gene of interest.

The first two steps have already been described. Listed below are some of the principal methods used to screen for a gene.

Subcloning by Recombination

New technological advances have facilitated the rapid transfer of genes into a variety of plasmids, allowing expression of a given gene of interest in different contexts (e.g., expression for protein purification from bacteria and baculovirus; mammalian or viral overexpression; two-hybrid or library screening). Traditional approaches of subcloning employ steps of low efficiency or infrequent biochemical events. A new technology uses recombination of specific DNA target sequences mediated by the λ integrase recombination proteins to provide higher efficiency rates of gene transfer into a variety of vectors. The DNA of interest is subcloned between λ recombination sites into an "entry" or "donor" vector, which is then mixed with a "destination" or "acceptor" vector that also contains λ recombination sites. Gene orientation and direction of DNA transfer are controlled by using different combinations of λ integrase recombination sites and proteins, eliminating the need for gene sequencing. If the gene of interest is already in a vector, this vector can be converted to an "entry" vector by the addition of the specific recombination sequences. Furthermore, the acceptor vector can contain several different features, including amino or carboxy terminal tags for protein analysis. Subcloning by recombination represents a powerful technique for increasing productivity.

Functional Complementation

This technique depends on the DNA segment producing its corresponding protein within the cell, thereby giving the host a specific and detectable

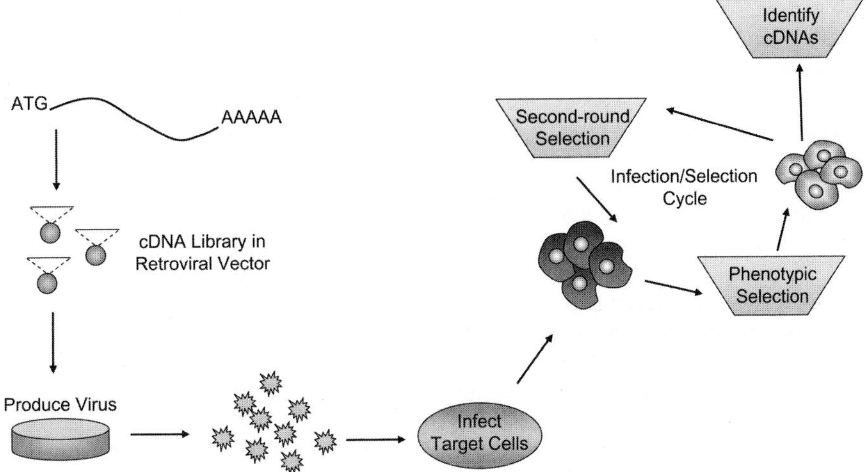

FIGURE 16.14 • Using a retroviral cDNA library to screen for functional complementation. A cDNA library is cloned into a retroviral vector and transfected into a host cell line to generate a viral library. The virus is added to target cells and the resulting transformants screened for phenotype. Virus is collected from the selected pool of cells and used to reinfect for another round of selection. The cDNAs are identified and infected as single clones to verify identity and function. (Adapted from Brummelkamp TR, Bernards R: New tools for functional mammalian cancer genetics. *Nature Reviews Cancer* 3:781–789, 2003.)

phenotype. For example, in screening for a repair gene that confers resistance to radiation or to a particular chemical agent (e.g., mitomycin C), a sensitive line of cells that lacks the functional gene is virally transduced or transfected with a library of cDNA or genomic DNA from cells containing the active gene (Fig. 16.14).

Only one in many thousands of cells takes up the gene of interest, but these cells acquire resistance and can be selected by long-term treatment with the cytotoxic agent (e.g., x-rays, mitomycin C).

During DNA transfection, many genes enter the cell, so it is necessary to first determine which of the introduced sequences contain the repair gene. The DNA fragment from the library can be identified by its association with the vector sequence. Once all of the library sequences are isolated, they must be screened individually to determine which contains the repair gene or genes. This can be done by reintroducing the purified vector genomic DNA clones into the sensitive cell line to determine which clone confers resistance.

Hybridization

Double-stranded DNA can be denatured; that is, the hydrogen bonds between the base pairs can be disrupted, causing the complementary strands to disassemble. DNA denatures under a variety of conditions, such as in the presence of high pH or high temperature. Under the right conditions, the two single-stranded molecules can reform the original duplex DNA molecule. This process of complementary single-stranded molecules lining up to form a double-stranded molecule is known as **hybridization**. Under "low stringency" conditions, partial hybridization takes place if the strands have a lesser degree of complementarity.

A genomic library, prepared as described previously, can be screened for the presence of a particular gene of interest by hybridization. The library consisting of bacteriophage or another suitable vector is grown on plates. A replica copy of each plate is made by transferring the colonies or plaques onto a filter disk, rather like a rubber stamp. The cells or bacteriophage are lysed and their DNA denatured, followed by screening with a probe that has a sequence complementary to the gene of interest. The probe is labeled with a β-emitting radionuclide (such as phosphorus-32) so that it can be detected easily. The filters are incubated under conditions that favor hybridization of the probe to its complementary sequence (neutral pH, presence of sodium ions to neutralize the negative charge on the DNA, and an elevated temperature). After removing the unhybridized probe, x-ray film is pressed tightly against the filters so that β-particles emitted from the phosphorus-32 expose the film; this is called **autoradiography**. After development, the exposed areas appear as black spots on the film, corresponding to the plaques/colonies that contain the gene of interest.

Oligonucleotide Probes

If it is possible to obtain a partial or complete amino acid sequence of the protein encoded by the gene under study, the coding sequence derived from these amino acids can be used to synthesize an oligonucleotide, a DNA sequence of a few nucleotides. This can be used as a probe for the gene of interest. A six-amino-acid sequence can be used to derive a series of 18 nucleotide DNA probes that take into consideration the redundancy of the genetic code. This mixture of oligonucleotides is labeled with a β-emitting radionuclide so that the plaques or lysed bacterial colonies to which it hybridizes in the DNA library can be identified readily by autoradiography.

Positional Cloning

Positional cloning is a strategy used to isolate a gene if no information is available about its protein product. This is the situation for many human inherited disorders in which the underlying biochemical defects are simply unknown.

The identification of genes responsible for inherited human disorders is an integral part of the Human Genome Project. Several approaches are combined to isolate genes by positional cloning. As its name implies, the first step in this procedure is to determine the chromosomal location of the gene. This information is used to clone DNA sequences from that location, and these sequences are used as probes to find the gene itself. Linkage analysis facilitates the localization of a gene by comparing within a family the inheritance of a mutant gene with the inheritance of DNA markers of known chromosomal location. This approach requires identification of several markers and an increase of the markers within the defined region of the chromosome. Coinheritance of the disease gene and the marker suggests that they are physically close together on the chromosome. This *linked DNA sequence* is used as the starting point to "walk" or "jump" to the gene by cloning DNA fragments that are even more tightly linked and therefore closer to the gene.

After the gene has been isolated, the DNA sequence can be determined and analyzed to predict the biochemical properties of the encoded protein. The technique of positional cloning has become a familiar component of modern human genetics research. After a halting start in the mid-1980s, the number of disease genes isolated by cloning efforts based solely on pinpointing their position in the genome is growing rapidly. More than 110 genes have been identified so far. The positional candidate approach, which combines knowledge of map position with the increasingly dense human transcript map, greatly expedites the search process and has become the predominant method of disease-gene discovery.

It is important to recognize the difference between positional cloning and functional complementation. Oncogenes were cloned and sequenced before tumor-suppressor genes because they act in a dominant fashion and so can be detected by functional complementation, which is by far the simpler procedure. Tumor-suppressor genes at a cellular level are recessive acting and so are not so easily detected by complementation; most of those discovered so far have been isolated by positional cloning. The other limitation of functional complementation becomes evident in the search for a very large gene. If the gene is so large that it is never contained in any of the DNA fragments used to complement, then the function of the gene is not recovered and the approach fails to identify the gene. An example is the cloned gene for ataxia telangiectasia, termed the *ATM* (AT-mutated) gene. This gene has 66 exons and is 150 kb in length; it was finally cloned by the positional cloning approach in 1995, after attempts by other means had failed for quite a few years.

GENE ANALYSES

Mapping

Southern Blotting

Southern blotting, named after its inventor, Ed Southern, is a method to detect specific fragments of DNA. The DNA to be analyzed, such as genomic DNA, is digested by restriction enzymes and separated by electrophoresis on an agarose gel. The fragmented DNA is denatured and transferred to a nitrocellulose or nylon membrane. This filter is then subjected to hybridization with a specific single-stranded DNA probe, which will complex to its complementary sequence. The DNA probe can be radioactive (^{32}P), bioluminescent, or biotin/streptavidin labeled. This complex can then be imaged by autoradiography, luminescence, or colorimetry, respectively. Southern blotting can detect mutations—specifically insertions, deletions, and sequence differences in DNA. The technique is illustrated in Figure 16.15.

Southern blotting is useful for analyzing the sizes of DNA fragments lost in radiation-induced mutations. It is also useful for detecting structural variations in DNA that result in restriction

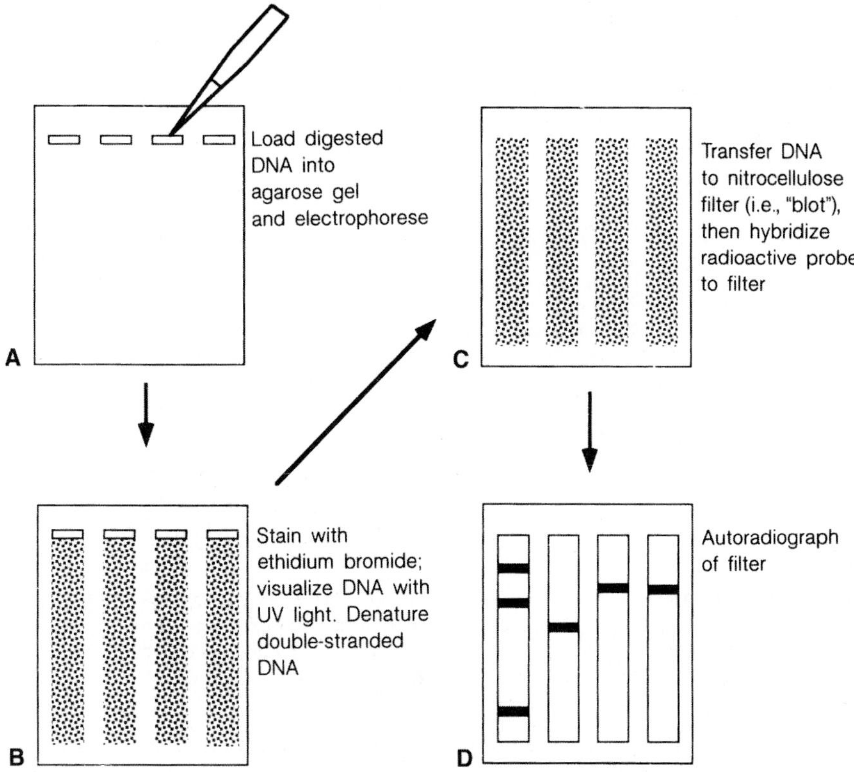

FIGURE 16.15 ● The technique of Southern blot analysis. **A:** Digested DNA fragments are loaded into the wells of an agarose gel and subjected to electrophoresis. **B:** DNA fragments move different distances according to their sizes and can be visualized under ultraviolet illumination after staining with ethidium bromide.**C:** The DNA is denatured and then transferred to a nitrocellulose filter by capillary action; that is, a "blot" is made. A probe labeled with a radionuclide is hybridized to the filter. **D:** An autoradiograph is made of the filter. Bands corresponding to DNA strands to which the probe hybridizes are visualized clearly.

fragments of different lengths, known as **restriction fragment length polymorphisms**, which can be used as genetic markers to map genes to specific chromosomal locations. The technique of Southern blotting has been used by human geneticists to localize and identify a number of disease genes and also has been used in "DNA fingerprinting."

Chromosome Walking

The chromosome-walking technique is necessary if a gene of interest has been mapped to a specific arm of a chromosome and one wants to isolate the gene. It is not needed if the gene of interest is already contained in a discrete DNA fragment obtained from a DNA library. The process is illustrated in Figure 16.16. The starting point is to identify a piece of DNA, a flanking marker, that is close to the gene. This is accomplished by making a genomic library of large DNA fragments (20,000–40,000 bp) that includes the gene of interest and identifying flanking markers by mapping or hybridization. Probes are then used to identify an overlapping fragment of DNA from the genomic library that contains the flanking marker and some other identifiable marker. The next step is to find a new probe from the genomic library that has the second marker at its 5′ end and that includes yet another identifiable marker (C). This process of identifying overlapping probes that span a chromosomal region containing a gene of interest is referred to as **chromosome walking** and is continued until the gene of interest is reached.

Contiguous Mapping

Mapping refers to the determination of the physical location of a gene or genetic marker on a chromosome. **Contiguous mapping** refers to the alignment of sequence data from large, adjacent regions of the genome to produce a continuous nucleotide sequence of a region of a chromosome. The basic idea is to orient physical markers, such as restriction

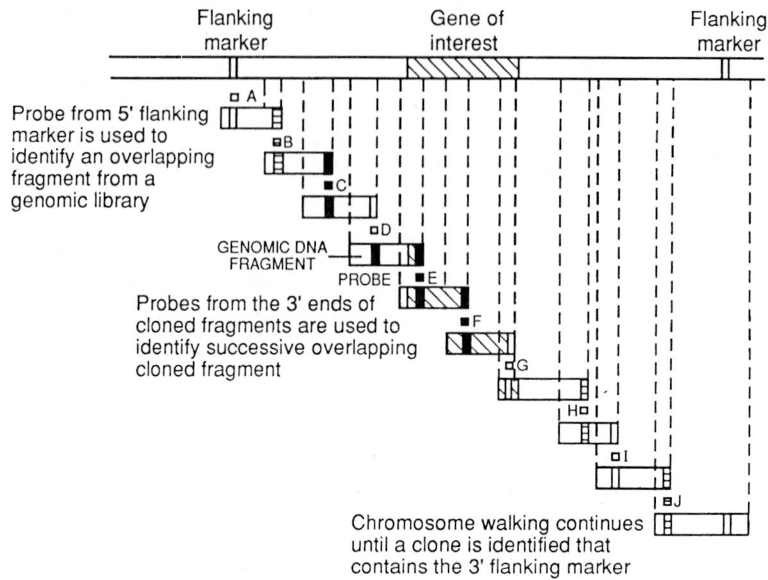

FIGURE 16.16 • Illustration of the technique of chromosome walking. Working from a flanking DNA marker, overlapping clones are successively identified that span a chromosomal region containing a gene of interest. (Courtesy of Dr. Greg Freyer.)

fragment length polymorphisms, on adjacent fragments so that they can be lined up and the nucleotide sequence can be made continuous. If, for example, restriction fragments from a DNA library are sequenced, relating these sequences to known physical markers eventually can produce the nucleotide sequence of the entire genome. This is the goal of the Human Genome Project, but the task is so massive that it cannot be accomplished without the development of automated sequencing technology and sophisticated computer strategies to store and handle the data.

DNA Sequence Analyses

DNA sequencing is the process of identifying the exact sequence of nucleotides in a given DNA sample, whether it is a particular gene or an entire genome. DNA sequencing is achieved by the dideoxynucleotide chain termination method (the Sanger method), which exploits the fact that DNA is composed of deoxynucleotides. Primers are used to amplify a given target of the single-stranded DNA to be sequenced. Dideoxynucleotides lack a hydroxyl (OH) group at the 3′ position. Thus, when a dideoxynucleotide is added, the chain is terminated. Using conditions similar to PCR, multiple rounds of primer extension incorporate deoxynucleotides and labeled dideoxynucleotides on the sequenced strand. In manual sequencing, four separate reactions are run in which only one radiolabeled dideoxynucleotide is added to the reaction. Each of the four dideoxynucleotides is electrophoresed on a gel and visualized by autoradiography. A more recent (and commonly used) innovation is automated sequencing, in which a single reaction is run with a mixture of all four dideoxynucleotides, each carrying a different-colored fluorescent label. The products are electrophoresed in one lane, separating the replication products based on size. A laser scans the bottom of the gel, detecting the four fluorescent tags of the dideoxynucleotide from which the original strand sequence of nucleotides can be determined.

Polymorphisms or Mutations

Restriction Fragment Length Polymorphisms

Relatively small differences in similar DNA sequences, or **polymorphisms**, as they are called, may result from point mutations, deletions or insertions, or varying numbers of copies of a DNA fragment (so-called tandem repeats). A Southern blot analysis can be used to detect DNA polymorphisms by using a probe that hybridizes to a polymorphic region of the DNA molecule. Other techniques also may be used to detect polymorphisms.

If a particular restriction enzyme is used to cut human DNA, a polymorphic locus yields restriction fragments of different sizes. These are restriction fragment length polymorphisms. Deletions, insertions, or tandem repeats involving more than about 30 nucleotides can be detected as recognizable shifts in the Southern blot hybridization pattern. Even a point mutation can be detected if the resultant change in sequence removes or adds a new recognition site at which a restriction endonuclease cuts.

Single-Stranded Conformation Polymorphism

Several methods have been developed to screen for an *unknown* mutation in a gene. Among them, single-stranded conformation polymorphism is particularly useful. A single base-pair difference between two short single-stranded DNA molecules (such as the difference between a wild-type gene and one that has suffered a point mutation) results in a difference in conformation between the two strands that, remarkably enough, can be detected by a difference in the molecule's electrophoretic mobilities on a neutral polyacrylamide gel. The same change would go undetected if electrophoresis were carried out under denaturing conditions in which strands separate only according to size, not base composition. This represents a powerful technique to screen for mutations in an oncogene (such as *ras*) or in a tumor-suppressor gene (such as *p53*).

Comparative Genome Hybridization (CGH)

Genomic DNA is harvested from a tumor or cancer cell line and digested with DpnII (a restriction endonuclease that cleaves DNA approximately every 256 base pairs), creating a random pool of DNA fragments. DNA is amplified with random primers and nucleotides labeled with the fluorescent dye Cy5 (red). As a control, DNA from a normal cell line is also fragmented and then amplified with the fluorescent dye Cy3 (green). The two samples are mixed and hybridized to a DNA microarray composed of a genome-wide sampling of cDNA. The microarray is scanned and the ratio of Cy5 to Cy3 (red to green) fluorescence calculated for each cDNA spot to generate a baseline fluorescent ratio. Individual spots with a Cy5:Cy3 ratio significantly higher than background correspond to regions of the genome that are amplified in that specific cancer cell, whereas those with lower than baseline correspond to chromosomal deletions (also called loss of heterozygosity). Spots corresponding to contiguous chromosomal regions should show similar alterations in enrichment and define a common locus. The genes residing in the altered loci are identified from the human genome database to generate a list of potential tumor suppressors or oncogenes.

GENE KNOCKOUTS

Homologous Recombination to Knock Out Genes

Homologous recombination is the cellular process that allows the eukaryotic cell to repair damage to one chromosome with the DNA from the homologous sister chromosome acting as a template (Chapter 5). This process also occurs during meiosis, where the DNA from the parental chromosomes is shuffled before segregation to gametes. Homologous recombination can be used to selectively delete or alter the endogenous gene in a cell line. A simplified version of this process is illustrated in Figure 16.17. Cloned DNA from a gene of interest (GOI) is modified to delete a key functional domain from the middle of the sequence and

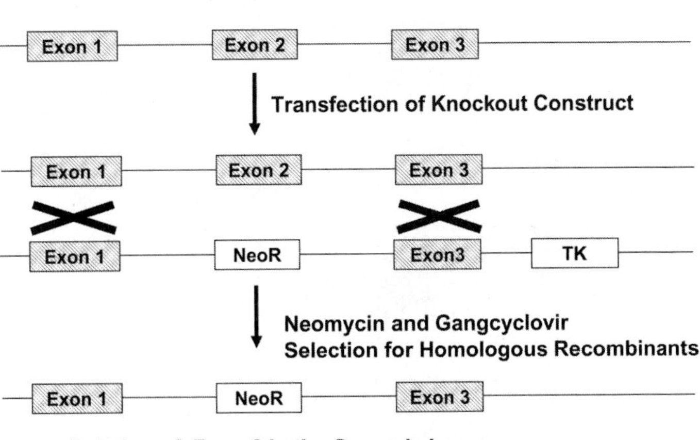

FIGURE 16.17 • Use of homologous recombination to delete function in a gene of interest (GOI). Exon 2 of GOI is known to be responsible for GOI's biologic activity. A knockout construct is cloned from a genomic fragment spanning GOI by replacing exon 2 with the neomycin antibiotic resistance gene (*neoR*). The gene for thymidylate kinase (*tk*) at the 5′ end of the construct is cloned. Cells are transfected with the knockout construct and treated with neomycin and gangcyclovir to select for homologous recombinants and against random integrants. The surviving colonies are screened by PCR or Southern blotting to verify deletion of exon 2.

replace it with a cDNA for neomycin resistance (*neoR*). A cDNA (*tk*) conferring sensitivity to another drug (gangcyclovir) is ligated to the end of the GOI-neo construct. The linearized construct is then transfected into cells, and the cells are treated with both neomycin and gangcyclovir. If the construct is randomly inserted into the cell's genome (a common event), both *neoR* and *tk* are inserted and expressed. These cells are resistant to neomycin, but will be killed by gangcyclovir. If homologous recombination occurs (a rare event), the GOI sequences flanking the *neoR* cassette will be recognized by the cellular recombination machinery and replace the original region of GOI with the *neoR* cassette, but will not incorporate the *tk* gene. These cells will then be neomycin resistant and survive gangcyclovir. The same process is repeated with a different antibiotic resistance marker to delete the other copy of the GOI. PCR or Southern blotting is then used to verify loss of the native gene and insertion of the *neoR* gene. A similar process can be used to swap native parts of a GOI with mutant forms.

Knockout Mice

Using homologous recombination, one copy of a GOI is deleted in mouse embryonic stem (ES) cells. The neomycin- and gangcyclovir-resistant ES cells are injected into early mouse embryos. The resultant chimeric mice that are heterozygous for GOI in their gametes are bred to generate male and female GOI heterozygous mice. The heterozygotes are subsequently bred, and of their offspring, one in four should be homozygous knockouts for GOI. PCR or Southern blotting is used to confirm homozygous GOI deletion. More sophisticated methods use the specialized recombination systems to delete a GOI in a tissue-specific and/or temporally regulated manner.

GENE EXPRESSION ANALYSIS

Northern Blotting

The name **Northern blot** was coined to describe the technique for separating RNA by gel electrophoresis and is analogous to the Southern blot technique used to study DNA. Both abundance and turnover of specific RNAs can be detected by Northern blot. Total cellular RNA is harvested from tissue or cells and then denatured to prevent hydrogen bonding between base pairs. Denatured RNA is in a linear, unfolded conformation, which allows fragments to be separated by gel electrophoresis according to size. This is then transferred to a membrane, made of either nitrocellulose or nylon, which can then be hybridized by a specific DNA probe.

RNA Interference

The expression of a given gene can be reduced through **RNA interference (RNAi).** In mammalian cells, gene silencing by RNAi is initiated in one of two ways, either short-interfering RNAs (siRNAs) or short-interfering RNA expression vectors (Fig. 16.18). Short-interfering RNAs utilize the fact that double-stranded RNA induces a potent antiviral response. Once introduced into a cell, siRNAs of 21 to 25 nucleotides in length interact with the RNA-induced silencing complex (RISC), composed of several proteins. The siRNA

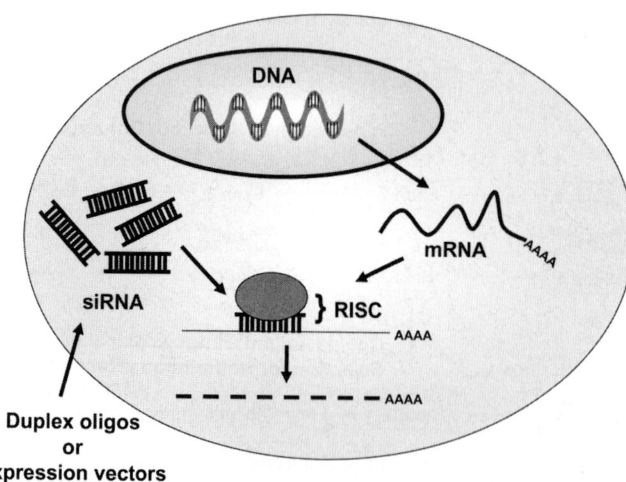

FIGURE 16.18 ● Short double-stranded RNA molecules (siRNA) are transfected into a cell as chemically synthesized oligo duplexes or hairpin expression vectors. Cellular RNA degradation machinery incorporates the siRNA to form the RNA-induced silencing complex (RISC). The sequences incorporated cause the RISC complex to selectively recognize the complementary sequences on target mRNAs. RISC cleaves the mRNA, leading to degradation and a functional loss of protein expression. (Adapted from Brummelkamp TR, Bernards R: New tools for functional mammalian cancer genetics. *Nature Reviews Cancer* 3:781–789, 2003.)

directs RISC to its complementary RNA target sequence, resulting in cleavage and subsequent silencing of the target RNA. Similarly, siRNA expression vectors can be used to introduce short hairpin RNAs, which are then cleaved into double-stranded RNAs by Dicer, a cytoplasmic nuclease. These RNAs of 21 to 25 nucleotides can then interact with RISC, leading to silencing of target RNA sequences.

Reverse Transcription PCR

While the Northern blot is the classical method to assay gene expression, it requires a rather large amount of RNA (5–10 μg), particularly if the RNA to assay is in low abundance. To circumvent this limitation, the researcher can effectively amplify RNA using reverse transcription (RT) followed by amplification of the resulting complementary DNA (cDNA) with conventional PCR techniques. A number of retroviruses express DNA polymerases that can reverse transcribe viral RNA into DNA prior to genomic insertion. RNA purified from cells is annealed with random primers and incubated with a reverse transcriptase (Moloney Murine Leukemia Virus RT or a commercial variant is most common) and deoxynucleotides. The cDNA is amplified by PCR with primers specific for the gene of interest and separated by electrophoresis for imaging. As long as the researcher takes care to use linear PCR conditions and to also amplify a control RNA (actin, GAPDH) for normalization, relative quantities can be determined and used to assay changes in gene expression. However, because this technique is subject to variation from primer efficiencies and PCR amplification, it is often referred to as semiquantitative RT-PCR.

Quantitative Real-Time PCR

The need to verify gene expression data from microarray studies led to the widespread use of **quantitative real-time PCR (qRT-PCR).** Originally developed for preimplantation diagnosis in fertility clinics, qRT-PCR makes it possible to accurately quantify data from very small amounts of starting sample. Amplification and measurement take place in the same reaction vessel, enabling high-throughput analysis. The qRT-PCR thermocyclers have extremely large dynamic ranges (greater than 5 orders of magnitude), allowing for quantitation of both high- and low-abundance RNAs from the same sample. RNA from cells or tissue is reverse transcribed into cDNA and then amplified with specific primers in the presence of a fluorescent oligo specific for a gene of interest (TaqMan, MGB probes, etc.) or a fluorescent intercalating dye (SYBR Green). At each PCR cycle, the change in fluorescence is recorded. After normalizing amplification of a gene of interest against that of a control RNA (typically 18S ribosomal RNA), it is then possible to calculate the differences in gene expression among samples.

Genetic Reporters

Genetic reporters are extremely useful tools for monitoring a broad range of cellular processes. Reporters can be used to assay the cellular microenvironment, to study protein-protein interactions, to study RNA processing, or to study regulation of gene transcription. Reporters are often plasmids that contain a sequence of DNA derived from a promoter or other transcriptional regulatory sequence, such as an enhancer or repressor, that is ligated to a gene that is not normally expressed in the mammalian cell. These reporter genes encode proteins that are easily detected by changes in enzymatic activity, by resistance to antibiotics, or by expression of a membrane protein. Common reporter genes are those that code for β-galactosidase, chloramphenicol acetyltransferase, firefly luciferase, *Renilla* luciferase, and a host of fluorescent proteins from aquatic organisms (GFP, RFP, etc.). There are many different types of promoter sequences that can be used to regulate the expression of a reporter gene: Some promoters are constitutively expressed (from housekeeping genes or viral genes), while others are artificial creations of a particular transcriptional regulatory sequence (i.e., the p53 tumor-suppressor binding sequence) and a basal promoter element. For example, to investigate the regulation of p53 in irradiated cells using a reporter gene, a promoter consisting of the p53 binding site and a basal regulatory element would be more appropriate than a large promoter that contains other radiation-responsive regulatory factors in addition to p53.

Promoter Bashing

A very common use of biologic reporters is the "promoter bash," where a promoter is dissected to determine which region is responsible for an interesting activity (such as induction during ionizing radiation or hypoxia, for example). Using conventional techniques, the promoter is cloned upstream of a bioluminescent reporter gene, such as the gene coding for firefly luciferase, and transfected into cells with a control plasmid constitutively expressing *Renilla* luciferase. This approach makes use of the differing substrate dependencies of luciferase enzymes from fireflies (*Photinus pyralis*)

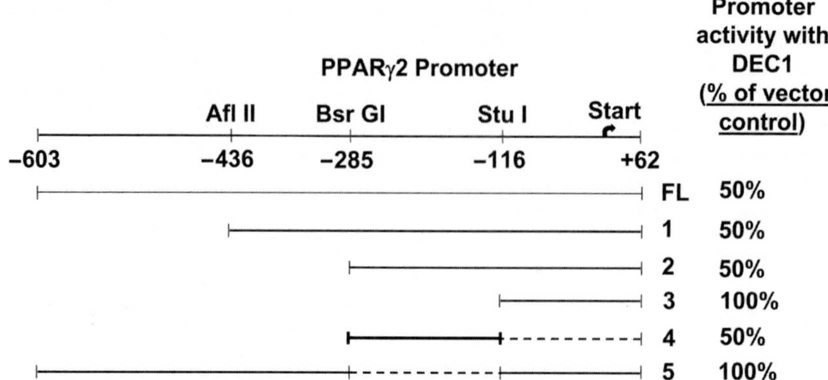

FIGURE 16.19 ● Example of a promoter-bashing experiment. *PPARγ2* expression has been shown to be repressed by the transcription repressor DEC1. 665 (the span from −603 to +62) base pairs of the *PPARγ2* promoter are cloned upstream of a firefly luciferase reporter (FL) and transfected into NIH3T3 mouse fibroblasts with either a *DEC1* expression construct or an empty vector. The activity of the FL construct is repressed to approximately 50% by DEC1. The FL construct was progressively truncated with restriction enzymes (constructs 1–3), demonstrating that deletion of a fragment spanning −285 through −116 (construct 3) removes the ability of DEC1 to repress transcription. Luciferase driven by the −285 through −116 fragment in isolation (construct 4) is still repressed by DEC1, confirming the location of a repressed region. This is confirmed by deletion of the region from the full-length promoter (construct 5), which is no longer repressed by DEC1. (Yun Z Maecker HL, Johnson RS, Giaccia AJ: Inhibition of *PPARγ2* gene expression by the HIF-1-regulated gene *DEC1/Stra13:* A mechanism for regulation of adipogenesis by hypoxia. *Dev Cell* 2:331–341, 2002.)

and jellyfish (*Renilla reniformis*). Using two distinct reagents, light emitted by the firefly construct that reflects promoter activity in response to ionizing radiation can be normalized with the signal from the *Renilla* construct that reflects promoter expression in unstressed cells to correct for transfection efficiency. By systematically deleting parts of the experimental promoter, one can isolate the DNA sequence that regulates expression (Fig. 16.19).

Electrophoretic Mobility Shift Assay (EMSA)

If a regulatory element in a promoter has been identified, the electrophoretic mobility shift assay (EMSA) is a powerful tool to identify the specific sequence bound by a transcription factor. A short fragment of double-stranded DNA (typically 40 bp in length) is radiolabeled and incubated with cellular extracts or purified protein and electrophoresed under nondenaturing conditions that maintain the protein and DNA interaction. If a transcription factor recognizes and binds the radiolabeled sequence, the DNA fragment migrates more slowly in the gel compared with the unbound fragment. This difference can be observed by exposure to x-ray film. Specificity of the interaction is verified by either mutating the fragment to destroy the protein-binding site, competing the protein away with excess unlabeled binding site, or reducing band mobility further by binding the transcription factor with a specific antibody. By comparing the ratios of bound to unbound fragment with titrations of purified transcription factor, it is also possible to determine binding constants and other biochemical properties.

Chromatin Immunoprecipitation (ChIP)

Methods to study transcriptional regulation in mammalian cells are generally limited to biochemical assays (cell-free transcription, electrophoretic mobility shift assays, etc.) or cellular assays (transiently transfected reporter assays). Although both approaches are useful, they are limited in that they can only approximate the interactions that occur in the cell, primarily because neither can completely duplicate the chromatin environment *as it exists in the cell.* On the other hand, *in vivo* footprinting can demonstrate that something is bound to native chromatin, but cannot identify the specific protein involved. Chromatin immunoprecipitation (ChIP) is a revolutionary advance that determines transcription factor interactions with a target promoter in the native chromatin environment (Fig. 16.20). Cells,

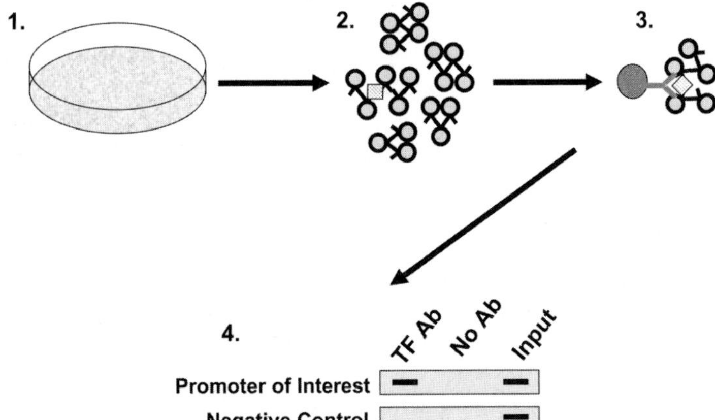

FIGURE 16.20 • Illustration showing key steps in chromatin immunoprecipitation. 1. Fix cells with formaldehyde. 2. Sonicate chromatin into 500- to 1,000-bp fragments. 3. Immunoprecipitate transcription factor (TF) with a specific antibody. 4. De-crosslink DNA, use PCR to verify specific interaction with target promoter, and visualize specific amplification by agarose electrophoresis.

tissues, or tumors are fixed with formaldehyde and sonicated to shear DNA into short fragments (typically 1 kb or less). Promoters and other regulatory regions are then immunoprecipitated with an antibody against a protein thought to bind to that region. DNA can then be identified and quantified by PCR or microarray analysis. Using this technique, it is possible to correlate the DNA-binding activity of a given transcription factor with corresponding changes in the surrounding chromatin environment and gene expression in cells exposed to different hormones, cellular stresses, and differentiation programs.

Protein-DNA Interaction Arrays (ChIP-Chips)

Surveying all of the interactions of the transcription apparatus with the human genome is a daunting task. ChIP-chips combines the power of the ChIP assay with the global nature of the microarray to investigate these interactions (the "Chips" are chips of glass slides on which the ChIP is placed). Immunoprecipitated chromatin is ligated to universal primers and amplified by PCR to generate a pool of DNA associated with a given transcription factor. DNA is fluorescently labeled, mixed with amplified and labeled unprecipitated DNA (input), and hybridized to a microarray of regulatory DNA. Higher relative fluorescence from the immunoprecipitated DNA on a spot compared with input indicates an interaction of the protein with that regulatory sequence. This technique has been used primarily to map transcription factor binding and histone modification across the entire yeast genome. The vastly larger size of the human genome has made it necessary to focus on more specific regions using arrays of either cloned promoter fragments or CpG islands (sequences of DNA that cluster around promoters and other regulatory regions). Production of high-density tiled microarrays spanning all promoters in the human genome will soon make possible the correlation of transcription factor binding, chromatin structure, and gene expression.

Microarrays to Assay Gene Expression

With the sequencing of the human genome, studying global changes in gene expression became possible in principle. Concurrently, efforts were being made to study the expression of as many genes as possible without resorting to individual Northern blots for each identified gene. In this way, the microarray was born. Expression arrays work like an inverse Northern blot: Cellular RNA is reverse transcribed, amplified with modified nucleotides that allow fluorescent detection, and hybridized to an array of sequences corresponding to the genes in an organism (Fig. 16.21). The arrays used for detection fall into two types: spotted and oligo arrays.

Spotted arrays consist of a glass microscope slide spotted with a grid of cDNAs for specific genes. RNA from two different samples are amplified with two different colored fluorescent dyes and scanned after hybridization. The ratio of fluorescence for each spot is calculated to generate a baseline ratio. Spots that differ from the baseline by a statistically determined amount correspond to genes whose expression differs between the two samples. Facilities to print spotted arrays can be found at most universities.

An alternative method is to use oligo arrays, like those offered by Affymetrix. Using photolithography, thousands of short DNA oligos corresponding to genes are printed in multiple places on an area about the size of a postage stamp. RNA is amplified

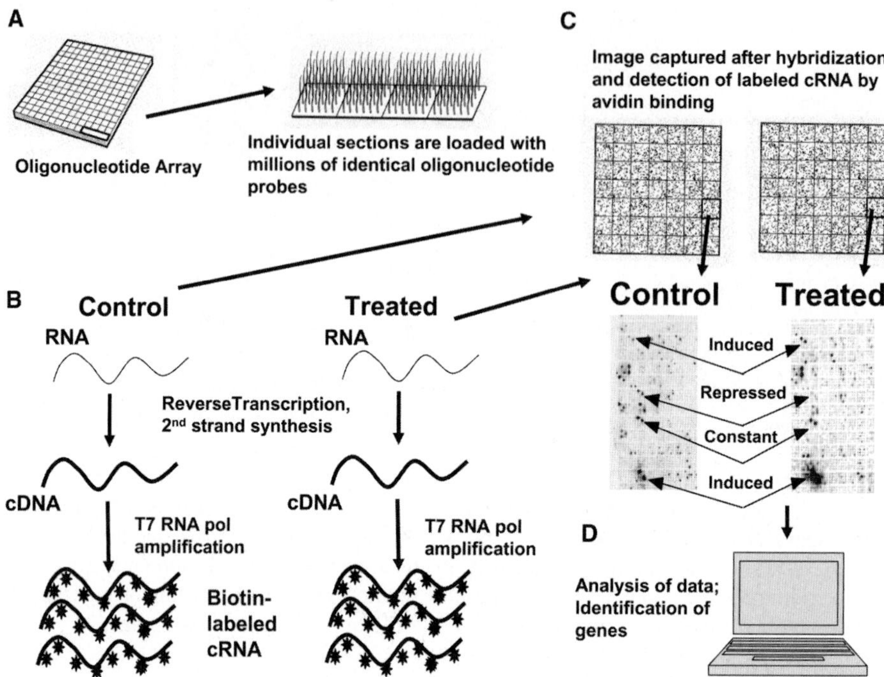

FIGURE 16.21 ● Oligonucleotide microarray analysis. **A:** Silicon wafers are divided into thousands of sectors, each contains millions of identical 20- to 50-bp oligonucleotides corresponding to a different unique gene sequence. **B:** RNA from cell samples is reverse transcribed to cDNA. cRNA is amplified from the cDNA using T7 RNA polymerase and biotinylated nucleotides. **C:** The labeled cRNA is hybridized to the arrays, bound with fluorescently labeled avidin, and detected by microscopy. **D:** Differences in intensity between experimental and control samples are quantified and analyzed with computer software.

with biotinylated nucleotides and hybridized. The hybridized RNA is then bound with fluorescently labeled avidin and visualized. Because of the large number of sequences printed with a high degree of redundancy, different samples can be compared with each other in separate hybridizations, removing the need to hybridize two samples on one slide.

With either type of array, the experiment needs to be repeated several times before the result can be relied upon. It is also necessary to verify selected expression differences using independent means, such as Northern blotting, reverse transcription PCR, or quantitative real-time PCR.

PROTEIN ANALYSIS

Western Blotting

The term *Western blot* is used for proteins, analogous to Southern blot for DNA and Northern blot for RNA. Western blot analysis is a method to detect the presence and abundance of a specific protein within a mixture of proteins. This is achieved by first separating the mixture of proteins based on both charge and size through polyacrylamide gel electrophoresis (PAGE). A membrane (nitrocellulose or vinyl) is then placed on top of the gel, and the proteins are transferred by electrophoresis toward the membrane. The membrane is incubated with a primary antibody, which specifically recognizes the protein of interest. Following a brief wash period to eliminate any excess primary antibody, the membrane is incubated with a secondary antibody, which specifically recognizes the primary antibody. The secondary antibody is conjugated to an enzyme to allow subsequent detection.

Antibody Production

Antibodies specific to a gene product of interest can be produced, provided there is a source of purified protein. This purified protein is then injected into an animal (e.g., mouse, rat, rabbit, goat, sheep, chicken or horse) with an adjuvant to stimulate the immune response to the purified protein. Monoclonal antibodies are made by injecting either mouse or rats with the protein of interest. The antibody-producing cells of the spleen are then fused to a specific tumor cell line to create a hybridoma. The hybridoma is then screened for antibody production and specificity. For polyclonal antibodies, an animal is injected with the protein of interest and adjuvant and then bled. The antibodies can then be purified out of the blood.

Immunoprecipitation

Immunoprecipitation is used to detect specific protein–protein interactions. An antibody against a specific protein is incubated with a sample that contains the target and allowed to form an immune complex. This complex is then captured and immobilized by the addition of proteins A and G agarose, which are used for the isolation and purification of the antibody and protein complex. Proteins A and G are derived from streptococcal groups A and G, respectively, and bind IgG antibodies with high affinity. Unbound proteins are washed away, and the bound immune complex are eluted and analyzed by Western blot.

Far Western Blotting

The Far Western blot is another useful method for probing protein–protein interactions. In this variation of the Western blot (or immunoblot), instead of using an antibody to detect a specific protein, purified recombinant protein is used to probe a membrane of electrophoresed cellular protein. The recombinant protein (sometimes called the "bait") binds to specific cellular proteins on the membrane and is detected by autoradiography or with a specific antibody. Various protein chemistry approaches can then be used to identify the interacting proteins on the membrane.

Fluorescent Proteins

A number of aquatic organisms express fluorescent proteins that make excellent reporters. The two most commonly used fluorescent proteins are green fluorescent protein (GFP) from the jellyfish *Aequorea coerulescens* and red fluorescent protein (RFP) from *Discosoma* reef coral. Because of their widely different spectral properties, they make excellent reagents for two-color labeling of cells. A common practice is to fuse GFP to a protein of interest and RFP to another to monitor intracellular protein activity either in cells in culture or in mice (Fig. 16.22). GFP has also been engineered to fluoresce in the cyan (CFP) and yellow (YFP) spectra. The emission spectrum of CFP overlaps with the excitation spectrum of YFP. By fusing CFP to a protein of interest and YFP to another protein, it is possible to observe interactions by exciting CFP with light and observing YFP fluorescence. This method, called fluorescence resonance energy transfer (FRET), is a useful way to observe the dynamic interactions of proteins in the cell. Fluorescence recovery after photobleaching (FRAP) can be used to determine intracellular dynamics of proteins. A GFP fusion protein is bleached with laser light in a specific region of a cell. Observing the rate of fluorescence recovery to the bleached spot with a microscope can reveal the mechanisms governing cellular trafficking of the labeled protein.

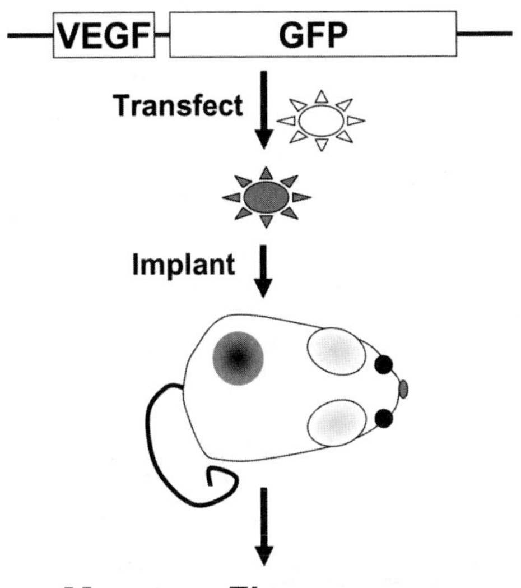

FIGURE 16.22 • Use of a genetic reporter to visualize biologic activity. The *VEGF* promoter is cloned upstream of the *GFP* gene in an expression vector and transfected into a tumor cell line. The tumor cells are implanted into a mouse and allowed to grow. The *VEGF* promoter becomes active in areas of hypoxia that will stimulate angiogenesis. Once new blood vessels are formed, hypoxia is decreased and GFP levels will decrease. The change in fluorescence reflects the change in hypoxia *in vivo*.

Two-Hybrid Screening

The two-hybrid screen, most frequently performed in the model organism *Saccharomyces cerevisiae* (budding yeast), is a powerful method for identifying factors that interact with a given protein. The cDNA for a protein of interest (POI) is cloned into an expression vector as a fusion to the DNA-binding domain of a transcription factor (GAL4-DBD) (Fig. 16.23). This construct is referred to as the " bait." A cDNA library is cloned into an expression vector as a fusion to the activation domain of a transcription factor. This library is referred to as the "prey." The

DNA-binding domain hybrid

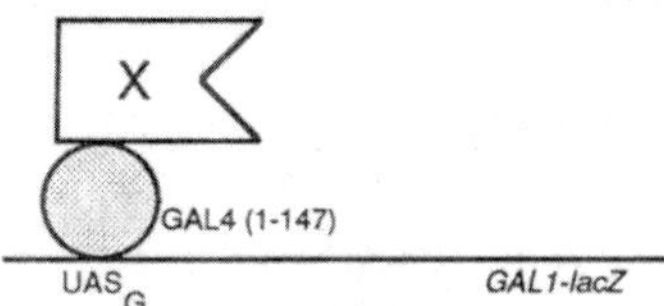

Activation domain hybrids encoded by a library

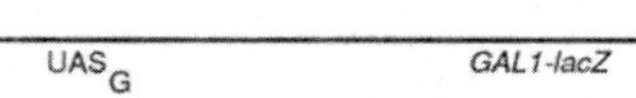

Interaction between DNA-binding domain hybrid and a hybrid from the library

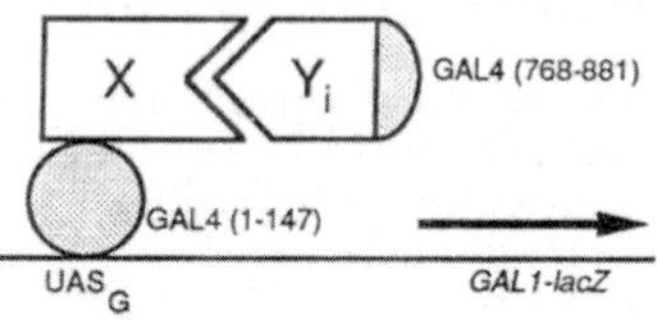

FIGURE 16.23 ● Scheme for a yeast two-hybrid screen. The cDNA for a protein X is cloned into a yeast expression vector as a fusion to the GAL4 DNA-binding domain and transformed into a line of yeast expressing the reporter gene *LacZ* under transcriptional control of GAL4 binding sites (UAS_G). Genes (Y) from a cDNA library are cloned into an expression vector as fusions to the GAL4 transcription activation domain and transformed into the *LacZ* reporter yeast line. When the two lines are crossed, any of the proteins from the cDNA library that interact with protein X will complete the GAL4 transcription factor and result in increased *LacZ* expression that can then be assayed by colorimetry. (From Chien CT, Bartel PL, Sternglanz R, Fields S: The two-hybrid system: A method to identify and clone genes for proteins that interact with a protein of interest. *PNAS* 88:9578–9582, 1991, with permission.)

bait is transformed into a line of yeast that expresses a selection reporter (HIS3, an enzyme required for histidine biosynthesis) only if a complete transcription factor binds GAL4 recognition sequences in the promoter. When the bait fusion is expressed, it binds to the HIS3 reporter with the GAL4-DBD, but cannot activate transcription and the yeast cannot grow on media lacking the amino acid histidine. If one of the "prey" constructs expresses a protein that interacts with the POI, it brings with it a transcription activation domain, HIS3 expression occurs, and a yeast colony grows on the selective media. The "prey" plasmid is recovered from the yeast colony and sequenced to identify the POI-interacting protein. The two-hybrid screen has been widely used to identify proteins that are involved in DNA repair complexes and radiation-induced signal transduction.

Proteomics

Just as the field of genomics seeks to catalog genes and transcriptional regulation, the field of proteomics seeks to catalog all of the proteins in the cell and their interactions with each other. This is a tremendous endeavor. While the genes in a genome are static, each gene can have different transcripts and splice variants, each of which may be translated into a distinct protein. Each protein may also be modified in multiple ways after translation, essentially creating a different protein with each modification. A given cell could contain several hundred thousand different proteins at a given instant. This phenomenal complexity has fed the innovation of a number of protein chemistry and detection technologies, including 2-D PAGE/MALDI-TOF, microfluidic separation, and protein microarrays. Proteomics is currently being heralded as the future of personalized medicine, where a tissue or blood sample can be used to direct the course of therapy or determine prognosis (Fig. 16.24).

Two-Dimensional Electrophoresis

Two-dimensional polyacrylamide electrophoresis (2-D PAGE) is a workhorse technique for molecular biologists studying posttranslational modification of proteins. Every protein has a distinct electrochemical charge that is a result of its unique amino acid composition. Using an electrophoresis technique known as isoelectric focusing (IEF), proteins can be separated by charge in tube gels or paper strips. The IEF tubes or strips are then laid across the top of an SDS-PAGE gel and separated by size. The gel is then stained to visualize proteins, which appear as slightly elongated spots. The identity (and modification) of the proteins in the spots can then be determined using Western blotting or mass spectrometry. High-throughput methods to automate this process are still in development.

DATABASES AND SEQUENCE ANALYSIS

Before completion of the large-scale genome-sequencing projects, when individual research groups cloned and sequenced a gene, they needed to know if the same or if homologous sequences had already been identified in other model organisms. This led to the development of databases, like

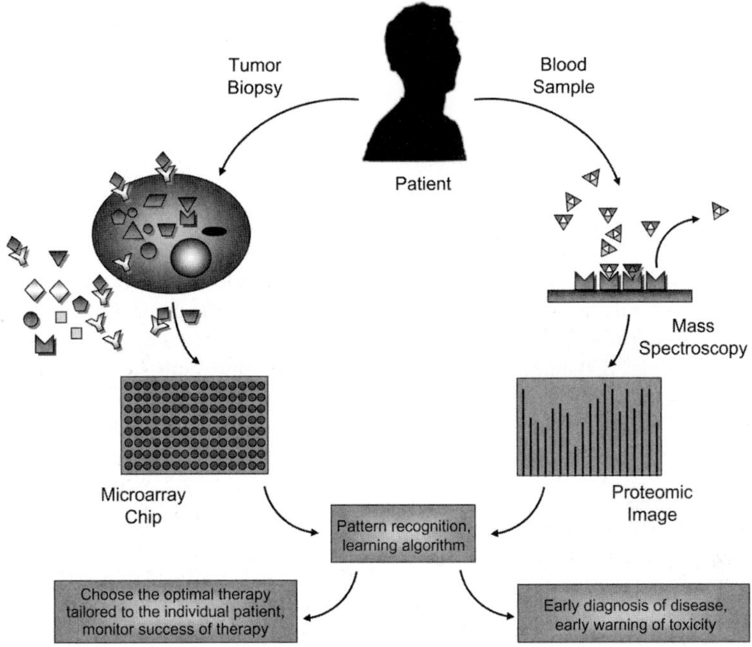

FIGURE 16.24 • Proteomics has two major uses for cancer therapy. First, it can be used to detect specific secreted proteins or fragments in the serum of cancer patients that reflect a disease state or response to therapy. Second, it can be used to determine the protein profile of tumor cells to aid in directing therapy. Proteomic microarrays are still in their early days and are in large part arrayed antibodies that detect protein binding. (Adapted from Petricoin E, Zoon K, Kohn E, Barrett J, Liotta L: Clinical proteomics: Translating benchside promise into bedside reality. *Nature Reviews Drug Discovery* 1:683–695, 2002.)

GenBank, a database at the National Center for Biotechnology Information (www.ncbi.nlm.nih.gov) for the deposition of individually cloned genomic, cDNA and protein sequences. At the same time, sequence analysis programs were developed to identify regions of similarity among different nucleotide or protein sequences. Related programs, called search engines, were developed to find similar sequences from the ever-growing list of identified genes contained in the databases. One of the most commonly used programs for finding related sequences from the genome databases is BLAST, found on the NCBI website. These approaches expanded in scope to include the genomes of organisms and the annotated coding sequences and their identified functions. It is now possible to take virtually any sequence and search for the identity of the corresponding gene in humans, mice, and an ever-expanding collection of model and agricultural organisms. Similar search engines can identify putative transcription factor binding sites from a gene promoter region or cluster proteins by related enzymatic functions. These databases and search engines are now the first step in designing strategies to study genes identified by microarray analysis.

HYPOTHETICAL PROBLEMS THAT ILLUSTRATE THE USE OF MOLECULAR TECHNIQUES TO UNDERSTAND TUMOR BIOLOGY

Hypothetical Problem #1: How Would You Identify a New Oncogene Involved in the Malignant Progression of Squamous Cell Carcinoma of the Head and Neck?

Genomic DNA is harvested from a panel of both squamous cell carcinoma tumors from the head and neck and established head and neck tumor cell lines. DNA from each sample is then processed for comparative genome hybridization (CGH) on a cDNA microarray that spans the human genome at a resolution of approximately 100 kb. At the same time, RNA from the samples is processed for expression analysis by oligonucleotide microarrays. Regions of chromosomal amplification or deletion are identified and correlated with expression changes to generate a list of genes with potential roles in the progression of squamous cell carcinoma of the head and neck. Using this approach on 100 samples, a limited number of genes with altered expression and copy number in head and neck tumors can be identified. The cDNAs of the identified genes can then be cloned in expression vectors so that they can be introduced into rodent cell lines to look for transforming potential. Transforming genes can then be analyzed further by comparing them with their normal cellular proto-oncogenes to look for mutations by DNA sequencing or single-stranded conformation polymorphisms.

Hypothetical Problem #2: How Is Your New Oncogene Regulated?

Once a gene (gene *X*) has been identified by either CGH or expression analysis as being an interesting candidate for head and neck squamous cell carcinoma progression, it is useful to characterize it at the level of RNA and protein. Information on gene *X* is gleaned from the literature and genome databases to determine suitability for further characterization. For example, a secreted protein with links to cell proliferation may be an attractive candidate for therapy. From the human genome database, the sequence of the gene *X* genomic locus and mRNA sequence can be obtained electronically. Based on this sequence information, RT-PCR primers are designed to amplify gene *X* cDNA for subcloning. This cDNA clone can also be used as a probe for Northern blotting. To determine the variation in gene *X* expression in different cancers and normal tissue, RNA from a number of different tumors and normal tissues is harvested and levels of gene *X* expression quantified by either Northern blotting, RT-PCR, or QRT-PCR. The same techniques are also applied to determine whether gene *X* is stress inducible by exposing squamous cell carcinoma–derived cell lines to a number of conditions (oxygen tensions, chemotherapeutic treatments, radiation, etc.). The transcription start site and promoter region are inferred from sequence data. High-fidelity PCR is then used to amplify parts of the genomic locus (like the promoter, 5′ untranslated region, or 3′ untranslated region) prior to insertion into a luciferase reporter vector. Alternatively, BAC clones covering the gene *X* locus can be acquired and digested with the appropriate restriction enzymes to isolate the genomic fragments of interest. Promoter-bashing techniques are employed to identify basal promoter and regulatory elements near the gene *X* promoter. Site-directed mutagenesis of the promoter-luciferase reporter confirms identity and importance of specific regulatory sequences. The sequence of the regulatory element is used to search a transcription factor database to identify the factor that regulates gene *X* expression. Chromatin immunoprecipitation (ChIP) using antibodies against the identified transcription factor and/or modified histones followed by PCR of the gene *X* promoter verifies the mechanism of gene *X* regulation in the context of a living cell.

While understanding the regulation of gene *X* RNA is interesting for academic and diagnostic purposes, characterizing gene *X* protein expression may be more useful for understanding its function. An antibody is generated against a peptide sequence in gene *X* and affinity purified. The antibody is used in immunohistochemistry experiments to determine expression and intracellular localization of gene *X* protein in squamous cell tumors. The antibody can also be used for Western blotting to quantify cellular protein expression in tumors, tissue culture, or serum. Inserting the 5′ untranslated region (5′ UTR) of gene *X* mRNA into a luciferase reporter vector reveals sequences regulating translational control (i.e., internal ribosome entry sites). Yeast two-hybrid screens are used to identify potential interacting proteins. Interaction is confirmed by immunoprecipitation of gene *X* from cell extracts and Western blotting for proteins identified from the two-hybrid screen. Posttranslational phosphorylation is determined by immunoprecipitating gene *X* from ^{32}P-labeled protein extracts followed by SDS-PAGE and autoradiography. Site-directed mutagenesis of serine, threonine, or tyrosine amino acid residues is used to determine the site of modification. Antibodies against the modified protein can also be generated for Western blot analysis and immunohistochemistry. Cellular localization and dynamics are determined by expressing gene *X* cDNA fused to a fluorescent reporter protein (e.g., GFP). Coexpressing an interacting protein fused to a different reporter (e.g., RFP) allows simultaneous detection of the two proteins by fluorescent microscopy. Countless reports in the literature have followed this approach to characterize cellular gene expression. It should be noted that this analysis will take years, but has been highly successful in understanding how oncogenes such as NF-κB work.

Hypothetical Problem #3: How Important Is Gene *X* for Tumor Formation?

The next step is to determine the functional importance of the identified gene. If gene *X* had been previously identified, the genome databases will report previously identified functions for the gene. If not, homologies to other proteins can be determined by sequence analysis and function inferred by similarities to related proteins in both humans and model organisms such as mice, *Drosophila melanogaster* (fruit flies), *C. elegans* (nematodes), or yeast. Inferred function is merely a starting point; the definitive proof in most cases is to selectively alter expression of the gene in the context of the cell or an organism. For mammalian cell studies, RNA interference is the method of choice to suppress expression of a gene. Short RNA duplexes corresponding to gene *X* are transfected into cells with liposomes. Alternatively, shRNA (stable hairpin RNA) expression constructs are stably integrated into the cellular DNA for long-term suppression. This can be done with either transfected plasmids or viral vectors. Alternatively, homologous recombination techniques can be used to create a somatic knockout in tissue culture. Decreased expression is confirmed by quantifying RNA and protein with Northern blotting, and Western blotting, respectively. The effect of gene loss is then determined in the context of growth of tumor implants in mice, response to drug treatment, cell survival, and so on. The inverse experiments are performed by overexpressing the wild-type or mutant forms of gene *X* in tissue culture. Expression of GFP-fusions are used to track cellular dynamics and interactions with other proteins (also discussed previously). Creation of a transgenic mouse expressing exogenous gene *X* illustrates the effect of overexpression in an intact organism. Luciferase or fluorescent reporter fusions enable visualization of gene *X* in whole organisms. Whereas studying the effects of gene deletions in humans is limited to epidemiological and tissue culture studies, creating a knockout mouse reveals the effects of a gene knockdown on tumor susceptibility.

Summary of Terms and Techniques

- **Restriction endonucleases** are enzymes that cleave DNA after recognizing a specific sequence. Those most useful for constructing recombinant molecules leave a "sticky" end, that is, a single-strand overhang of two to four nucleotides that can pair with a complementary strand.
- A **vector** is an autonomously replicating DNA molecule into which foreign DNA fragments are inserted and then propagated in a host cell. Vectors include plasmids, bacteriophage, bacterial artificial chromosomes, and viruses.
- A **library** is a collection of cells, usually bacteria or yeast, containing recombinant vectors, carrying DNA inserts from a different species. The inserts may be constructed by using restriction enzyme–digested genomic DNA or cDNA.
- A **host** is used to grow (i.e., to multiply) or to express a DNA fragment containing a gene of interest.
- In **agarose gel electrophoresis**, DNA or RNA molecules can be separated according to size by causing them to move through a matrix composed of purified agar under the influence of an electrical field.
- **Polymerase chain reaction (PCR)** is a procedure that enzymatically amplifies the number of copies of a DNA sequence, up to several thousand base pairs, through repeated replication by DNA polymerase. (A DNA polymerase is an enzyme that catalyzes the addition of nucleotides to a growing DNA molecule.) PCR has been adapted to analyze RNA expression through the use of **reverse transcription PCR** (RT-PCR). Use of a specialized thermocycler enables **quantitative real-time PCR** (qRT-PCR), a very sensitive PCR technique that enables high-throughput nucleic acid analysis and quantitation.
- Genes may be cloned by **functional complementation** (i.e., putting a functional version of a defective gene into cells to correct the phenotype associated with the defect) by **hybridization** to **oligonucleotide probes, microarrays, or sequencing**.
- **Positional cloning** is a strategy used to clone a gene for which no information is available about its protein product. This is true of most human inherited diseases, and so this strategy has been used to clone, for example, many of the tumor-suppressor genes.
- **Comparative genomic hybridization** (CGH) is a more modern refinement that starts by identifying regions of chromosomal

(continued)

Summary of Terms and Techniques (Continued)

duplication or deletion. The genes in the abnormal region can then be analyzed by expression or functional studies to identify candidate genes in the region.

- RNA transcription can be measured by **Northern blotting**, **RT-PCR** methods, or hybridization to microarrays.
- The **microarray** is a useful platform for studying gene expression changes (RNA), gene aneuploidy (CGH), and DNA–protein interactions (ChIP-chips). The primary advantage of the microarray is the sheer number of sequences that can be analyzed at one time.
- Genes may be "mapped," that is, their position in the genome identified by ***in situ* hybridization**, by **Southern blotting**, by **chromosome walking** if a flanking sequence is identified, and by **contiguous mapping** if sequence data from large adjacent regions of the genome are aligned.
- The completion of whole **genome-sequencing projects** for humans, mice, fruit flies, nematodes, and yeast has made the above process gene mapping largely obsolete. Virtually any genomic sequence can now be accessed from the international databases. **BACs** used in the sequencing projects can be acquired for use in cloning experiments.
- Once a gene is cloned, it can be **sequenced** by one of several methods, the most common of which is the **chain termination method**. Use of fluorescently labeled dyes on the dideoxynucleotides enables automated laser scanners to acquire sequence from a single lane.
- The amino acid sequences within a protein can be determined from the corresponding DNA sequence using the known genetic triplet code.
- A newly acquired sequence can be compared with the international database to seek **homologies** with known genes or proteins.
- Structural variations in DNA caused by point mutations, deletions, or insertions can result in restriction fragments of different lengths, which can often be detected by Southern blotting. These are known as **restriction fragment length polymorphisms**, which can be used as genetic markers to map genes to specific chromosomal locations and identify aberrant genes causing disease.
- A mutation involving only a single base-pair difference between two short single-stranded DNA molecules can be detected by the technique of **single-stranded conformation polymorphism**.
- A useful approach to studying a gene of interest is to introduce it into a cell or organism (typically a mouse), overexpress it, and observe the biologic effect.
- Another useful approach for studying the function of an identified gene is to "knock out" expression of a gene. This can be done by using either **homologous recombination** or **RNA interference** (RNAi).
- Genetic reporters are useful tools for studying biologic phenomena like transcriptional regulation, protein dynamics, and intracellular location. Reporters have easily assayable activities (light emission, fluorescence, or colorimetric substrates), providing flexibility to suit a given experimental system.
- The **chromatin immunoprecipitation** (ChIP) assay can be used to study promoter function in intact cells, either to identify transcription factor interactions with promoters or to dissect mechanisms of regulation. DNA purified by ChIP can be analyzed individually by PCR or by hybridization to promoter microarrays.
- The field of **proteomics** seeks to define the quantities and interactions of the vast number of proteins in a given cell at a given instant in time. Proteomics uses established technology like **2-D electrophoresis**, **Western blotting**, **immunoprecipitation**, and mass spectroscopy but uses more advanced high-throughput technology to expedite the process.
- Protein–protein interactions can be identified by **coimmunoprecipitation** or **two-hybrid** analysis. Fluorescent protein fusion proteins are useful tools for further study of intracellular interactions and dynamics.

GLOSSARY OF TERMS

alleles Alternate forms of a gene or DNA sequence on the two homologous chromosomes of a pair.

amino acids The 20 basic building blocks of proteins.

amplify To increase the number of copies of a DNA sequence by inserting into a cell *in vivo* or *in vitro* by the polymerase chain reaction.

anneal To pair complementary DNA or RNA sequences, via hydrogen bonding, to form a double-stranded polynucleotide.

antibiotic A compound such as ampicillin, that inhibits the growth of or kills microorganisms.

antibiotic resistance The ability of a microorganism to disable an antibiotic or prevent transport of the antibiotic into the cell.

antibody An immunoglobulin protein produced by B lymphocytes that binds to a specific antigen.

monoclonal antibodies Immunoglobulin molecules of single-epitope specificity.

polyclonal antibodies A mixture of immunoglobulin molecules secreted against a specific antigen, each recognizing a different epitope.

antigen Any foreign substance that elicits an immune response by stimulating the production of antibodies.

bacterial artificial chromosome A vector used to clone DNA fragments of up to 300,000 bp, which contains the minimum chromosomal sequences needed to replicate at a low copy number in bacteria.

bacteriophage A virus that infects bacteria. Altered forms are used as vectors for cloning DNA.

bacterium A single-cell prokaryotic organism.

base pair A pair of complementary nitrogenous bases in a DNA molecule: adenine–thymine or guanine–cytosine. It is also a measure of the length of DNA.

B lymphocyte A white blood cell responsible for production of antibodies in the humoral immune response.

cDNA See **DNA**.

cDNA library See **library**.

centromere The central portion of the chromosome to which the spindle fibers attach during mitotic and meiotic division.

chromatin immunoprecipitation The selective purification of transcription factors bound to DNA that provides information on transcriptional regulation inside cells.

codon A group of three nucleotides that specifies the addition of one of the 20 amino acids during translation of mRNA into a polypeptide.

initiation codon The mRNA sequence AUG, which codes for methionine and which initiates translation.

termination (stop) codon Any of three mRNA sequences (UGA, UAG, UAA) that do not code for an amino acid and thus signal the end of protein synthesis.

colony A group of identical cells derived from a single ancestor cell.

contig A collection of DNA sequences that overlap at portions of their ends.

digest To cut DNA molecules with one or more restriction endonucleases.

DNA (deoxyribonucleic acid) An organic acid composed of four nitrogenous bases (adenine, thymine, cytosine, and guanine) linked via sugar and phosphate units. DNA is the genetic material of most organisms and usually exists as a double-stranded molecule in which two antiparallel strands are held together by hydrogen bonds between adenine–thymine and cytosine–guanine base pairs.

cDNA (complementary DNA) DNA synthesized from an RNA template using reverse transcriptase.

DNA fingerprint A unique pattern of DNA fragments identified by Southern hybridization or by polymerase chain reaction.

DNA polymorphism Two or more alternate forms of a chromosomal locus that differ in nucleotide sequence or have variable numbers of repeated nucleotide units.

DNA sequencing Procedures for determining the nucleotide sequence of a DNA fragment.

electrophoresis The technique of separating charged molecules in a matrix to which an electrical field is applied.

agarose gel electrophoresis Electrophoresis in which a matrix composed of purified agarose is used to separate larger DNA and RNA molecules (ranging from 100 to 20,000 nucleotides).

polyacrylamide gel electrophoresis Electrophoresis through a matrix composed of synthetic polymer, used to separate small DNA or RNA molecules (up to 1,000 nucleotides) or proteins.

pulsed-field electrophoresis Electrophoresis in which the current is alternated between pairs of electrodes set at angles to one another to separate very large DNA molecules (up to 10 million nucleotides).

two-dimensional gel electrophoresis Separation of cellular proteins in one dimension based on changes in protein charge followed by separation based on size using 2-D PAGE.

electroporation Process in which high-voltage pulses of electricity are used to open pores in the cell membrane through which foreign DNA can pass.

Escherichia coli A bacterium that is found in the human colon and is widely used as a host for molecular cloning experiments.

ethidium bromide A fluorescent dye used to stain DNA and RNA that intercalates between nucleotides and fluoresces if exposed to ultraviolet light.

exon That portion of a gene expressed in mature mRNA.

flanking region The DNA sequences extending on either side of a specific locus or gene.

gene A locus on a chromosome that encodes a specific protein or several related proteins.

dominant gene A gene whose phenotype is expressed if it is present in a single copy.

recessive gene A gene whose phenotype is expressed only if both copies of the gene are mutated or missing.

gene amplification The presence of multiple copies of a gene. This is one mechanism by which proto-oncogenes are activated to result in neoplasia.

gene expression The process of producing a protein from its DNA- and mRNA-coding sequences.

genetic code The three-letter code that translates a nucleic acid sequence into a protein sequence.

genome The genetic complement contained in the chromosomes of a given organism.

GFP Green fluorescent protein—a naturally fluorescent protein that can be used as a bioluminescent marker in cell culture studies and in mice.

hybrid The offspring of two parents differing in at least one genetic characteristic.

hybridization The hydrogen bonding of complementary DNA or RNA sequences to form a duplex molecule.

Northern blotting A procedure in which RNA fragments are transferred from an agarose gel to a nitrocellulose filter, where the RNA is then hybridized to a radioactive probe.

Southern blotting A procedure in which DNA restriction fragments are transferred from an agarose gel to a nitrocellulose filter, where the denatured DNA is then hybridized to a radioactive probe.

immunoprecipitation Detection of cellular proteins or protein complexes by the binding to antibodies immobilized on beads.

library A collection of cells (usually bacteria or yeast) that have been transformed with recombinant vectors carrying DNA inserts from a single species.

cDNA library A library composed of complementary copies of cellular mRNAs (i.e., the exons without the introns).

expression library A library of cDNAs whose encoded proteins are expressed by specialized vectors.

genomic library A library composed of fragments of genomic DNA.

ligase An enzyme that catalyzes a reaction that links two DNA molecules by the formation of a phosphodiester bond.

ligation The process of joining two or more DNA fragments.

microarray A slide coated with thousands of oligonucleotides or cDNAs that is hybridized with labeled cRNA from cells to monitor expression changes.

microinjection Introducing DNA into a cell using a fine microcapillary pipette.

mitosis Replication of a cell to form two identical daughter cells.

mutation An alteration in DNA structure or sequence of a gene.

point mutation A change in a single base pair in a gene.

nucleotide A building block of DNA and RNA.

complementary nucleotides Members of the pairs adenine–thymine, adenine–uracil, and guanine–cytosine that have the ability to hydrogen-bond to each other.

oncogene A gene that contributes to cancer formation when mutated or inappropriately expressed.

cellular oncogene (proto-oncogene) A normal gene that if mutated or improperly expressed contributes to the development of cancer.

myc A nuclear oncogene involved in immortalizing cells.

ras An oncogene that can induce the malignant phenotype; it converts guanosine triphosphate to guanosine diphosphate, a step in signal transduction.

plaque A clear spot on a lawn of bacteria or cultured cells where cells have been lysed by viral infection and replication.

plasmid A circular DNA molecule that is capable of autonomous replication and may typically carry one or more genes encoding antibiotic resistance.

polymerase An enzyme that catalyzes the addition of multiple subunits to a substrate molecule.

DNA polymerase An enzyme that synthesizes a double-stranded DNA molecule using a primer and DNA as a template.

RNA polymerase An enzyme that transcribes RNA from a DNA template.

***Taq* polymerase** A heat-stable DNA polymerase used in the polymerase chain reaction.

polymerase chain reaction A procedure that enzymatically amplifies a DNA sequence through repeated replication by DNA polymerase.

quantitative real-time PCR A very sensitive PCR technique to quantify changes in DNA or RNA accurately in a high-throughput manner.

positional cloning A strategy to clone a gene where the protein product is not known.

primer A short DNA or RNA fragment annealed to single-stranded DNA.

probe A single-stranded DNA (or RNA) that has been radioactively labeled and is used to identify complementary sequences.

reading frame A series of triplet codons beginning from a specific nucleotide.

open reading frame A long DNA sequence, uninterrupted by a stop codon, that encodes part or all of a protein.

recombinant DNA The process of cutting and recombining DNA fragments.

restriction endonuclease (enzyme) An enzyme that cleaves DNA after recognizing a specific sequence.

restriction fragment length polymorphism Differences in nucleotide sequence between alleles that result in restriction fragments of varying lengths.

retrovirus A type of virus whose genome consists of RNA and which utilizes the enzyme reverse transcriptase to copy its genome into a DNA intermediate, which integrates into the chromosome of a host cell.

reverse transcriptase An enzyme that synthesizes a complementary DNA strand from an RNA template.

RNA (ribonucleic acid) An organic acid composed of repeating nucleotide units of adenine, guanine, cytosine, and uracil and whose ribose components are linked by phosphodiester bonds.

cRNA (complementary RNA) RNA synthesized from a cDNA template using T7 RNA polymerase for the purpose of microarray hybridization.

messenger RNA (mRNA) The class of RNA molecules that copies the genetic information from DNA, in the nucleus, and carries it to ribosomes, in the cytoplasm.

transfer RNA (tRNA) Small RNA molecules that transfer amino acids to the ribosomes during protein synthesis.

Saccharomyces cerevisiae Brewer's yeast.

selectable marker A gene whose expression makes it possible to identify cells that have been transformed or transfected with a vector containing the marker gene. It is usually a gene for resistance to an antibiotic.

shRNA A complementary hairpin expressed from a vector that causes target cellular RNA to be degraded.

siRNA A short inhibitory double-stranded RNA molecule that causes target cellular RNA to be degraded.

somatic cell Any cell other than a germ cell in the body of an organism, possessing a set of multiploid chromosomes.

stem cell An undifferentiated cell that gives rise to one or more types of specialized cells.

sticky end A single-stranded nucleotide sequence produced if a restriction endonuclease cleaves off-center in its recognition sequence.

stringency Reaction conditions, such as temperature, salt, and pH, that dictate the annealing of single-stranded DNA/DNA, DNA/RNA, and RNA/RNA hybrids. At high stringency, duplexes form only between strands with perfect one-to-one complementarity. Lower stringency allows annealing between strands with less than a perfect match between bases.

template An RNA or single-stranded DNA molecule on which a complementary nucleotide strand is synthesized.

transcription The process of creating a complementary RNA copy of DNA.

transfection The uptake and expression of foreign DNA by cultured eukaryotic cells.

transformation In higher eukaryotes, the conversion of cultured cells to a malignant phenotype. In prokaryotes, the natural or induced uptake and expression of a foreign DNA sequence.

translation The process of converting the genetic information of an mRNA on ribosomes into a polypeptide.

vector An autonomously replicating DNA molecule into which foreign DNA fragments are inserted and then propagated in a host cell.

Western blotting The detection of proteins and modifications of proteins immobilized on membranes by probing with specific antibodies.

yeast artificial chromosome A vector used to clone DNA fragments of up to 400,000 bp, which contains the minimum chromosomal sequences needed to replicate in yeast.

BIBLIOGRAPHY

Aguirre AJ, Brennan C, Bailey G, et al.: High-resolution characterization of the pancreatic adenocarcinoma genome. *Proc Natl Acad Sci USA* 101(24):9067–9072, 2004

Altschul SF, Gish W, Miller W, Myers EW, Lipman DJ: Basic local alignment search tool. *J Mol Biol* 215(3):403–410, 1990

Arya M, Shergill I, Williamson M, et al.: Basic principles of real-time quantitative PCR. *Expert Rev Mol Diagn* 5(2):209–219, 2005

Berns K, Hijmans EM, Mullenders J, Brummelkamp TR, et al.: A large-scale RNAi screen in human cells identifies new components of the p53 pathway. *Nature* 428:431–437, 2004

Brummelkamp TR, Bernards R: New tools for functional mammalian cancer genetics. *Nature Reviews Cancer* 3:781–789, 2003

Capecchi MR: Altering the genome by homologous recombination. *Science* 244(4910):1288–1292. 1989

Chalfie M, Tu Y, Euskirchen G, Ward WW, Prasher DC: Green fluorescent protein as a marker for gene expression. *Science* 263(5148):802–805, 1994

Chien C, Bartel P, Sternglanz R, Fields S: The two-hybrid system: A method to identify and clone genes for proteins that interact with a protein of interest. *Proc Natl Acad Sci USA* 88(21):9578–9582, 1991

Copeland NG, Jenkins NA, Court DL: Recombineering: A powerful new tool for mouse functional genomics. *Nat Rev Genet* 2:769–779, 2001

Das PM, Ramachandran K, vanWert J, Singal R: Chromatin immunoprecipitation assay. *Biotechniques* 37:961–969, 2004

Eckel-Passow JE, Hoering A, Therneau TM, Ghobrial I: Experimental design and analysis of antibody microarrays: Applying methods from cDNA arrays. *Cancer Res* 65:2985–2989, 2005

Elbashir SM, Harborth J, Lendeckel W, Yalcin A, Weber K, Tuschl T, et al.: Duplexes of 21-nucleotide RNAs mediate RNA interference in cultured mammalian cells. *Nature* 411(6836):494–498, 2001

Fire A, Xu S, Montgomery MK, Kostas SA, Driver SE, Mello CC: Potent and specific genetic interference by double-stranded RNA in *Caenorhabditis elegans. Nature* 391(6669):806–811, 1998

Fukumura D, Xavier R, Sugiura T, et al.: Tumor induction of *VEGF* promoter activity in stromal cells. *Cell* 94(6):715–725, 1998

Fukumura D, Xu L, Chen Y, Gohongi T, Seed B, Jain RK: Hypoxia and acidosis independently up-regulate vascular endothelial growth factor transcription in brain tumors in vivo. *Cancer Res* 61(16):6020–6024, 2001

Gordon JW, Ruddle FH: Integration and stable germ line transmission of genes injected into mouse pronuclei. *Science* 214:1244–1246, 1981

Gordon JW, Scangos GA, Plotkin DJ, BapRbosa JA, Ruddle FH: Genetic transformation of mouse embryos by microinjection of purified DNA. *Proc Natl Acad Sci USA* 77:7380–7384, 1980

Hardiman G: Microarray platforms—comparisons and contrasts. *Pharmacogenomics* 5(5):487–502, 2004

Joyner AL, Skarnes WC, Rossant J: Production of a mutation in mouse En-2 gene by homologous recombination in embryonic stem cells. *Nature* 338:153–156, 1989

Kuo M, Allis C: *In vivo* cross-linking and immunoprecipitation for studying dynamic Protein: DNA associations in a chromatin environment. *Methods* 19(3):425–433, 1999

Lander ES, Linton LM, Birren B, et al.: Initial sequencing and analysis of the human genome. *Nature* 409(6822):860–921, 2001

Micklos DA, Freyer GA: *DNA Science: A First Course in Recombinant DNA Technology.* Burlington, NC, Cold Spring Harbor Laboratory Press and Carolina Biological Supply Company, 1990

Murray JM, Carr AM, Lehmann AR, Watts Z: Cloning and characterization of the *rad9* DNA repair gene from *Schizosaccharomyces pombe Nucleic Acids Res* 19:3525–3531, 1991

Olive KP, Tuveson DA, Ruhe ZC, Yin B, Willis NA, Bronson RT, Crowley D, Jacks T: Mutant p53 gain of function in two mouse models of Li-Fraumeni syndrome. *Cell* 119:847–60, 2004

Palapattu GS, Bao S, Kumar TR, Muatzuk MM: Transgenic mouse models for tumor suppressor genes. *Cancer Detect Prev* 22:75–86, 1998

Palmiter RD, Brinster RL, Hammer RE, et al.: Dramatic growth of mice that develop from eggs microinjected with metallothionein-growth hormone fusion genes. *Nature* 300:611–615, 1982

Palmiter RD, Chen HY, Brinster RL: Differential regulation of metallothionein-thymidine kinase fusion genes in transgenic mice and their offspring. *Cell* 29:701–710, 1982

Petricoin E, Zoon K, Kohn E, Barrett J, Liotta L: Clinical proteomics: Translating benchside promise into bedside reality. *Nature Reviews Drug Discovery* 1:683–695, 2002

Sambrook J, Fritsch EF, Maniatis T: *Molecular Cloning: A Laboratory Manual*, 2nd ed. New York, Cold Spring Harbor Press, 1989

van Duin M, deWit J, Odijk H, et al.: Molecular cloning and characterization of the human excision repair gene *ERCC-I:* cDNA cloning and amino acid homology with the yeast DNA repair gene. *Radio Cell* 44:913–923, 1986

Venter JC, Adams MD, Myers EW, et al.: The sequence of the human genome. *Science* 291(5507):1304–1351, 2001

Vijg J, van Steeg H: Transgenic assays for mutations and cancer: Current status and future perspectives. *Mutat Res* 400:337–354, 1998

Watson JD, Gilman M, Witkowski J, Zoller M: *Recombinant DNA,* 2nd ed. New York, Scientific American Books, 1992

Yu JY, DeRuiter SL, Turner DL: RNA interference by expression of short-interfering RNAs and hairpin RNAs in mammalian cells. *Proc Natl Acad Sci USA* 99(9):6047–6052, 2002

Yun Z, Maecker HL, Johnson RS, Giaccia AJ: Inhibition of *PPARγ2* gene expression by the HIF-1-regulated gene *DEC1/Stra13:* A mechanism for regulation of adipogenesis by hypoxia. *Dev Cell* 2:331–341, 2002

Zimmer A, Gruss P: Production of chimaeric mice containing embryonic stem (ES) cells carrying a homoeobox *Hox 1.1* allele mutated by homologous recombination. *Nature* 338:150–153, 1989

CHAPTER 17

Cancer Biology

Tissue homeostasis depends on the regulated cell division and self-elimination (programmed cell death) of each of its constituent members except its stem cells. In fact, a tumor arises as a result of uncontrolled cell division and failure for self-elimination. One can consider cancer as a Darwinian-like process whereby the fittest cells reproduce to become the dominant population of a tumor. Alterations in three groups of genes are responsible for the deregulated control mechanisms that are the hallmarks of cancer cells:

- Proto-oncogenes are components of signaling networks that act as positive growth regulators in response to mitogens, cytokines, and cell-to-cell contact. A gain-of-function mutation in only one copy of a proto-oncogene results in a dominantly acting oncogene that often fails to respond to extracellular signals.
- Tumor-suppressor genes are also components of the same signaling networks as proto-oncogenes, except that they act as negative growth regulators. They modulate proliferation and survival by antagonizing the biochemical functions of proto-oncogenes or responding to unchecked growth signals. In contrast to oncogenes, inactivation of both copies of tumor-suppressor genes is required for loss of function in most cases.

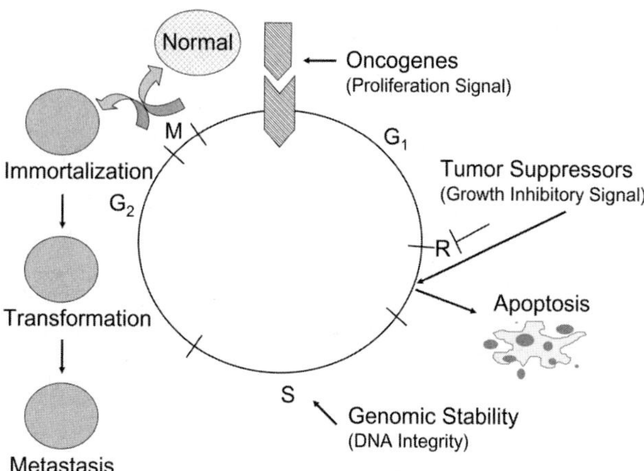

FIGURE 17.1 ● The process of malignant transformation results from mutations in three groups of genes: gain-of-function mutations that activate oncogenes, loss-of-function mutations that inactivate tumor-suppressor genes, and loss of activity of DNA stability (e.g., repair) genes that increase the probability for genomic instability. This figure depicts how the stimulatory effects of oncogenes on the cell cycle are opposed by the inhibitory effects of tumor-suppressor genes on the cell cycle that can lead to apoptosis. R indicates the restriction point that is regulated by the *p53* and *pRb* tumor-suppressor genes. The consequences of oncogene activation and tumor-suppressor gene and DNA integrity gene inactivation are immortalization, transformation, and metastasis.

- DNA stability genes form a class of genes involved in both monitoring and maintaining the integrity of DNA. Loss of these genes results in defective sensing of DNA lesions as well as improper repair of the damaged template.

The malignant progression from normal tissue to tumor to metastasis occurs in a number of discrete "steps" over a period of time. These steps, which are the result of mutations, deletions, or gene changes in the three groups of genes described here, may occur spontaneously as a consequence of random errors or result from exposure to agents as diverse as chemical mutagens, ionizing radiations, ultraviolet light, and viruses and provide a growth or survival advantage that allows the cells to become the clonal origin of the tumor. To summarize, tumor evolution results from the accumulation of gene mutations that arise in a single cell that has suffered a disruption in its regulatory mechanisms for proliferation, self-elimination, immortalization, and genetic stability. This is illustrated in Figure 17.1.

MECHANISMS OF CARCINOGENESIS

A single genetic alteration that leads to the activation of an oncogene or loss of a tumor-suppressor gene does not by itself lead to the formation of a solid tumor. Instead, carcinogenesis appears to be a multistep process with multiple genetic alterations occurring over an extended period of time; at least, that is how it appears. Sometimes these genetic alterations are carried in the germ line, as, for example, in the cancer-predisposing syndrome retinoblastoma; however, heritable mutations are rare. Most alterations that lead to cancer are acquired in the form of somatic mutations: chromosomal translocations, deletions, inversions, amplifications, or simple point mutations.

Initially, it was thought that cancer was the result of deregulated growth signals by oncogenes, a concept supported by increased proliferation in many types of cancer. In the last decade, the finding that many cancers possess diminished apoptotic (programmed cell death) programs or loss of cell-cycle control has led to the concept that mutations in proto-oncogenes and tumor-suppressor genes that inhibit apoptosis provide a selective growth advantage to a premalignant cell that allows it to clonally expand. Mutations in DNA stability genes increase the rate of acquiring genetic mutations that will result in a malignant tumor. Thus, while tumor cells are considered clonal in origin, most tumors contain heterogeneous populations of cells that differ in their ability to repopulate the tumor or form metastasis. In fact, only a small percentage of tumor cells possess the ability to form a tumor, leading to the concept that tumors possess "stem cells" and that elimination of these stem cells is essential for controlling tumor growth.

ONCOGENES

The first demonstration that a tumor was initiated by a cellular component found in tumor cells but not normal cells was shown by Rous in the early 1900s. His landmark studies demonstrated that cell-free extracts derived from chicken sarcomas could cause a new sarcoma if injected into healthy chickens. In the 1970s, with the advent of molecular biology, several groups identified the etiological agent for sarcoma formation in chickens as an RNA virus, designated the Rous sarcoma virus (RSV), which belongs to a group of viruses designated retroviruses—viruses whose genomes are

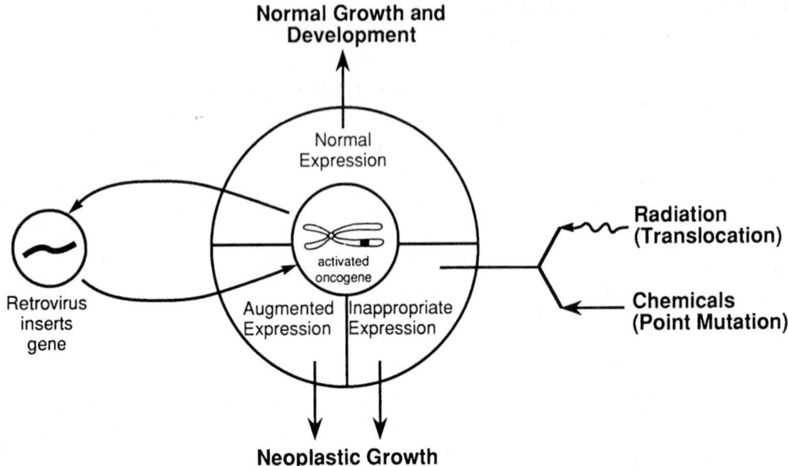

FIGURE 17.2 ● How the concept of oncogenes provides a ready answer for how agents as diverse as viruses, radiations, and chemicals all can induce tumors that are essentially indistinguishable one from another. The retrovirus inserts a gene; a chemical may activate an endogenous oncogene by a point mutation; radiation may do the same by causing, for example, a translocation. (Adapted from Bishop JM: Cellular oncogene retroviruses. *Ann Rev Biochem* 52:301–354, 1983, with permission.)

composed of RNA. Thus, oncogenes were first discovered from a study of retroviruses that cause cancers in animals. Although the virus had been identified, it still remained to be elucidated how this retrovirus causes a sarcoma, since another virus belonging to this same group of RNA viruses, avian leukosis virus (ALV), does not transform cells in culture or induce sarcomas. Analysis of the genomes of ALV and RSV revealed that RSV contains approximately 1,500 more base pairs of DNA than ALV. It was hypothesized, therefore, that these extra base pairs of DNA in the RSV genome are responsible for the tumorigenic activity. This was supported by the observation that deletion mutants of RSV that are missing this 1,500-bp region lose their transformation potential but can still replicate and produce viral progeny normally. This led to the conclusion that the transforming activity and replicative activity of RSV are encoded by genetically distinct regions of the virus and that only a small portion of the RSV genome is needed for transformation.

From these early studies, several important conclusions could be derived: (1) Cancer can be caused by a genetically transmissible agent—in the case of chicken sarcoma, by a retrovirus containing a unique piece of genetic information that was latter designated the *src* gene; (2) only a certain region of a retrovirus is needed for transformation; and (3) the region of the viral genome necessary for transformation is not involved in the normal replicative life cycle.

Huebner and Todaro later proposed that cancer-causing viral genes such as *src* are normally inactive but can be activated when they recombine with a retroviral genome. Once they do so, they pass from being a benign proto-oncogene (i.e., c-*src*) to a malignant form (v-*src*) capable of causing cancer when introduced into the appropriate host cell. Although we now know that viruses represent only one of several mechanisms that cause the deregulated expression of a proto-oncogene, these studies helped to define oncogenes as mutant forms of normal cellular genes that are altered in expression and/or function by various agents, including radiation, chemicals, and viruses. Consequently, very different agents produce tumors that are indistinguishable one from another. This is illustrated in Figure 17.2.

MECHANISMS OF ONCOGENE ACTIVATION

Although many mechanisms are involved in oncogene activation, transcriptional deregulation by overexpression or abnormal expression of the mRNA of a proto-oncogene is a common theme. At least four mechanisms exist for oncogene activation in human neoplasms (Fig. 17.3).

Retroviral Integration through Recombination

Retroviral integration of proto-oncogene sequences in retroviral genomes occurs through two possible recombinational mechanisms. In the first,

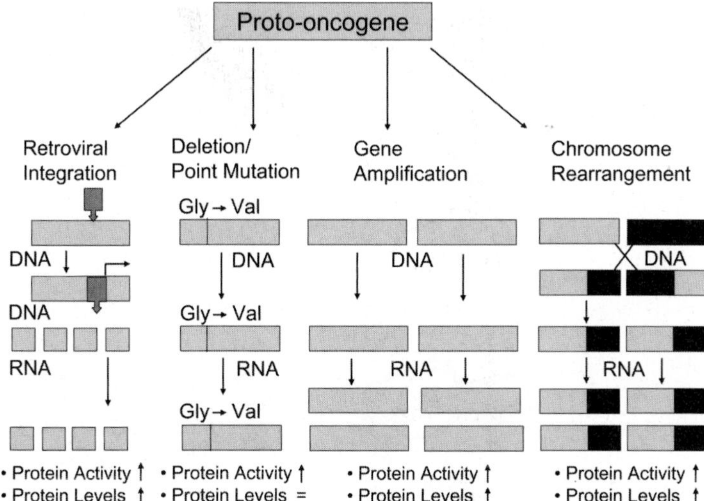

FIGURE 17.3 ● Four basic mechanisms of how a proto-oncogene can become an activated oncogene. Retroviral integration in close proximity to a proto-oncogene results in transcriptional control of the proto-oncogene by the viral promoter, resulting in increased proto-oncogene protein and activity. Deletion or point mutations in the proto-oncogene result in increased activity of the proto-oncogene without necessarily changing transcription or protein levels of the proto-oncogene. Increased copy number of a proto-oncogene by gene amplification results in increased transcription, protein levels, and activity of the proto-oncogene. Chromosome translocation results in an altered proto-oncogene product that can have increased transcription, protein levels, and activity. All of these alterations in a proto-oncogene that occur at the DNA level manifest themselves at the protein level as increased activity and in some cases increased protein levels.

mRNAs from a proto-oncogene recombine with viral genomic RNAs. During the recombination process, the proto-oncogene mRNA becomes deregulated as it comes under the control of the viral promoter, termed LTR. However, the probability of RNA recombination events between proto-oncogene mRNA and viral mRNA generating an oncogenic retrovirus is quite low and undermines the importance of this mechanism.

A second more probable mechanism is as follows: First a retroviral genome integrates in close proximity to a proto-oncogene, where the proto-oncogene is under the transcriptional control of the retrovirus LTR promoter. Then the viral and proto-oncogene sequences become closely associated through a DNA recombination event that permits the production of mRNAs that contain both viral and proto-oncogene sequences. In this scenario, the proto-oncogene becomes transcriptionally deregulated as it is under the control of the viral promoter LTR. In addition, it can acquire mutations in its coding sequence. Although the proto-oncogene can become mutated during the recombination process, the key point is that its deregulated expression by the viral LTR increases its expression and promotes cell growth.

DNA Mutation of Regulatory Sites

The union of the technique for gene transfer with mouse transformation assays facilitated the isolation of human oncogenes that were activated by DNA mutation. Transfection of human DNA into immortalized but untransformed mouse cells was first used to isolate the H-*ras* oncogene from bladder carcinoma cells. The key to this approach is that only transformed cells possess the ability to grow in soft agar (Fig. 17.4). The implicit assumption is that a specific gene (or more than one) is responsible for causing the bladder carcinoma and that it will act in a dominant fashion to induce a tumor. Indeed, multiple groups were successful in isolating the H-*ras* oncogene by this approach.

Several steps are needed for the molecular cloning of an oncogene from transformed rodent cells using the rodent fibroblast transformation assay. First, human DNA containing the transforming oncogene is transfected into mouse cells, and then DNA from the transformed mouse cells is serially transfected to reduce the amount of human DNA that is not associated with the transforming oncogene. After several rounds of transfection, the DNA is isolated from a soft agar colony and

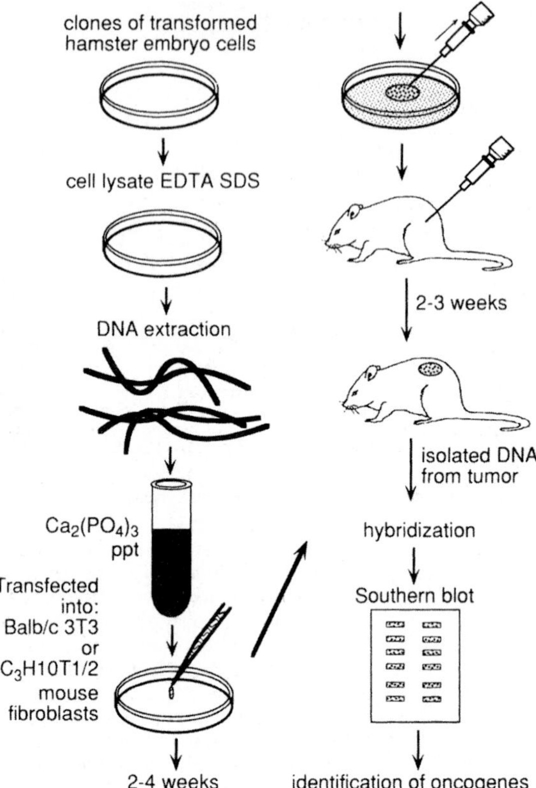

FIGURE 17.4 ● Schematic diagram of a typical DNA transfection protocol, in which oncogenes can be isolated from cells transformed *in vitro* by either radiation or chemical carcinogens. DNA sequences are then characterized using Southern blot hybridization.

digested with restriction enzymes to make a genomic DNA library. The library is then screened with a human-specific repetitive probe that does not cross-react with mouse DNA, thereby identifying human sequences in a mouse background. Clones that possess human repetitive sequences are then isolated and digested with restriction enzymes to identify a similar-length fragment that is common to all transformants. Finally, DNA from the clones is transfected into mouse cells to confirm its oncogenic potential. If the oncogene is present in this genomic clone, then a significant percentage of the transfected mouse cells should be transformed when compared with transfecting genomic DNA from untransformed cells.

Perhaps the prototypical example of oncogene activation by DNA mutation is the H-*ras* oncogene. The H-*ras* oncogene was isolated by the approach just described, and its DNA sequence was compared with its normal cellular counterpart. At first comparison, there did not seem to be any difference between oncogenic and proto-oncogenic forms. However, because H-*ras* is a relatively small oncogene, it was possible to sequence the entire gene to rigorously search for small mutations. It did not take long to find the difference between the two forms of the gene. The transforming, oncogenic H-*ras* gene possesses a single base-pair mutation that changes the 12th amino acid from glycine to valine. This single DNA mutation is responsible for changing H-*ras* from a benign proto-oncogene into a malignant oncogene. We now know that mutations in codons 13 and 61 will also produce oncogenic H-*ras* genes that are constitutively locked in an active state.

Gene Amplification

Oncogene amplification occurs through bridge breakage fusion cycles in anaphase during mitosis. In contrast to the other mechanisms discussed that involve transcriptional deregulation as a key mechanism of oncogene activation, gene amplification represents an alternative means of increasing proto-oncogene expression by increasing the number of DNA copies of the proto-oncogene. Gene amplification can result in an increased number of copies of extrachromosomal molecules called

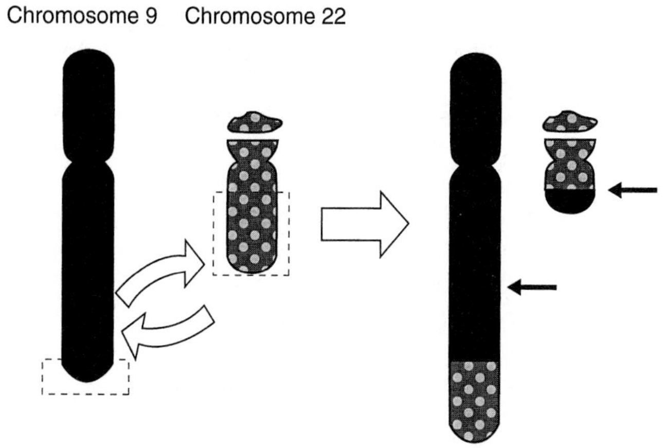

Chromosome 9 Chromosome 22

FIGURE 17.5 • A symmetric translocation between chromosomes 9 and 22 brings together the *bcl* and *abl* genes to form a fusion gene associated with over 90% of cases of chronic myelogenous leukemia (CML).

double minutes or can result in intrachromosomal amplified regions called homogeneously staining regions (HSRs), both of which are detectable by fluorescence *in situ* hybridization or Giemsa banding of chromosomes. The N-*myc* oncogene is a classic example of an oncogene amplified in leukemia, neuroblastoma, and breast cancer.

Chromosome Translocation

It had long been known that tumors possessed abnormal karyotypes. However, the chromosome content of many solid tumors is unstable, making it difficult to determine which cytogenetic alterations are causative for tumorigenesis and which are the consequence of the neoplastic process. The first real breakthrough in identifying tumor-specific chromosome alterations occurred in the late 1950s when Dr. Peter Nowell found a consistent shortened version of chromosome 22 in individuals afflicted with chronic myelogenous leukemia (CML). Because many patients with CML possess an abnormal chromosome 22 in their leukemic cells, this was a strong indication that a specific chromosome alteration is involved in the pathogenesis of this malignancy. With the advent of more sophisticated cytogenetic and molecular techniques, it was discovered that this shortened version of chromosome 22 is due to a symmetric translocation with chromosome 9. It was hypothesized, therefore, that the translocation between chromosomes 9 and 22 gives rise to CML. Further molecular analysis revealed that the *bcr* gene on chromosome 9 translocates in front of the *abl* gene on chromosome 22, producing a fusion transcript with abnormal expression (Fig. 17.5).

With the recent advent of molecular cytogenetics—that is, fluorescent *in situ* hybridization (FISH)—many translocation partners have been identified. In fact, a common strategy has been to use proto-oncogenes, which chromosomally map near translocation breakpoints, as markers to identify potential translocation partners. Although numerous translocation breakpoints have been identified in hematopoietic neoplasms, few consistent translocations have been found in solid-tissue tumors. The reason for this is still unclear, but may be attributed to the fact that hematopoietic cancers require fewer alterations for neoplasia than solid tumors. Table 17.1 provides examples of the chromosomal changes that result in oncogene activation and the associated human malignancies. Interestingly, there are no known examples of oncogenes activated by retroviruses in human malignancies.

MUTATION AND INACTIVATION OF TUMOR-SUPPRESSOR GENES

The Retinoblastoma Paradigm

Oncogenes result from a mutation, deletion, or alteration in the expression of one copy of a gene. Thus, oncogenes are dominant genes, because a mutation in only one copy will cause their activation, even though the other copy of the gene is unchanged. This concept led to speculation that another class of genes, termed "anti-oncogenes," suppress the effect of oncogenes on transformation and tumor formation. The existence of tumor-suppressor genes was supported by cell fusion studies between tumor cells and normal cells and by the family history studies of people afflicted with inherited cancer-prone disorders such as retinoblastoma or Li–Fraumeni syndrome. Although one mutated version of an oncogene is sufficient to drive malignant progression, one functional copy of a tumor-suppressor gene is sufficient to suppress transformation, suggesting that both copies of a tumor suppressor gene must be inactivated to inhibit tumor growth (Fig. 17.6). Insight into the mechanism of tumor-suppressor gene inactivation came from Knudson's epidemiological studies of families in

TABLE 17.1

Examples of Chromosomal Changes Leading to Oncogene Activation and Their Associated Murine or Human Malignancies[a]

Oncogene	Chromosomal Change	Cancer
int-1	Proviral insertion	Murine breast carcinoma
int-2	Proviral insertion	Murine breast carcinoma
pim-1	Proviral insertion	Murine T cell lymphoma
N-*ras*	Point mutation (1)	Melanoma
K-*ras*	Point mutation (12)	Pancreas carcinoma
H-*ras*	Point mutation (11)	Colon carcinoma
neu	Point mutation (17)	Neuroblastoma
N-*myc*	Gene amplification (8)	Neuroblastoma
L-*myc*	Gene amplification (8)	Lung carcinoma
neu	Gene amplification (17)	Breast carcinoma
EGFR	Gene amplification (7)	Squamous cell carcinoma
bcr-abl	Translocation (9–22)	Chronic myelogenous leukemia
c-*myc*	Translocation (8–14)	Burkitt's lymphoma
c-*myc*	Translocation (2–8)	Burkitt's lymphoma
c-*myc*	Translocation (8–22)	Burkitt's lymphoma
bcl-2	Translocation (14–18)	Diffuse large B cell lymphoma

[a] Human oncogenes activated by retroviruses have not yet been found in human malignancies, only murine cancers.

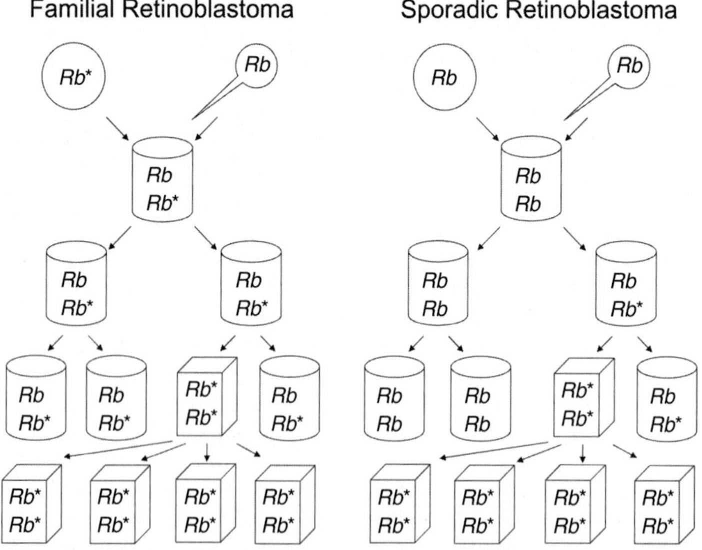

FIGURE 17.6 ● *Rb* mutations in familial and sporadic retinoblastoma. In familial retinoblastoma, one normal allele (*Rb*) and one mutated allele (*Rb**) are inherited from either parent, resulting in a heterozygous individual containing *Rb/Rb** retinal cells. Subsequent mutation in any retinal cell inactivates the remaining normal *Rb* allele, leading to loss of growth control and expansion of the homozygous mutant *Rb*/Rb** retinal cells that leads to retinoblastoma. In sporadic retinoblastoma, two normal *Rb* alleles are inherited from each parent. First, a mutation inactivates one copy, resulting in heterozygous *Rb/Rb** retinal cells. A subsequent mutation within the same retinal cell inactivates the remaining copy of normal *Rb*, leading to loss of growth control and expansion of homozygous *Rb*/Rb** retinal cells that leads to retinoblastoma. (Illustrating the concepts proposed by Knudson AG: Mutation and cancer: Statistical study of retinoblastoma. *Proc Natl Acad Sci USA* 68:820–823, 1971.)

which retinoblastoma appeared to be inherited in an autosomal dominant manner. Patients with familial retinoblastoma develop bilateral or multifocal disease at an earlier age than patients with sporadic retinoblastoma. Based on these observations, Knudson proposed that in the inherited form of retinoblastoma, individuals possess a germ-line mutation of the retinoblastoma gene (*Rb*) in all the cells of their body, but inactivation of one *Rb* allele does not give rise to retinoblastoma. Thus, the disease appeared to be autosomal dominant because individuals are born with one mutated allele. However, a second mutation in a retinal cell is required to develop retinoblastoma. In the sporadic form of the disease, an individual has to acquire two *Rb* mutations in the same retinal cell to develop retinoblastoma. The "two-hit hypothesis" by Knudson provided a genetic basis to understand the differences in inherited and sporadic mutations in the onset of tumors and to advance the concept that both alleles of a tumor-suppressor gene need to be inactivated to promote tumor development. Thus, tumor-suppressor genes are recessive genes that require the inactivation of both functional gene copies before malignancies develop, whereas loss of one functional copy results only in increased cancer susceptibility. In addition, it is often the case that the same tumor-suppressor gene involved in hereditary cancer syndromes, such as retinoblastoma, is also inactivated in other forms of cancer. The *Rb* gene itself has now been implicated in several other human cancers, which indicates that it may play a generalized role in tumor growth suppression in a variety of tissues. For example, patients who are cured of familial retinoblastoma are at increased risk of osteosarcoma, small-cell lung cancer, and breast cancer; although the loss of the *Rb* gene alone is sufficient for retinoblastoma, further changes are required for the development of these other tumors.

The Li–Fraumeni Paradigm

The Li–Fraumeni syndrome (LPS) is a rare autosomal dominantly inherited disease that predisposes individuals to develop osteosarcomas, soft-tissue sarcomas, rhabdomyosarcomas, leukemias, brain tumors, and carcinomas of the lung and breast (Fig. 17.7). Initial attempts to identify the genetic mutations that underlie LPS were unsuccessful because of the rarity of the syndrome and the high mortality of the patients. The major insight into the underlying cause of Li–Fraumeni came when it was found that mice that overexpress a mutant version of the *p53* tumor-suppressor gene in the presence of the wild-type *p53* gene develop a spectrum of tumors similar to that seen in Li–Fraumeni patients. Sequencing of *p53* in affected family members revealed germ-line missense mutations in the *p53* tumor-suppressor gene located on chromosome 17p13 that resulted in its inactivation, and tumors derived from affected individuals had lost the remaining wild-type allele of *p53*. Similar to retinoblastoma, loss or inactivation of both wild-type copies of *p53* is needed for tumor formation.

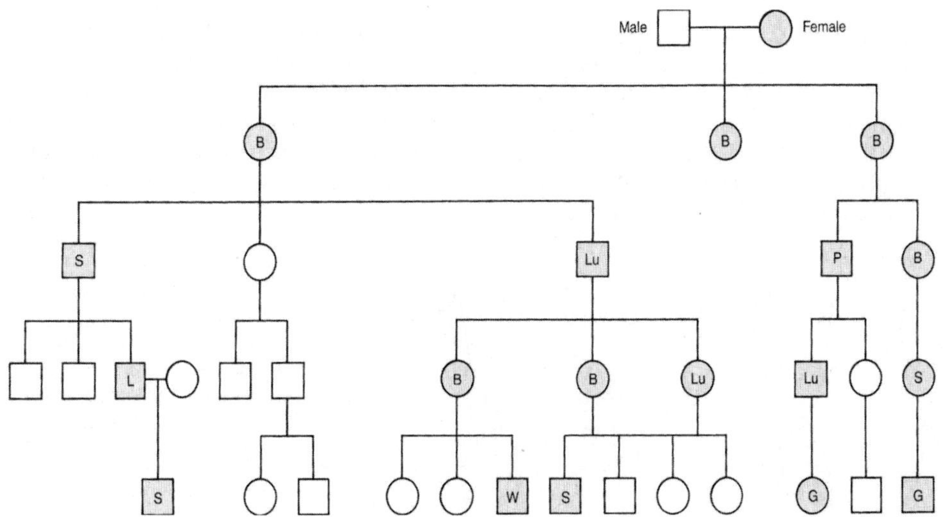

FIGURE 17.7 • Pedigree analysis of familial cancer history of Li–Fraumeni syndrome. Symbols: B = breast cancer; G = glioblastoma; L = leukemia; Lu = lung cancer; P = pancreatic cancer; S = sarcoma; W = Wilms' tumor. (From Li FP, Fraumeni JF: Prospective study of a family cancer syndrome. *J Amer Med Assoc* 247:2692–2694, 1982.)

TABLE 17.2

Examples of Cancer Predisposition Genes and Their Associated Syndromes

Tumor-Suppressor Gene	Syndrome	Tumor
Rb	Retinoblastoma	Retinoblastoma
WT1	Familial Wilms' tumor	Wilms' tumor
NFI	Neurofibromatosis type 1	Neurofibroma, sarcoma
NF2	Neurofibromatosis type 2	Schwannoma, meningioma
APC	Familial adenomatosis polyposis	Tumor of colon, stomach, intestine
p53	Li–Fraumeni Syndrome	Breast, lung, brain tumors, sarcoma
VHL	von Hippel-Lindau disease	Tumor of kidney, adrenal
E-CAD	Familial gastric cancer	Tumor of stomach, breast
PTCH	Gorlin syndrome	Basal cell carcinoma
PTEN	Cowden syndrome	Hamartoma
MEN1	Multiple endocrine neoplasia	Tumor of pituitary, pancreas, parathyroid

However, functional loss of one germ-line inherited copy of mutant *p53* accelerates the onset of spontaneous tumor formation. Therefore, Li–Fraumeni patients follow a similar paradigm as retinoblastoma patients in developing spontaneous tumors, but unlike retinoblastoma, in which germ-line mutations mainly give rise to retinal tumors, loss of *p53* results in a wide spectrum of tumors. Table 17.2 provides examples of other cancer predisposition genes and their associated syndromes.

SOMATIC HOMOZYGOSITY

How are recessive tumor-suppressor genes lost? Cytogenetic studies are used to identify chromosomal changes in peripheral blood lymphocytes or fibroblasts from cancer patients, especially those with a family history of cancer, to identify chromosomal rearrangements or deletions. At the subchromosomal level, genome-wide linkage analysis is used to determine that a certain chromosome region is tightly linked with cancer predisposition. Both copies of a suppressor gene in the sporadic form of retinoblastoma and other solid tumors may result from two independent allelic mutations, but in practice, it occurs more often by the process of *somatic homozygosity*. The steps appear to be as follows: One chromosome of a pair is lost, a deletion occurs in the remaining chromosome, and the chromosome with the deletion replicates. Instead of having each of the two alleles contributed by different parents, the cell has both alleles from the same parent, with loss of a vital piece containing the tumor-suppressor gene (Fig. 17.8). This process has been documented for chromosome 13 in the case of retinoblastoma, chromosome 11 in Wilms' tumor, chromosome 3 for small-cell lung cancer, and chromosome 5 for colon cancer. Most interesting of all, perhaps, is the case of astrocytomas, in which somatic homozygosity is observed for chromosome

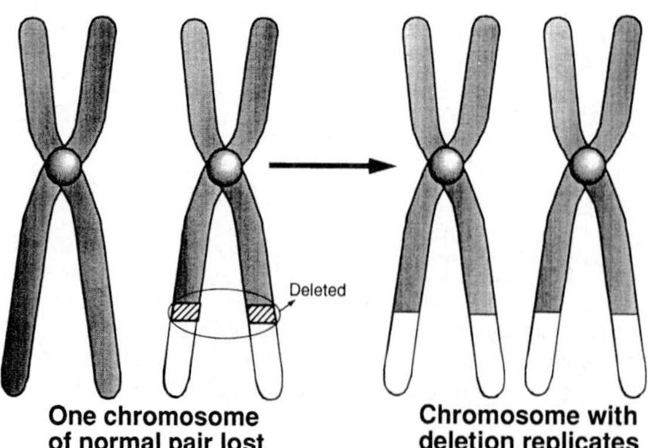

FIGURE 17.8 • The process of somatic homozygosity. In a normal cell, there are two copies of each chromosome, one inherited from each parent. For a given suppressor gene to be inactivated, the copy must be lost from both chromosomes. This could, of course, occur by independent deletions from the two chromosomes; but in practice, it is more common for a single deletion to occur in one chromosome while the second chromosome is lost completely. The remaining chromosome, with the deletion, then replicates. The cell is thus homozygous, rather than heterozygous, for that chromosome.

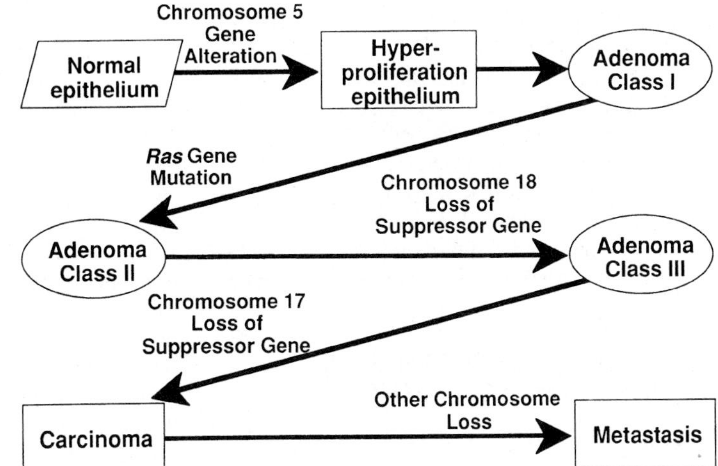

FIGURE 17.9 • Cancer has long been thought to be a multistep process and has been described with operational terms such as *initiation*, *promotion*, and *progression*. In at least one human malignancy, namely, colon cancer, the molecular events during the progress of the disease have been identified. (Based on the work of Vogelstein.)

10 in grade II and III astrocytoma and for both chromosomes 10 and 17 for grade IV glioblastoma.

THE MULTISTEP NATURE OF CANCER

Perhaps the most pervasive dogma in cancer research is that carcinogenesis is a multistage process. The implication is that there are a number of distinct events that may be separated in time. This idea is almost 70 years old and is exemplified by the skin cancer experiments in mice that introduced the concepts of *initiation, promotion, and progression* as stages in tumor development.

Genetic analysis of cells from solid tumors, too, suggests alterations, mutations, or deletions in multiple signaling genes, either oncogenes or suppressor genes; 6 to 12 mutations have been suggested for the formation of a carcinoma. In the case of colorectal cancer, a model has been proposed that correlates a series of chromosomal and molecular events with the changes in the histopathology of normal epithelium during the multistage formation of colorectal cancer and metastatic carcinoma. This concept is illustrated in Figure 17.9.

A more general model of the series of events in carcinogenesis is shown in Figure 17.10. The first event, from whatever cause (including ionizing radiation), causes a mutation in a gene in one of the families responsible for the stability of the genome. This leads to a mutator phenotype, so that with many cells dividing, multiple mutations are likely in cancer-associated genes, both oncogenes and tumor-suppressor genes. This in turn leads to

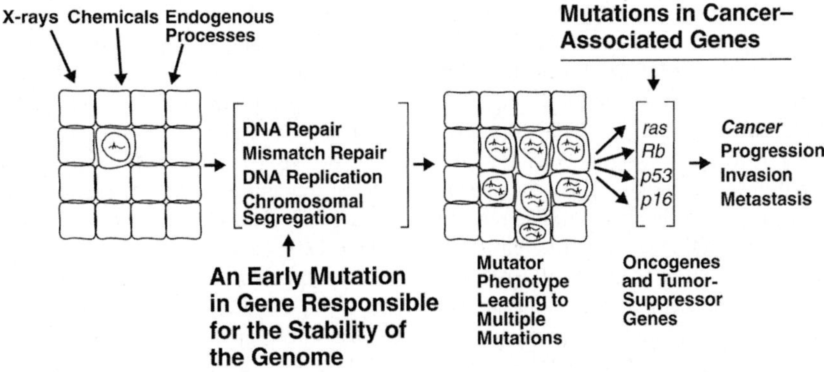

FIGURE 17.10 • Illustrating the multistep nature of carcinogenesis and the concept of the mutator phenotype. The first step in carcinogenesis by radiation or any other agent may be a mutation in one of the gene families responsible for the stability of the genome. This may be a DNA repair gene, a mismatch repair gene, or a gene in a family as yet unidentified. This leads to the mutator phenotype, with multiple mutations possible in both oncogenes and tumor-suppressor genes. This leads to a series of steps that result in an invasive metastatic cancer. Not all the same mutations need to be present in every case.

progression of the cancer and ultimately its invasive and metastatic properties.

Therefore, it is not surprising that restoration of one copy of a tumor-suppressor gene is sometimes not sufficient to restore tumor-suppressor activity, as solid tumors accumulate mutations that can make them refractory to the restoration of a single tumor-suppressor gene. Although tumor-suppressor genes are functionally quite different from oncogenes, they modulate similar cellular targets as oncogenes.

FUNCTION OF ONCOGENES AND TUMOR-SUPPRESSOR GENES

The myriad of genetic and epigenetic changes that drive tumor evolution is a systems biology problem in which cells can be thought of as circuits, where an alteration of the circuit can lead to increased output, decreased output, complete loss of output, or no change. Therefore, cancer biologists attempt to determine how a specific gene, when mutated, alters normal tissue function. To understand how oncogenes and tumor-suppressor genes lead to neoplasia, we need to understand how each of these circuits impacts normal cellular physiology. What cellular functions are disrupted by oncogene activation and tumor-suppressor gene inactivation, and how do these disrupted functions affect the differentiation, growth, and death of cells? What follows is a description of the general categories of cell functions that are perturbed by deregulation of these two classes of genes during malignant progression.

Deregulated Proliferation

The loss of proliferative control of cancer cells is evident to all who study cancer. In fact, the earliest concept suggested by tumor biologists was that cancer was a disease of uncontrolled proliferation. Untransformed cells respond to extracellular growth signals known as mitogens through a transmembrane receptor that signals to intracellular circuits that increase growth. Thus, the growth factor, the receptor, and the intracellular circuits can all lead to self-sufficiency when deregulated. Typically, one cell secretes a mitogenic signal to stimulate the proliferation of another cell type. For example, an epithelial cell can secrete a signal to stimulate fibroblasts to proliferate. In contrast to untransformed cells, transformed cells have become autonomous in regulating their growth by responding to the mitogenic signals they themselves produce. In this manner, they use an autocrine circuit to escape the need for other cell types. For example, mesenchymal cells are responsive to transformation by v-*sis*, as they possess receptors for PDGF, and breast epithelial cells are responsive to *int-2*, as they possess receptors for FGF.

If overexpression of growth factors can lead to uncontrolled proliferation, then continuous activation or overexpression of growth-factor receptors will do the same. Several well-known oncogenes, such as v-*erb-2* (*HER-2/neu*) and v-*fms*, encode growth-factor receptors. These receptors are mutated at their amino terminal residues so that they no longer require their respective growth factor (ligand) to signal induction of their kinase activity. Growth-factor receptors can structurally be divided into extracellular ligand-binding domains, transmembrane-spanning domains, and intracellular kinase domains. Although mutations have been found in all three domains, mutations in the ligand-binding domains are a common alteration that results in constitutive kinase activity that transduces the signal for the cell to proliferate. In addition to structural alterations in the receptor, some tumors overexpress growth-factor receptors that make them hyperresponsive to physiologic levels of growth-factor stimulation. In contrast to mitogenic-responsive growth-factor receptors, a second class of receptors that transmit signals from the extracellular matrix can also regulate proliferation. Integrin receptors are the prototypical example of this class of regulators that transmit signals from different components of the ECM to signal proliferation or quiescence.

There are numerous intracellular circuits that transduce the signal from the cell surface to the nucleus of the cell. The Src, Ras and Abl proteins are all members of this group. By and large, most members of this group are tyrosine–kinases or serine/threonine–kinases. Src and Abl are tyrosine–kinases located on the cytoplasmic side of the cell membrane. H-ras, K-ras and N-ras are a family of GTP-binding proteins also located on the cytoplasmic side of the cell membrane and are the most frequently mutated oncogene family in human cancers. The Ras-Raf-ERK, Ras-RalGDS-Ral, and Ras-PI(3)K-Akt-TOR pathways play critical roles in transducing signals from growth-factor receptors at the cell surface to the nucleus in untransformed cells. Oncogenic forms of ras bypass the normal growth regulatory signals of a cell by being locked in an "on" state, obviating the need for external signals from growth factors to activate them (Fig. 17.11).

Failure to Respond to Growth-Restrictive Signals

If signal transduction cascades initiate at the cell membrane, then they end in the nucleus. Normally,

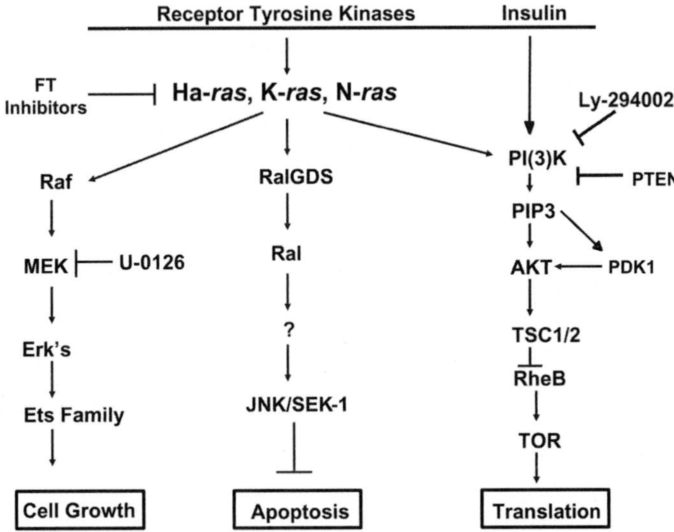

FIGURE 17.11 ● The Ras family (H-Ras, K-Ras and N-Ras) are proteins that act as GDP/GTP-regulated binary switches that reside at the inner surface of the plasma membrane and act to relay extracellular ligand-stimulated signals to cytoplasmic signaling cascades. However, oncogenic forms of Ras lose their responsiveness to growth receptor tyrosine–kinases and consitituively activate cascades of serine–threonine kinases that control cell proliferation, inhibit apoptosis, and increase protein translation. These pathways are depicted in a linear fashion, but are more complex and are regulated by positive and negative feedback loops. This illustration depicts three direct effectors of Ras that have been shown to mediate these events. Ras stimulates proliferation by activating the Raf–MEK–Erk pathway that phosphorylates and activate the Ets transcription factor that leads to increased levels of cyclin D_1, mRNA, and protein. Increased levels of cyclin D_1 result in increased Rb phosphorylation and transition of cells from G_1 to S phase of the cell cycle. A second direct effector of Ras, RalGDS, is a guanine nucleotide exchange factor that activates Ral A and B GTPases and promotes tumor cell survival through the JNK/SEK (Jun kinase/stress kinase) pathway. The third major pathway that Ras directly regulates is the PI(3)K pathway. This pathway has long been known to be important in regulating cell growth through insulin signaling. Like Raf and RalGDS, oncogenic forms of Ras increase PI(3)K activity that leads to increased phosphorylation of the lipid kinase PIP3, which in turn inhibits the negative regulation of TOR by TSC1/2 and RheB. Increased TOR leads to increased translational initiation of mRNAs that possess a structured 5′ region known as a "cap." This is an oversimplified illustration, because there are at least three other signaling pathways that lie downstream of Ras. The Ras pathway can be disrupted using pharmacologic inhibitors of farnesyltransferases (FT), PI(3)K (Ly-294002), or MEK (U-0126). (Adapted from Marianne Powell with permission.)

the majority of cells in the body are at rest in a nonproliferative state (G_0). The oncogenic activation of these nuclear oncogenes stimulates the cell into the synthetic phase (S phase), where it duplicates its genetic material before cell division. Nuclear control proteins that regulate entry into S phase include transcription factors, such as c-myc, c-rel, c-jun and c-fos, and cell-cycle regulatory proteins, such as E2F and cyclin D_1 (PRAD1). These nuclear proto-oncogenes can work as transcription factors by binding to DNA in a sequence-specific manner and forming complexes with themselves or other proteins that will increase mRNA transcription of genes such as *cyclin D* that promotes cell division.

To understand how tumor cells evade antiproliferative signals, one must appreciate how the cell cycle is regulated—in particular, the G_1 phase. It is during a cell's transit through the G_1 phase that it makes the decision to continue to the S phase and duplicate its genetic material or enter into a reversible state of quiescence (reversible growth arrest) or enter a permanent state of senescence (irreversible growth arrest). The Rb family of proteins are the most critical determinants of the fate of a G_1 phase cell. When Rb protein is in a hypophosphorylated state, Rb protein blocks progression into S phase by sequestering E2F transcription factors that regulate the expression of genes that are essential for the transition from G_1 to S phase. As previously discussed, the ECM can signal cell proliferation through integrin receptors. In addition, it can also produce antiproliferative signals through the secreted protein TGF-β. At the molecular level, TGF-β inhibits Rb protein phosphorylation and prevents the release and activation of the E2F family of transcription factors. It does this through the induction of inhibitors such as p21 and $p15^{INK4B}$ that inhibit the activity of the kinases that are essential to phosphorylate Rb protein. Thus, loss of *Rb* or failure to induce p21 and $p15^{INK4B}$ will aid cells in escaping antiproliferative signals.

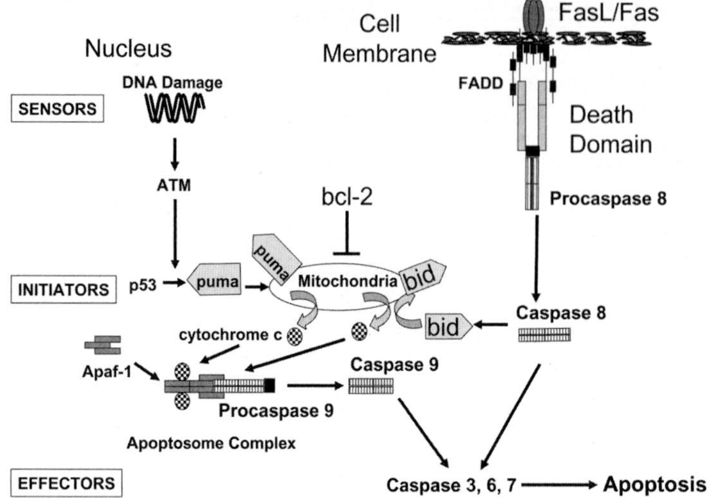

FIGURE 17.12 • Two major pathways that mediate cell death. Pathways initiate at either the cell membrane with a death receptor or in the nucleus with the detection of DNA-damaging stresses. Each pathway can be divided into sensors (e.g., Fas ligand binding to Fas receptor), initiators (e.g., caspases 8 and 9) and effectors (e.g., caspases 3, 6, and 7). See text for further details.

In addition to extracellular antiproliferation signals, endogenous proteins that down-regulate signal-amplifying kinases are also important in keeping signal transduction cascades in check. For example, the NF1 protein is a GTPase-activating protein that facilitates the hydrolysis of GTP by Ras. When Ras protein is complexed with GDP, it is inactive; when it is bound to GTP, it is active. Individuals afflicted with neurofibromatosis lack NF1 protein and have lower levels of GTPase activity and more Ras protein complexed with GTP, resulting in a more active Ras protein. Therefore, lack of NF1 protein activity will result in enhanced activity of Ras protein similar to what is found in Ras-transformed cells as already described. The NF1 protein and the Ras protein are excellent examples of how a tumor-suppressor gene and an oncogene work in unison to control a signal transduction pathway.

Failure to Commit Suicide (Apoptosis)

Two major pathways that mediate cell death emanate either from the cell membrane or from the mitochondrion (Fig. 17.12). The signals transmitted by each pathway results in the activation of intracellular cysteine proteases, termed caspases, that cleave a diverse and ever-increasing number of substrates, including themselves, at aspartic acid residues. Caspases can broadly be divided into initiator caspases and effector caspases. The binding of ligands such as Fas to specific death receptors on the cell surface induces receptor activity and the recruitment of the initiator procaspase 8. The recruitment of procaspase 8 proteins in close proximity to each other results in active caspase 8 and effector caspases, such as caspases 3, 6, and 7, that are responsible for the ultrastructural changes in the cell. In response to mitochondrial-dependent cell death, activation of initiator caspases (e.g., caspase 9) is achieved by proteolytic cleavage of their inactive pro-forms through their recruitment and interaction with specific adapter proteins. The adapter proteins are in turn regulated by the mitochondria through the release of cytochrome *c*. The release of cytochrome *c* from the mitochondria is controlled by the Bcl-2 protein family, which is composed of proapoptotic regulators such as Bax, Bak, Bid, and Bim and antiapoptotic family members Bcl-2, Bcl-xl, and Mcl-1. The *bcl-2* oncogene is the prototypical example of a membrane-associated oncogene whose overexpression protects the cell from death-inducing stimuli by a wide variety of agents.

How does Bcl-2 protect cells from undergoing apoptosis? Both proapoptotic and antiapoptotic Bcl-2 family members can form dimers with themselves (homodimers) or with other family members (heterodimers). This ability to form dimers with a pro-death-promoting family member has been proposed as one mechanism of how Bcl-2 prevents apoptotic cell death that is signaled by the release of cytochrome *c* from the mitochondria. In the cytoplasm, cytochrome *c* forms a complex with the adapter protein Apaf-1, and together they recruit the inactive form of the initiator caspase, Procaspase 9. In this complex, Caspase 9 becomes activated and in turn activates effector caspases such as Caspases 3, 6, and 7 through proteolytic cleavage. Cell lines deficient in Caspases 3 and 9 exhibit substantially reduced levels of apoptosis during development and in response to exogenous stress-inducing stimuli (Fig. 17.13).

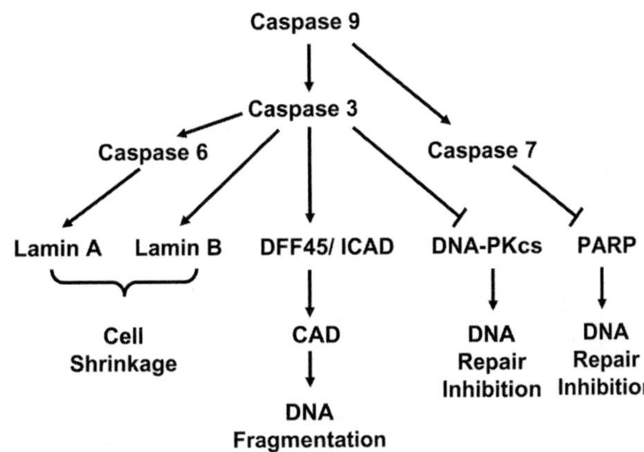

FIGURE 17.13 • Examples of caspase substrates that are responsible for the cellular ultrastructural changes that result in classic apoptotic morphology. Caspases degrade Lamin and structural components of the cytoskeleton, fragment DNA, and inhibit DNA repair processes by degrading DNA repair proteins. Abbreviations: ICAD = inhibitor of caspase-activated DNase; DNA-PK = DNA-directed protein kinase; PARP = poly-ADP ribose polymerase.

The *p53* tumor-suppressor gene is an important modulator of oncogene-induced apoptosis. Levels of p53 are kept low in unstressed cells through the binding of a specific E3-like ubiquitin ligase, Mdm2. Binding of Mdm2 to the N-terminus of p53 results in the complex being shuttled to the cytoplasm, where it is quickly degraded by the proteosome. However, in response to a variety of stresses, including ionizing radiation, serum starvation, and hypoxia, p53 protein levels increase both through protein stabilization and increased protein synthesis. Stabilization of p53 in response to stress is thought to occur through a number of mechanisms, including prevention of Mdm2 binding and phosphorylation of p53. Once stabilized, p53 is a powerful proapoptotic molecule capable of transcriptionally activating gene expression by sequence-specific DNA binding to regulatory sequences. Transcriptional targets of p53 that induce apoptosis include *bax, puma, noxa,* and *perp* and provide a link between the tumor-suppressor activity of p53 and apoptosis. This list of p53-regulated apoptotic genes is always growing and very dependent on the cell type and stress. Many of the mutations in the *p53* gene found in human tumors are found within the DNA-binding domain, highlighting the importance of this region to the role of p53 as a tumor suppressor and its ability to induce apoptosis. However, recent reports in the literature indicate a new role for p53 in the cytoplasm and specifically at the mitochondria, where it may function directly to release cytochrome *c* to initiate the caspase cascade and apoptosis, bypassing the need for its transcriptional activity.

Seemingly paradoxical to its role in proliferation and oncogenic transformation is the fact that overexpression of the *myc* oncogene primes cells for apoptotic cell death under growth-restrictive conditions generated by nutrient deprivation or

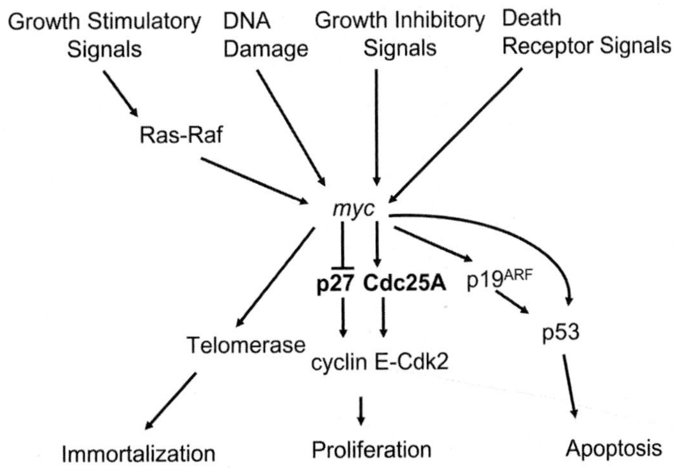

FIGURE 17.14 • The *myc* oncogene can stimulate cell proliferation and primes the cell for apoptotic cell death. Depending on the cellular context, *myc* can stimulate proliferation through the activation of cyclin E–cdk2, which phosphorylates pRb and drives cells into S phase in response to mitogenic signals, and *myc* can prime cells for apoptosis by increasing the levels of p53 through ARF (p19). Also, *myc* can promote the inactivation of the cyclin–cdk inhibitor p27 as well as increase Cdc25A phosphastase activity. Also *myc* can induce immortalization through regulating telomerase activity. Therefore, *myc* is the prototypical example of how one oncogene can affect cell proliferation, cell death, and immortalization.

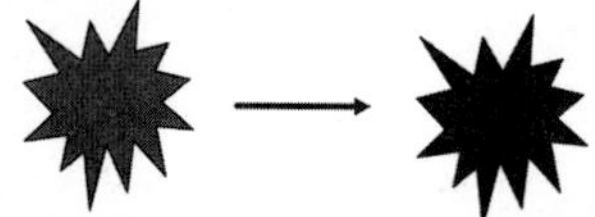

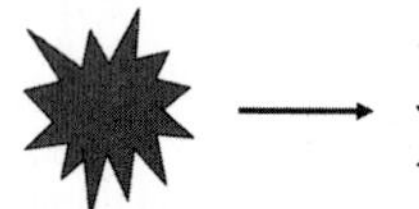

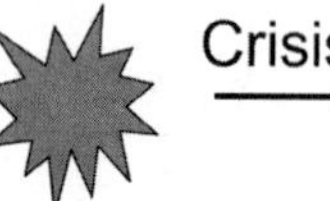

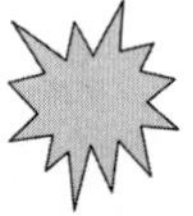

FIGURE 17.15 • *In vitro* senescence has been classically defined in fibroblasts that go through a defined number of generations before they stop proliferating. This permanent arrest has been termed senescence. It is characterized biochemically by increased SA-β-galactosidase activity in the lysosomes and shortened telomeres (telomere restriction fragments). Primary cells on the way to immortalization must overcome the crisis of shortened telomeres by reactivating telomerase and losing the p53 and pRb (p16 loss) control over the cell cycle and apoptosis to survive.

low-oxygen conditions (Fig. 17.14). It is this paradox that has set forth the hypothesis that *myc* deregulation results in a cellular state where increased proliferation or apoptotic death are both equally possible, depending on the cellular microenvironment and the activity of certain crucial genetic determinants, such as the *p53* tumor-suppressor gene. Evidence has accumulated that oncogenes such as *myc* and the adenovirus *E1A* gene increase p53 protein stabilization and sensitize cells to killing by growth-restrictive conditions. Loss of *p53* through mutation or functional inactivation severely attenuates the sensitivity of these same oncogene-expressing cells to stress-induced apoptosis. Analysis of cells deficient in $p19^{ARF}$ (a cell-cycle inhibitor protein) indicates that myc signals to p53 through $p19^{ARF}$. Loss of $p19^{ARF}$ attenuates the sensitivity of *myc*-expressing cells to apoptosis even in the presence of wild-type p53, suggesting that myc needs to signal $p19^{ARF}$ to activate p53-dependent apoptosis. Furthermore, genetic analysis of tumor cells indicates that they possess either *p53* mutations or $p19^{ARF}$ mutations, but rarely both. Implicit in this observation is that *myc* deregulation favors proliferation and that a growth-restrictive state induced by DNA damage, lack of nutrients, or oxygen starvation is needed to substantially tip the cellular balance to favor apoptotic cell death. Therefore, increased sensitivity to growth-restrictive conditions that induce apoptotic cell death will result in a selective pressure for the loss or inactivation of $p19^{ARF}$, *p53*, or other components of this stress-induced pathway. In addition to inactivating *p53*, overexpression of antiapoptotic proteins such as Bcl-2 can accelerate tumor expansion. Myc and bcl-2 cooperate in lymphomagenesis *in vivo*, suggesting that overcoming apoptosis is an important step in stimulating tumor growth by the *myc* oncogene.

Escaping Senescence

Just like Janus, the mythological Roman god who had two faces, oncogenes that stimulate transformation, such as *ras*, can also drive cells into senescence. The observations that led to this discovery were based on the ability of the *ras* oncogene alone to transform and immortalize primary rodent fibroblasts only if they lacked the *p53* tumor-suppressor gene or the cell-cycle inhibitor *p16* that regulates the *Rb* pathway. The loss of *p53* and *p16* is also important for human cell immortalization. In addition, senescent cells have elevated levels of p53 or p16, suggesting that senescence is ultimately an irreversible cell-cycle arrest. In primary cells, such as fibroblasts, the activation of the constitutive growth signal by the *ras* oncogene will induce the activity of p16 and p53 that will counter this signal and result in the induction of cellular senescence. Therefore, for a cell to develop independence of extracellular mitogenic growth signals, it must develop mutations in pathways that send a continuous proliferation signal as well as in pathways that attempt to restrict this signal. Cell immortalization can be viewed as a competing process that requires both the activation of dominant activating oncogenes to induce proliferation and the loss of recessive tumor-suppressor genes that induce a cell-cycle arrest in response to this constitutive activating signal.

Although cellular senescence can be delayed by mutations in the *p53* and *Rb* pathways, cells will ultimately encounter another junction in their road to transformation, namely, crisis (Fig. 17.15). This term *crisis* is highly appropriate, as this roadblock to cell immortalization results in chromosomal rearrangements and cell death. Less than 1 in 10 million cells that enter crisis survives and gains the ability to replicate indefinitely. One clue to what drives cells to the crisis stage comes from the end-to-end fusions of chromosomes. From this it is apparent that crisis results from the progressive shortening of the protective caps (telomeres) on the ends of chromosomes.

Mammalian telomeres consist of long arrays of the repeat sequence TTAGGG that range in length anywhere from 1.5 to 150 kb. Each time a normal somatic cell divides, the terminal end of the telomere is lost; successive divisions lead to progressive shortening, and after 40 to 60 divisions, vital DNA sequences are lost. At this point, the cell cannot divide further and undergoes senescence. Telomere length has been described as the "molecular clock," because it shortens with age in somatic tissue cells during adult life. Stem cells in self-renewing tissues, and cancer cells in particular, avoid this process of aging by activating the enzyme telomerase. Telomerase is a reverse transcriptase that polymerizes TTAGGG repeats to offset the degradation of chromosome ends that occurs with successive cell divisions; in this way, the cell becomes immortal. Telomere shortening inhibits tumor expansion when the p53 tumor-suppressor gene is intact. Although it has not been proven, telomeres seem to engage the p53 pathway by inducing a damage response signaled through the ATM pathway (Chapter 5). Studies have shown that telomere shortening leads to senescence and tumor suppression in cells with an intact *p53* pathway. Surprisingly, telomere shortening accelerates tumorigenesis in cells that were deficient in p53 activity. The ability of shortened telomeres to accelerate tumorigenesis in *p53*-deficient cells results from increased chromosomal instability and rearrangements and gene amplification.

Angiogenesis

Angiogenesis, the recruitment of new blood vessels to regions of chronically low blood supply, is essential for the progression of solid tumors to malignancy. Increasing evidence supports the hypothesis that tumor angiogenesis is controlled by an "angiogenic switch," a physiologic mechanism involving a dynamic balance of angiogenic factors that include both inhibitors and inducers. Numerous angiogenic factors have been identified, including specific endothelial cell growth factors (e.g., vascular endothelial growth factor, or VEGF), cytokines and inflammatory agents (e.g., tumor necrosis factor α, or TNF-α, and interleukin-8, or IL-8), fragments of circulatory system proteins (e.g., angiostatin and endostatin), and extracellular matrix components (e.g., thrombospondins, or TSPs). Presumably, this diversity of angiogenic factors reflects a strict requirement for controlling angiogenesis under normal physiologic conditions and in response to oncogenic events by modulating the expression of both angiogenic inducers and inhibitors.

Although the list of proangiogenic growth factors is expanding, VEGF was the first growth factor isolated that could stimulate endothelial proliferation and migration. In tumors, VEGF can be regulated by oncogenic stimuli such as *ras* and *raf*, hypoxia, and deregulated growth-factor receptor signaling. Both tumor cells and host stromal cells produce VEGF. However, the target for VEGF lies on the cell surface of endothelial cells. These cells possess several specific transmembrane receptor tyrosine–kinases that bind VEGF, which in turn initiate endothelial migration and proliferation. In regard to neoangiogenesis, VEGF receptor II is the most important for stimulating new blood vessel formation. Studies have shown that blocking the binding of VEGF to its receptor inhibits tumor angiogenesis and tumor growth. These findings have led to the development of new antibody approaches for antiangiogenesis therapy for clinical use.

Tumors such as renal cell carcinomas that possess mutations in the von Hippel-Lindau gene (*VHL*) exhibit high aerobic expression of proangiogenic genes such as VEGF, whereas reintroduction of wild-type *VHL* substantially reduces VEGF levels to those found in untransformed cells. The mechanism underlying this observation is that VHL inhibits HIF levels under aerobic conditions by targeting HIF for ubiquitin-mediated degradation. Cells that have lost VHL are impaired in their ability to degrade HIF and have constitutive elevated levels of HIF and HIF target genes, of which *VEGF* is one under aerobic conditions (see Chapter 6 for further explanation).

TSP-1 is a secreted adhesive glycoprotein that has been shown to have antiangiogenic activity by preventing angiogenic factors such as VEGF from binding to their target receptors. Compelling evidence of an antiangiogenic function for TSP-1 is provided by studies showing that activation of the angiogenic switch in Li–Fraumeni fibroblasts lacking functional *p53* is associated with diminished TSP-1 expression. Furthermore, introduction of functional *p53* into carcinoma cells generates an antiangiogenic activity involving induction of TSP-1 expression. Reports that endogenous TSP-1 expression can be induced by p53, repressed by oncogenic signals such as c-*jun* overexpression, and silenced by DNA methylation, indicate that downregulation of TSP-1 contributes to oncogenesis. As

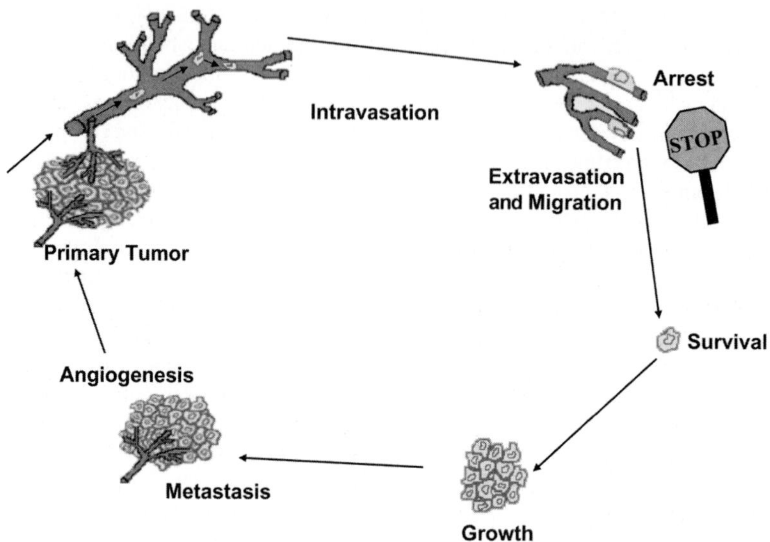

FIGURE 17.16 ● Critical steps in the metastatic process. Tumor cells acquire the ability to disrupt the extracellular matrix of the basement membrane, allowing them to intravasate into local blood or lymph vessels. To form metastases at remote locations, they must migrate and extravasate through the host tissue, blood or lymph supply and survive and proliferate in the new soil. All of these processes are depicted in this figure. (From Le Q, Denko NC, Giaccia AJ: Hypoxic gene expression and metastasis. *Cancer and Metastasis Rev* 23:293–310, 2004.)

both *p53* and c-*jun* are inducible by hypoxia, the regulation of TSP-1 expression by these proteins suggests that it is also a hypoxia-responsive angiogenic inhibitor.

In summary, TSP-1 and VEGF are genetically controlled by both tumor-suppressor gene and proto-oncogene activity, providing molecular mechanisms that could contribute to the switch to the angiogenic phenotype when these controls are deregulated during oncogenesis.

Invasion and Metastasis

Many years ago, Paget realized that cancer spreads in defined patterns and is influenced by both lymph and blood flow patterns as well as the tissue being invaded. He proposed that a metastatic cell is analogous to a vegetable seed, in that without the right soil conditions, it would never grow. Malignant tumor cells become locally invasive and escape their tissue confines by invading the substratum beneath them, before they can colonize to distant tissues (Fig. 17.16). Local invasion necessitates the breakdown of epithelial integrity that is influenced by cell–cell and cell–matrix interactions through the loss of adhesion molecules such as *E-cadherin*. Decreased expression or impaired function of *E-cadherin* (*E-CAD*) leads to deregulated intercellular adhesion and increases the invasive growth and spread of the primary tumor, whereas overexpression of reduces the invasive and metastatic growth of transformed cells. In gastric carcinomas and lobular breast carcinomas, *E-CAD* has been found to be mutated and functionally inactivated. Thus, loss of *E-CAD* can permit local invasion of tumor cells and may be a common step in invasion. In addition to E-cadherin, cell adhesion molecules such as N-CAM also appear to play an important role in invasion. Their expression is decreased in invasive cells and when overexpressed can decrease invasion and metastasis. One final group of proteins that contribute to the invasive capability of tumor cells are integrins, which relay signals from the ECM to epithelial cells. In this case, the cell-surface repertoire of integrins changes when tumor cells become invasive.

The genetic circuits that regulate metastasis remain mainly undiscovered and elusive. Some broad concepts about metastasis have been proposed, such as the need for proteases to degrade the ECM. However, which proteases and how they are regulated differently in tumor cells compared with untransformed cells are unknown. An important question is whether or not tumor cells must acquire additional mutations to invade and metastasize. In returning to Paget's concept of the seed and the soil, only a small percentage of tumor cells are able to metastasize. Some die rapidly by apoptosis, some remain

TABLE 17.3

DNA Repair and Stability Genes and Their Associated Syndromes

Suppressor	Syndrome	Tumor
ATM	Ataxia-telangiectasia	Leukemia, lymphoma
XP	Xeroderma pigmentosum	Skin
BRCA1	Hereditary breast cancer 1	Breast
BRCA2	Hereditary breast cancer 2	Breast, ovary
FANC	Fanconi's anemia	Leukemia
NBS	Nijmegen breakage syndrome	Lymphoma
hMSH2	Hereditary nonpolyposis colorectal cancer	Colon
hMLH1	Hereditary nonpolyposis colorectal cancer	Colon
hMSH6	Hereditary nonpolyposis colorectal cancer	Colon
hPMS1	Hereditary nonpolyposis colorectal cancer	Colon
hPMS2	Hereditary nonpolyposis colorectal cancer	Colon

in the circulation, and a small number invade and colonize other tissues. One noteworthy point is that loss of apoptosis in response to detachment from neighboring cells and the ECM (anoikis) is essential for metastatic spread. Metastasis represents a major challenge in the treatment of cancer, especially as the ability to control local tumor growth is increasing though the combination of surgery and radiotherapy. Metastasis research represents the most critical frontier in cancer research.

THE CONCEPT OF GATEKEEPERS AND CARETAKERS

It appears that most tumor-suppressor genes can be broadly divided into two classes that have been called "gatekeepers" and "caretakers." Gatekeepers are genes that directly regulate the growth of tumors by inhibiting cell division or promoting cell death. The function of these genes, therefore, is rate limiting for tumor growth; both alleles (maternal and paternal) must be lost or inactivated for a tumor to develop. Predisposed individuals inherit one damaged copy of such a gene and so require only one additional mutation for tumor initiation. The identity of gatekeepers varies with each tissue, such that inactivation of a given gene predisposes to specific forms of cancer; inherited mutations in APC predispose to colon cancer, for example; mutations in VHL predispose to kidney cancers; and so on. Because these gatekeeper genes are rate limiting for tumor initiation, they tend to be mutated in many cancers. They can arise both through somatic or germ-line mutations.

By contrast, inactivation of caretaker genes does not directly promote the growth of tumors, but leads instead to genomic instability that only indirectly promotes growth by causing an increase in mutation rate. This increase in genetic instability can greatly accelerate the development of cancers, especially those that require numerous mutations for their full development. Colon cancer is a good example. The targets of the accelerated mutation rate that occurs in cells with defective caretakers are the gatekeeper tumor-suppressor genes, oncogenes, or both. Table 17.3 provides examples of cancer predisposition syndromes caused by mutations in DNA repair and stability genes. The evidence is highly suggestive that mutations in these predisposition genes increases the rate of acquiring cancer after exposure to DNA-damaging agents such as ionizing radiation.

Evidence for this comes from a review by Swift of 161 families affected by AT. In this prospective study, new cases of cancers were observed in blood relatives of persons with AT (of whom about half may be heterozygotic), in those who are definite heterozygotes (obligates), and in spouses who were assumed to be normal but who lived in the same environment. This extensive study also divided blood relatives of AT homozygotes into those with and those without a "radiation history." A radiation history was interpreted loosely as fluoroscopy of the chest, back, or abdomen, therapeutic irradiation, or occupational exposure. Table 17.4 shows the results of the survey: 53% of blood relatives with cancer had a radiation history, compared with 19% of those without cancer.

TABLE 17.4

Breast Cancer and Radiation in 161 Families with Ataxia Telangiectasia

	Blood Relatives with Cancer	Blood Relatives without Cancer
Number	19	57
With Radiation History[a]	10/19 = 53%	11/57 = 19%

[a] Radiation history includes fluoroscopy of chest, back, or abdomen; therapeutic radiation; and occupational exposure.
From Swift M, Morrell D, Massey RB, Chase CL: *N Engl J Med* 325:1831–1836, 1991, with permission.

TABLE 17.5

Human Mismatch Repair Genes

Gene	Chromosomal Location	Germ-Line Mutations in HNPCC Cases (Reported Family Studies), %
hMSH2	2p21–22 (2p16?)	60
hMLH1	3p21	30
hPMS1	2q31–33	4
hPMS2	7p21	4
GTBP	2p16 (2p21–22?)	0

From these data, the study purported to show that AT heterozygotes are very sensitive to radiation-induced cancer; a control study of this kind does not provide proof of this, but the possibility certainly exists. It is a challenging and sobering thought to diagnostic radiologists that a proportion of the women routinely screened by mammography may be exquisitely sensitive to radiation-induced carcinogenesis because of repair deficiencies associated with being heterozygotic for AT.

MISMATCH REPAIR

Interest in **mismatch repair genes** heightened with the discovery that they were responsible for the mutator phenotype associated with a predisposition for hereditary nonpolyposis colon cancer (HNPCC) and possibly other familial cancers. The initial clue to this novel molecular mechanism was the discovery of deletions of long monotonic (dA-dT) runs in a subset of human colon cancers. Soon after, insertions or deletions at mono-, di-, and trinucleotide repeat sequences were discovered in subsets of colon tumors as well as in a majority of colon cancers from individuals with HNPCC. This phenotype also has been detected in several other types of human malignancies, especially those associated with type 2 Lynch syndrome. These various investigations culminated in the identification and cloning of the human *hMSH2* gene, which maps to a locus linked to HNPCC on chromosome 2p21–22 and whose homologues in *Saccharomyces cerevisiae* and *Escherichia coli* are involved in the process of DNA mismatch repair.

The primary function of mismatch repair genes in *E. coli* appears to be to scan the genome as it replicates and to spot errors of mismatch as the DNA is replicated, that is, as the new strand is laid down using the stable methylated strand as a template. A growing number of human genes have been associated with HNPCC by means of linkage analysis and studies of mutational mapping. Table 17.5 lists human mismatch repair genes associated with HNPCC. The mismatch repair process in yeast and bacteria involves a large number of proteins, and so it is likely that additional causes of HNPCC remain to be uncovered.

Cells with defective or nonfunctioning mismatch repair genes can be identified by two quite different techniques:

1. By using a selectable reporter system that inserts an exogenous long repeat sequence into the cells in question and measures the mutation rate in it.
2. By measuring the mutation rate in one or more of the many endogenous repeat sequences that already exist in every human cell—the so-called microsatellite instability assay. Microsatellite instability appears to be a factor of some importance in a wide variety of human tumors.

Both techniques have strengths and weaknesses and are far from perfect.

RADIATION-INDUCED SIGNAL TRANSDUCTION

Ionizing radiation can regulate the expression of early-response genes such as c-*fos*, c-*jun*, and c-*myc*, genes that control lipid signaling such as acid sphingomyelinase, and the PIKK family that includes *ATM* and *DNA-PK*.

Early-Response Genes

The activation of early-response genes by ionizing radiation suggests that radiation in some way mimics the mitogenic activation of quiescent cells. Evidence for the importance of such effects is that the overexpression of proto-oncogenes such as c-*ras* and c-*raf*, whose products are intermediates in the pathways of mitogenic signal transduction, is associated with radiation resistance. The induction of these pathways results in gene activation through elements such as AP-1, serum response element, and CREB.

The role of these early-response genes is not clear at the present time, but the stimulation of signal transduction pathways and activation of transcription factors may enhance secondarily the response of the cell to radiation in terms of repair and cell-cycle arrest. In addition, the activation of these early-response genes in turn could provide a mechanism for secondary stimulation of various late-response genes such as *TNF-α*, *PDGF*, *FGF*, and *IL-1*. Activation of these genes may allow the cell to adapt to acute changes in the microenvironment and may be responsible for some of the chronic responses of the cell to ionizing radiation, including apoptosis.

Phosphatidyl-Inositol-3-OH Kinase-Like Kinases (PIKK)

A cell's response to DNA damage depends on the type of damage. The PIKK family is comprised of proteins such as ATM and DNA-PK that sense and respond to DNA strand breaks. In unstressed cells, ATM exists as a homodimer in which the kinase domain is sterically blocked by its tight binding to a region that includes serine 1981. Recruitment of ATM to sites of DNA damage is still under investigation and may involve the MRE11/RAD50/NBS (MRN) complex. In response to DNA strand breaks, ATM changes conformation and autophosphorylates at serine 1981, resulting in dissociation of the inactive dimer into a monomer. The resulting ATM monomer is the active species that in turn phosphorylates target proteins involved in cell-cycle control and DNA repair such as Nijmegen breakage syndrome (NBS), breast cancer 1 (BRCA1), structural maintenance of chromosome 1 (SMC1), H2AX, and p53BP1 (Fig. 17.17). The p53 protein is also an ATM target that plays a major role in the regulation of the mammalian cellular stress response, in part through the transcriptional activation of genes involved in cell-cycle control, DNA repair, and apoptosis. Past studies indicate that the p53 protein can also be phosphorylated by other PIKK family members, such as DNA-PK and ATR, various cyclin-dependent kinases, and the c-*abl* proto-oncogene product under different cell-cycle phases in different cell types. It has been proposed that changes in p53 phosphorylation status and protein–protein interactions are important for p53 protein stability and function.

The Ceramide Pathway

Exposure of cells to DNA damage induces the production of ceramide through two major pathways.

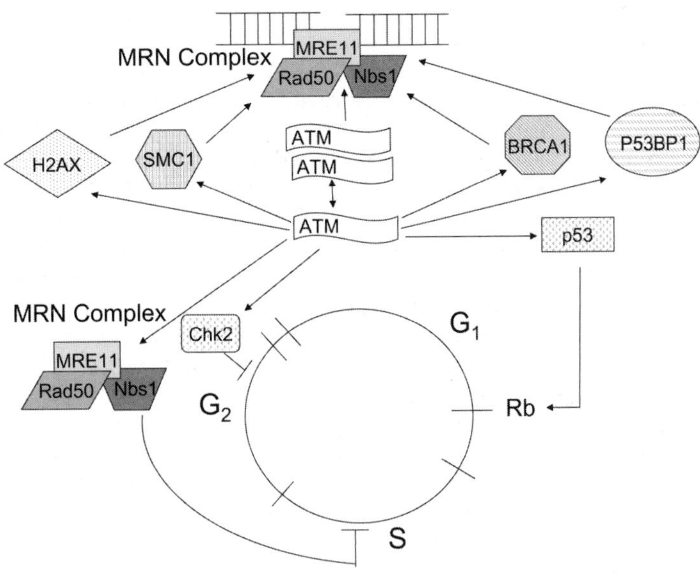

FIGURE 17.17 • Activation of the ATM pathway by an ionizing radiation-induced DNA double-strand break. The model proposed by Kastan and Bakkenist indicates that ATM exists as a dimer and undergoes rapid autophosphorylation in response to DNA strand breaks and chromatin conformation changes. This results in dissociation of the dimer into a monomer and the phosphorylation of numerous substrates involved in DNA repair (H2AX, SMC1, BRCA1, and p53BP1) and cell-cycle control (p53 and Chk2). Recent studies have shown that the MRN complex can function upstream of ATM by sensing and localizing to DNA breaks and can also be a target of ATM.

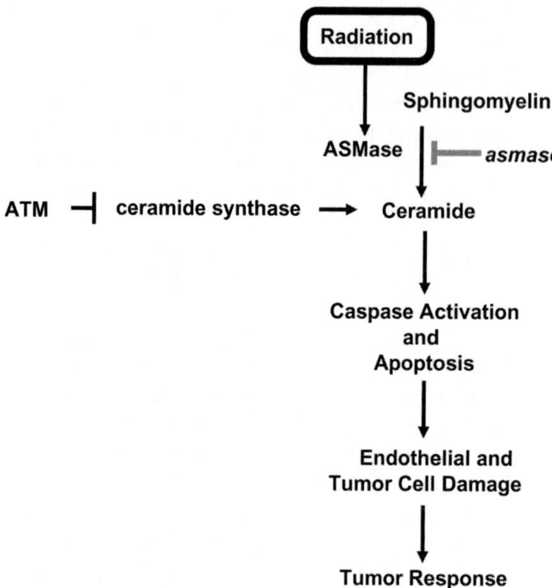

FIGURE 17.18 • The acid sphongomyelinase (ASMase) pathway for the generation of ceramide. When cells are irradiated, ASMase activity increases and converts sphingomyelin to ceramide. The intracellular production of ceramide acts as a potent activator of the caspase cascade to induce apoptosis in endothelial cells as well as tumor cells. Cells deficient in acid sphingomyelinase (*asmase*$^{-/-}$) can only generate ceramide from ceramide synthase, which is negatively regulated by ATM. (Figure provided courtesy of Richard Kolesnick, Memorial Sloan Kettering Cancer Center.)

In one pathway that is activated by ionizing radiation and DNA-damaging agents, ceramide is generated from sphingomyelin hydrolysis by the enzyme acid sphongomyelinase (Fig. 17.18). This results in the catalysis of up to one half of total cellular sphingomyelin, the majority of which would be presumably associated with the plasma membrane. Ceramide can also be generated by ceramide synthase, which is inhibited by the *ATM* kinase. Therefore, in response to ionizing radiation, individuals who have lost ATM have elevated levels of ceramide synthase and increased apoptosis of certain cell types (e.g., crypt cells). It is important to note that ionizing radiation can activate both nuclear and membrane–cytoplasmic signal transduction pathways, which can lead to either cell-cycle arrest or, alternatively, apoptosis.

In summary, although there is little doubt that the lethal effects of ionizing radiation result from extensive DNA damage leading to chromosomal aberrations, radiation can also stimulate signal transduction pathways that can lead to cell-cycle arrest or cell death by apoptosis, depending on the dose of radiation and genetic background of the cell.

THERAPEUTIC EXPLOITATION OF RADIATION-ACTIVATED SIGNAL TRANSDUCTION PATHWAYS

The molecular exploitation of oncogenic protein products should soon be possible. For example, it is still controversial whether the Erb-2 receptor is predictive of a poor prognosis for breast cancer. However, as already stated, many growth-factor receptors possess truncated extracellular ligand-binding domains. Therefore, it is possible to specifically target monoclonal antibodies coupled to radionuclides or chemotherapeutic agents to these truncated receptors. It also seems possible to reverse or decrease the oncogenic effects of certain oncogenes by altering essential interactions with subcellular compartments. For example, the *ras* oncogene protein product requires the addition of an isoprenoid lipid (a process termed prenylation) so that it can attach to the cell membrane where it is active. Prenylation of ras is performed by farensyltransferase or geranylgeranyltransferase. Recent studies have shown that the first generation of farensyltransferase inhibitors is able to alter ras activity and decrease growth of transformed cells. Since *ras* is found to be mutated in a wide variety of human tumors, and ras requires this modification for activity, the farensyltransferase would therefore be an excellent candidate enzyme to inhibit.

A second example of an oncogenic target is the NF-κB transcription factor (a member of the *c-rel* family of proto-oncogenes), which is found to be constitutively active in a wide variety of tumor cells by multiple mechanisms (Fig. 17.19). If NF-κB activity is inhibited in these tumor cells, they fail to proliferate in soft agar, become more sensitive to apoptotic cell death induced by ionizing radiation or chemotherapy, and exhibit decreased migration and apoptosis. What makes this transcription factor

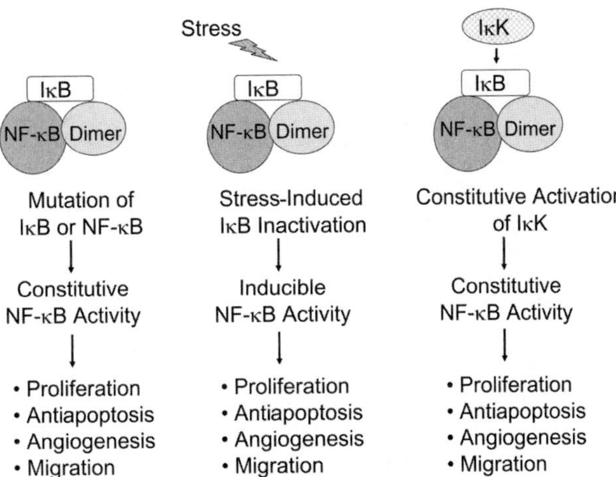

FIGURE 17.19 • Mechanisms and consequences of NF-κB activation in tumor cells. All three pathways converge on the important role of IκB in maintaining NF-κB in the cytoplasm and not in the nucleus. Loss of IκB results in the NF-κB dimer translocating into the nucleus and activating target genes involved in proliferation, antiapoptosis, angiogenesis, and migration. IκK = IκB kinase; IκB = inhibitor of κB; NF-κB = nuclear factor κB. (Based on work of Nakanishi C, Toi M: Nuclear factor-kappa B inhibitors as sensitizers to anticancer drugs. *Nat Rev Cancer* 5:297–309, 2005.)

a good target for therapy is that it is normally held in the cytoplasm by an inhibitory molecule called IκB (inhibitor of κB). If IκB is overexpressed or prevented from degradation, then NF-κB will be held in check in the cytoplasm, where it is inactive and kept out of the nucleus. At present, several drugs exist that could therapeutically inhibit IκB degradation. These are but several examples of molecular strategies that target key components of oncogene regulation for the treatment of cancer.

THE CELL CYCLE

The ability of cells to produce exact, accurate copies of themselves is essential to the continuance of life; it is accomplished through highly organized processes, well conserved through evolution. Lack of fidelity in cellular reproduction as manifested by DNA and chromosome alterations is a hallmark of cancer.

The only event in the cell cycle that can be identified with a simple light microscope is the condensation of the chromosomes during mitosis (M); this was observed in the late 19th century. Using autoradiography, Howard and Pelc in the early 1950s divided up the cell cycle by showing that DNA was synthesized only during a discrete time interval, which they called S phase. Between mitosis and the S phase was the "first gap in activity" (G_1), and between S phase and the next mitosis was the "second gap in activity" (G_2). If the cells stop progressing through the cycle—that is, if they are arrested—they are said to be in G_0. The cell cycle was discussed in detail in Chapter 4.

Howard and Pelc also showed that it was in these gaps that radiation affects cell-cycle progression, because in their early studies it was obvious that cells arrest cell-cycle progression after low-dose radiation damage not in S or M but in either G_1 or G_2. It was subsequently recognized that these arrests also were related to the process of malignancy, because primary cells would arrest in both G_1 and G_2, but tumor cells often would show only the G_2 arrest point. Breakthroughs in understanding these events and the nature of the cell cycle itself came with the discovery of the cyclins, the cyclin-dependent kinases, and the cyclin–kinase inhibitors and with the elaboration by Weinert and Hartwell of the concept of cell-cycle checkpoints. The current concept of the cell cycle and its regulation is illustrated in Figure 17.20.

CYCLINS AND KINASES

Regulation of the complex processes that occur as a cell passes through the cycle is a result of a series of changes in the activity of intracellular enzymes known as **cyclin-dependent kinases (Cdks)**. The active forms of these enzymes exist in protein complexes with a cell-cycle phase-specific protein known as a cyclin. Transitions from one phase to the next in the cycle occur only if the enzymatic activity of a given kinase activates the proteins required for progression.

In mammals, cyclins A through H have been described. Each cyclin protein is synthesized at a discrete phase of the cycle: cyclin D and E in G_1, cyclin A in S and G_2, and cyclin B in G_2 and M. Cyclin levels oscillate with phase of the cycle.

Seven Cdks have been described. Cdk levels are constant throughout the cell cycle, but their activity is regulated by cyclin-dependent activating kinases, the protein level of cyclin regulatory subunits, and association with Cdk inhibitors.

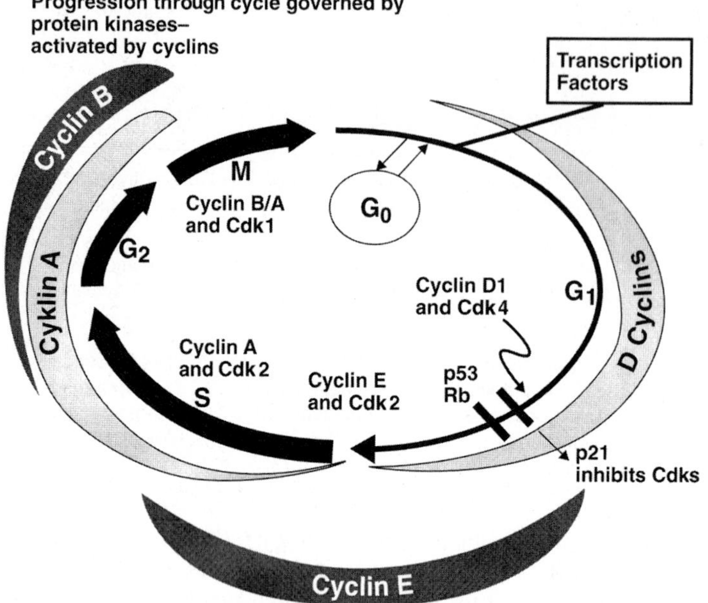

FIGURE 17.20 ● The current concept of the cell cycle and its regulation by protein kinases, activated by cyclins.

Molecular events in G_1 prepare the cell for DNA synthesis. There is a stage in G_1, known as the G_1 restriction point, after which cells are committed to enter the S phase and no longer respond to growth conditions. Prior to this point, cells may take several routes: They may progress, differentiate, senesce, or die, depending on external signals. Key players in the G_1 restriction point include the protein of the *Rb* gene, D-type cyclins, and Cdk4 and Cdk6, as well as Cdk inhibitors (Fig. 17.21). If extracellular signals stimulate a cell to enter the cycle from quiescence, D-type cyclins are stimulated and continue through G_1 and form a complex with Cdk4 or Cdk6. The activated cyclin–Cdk4 or cyclin–Cdk6 complex then phosphorylates the Rb protein, which releases it from E2F and its growth-suppressive function. E2F that is released from the Rb protein binds to the promoter of the cyclin E gene, resulting in increased cyclin E mRNA and protein. There is more cyclin E available to bind Cdk2 and phosphorylate Rb, resulting in a positive feedback loop that is now refractory to mitogenic signals. Although numerous studies have documented the importance of all three D-type cyclins, two E-type cyclins, and Cdk2, Cdk4, and Cdk6, gene knockout studies in mice have indicated that all of these

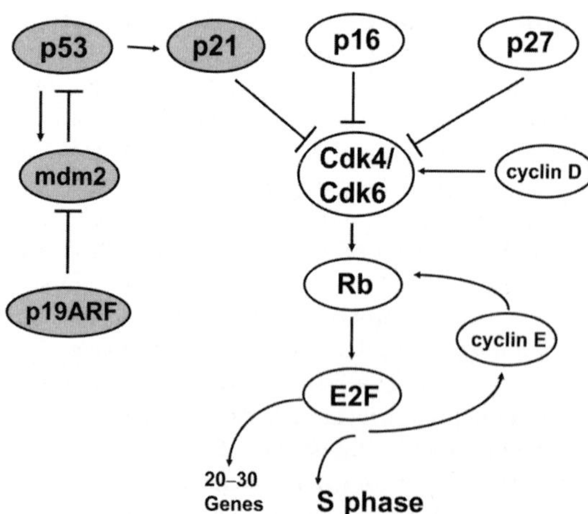

FIGURE 17.21 ● The Rb growth suppression pathway. The events depicted represent the criticial steps in the phosphorylation of Rb by cyclin-dependent kinases to allow cells to progress through the G_1 restriction point into S phase. Irradiated cells exhibit a G_1 checkpoint arrest at this restriction point when the p53 tumor-suppressor gene is induced to activate the p21 cyclin-dependent kinase inhibitor.

cyclins and their dependent kinases are not essential for normal cell-cycle progression. However, the ability of cells to be transformed by oncogenes is dependent on G_1 cyclins and their dependent kinases. The current thinking is that untransformed cells require a lower level of G_1 cyclins to proliferate and differentiate, whereas transformation requires a quantitatively different level of G_1 cyclins. Thus, if increased G_1 cyclin activity is needed for transformation, then loss or diminished G_1 cyclin activity could act to suppress tumor formation.

Once a cell has committed to entering S, it must begin the incredibly difficult task of accurately copying over 3 billion bases of the genome; this feat is completed in a matter of a few hours. DNA polymerases are the enzymes involved in this copying process, which must be completed with high fidelity, aided by repair and misrepair genes that remove and replace mismatched DNA bases. Cyclin A is maximally expressed in S phase and enhances transition of the cell through this phase of the cycle.

After the cell has copied its entire genome, the next important task is to segregate the two copies of the DNA equally into the progeny cells. There is a gap (G_2), however, between the end of all detectable DNA synthesis and the beginning of cell division, at which the process of condensing and segregating the chromosomes begins. Events during this period are controlled by Cdk activity analogous to that occurring at the G_1/S transition, but this time it is a complex of cyclins B and A with Cdk1.

Although the cell is progressing through this complicated process of DNA replication and division, it must respond constantly to extracellular signals concerning nutrient status, cell-to-cell contact, and so forth, that arrive at the nucleus through one or another signal transduction pathway.

CHECKPOINT PATHWAYS

Events in the cell cycle must take place in a specific order, and it is the function of a number of checkpoint genes to ensure that the initiation of late events is delayed until earlier events are complete.

There are three principal places in the cell cycle at which checkpoints function:

1. G_1/S checkpoint
2. S phase checkpoint
3. G_2/M checkpoint

If DNA is damaged, normal cells stop progressing through the cycle and are arrested at one of these checkpoints, depending on their position in the cell cycle at the time at which the damage occurs.

Cells with damaged DNA in G_1 avoid replicating that damage by arresting at the G_1/S interface, or if they have already passed the restriction point governed by phosphorylation of Rb, they will transiently arrest in the S phase. Avoiding the replication of damaged DNA and allowing time for repair prevents cell death and the accumulation of heritable mutations. The tumor-suppressor gene *p53* is critical in the pathway that leads to G_1 arrest. DNA damage initiates a chain of events: First ATM autophosphorylates and releases an active monomer that can directly phosphorylate p53 and Mdm2, the ubiquitin ligase that targets p53 for degradation. In addition, the checkpoint kinases (Chk), also targets of ATM, can also phosphorylate p53 and Mdm2. Phosphorylation of both p53 and Mdm2 results in increased levels of p53 protein. Activated p53 enhances $p21^{WAF1/CIPI}$ gene expression, which results in a sustained inhibition of G_1 cyclin/Cdks. G_1 cyclin inhibition prevents phosphorylation of Rb and progression from G_1 into S. Mutations in *p53* (which are present in so many human tumors) clearly compromise this checkpoint function. A second more rapid but transient checkpoint is also induced by DNA damage through Chk1 phosphorylation of the Cdc25A phosphatase and the inhibition of cyclin E–Cdk2 and cyclin A–Cdk2 complexes. This later checkpoint works independently of p53.

Control of the S phase checkpoint is in part mediated by the Cdc25A phosphatase inhibiting Cdk2 activity and the loading of Cdc45 onto chromatin. Failure to load Cdc45 onto chromatin prevents the recruitment of DNA polymerase α and replicon initiation. A second mechanism for S phase arrest is signaled by phosphorylation of NBS by ATM. The importance of the S phase checkpoint is in protecting replication forks from trying to replicate through DNA strand breaks.

The arrest of cells in G_2 following DNA damage is observed readily in mammalian cells and was studied by radiation biologists for decades before checkpoints were understood at the molecular level. The arrest occurs after the levels of cyclin A increase in quantity but before cyclin B increases. The function of this checkpoint in normal cells is to prevent cells with damaged chromosomes from attempting the complex process of mitosis; they are arrested in G_2 to allow DNA repair to be completed. It follows, therefore, that cells lacking the G_2 checkpoint are radiosensitive, because they cannot repair all of their damaged chromosomes before entering mitosis. At the molecular level, multiple kinase signaling pathways have been implicated in regulating this checkpoint. For example, ATM and Chk target the Cdc25C phosphatase and prevent cyclin B/A–Cdk1 activation. In addition, other regulatory proteins have been implicated in G_2 arrest, such as polo-like kinases, Brca1 and p53bp1. It appears that the G_2 checkpoint is the most regulated of all checkpoints and probably the most important in preventing the inappropriate entry of damaged cells into mitosis. Consequently, targeting the inhibition of key components of the G_2 checkpoint could increase radiosensitization.

The hallmark of cancer is a lack of the ability to respond to signals that normally would cause the cell to stop progressing through the cycle and dividing. Checkpoint proteins provide an important mechanism by which a cell can temporarily halt its transit through the cell cycle and attempt to restore chromosome integrity.

GENOMIC IMPRINTING

With the notable exception of the sex chromosomes, both parents contribute equally to the genetic makeup of their offspring. Although two copies of each gene are present, there are certain instances in which only one allele is expressed. This is termed **genomic imprinting**.

The imprinting that results in the inhibition of gene expression results from either DNA methylation or a chromatin structure change. It is parent-of-origin specific, and it is erased if passed through the opposite sex. Imprinting varies with the species, the individual, the tissue, and the time. It plays a critical role in fetal development; it can be turned on and off at different times.

Genomic imprinting is important in oncology because it leads to loss of heterozygosity and therefore to the inheritance of cancer susceptibility in a non-Mendelian fashion. Presently, about 20 imprinted genes are known in the human, but it is suspected that there are many more. Several are implicated in carcinogenesis, including one oncogene and several tumor-suppressor genes. For example, in the case of a paternally imprinted, maternally expressed gene (such as the one involved in Wilms' tumor), males *always* would pass on an inactive gene; females *always* would pass on an expressed gene.

Summary of Pertinent Conclusions

- Cancer is thought to be a clonal disorder.
- The control of cell proliferation is the consequence of signals that may be positive or negative.
- Gain-of-function mutations can activate oncogenes, which are positive growth regulators; tumor-suppressor genes are a negative growth regulator.
- Oncogenes are genes found in either a mutant or an abnormally expressed form in many human cancers.
- Oncogenes can be activated by retroviral integration, point mutation, a chromosomal rearrangement such as a translocation, or gene amplification.
- Some human leukemias and lymphomas appear to be caused by specific chromosomal translocations that lead to oncogene activation in several different ways.
- Knudson postulated that all types of retinoblastoma involve two separate mutations. In sporadic retinoblastoma, both mutations occur somatically in the same retinal cell; therefore, this condition is rare. In the heritable form, one of the two mutations is inherited from a parent and is present in all retinal cells, so that the second mutation would occur somatically in any of these cells; hence, the incidence is close to 100%.
- There are many tumor-suppressor genes whose location and function are known; the two most intensively studied are *p53* and *Rb*.
- Because oncogenes are gain-of-function mutations, only one copy needs to be activated; that is, they act in a dominant fashion. Tumor-suppressor genes involve loss-of-function mutations, so that both copies must be lost; that is, they act in a recessive fashion.
- Somatic homozygosity is the process by which one chromosome of a pair is lost, a deletion occurs in the remaining chromosome, and the chromosome with the deletion replicates.
- Carcinogenesis appears to be a multistep process with multiple genetic alterations occurring. An attractive model of carcinogenesis includes the idea that an early step causes a mutation in a gene in one of the families responsible for the stability of the genome. This leads to a mutator phenotype, so that multiple further changes are likely in the progression of the cancer.

(continued)

Summary of Pertinent Conclusions (Continued)

- Telomeres cap the ends of chromosomes; they are long arrays of TTAGGG repeats. Each time a normal somatic cell divides, the terminal end of the telomere is lost; after 40 to 60 divisions, the cell undergoes senescence. Stem cells and cancer cells activate telomerase, which maintains telomere length, so the cell becomes immortal.
- Signal transduction refers to the flow of information from the outer membrane of the cell into the nucleus. Multiple signal transduction pathways can operate simultaneously in tandem. One pathway includes the GTP-binding proteins, including the *ras* family; this is important because *ras* is frequently mutated in human cancers. Another example is the protein kinase C signal transduction pathway.
- Low doses of ionizing radiation can up-regulate or down-regulate a host of early-responding genes.
- The transcriptional activity of p53 is modulated in response to DNA damage by the activity of a number of kinases, as well as by protein–protein interactions resulting in either cell-cycle arrest or apoptosis.
- Ionizing radiations can activate both nuclear and membrane–cytoplasmic signal transduction pathways. This can lead to cell-cycle arrest or apoptosis.
- The division of the cell cycle into its constituent phases, M, G_1, S, and G_2 was accomplished in the 1950s.
- The arrest of cells at various positions in the cycle by the action of "checkpoint genes" is an important response to DNA damage. The two principal checkpoints are the G_1/S and the G_2/M boundary, but there is also a checkpoint in S. G_2/M is the most important checkpoint following radiation damage; cells pause at G_2/M to repair radiation-induced damage before attempting the complex process of mitosis.
- Progression through the cell cycle is governed by protein kinases, activated by cyclins. Each cyclin protein is synthesized at a discrete phase of the cycle: cyclin D and E in G_1, cyclin A in S and G_2, and cyclin B in G_2 and M. Transitions in the cycle occur only if a given kinase activates the proteins required for progression.
- Hereditary disorders predisposing to cancer may result from a germ-line mutation in a tumor-suppressor gene or a DNA repair defect.
- Genomic imprinting is the term used if only one allele is expressed, although both copies of the gene are present. It can lead to inheritance of cancer susceptibility in a non-Mendelian fashion.

BIBLIOGRAPHY

Signal Transduction

Amundsen SA, Myers TG, Fornace AJ: Roles of p53 in growth arrest and apoptosis: Putting on the brakes after genotoxic stress. *Oncogene* 17:3287–3299, 1998

Datta R, Rubin E, Sukhatme V, et al.: Ionizing radiation activates transcription of the *EGR1* gene via CArG elements. *Proc Natl Acad Sci USA* 89:10149–10153, 1992

Dent P, Yacoub A, Contessa J, Caron R, Amorino G, Valerie K, Hagan MP, Grant S, Schmidt-Ullrich R: Stress and radiation-induced activation of multiple intracellular signaling pathways. *Radiat Res* 159:283–300, 2003

Folkman J: Role of angiogenesis in tumor growth and metastases. *Semin Oncol* 29:15–18, 2002

Fornace AJ, Fuks Z, Weichselbaum RR, Milas L: Radiation therapy. In Mendelsohn J, Howley PM, Israel MA, Liotta LA (eds): *The Molecular Basis of Cancer*. Philadelphia, WB Saunders, 1998

Hunter T: Signaling-2000 and beyond. *Cell* 100:113–127, 2000

Jones HA, Hahn SM, Bernhard E, McKenna WG: Ras inhibitors and radiation therapy. *Semin Radiat Oncol* 11:328–337, 2001

Malumbres M, Pellicer A: Ras pathways to cell cycle control and cell transformation. *Frontiers in Bioscience* 3:887–912, 1998

McCormick F: Signaling networks that cause cancer. *Trends Cell Biol* 9:53–56, 1999

Reynolds CP, Maurer BJ, Kolesnick RN: Ceramide synthesis and metabolism as a target for cancer therapy. *Can Let* 206:169–180, 2004

Savitsky K, Bar-Shira A, Gilad S, et al.: A single ataxia telangiectasia gene with a product similar to PI-3 Kinase. *Science* 268:1749–1753, 1995

Sebolt-Leopold JS, Herrera R: Targeting the mitogen-activated protein kinase cascade to treat cancer. *Nat Rev Cancer* 4:937–947, 2004

Stevenson MA, Pollock SS, Coleman CN, et al.: X-irradiation phorbol esters and H_2O_2 stimulate mitogen-activated protein kinase activity in NIH-3T3 cells through the formation of reactive oxygen intermediates. *Cancer Res* 54:12–15, 1991

Vogelstein B, Lane D, Levine AJ: Surfing the p53 network. *Nature* 408:307–310, 2000

Vojtek AB, Der CJ: Increasing complexity of the ras signaling pathway. *J Biol Chem* 273:19925–19928, 1998

Xia Z, Dickens M, Raingeaud J, et al.: Opposing effects of ERK and JNK-p38 map kinase on apoptosis. *Science* 270:1326–1331, 1995

The Cell Cycle

Abraham RT: Cell cycle checkpoint signaling through the ATM and ATR kinases. *Genes Dev* 15:2177–2196, 2001

Bakkenist CJ, Kastan MB: DNA damage activates ATM through intermolecular autophosphorylation and dimer dissociation. *Nature* 421:499–506, 2003

Bartek J, Lukas J: Chk1 and Chk2 kinases in checkpoint control and cancer. *Cancer Cell* 3:421–429, 2003

El-Deiry WS, Kern SE, Pietenpol JA, Kinzler KW, Vogelstein B: Definition of a consensus binding site for p53. *Nat Genet* 1:45–49, 1992

Elkind M, Han A, Volz K: Radiation response of mammalian cells grown in culture: IV. Dose dependence of division delay and post irradiation growth of surviving and non-surviving Chinese hamster cells. *J Natl Cancer Inst* 30:705–711, 1964

Fornace AJ, Nebert DW, Hollander MC, et al.: Mammalian genes coordinately regulated by growth arrest signals and DNA-damaging agents. *Mol Cell Biol* 9:4196–4203, 1989

Hartwell LH, Weinert TA: Checkpoints: Controls that ensure the order of cell cycle events. *Science* 246:629–634, 1989

Howard A, Pelc SR: The synthesis of desoxyribose nucleic acid and its relationship to the chromosome damage induced by x-rays. *Heredity* 6(suppl):261–273, 1953

Kastan MB, Bartek J: Cell-cycle checkpoints and cancer. *Nature* 432:316–323, 2004

Kastan MB, Onyekwere O, Sidransky D, Vogelstein B, Craig R: Participation of p53 protein in the cellular response to DNA damage. *Cancer Res* 511:6304–6311, 1991

Kastan MB, Zhan Q, El-Deiry WS, et al.: A mammalian cell cycle checkpoint pathway utilizing p53 and GADD45 is defective in ataxia-telangiectasia. *Cell* 71:587–597, 1992

Kitagawa R, Bakkenist CJ, McKinnon PJ, Kastan MB: Phosphorylation of SMC1 is a critical downstream event in the ATM-NBS1-BRCA1 pathway. *Genes Dev* 18:1423–1438, 2004

Kuerbitz SJ, Plunkett BS, Walsh WV, Kastan MB: Wild-type p53 in a cell cycle checkpoint determinant following irradiation. *Proc Natl Acad Sci USA* 89:7491–7495, 1992

Lee JH, Paull TT: ATM activation by DNA double-strand breaks through the Mre11-Rad50-Nbs1 complex. *Science* 308:551–554, 2005

McKenna W, Iliakis G, Weiss MC, Bernhard EJ, Muschel RJ: Increased G_2 delay in radiation-resistant cells obtained by transformation of primary rat embryo cells with the oncogens H-*ras* and v-*myc*. *Radiat Res* 125:283–287, 1991

Muschel RJ, Zhang HB, Illiakis G, McKenna WG: Cyclin B expression in HeLa cells during the G_2 block induced by radiation. *Cancer Res* 51:5113–5117, 1991

Muschel R, Zhang HB, Iliakis G, McKenna WG: Effects of ionizing radiation on cyclin expression HeLa cells. *Radiat Res* 132:153–157, 1992

Norbury C, Nurse P: Animal cell cycles and their control. *Annu Rev Biochem* 61:441–470, 1992

Pines J, Hunter T: Isolation of a human cyclin cDNA: Evidence for cyclin mRNA and protein regulation in the cell cycle and for interaction with p34cdc2. *Cell* 58:833–846, 1989

Sherr CJ, Roberts JM: Living with or without cyclins and cyclin-dependent kinases. *Genes Dev* 18:2699–2711, 2004

Shiloh Y: ATM and related protein kinases: Safeguarding genome integrity. *Nat Rev Cancer* 3:155–168, 2003

Oncogenes and Tumor-Suppressor Genes

Adams JM, Harris AW, Pinktert CA, et al.: The c-*myc* oncogene driven by immunoglobulin enhancers induces lymphoid malignancy in transgenic mice. *Nature* 318:533–538, 1985

Barbacid M: *RAS* genes. *Ann Rev Biochem* 56:779–827, 1987

Bishop JM: Cellular oncogene retroviruses. *Ann Rev Biochem* 52:301–354, 1983

Bishop JM, Varmus HE: Functions and origins of retroviral transforming genes. In Weiss R, Teich N, Varmus H, Coffinm J (eds): *RNA Tumor Viruses: Molecular Biology of Tumor Viruses*, 2nd ed, pp 990–1108. Cold Spring Harbor, NY, Cold Spring Harbor Laboratory, 1984

Bos J, Fearon E, Hamilton S, et al.: Prevalence of *RAS* gene mutations in human colorectal cancers. *Nature* 327:293–297, 1987

Cavanee WK, Hansen MF, Nordenskjold M, et al.: Genetic origin of mutations predisposing to retinoblastoma. *Science* 228:501–503, 1985

Cavenee WT, Dryja T, Phillips R, et al.: Expression of recessive alleles by chromosomal mechanisms in retinoblastoma. *Nature* 305:779–784, 1983

Cole M: The *myc* oncogene: Its role in transformation and differentiation. *Annu Rev Genet* 20:361–384, 1986

Der C, Krontiris T, Cooper G: Transforming genes of human bladder and lung carcinoma cell lines are homologous to the *ras* gene of Harvey and Kirsten sarcoma viruses. *Proc Natl Acad Sci USA* 79:3637–3640, 1982

El-Deiry W, Tokino T, Velculescu V, et al.: WAFI, a potential mediator of p53 tumor expression. *Cell* 75:817–825, 1993

Fernandez-Sarabia M, Bischoff J: Bcl-2 associates with the ras-related protein R-ras p23. *Nature* 366:274–275, 1993

Fidler IJ: Critical determinants of metastases. *Semin Cancer Biol* 12:89–96, 2002

Grignani F, Ferrucci P, Testa U, et al.: The acute promyelocytic leukemia-specific PML-RAR alpha fusion protein inhibits differentiation and promotes survival of myeloid precursors. *Cell* 74:423–431, 1993

Harley C, Futcher A, Greider C: Telomeres shorten during aging of human fibroblasts. *Nature* 345:458–460, 1990

Harris C, Hollstein M: Clinical implications of the *p53* tumor-suppressor gene. *N Engl J Med* 329:1318–1327, 1993

Hartwell LH, Kastan MB: Cell cycle control and cancer. *Science* 266:1821–1828, 1994

Jiang W, Kahn S, Guillem J, Lu S, Winstein IB: Rapid detection of *ras* oncogenes in human tumors: Applications to colon, esophageal, and gastric cancer. *Oncogene* 4:923–928, 1989

Kastan M, Zhan Q, El-Deiry W, et al.: A mammalian cell cycle checkpoint pathway utilizing p53 and GADD45 is defective in ataxia-telangiectasia. *Cell* 71:587–597, 1992

Kelly K, Cochran B, Stiles C, et al.: Cell-specific regulation of the c-*myc* gene by lymphocyte mitogens and platelet-derived growth factor. *Cell* 35:603–610, 1983

Knudson A: Anti-oncogenes and human cancer. *Proc Natl Acad Sci USA* 90:10914–10921, 1993

Knudson AG: Mutation and cancer: Statistical study of retinoblastoma. *Proc Natl Acad Sci USA* 68:820–823, 1971

Land H, Parada L, Weinberg R: Tumorigenic conversion of primary embryo fibroblasts requires at least two cooperating oncogenes. *Nature* 304:596–602, 1983

Lengauer C, Kinzler KW, Vogelstein B: Genetic Instabilities in human cancers. *Nature* 396:643–649, 1998

Lynch D, Watson M, Alderson M, et al.: The mouse Fas-ligand gene is mutated in gld mice and is part of a TNF family gene cluster. *Immunity* 1:131–136, 1995

Nagata S, Golstein P: The Fas death factor. *Science* 267:1449–1456, 1995

Nowell PC: Tumor progression: A brief historical perspective. *Sem Cancer Biol* 12:261–266, 2002

Prives C, Hall PA: The p53 pathway. *J of Path* 187:112–126, 1999

Rous P: A sarcoma of fowl transmissible by an agent separable from the tumor cells. *J Exp Med* 13:397, 1911

Rowley J: Molecular cytogenetics: Rosetta stone for understanding cancer. Twenty-ninth GHA Clowes Memorial Award Lecture. *Cancer Res* 50:3816–3825, 1990

Sabbatini P, Lin J, Levine A, et al.: Essential role for p53-mediated transcription in E1A-induced apoptosis. *Genet Dev* 9:2184–2192, 1995

Schwab M, Varmus H, Bishop J, et al.: Chromosome localization in normal cells and neuroblastomas of a gene related to c-*myc*. *Nature* 308:288–291, 1984

Shay JW, Roninson IB: Hallmarks of senescence in carcinogenesis and cancer therapy. *Oncogene* 23:2919–2933, 2004

Sherr CJ, McCormick F: The RB and p53 pathways in cancer. *Cancer Cell* 2:103–112, 2002

Sklar M, Thompson E, Welsh M, et al.: Depletion of c-*myc* with specific antisense sequences reverses the transformed phenotype in *ras* oncogene-transformed NIH 3T3 cells. *Mol Cell Biol* 11:3699–3710, 1991

Spector D, Varmus H, Bishop J: Nucleotide sequences related to the transforming gene of avian sarcoma virus are present in the DNA of uninfected vertebrates. *Proc Natl Acad Sci USA* 75:4102–4106, 1978

Stanbridge EJ: Suppression of malignancy in human cells. *Nature* 260:17–20, 1976

Stewart T, Pattingale P, Leder P: Spontaneous mammary adenocarcinomas in transgenic mice that carry and express *MTV/myc* fusion genes. *Cell* 38:627–637, 1984

Tabin CJ, Bradley SM, Bargmann CI, et al.: Mechanism of activation of a human oncogene. *Nature* 300:143–159, 1982

Temin HM, Rubin H: Characteristics of an assay for Rous sarcoma virus and Rous sarcoma cells in tissue culture. *Virology* 6:669–688, 1958

Vogelstein B, Kinzler KW: Cancer genes and the pathways they control. *Nat Med* 10:789–799, 2004

Weiss R, Teich N, Varmus H, et al.: *RNA Tumor Viruses*. Cold Spring Harbor, NY, Cold Spring Harbor Laboratories, 1982

Cancer Genetics

Donis-Keller H, Dou S, Chi D, et al.: Mutations in the RET proto-oncogene are associated with MEN 2A and FMTC. *Hum Mol Genet* 2:851–856, 1993

Evans DGR, Farndon PA, Burnell LD, Gattamaneni HR, Birch JM: The incidence of Gorlin syndrome in 173 consecutive cases of medulloblastoma. *Br J Cancer* 64:959–961, 1991

Garber JE, Goldstein AM, Kantor AF: Follow-up study of twenty-four families with Li Fraumeni syndrome. *Cancer Res* 51:6094–6097, 1991

Gorlin RJ, Goltz RW: Nevoid basal-cell carcinoma syndrome. *Medicine* 66:98–113, 1987

Gruis NA, van der Velden PA, Sandkuijl LA, et al.: Homozygotes for CDKN2 (p16) germline mutation in Dutch familial melanoma kindreds. *Nat Genet* 10:351–353, 1995

Kim WY, Kaelin WG: Role of VHL gene mutation in human cancer. *J Clin Oncol* 22:4991–5004, 2004

Knudson AG: Mutation and cancer: Statistical study of retinoblastoma. *Proc Natl Acad Sci USA* 68:820–823, 1971

Knudson AG, Strong LC: Mutation and cancer: A model for Wilms' tumour of the kidney. *J Natl Cancer Inst* 48:313–324, 1972

Li FP: Familial cancer syndromes and clusters. *Curr Probl Cancer* 14:77–113, 1990

Li FP, Fraumeni JF Jr: Familial breast cancer, soft-tissue sarcomas, and other neoplasms. *Ann Intern Med* 83:833–834, 1975

Li FP, Garber JG, Friend SH, et al.: Recommendations on predictive testing for germ line *p53* mutations among cancer-prone individuals. *J Natl Cancer Inst* 84:1156–1160, 1992

Malkin D, Jolly KW, BapRbier N, et al.: Germline mutations of the *p53* tumor-suppressor gene in children and young adults with second malignant neoplasms. *N Engl J Med* 326:1309–1315, 1992

McGlynn KA, Rosvold EA, Lustbader ED, et al.: Susceptibility to hepatocellular carcinoma is associated with genetic variation in the enzymatic detoxification of aflatoxin B1. *Proc Natl Acad Sci USA* 92:2384–2387, 1995

Miller RW, Fraumeni JF, Manning MD: Association of Wilms' tumor with aniridia, hemihypertrophy, and other congenital malformations. *N Engl J Med* 270:922–927, 1964

Parry DM, Eldridge R, Kaiser-Kupfer MI, Bouzas EA, Pikus A, Patronas N: Neurofibromatosis 2 (NF2): Clinical characteristics of 63 affected individuals and clinical evidence for heterogeneity. *Am J Med Genet* 52:450–461, 1994

Pelletier J, Bruening W, Li FP, Haber DA, Glaser T, Housman DE: WTI mutations contribute to abnormal genital system development and hereditary Wilms' tumour. *Nature* 353:431–434, 1991

Seizinger BR, Rouleau GA, Ozelius LJ, et al.: Genetic linkage of von Recklinghausen neurofibromatosis to the nerve growth factor receptor gene. *Cell* 49:589–594, 1987

Sparkes RS, Murphree AL, Lingua RW, et al.: Gene for hereditary retinoblastoma assigned to human chromosome 13 by linkage to esterase D. *Science* 219:971–973, 1983

Strong LC, Williams WR, Trainsky MA: The Li Fraumeni syndrome: From clinical epidemiology to molecular genetics. *Am J Epidemiol* 135:190–199, 1992

van Heyningen V, Hastie ND: Wilms' tumour: Reconciling genetics and biology. *Trends Genet* 8:16–21, 1992

Multistep Nature of Cancer and Mismatch Repair

Aaltonen L, Peltomaki P, Leach F, et al.: Clues to the pathogenesis of familial colorectal cancer. *Science* 260:812–816, 1993

Armitage P, Doll R: The age distribution of cancer and a multi-stage theory of carcinogenesis. *Br J Cancer* 8:1–12, 1954

Bronner C, Baker S, Morrison P, et al.: Mutation in the DNA mismatch repair gene homologue hMLH1 is associated with hereditary non-polyposis colon cancer. *Nature* 368:258–261, 1994

Eshleman JR, Lang EZ, Bowerfind GK, et al.: Increased mutation rate at the *hprt* locus accompanies microsatellite instability in colon cancer. *Oncogene* 10:33–37, 1995

Fearon ER, Vogelstein B: A genetic model for colorectal tumorigenesis. *Cell* 61:759–767, 1990

Fishel R, Lescoe MK, Rao M, et al.: The human mutator gene homolog MSH2 and its association with hereditary nonpolyposis colon cancer. *Cell* 75:1027–1038, 1993

Hanahan D, Weinberg RA: The hallmarks of cancer. *Cell* 100:57–70, 2000

Ionov Y, Peinado M, Malkhosyan S, Shibata D, Perucho M: Ubiquitous somatic mutations in simple repeated sequences reveal a new mechanism for colonic carcinogenesis. *Nature* 263:558–561, 1993

Leach F, Nicolaides N, Papadopoulos N, et al.: Mutations of a mutS homolog in hereditary nonpolyposis colorectal cancer. *Cell* 75:1215–1225, 1993

Lindblom A, Tannergard P, Werclius B, Nordenskjold M: Genetic mapping of a second locus predisposing to hereditary non-polyposis colon cancer. *Nat Genet* 5:279–282, 1993

Luo J, Kahn S, O'Driscoll K, Weinstein IB: The regulatory domain of protein kinase beta 1 contains phosphatidylserine- and phorbol ester-dependent calcium binding activity. *J Biol Chem* 268:3715–3719, 1993

Lynch H, Smyrk T, Watson P, et al.: Genetics, natural history, tumor spectrum, and pathology of hereditary nonpolyposis colorectal cancer: An updated review. *Gastroenterology* 104:1535–1549, 1993

Maity A, McKenna W, Muschel R: The molecular basis for cell cycle delays following ionizing radiation: A review. *Radiother Oncol* 31:1–13, 1994

Marx J: New link found between p53 and DNA repair. *Science* 266:1321–1322, 1994

McCann J, Dietrich F, Rafferty C, Martin A: A critical review of the genotoxic potential of electric and magnetic fields. *Mutat Res* 297:61–95, 1993

Nicolaides N, Papadopoulos N, Liu B, et al.: Mutations of two PMS homologues in hereditary nonpolyposis colon cancer. *Nature* 371:75–80, 1994

Papadopoulos N, Nicolaides N, Wei Y-F, et al.: Mutation of a mutL homolog in hereditary colon cancer. *Science* 263:1625–1629, 1994

Peltomaki P, Aaltonen L, Sistonen P, et al.: Genetic mapping of a locus predisposing to human colorectal cancer. *Science* 260:810–812, 1993

Ridley AJ, Schwartz MA, Burridge K, Firtel RA, Ginsberg MH, Borisy G, Parsons JT, Horwitz AR: Cell migration: Integrating signals from front to back. *Science* 302:1704–1709, 2003

Genes and Ionizing Radiation

Amundson SA, Bittner M, Fornace AJ Jr: Functional genomics as a window on radiation stress signaling. *Oncogene* 22:5828–5833, 2003

Burns TF, El-Deiry WS: Microarray analysis of p53 target gene expression patterns in the spleen and thymus in response to ionizing radiation. *Cancer Biol Ther* 2:431–443, 2003

Chaudhry MA, Chodosh LA, McKenna WG, Muschel RJ: Gene expression profile of human cells irradiated in G_1 and G_2 phases of cell cycle. *Cancer Lett* 195:221–233, 2003

Datta R, Hass R, Gunji J, Weichselbaum R, Kufe D: Down regulation of cell cycle control genes by ionizing radiation. *Cell Growth Differ* 3:637–644, 1992

Woloschak G, Chang C: Differential modulation of specific gene expression following high-low-LET radiations. *Radiat Res* 124:183–187, 1990

Woloschak G, Chang C: Effects of low-dose radiation on gene expression in Syrian hamster embryo cells: Comparison of JANUS neutrons and gamma rays. In Sugahara T, Sagan L, Aoyama T (eds): *Low Dose Irradiation and Biological Defense Mechanisms*, pp 239–242. Amsterdam, Excerpta Medica, Elsevier Science Publishers, 1992

Woloschak G, Chang C, Jones P, Jones C: Modulation of gene expression in Syrian hamster embryo cells following ionizing radiation. *Cancer Res* 50:339–344, 1990

CHAPTER 18

Dose–Response Relationships for Model Normal Tissues

DOSE–RESPONSE RELATIONSHIPS

Radiation biology applied to clinical radiotherapy is concerned with the relationship between a given absorbed dose of radiation and the consequent biologic response; of particular interest are factors that modify this relationship. With increasing radiation dose, radiation effects may increase in severity (i.e., grade), in frequency (i.e., incidence), or both. In most cases, it is the relation between dose and incidence that is important. Such dose–response curves have a sigmoid (S) shape, with the incidence tending to zero as dose tends to zero and the incidence tending to 100% at very large doses. This applies to both tumor control and normal-tissue complications.

A simple example is shown in Figure 18.1. Tumor control probability is plotted as a function of total dose, and the incidence of normal-tissue complications is also plotted as a function of dose. What is illustrated is a favorable situation where the tumor is more radiosensitive than the normal tissue. In the case of tumor control, the shape can be explained solely from the random nature of cell killing (or clonogen survival) after irradiation and the need to kill every single cell.

For most normal-tissue end points, the biologic interpretation of the sigmoid shape of the relationship is not obvious. Some researchers have evoked a hypothetical *tissue rescue unit* (*TRU*), arguing that tissue breakdown occurs when the number of TRUs falls below a critical level; however, this explanation is questionable.

Therapeutic Ratio (Therapeutic Index)

The ratio of the tumor response for a fixed level of normal-tissue damage has been variously called the *therapeutic ratio* or *therapeutic index*. In the hypothetical example in Figure 18.1, there is a favorable therapeutic ratio, because a 30% probability of tumor control is possible for a 5% incidence of complications.

The time factor is the one parameter that has been most often manipulated to increase this ratio; hyperfractionation, for example, produces a greater

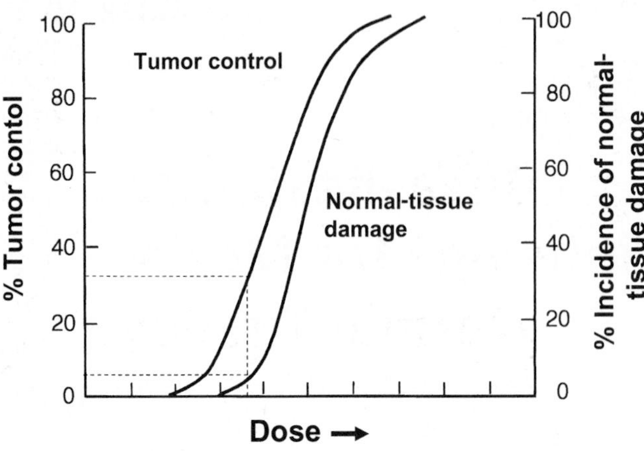

FIGURE 18.1 ● The dose–response relationship is sigmoid in shape for both tumor control and normal-tissue damage. That for normal-tissue damage may be steeper than for tumor control. The therapeutic ratio (or index) is the percent of tumor control that can be achieved for a given level of normal-tissue damage. In this hypothetical example, about 30% tumor control can be achieved for a 5% incidence of normal-tissue damage.

sparing of late-responding normal tissue than tumor control. Another strategy often quoted, though seldom achieved in practice, is to add a drug or radiosensitizer that potentiates the tumor control without potentiating the radiation damage to normal tissue. In practice, it does not need to be as clear-cut as this; it would suffice for the drug to increase tumor control to a greater extent than it increases normal tissue damage. This would result in a therapeutic gain. This is illustrated in Figure 18.2. The addition of the drug moves the tumor control curve to the left to a greater extent than the normal-tissue damage curve; that is, the drug has a larger cytotoxic effect on the tumor than on the normal tissue. Consequently, with the combined modalities, an improved tumor control probability is possible for the same probability of normal-tissue injury.

MITOTIC DEATH AND APOPTOSIS: HOW AND WHY CELLS DIE

Most cell lines cultured *in vitro* die a **mitotic death** after irradiation; that is, they die attempting to divide. This does not necessarily occur at the first postirradiation mitosis; the cell may struggle through one, two, or more mitoses before the damaged chromosomes cause cell death while attempting the complex task of cell division. Time-lapse films of irradiated cells cultured *in vitro* clearly show this process of mitotic death, which is the dominant cause of death if reproductive integrity is assessed *in vitro* as described in Chapter 3.

Mitotic death, however, is not the only form of cell death. Programmed cell death, or **apoptosis**, occurs in normal tissues and neoplasms, in

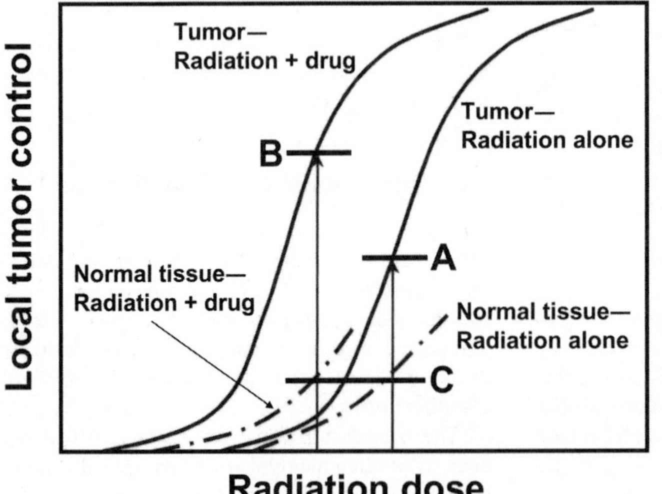

FIGURE 18.2 ● Illustrating how the addition of a drug, a chemotherapy agent or a radiosensitizer, may improve the therapeutic ratio (index). With radiation alone, a given level (**A**) of tumor control is possible for a maximum tolerable level of normal tissue damage (**C**). The addition of the drug moves the dose–response curve for both tumor and normal tissue to the left. If the addition of the drug has a greater effect on tumor control than on normal-tissue morbidity (i.e., it moves the curve further to the left), then a higher local tumor control (**B**) is possible for the same level of normal-tissue injury (**C**).

mammals and amphibians, in the embryo and the adult. It is implicated, for example, in tissue involution, such as the regression of the tadpole tail during metamorphosis, and it is common during embryonic development. It also can occur after irradiation. *Apoptosis* means "falling off," as of petals from flowers or leaves from trees. (Like the word *mitosis*, it comes from the Greek.)

Apoptosis is characterized by a stereotyped sequence of morphologic events that take place in two discrete phases. In the first phase, cells condense and bud to produce many membrane-enclosed bodies. In the second phase, these bodies are phagocytized and digested by nearby tissue cells. The characteristic "laddering" of DNA that occurs during apoptotic death is illustrated in Chapter 3. Apoptosis characteristically affects scattered individual cells. If apoptosis affects cells in tissues, the resulting apoptotic bodies are squeezed along the intercellular spaces and are either shed from the epithelial surface or rapidly phagocytized by nearby cells. The cells surrounding those being deleted merely close ranks, and there is no tissue disorganization such as occurs after necrosis.

ASSAYS FOR DOSE–RESPONSE RELATIONSHIPS

A number of experimental techniques are available to obtain dose–response relationships for the cells of normal tissues. First, there are a limited number of clonogenic assays—techniques in which the end point observed depends directly on the reproductive integrity of individual cells. These systems are directly analogous to cell survival *in vitro*. The techniques developed by Withers and his colleagues are based on their observation of a clone of cells regenerating *in situ* in irradiated tissue. Skin colonies, regenerating crypts in the jejunum, testes stem cells, and kidney tubules are described briefly later in this chapter. It is also possible to obtain dose–response curves for the cells of the epithelial lining of the colon or stomach, but the method used is essentially the same as for the jejunum. Kember described a system for scoring regenerating clones in cartilage at about the same time as the Withers' skin colony system, but it has not been used widely and is not discussed here.

The assay system for the stem cells in the bone marrow or cells of the thyroid and mammary gland depends on the observation of the growth of clones of cells taken from a donor animal and transplanted into a different tissue in a recipient animal. In Till and McCulloch's bone-marrow assay, colonies of bone marrow cells are counted in the spleens of recipient animals. Dose–response curves for mammary and thyroid cells have been obtained by Gould and Clifton by observing colonies growing from cells transplanted into the fat pads of recipient animals.

Second, dose–response relationships can be obtained that are repeatable and quantitative but that depend on functional end points. These include skin reactions in rodents or pigs (e.g., erythema and desquamation), pneumonitis or fibrosis in mouse lungs reflected in an increased breathing rate, myelopathy of the hind limbs from damage to the spinal cord, and deformities to the feet of mice. The end points observed tend to reflect the minimum number of functional cells remaining in a tissue or organ, rather than the fraction of cells retaining their reproductive integrity.

Finally, one can *infer* a dose–response curve for a tissue in which it cannot be observed directly by assuming the form of the dose–response curve (linear-quadratic) and performing a series of multifraction experiments. This procedure, first suggested by Douglas and Fowler, has been used widely to infer values for α and β in the dose–response relationships for normal tissues in which the parameters cannot be measured directly.

This chapter includes assays for both early- and late-responding tissues. The skin, intestinal epithelium, and bone-marrow cells, for example, are rapidly dividing self-renewal tissues and respond early to the effects of radiation. The spinal cord, lung, and kidney, by contrast, are late-responding tissues. This reflects the current philosophy that the radiation response of *all* tissues results from the depletion of the critical parenchymal cells and that the difference in time at which early- and late-responding tissues express radiation damage is a function simply of different cell turnover rates. Many older papers in the literature ascribe the response of late-responding tissues to vascular damage rather than to depletion of parenchymal cells, but this thesis is becoming increasingly difficult to accept.

The various types of normal-tissue assay systems are described briefly. The reader who is content with the summary already given may wish to skip the remainder of this chapter.

CLONOGENIC END POINTS

Clones Regrowing *in Situ*

Skin Colonies

Withers developed an ingenious technique (Fig. 18.3) to determine the survival curve for mouse skin cells. The hair was plucked from an area on the back of the mouse, and a superficial x-ray

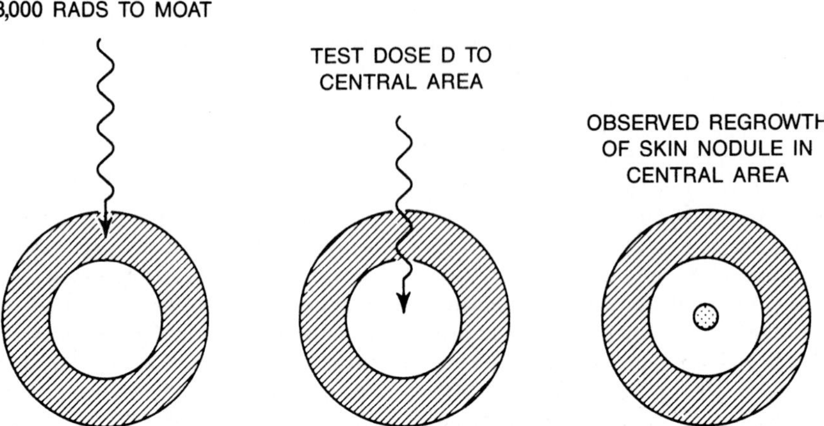

FIGURE 18.3 ● Technique used to isolate an area of skin for experimental irradiation. A superficial (30-kV) x-ray machine is used to irradiate an annulus of skin to a massive dose of about 3,000 rad (30 Gy). An isolated island of intact skin in the center of this "moat" is protected from the radiation by a metal sphere. The intact skin is then given a test dose (D) and observed for nodules of regrowing skin. (Adapted from Withers HR: The dose-survival relationship for irradiation of epithelial cells of mouse skin. *Br J Radiol* 40:187–194, 1967, with permission.)

machine was used to irradiate an annulus of skin to a massive dose of 30 Gy (3,000 rad). This produced a "moat" of dead cells, in the center of which was an isolated island of intact skin that had been protected during the first exposure to low-voltage x-rays by a small metal sphere. This small area of intact skin was then given a test dose (D) and subsequently observed for regrowth of skin. If one or more stem cells survived in this small area, nodules of regrowing skin could be seen some days later. If no cells survived in this small area, the skin would heal much later by infiltration of cells crossing the moat. Figure 18.4 shows nodules regrowing in mouse skin. To obtain a survival curve, it was necessary to repeat this operation with a number of different areas of skin. A range of ball bearings was used to shield a small area of skin in the middle of the "moat." The resulting survival data are shown in Figure 18.5, in which the dose (D) to the control area is plotted against the number of surviving cells per square centimeter of skin.

There are practical limits to the range in which the dose–response relationship can be determined. At one extreme, it is not possible to irradiate too large an area on the back of the mouse to produce the moat of sterilized skin. At the other extreme,

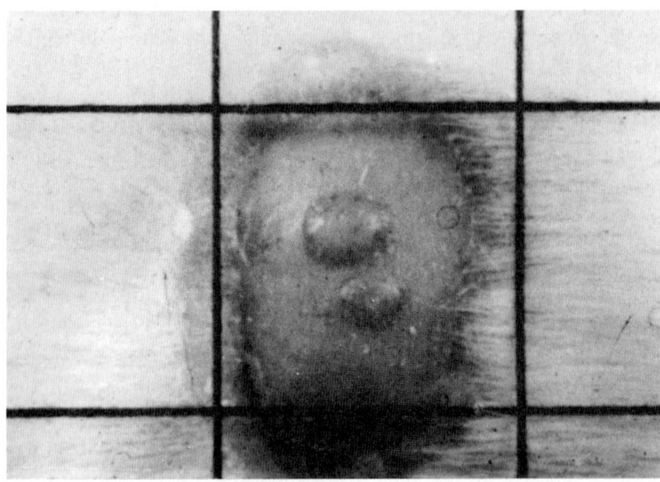

FIGURE 18.4 ● Photograph of nodules of mouse skin regrowing from a single surviving cell in the treated area. (Courtesy of Dr. H.R. Withers.)

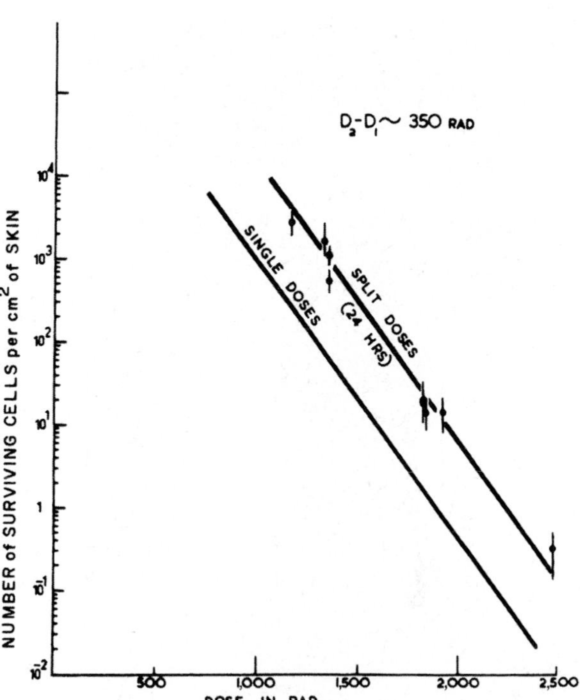

FIGURE 18.5 ● Single-dose and two-dose survival curves for epithelial cells of mouse skin exposed to 29-kVp x-rays. The 37% dose slope (D_0) is 1.35 Gy (135 rad). The ordinate is not the surviving fraction, as in the survival curves for cells cultured *in vitro*, but is the number of surviving cells per square centimeter of skin. In the two-dose survival curve, the interval between dose fractions was always 24 hours. The curves are parallel, their horizontal separation being equal to about 3.5 Gy (350 rad); this corresponds to $\mathbf{D_q}$. From a knowledge of $\mathbf{D_q}$ and the slope of the survival curve, D_0, the extrapolation number, n, may be calculated. (From Withers HR: Recovery and repopulation in vivo by mouse skin epithelial cells during fractionated irradiation. *Radiat Res* 32:227–239, 1967; and Withers HR: The dose-survival relationship for irradiation of epithelial cells of mouse skin. *Br J Radiol* 40:187–194, 1967, with permission.)

the smallest area that can be used is determined by the fact that even 30-kV radiation scatters laterally to some extent. As can be seen in Figure 18.5, the technique results in a single-dose survival curve that extends from about 8 to 25 Gy (800–2,500 rad); over this range, with dose plotted on a linear scale and the number of surviving cells per square centimeter plotted on a logarithmic scale, the survival curve is straight and has a D_0 of 1.35 Gy (135 rad). This D_0 value is very similar to that obtained with mammalian cells cultured *in vitro*.

The extrapolation number cannot be obtained directly with this technique; the ordinate is the number of surviving cells per square centimeter of skin, and this cannot be converted to the surviving fraction because it is not known with any accuracy how many skin stem cells there are per unit area. It is, however, possible to make an indirect estimate of the extrapolation number by obtaining the survival curve for doses given in two fractions separated by 24 hours. The survival curve obtained in this way also is shown in Figure 18.5. It is parallel to that obtained for single doses but is displaced from it toward higher doses. As explained in Chapter 3, this lateral displacement in a direction parallel to the dose axis is a measure of $\mathbf{D_q}$, the *quasithreshold dose*. The D_q for mouse skin is about 3.5 Gy (350 rad), which is very similar to the value for human skin estimated from split-dose experiments.

Crypt Cells of the Mouse Jejunum

A technique perfected by Withers and Elkind makes it possible to obtain the survival characteristics of the crypt cells of the mouse jejunum. The lining of the jejunum is a classic example of a self-renewal system. The cells in the crypts divide rapidly and provide a continuous supply of cells that move up the villi, differentiate, and become the functioning cells. The cells at the top of the folds of the villi are slowly but continuously sloughed off in the normal course of events and are replaced continuously by cells that originate from mitoses in the crypts.

Figure 18.6, an electron micrograph, dramatically shows the three-dimensional structure of the lining of the intestinal epithelium. Mice are given a total-body dose of 11 to 16 Gy (1,100–1,600 rad), which sterilizes a significant proportion of the dividing cells in the crypts but has essentially no effect on the differentiated cells in the villi. Consequently, crypt degeneration appears early after irradiation, and the villi remain long and their epithelial covering of differentiated cells shows little change. With the further passage of time, the tips of the villi continue to be sloughed away by normal use, but no replacement cells are available from the depopulated crypts, and so the villi begin to shorten and shrink. At sufficiently high doses, the surface lining of the jejunum is completely denuded of villi.

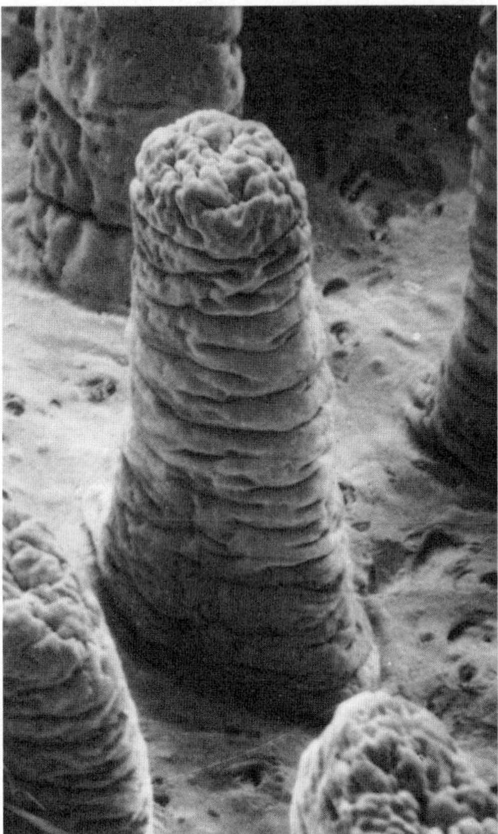

FIGURE 18.6 ● Scanning electron micrograph that allows three-dimensional visualization of the jejunal villi from the hamster. (Magnification ×175.) (From Taylor AB, Anderson JH: Scanning electron microscope observations of mammalian intestinal villi, intervillus floor and crypt tubules. *Micron* 3:430–453, 1972, with permission.)

To obtain a survival curve for the jejunal crypt cells, groups of animals are exposed to graded total-body doses of radiation. After 3.5 days, each animal is sacrificed and sections are made of the jejunum (Fig. 18.7**A**). At this time, crypts are just beginning to regenerate and it is relatively simple to identify them. Figure 18.7**B** shows a number of regenerating crypts at a higher magnification. These pictures also show the shortened villi and the greatly reduced density of cells lining the surface. The score of radiation damage is the *number of regenerating crypts per circumference* of the sectioned jejunum. This quantity is plotted as a function of dose and yields a survival curve as shown in Figure 18.8. The single-dose survival curve has a D_0 (for γ-rays) of about 1.3 Gy (130 rad). Also shown in Figure 18.8 are survival curves for radiation delivered in multiple fractions, from 2 to 20. The separation between the single- and two-dose survival curves gives a measure of D_q, which has the very large value of between 4 and 4.5 Gy (400–450 rad).

This technique has two limitations. First, the quantity plotted on the ordinate is the number of surviving crypts per circumference, not the surviving fraction. Second, experiments can be done only at doses of about 10 Gy (1,000 rad) or more, at which there is a sufficient level of biologic damage for individual regenerating crypts to be identified. The doses can be delivered, however, in a number of smaller fractions, as long as the total results in enough biologic damage to be scored. The shape of the entire survival curve then can be reconstructed from the multifraction data if it is assumed that in a fractionated regimen each dose produces the same amount of cell killing and if an estimate is made of the number of clonogens at risk per crypt. This has been done by Withers and his colleagues; the resultant survival curve is shown in Figure 18.9.

Testes Stem Cells

A technique to measure the radiation response of testicular cells capable of sustaining spermatogenesis (i.e., the stem cells) was devised by Withers and his colleagues. About 6 weeks after irradiation, mouse testes are sectioned and examined histologically. Sections of normal and irradiated testes are shown in Figure 18.10. The proportion of tubules containing spermatogenic epithelium is counted and plotted as a function of dose in Figure 18.11. As in many *in vivo* assays, relatively high single doses of 8 to 16 Gy (800–1,600 rad) are necessary so that the level of damage is sufficient to be scored. In this dose range, D_0 is about 1.68 Gy (168 rad). If the split-dose technique is used, the D_q is about 2.7 Gy (270 rad). It is possible to estimate the effect of small doses and reconstruct a complete survival curve by giving large doses in multiple small fractions and assuming that the response to each fraction is the same. The result of this reconstruction is shown in Figure 18.12.

Kidney Tubules

A technique using kidney tubules, again developed by Withers and his colleagues, is the first clonal assay for a late-responding tissue. One kidney per mouse is irradiated with a small field and removed for histologic examination 60 weeks later. Figure 18.13 shows sections of normal and irradiated kidneys. For ease of scoring, only those tubules touching the renal capsule are scored, and a tubule is considered fully regenerated only if it is lined with well-differentiated cuboidal or columnar cells with a large amount of eosinophilic cytoplasm. By 60 weeks, tubules either have no surviving epithelial

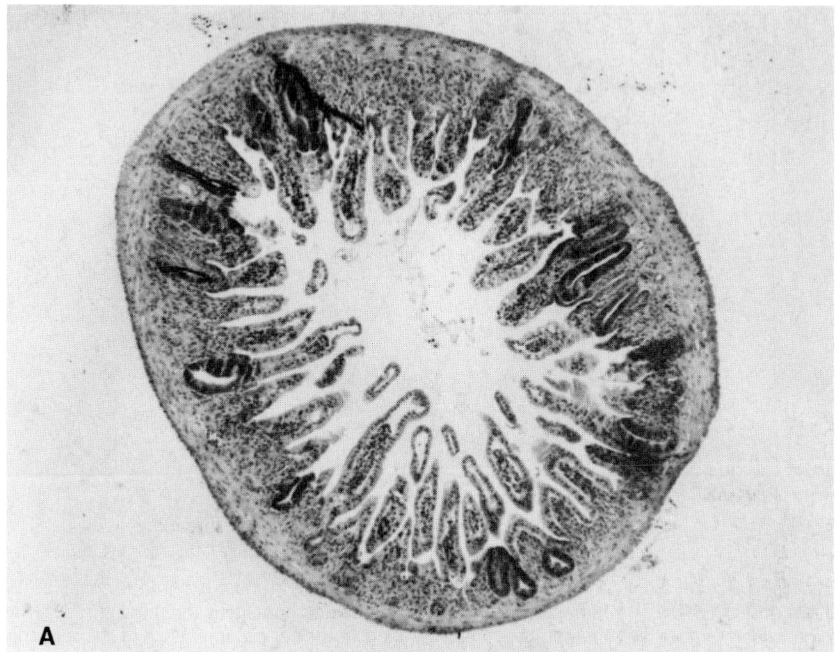

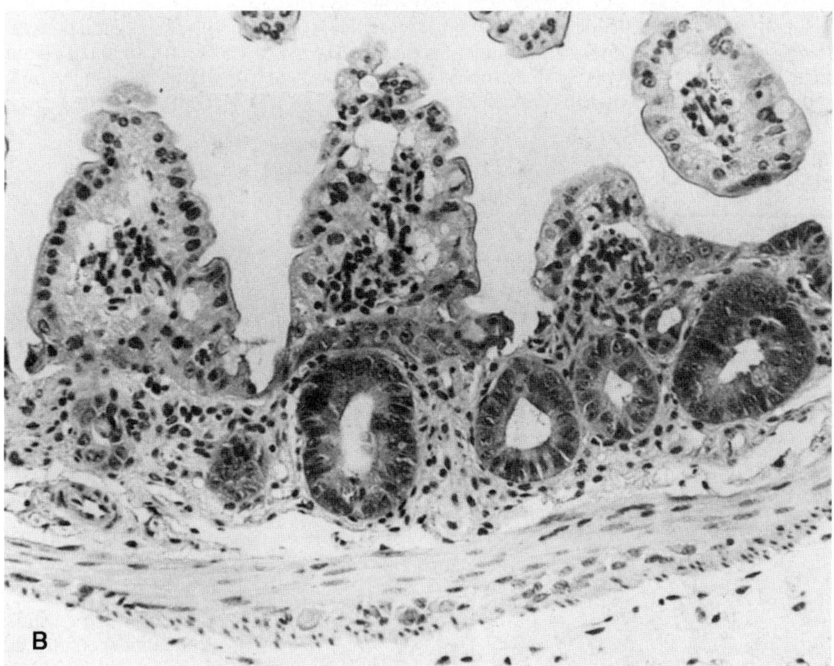

FIGURE 18.7 • **A:** Section of mouse jejunum taken 3.5 days after a total-body dose in excess of 10 Gy (1,000 rad). Note the shortened villi and the regenerating crypts. **B:** Regenerating crypts shown at a higher magnification. (From Withers HR: Regeneration of intestinal mucosa after irradiation. *Cancer* 28:78–81, 1971, with permission.)

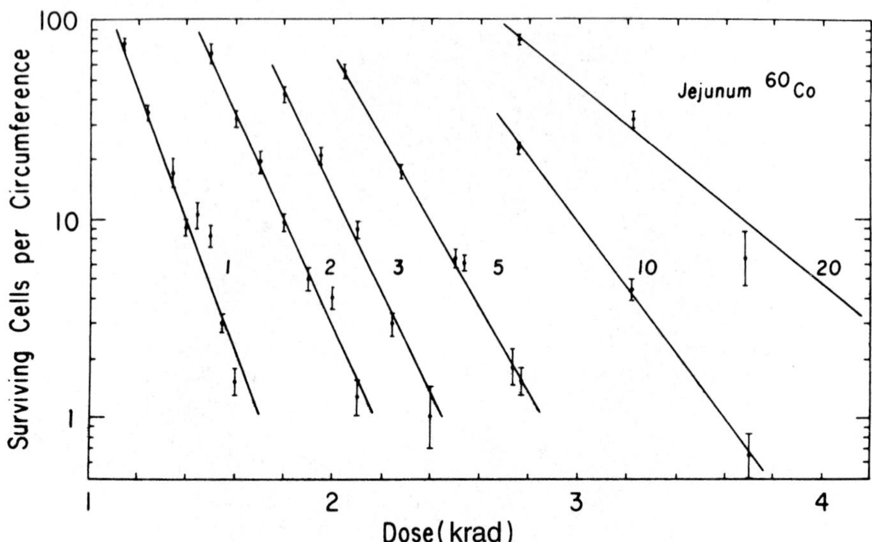

FIGURE 18.8 ● Survival curves for crypt cells in the mouse jejunum exposed to single or multiple doses of γ-rays (1–20 fractions). The score of radiation damage is the number of surviving cells per circumference (i.e., the number of regenerating crypts per circumference of the sectioned jejunum) counted from sections such as those shown in Figure 18.7. This quantity is plotted on a logarithmic scale against radiation dose on a linear scale. The D_0 for the single-dose survival curve is about 1.3 Gy (130 rad). The shoulder of the survival curve is very large. The separation between the single- and two-dose survival curves indicates that the $\mathbf{D_q}$ is 4 to 4.5 Gy (400–450 rad). (From Withers HR, Mason K, Reid BO, et al.: Response of mouse intestine to neutrons and gamma rays in relation to dose fractionation and division cycle. *Cancer* 34:39–47, 1974, with permission.)

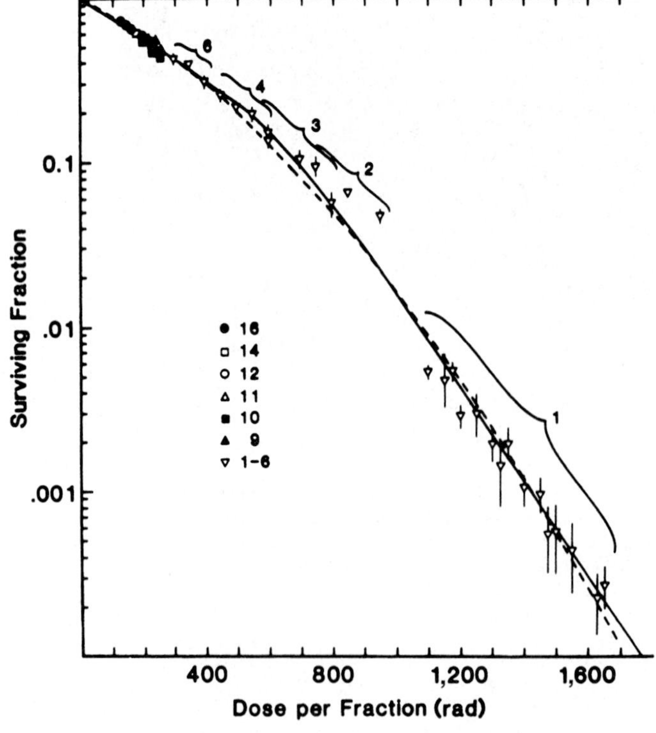

FIGURE 18.9 ● Effective single-dose survival curve reconstructed from multifraction experiments for clonogenic cells of the jejunal crypts of mice. The numbers on the curve refer to the number of fractions used to reconstruct that part of the curve. The initial and final slopes are about 3.57 and 1.43 Gy (357 and 143 rad), respectively. The quasithreshold dose is 4.3 Gy (430 rad). The data are equally well fitted by the linear-quadratic formulation. (From Thames HD, Withers R, Mason KA, Reid BO: Dose survival characteristics of mouse jejunal crypt cells. *Int J Radiat Oncol Biol Phys* 7:1591–1597, 1981, with permission.)

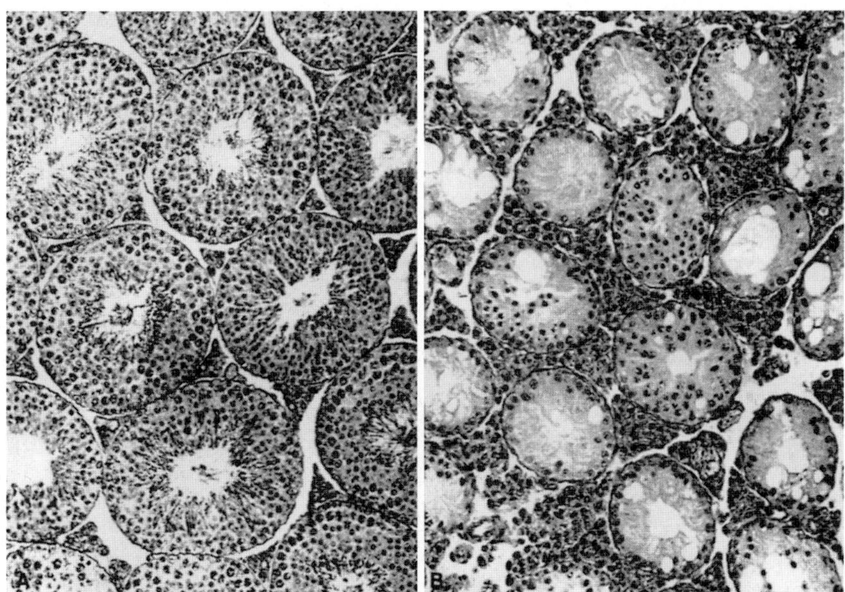

FIGURE 18.10 ● **Left:** Histology of normal testis. **Right:** Histology of testis 35 days after a dose of 9 Gy (900 rad) of γ-radiation. Some tubules are completely devoid of spermatogenic epithelium and some are not. (Sertoli's cells persist in the tubules sterilized of spermatogenic cells.) Foci of spermatogenesis can be derived from single surviving stem cells. (Magnification × 200.) (From Withers HR, Hunter N, Barkley HT Jr, Reid BO: Radiation survival and regeneration characteristics of spermatogenic stem cells of mouse testis. *Radiat Res* 57:88–103, 1974, with permission.)

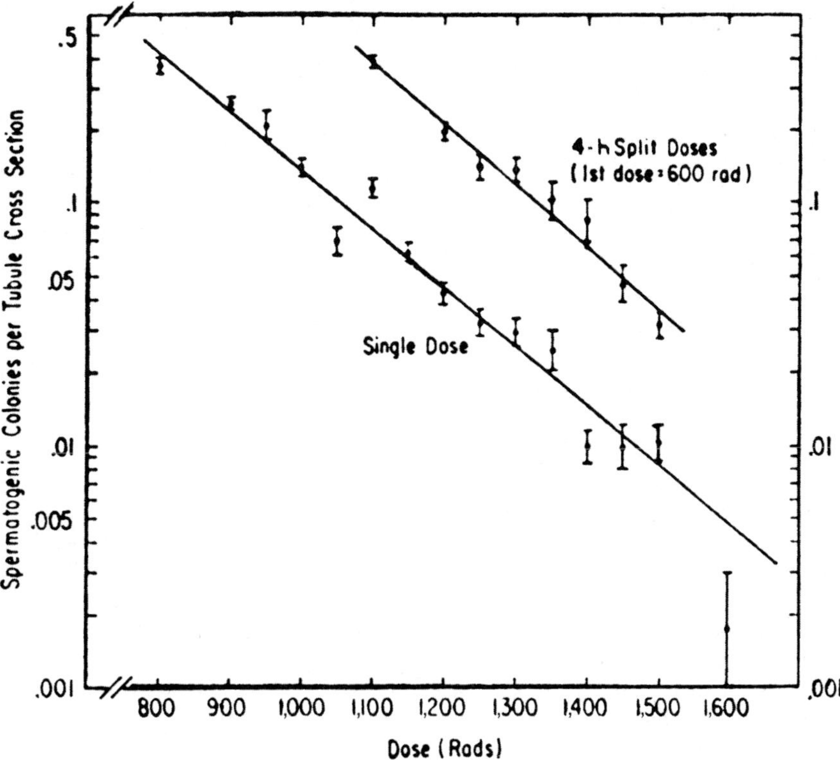

FIGURE 18.11 ● Single- and split-dose survival curves for spermatogenic stem cells of the mouse testis. The D_0 is about 1.68 Gy (168 rad). The $\mathbf{D_q}$, assessed from the horizontal separation of the single- and split-dose curves, is about 2.7 Gy (270 rad). (From Withers HR, Hunter N, Barkley HT Jr, Reid BO: Radiation survival and regeneration characteristics of spermatogenic stem cells of mouse testis. *Radiat Res* 57:88–103, 1974, with permission.)

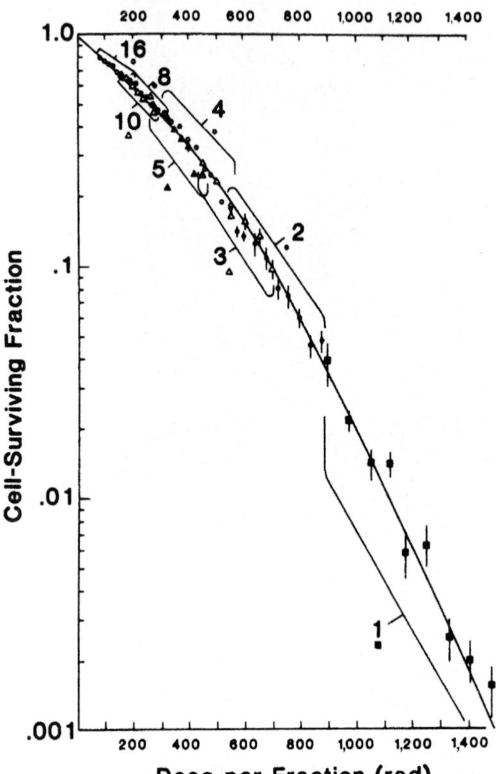

FIGURE 18.12 ● Survival curve for testis stem cells reconstructed from multifraction experiments, assuming that each fraction produces the same biologic effect. The numbers on the curve refer to the number of fractions used to reconstruct that portion of the curve. The D_0 is about 1.6 Gy (160 rad), and the $\mathbf{D_q}$ is about 3.92 Gy (392 rad). (From Thames HD, Withers HR: Test of equal effect per fraction and estimation of initial clonogen number in microcolony assays of survival after fractionated irradiation. *Br J Radiol* 53:1071–1077, 1980, with permission.)

cells or are lined completely with epithelium that has regenerated from a small number of surviving cells, usually one. The number of tubules regenerating in an arbitrary number of sections counted is plotted as a function of radiation dose. The result is shown in Figure 18.14; D_0 is about 1.53 Gy (153 rad).

The radiosensitivity of the cells of this late-responding tissue is not very different from that of early-responding tissues, such as the skin or intestinal epithelium. The *rate* of response, however, is quite different. The time required for depletion of the epithelium after a single dose of 14 Gy (1,400 rad) is about 3 days in the jejunum, 12 to 24 days in the skin, and 30 days in the seminiferous tubules of the testes, but 300 days in the kidney tubules. These results argue strongly that radiation injury in the kidney results from depletion of parenchymal cells and that the slow expression of injury merely reflects the slow turnover of this cell population. Vascular injury is unlikely to be the mechanism underlying the destruction of renal tubules.

Cells Transplanted to Another Site

Bone Marrow Stem Cells

Till and McCulloch developed a system to determine a survival curve for colony-forming bone marrow cells (Fig. 18.15). Recipient animals first are irradiated supralethally with a dose of 9 to 10 Gy (900–1,000 rad), which sterilizes their spleens. Nucleated isologous bone marrow cells taken from another animal are then injected intravenously into the recipient animals. Some of these cells lodge in the spleen, where they form nodules, or colonies, 10 to 11 days later, because the spleen cells of the recipient animals have been sterilized previously by the large dose of radiation. At this time, the spleens are removed and the colonies counted. Figure 18.16 is a photograph of a spleen showing the colonies to be counted.

About 10^4 cells must be injected into a recipient animal to produce one spleen colony, because the majority of the cells in the nucleated isologous bone marrow are fully differentiated cells and would never be capable of forming a colony. To obtain a surviving fraction for bone marrow cells, a donor animal is irradiated to some test dose, and the suspension of cells from the bone marrow is inoculated into groups of recipient animals that previously had been irradiated supralethally. By counting the colonies in the spleens of the recipient animals, and with a knowledge of the number of cells required to produce a colony in an unirradiated animal (plating efficiency), the surviving fraction may be calculated as follows:

$$\text{Surviving fraction for a dose D} = \frac{\text{colonies counted}}{\text{cells inoculated} \times \text{plating efficiency}}$$

This procedure is repeated for a range of doses, and a survival curve is obtained (Fig. 18.17). These bone marrow stem cells are very sensitive with a D_0 of about 0.95 Gy (95 rad) and little or no shoulder to the survival curve.

Mammary and Thyroid Cells

Clifton and Gould and their colleagues developed very useful clonogen transplant assays for epithelial cells of the mammary and thyroid glands. They have

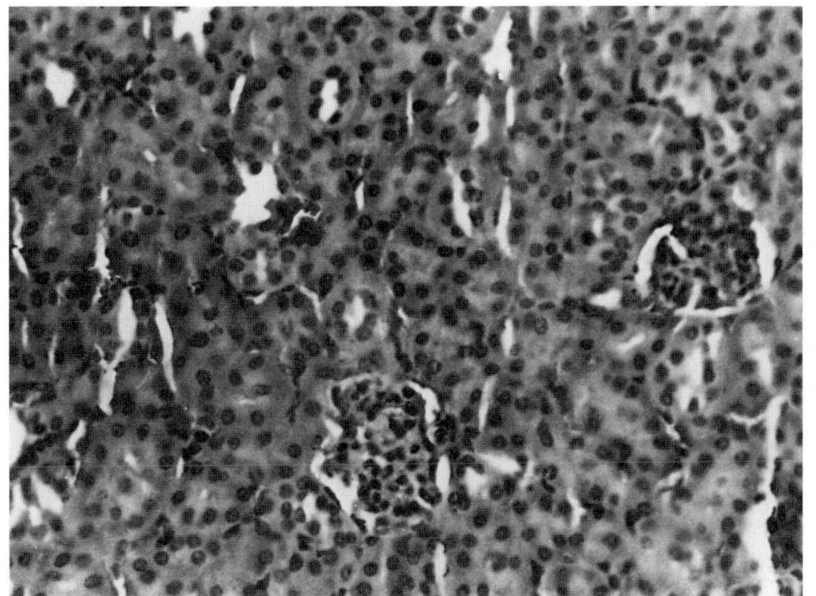

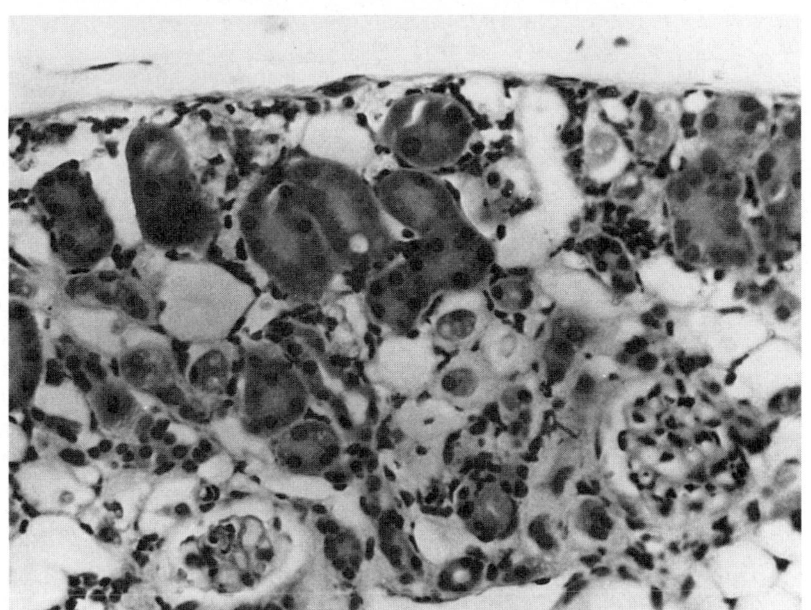

FIGURE 18.13 • Photomicrographs of mouse kidney. **A:** Normal, showing proximal tubules in contact with the capsule. (Hematoxylin–eosin stain, magnification ×400.) **B:** Sixty weeks after irradiation with 13 Gy (1,300 rad). Note normal proximal tubules and glomeruli amid ghosts of deepithelialized tubules. One epithelialized tubule is in contact with the capsule. (Hematoxylin–eosin stain, magnification ×200.) (From Withers HR, Mason KA, Thames HD: Late radiation response of kidney assayed by tubule cell survival. *Br J Radiol* 59:587–595, 1986, with permission.)

been used largely for cell survival studies, described later, but the initial motivation for their development was to study carcinogenesis in a quantitative system. Most *in vitro* transformation assays involve fibroblasts, and the bulk of human cancers arise in epithelial cells—hence, the importance and interest in these two systems.

The techniques for these two systems are much the same. To generate a survival curve for mammary or thyroid gland cells in the rat, cells may be

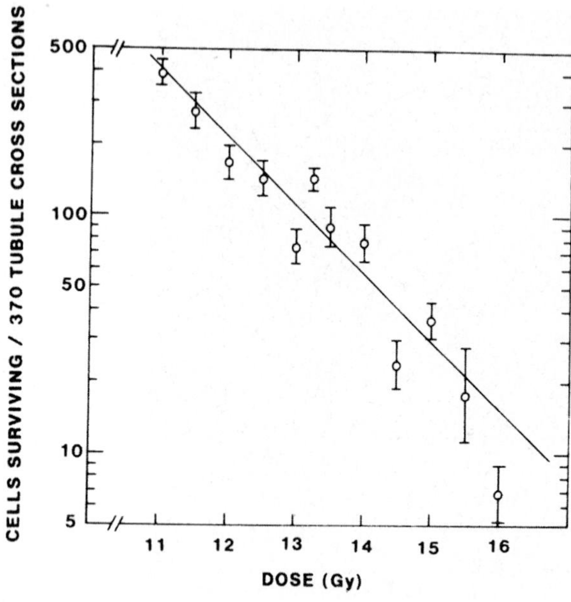

FIGURE 18.14 ● Dose–survival curve for tubule-regenerating cells. The D_0 is 1.53 Gy (153 rad). (From Withers HR, Mason KA, Thames HD Jr: Late radiation response of kidney assayed by tubule cell survival. *Br J Radiol* 59:587–595, 1986.)

irradiated *in vivo* before the gland is removed from donor animals and treated with enzymes to obtain a monodispersed cell suspension. Known numbers of cells are injected into the inguinal or interscapular white fat pads of recipient animals.

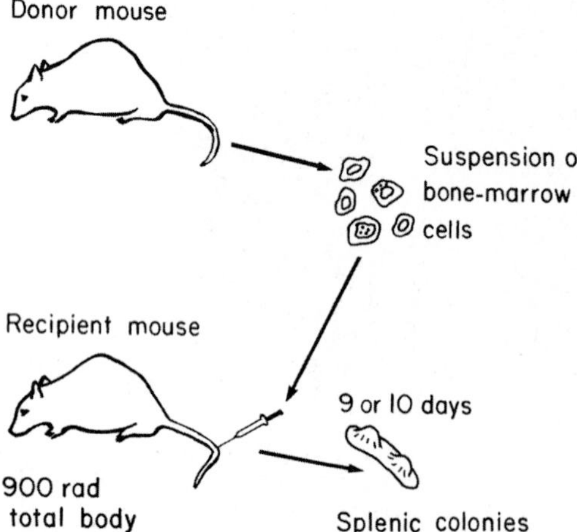

FIGURE 18.15 ● Till and McCulloch's technique. From the donor mouse a cell suspension is made of nucleated isologous bone marrow. A known number of cells are injected into recipient mice previously irradiated with a 9-Gy (900-rad) total-body dose. The spleen is removed from each recipient mouse 9 or 10 days later, and the number of nodules are counted. (Adapted from Till JE, McCulloch EA: In Cameron IL, Padilla GM, Zimmerman AM [eds]: *Developmental Aspects of the Cell Cycle*, pp 297–313. New York, Academic Press, 1971, with permission.

Under appropriate host conditions and grafted cell numbers, the injection of mammary cells gives rise to mammary structures that are morphologically and functionally normal. One such mammary structure may develop from a single cell. By 3.5 weeks after the injection of mammary cells, positive growth is indicated by alveolar units. An example of a milk-filled alveolar unit is shown as an inset in Figure 18.18. If thyroid cells are injected, thyroid follicular units develop (Fig. 18.19).

With either type of cell, a larger number must be injected to produce a growing unit if the cells first are irradiated to a given dose. In practice, some fancy statistics are involved, a discussion of which is beyond the scope of this chapter; in essence, the ratio of the number of irradiated to unirradiated cells required to produce one growing unit (thyroid follicular unit or alveolar unit) is a measure of the cell-surviving fraction corresponding to the dose. This procedure must be repeated for a range of graded doses to generate a survival curve. The resultant survival curve for mammary cells is shown in Figure 18.18. The characteristics of the curve are unremarkable: D_0 is about 1.27 Gy (127 rad), and the extrapolation number is about 5, quite typical of rodent cells cultured *in vitro*. The corresponding survival curve for thyroid cells is shown in Figure 18.19. D_0 is a little larger than for mammary glands assayed in a similar way, implying that the cells are a little more resistant. Figures 18.18 and 18.19 also show data for cells left *in situ* for 24 hours after irradiation before being removed and assayed. If this is done, the shoulder of the survival curve

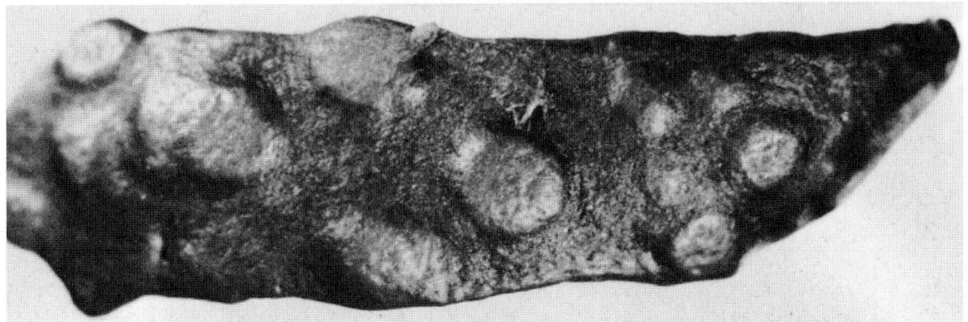

FIGURE 18.16 ● Photograph of a mouse's spleen. The mouse was irradiated supralethally to sterilize all the cells of the spleen. The nodules of regrowth originate from intravenously injected bone-marrow cells from another animal. (Courtesy of Dr. A. Carsten, Brookhaven National Laboratory.)

is larger because of the repair of potentially lethal damage. This is discussed in more detail in Chapter 5.

An interesting use of these clonogen transplant assays is that the physiologic states of either donor or recipient animals can be manipulated hormonally. For the mammary cell assay, cells may be taken from inactive, slowly dividing glands of virgin rats, from rapidly dividing glands of rats in midpregnancy, or from milk-producing glands of lactating rats. For the thyroid cell assay, the physiologic states of both donor and recipient can be manipulated by control of the diet or by partial thyroidectomy.

SUMMARY OF DOSE–RESPONSE CURVES FOR CLONOGENIC ASSAYS IN NORMAL TISSUES

The survival curves for all of the clonogenic assays in normal tissues are plotted together in Figure 18.20. There is a substantial range of radiosensitivities, with shoulder width being the principal variable. *In vitro* curves for cells from patients with

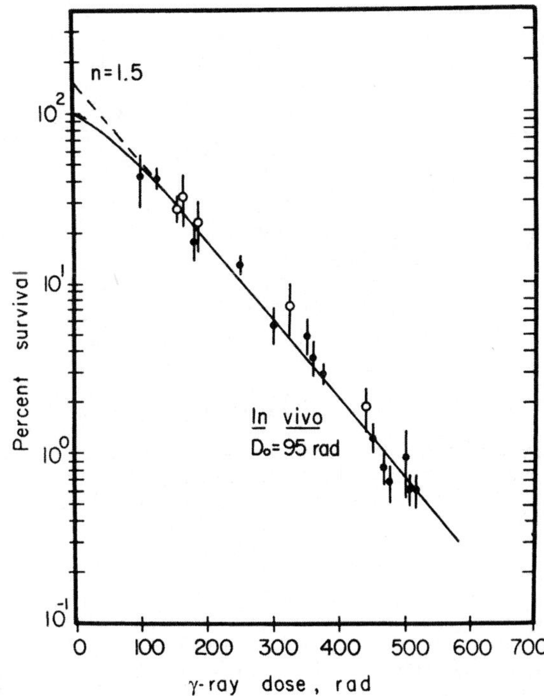

FIGURE 18.17 ● γ-Ray survival curve for the colony-forming ability of mouse bone-marrow cells. The cells are irradiated *in vivo* in the donor animal and grow into colonies in the spleens of supralethally irradiated recipient animals. (Adapted from McCulloch EA, Till JE: The sensitivity of cells from normal mouse bone marrow to gamma radiation *in vitro* and *in vivo*. *Radiat Res* 16:822–832, 1962, with permission.)

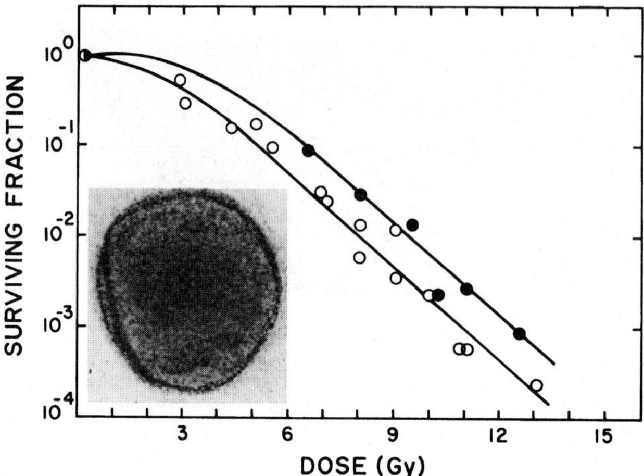

FIGURE 18.18 ● Dose–response relationship for rat mammary cells assayed by transplantation into the fat pads of recipient animals. (Adapted from Gould MN, Clifton KH: Evidence for a unique *in situ* component of the repair of radiation damage. *Radiat Res* 77:149–155, 1979, with permission.) **Inset:** A milk-filled spherical alveolar unit developed from a transplanted cell. (From Gould MN, Biel WF, Clifton KH: Morphological and quantitative studies of gland formation from inocula of monodispersed rat mammary cells. *Exp Cell Res* 107:405–416, 1977, with permission.)

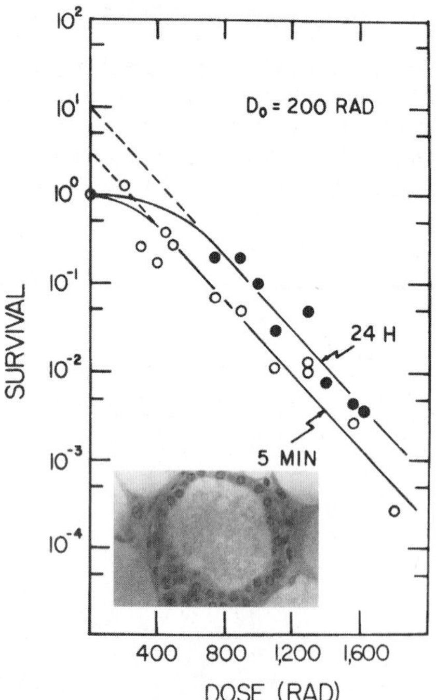

FIGURE 18.19 ● Dose–response relationship for rat thyroid cells assayed by transplantation into the fat pads of recipient animals. (From Mulcahy RT, Gould MN, Clifton KH: The survival of thyroid cells: *in vivo* irradiation and *in situ* repair. *Radiat Res* 84:523–528, 1980, with permission.) **Inset:** A single thyroid follicle that developed 4 weeks after the inoculation of thyroid cells into the fat pads of recipient animals. (From Clifton KH, Gould MN, Potten CS, Hendry J [eds]: *Cell Clones*, pp 128–138. New York, Churchill Livingstone, 1985, with permission.)

ataxia-telangiectasia also are shown because these are probably the most radiosensitive mammalian cells.

DOSE–RESPONSE RELATIONSHIPS FOR FUNCTIONAL END POINTS

Pig Skin

Pig skin has been used widely in radiobiologic studies because it has many features in common with human skin, such as color, hair follicles, sweat glands, and a layer of subcutaneous fat. In view of these structural similarities, it is not surprising that the response of pig skin to radiation closely resembles that of human skin, both qualitatively and quantitatively.

Fowler and his colleagues pioneered the use of pig skin as a radiobiologic test system. A number of small rectangular fields on the pig's flank were irradiated with graded doses of x-rays, and the reactions were scored daily using the arbitrary scale shown in Table 18.1. After a single dose of radiation, the reaction becomes apparent after about 15 days and develops as shown in Figure 18.21.

Two phases of the reaction can be distinguished. First, an early wave of erythema occurred (at 10–40 days), which was variable from one animal to another. This represents the uncomfortable "acute" reaction sometimes seen in patients on radiotherapy at about the end of a course of treatment. Second, a more gradual increase to a second broad wave of moderately severe reactions took place (at 50–100 days), representing a more permanent kind of damage. This second wave shows the tolerance of skin to a more serious type of long-term damage and is also a more repeatable and consistent index of radiation damage. It was subsequently found to

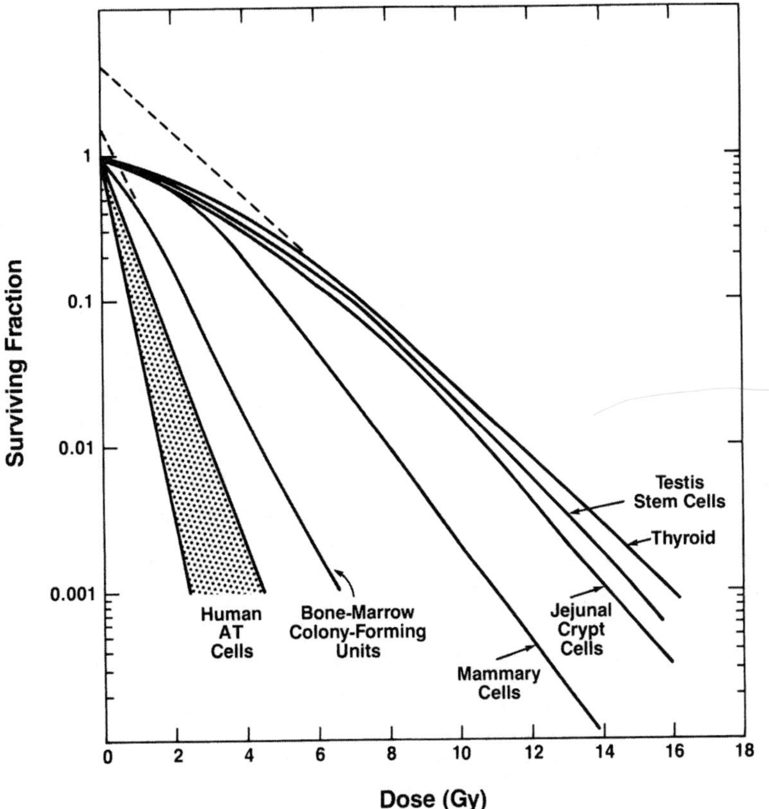

FIGURE 18.20 • Summary of survival curves for clonogenic assays of cells from normal tissues. The human ataxia-telangiectasia (AT) cells are included because they are the most sensitive mammalian cells. The bone-marrow colony-forming units, together with the mammary and thyroid cells, represent systems in which cells are irradiated and assayed by transplantation into a different tissue in recipient animals. The jejunal crypt and testis stem cells are examples of systems in which cells are assayed for regrowth *in situ* after irradiation.

TABLE 18.1

Radiation Reactions in Pig Skin

Arbitrary Score	Reaction
0	No visible reaction
1	Faint erythema
2	Erythema
3	Marked erythema
4	Moist desquamation of less than half the irradiated area
5	Moist desquamation of more than half the Irradiated area

From Fowler JR, Morgan RL, Silvester JA, Bewley DK, Turner BA: Experiments with fractionated x-ray treatment of the skin of pigs: 1. Fractionation up to 28 days. *Br J Radiol* 36:188–196, 1963, with permission.

correlate well with longer-term damage (up to 2 years) and with subcutaneous damage.

The "score" of radiation damage is taken to be the average skin reaction occurring between certain time limits that encompass the medium-term reactions. After a single dose, this might be a 35-day period between 50 and 85 days after irradiation. For a protracted fractionated regimen, this period of reaction may come later, between days 65 and 100. The average skin reaction in the chosen time period then is plotted as a function of dose; examples of dose–response curves obtained this way are shown in Figure 18.22 for single and fractionated doses.

Late effects also have been studied in pig skin by measuring the contraction that results from fibrosis a year or more after irradiation. A square is tattooed on the skin of the animal in the irradiated field, and the dimensions of this square are recorded as a function of dose as the contraction occurs. This is a primitive but effective measure of late effects.

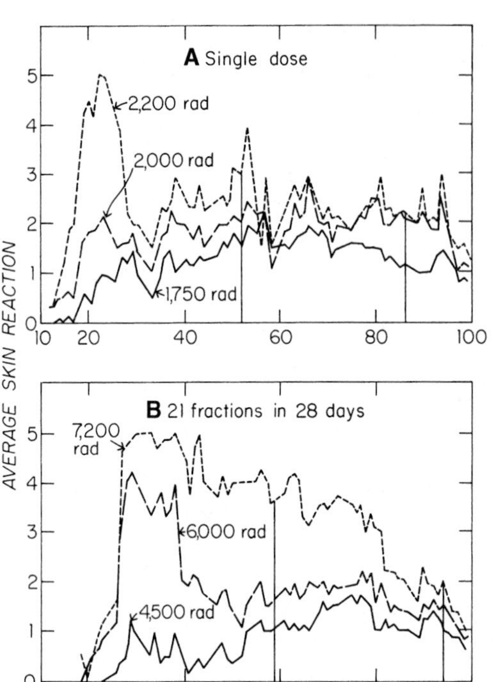

FIGURE 18.21 ● Development of skin reactions in the pig after graded doses of x-rays, delivered as a single exposure (**A**) or as multiple fractions spaced over time (**B**). (Adapted from Fowler JF, Morgan RL, Silvester JA, Bewley DK, Turner BA: Experiments with fractionated x-ray treatment of the skin of pigs: 1. Fractionation up to 28 days. *Br J Radiol* 36:188–196, 1963, with permission.)

Many of the important early studies on the fractionation effects of x-rays and the comparison of x-rays with fast neutrons were performed with this biologic system. One overwhelming advantage is that data obtained this way can be extrapolated to the human with a high degree of confidence. The disadvantage is that the animals are large and awkward to work with, and their maintenance involves a considerable expense.

Rodent Skin

Because of the inconvenience and expense of using pigs, the skin of the mouse leg and foot is commonly used instead. One hind leg of each animal is irradiated; the other serves as a control. The skin response is observed each day after irradiation and is scored according to the arbitrary scale shown in Table 18.2. Various doses are used. The progressive development of the reaction after ten doses of 6 Gy (600 rad) each is illustrated in Figure 18.23; each point represents the mean of several animals. Reactions appear by about the 10th day, peak by 20 to 25 days, and then subside. The second wave of the reaction, noted for pig skin, is not seen in mice but is observed in rats. A dose–response curve is obtained by averaging the skin reaction over a period of time and plotting this average as a function of dose.

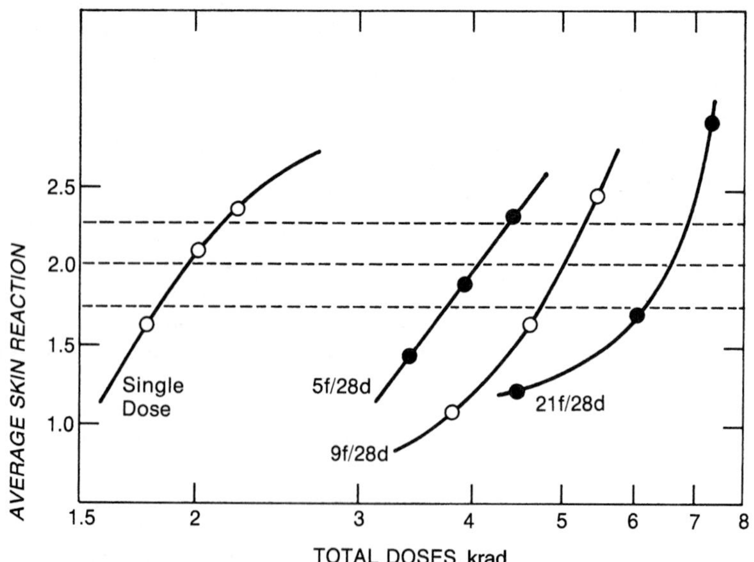

FIGURE 18.22 ● Average skin reaction as a function of total dose for medium-term skin reactions in pigs exposed to a single dose of x-rays or to fractionated doses given over 28 days. (Adapted from Fowler JF, Morgan RL, Silvester JA, Bewley DK, Turner BA: Experiments with fractionated x-ray treatment of the skin of pigs: 1. Fractionation up to 28 days. *Br J Radiol* 36:188–196, 1963, with permission.)

TABLE 18.2

Radiation Reactions in Mouse Leg Skin

Arbitrary Score[a]	Observations
0.5	50/50; doubtful if any difference from normal or not
1−	Because 1 covers a wide range of reddening, even before reaching the severity or additional factors requiring 1+, it is necessary to have 1− for "definite reddening (i.e., definitely not normal), but only a very slight degree"
1	Definite abnormality; definite reddening, top or bottom of leg; "clean" appearance means not greater than 1
1+	Severe reddening or reddening with definite white marks in creases under foot; query breakdown; query puffiness
1.5	Some breakdown of skin (usually seen on bottom of foot first); scaly or crusty appearance; definite puffiness, plus (query) breakdown; very marked white marks in creases plus puffiness or severe redness
1.5+	Query possibly moist desquamation in small areas
2	Breakdown of large areas of skin or toes stuck together; possibly moist in places but not all moist
2.5	Breakdown of large areas of skin with definite moist exudate
3	Breakdown of most of the skin with moist exudate
3.5	Complete necrosis of limb (rarely seen so far)

[a] + and − are equivalent to 0.25.

From Fowler JF, Kragt K, Ellis RE, Lindop PJ, Berry RJ: The effect of divided doses of 15 MeV electrons on the skin response of mice. *Int J Radiat Biol* 9:241–252, 1965, with permission.

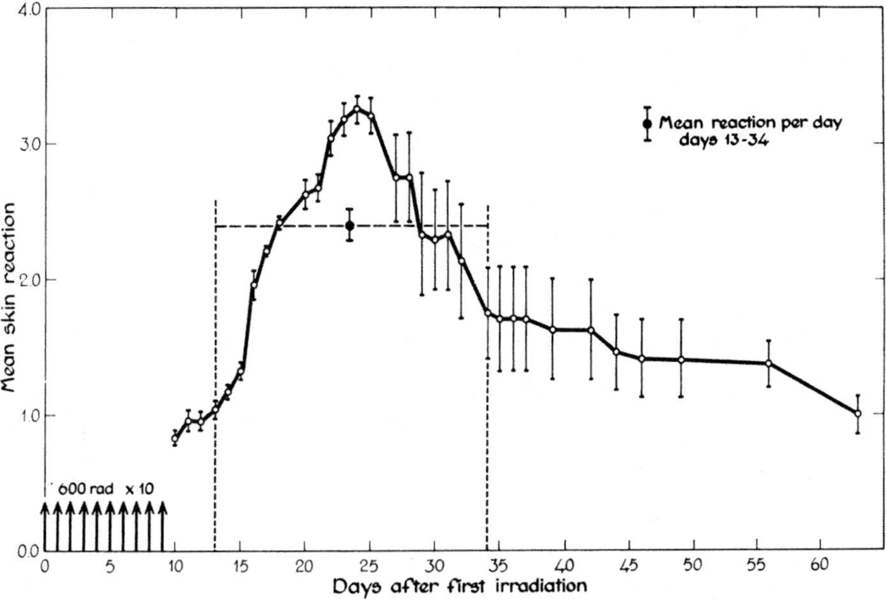

FIGURE 18.23 • Daily skin reaction scores for mice receiving 60 Gy (6,000 rad) in ten equal fractions to the right hind leg. Each point represents the mean score of six animals; the vertical lines represent the standard errors of the mean. (From Brown JM, Goffinet DR, Cleaver JE, Kallman RF: Preferential radiosensitization of mouse sarcoma relative to normal skin by chronic intra-arterial infusion of halogenated pyrimidine analogs. *JNCI* 47:75–89, 1971, with permission.)

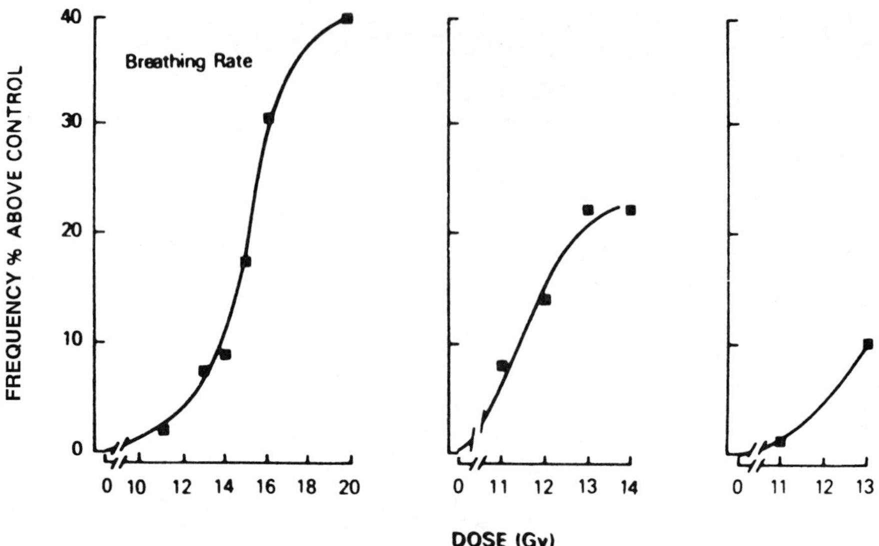

FIGURE 18.24 ● Breathing frequency in mice as a function of dose measured (left to right) 16, 36, and 52 weeks after irradiation with x-rays. Breathing frequency is expressed as a percentage increase above the age-related control value. (From Travis EL, Down JD, Holmes SJ, Hobson B: Radiation pneumonitis and fibrosis in mouse lung assayed by respiratory frequency and histology. *Radiat Res* 84:133–142, 1980, with permission.)

Early and Late Response of the Lung Based on Breathing Rate

Travis and her colleagues developed a noninvasive assay of breathing frequency to assess both early and late damage in mouse lungs. Breathing frequency increases progressively with dose after a threshold of about 11 Gy (1,100 rad) (Fig. 18.24). The increased breathing frequency in rodent lungs at 16 and 36 weeks is associated with the early response (i.e., pneumonitis); by 52 weeks, the elevated breathing frequency is associated with the late response (i.e., fibrosis). This is a simple but highly quantitative and reproducible system.

Spinal Cord Myelopathy

A dose–response relationship can be determined for late damage caused by local irradiation of the spinal cords of rats. A number of investigators have worked with this system, notably van der Kogel. After latent periods of 4 to 12 months, symptoms of myelopathy develop, the first signs of which are palpable muscle atrophy, followed some time later by impaired use of the hind legs. Figure 18.25 shows the steep dose–response relationship for hind-limb paralysis following the irradiation of a section of the spinal cord in rats. These data also show the dramatic sparing that results from fractionation; this is discussed further in another section of this chapter.

The various syndromes of radiation-induced injury in rodent brain and spinal cord are very similar to those described in humans. Lesions observed within approximately the first 6 months after irradiation are limited primarily to the white matter and range between early diffuse or focal demyelination and extensive necrosis. Different pathogenic pathways toward the development of white-matter necrosis have been proposed, with the glial and vascular tissue components the major targets. The most common type of late delayed injury peaks at 1 to 2 years postirradiation and almost certainly has a vascular basis. Another type of late injury that has been described more recently in various species, including humans, is slowly progressive glial atrophy. This lesion is not associated with necrosis but occurs diffusely and at lower doses. With improvements in diagnostic procedures such as magnetic resonance imaging, glial atrophy may become a more frequently recognized adverse effect of brain tumor therapy.

Latency

Over a dose range of about 25 to 60 Gy (2,500–6,000 rad), delivered in single doses, the general tendency is a decreasing latency with increases in dose of approximately 2 days/Gy (2 days/100 rad). There is a considerable variation with animal strain, as well as with the region of the cord irradiated.

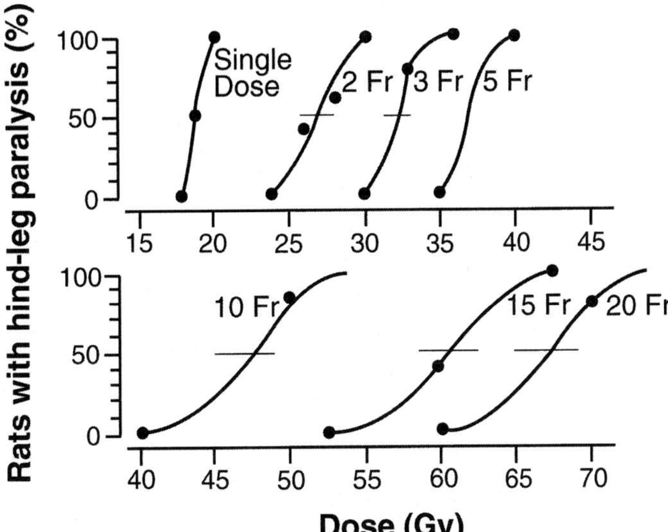

FIGURE 18.25 • Dose–response curves for the induction of hind-leg paralysis in rats following irradiation of a section of the spinal cord (L2–L5). Note how the dose necessary to produce paralysis increases rapidly with increasing numbers of fractions. (Redrawn from van der Kogel AJ: *Late Effects of Radiation on the Spinal Cord*, pp 1–160. Rijswik, the Netherlands, the Radiobiological Institute of the Organization for Health Research TNO, 1979, with permission.)

In terms of mechanisms, demyelination or slowly progressive atrophy is probably a consequence of interference with the slow continuous turnover of oligodendrocytes by killing of glial progenitor cells. Vascular injury may accelerate, precipitate, or even initiate the white-matter changes leading to necrosis. This is an area of some controversy.

Fractionation and Protraction

The effect of dose fractionation and protraction on tolerance to radiation has been investigated extensively in the rat spinal cord and to a lesser extent in the mouse, monkey, and guinea pig. Because these systems turn over slowly, there is little influence of overall treatment time up to any conventional clinical regimen of 6 to 8 weeks. On the other hand, dose per fraction is very important (Fig. 18.25), with the dose to produce paralysis increasing dramatically with number of fractions. The effect of a large number of very small fractions also has been investigated. Figure 18.26 shows the relation between total dose and dose per fraction to produce paralysis in 50% of rats from irradiation of a short length of cervical spine. The smooth curve is an isoeffect curve calculated for the very low α/β value of 1.5 Gy (150 rad). The experimental data suggest that the linear-quadratic (LQ) model overestimates the tolerance for small doses per fraction of less than 2 Gy (200 rad). However, this may be a result of incomplete repair, because in these experiments, the interfraction interval was only 4 hours. There is good reason to believe that repair of sublethal damage takes place slowly in this normal tissue, and indeed, repair may be biphasic, with "fast" and "slow" components. For this reason, if multiple doses per day are used to the spinal cord, the interfraction interval should be at least 6 to 8 hours.

Volume Effects

The total volume of irradiated tissue usually is assumed to have an influence on the development of tissue injury. The spinal cord is perhaps the clearest case in which the functional subunits (FSUs) are arranged in linear fashion, like links in a chain. Figure 18.27 shows the relation between tolerance dose and the length of cord irradiated in the rat. For short lengths of cord, below 1 cm, tolerance in terms of white-matter necrosis shows a marked dependence on the length of cord irradiated. Late vascular injury shows less dependence on cord length. Beyond a few centimeters, the tolerance is virtually independent of the length of cord irradiated. This would be predicted from the linear arrangement of the functional subunits. A chain is broken whether one, two, three, or more links are removed.

Retreatment after Long Time Intervals

The spinal cord does recover to some extent after long time periods following irradiation. The extent of the recovery depends, of course, on the first treatment—that is, what fraction of tolerance was involved. Experiments with rats indicate that after an initial treatment to 50% tolerance, the retreatment tolerance approaches 90% of the tolerance of the untreated control group by about a year after the initial irradiation. If the initial treatment represented a larger fraction of tolerance, the retreatment that can be tolerated is reduced.

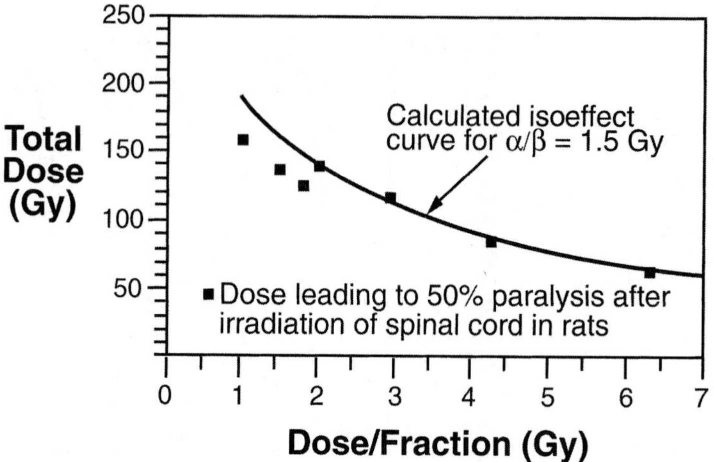

FIGURE 18.26 ● The data points show total dose, as a function of dose per fraction, to produce paralysis in 50% of rats after irradiation of the spinal cord. The curve is an isoeffect relationship based on the linear-quadratic equation with an α/β value of 1.5 Gy (150 rad). The experimental data suggest that the linear-quadratic model overestimates tolerance for dose-per-fraction values less than 2 Gy (200 rad). This may be a result of incomplete repair, because the interfraction interval was only 4 hours. (Adapted from van der Kogel AJ: Central nervous system radiation injury in small animal models. In Gutin PH, Leibel SA, Sheline GE [eds]: *Radiation Injury to the Nervous System*, pp 91–112. New York, Raven Press, 1991, with permission.)

INFERRING THE RATIO α/β FROM MULTIFRACTION EXPERIMENTS IN NONCLONOGENIC SYSTEMS

The parameters of the dose–response curve for any normal tissue system for which a functional end point can be observed may be inferred by performing a multifraction experiment. Take, for example, an experiment in which mouse foot skin reaction is scored. Doses that result in the same skin reaction (e.g., moist desquamation over 50% of the area irradiated) if delivered as a single exposure in a multifraction regimen (e.g., 5, 10, or 20 fractions) must be determined experimentally. A number of assumptions must be made:

1. The dose–response relationship is represented adequately by the linear-quadratic formulation:

$$S = e^{-\alpha D - \beta D^2}$$

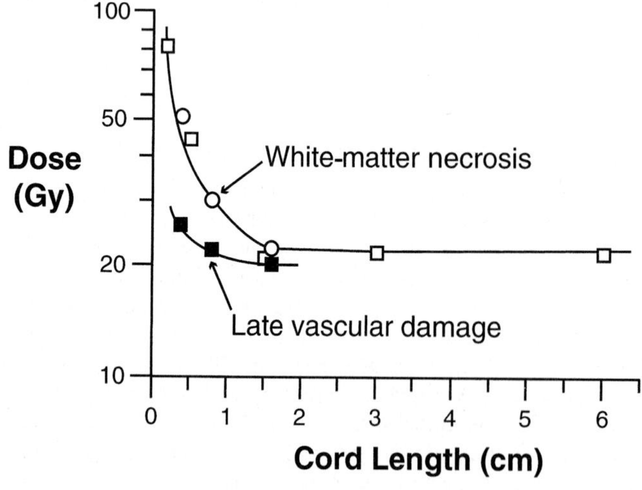

FIGURE 18.27 ● The dependence of spinal cord tolerance on the length of cord irradiated in the rat. For short lengths of cord, shorter than about 1 cm, tolerance for white-matter necrosis shows a marked dependence on the length of cord irradiated. Late vascular injury shows less dependence on cord length. Beyond a few centimeters, the tolerance dose is virtually independent of the length of cord irradiated. (Adapted from van der Kogel AJ: Central nervous system radiation injury in small animal models. In Gutin PH, Leibel SA, Sheline GE [eds]: *Radiation Injury to the Nervous System*, pp 91–112. New York, Raven Press, 1991, with permission.)

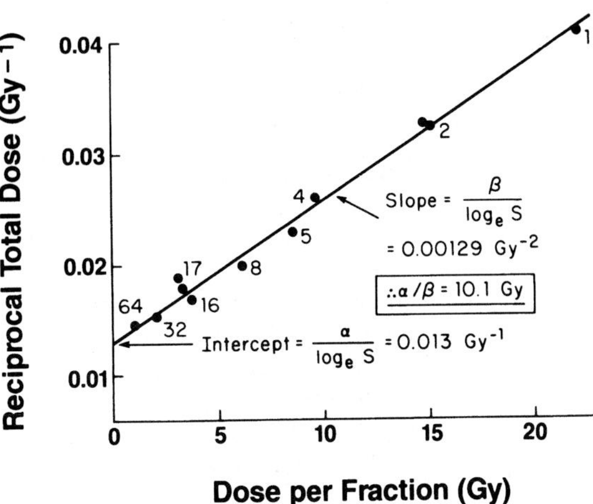

FIGURE 18.28 • Reciprocal of the total dose required to produce a given level of injury (acute skin reaction in mice) as a function of dose per fraction in multiple equal doses. The overall time of these experiments was sufficiently short so that proliferation could be neglected. Numbers of fractions are shown by each point. From the values of the "intercept" and "slope" of the best-fit line, the values of α and β and the ratio α/β for the dose–response curve for organ function can be determined. (Adapted from Douglas BG, Fowler JR: The effect of multiple small doses of x rays on skin reactions in the mouse and a basic interpretation. *Radiat Res* 66:401–426, 1976, with permission.)

in which S is the fraction of cells surviving a dose, D, and α and β are constants.

2. Each dose in a fractionated regimen produces the same biologic effect.
3. Full repair of sublethal damage takes place between dose fractions, but no cell proliferation occurs.

Suppose the total dose, D, is divided into n equal fractions of dose d. The previous equation then can be rewritten:

$$S = (e^{-\alpha d - \beta d^2})^n$$

or

$$-\log_e S/nd = \alpha + \beta d$$

If the reciprocal of the total dose (1/nd) is plotted against the dose per fraction (d), a straight line results, as shown in Figure 18.28. The intercept on the ordinate gives $\alpha/\log_e S$; the slope gives $\beta/\log_e S$. In general, the value of $\log_e S$ is not known unless other cell survival studies are available, but the ratio of the intercept to the slope provides an estimate of α/β.

Multifraction experiments have been performed and estimates of α/β made for essentially all of the normal-tissue end points described in this chapter. One of the important conclusions arrived at is that the value of α/β tends to be larger for early-responding tissues, about 10 Gy (1,000 rad), than for late-responding tissues, about 2 Gy (200 rad).

Because α/β is the dose at which cell killing by linear and by quadratic components of radiation damage are equal (Chapter 3), the implication is that dose–response relationships for late-responding tissues are "curvier" than for early-responding tissues. The importance of this conclusion becomes evident in the discussion of fractionation in radiotherapy in Chapter 22.

Summary of Pertinent Conclusions

- The relationship between dose and incidence is sigmoid for both tumor control and normal-tissue damage.
- The ratio of tumor response to normal-tissue damage is called the therapeutic ratio or therapeutic index.
- The therapeutic index can be manipulated by dose fractionation or by the use of drugs that preferentially increase tumor response.
- After irradiation, most cells die a mitotic death; that is, they die in attempting the next or a later mitosis. In some tissues, cells die by apoptosis, which is a programmed cell death.
- Systems involving clonogenic end points (i.e., cell survival) for cells of normal tissues include some in which cells regrow *in situ* and some in which cells are transplanted to another site.
- *In situ* regrowth techniques include skin colonies, crypts in the jejunum, testes stem cells, and kidney tubules. Single-dose experiments can yield the slope (D_0) of the dose–response curve over a range of high doses. Multifraction experiments allow the whole dose–response curve to be reconstructed.

(continued)

Summary of Pertinent Conclusions (Continued)

- Systems in which cell survival is assessed by transplantation into another site include bone-marrow stem cells, thyroid cells, and mammary cells.
- A dose–response curve for bone-marrow stem cells can be obtained by allowing cells from the donor animal to lodge and grow in the spleens of recipient animals. These are very sensitive cells with a D_0 close to 1 Gy (100 rad), with little or no shoulder.
- Dose–response curves for mammary and thyroid cells can be obtained by transplanting them into fat pads of recipient animals.
- The radiosensitivity of cells from normal tissues varies widely. The width of the shoulder of the curve is the principal variable. Jejunal crypt cells have a very large shoulder; bone-marrow stem cells have little, if any, shoulder. Most other cell types studied in clonogenic assays fall in between.
- Dose–response curves for functional end points, distinct from cell survival, can be obtained for:

  1. Pig skin and rodent skin by measuring skin reactions
  2. Early and late response of the lung by measuring breathing rate
  3. Spinal cord by observing myelopathy:
     a. Paralysis develops after a latency of months to years.
     b. Early lesions are limited to white matter; late delayed injury may have a vascular basis.
     c. Spinal cord damage is very sensitive to fractionation; α/β of about 1.5 Gy (150 rad).
     d. Sublethal damage repair probably has "fast" and "slow" components.
     e. If multiple fractions per day are used, the interfraction interval should be at least 6 to 8 hours.
     f. Functional subunits are arranged serially like links in a chain.
     g. For short lengths of cord, tolerance dose varies markedly with cord length irradiated; for cord lengths greater than a few centimeters, tolerance dose is virtually independent of cord length.

- The shape of the dose–response relationship for functional end points, obtained from multifraction experiments, is more pertinent to radiotherapy than clonogenic assays.
- The ratio α/β (the dose at which the linear and quadratic components of radiation damage are equal) may be inferred from multifraction experiments in systems scoring nonclonogenic end points.

BIBLIOGRAPHY

Andrews JR: *The Radiobiology of Human Cancer Radiotherapy*. Philadelphia, WB Saunders, 1968

Ang KK, Thames HD Jr, van der Kogel AJ, van der Schueren E: Is the rate of repair of radiation-induced sublethal damage in rat spinal cord dependent on the size of the dose per fraction? *Int J Radiat Oncol Biol Phys* 13:552–562, 1987

Ang KK, van der Kogel AJ, van der Schueren E: The effect of small radiation doses on the rat spinal cord: The concept of partial tolerance. *Int J Radiat Oncol Biol Phys* 9:1487–1491, 1983

Ang KK, van der Kogel AJ, van der Schueren E: Lack of evidence for increased tolerance of rat spinal cord with decreasing fraction doses below 2 Gy. *Int J Radiat Oncol Biol Phys* 11:105–110, 1985

Barendsen GW, Broerse JJ: Experimental radiotherapy of a rat rhabdomyosarcoma with 15 MeV neutrons and 300 kV x-rays: 1. Effects of single exposures. *Eur J Cancer* 5:373–391, 1969

Bradley WG, Fewings JD, Cumming WJK, Harrison RM, Faulds AJ: Delayed myeloradiculopathy produced by spinal X-irradiation in the rat. *J Neurol Sci* 31:63–82, 1977

Brown JM, Goffinet DR, Cleaver JE, Kallman RF: Preferential radiosensitization of mouse sarcoma relative to normal skin by chronic intra-arterial infusion of halogenated pyrimidine analogs. *JNCI* 47:75–89, 1971

Clifton KH, Briggs RC, Stone HB: Quantitative radiosensitivity studies of solid carcinomas *in vivo*: Methodology and effect of anoxia. *JNCI* 36:965–974, 1966

Clifton KH, Gould MN, Potten CS, Hendry J (eds): *Cell Clones*, pp 128–138. New York, Churchill Livingstone, 1985

DeMott RK, Mulcahy RT, Clifton KH: The survival of thyroid cells following irradiation: A directly generated single-dose survival curve. *Radiat Res* 77:395–403, 1979

Douglas BG, Fowler JR: The effect of multiple small doses of x-rays on skin reactions in the mouse and a basic interpretation. *Radiat Res* 66:401–426, 1976

Field SB, Jones T, Thomlinson RH: The relative effects of fast neutrons and x-rays on tumor and normal tissue in the rat.*Br J Radiol* 40:834–842, 1967

Fowler JF, Denekamp J, Page AL, Begg AC, Field SB, Butler K: Fractionation with x-rays and neutrons in mice: Response of skin and C3H mammary tumors. *Br J Radiol* 45:237–249, 1972

Fowler JF, Kragt K, Ellis RE, Lindop PJ, Berry RJ: The effect of divided doses of 15 MeV electrons on the skin response of mice. *Int J Radiat Biol* 9:241–252, 1965

Fowler JF, Morgan RL, Silvester JA, Bewley DK, Turner BA: Experiments with fractionated x-ray treatment of the skin of pigs: 1. Fractionation up to 28 days. *Br J Radiol* 36:188–196, 1963

Goffinet DR, Marsa GW, Brown JM: The effects of single and multifraction radiation courses on the mouse spinal cord. *Radiology* 119:709–713, 1976

Gould MN, Biel WF, Clifton KH: Morphological and quantitative studies of gland formation from inocula of monodispersed rat mammary cells. *Exp Cell Res* 107:405–416, 1977

Gould MN, Clifton KH: Evidence for a unique *in situ* component of the repair of radiation damage. *Radiat Res* 77:149–155, 1979

Gould MN, Clifton KH: The survival of mammary cells following irradiation *in vivo*: A directly generated single-dose survival curve. *Radiat Res* 72:343–352, 1977

Hermens AF, Barendsen GW: Cellular proliferation patterns in an experimental rhabdomyosarcoma in the rat. *Eur J Cancer* 3:361–369, 1967

Hermens AF, Barendsen GW: Changes of cell proliferation characteristics in a rat rhabdomyosarcoma before and after irradiation. *Eur J Cancer* 5:173–189, 1969

Hewitt HB: Studies on the quantitative transplantation of mouse sarcoma. *Br J Cancer* 7:367–383, 1953

Hewitt HB, Chan DPS, Blake ER: Survival curves for clonogenic cells of a murine keratinizing squamous carcinoma irradiated *in vivo* or under hypoxic conditions. *Int J Radiat Biol* 12:535–549, 1967

Hewitt HB, Wilson CW: A survival curve for mammalian leukaemia cells irradiated *in vivo*. *Br J Cancer* 13:69–75, 1959

Hewitt HB, Wilson CW: Survival curves for tumor cells irradiated *in vivo*. *Ann NY Acad Sci* 95:818–827, 1961

Hill RP, Bush RS: A lung colony assay to determine the radiosensitivity of the cells of a solid tumor. *Int J Radiat Biol* 15:435–444, 1969

Hopewell JW: Late radiation damage to the central nervous system: A radiobiological interpretation. *Neuropathol Appl Neurobiol* 5:329–343, 1979

Hopewell JW, Morris AD, Dixon-Brown A: The influence of field size on the late tolerance of the rat spinal cord to single doses of X rays. *Br J Radiol* 60:1099–1108, 1987

Kerr JFR, Searle J: Apoptosis: Its nature and kinetic role. In Meyn RE, Withers HR (eds): *Radiation Biology in Cancer Research*, pp 367–384. New York, Raven Press, 1980

McCulloch EA, Till JE: The sensitivity of cells from normal mouse bone marrow to gamma radiation *in vitro* and *in vivo*. *Radiat Res* 16:822–832, 1962

McNally NJ: A comparison of the effects of radiation on tumor growth delay and cell survival: The effect of oxygen. *Br J Radiol* 46:450–455, 1973

McNally NJ: Recovery from sublethal damage by hypoxic tumor cells *in vivo*. *Br J Radiol* 45:116–120, 1972

Mulcahy RT, Gould MN, Clifton KH: The survival of thyroid cells: *In vivo* irradiation and *in situ* repair. *Radiat Res* 84:523–528, 1980

Peters LJ, Brock WA, Travis EL: Radiation biology at clinically relevant doses. In DeVita VT, Hellman S, Rosenberg SA (eds): *Important Advances in Oncology*, pp 65–83. Philadelphia, JB Lippincott Co, 1990

Reinhold HS: Quantitative evaluation of the radiosensitivity of cells of a transplantable rhabdomyosarcoma in the rat. *Eur J Cancer* 2:33–42, 1966

Rockwell SC, Kallman RF: Cellular radiosensitivity and tumor radiation response in the EMT6 tumor cell system. *Radiat Res* 53:281–294, 1973

Rockwell SC, Kallman RF, Fajardo LF: Characteristics of a serially transplanted mouse mammary tumor and its tissue-culture-adapted derivative. *J Natl Cancer Inst* 49:735–749, 1972

Scalliet P, Landuyt W, van der Schueren E: Repair kinetics as a determining factor for late tolerance of central nervous system to low dose rate irradiation. *Radiother Oncol* 14:345–353, 1989

Stephen LC, Arg KK, Schultheiss TE, Milas L, Meyn R: Apoptosis in irradiated murine tumors. *Radiat Res* 127:308–316, 1991

Suit HD, Maeda M; Hyperbaric oxygen and radiobiology of the C3H mouse mammary carcinoma. *J Natl Cancer Inst* 39:639–652, 1967

Suit H, Wette R: Radiation dose fractionation and tumor control probability. *Radiat Res* 29:267–281, 1966

Suit HD, Wette R, Lindberg R: Analysis of tumor recurrence times. *Radiology* 88:311–321, 1967

Sutherland RM, Durand RE: Radiation response of multicell spheroids: An In vitro tumor model. *Curr Top Radiat Res Q* 11:87–139, 1976

Sutherland RM, McCredie JA, Inch WR: Growth of multicell spheroids in tissue culture as a model of nodular carcinomas. *J Natl Cancer Inst* 46:113– 120, 1971

Taylor AB, Anderson JH: Scanning electron microscope observations of mammalian intestinal villi, intervillus floor and crypt tubules. *Micron* 3:430–453, 1972

Tannock IF: The relation between cell proliferation and the vascular system in a transplanted mouse mammary tumour. *Br J Cancer* 22:258–273, 1968

Thames HD, Withers HR: Test of equal effect per fraction and estimation of initial clonogen number in microcolony assays of survival after fractionated irradiation. *Br J Radiol* 53:1071–1077, 1980

Thames HD, Withers R, Mason KA, Reid BO: Dose survival characteristics of mouse jejunal crypt cells. *Int J Radiat Oncol Biol Phys* 7:1591–1597, 1981

Till JE, McCulloch EA: In Cameron IL, Padilla GM, Zimmerman AM (eds): *Developmental Aspects of the Cell Cycle*, pp 297–313. New York, Academic Press, 1971

Travis EL, Down JD, Holmes SJ, Hobson B: Radiation pneumonitis and fibrosis in mouse lung assayed by respiratory frequency and histology. *Radiat Res* 84:133–142, 1980

Travis EL, Vojnovic B, Davies EE, Hirst DG: A plethysmographic method for measuring function in locally irradiated mouse lung. *Br J Radiol* 52:67–74, 1979

van der Kogel AJ: Central nervous system radiation injury in small animal models. In Gutin PH, Leibel SA, Sheline GE (eds): *Radiation Injury to the Nervous System*, pp 91–112. New York, Raven Press, 1991

van der Kogel AJ: Effect of volume and localization on rat spinal cord tolerance. In Fielden EM, Fowler JF, Hendry JH, Scott D (eds): *Radiation Research*, vol 1 (*Proceedings of the 8th International Congress of Radiation Research*), p 352, New York, Taylor & Francis, 1987

van der Kogel AJ: *Late Effects of Radiation on the Spinal Cord*, pp 1–160. Rijswik, the Netherlands, the Radiobiological Institute of the Organization for Health Research TNO, 1979

van der Kogel AJ: Radiation tolerance of the rat spinal cord: Time-dose relationships. *Radiology* 122:505–509, 1977

van der Kogel AJ: Radiation-induced damage in the central nervous system: An interpretation of target cell responses. *Br J Cancer* 53(suppl VII):207–217, 1986

van der Schueren E, Landuyt W, Ang KK, van der Kogel AJ: From 2 Gy to 1 Gy per fraction: Sparing effect in rat spinal cord? *Int J Radiat Oncol Biol Phys* 14:297–300, 1988

Wara WM, Phillips TL, Margolis LW, Smith V: Radiation pneumonitis: A new approach to the derivation of time-dose factors. *Cancer* 32:547–552, 1973

White A, Hornsey S: Radiation damage to the rat spinal cord: The effect of single and fractionated doses of x-rays. *Br J Radiol* 51:515–523, 1978

Williams GT: Programmed cell death: Apoptosis and oncogenesis. *Cell* 65:1097–1098, 1991

Withers HR: The dose-survival relationship for irradiation of epithelial cells of mouse skin. *Br J Radiol* 40:187–194, 1967

Withers HR: Recovery and repopulation *in vivo* by mouse skin epithelial cells during fractionated irradiation. *Radiat Res* 32:227–239, 1967

Withers HR: Regeneration of intestinal mucosa after irradiation. *Cancer* 28:78–81, 1971

Withers HR, Hunter N, Barkley HT Jr, Reid BO: Radiation survival and regeneration characteristics of spermatogenic stem cells of mouse testis. *Radiat Res* 57:88–103, 1974

Withers HR, Mason K, Reid BO, et al.: Response of mouse intestine to neutrons and gamma rays in relation to dose fractionation and division cycle. *Cancer* 34:39–47, 1974

Withers HR, Mason KA, Thames HD: Late radiation response of kidney assayed by tubule cell survival. *Br J Radiol* 59:587–595, 1986

CHAPTER 19

Clinical Response of Normal Tissues

CELLS AND TISSUES

The majority of the effects of radiation therapy on normal tissues can be attributed to cell killing, but there are some that cannot. Examples include:

- Nausea or vomiting that may occur a few hours after irradiation of the abdomen.
- Fatigue felt by patients receiving irradiation to a large volume, especially within the abdomen.
- Somnolence that may develop several hours after cranial irradiation.
- Acute edema or erythema that results from radiation-induced acute inflammation and associated vascular leakage.

It is thought that these effects are mediated by radiation-induced inflammatory cytokines. These effects aside, most effects of radiation on normal tissues result from the depletion of a cell population by cell killing.

The cells of normal tissues are not independent but form a complete integrated structure. There is a delicate balance between cell birth and cell death to maintain tissue organization and the number of cells. The response to damage is governed by (1) the inherent cellular radiosensitivity, (2) the kinetics of the tissue, and (3) the way cells are organized in that tissue.

If the fate of individual cells is studied, as described in Chapter 3, there is a continuous monotonic relationship between the magnitude of the dose and the fraction of cells that are "killed" in the sense that they lose their reproductive integrity—the ability to divide indefinitely. By contrast, no effects are seen in tissues after small doses, though effects of increasing severity become apparent if the dose rises above a threshold level. The reason is, of course, that killing a small number of cells in a tissue matters very little; visible damage is evident only if a large enough proportion of the cells are killed and removed from the tissue. The threshold dose below which no effect is seen and the delay between irradiation and the time at which the damage becomes observable vary greatly among different tissues.

Cell death after irradiation occurs mostly as cells attempt to divide. In tissues with a rapid turnover rate, damage becomes evident quickly—in a matter of hours in the intestinal epithelium and bone marrow, in a matter of days in the skin and mucosa. In tissues in which cells divide rarely, radiation damage to cells may remain latent for a long period of time and be expressed very slowly. Radiation damage to cells that are already on the path to differentiation (and would not have divided many times anyway) is of little consequence. By contrast, radiation damage to stem cells has serious repercussions because they were programmed to divide many times to maintain a large population, and if they lose their reproductive integrity, both they and their potential descendants are lost from the population. Thus, cells on the road to differentiation appear to be more **radioresistant** than stem cells. In fact, the fraction of cells surviving a given dose may be identical at the single-cell level, so strictly speaking, it is their **radioresponse** that is different, not their **radiosensitivity**. This explains the so-called law of Bergonié and Tribondeau (1906), who noted that tissues appear to be more "radiosensitive" if their cells are less differentiated, have a greater proliferative capacity, and divide more rapidly.

EARLY (ACUTE) AND LATE EFFECTS

Radiation effects are commonly divided into two categories, **early** and **late**, which show quite different patterns of response to fractionation; their dose–response relations are characterized by different α/β ratios, as described in more detail in Chapter 22. **Late effects** are much more sensitive to changes in fractionation than early effects. **Early**, or **acute, effects** result from the death of a large number of cells and occur within a few days or weeks of irradiation in tissues with a rapid rate of turnover. Examples include effects in the epidermal layer of the skin, gastrointestinal epithelium, and hematopoietic system, in which the response is determined by a hierarchical cell lineage composed of stem cells and their differentiating offspring. The time of onset of early reactions correlates with the relatively short life span of the mature functional cells; the identity of the target cells is usually obvious.

Late effects appear after a delay of months or years and occur predominantly in slowly proliferating tissues, such as tissues of the lung, kidney, heart, liver, and central nervous system. The difference between the two types of lesions lies in their progression: Acute damage is repaired rapidly because of the rapid proliferation of stem cells and may be completely reversible. By contrast, late damage may improve but is never completely repaired. A late effect may result from a combination of vascular damage and loss of parenchymal cells. Clearly, vascular damage is not the dominant factor in every case, because if it were, the dose–effect relationship would be the same for all tissues, and that is not the case. It may be true for some tissues, however, including the spinal cord. If intensive fractionation protocols deplete the stem-cell population below levels needed for tissue restoration, an early reaction in a rapidly proliferating tissue may persist as a chronic injury. This has been termed a **consequential late effect**, that is, a late effect consequent to, or evolving out of, a persistent severe early effect. The earlier damage is most often attributable to an overlying acutely responding epithelial surface—for example, fibrosis or necrosis of skin consequent to desquamation and acute ulceration.

FUNCTIONAL SUBUNITS (FSUs) IN NORMAL TISSUES

The fraction of cells surviving determines the success or failure of a treatment regimen as far as the tumor is concerned, because a single surviving cell may be the focus for the regrowth of the tumor. For normal tissues, however, this is not the whole story. The tolerance of normal tissues for radiation depends on the ability of the clonogenic cells to maintain a sufficient number of mature cells suitably structured to maintain organ function. The relationship between the survival of clonogenic cells and organ function or failure depends also on the structural organization of the tissue. Many tissues may be thought of as consisting of **functional subunits (FSUs)**.

In some tissues, the FSUs are discrete, anatomically delineated structures whose relationship to tissue function is clear. Obvious examples are the nephron in the kidney, the lobule in the liver, and perhaps the acinus in the lung. In other tissues, the FSUs have no clear anatomic demarcation. Examples include the skin, the mucosa, and the spinal cord. The response to radiation of these two types of tissue—with structurally defined or structurally undefined FSUs—is quite different.

The survival of **structurally defined FSUs** depends on the survival of one or more clonogenic cells within them, and tissue survival in turn depends on the number and radiosensitivity of these clonogens. Although such tissues are composed of a large number of FSUs, each is a small self-contained entity independent of its neighbors. Surviving clonogens cannot migrate from one to the other. Because each FSU is both small and autonomous, low doses deplete the clonogens in it. Each kidney, for example, is composed of a large number of relatively small FSUs, each of which is a self-contained structural entity independent of its neighbors. Consequently, survival of a nephron after irradiation depends on the survival of at least one clonogen within it and therefore on the initial number of renal tubule cells per nephron and their radiosensitivity. Because this FSU is relatively small, it is completely depleted of clonogens by low doses, which accounts for the low tolerance to radiation of the kidney. Other organs that resemble the kidney in having structurally defined FSUs not repopulated from adjacent FSUs may be those with a branching treelike system of ducts and vasculature that ultimately terminate in "end structures" or lobules of parenchymal cells. These can be visualized as independent structurally defined FSUs. Examples of organs with this tissue architecture include the lung, liver, and exocrine organs. At least some of these also have low tolerance to radiation.

By contrast, the clonogenic cells that can repopulate the **structurally undefined FSUs** after depletion by radiation are not confined to one particular FSU. Rather, clonogenic cells can migrate from one FSU to another and allow repopulation of a depleted FSU. For example, reepithelialization of a denuded area of skin can occur either from surviving clonogens within the denuded area or by migration from adjacent areas.

A concept proposed to link the survival of clonogenic cells and functional survival is the **tissue rescue unit**, defined as the minimum number of FSUs required to maintain tissue function. This model assumes that the number of tissue rescue units in a tissue is proportional to the number of clonogenic cells, that FSUs contain a constant number of clonogens, and that FSUs can be repopulated from a single surviving clonogen.

Some tissues defy classification by this system. The crypts of the jejunum, for example, are structurally well-defined subunits, but surviving crypt cells can and do migrate from one crypt to another to repopulate depleted neighbors.

THE VOLUME EFFECT IN RADIOTHERAPY: TISSUE ARCHITECTURE

It is generally observed in clinical radiotherapy that the total dose that can be tolerated depends on the volume of tissue irradiated. **Tolerance dose** has been defined as the dose that produces an acceptable probability of a treatment complication. This definition includes objective criteria, such as the radiobiology involved, and subjective factors that may be socioeconomic, medicolegal, or psychological.

The spatial arrangement of the FSUs in the tissue is critical. In the case of tissues in which the FSUs are arranged in a series, like the links of a chain, the integrity of each is critical to organ function, and elimination of any one FSU results in a measurable probability of a complication. The spinal cord is the clearest example in which specific functions are controlled by specific segments arranged linearly, or serially. Because impulses must pass along the cord, death of critical cells in any one segment results in complete failure of the organ. Radiation damage to such tissues is expected to show a binary response, with a threshold dose below which there is normal function and above which there is loss of function (e.g., radiation-induced myelopathy). This is illustrated in Figure 19.1. As the field size increases to include a greater number of FSUs—1,

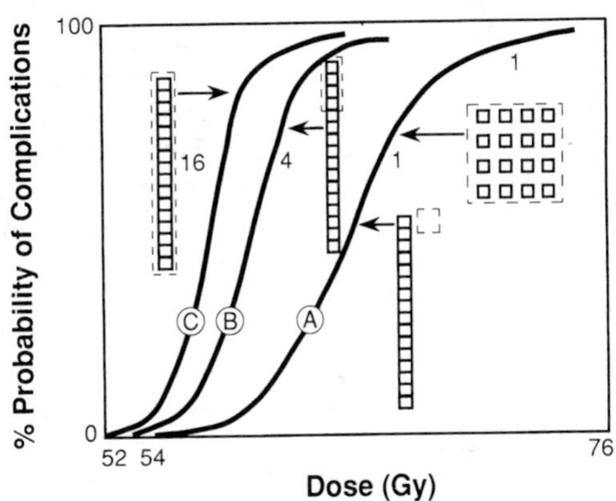

FIGURE 19.1 • Relationship between dose and probability of complications for different types of normal tissues. Curve A relates to a normal tissue in which the functional subunits are not arranged serially regardless of whether one or all subunits are exposed (i.e., regardless of field size). It also applies to a normal tissue in which functional subunits are arranged serially if only one subunit is exposed (i.e., if the field is small). Note that the curve is relatively shallow (i.e., the probability of a complication rises relatively slowly with dose). Curves B and C refer to a tissue with serially arranged functional subunits; the complication curve gets steeper and moves to lower doses as the treatment field size increases. For example, curves B and C, respectively, relate to 4 or 16 functional subunits exposed. (Note that the position of the curves in relation to the abscissae is arbitrary, resulting from two assumptions: that there is an effective D_0 of 4 Gy for a survival curve for cells exposed to multiple doses of 2 Gy and that 58 Gy in 2-Gy fractions sterilizes 10% of the functional subunits.) (Adapted from Withers HR, Taylor JMG, Maciejewski B: Treatment volume and tissue tolerance. *Int J Radiat Oncol Biol Phys* 14:751–759, 1988, with permission.)

4, or 16 in this example—the curve relating probability of a complication to dose rises much more steeply with dose and moves to lower doses. This explains the important volume effect found in, for example, the spinal cord, in which FSUs are arranged in series and loss of any one may result in myelopathy.

Clinical tolerance also depends strongly on the volume irradiated in the kidney and lung; both of these organs are very sensitive to irradiation of their entire volume, but small volumes can be treated to much higher doses. This is because there is considerable functional reserve capacity, with only about 30% of the organ required to maintain adequate function under normal physiologic conditions. The large reserve capacity and increased tolerance to partial-volume irradiation are due to the parallel organization of functional nephrons and alveolar subunits. Inactivation of a small number of FSUs does not lead to loss of organ function. Functional damage will not occur until a critical number of FSUs are inactivated by irradiation. This implies that there should also be a threshold volume of irradiation below which no functional damage will develop, even after high-dose irradiation. Above this threshold, damage is usually exhibited as a graded response—increasing severity of functional impairment with increasing dose—rather than a binary, all-or-nothing response.

Skin and mucosa have no well-defined FSUs, but respond in a way similar to tissues where the FSUs are in parallel. They do not show a volume effect at lower levels of injury at which healing can occur from surviving clonogens scattered throughout the treatment volume. This seemingly should be true for the skin or mucosa, in which a volume effect would not be expected on radiobiologic grounds; however, this is never quite true in practice, because if a larger area of skin or mucosa is ulcerated, the prolonged healing time plus the increased potential for infection are more debilitating than similarly severe ulceration in a smaller area. In other words, although the severity of a skin reaction is relatively independent of the area irradiated because healing occurs by regeneration of surviving clonogens scattered throughout the treated area, the tolerability is not. Therefore, there is a volume effect in clinical practice, but it is not based on an increased probability of injury as it is in tissues in which FSUs are arranged serially.

RADIATION PATHOLOGY OF TISSUES

As previously stated, the response of a tissue or organ to radiation depends primarily on three factors: (1) the inherent sensitivity of the individual cells; (2) the kinetics of the tissue as a whole of which the cells are a part; and (3) the way the cells are organized in that tissue. These factors combine to account for the substantial variation in response to radiation characteristic of different tissues.

In the case of tissues composed of highly differentiated cells performing specialized functions, cell survival curves (Chapter 3) are largely irrelevant, because these cells have no mitotic future. Little information is available at the cellular level concerning the effects of radiation on differentiated cells. All that can be said is that in general, the amount of radiation needed to destroy the functioning ability of a differentiated cell is far greater than that necessary to stop the mitotic activity of a dividing cell.

A closed static population, composed entirely of mature differentiated cells, is therefore very resistant to radiation. In the case of self-renewing tissues, the Achilles heel is the dividing cell: Loss of reproductive ability in an appreciable fraction of these cells occurs after a moderate dose of a few gray (a few hundred rad). Whether the tissue or organ as a whole appears to be affected to a small or large extent—and is consequently labeled as sensitive or resistant—depends on the extent to which the tissue involved can continue to function adequately with a reduced number of cells.

Another factor that is evident from even this most elementary consideration of population kinetics is that the time interval between the delivery of the radiation insult and its expression in tissue damage is very variable for different populations. This time interval is determined by the normal life span of the mature functional cells and the time it takes for a cell "born" in the stem-cell compartment to mature to a functional state. For example, mature erythrocytes in circulating blood have a relatively long life span and are separated from the primitive stem-cell compartment by a number of transit compartments, so that time is required for a cell to pass through the various stages of differentiation and maturation. Consequently, a considerable time interval elapses between the depopulation of the stem-cell compartment and the final expression of this injury in terms of a reduced peripheral blood cell count. By contrast, in the case of the intestinal epithelium, the mature functional cells on the surface of the villi have a short life span, and the time interval between the "birth" of a new cell in the stem compartment of the crypt and its appearance as a mature functional cell is very short, on the order of a few days. As would be expected, therefore, radiation damage is expressed correspondingly quickly in this tissue. Two systems are typically used to classify tissue radiosensitivity in terms of population kinetics and tissue architecture: Casarett's classification and Michalowski's classification.

CASARETT'S CLASSIFICATION OF TISSUE RADIOSENSITIVITY

The limitations of our knowledge of cellular population kinetics is remedied to some extent by a wealth of information on the relative sensitivities of various tissues based on histopathologic observations. It must be emphasized that these data are based on entirely different end points than those with which previous chapters have been concerned. To score a cell as "dead" by observing a fixed and stained section of tissue through a microscope is quite different from the experimental test of cell death in terms of loss of reproductive capacity, which has been used previously. Nevertheless, the study of radiation pathology provides data that are highly relevant to clinical radiotherapy.

Casarett has suggested a classification of mammalian cell radiosensitivity based on histologic observation of early cell death. He divided parenchymal cells into four major categories, numbered I through IV (Table 19.1). The supporting structures, such as the connective tissue and the endothelial cells of small blood vessels, are regarded as intermediate in sensitivity between groups II and III of the parenchymal cells.

One of the most sensitive cells to radiation in fact defies all the "laws" and systems of classification; it is the small lymphocyte. This cell, it is believed, never divides at all, or at least only in exceptional circumstances. Small lymphocytes disappear from circulating blood after very small doses of radiation, and it is believed that they suffer an interphase death (by the process of apoptosis). Most sensitive cells die a mitotic death after irradiation; most cells that never divide require very large doses to kill them. The small lymphocyte breaks both of these rules, inasmuch as it does not usually divide, dies of interphase death, and yet is one of the most sensitive mammalian cells.

Group I of Casarett's classification, the most sensitive group, consists of vegetative intermitotic cells and includes the stem cells of the classic self-renewing systems, such as the basal layers of the epidermis and the intestine, the erythroblasts (precursors of red blood cells), intestinal crypt cells, and the primitive cells of the spermatogenic series. The stem cells divide regularly and provide a steady and abundant supply of progeny, some of which differentiate and mature into functioning cells. A reservoir of primitive dividing stem cells is maintained and in some cases can be triggered to divide more rapidly in response to a need. The primitive dividing stem cells are vulnerable to radiation; a moderate dose causes a proportion of them to "die" in attempting the next or a subsequent mitosis. The time of crisis for the organism as a whole occurs if the supply of functioning cells is inadequate: a shortage of circulating red and white blood cells in the case of the blood, and a shortage of mature covering dermal cells in the case of the skin. The time interval between irradiation and the crisis is about equal to the life span of the mature functioning cells. As the functioning cells die off at the end of their natural life span, there are none to take their place if a dose of radiation previously has

TABLE 19.1

Categories of Mammalian Cell Sensitivity

Cell Type	Properties	Examples	Sensitivity[a]
I Vegetative intermitotic cells	Divide regularly; no differentiation	Erythroblasts Intestinal crypt cells Germinal cells of epidermis	High
II Differentiating intermitotic cells	Divide regularly; some differentiation between divisions	Myelocytes	
Connective tissue cells[b]			
III Reverting postmitotic cells	Do not divide regularly; variably differentiated	Liver	
IV Fixed postmitotic cells	Do not divide; highly differentiated	Nerve cells Muscle cells	Low

[a] Sensitivity decreases for each successive group.
[b] Intermediate in sensitivity between groups II and III.
Based on Rubin P, Casarett GW: *Clinical Radiation Pathology*, vol 1. Philadelphia, WB Saunders, 1968, with permission.

depopulated the stem-cell compartment. Depending on the size of the dose, the organ or tissue may not survive the critical time at which the number of functioning cells reaches a minimum value.

Group II consists of cells that divide regularly but that also mature and differentiate between divisions. Cells in this category are relatively short-lived as individuals and are produced by division of vegetative intermitotic cells. These cells usually complete a limited number of divisions and differentiate to some extent between successive mitoses. This group includes cells of the hematopoietic series in the intermediate stages of differentiation and likewise the more differentiated spermatogonia and spermatocytes.

Group III, the reverting postmitotic cells, are relatively resistant and as individuals have relatively long lives. Ordinarily, they do not undergo mitosis, but they are capable of dividing with the appropriate stimulus, which is usually damage or loss of many of their own kind. The liver cells are a good example of this category. In the adult, there is normally little or no cell division, but if a large part of the liver is removed by surgery, the remaining cells are triggered to divide and make good the loss. Other examples in this category include the cells of the kidney and pancreas and of various glands, such as the adrenal, thyroid, and pituitary.

Group IV consists of the fixed postmitotic cells. These generally are considered the most resistant to radiation. They are highly differentiated and appear to have lost the ability to divide. Some have a long lifespan, such as the neurons. Others have a short lifespan, such as the granulocytes, which have to be continually replaced by the division of more primitive cells. The superficial epithelial cells of the gut also fall into this category. In the normal course of events, they are sloughed off the tops of the villi and replaced by cells dividing in the crypts.

MICHALOWSKI'S H- AND F-TYPE POPULATIONS

Michalowski classified tissues as following either a "hierarchical" model or a "flexible" model. Within tissues, three distinct categories of cells can be identified. First are the **stem cells**, which are capable of unlimited proliferation and escape senescence because of telomere shortening by the enzyme telomerase. Examples include the crypt cells in the intestinal mucosa. The cells produced by stem-cell proliferation both maintain the stem-cell pool and provide candidates for differentiation. Second, at the other extreme, are **functional cells**, which are fully differentiated; they are usually incapable of further division and die after a finite lifespan, though the lifespan varies enormously between different cell types. Examples include circulatory granulocytes and the cells that make up the villi of the intestinal mucosa. Between these two extremes are **maturing partially differentiated cells**; these are descendants of the stem cells, still multiplying as they complete the process of differentiation. In the bone marrow, for example, the erythroblasts and granuloblasts represent intermediate compartments. Many tissues represent this **hierarchical** model (**H-type** populations), including the hematopoietic bone marrow, intestinal epithelium, and epidermis.

Other tissues, such as liver, thyroid, and dermis, are composed of cells that rarely divide under normal conditions but can be triggered to divide by damage to the tissue or organ. These **flexible** tissues (**F-type** populations) have no compartments and no strict hierarchy. After damage to the tissue, all cells, including those that are functional, enter the cell cycle. The time interval before damage becomes evident is a function of dose. If the dose is small, the expression of damage is delayed because cells divide infrequently. Consequently, the damage may be hidden for a long time.

Many tissues are hybrids of these two extreme models, with most cells able to make a few divisions and a minority of the population behaving as stem cells.

GROWTH FACTORS

Radiation induces interleukin-1 as well as interleukin-6. Interleukin-1 acts as a radioprotectant of hematopoietic cells by increasing both the shoulder and the D_0 of the survival curve. **Basic fibroblast growth factor** induces endothelial cell growth, inhibits radiation-induced apoptosis, and therefore protects against microvascular damage. This growth factor is produced in response to stress (heat, hypoxia, chemicals, radiation) and tends to reduce late effects. Microvascular protection is more effective in branching midsize capillaries (in which higher concentrations of basic fibroblast growth factor are seen) than in nonbranching capillaries. To the extent that radiation-induced late effects are mediated by damage to blood vessels, radiation tolerance is high in organs with large blood vessels (corresponding to high levels of growth factors) and lower near nonbranching capillaries.

Platelet-derived growth factor β increases damage to vascular tissue. **Transforming growth factor β (TGF-β)** induces a strong inflammatory response—for example, in pneumonitis. It stimulates the growth of connective tissue and tends to inhibit epithelial cell growth. Consequently, fibrosis and vascular changes associated with late radiation effects are linked with this factor. TGF-β may down-regulate interleukin-1 and **tumor necrosis factor (TNF)** and increase damage to hematopoietic tissue.

TNF is a cytotoxic agent that mediates the inflammatory response produced by monocytes and tumor cells by binding to cell-surface receptors that initiate signal transduction pathways. TNF induces proliferation of fibroblasts, inflammatory cells, and endothelial cells and so is associated with complications. In clinical trials, the administration of TNF causes fatigue, anorexia, weight loss, and transient leukopenia. TNF protects hematopoietic cells and sensitizes tumor cells to radiation. Serum concentrations of TNF correlate with severity of pneumonitis, hepatic dysfunction, renal insufficiency, and demyelination. TNF may contribute to the pathophysiology of radiation-induced central nervous system symptoms. The expression of TNF following radiation is believed to be regulated at the transcriptional level and involves the protein kinase C–dependent pathway.

SPECIFIC TISSUES AND ORGANS

Table 19.2 is a compilation of tissue and organ sensitivities. Important examples will be discussed in turn.

Skin

The skin is composed of the outer layer, the epidermis, which is the site of early radiation reactions, and the deeper layer, the dermis, which is the site of late radiation reactions (Fig. 19.2).

The epidermis (30–300 μm thick) is derived from a basal layer of actively proliferating cells, which is covered by several layers of nondividing differentiating cells to the surface, at which the most superficial keratinized cells are desquamated. It takes about 14 days from the time a newly formed cell leaves the basal layer to the time it is desquamated from the surface. The target cells for radiation damage are the dividing stem cells in the basal layer.

The dermis is a dense connective tissue (1–3 mm thick) within which scattered fibroblasts produce most of the dermal proteins. The vasculature of the dermis plays a major role in the radiation response. The target cells are thus the fibroblasts and the vascular endothelial cells.

A few hours after doses greater than 5 Gy (500 rad), there is an early erythema similar to sunburn, which is caused by vasodilation, edema, and loss of plasma constituents from capillaries. Reactions resulting from stem-cell death take longer to develop. When orthovoltage (250-kV) x-rays were the modality commonly used, skin was frequently dose limiting, because the full dose is deposited in the superficial layers. In this case, an erythema develops in the 2nd to 3rd week of a fractionated regimen, followed by dry or moist desquamation resulting from depletion of the basal cell population. At lower doses, islets of skin may regrow from surviving stem cells (see the model scoring system in mouse skin developed and described by Withers, described in Chapter 18); at higher doses, at which there are no surviving stem cells within the area treated, moist desquamation is complete, and healing must occur by migration of cells from outside the treated area.

With megavoltage x-ray equipment presently being used, the maximum dose (D_{max}) occurs at a depth from several millimeters to several centimeters below the skin surface, depending on the energy. Consequently, epidermal reactions usually are limited to dry desquamation and increased pigmentation. Conventional doses of 60 Gy (6,000 rad) or more are tolerated by the skin readily if they are spread out over 6 to 8 weeks, because a substantial amount of stem-cell proliferation can occur during this time. For skin, as for oral mucosa, the total dose tolerated depends more on overall time than on fraction size. Because for high-energy x-rays D_{max} occurs at a depth below the surface, late damage may occur in the dermis in the absence of early reactions in the epidermis. The clinical appearance of radiation fibrosis results from atrophy leading to contraction of the irradiated area. Telangiectasia developing more than a year after irradiation reflects late-developing vascular injury.

Skin Appendages: A Special Case

Within a few days after irradiation, the death of germinal cells results in hair dysplasia (i.e., short, thin hair). The proportion of dysplastic hair is dose dependent. Epilation occurs during the 3rd week, and regrowth may occur after 1 to 3 months. Sebaceous glands are as sensitive as hair, but sweat glands are less radiosensitive. Regenerated skin may be dry and hairless. An objective measure of skin damage may be obtained by a determination of electrical conductivity, which is influenced by sweat production.

Hematopoietic System

Hematopoietic tissues are located primarily in the bone marrow, with 60% located in the pelvis and vertebrae and the remainder in the ribs, skull, sternum, scapula, and proximal sections of the femur and humerus. A tiny fraction of stem cells are found

TABLE 19.2

A Compilation of Tissue and Organ Sensitivities

	Injury	$TD_{5/5}$, Gy	$TD_{50/5}$, Gy	Field Size
Class I organs				
Bone marrow	Aplasia, pancytopenia	2.5	4.5	Whole segment
Liver	Acute and chronic hepatitis	30	40	Whole
		50	55	1/3
Intestine	Obstruction, perforation, fistula	40	55	Whole
		50	65	1/3 or 1/2
Stomach	Perforation, ulcer, hemorrhage	50	65	Whole
		60	70	1/3
Brain	Infarction, necrosis	45	60	Whole
		60	75	1/3
Spinal cord	Infarction, necrosis	47	—	20 cm
		50	70	5 or 10 cm
Heart	Pericarditis and pancarditis	40	50	Whole
		60	70	1/3
Lung	Acute and chronic pneumonitis	17.5	24.5	Whole
		45	65	1/3
Kidney	Acute and chronic nephrosclerosis	23	28	Whole
		50(1/3)	45(2/3)	1/3 or 2/3
Class II organs				
Oral cavity and pharynx	Ulceration, mucositis	60	75	50 cm^2
Skin	Acute and chronic dermatitis, telangiectasia	55	65	100 cm^2
Esophagus	Esophagitis, ulceration	55	68	Whole
		60	72	1/3
Rectum	Ulcer, stenosis, fistula	60	80	No vol effect
Salivary glands	Xerostomia	32	46	1/3 or 1/2
Bladder	Contracture	65	80	2/3
		80	85	1/3
Ureters	Stricture	70	100	5–10 cm length
Testes	Sterilization	1	2	Whole
Ovaries	Sterilization	2–3	6–12	Whole (age dep.)
Growing cartilage, child bone	Growth arrest, dwarfing	10	30	Whole
Mature cartilage, adult bone	Necrosis, fracture, sclerosis	60	100	Whole
		60	100	10 cm^2
Eye				
Retina	Blindness	45	65	Whole
Cornea		50	60	Whole
Lens	Cataract	10	18	Whole
Endocrine				
Thyroid	Hypothyroidism	45	150	Whole
Adrenal	Hypoadrenalism	60		Whole
Pituitary	Hypopituitarism	45	200	Whole
Peripheral nerves	Neuritus	60	100	

(Continued)

TABLE 19.2

(Continued)

	Injury	$TD_{5/5}$, Gy	$TD_{50/5}$, Gy	Field Size
Ear				
Middle	Serous otitis	30	40	No vol effect
Vestibular	Meniere's syndrome	60	70	
Class III organs				
Muscle				
Child	Atrophy	20	40	Whole
Adult	Fibrosis	60	80	Whole
Lymph nodes and lymphatics	Atrophy, sclerosis	50	70	Whole node
Large arteries and veins	Sclerosis	80	100	10 cm^2
Articular cartilage	None	500	5,000	Joint surface (mm^2)
Uterus	Necrosis, perforation	100	200	Whole
Vagina	Ulcer, fistula	90	100	Whole
Breast				
Child	No development	10	15	Whole
Adult	Atrophy, necrosis	50	100	Whole

Based on a combination of Rubin P, Casarett GW: *Clinical Radiation Pathology*, vol 1. Philadelphia, WB Saunders, 1968; and Emami B, Lyman J, Broun A, et al.: Tolerance of normal tissue to therapeutic irradiation. *Int J Radiat Oncol Biol Phys* 21:109–122, 1991, with permission. Table compiled by Dr. Richard Miller. The figures in this table are a guide only.

in the circulation. In the normal healthy adult, the liver and spleen have no hematopoietic activity, but they can become active in some circumstances—for example, after partial-body irradiation. The pluripotent stem cells go through a period of multiplication and maturation, followed by differentiation without division, before they become mature circulating blood elements of the various types.

The stem cells are particularly radiosensitive. The survival curve has little or no shoulder and a D_0 of slightly less than 1 Gy (100 rad) (Chapter 18). There is little sparing from either fractionating the dose or lowering the dose rate. The transit time from stem cell to fully functioning cell, however, differs for the various circulatory blood elements, and these differences account for the complex changes in blood count seen after irradiation.

Blood Cell Counts after Total-Body Irradiation

A dose as low as 0.3 Gy (30 rad) leads to a reduction in the number of lymphocytes, because they are among the most sensitive cells in the body. After larger doses, the number of all blood cells is altered; lymphopenia is followed by granulopenia, then thrombopenia, and finally anemia.

Following a total-body dose of 4 to 6 Gy (400–600 rad), there is a temporary increase in the number of granulocytes because of the mobilization of the reserve pool, followed by a rapid fall by the end of the 1st week. The number then remains almost constant before falling again to a minimum value at 18 to 20 days after irradiation. After 1 week of aplasia, regeneration is rapid and takes place more or less simultaneously in platelets, reticulocytes, and granulocytes. After higher doses, the cell minimum is reached earlier and the period of aplasia lasts longer, increasing the possibility of hemorrhage and/or infection, which could prove fatal. At lower doses, around 1 Gy (100 rad), the depression in granulocyte count is less marked and regeneration less rapid. The general pattern of the blood counts after a modest dose of radiation is illustrated in Figure 19.3.

The survival of stem cells determines the subsequent performance of the bone marrow after total-body irradiation, because in the first few hours there is a sudden decrease in the number of pluripotent stem cells and progenitor cells. If the number of stem cells falls below a critical level, production of functional cells essentially stops until partial regeneration of the stem-cell compartment occurs and differentiation is allowed to resume. Administration of hematopoietic growth factors can shorten the period of aplasia markedly and accelerate regeneration of all blood cells.

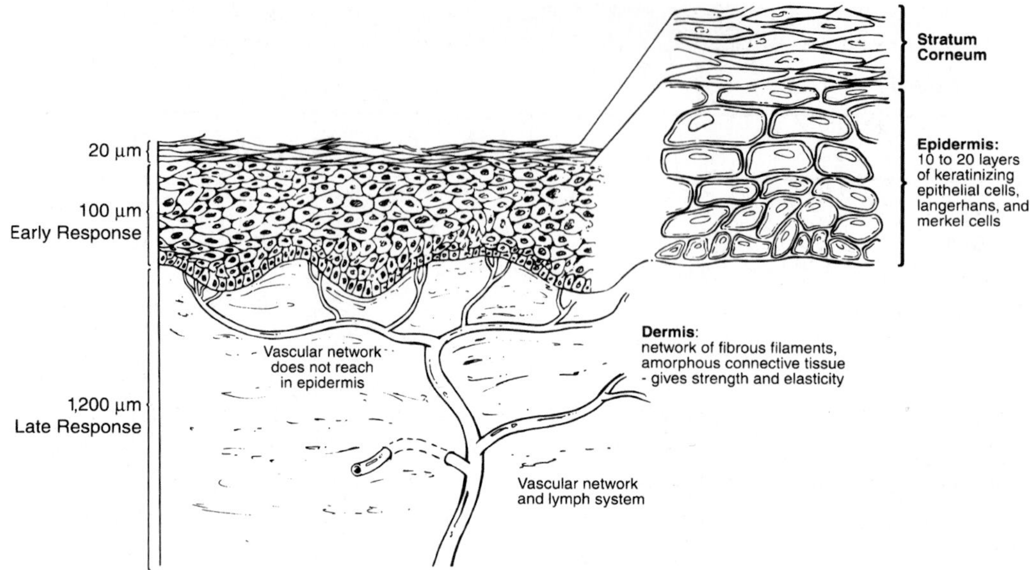

FIGURE 19.2 ● The skin from the perspective of a radiation biologist. The epidermis has a thickness of about 100 μm, though it varies with body site (30–300 μm). It consists of 10 to 20 layers of keratinizing epithelial cells. This is a self-renewing tissue. The stem-cell compartment forms part of the basal layer and has an unlimited capacity for proliferation. Cells produced in the basal layer migrate to the surface, differentiating as they do so, but retaining some proliferative potential. Cells in the surface layer are fully differentiated and keratinized and gradually are sloughed off and lost. The transit time for an epidermal cell to pass from the basal layer to the surface is 12 to 48 days, depending on skin thickness. The dermis is about 1,200 μm thick (1,000–3,000 μm) and consists of a dense network of fibrous filaments and connective tissue. The vascular network, capillaries, and lymph system are in the dermis. The vascular network does not extend into the epidermis. Two distinct waves of reactions are observed in the skin following irradiation. An early, or acute, reaction is observed about 10 days after a single dose and results from damage to the epidermis. Late reactions occur months later, mediated through damage to the dermis, principally to the vasculature. In clinical radiation therapy, late damage is now the dose-limiting reaction, because the buildup associated with megavoltage beams spares the epidermis.

Partial-Body Irradiation

In the irradiated volume, the effects of partial-body irradiation are analogous to those following total-body irradiation. In the unirradiated marrow, the stem cells start dividing within a few hours, and a compensatory hyperplasia attempts to maintain the total production of blood elements. There also may be an extension of hemopoiesis into the long bones, spleen, and liver, which are not normally hemopoietic in the adult human.

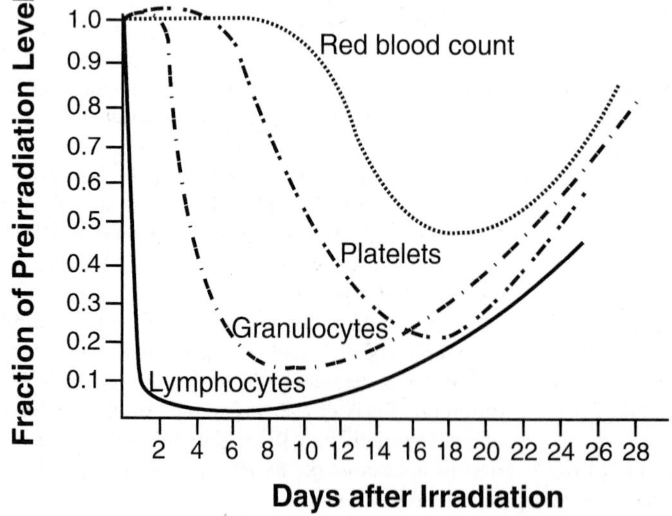

FIGURE 19.3 ● The pattern of depletion and recovery of the principal circulating elements of the blood following an intermediate dose of total-body radiation. The curves are purely illustrative: The time at which the nadir occurs is a combination of the radiosensitivity of the stem cells and the lifetime of the mature functional cells.

With fractionated radiation therapy, the pool of stem cells in the unirradiated volume falls progressively as differentiation is accelerated in an attempt to maintain the circulating blood count. Doses greater than about 30 Gy (3,000 rad) may cause permanent aplasia in the irradiated volume; hyperplasia and extension of the active bone marrow in the unirradiated volume may persist indefinitely.

Irradiation always reduces the number of stem cells in the bone marrow, and the return to normal may take a long time. This explains why patients remain sensitive to a new insult for months or even years following irradiation.

Radiation and Chemotherapy Agents

Some cytotoxic drugs act essentially on only those cells in cycle, and they have little effect on hematopoietic stem cells, because 90% of them are out of cycle unless the marrow is regenerating following a previous insult. This explains why these drugs show extra toxicity if administered shortly after radiotherapy. The marrow of patients irradiated to a large volume is always more sensitive to cytotoxic drugs, partly because the pool of stem cells is reduced and partly because a greater proportion of stem cells are dividing actively.

The addition of chemotherapy may also have different effects on acute and late reactions. Although many chemotherapeutic agents are dose limited by their toxicity to rapidly proliferating tissues, such as gut mucosa and bone marrow, others (bleomycin, doxorubicin, *cis*-platinum) have specific toxicities to slow turnover tissues, such as lung, heart, or kidney. The additive toxicities may therefore also differ for acute and late reactions of tissues included in the irradiated volume. (For more on chemotherapy, see Chapter 27.)

Lymphoid Tissue and the Immune System

The immune system is composed of macrophages and lymphocytes. Macrophages are derived from the same progenitors as granulocytes. These give rise to monocytes, which are transformed into macrophages. This cell line is less radiosensitive than lymphocytes, which are derived, however, from the same pluripotent stem cells.

The B line gives rise to B lymphocytes and plasmocytes, which are responsible for humoral immunologic responses and have life spans of 7 weeks and 2 to 3 days, respectively. Cells of the T line pass through the thymus, where they mature to become T lymphocytes. These cells have a life span of about 5 months and are responsible for cellular immunity and for secreting lymphokines. There are also other types of lymphocytes, including killer cells, responsible for antibody-dependent cytotoxic reactions, and natural killer cells, the function of which is not fully understood.

Total-body irradiation leads to a rapid fall in the number of circulating B and T lymphocytes, with the number returning to normal in a few weeks, depending on the dose. The lymphoid tissues (e.g., nodes, spleen) are very radiosensitive and are depleted of cells by quite small radiation doses. Lymphocytes are very radiosensitive, largely because of apoptosis. B cells are more radiosensitive than T cells, and overall, their radiosensitivity, as measured by a clonogenic assay, is similar to that of hematopoietic stem cells.

The effect of irradiation on immune function is complex, depending on the volume irradiated and the number of surviving cells, as well as their capacity to migrate and become lodged in the microenvironment. Total-body irradiation is used to inhibit the immune system in preparing patients for an organ transplant, such as a kidney or bone-marrow transplant. A total-body dose of 3.5 to 4.5 Gy (350–450 rad) inhibits the immune response against a new antigen, though it is much less effective against an antigen to which the individual is already sensitized. The graft-versus-host reaction after bone-marrow transplantation is relatively radioresistant. Partial-body irradiation, characteristic of ordinary radiation therapy, has only a limited effect on the immune response, and whether it influences metastatic dissemination is controversial. Total lymphoid irradiation to a dose of 30 to 40 Gy (3,000–4,000 rad) is used for the treatment of lymphomas and leads to a long-lasting T cell lymphopenia. It can be used to treat autoimmune diseases and also to prepare patients for organ transplants.

The Digestive Tract

Oral Mucosa

The cellular organization of the mucosa is similar to that of the skin in that cells multiply in the basal layer and then migrate toward the surface as they differentiate. The life span of the differentiated cells, however, is much shorter than in the epidermis, so there is a more rapid reaction to radiation. The intensity of early mucous membrane reactions is a major factor limiting daily and weekly dose accumulation in the treatment of cancer of the head and neck (Table 19.2). For example, a schedule of 70 Gy (7,000 rad) delivered in 2-Gy (200-rad) fractions over 7 weeks leads to spotted-confluent mucositis in most patients, which approaches maximum tolerance if the schedule is accelerated to 5.5 weeks by, for example, the use of a concomitant boost technique.

The oral cavity contains a variety of tissue types as well as the mucous membrane. The tongue consists of muscle bundles as well as mucosa with taste buds. The muscles undergo mild progressive fibrosis and fiber atrophy after irradiation. The tonsils are lymphatic tissues and function as sites of antigen process and recognition. Following radiation exposure to a maximum tolerance dose, desquamation of the oral cavity occurs by about day 12, with recovery in 2 to 3 weeks. Desquamation occurs first in the soft palate, followed by the hypopharynx, vallecula, floor of the mouth, cheeks, epiglottis, base of tongue, vocal chords, and dorsum of tongue.

The sequence of events that occurs during radiation therapy for head and neck cancer is so important for the comfort and welfare of the patient that it is worth spelling out in detail. The order of events reflects the different kinetics of the cell populations involved:

1st week: Asymptomatic to slight focal hyperemia and edema caused by dilatation of capillaries in sensitive patients. Sensitivity may be associated with alcohol or tobacco use, chemotherapy, infection (oral candidiasis, herpes simplex virus), or immunosuppression (HIV).

2nd week: Increasing pain and loss of desire to eat. Sense of taste is altered; bitter and acid flavors are most changed, with less change with salty and sweet tastes. Erythema and edema increase, and early desquamative mucositis occurs. Basal cell division has been affected; this layer is being denuded, and vasculoconnective tissue damage becomes apparent. Mucositis is patchy.

3rd week: Mucositis and swelling with depletion of gland secretions leading to difficulty in swallowing. Mucositis plaques are confluent.

4th week: Progression of signs. Confluent mucositis sloughs, resulting in denuded lamina propria. Mucosa becomes covered by fibrin and polymorphonuclear leukocytes.

5th week: Maximum radiation damage apparent by this time. Extreme sensitivity to touch, temperature, and grainy food. Recovery of epithelial layer may begin during therapy.

Post-therapy, the basal cells migrate into the area and proliferate. In 2 to 4 weeks, complete resolution is observed. The serous acinar cells of the parotid and submaxillary salivary glands undergo interphase death, and hence salivary dysfunction appears after irradiation, with no threshold dose and little sparing by fractionation. Xerostomia is the main clinical effect that can interfere with nutrition, deteriorate oral hygiene, and predispose a patient to dental problems. $TD_{5/5}$ (the tolerance dose for 5% complication in 5 years) is 32 Gy (3,200 rad), and $TD_{50/5}$ (the tolerance dose for 50% complications in 5 years) is 46 Gy (4,600 rad). Impairment of taste acuity occurs during the 3rd week of a multifraction radiotherapy regime.

Esophagus

The mucosa consists of rapidly dividing cells. After radiation, the esophagus displays an acute mucosal response of esophagitis and increased thickness of the squamous layer. Symptoms appear that include substernal burning with pain on swallowing at about 10 to 12 days after the start of therapy, with a return to normal within a week of the end of therapy. Late effects are related to the muscle layer; they include necrosis and a thickening of the epithelium. This leads to symptoms of difficulty on swallowing and possibly ulcerations after high doses. The tolerance dose is 57.5 Gy (5,750 rad) in 10 fractions (acute effects limit).

Stomach

Irradiation of the stomach often causes nausea and vomiting immediately afterward. The precursor cells of the gastric glands give rise to mucin-secreting surface columnar cells with short life-spans (about 3 or 4 days) and to acid-secreting parietal and pepsinogen-secreting chief cells that have long life spans (hundreds of days). The precursor cells are radiosensitive, and their death leads to early depletion of the surface columnar cell epithelium. Delayed gastric emptying and epithelial denudement are the two main early radiation effects. Peptic ulceration is seen in patients receiving more than 40 Gy (4,000 rad) to the upper abdomen.

Dyspepsia may be evident in 6 months to 4 years and gastritis in 1 to 12 months. Acute ulceration may occur shortly after the completion of treatment but rarely leads to perforation. At about 5 months, late ulceration and submucosal fibrosis leading to antral fibrosis may occur. Tolerance doses range from 40 to 50 Gy (4,000–5,000 rad).

Small and Large Intestines

As with the skin and oral mucosa, both early and late complications are observed in the gastrointestinal tract. Acute mucositis frequently occurs, with symptoms such as diarrhea or gastritis, depending on the treatment field. If the dose is limited to 50 to 54 Gy (5,000–5,400 rad) in 2-Gy (200-rad) fractions, acute reactions are seldom dose limiting, and if they do occur, interruption of treatment for a few days usually alleviates the problem. Much more serious are the long-term late sequelae, which may develop either from persistent severe early reactions (consequential late effects) or independently of acute damage in the submucosal, muscular, or serosal layers.

In the small intestine, stem cells are located toward the bottom of the crypts of Lieberkühn. Atrophy of the villus occurs about 2 to 4 days postirradiation. Epithelial denudation is responsible for the acute gut reactions. A regenerative response appears rapidly, and within 2 to 4 days, micro- and macrocolonies are detectable. The surviving crypts have at least the same radiosensitivity to reirradiation as the unirradiated crypts, and very little dose is "remembered."

Late bowel reactions involve all tissue layers and are caused by atrophy of the mucosa caused by vascular injury, with subsequent breakdown resulting from mechanical irritation and bacterial infection, which leads to an acute inflammatory response. Also, overgrowth of the fibromuscular tissue with stenosis and serosal breakdown and adhesion formation may occur, which may be predisposed to by previous surgery and is related to inflammatory mediators. Fibrosis and ischemia are typical late effects. Tolerance dose is about 50 Gy (5,000 rad) for the small intestine and slightly higher for the large intestine. Rectal tolerance is about 70 Gy (7,000 rad).

Lungs

The lung is an intermediate- to late-responding tissue. Two waves of damage can be identified: acute pneumonitis at 2 to 6 months after treatment, and fibrosis, which may develop slowly over a period of several months to years. The only symptom of early acute pneumonopathy may be an opacity on a chest x-ray, though it may be accompanied by functional signs, including cough, dyspnea, and respiratory difficulties. Progressive pulmonary fibrosis develops in most patients, including those who previously were asymptomatic, beginning about a year after irradiation.

Difficulties in respiratory function increase in severity with time and are generally irreversible. Their severity depends on three factors: volume irradiated, dose, and fraction size. The lung is particularly sensitive to fractionation, with an α/β estimated to be about 3 Gy (300 rad). The most likely target cells are the pulmonary endothelial cells and the type II pneumocytes (cells of the alveolar wall). Type II cells are associated with the production of surfactant during the first few days after irradiation.

The lung is among the most sensitive of late-responding organs. The FSU in the lung is the pulmonary lobule, consisting of the terminal bronchioli and respiratory parenchyma that it serves. The FSUs are arranged in parallel, with a large number of bronchi and alveoli working together; consequently, volume as well as dose is important. Because of this organization of the functional subunits, the lung is only dose limiting if large volumes are irradiated and if the remaining lung is not capable of providing adequate function.

Pulmonary damage also may occur following use of chemotherapy agents, notably bleomycin, cyclophosphamide, and mustine. Combining radiation with these drugs reduces lung tolerance.

Kidneys

Together with the lung, the kidney is among the more radiosensitive late-responding critical organs (Table 19.2). Irradiation of both kidneys to a modest dose of about 30 Gy in 2-Gy fractions (3,000 rad in 200-rad fractions) results in nephropathy with arterial hypertension and anemia. Radiation damage develops slowly and may not become evident for years. Parts of one or even both kidneys can receive much higher doses. In contrast to most organs or tissues, increasing treatment time does not allow higher doses to be tolerated. Functional subunits are arranged in parallel, with each containing only about 1,000 stem cells. Damage to tubules, therefore, may result from sterilization of all the cells in a tubule.

Liver

In terms of radiosensitivity, the liver ranks immediately below the kidney and lung. It shares with these organs the fact that its functional subunits are arranged in parallel, so that much larger doses are tolerated if only part of the organ is exposed.

Liver tolerance is dose limiting only if the whole organ is irradiated, as in, for example, total-body irradiation prior to bone-marrow transplantation. The lifespan of a hepatocyte is about 1 year, so that under normal conditions the cell renewal rate in the liver is very slow. Even large doses apparently are tolerated for a few months, but then hepatic function deteriorates progressively. Fatal hepatitis may result from a fractionated protocol of only 35 Gy (3,500 rad) if the whole organ is irradiated.

Bladder Epithelium

The epithelium of the bladder consists of a basal layer formed of small diploid cells, covered by several layers of larger transitional cells and at the surface by a layer of very large polyploid cells with a thick membrane designed to resist the irritation caused by urine. Cell renewal rate is low, the superficial cells having a lifespan of several months. Because of this long lifespan, accelerated proliferation following irradiation does not begin for months. Senescence of the differentiated functional cells then reveals latent damage in the basal layer. Frequency of urination increases in parallel with bladder damage and loss of surface cells. The absence of these surface cells explains the irritation by urine of the deeper cellular layers, leading to stimulation of cellular proliferation. Subsequent late effects are related to fibrosis and reduction in bladder capacity.

Central and Peripheral Nervous Systems

The nervous system is less sensitive to radiation than other late-responding organs and tissues such as the kidney or lung. Although tolerance doses are frequently quoted at the 5% complication level (i.e., TD_5), wide margins of safety in dose usually are included, because damage to these tissues results in severe consequences, including paralysis.

Brain

Three main categories of cells are involved: neurons, vascular endothelial cells, and glial cells. Neurons are nonproliferating end cells in adults; glial cells have a slow rate of turnover, with a small precursor (stem-cell) compartment of only about 1%. Endothelial cells also have a slow turnover but can proliferate rapidly after injury. The most important injuries to the brain by radiation are all late syndromes, developing months to years after exposure. Some reactions occur within the first 6 months, including transient demyelination (somnolence syndrome) or the much more serious leukoencephalopathy. Typical radiation necrosis may become evident as early as 6 months, but may be delayed as long as 2 to 3 years. Histopathologic changes that occur within the first year are most likely to involve white matter, whereas for times beyond 6 to 12 months, the gray matter usually shows changes accompanied by vascular lesions such as telangiectasia and focal hemorrhages. A mixture of histologic characteristics is likely to be associated with radionecrosis manifest from 1 to 2 years postirradiation, accompanied by cognitive defects.

Spinal Cord

Radiation-induced changes in the spinal cord are similar to those seen in the brain as far as latency, tolerance dose, and histology are concerned. Lhermitte's sign is a demyelating injury that develops early, by several months after treatment, persists for a few months to a year, but is usually reversible. It may occur at doses as low as 35 Gy (3,500 rad), well below the tolerance dose for permanent radiation myelopathy, and its appearance does not predict later more serious problems.

Late damage includes two principal syndromes. The first, occurring from about 6 to 18 months, involves demyelination and necrosis of the white matter; the second is mostly a vasculopathy and has a latency of 1 to 4 years.

For the spinal cord, the $TD_{5/5}$ is about 50 Gy (5,000 rad) for a 10-cm length irradiated and 55 Gy (5,500 rad) for a 5-cm length. By 70 Gy (7,000 rad), the incidence of myelopathy would be about 50%.

The tolerance dose to the spine shows little dependence on overall treatment time, at least for protocols of conventional length up to 10 weeks. By contrast, tolerance depends critically on dose per fraction. Lower doses per fraction reduce the risk of late effects, but if two doses per day are used, the time between fractions must be at least 6 hours (and preferably more), because the repair of sublethal damage is slow in this tissue. There is evidence of two components of repair, one with a half-time less than 1 hour and one with a half-time close to 4 hours. The spinal cord is the clearest example of a tissue in which FSUs are arranged in series. The probability of a myelopathy depends critically on the length irradiated for very small lengths, but once the length of the field exceeds a few centimeters, the treatment volume has little effect.

Caution must be exercised in combining radiation with chemotherapy agents, because neurotoxic agents such as methotrexate, *cis*-platinum, vinblastine, and AraC reduce the tolerance to radiation delivered simultaneously or sequentially.

As far as retreatment is concerned, animal data suggest that by about 2 years the majority of the damage from a prior exposure has been repaired; the extent of the repair depends very much on the level of the initial injury.

Peripheral Nerves

Radiation injury of peripheral nerves probably is more common than effects on the spinal cord. It is often said that peripheral nerves are more radioresistant than the cord or brain, but there are few quantitative data to support this. A dose of 60 Gy (6,000 rad) in a conventional regimen of 2-Gy (200-rad) fractions may lead to a 5% probability of injury, with the probability rising steeply thereafter with increasing dose.

Testes

The seminiferous tubules are composed of two types of cells: sertoli cells, which secrete a hormone that controls the secretion of FSH by the hypophysis; and the germinal cells, the hierarchy of which is strictly defined. The stem cells, the type A spermatogonia, have a long cell cycle and divide infrequently. The process of differentiation proceeds through several types of spermatogonia to the spermatocytes, which are the cells in which meiosis occurs. Each spermatocyte gives rise to four spermatids, which finally result in spermatozoa. In humans, the transit time from stem cell to spermatozoa is about 74 days. There is considerable cell loss along the way, so that the amplification factor is much less than might be calculated from the number of divisions that occur.

Leydig cells, which secrete testosterone, also are found in the testis, and their function is regulated by pituitary gonadotropins, prolactin, and luteinizing hormone. This is important in the use of neoadjuvant hormone therapy during the treatment of prostatic cancer.

In humans, a dose as low as 0.1 Gy (10 rad) leads to a temporary reduction in the number of spermatozoa, and 0.15 Gy (15 rad) leads to temporary sterility. Azoospermia lasting for several years occurs after 2 Gy (200 rad), and permanent azoospermia occurs after about 6 to 8 Gy (600–800 rad) in 2-Gy (200-rad) fractions. On the other hand, even much larger doses have little effect on the Leydig cells in the adult, so that although irradiation of the testes may lead to sterility, it has little or no effect on the libido.

The stem cells appear to be more radiosensitive than the differentiating spermatogonia, which explains why the duration of azoospermia increases as the dose is increased. Fractionated or continuous low-dose-rate irradiation is more effective than a single acute exposure, because a large proportion of the stem cells are in a radioresistant phase of the cell cycle. If irradiation is protracted, it affects stem cells as they move through the cell cycle into more radiosensitive phases. This accounts for the long-lasting azoospermia seen after relatively low daily doses of scattered radiation reaching the testes during irradiation of the pelvis and also the occurrence of testicular dysfunction seen after years of occupational exposure to ionizing radiation.

A number of cytotoxic drugs have substantial effects on spermatogenesis. For example, the alkylating agents included in MOPP [mechlorethamine (Mustargen), vincristine (Oncovin), procarbazine, and prednisone], the combination of chemotherapy agents used at one time for the treatment of Hodgkin's lymphoma, led to sterility in almost all patients. Of course, the drug treatment was prolonged and simulated low-dose-rate irradiation, killing stem cells as they came into cycle.

Ovaries

The effects of radiation on the ovaries are quite different from those on the testes, because after the fetal stage, the oocytes no longer divide. They are all present at birth, and their number diminishes steadily with age, reaching zero by the time of menopause. Oocytes are extremely radiosensitive to cell killing; like lymphocytes, they die an interphase death, with D_0 of only 0.12 Gy (12 rad). There is little effect of fractionation. Mature follicles and those in the process of maturation are damaged equally by radiation, so that sterilization is immediate (i.e., there is no latent period, as in the male). Because hormonal secretion is associated with follicular maturation, sterilization by radiation leads to a loss of libido and all of the changes associated with menopause.

Female Genitalia

The skin of the vulva reacts like skin elsewhere, but because of moisture and friction, a tolerance dose of 50 to 70 Gy (5,000–7,000 rad) in conventional fractions is considered on the high side.

Acute effects of irradiation of the vagina include erythema, moist desquamation, and confluent mucositis, leading to the loss of vaginal epithelium that may persist for 3 to 6 months. Gross abnormalities in the vagina may include pale color, a thin atrophic mucosa, inflammation, and tissue necrosis with ulceration leading to a fistula. Tolerance doses, however, are high: 90 Gy (9,000 rad) before ulceration and 100 Gy (10,000 rad) for the development of a fistula. From intracavitary treatments, doses to the cervix and uterus may reach as high as 200 Gy (20,000 rad). Effects seen include atrophy of the endometrial glands and stroma as well as ulceration.

Blood Vessels and the Vascular System

The effects of radiation on blood vessels is particularly important, because late damage to many different tissues and organs is mediated to some extent by effects on the vasculature. Blood vessels have a complex structure. A monolayer of endothelial cells lines the interior surface, resting on connective tissue, the thickness of which depends on the type of vessel. Under normal circumstances, the rate or proliferation of endothelial cells is low, so that following exposure to radiation, cell loss occurs over a period of time as cells enter mitosis. Regions of constriction appear because of the abnormal proliferation of surviving cells. Denudation of the surface of blood vessels leads to the formation of thromboses and capillary necroses. In the smooth muscle cells that make up the wall of blood vessels, the proportion of cells cycling is very low, so that it takes several years for the number of cells to diminish significantly following irradiation. The loss of muscular fibers plays an important role in the development of late damage that may become evident several years later. Muscle cells are replaced by collagen fibers, vessel walls lose their elasticity, and blood flow is diminished.

Arterial damage may occur after doses of 50 to 70 Gy (5,000–7,000 rad) delivered in conventional fractionation patterns, but capillaries are damaged by doses above about 40 Gy (4,000 rad). In general, veins are less sensitive to radiation than arteries.

Heart

In its tolerance to radiation, the heart is intermediate between the kidney or lung and the central nervous system. The most common radiation-induced heart injury is acute pericarditis, which seldom occurs during the first year posttherapy. It varies in severity from transient pericarditis, which runs a benign course, to dense sclerosis with cardiac constriction. Anterior chest pain with shortness of breath and low-grade fever may be observed. The threshold dose may be as low as 20 Gy (2,000 rad) if more than 50% of the heart is irradiated, but higher for partial exposure. A dose of 45 to 50 Gy (4,500–5,000 rad) in conventional fractions produces an 11% incidence. The α/β ratio for the heart is low (about 1 Gy, or 100 rad), so that fractionation results in a substantial sparing effect.

Radiation-induced cardiomyopathy results from dense and diffuse fibrosis; it is a slowly evolving lesion that develops over a period of many years and leads to impaired function. Reduced cardiac function is seen in some patients with Hodgkin's disease who receive a dose of about 30 Gy (3,000 rad) to most of the heart. Protection of part of the heart greatly reduces the incidence of symptoms.

The chemotherapy agent Adriamycin (doxorubicin) increases the severity of radiation-induced complications. In addition, Adriamycin may reveal latent radiation damage many years after radiation therapy.

Bone and Cartilage

In children, growing cartilage is particularly radiosensitive. Doses as low as 10 Gy (1,000 rad) can slow growth because of the death of chondroblasts. Above about 20 Gy (2,000 rad), the deficit in growth is irreversible. The effects of radiation on bone growth are more serious for higher doses and for younger ages. Sequelae are particularly serious in children younger than 2 years of age, and radiation can affect stature adversely up to the time of puberty.

In the adult, osteonecrosis of the lower maxilla may be a serious complication following radiation therapy for cancer of the buccal cavity. The $TD_{5/5}$ is 50 to 60 Gy (5,000–6,000 rad); the $TD_{50/5}$ is about 70 Gy (7,000 rad) for large irradiated volumes. Fractures of the humeral and femoral head are observed if the dose, in conventional fractions, is high. The $TD_{5/5}$ is 52 Gy (5,200 rad), and the $TD_{50/5}$ is 65 Gy (6,500 rad). Fractures of the ribs and clavicle are sometimes seen in patients receiving radiotherapy for breast cancer but are generally not serious complications.

LENT AND SOMA

The two large organizations that initiate and coordinate multicenter clinical trials in Europe and North America, namely, the European Organization for Research and Treatment of Cancer (EORTC) and the Radiation Therapy Oncology Group (RTOG), formed working groups to update their system for assessing late injury to normal tissues. This led to the **Late Effects of Normal Tissue (LENT)** conference in 1992. This conference led to the introduction of the **SOMA** classification for late toxicity. SOMA is an acronym for ***S***ubjective, ***O***bjective, ***M***anagement criteria with ***A***nalytic laboratory and imaging procedures. These scales, specific for each organ, form a scaffold for understanding the expression of later injury because they are the substance of LENT expression. The SOMA scales have been formulated for all anatomic sites listed in Table 19.3. An example for the central nervous system is given in Table 19.4.

The SOMA Scoring System

The SOMA scales have been designed to allow the acquisition of data by several different methods, which it is hoped are not inevitably dependent one upon the other:

- **S**ubjective—in which the injury, if any, will be recorded from the subject's point of view, that is, as perceived by the patient. This information can be elicited during interviews or derived by asking the patient to complete a carefully designed questionnaire or diary.
- **O**bjective—in which the morbidity is assessed as objectively as possible by the clinician during a clinical examination. In this case, the clinician may be able to detect signs of tissue dysfunction that are still below the threshold that will give the patient symptoms but are an indication of how close to tissue tolerance the treatment is or that may be early indicators of more serious problems that are developing and will be expressed later.
- **M**anagement—which indicates the active steps that may be taken in an attempt to ameliorate the symptoms.
- **A**nalytic—involving tools by which tissue function can be assessed even more objectively or with more biologic insight than by simple clinical examination. It is recognized that the tools available for such analysis may differ widely from one center to another and may evolve as the clinical trials progress. The invasiveness and cost of any tool used to quantify the late effects must

TABLE 19.3

Anatomic Sites for Which There Are LENT and SOMA Scales

Central nervous system
- Brain
- Spinal cord
- Male hypothalamic/pituitary/gonadal axis
- Female hypothalamic/pituitary/gonadal axis

Head and neck
- Eye
- Ear
- Mucosa
- Mandible
- Teeth
- Larynx
- Thyroid and hypothalamic/pituitary/thyroid axis

Breast

Heart
- Blood vessels

Lung

Gastrointestinal system
- Esophagus
- Stomach
- Small intestine/colon
- Rectum

Major digestive glands
- Liver

Genitourinary system
- Kidney
- Ureter
- Bladder/urethra
- Testes
- Male sexual dysfunction

Gynecologic system
- Vulva
- Vagina
- Uterus/reproductive organs
- Female sexual dysfunction

Bone, muscle, and skin
- Muscle/soft tissue
- Peripheral nerves
- Growing bone
- Mature bone (excluding mandible)
- Bone marrow
- Skin/subcutaneous tissue

Based on *Late Effects of Normal Tissues Consensus Conference*, San Francisco, CA, Aug 26–28, 1992. Rubin P, Constine LS, Fajardo LF, Phillips TL, Wasserman TH (eds). Published as a special issue of *Int J Radiat Oncol Biol Phys* 31:1049–1081, 1995.

TABLE 19.4

Central Nervous System SOMA

Subjective	Objective	Management	Analytic
Headache	Neurologic deficit	Anticonvulsives	MRI
Somnolence	Cognitive function	Steroids	CT
Intellectual deficit	Mood and personality changes	Sedation	MRS
			PET
Functional competence	Seizures		Magnetic mapping
Memory			Serum
			Cerebrospinal fluid

Based on Late Effects of Normal Tissues Consensus Conference, San Francisco, CA, Aug 26–28, 1992. Rubin P, Constine LS, Fajardo LF, Phillips TL, Wasserman TH (eds). Published as a special issue of *Int J Radiat Oncol Biol Phys* 31:1049–1081, 1995.

TABLE 19.5

LENT and SOMA Scoring System and Grading Categories

Grade 1	Grade 2	Grade 3	Grade 4
Subjective: *Ascending order of severity of symptoms perceived by patient (e.g., pain)*			
Occasional and minimal	Intermittent and tolerable	Persistent and intense	Refractory and excruciating
Objective: *Signs that can be assessed by clinician (e.g., neurologic deficit)*			
Barely detectable	Easily detectable	Focal motor signs, vision disturbances, etc.	Hemiplegia, hemisensory deficit, etc.
Management: *Active steps taken to ameliorate symptoms (e.g., pain)*			
Occasional nonnarcotic	Regular nonnarcotic	Regular narcotic	Surgical intervention
Analytic: *Findings that are quantifiable (e.g., CT and MRI, special laboratory tests)*			

Based on Late Effects of Normal Tissues Consensus Conference, San Francisco, CA, Aug 26–28, 1992. Rubin P, Constine LS, Fajardo LF, Phillips TL, Wasserman TH (eds). Published as a special issue of *Int J Radiat Oncol Biol Phys* 31:1049–1081, 1995.

be reasonable and proportional to the severity of the symptoms and the possible therapeutic consequences. The scales list the techniques that could yield valuable data, but it is not envisaged that all such tests would be feasible or even desirable in all studies.

The grading categories in the LENT and SOMA scoring system are shown in Table 19.5. There is no grade 0, because that would indicate no effect, and no grade 5, because that would indicate totality, or loss of an organ or function.

Summary of Pertinent Conclusions

- Most effects of radiation on normal tissues are due to cell killing, but some, such as nausea, vomiting, or fatigue experienced by patients following irradiation of large volumes including the abdomen, may be mediated by radiation-induced inflammatory cytokines.
- Apparent radioresponsiveness of a tissue depends on inherent sensitivity of cells, kinetics of the tissue or cell population, and the way cells are organized in that tissue.
- Sensitivity of actively dividing cells is expressed by their survival curve for reproductive integrity.
- The radiation dose needed to destroy the functioning ability of a differentiated cell is far greater than that necessary to stop the mitotic activity of a dividing cell.
- The shape of the dose–response relationship for functional end points, obtained from multifraction experiments, is more pertinent to radiotherapy than clonogenic assays.
- The time interval between irradiation and its expression in tissue damage depends on the life span of mature functional cells and the time it takes for a cell born in the stem compartment to mature.
- Hyperthermia damage is expressed early compared with radiation damage (Chapter 28).
- Both early and late effects may develop in one organ system because of injury to different target cell populations or tissue elements.
- The ratio α/β (the dose at which the linear and quadratic components of radiation damage are equal) may be inferred from multifraction experiments in systems scoring nonclonogenic end points.

(continued)

Summary of Pertinent Conclusions (Continued)

- Tolerance doses for late effects are more sensitive to changes in dose per fraction (low α/β value) compared with tolerance doses for early effects.
- Spatial arrangement of functional subunits (FSUs) is critical to the tolerance of some normal tissues.
- In some tissues (e.g., spinal cord), the FSUs are arranged serially (like links in a chain), and the integrity of each is critical to organ function.
- Tissues with a serial organization (e.g., spinal cord) have little or no functional reserve, and the risk of developing a complication is less dependent on volume irradiated than for tissues with a parallel organization. The risk of complication is strongly influenced by high-dose regions and hot spots.
- A tissue with intrinsically high tolerance may fail as a result of the inactivation of a small segment (as in the spinal cord); a tissue with an intrinsically low tolerance (kidney, lung) may lose a substantial number of its functional units without impact on clinical tolerance.
- Casarett's classification of tissue radiosensitivity is based on histopathologic observations.
- In terms of radiosensitivity based on histologic observation of cell death, parenchymal cells fall into four categories, from most sensitive to most resistant:

  I. Stem cells of classic self-renewal tissues, which divide regularly
  II. Differentiating intermitotic cells, which divide regularly but in which there is some differentiation between divisions, and which are variably differentiated
  III. Reverting postmitotic cells, which do not divide regularly but can divide under the appropriate stimulus
  IV. Fixed postmitotic cells, which are highly differentiated and appear to have lost the ability to divide

- Connective tissue and blood vessels are intermediate in radiosensitivity between groups II and III.
- Michalowski's classification divides tissues into hierarchical (H-type) and flexible (F-type) populations, which respond differently to radiation.
- Many tissues are a hybrid of H-type and F-type.
- The response of a tissue is influenced greatly by a host of growth factors, including interleukin-1 and 6, basic fibroblast growth factor, platelet-derived growth factor β, transforming growth factor β, and tumor necrosis factor.
- Early radiation response in the skin is caused by damage to the epidermis; the late response reflects damage to the dermis.
- The hematopoietic system is very sensitive to radiation, especially the stem cells. The complex changes seen in peripheral blood count after irradiation reflect differences in transit time from stem cell to functioning cell for the various circulatory blood elements.
- The effect of irradiation on the immune function is complex, depending on the volume irradiated and the number of surviving cells. A total-body dose of 3.5 to 4.5 Gy (350–450 rad) inhibits the immune response against a new antigen.
- The cellular organization of the lining of the gastrointestinal tract is similar to that of the skin, but the life span of the differentiated cells is shorter. Both early and late sequelae can occur.

  Oral mucosa: Damage to the oral mucosa during radiotherapy for head and neck cancer is very important for both the comfort and welfare of the patient. Xerostomia can interfere with nutrition and dental health.

  Esophagus: Early and late effects can occur and lead to difficulty in swallowing. Tolerance is 57.5 Gy (5,750 rad) in 10 fractions (acute effects limit).

  Stomach: Irradiation of the stomach often leads to nausea and vomiting. Tolerance doses range from 40 to 50 Gy (4,000–5,000 rad).

  Small and large intestines: Both early and late complications can occur. Tolerance dose is about 50 Gy (5,000 rad) for the small intestine, slightly higher for the large intestine, and 70 Gy (7,000 rad) for the rectum.

- The lung is an intermediate- to late-responding tissue. Two waves of damage can be

(continued)

Summary of Pertinent Conclusions (Continued)

identified, an acute pneumonitis and a later fibrosis. The lung is among the most sensitive late-responding organs. Pulmonary damage also may occur following chemotherapy.

- Together with the lung, the kidney is among the more radiosensitive late-responding critical organs. FSUs are in parallel, with only about 1,000 stem cells in each. Thirty gray (3,000 rad) in 2-Gy (200-rad) fractions to both kidneys results in nephropathy.
- In terms of radiosensitivity, the liver ranks immediately below kidney and lung. FSUs are in parallel, so that much larger doses are tolerated if only part of the organ is exposed. Fatal hepatitis may result from 35 Gy (3,500 rad) (conventional fractionation) to the whole organ.
- Cell renewal is low in the bladder epithelium, so proliferation following irradiation is delayed. Frequency of urination increases in parallel with loss of surface cells. Absence of surface cells explains irritation by urine.
- The nervous system is less sensitive to radiation than other late-responding organs, such as the kidney or lung.

  Brain: Histopathologic changes that occur in the first year are most likely to involve white matter; at later times, gray matter usually shows changes accompanied by vascular lesions. Radionecrosis may occur accompanied by cognitive defects.

  Spinal cord: Early demyelating injuries may develop after doses as low as 35 Gy (3,500 rad) but are usually reversible. For late damage, the $TD_{5/5}$ is about 50 Gy (5,000 rad) for a 10-cm length of cord. By 70 Gy (7,000 rad) in conventional fractions, the incidence of myelopathy would be 50%. FSUs are in series, but once the field exceeds a few centimeters, the treatment volume has little effect. Tolerance dose shows little dependence on overall time but depends critically on dose per fraction (α/β is low). If two doses per day are used, the interfractionation interval must be more than 6 hours, because there is a slow component of repair.

- In the testes, a dose of 0.1 to 0.15 Gy (10–15 rad) leads to temporary sterility. A dose of 6 to 8 Gy (600–800 rad) in 2-Gy (200-rad) fractions leads to permanent sterility. Such doses have little effect on libido. The stem cells are more radiosensitive than the differentiated cells, so continuous or fractionated radiation is more effective than a single acute dose.
- Sterilization by radiation to the ovaries is immediate (no latent period, as in the male) and leads to all the changes associated with menopause.
- Among the female genitalia, tolerance doses for the vagina are high: 90 Gy (9,000 rad) before ulceration and 100 Gy (10,000 rad) for the development of a fistula. For intracavitary treatment, doses to the cervix and uterus may reach 200 Gy (20,000 rad).
- Late damage to many different tissues and organs is mediated to some extent by effects on the vasculature. Arterial damage may occur after fractionated doses of 50 to 70 Gy (5,000–7,000 rad), but capillaries are damaged by doses above about 40 Gy (4,000 rad).
- In its tolerance to radiation, the heart is intermediate between the kidney or lung and the central nervous system. The most common radiation-induced heart injury is acute pericarditis, which seldom occurs in the first year posttherapy. A dose of 40 to 50 Gy (4,500–5,000 rad) in conventional fractions induces about an 11% incidence. The α/β ratio is low (1 Gy, or 100 rad), so that fractionation results in a substantial sparing. Protection of part of the heart reduces symptoms.
- Growing cartilage is particularly radiosensitive in children: 10 Gy (1,000 rad) can slow growth, and deficits in growth are irreversible above about 20 Gy (2,000 rad). In the adult, osteoporosis of the lower mandible may be a serious complication following radiotherapy for cancer of the buccal cavity. Fractures of the humeral or femoral head may occur; the $TD_{50/5}$ is about 65 Gy (6,500 rad).
- The RTOG and EORTC introduced the SOMA classification for late effects of normal tissues (LENT): SOMA is an acronym for *S*ubjective, *O*bjective, *M*anagement criteria with *A*nalytic laboratory and imaging procedures.

BIBLIOGRAPHY

Al-Barwari SE, Potten CS: A cell kinetic model to explain the time of appearance of skin reaction after *X*-rays or ultraviolet light irradiation. *Cell Tissue Kinet* 12:281–289, 1979

Blackett N, Aguado M: The enhancement of haemopoietic stem cell recovery in irradiated mice by prior treatment with cyclophosphamide. *Cell Tissue Kinet* 12:291–298, 1979

Botnik LE, Hannon ECM, Hellman S: Late effects of cytotoxic agents on the normal tissue of mice. *Front Radiat Ther Oncol* 13:36–47, 1979

Clifton KF: Thyroid and mammary radiobiology: Radiogenic damage to glandular tissues. *Br J Cancer* 53(suppl VII):237–250, 1986

Croizat H, Frindel E, Tubiana M: The effect of partial body irradiation on haemopoietic stem cell migration. *Cell Tissue Kinet* 13:309–317, 1980

Croizat H, Frindel E, Tubiana M: Long term radiation effects on the bone marrow stem cells of C3H mice. *Int J Radiat Biol* 36:91–99, 1979

Denekamp J: Cell kinetics and radiation biology. *Int J Radiat Biol* 49:357–380, 1986

Emami B, Lyman J, Brown A, et al.: Tolerance of normal tissue to therapeutic irradiation. *Int J Radiat Oncol Biol Phys* 21:109–122, 1991

Fajardo LF: *Pathology of Radiation Injury*. New York, Masson, 1982

Frindel E, Croizat H, Vassort F: Stimulating factors liberated by treated bone marrow: *In vitro* effect on CFU kinetics. *Exp Hematol* 4:56–61, 1976

Frindel E, Hahn C, Robaglia D, Tubiana M: Responses of bone marrow and tumor cells to acute and protracted irradiation. *Cancer Res* 32:2096–2103, 1972

Hegazy MAH, Fowler JF: Cell population kinetics and desquamation: Skin reactions in plucked and unplucked mouse skin: II. Irradiated skin. *Cell Tissue Kinet* 6:587–602, 1973

Hendry JH, Thames HD: The tissue-rescuing unit. *Br J Radiol* 59:628–630, 1986

Hopewell JW: Mechanisms of the action of radiation on skin and underlying tissues. *Br J Radiol* (suppl 19):39–51, 1986

Hopewell JW, Campling D, Calvo W, Reinhold HS, Wilkinson JH, Yeung TK: Vascular irradiation damage: Its cellular basis and likely consequences. *Br J Cancer* 53(suppl VII):181–191, 1986

Hopewell JW, Morris AD, Dixon-Brown A: The influence of field size on the late tolerance of the rat spinal cord to single doses of X-rays. *Br J Radiol* 60:1099–1108, 1987

Job G, Preundschuh M, Bauer M, zum Winkel J, Hunstein W: The influence of radiation therapy on T-lymphocyte subpopulations defined by monoclonal antibodies. *Int J Radiat Oncol Biol Phys* 10:2077–2081, 1984

Joiner MC, Denekamp J: The effect of small radiation doses on mouse skin. *Br J Cancer* 53(suppl VII):63–66, 1986

Kaanders JHAM, van Daal WAAJ, Hoogenraad WJ, van der Kogel AJ: Accelerated fractionation radiotherapy for larynegeal cancer, acute and late toxicity. *Int J Radiat Oncol Biol Phys* 24:497–503, 1992

Kotzin BL, Kansas GS, Engleman EG, Hoppe RT, Kaplan HS, Strober S: Changes in T-cell subsets in patients with rheumatoid arthritis treated with total lymphoid irradiation. *Clin Immunol Immunopathol* 27:250–260, 1983

LeBourgeois JP, Meignan M, Parmentier C, Tubiana M: Renal consequences of irradiation of the spleen in lymphoma patients. *Br J Radiol* 52:56–60, 1979

Meistrich MD: Relationship between spermatogonial stem cell survival and testis function after cytotoxic therapy. *Br J Cancer* 53(suppl VII):89–101, 1986

Michalowsli A: A critical appraisal of clonogenic survival assays in the evaluation of radiation damage to normal tissues. *Radiother Oncol* 1:241–246, 1984

Michalowski A: Effects of radiation on normal tissues: Hypothetical mechanisms and limitations of *in situ* assays of clonogenicity. *Radiat Environ Biophys* 19:157–172, 1981

Parmentier C, Morardet N, Tubiana M: Late effects on human bone marrow after extended field radiotherapy. *Int J Radiat Oncol Biol Phys* 9:1303–1311, 1983

Potten CS, Hendry JH (eds): *Cytotoxic Insult to Tissue: Effects on Cell Lineages*. Edinburgh, Churchill Livingstone, 1983

Rubin P: Late effects of chemotherapy and radiation therapy: A new hypothesis. *Int J Radiat Oncol Biol Phys* 10:5–34, 1984

Rubin P, Casarett GW: *Clinical Radiation Pathology*, vol 1. Philadelphia, WB Saunders, 1968

Rubin P, Constine LS, Fajardo LF, Phillips TL, Wasserman TH (eds): *Late Effects of Normal Tissues Consensus Conference*, San Francisco, CA, Aug 26–28, 1992. Published as a special issue of *Int J Radiat Oncol Biol Phys* 31:1049–1081, 1995

Schofield R: Assessment of cytotoxic injury to bone marrow. *Br J Cancer* 53(suppl VII):115–125, 1986

Schultz-Hector S: Heart. In Scheerer E, Streffer C, Trott KR (eds): *Radiopathology of Organs and Tissues*, pp 347–368. Berlin, Springer-Verlag, 1981

Stewart FA: Mechanism of bladder damage and repair after treatment with radiation and cytostatic drugs. *Br J Cancer* 53(suppl VII):280–291, 1986

Travis EL: The tissue rescuing unit. In Fielden EM, Fowler JF, Hendry JH, Scott D (eds): *Proceedings of the 8th International Congress of Radiation Research*, Edinburgh, July 1987. *Radiat Res* 2:795–800, 1987

Travis EL, Down JD: Repair in mouse lung after split doses of X-rays. *Radiat Res* 87:166–174, 1981

Travis EL, Liao Z-X, Tucker SL: Spatial heterogeneity of the volume effect for radiation pneumonitis in mouse lung. *Int J Radiat Oncol Biol Phys* 38:1045–1054, 1997

Travis EL, Tucker SL: Relationship between functional assays of radiation response in the lung and target cell depletion. *Br J Cancer* 53(suppl VII):304–319, 1986

Trott KR: Chronic damage after radiation therapy: Challenge to radiation biology. *Int J Radiat Oncol Biol Phys* 10:907–913, 1984

Tubiana M: Cell kinetics and radiation oncology. *Int J Radiat Oncol Biol Phys* 8:1471–1489, 1982

Turesson I, Notter G: Dose-response and dose-latency relationships for human skin after various fractionation schedules. *Br J Cancer* 53(suppl VII):67–72, 1986

Turesson I, Thames HD: Repair capacity and kinetics of human skin during fractionated radiotherapy: Erythema, desquamation, and telangiectasia after 3 and 5 years' follow-up. *Radiother Oncol* 15:169–188, 1989

van der Kogel AJ: Central nervous system radiation injury in small animal models. In Gutin PH, Leibel SA, Sheline GE (eds): *Radiation Injury to the Nervous System*, pp 91–112. New York, Raven Press, 1991

van der Kogel AJ: Mechanisms of late radiation injury in the spinal cord. In Meyn RE, Withers HR (eds): *Radiation Biology in Cancer Research*, pp 461–470. New York, Raven Press, 1980

van der Kogel AJ: Radiation-induced damage in the central nervous system: An interpretation of target cell responses. *Br J Cancer* 53(suppl VII):207–217, 1986 van der Kogel AJ, Ang KK: Complications related to radiotherapy. In Peckham M, Pinedo H, Veronesi U (eds): *Oxford Textbook of Oncology*, vol 2, pp 2295–2306. Oxford, Oxford University Press, 1995

van der Kogel AJ, Sissingh HA, Zoetelief J: Effect of x-rays and neutrons on repair and regeneration in the rat spinal cord. *Int J Radiat Oncol Biol Phys* 8:2095–2097, 1982

Vassort F, Wintherholer M, Frindel E, Tubiana M: Kinetic parameters of bone marrow stem cells using *in vivo* suicide. *Blood* 41:789–796, 1973

Wheldon TE, Michalowski AS: Alternative models for the proliferative structure of normal tissues and their response to irradiation. *Br J Cancer* 53(suppl VII):382–385, 1986

Withers HR, Taylor JMG, Maciejewski B: Treatment volume and tissue tolerance. *Int J Radiat Oncol Biol Phys* 14:751–759, 1988

Withers HR, Thames HD, Peters LJ, Fletcher GH: Keynote address: Normal tissue radioresistance in clinical radiotherapy. In Fletcher GH, Nervi C, Withers HR (eds): *Biological Bases and Clinical Implications of Tumor Radioresistance*, pp 139–152. New York, Masson, 1983

CHAPTER 20

Model Tumor Systems

TRANSPLANTABLE SOLID-TUMOR SYSTEMS IN EXPERIMENTAL ANIMALS

A wide range of experimental tumors of various histologic types have been developed for radiobiologic studies. To produce a large number of virtually identical tumors, propagation by transplantation from one generation of animals to the next is used, which makes it mandatory that the animals be isologous. In practice, pure inbred strains of rats or mice are used and are maintained by brother–sister mating, which also serves the function of reducing the variability among animals to a minimum.

The tumor from a donor animal is removed aseptically and, if possible, prepared into a single-cell suspension; this is accomplished by separating the cells with an enzyme such as trypsin and then forcing them through a fine wire mesh. To effect a transplant, 10^4 to 10^6 cells are inoculated subcutaneously into each of a large group of recipient animals of the same strain. The site of transplantation varies widely; the flank or back commonly is used, but sometimes a special tumor requires a particular site, such as the brain. Some tumors cannot be handled in this way and must be propagated by transplanting a small piece of tumor rather than a known number of single cells; this is obviously less quantitative. Within days or weeks, depending on the type of tumor and the strain of animals, palpable tumors appear in the recipient animals that are uniform in size, histologic type, and so on. Hundreds to thousands of animals can be used, which makes it possible to design highly quantitative studies of tumor response to different radiations, fractionation regimens, sensitizers, and combinations of radiation and chemotherapeutic agents.

There are five commonly used techniques to assay the response of solid tumors to a treatment regimen:

1. Tumor growth measurements.
2. Tumor cure (TCD_{50}) assay.
3. Tumor cell survival determined *in vivo* by the dilution assay technique.
4. Tumor cell survival assayed by the lung colony assays.
5. Tumor cell survival using *in vivo* treatment followed by *in vitro* assay.

Each of these methods is discussed briefly.

TUMOR GROWTH MEASUREMENTS

Tumor growth measurement is possibly the simplest end point to use and involves the daily measurement

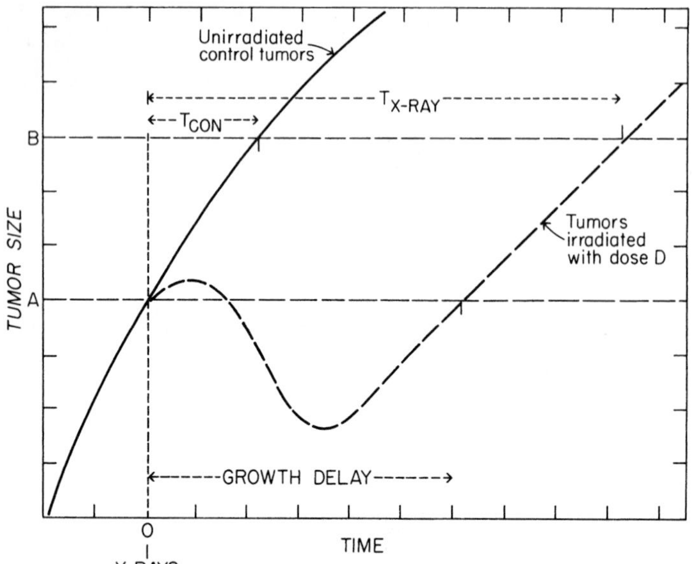

FIGURE 20.1 • The pattern of response of a tumor to a dose of x-rays. The size of the tumor, either the mean diameter or the volume, is plotted as a function of time after irradiation. Two different indices of tumor responses have been used by different investigators. Growth delay represents the time after irradiation that it takes for the tumor to regrow to the size at the time of irradiation. Alternatively, the index of radiation damage may be the time taken for the tumor to grow from a specified size A at the time of irradiation to some specified larger size B. Typically, this may be from 9 to 25 mm in diameter for rat tumors. This quantity is shown as T_{CON} for unirradiated control animals and $T_{X\text{-}RAY}$ for tumors irradiated with a dose (D) of x-rays. Either index of tumor response may be plotted as a function of radiation dose.

of each tumor to arrive at a mean diameter. For tumor growth experiments, a large number of transplanted tumors are prepared as previously described. When they have grown to a specified size (e.g., a diameter of 8 to 10 mm in rats or 2 to 4 mm in mice), they are treated according to the plan of the particular experiment. Figure 20.1 illustrates the variation of tumor size with time for unirradiated controls and tumors given a single dose of x-rays. The untreated tumors grow rapidly at a relatively uniform rate; the radiation treatment causes a temporary shrinkage of the tumor, followed by regrowth.

Two different methods have been used to score the tumor response. Barendsen and his colleagues have used growth delay, illustrated in Figure 20.1, as the time taken after irradiation for the tumor to regrow to the size it was at the time of irradiation. Clearly, this index of response is only suitable for tumors that shrink significantly after irradiation. For tumors that do not shrink so obviously, a more convenient index of growth delay is the time taken for the irradiated tumor to grow to some specified size after exposure, compared with controls. Either index of growth delay increases as a function of radiation dose. Figure 20.2**A** shows growth curves for a rat rhabdomyosarcoma irradiated with various doses of x-rays or fast neutrons. In Figure 20.2**B**, growth delay is expressed as a function of radiation dose.

TUMOR CURE (TCD_{50}) ASSAY

Tumor control provides data of most obvious relevance to radiotherapy. In experiments of this kind, a large number of animals with tumors of uniform size are divided into separate groups, and the tumors are irradiated locally with graded doses. The tumors subsequently are observed regularly for recurrence or local control. The proportion of tumors that are locally controlled can be plotted as a function of dose, and data of this kind are amenable to a sophisticated statistical analysis to determine TCD_{50}, the dose at which 50% of the tumors are locally controlled. This quantity is highly repeatable from one experiment to another in an inbred strain of animals.

Suit and his colleagues, over a period of more than 30 years, have made an extensive study of the response to radiation of a mammary carcinoma in C_3H mice. Data from a typical experiment are presented in Figure 20.3. Tumors were propagated by transplanting 4×10^4 cells into the outer portion of the mouse ear, and irradiations were performed when the tumors had grown to a volume of about 4 mm^3. A brass circular clamp was fitted across the base of the ear and maintained for at least a minute before the initiation of the irradiation, so that the tumors were uniformly hypoxic. Single-dose, two-dose, and ten-dose experiments were performed, with a 24-hour interval between dose fractions. Tumor control results are shown in Figure 20.3. The TCD_{50} for a single treatment is 45.75 Gy (4,575 rad), rising to 51.1 Gy (5,110 rad) for two fractions and to 84 Gy (8,400 rad) if the radiation is delivered in ten equal fractions. This indicates that a marked and extensive repair of sublethal damage has taken place during a multifraction regimen.

DILUTION ASSAY TECHNIQUE

The dilution assay technique was devised by Hewitt and Wilson, who used it to produce the first *in vivo*

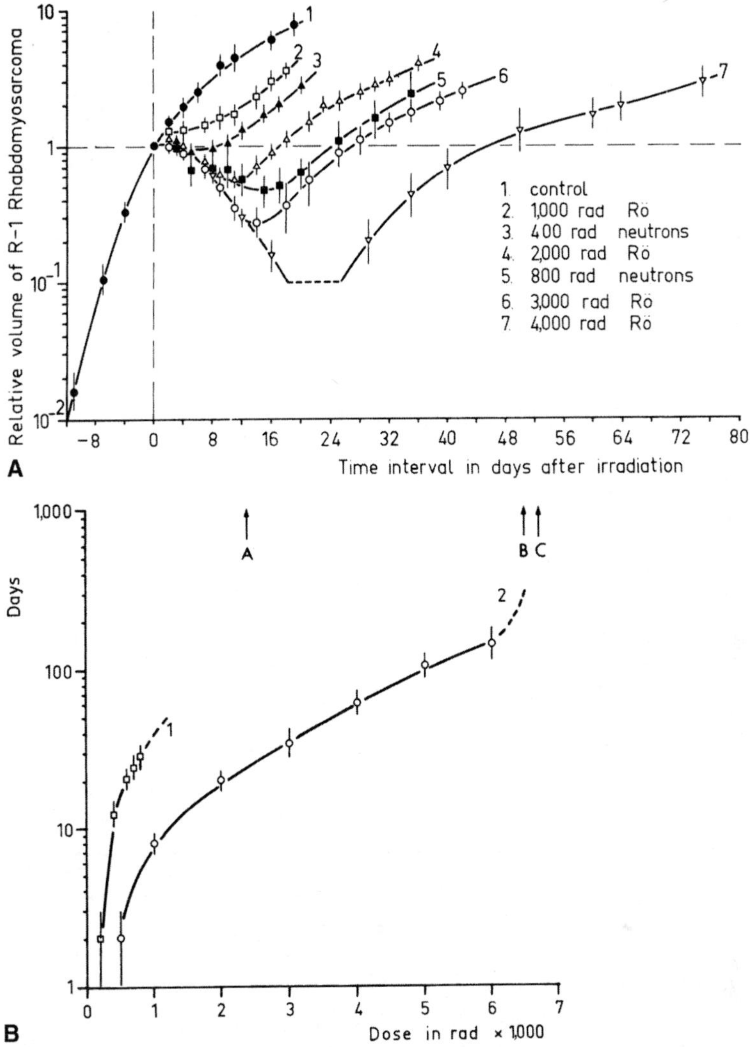

FIGURE 20.2 • **A:** Volume changes of rhabdomyosarcomas in rats after irradiation. Curve 1 represents the growth of the unirradiated control tumors. Curves 2, 4, 6, and 7 refer to tumors irradiated with 10 to 40 Gy (1,000–4,000 rad) of 300-kV x-rays. Curves 3 and 5 refer to tumors irradiated with 4 and 8 Gy (400 and 800 rad) of 15-MeV $d^+ \rightarrow T$ fast neutrons. **B:** Growth delay of rhabdomyosarcomas in rats as a function of dose of x-rays (curve 2) or fast neutrons (curve 1). A and C indicate the doses of neutrons and x-rays, respectively, required to "cure" 90% of the tumors, calculated on the basis of cell survival curves. B indicates the observed TCD_{90} for x-rays. Note the good agreement between calculated and observed values of the TCD_{90} for x-rays. (From Barendsen GW, Broerse JJ: Experimental radiotherapy of a rat rhabdomyosarcoma with 15 MeV neutrons and 300 kV x-rays: I. Effects of single exposures. *Eur J Cancer* 5:373–391, 1969, with permission.)

survival curve in 1959. They used a lymphocytic leukemia of spontaneous origin in mice. A single-cell suspension can be prepared from the infiltrated liver of an animal with advanced disease and the tumor transplanted by injecting known numbers of cells into the peritoneal cavities of recipient mice, which subsequently develop leukemias. The leukemia can be transmitted, on average, by the injection of only two cells; this quantity—the number of cells required to transmit the tumor to 50% of the animals—is known as TD_{50}. The dilution assay technique became the basis for obtaining an *in vivo* cell survival curve.

The procedure used, illustrated in Figure 20.4, is as follows. An animal containing the tumor may be irradiated to a given dose of radiation, for

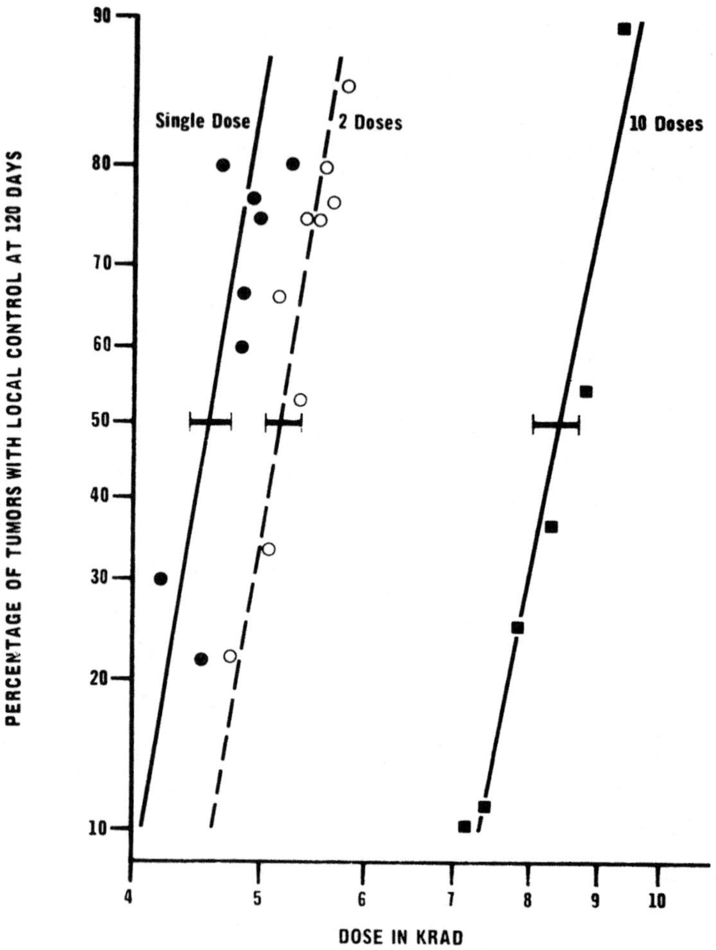

FIGURE 20.3 • Percentage of mouse mammary tumors locally controlled as a function of x-ray dose, for single exposures and for two different fractionation patterns. The tumors were isotransplants derived from a spontaneous mammary carcinoma in a C_3H mouse. The transplantation was made into the outer portion of the ear with 4×10^4 viable cells. The tumors were treated when they reached a diameter of 2 mm (i.e., a volume of about 4 mm^3). (From Suit H, Wette R: Radiation dose fractionation and tumor control probability. *Radiat Res* 29:267–281, 1966, with permission.)

example, 10 Gy (1,000 rad). A single-cell suspension then is prepared from the infiltrated liver, the cells are counted and diluted, and various numbers of these cells are injected intraperitoneally into groups of recipient animals. It is then a matter of observation and calculation to determine how many irradiated cells are required to produce a tumor in half of the animals inoculated with that given number of cells. Suppose, for instance, that it takes 20 irradiated cells, on average, to transmit the tumor; because it is known that only 2 clonogenic cells are needed to transmit the tumor, it is a simple matter to decide that in the irradiated population of cells, 2 of 20, or 10%, were clonogenic and survived the dose of 10 Gy (1,000 rad). That is,

$$\text{Surviving fraction} = \text{TD}_{50}\ \text{controls}/\text{TD}_{50}\ \text{irradiated}$$

If this process is repeated for a number of doses of radiation, and the corresponding surviving fractions are determined by this assay technique, a survival curve for cells irradiated and assayed *in vivo* can be constructed.

This technique is a true *in vivo* system, but it involves a leukemia as opposed to a solid tumor. The cells, after reinoculation into the mouse, grow in the peritoneal cavity in much the same way that

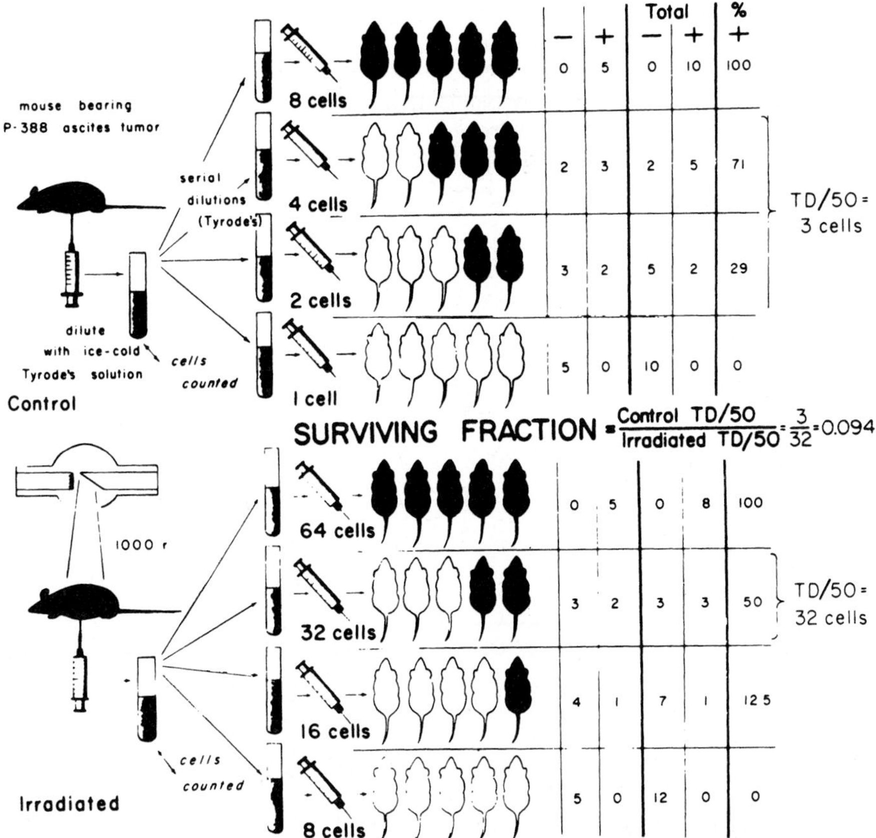

−	+	Total −	Total +	% +
0	5	0	10	100
2	3	2	5	71
3	2	5	2	29
5	0	10	0	0

−	+	Total −	Total +	% +
0	5	0	8	100
3	2	3	3	50
4	1	7	1	12 5
5	0	12	0	0

FIGURE 20.4 ● Schematic representation to show the general features of the dilution assay technique. Various numbers of tumor cells from the donor animal are injected into groups of recipients, and a determination is made of the number of cells required for a tumor to take in half of the animals of the group (TD_{50}). The ratio of this quantity for control and irradiated donors is the surviving fraction. (From Andrews JR, Berry RJ: Fast neutron irradiation and the relationship of radiation dose and mammalian tumor cell reproductive capacity. *Radiat Res* 16:76–81, 1962, with permission.)

the cells grow in a petri dish in the *in vitro* technique; the mice are in fact being used as small portable incubators.

Since these pioneering efforts, the dilution assay technique has been applied by many different workers to measure survival curves for a number of leukemias and solid tumors if the tumors can be removed and prepared into a single-cell suspension; some collected results are shown in Figure 20.5. The survival curves obtained have a D_0 of about 4 Gy (400 rad), because the cells in the peritoneal cavity of the mouse are so numerous and so closely packed that they are deficient in oxygen. This technique, therefore, produces a "hypoxic" survival curve. To obtain a survival curve characteristic of aerated conditions, it is necessary either to remove the cells from the donor animal and irradiate them in a petri dish in which they are in contact with air or to inject hydrogen peroxide into the peritoneal cavity of the mouse before irradiation so that oxygen is available to the tumor cells during the irradiation. If this is done, D_0 is about 1.3 to 1.6 Gy (130–160 rad).

LUNG COLONY ASSAY

Hill and Bush have devised a technique to assay the clonogenicity of the cells of a solid tumor irradiated *in situ* by injecting them into recipient animals and counting the number of lung colonies produced. The general principles of the method are illustrated in Figure 20.6. The tumor used in these studies was the KHT sarcoma, which is a transplantable tumor that arose originally in a C_3H mouse, and which has been propagated serially through many generations. Tumors are irradiated *in situ*, after which they are removed and made into a preparation of

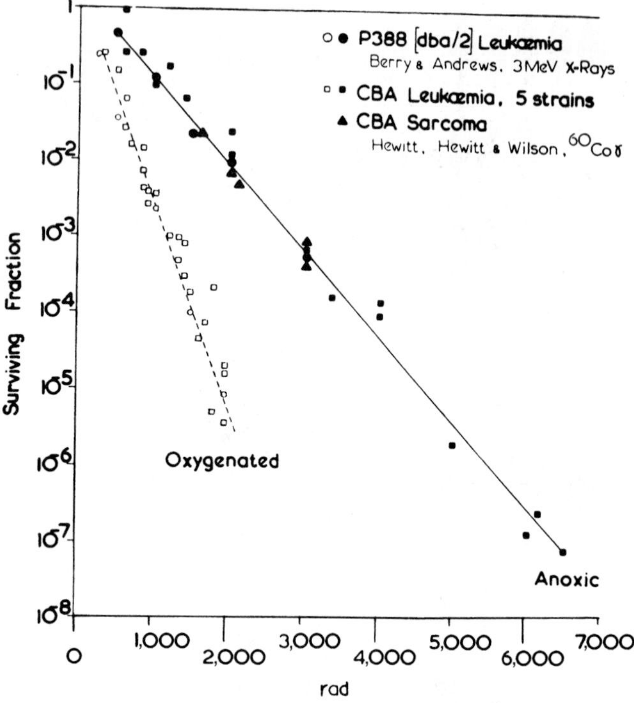

FIGURE 20.5 • Dose–response curves *in vivo*, using the dilution assay technique, for various murine tumors under oxygenated and hypoxic conditions. (From Berry RJ: On the shape of x-ray dose-response curves for the reproductive survival of mammalian cells. *Br J Radiol* 37:948–951, 1964, with permission.)

single cells by a combined trypsinization and mechanical procedure. A known number of cells then is mixed with a large number of heavily irradiated tumor cells and injected intravenously into recipient mice. About 3 weeks later these mice are sacrificed, and the colonies formed in the lungs are readily countable. The number of lung colonies is a measure of the number of surviving clonogenic cells in the injected suspension.

The lung colony technique is not confined to the KHT sarcoma but has been used with other tumor cells. For example, the demonstration of the absence of repair of potentially lethal damage after neutron irradiation involved the use of the Lewis lung carcinoma, and the fraction of surviving cells was assayed by counting lung colonies.

IN VIVO/IN VITRO ASSAY

A limited number of cell lines have been adapted so that they grow either as a transplantable tumor in an animal or as clones in a petri dish. These cells can be readily transferred from *in vivo* to *in vitro* and back. In one generation they may grow as a solid tumor in an animal, and in the next as a monolayer in a petri dish. The three most commonly used systems are a rhabdomyosarcoma in the rat (Hermens and Barendsen), a fibrosarcoma in the mouse (McNally), and the EMT6 mammary tumor, also in the mouse (Rockwell and Kallman).

The steps involved in this method are illustrated in Figure 20.7. This method combines many of the advantages of the *in vitro* and *in vivo* techniques.

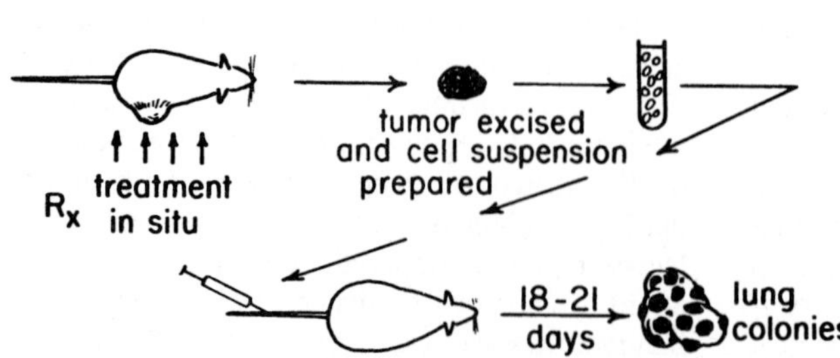

FIGURE 20.6 • The lung colony assay system. The tumor is irradiated *in situ*, after which it is excised and made into a single-cell suspension. A known number of cells are then injected intravenously into recipient animals. About 3 weeks later, the recipient animals are sacrificed and the colonies that have formed in the lungs are counted. The number of lung colonies is a measure of the number of surviving clonogenic cells in the injected suspension. (From Hill RP, Bush RS: The effect of continuous or fractionated irradiation on a murine sarcoma. *Br J Radiol* 46:167–174, 1973, with permission.)

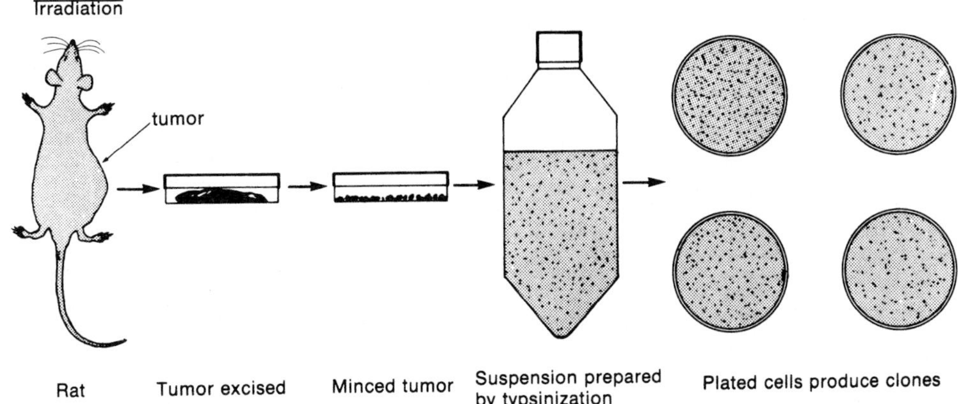

FIGURE 20.7 • The principle of the *in vivo/in vitro* assay system using the rhabdomyosarcoma in the rat. The solid tumor in the animal can be removed and the tumor cells assayed for colony formation in petri dishes. This cell line can be transferred back and forth between the animal and the petri dish. (Courtesy of Drs. G.W. Barendsen and J.J. Broerse.)

The tumors are treated *in vivo* in a natural environment, so that the cellular response is modified by the various factors that are important in determining gross tumor response. After treatment, each tumor is removed and prepared into a single-cell suspension, and the cell concentration is counted in a hemocytometer or electronic cell counter. Known numbers of cells then can be transferred to petri dishes containing fresh growth medium, and the proportion of clonogenic cells can be determined by counting colonies 10 days later. The speed, accuracy, and relative economy of the *in vitro* system replaces the expense and inconvenience of the recipient animals in the dilution assay technique.

XENOGRAFTS OF HUMAN TUMORS

A **xenograft** is a transplant from one species to another. In the cancer field, this usually refers to a human tumor growth transplanted in a laboratory animal. If the recipient animal has a normal immune system, a xenograft should not grow, but there are two main ways in which growth has been achieved. First, animal strains have been developed that are congenitally immune deficient. Best known are nude mice, which in addition to being hairless also lack a thymus. Many human tumors grow under the skin of nude mice. More recently there have been nude rats and SCID mice, which suffer from the severe combined immunodeficiency syndrome and are deficient in both B cell and T cell immunity. Second, it is possible to severely immune-suppress mice by the use of radiation or drugs or a combination of both, to the point at which they accept human tumor grafts. It is important to recognize that neither type of host completely fails to reject the human tumor cells: Rejection processes are still present, and these complicate the interpretation of *in situ* tumor therapeutic studies.

Despite the limitations, a wide variety of human tumor cells have been grown as xenografts in immune-deficient animals. Steel has estimated that more than 300 individual human tumors have been investigated in this way. Breast and ovarian tumors generally have been difficult to graft, with grafting of melanomas and tumors of the colon and bronchus being relatively successful.

Xenografts retain human karyotypes through serial passages and maintain some of the response characteristics of the individual source human tumors; to this extent, they have great advantages over mouse tumors. There are, however, certain drawbacks. First, there is a tendency for the tumor to be rejected, so that observing tumor control as an end point can be misleading. Growth delay and cell survival studies, on the other hand, are probably less affected. Second, human tumor cells do undergo kinetic changes and cell selection if transplanted into mice. For example, xenografts commonly have doubling times about one fifth of the values observed in humans, so that increased responsiveness should be expected to proliferation-dependent chemotherapeutic agents. Third, although the histologic characteristics of the human source tumors are usually well maintained by xenografts, the stromal tissue is of mouse origin. Consequently, xenografts of human tumor cells are not much more valid than murine tumors for any studies in which the vascular supply plays an important role. For example, the

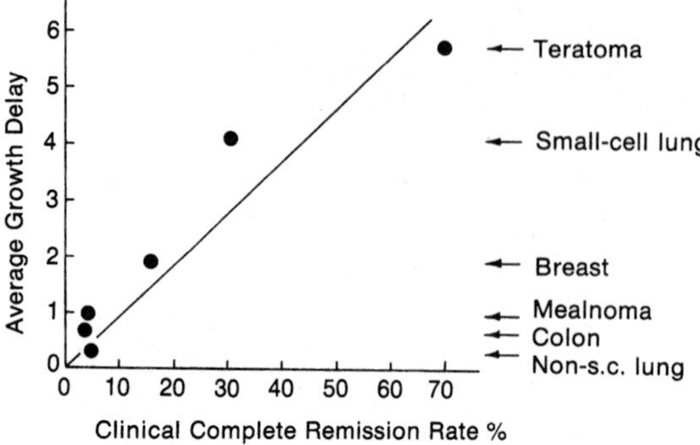

FIGURE 20.8 • Correlation between response of human tumor xenografts and clinical complete remission rates to chemotherapy. The ordinate is the growth delay observed in three to ten xenograft lines treated with the clinically used drugs that proved most effective in the xenografts. (Steel GG: How well do xenografts maintain the therapeutic response characteristics of the source tumor in the donor patient? In Kallman RF [ed]: *Rodent Tumors in Experimental Cancer Therapy*. New York, Pergamon, 1987, with permission.)

fraction of hypoxic cells in xenografts is much the same as in mouse tumors.

Steel and colleagues reviewed the field in 1983 and concluded that xenografts generally maintain the chemotherapeutic response characteristics of the class of tumors from which they are derived. There is good evidence, too, for individuality of response among xenografts. For example, in studying melanomas, one was responsive clinically, but another was not, and the cell survival curve after therapy with melphalan was twice as steep in the xenograft of the cells from the responsive tumor.

Figure 20.8 summarizes the correlation between growth delay in the xenograft and clinical remission of the donor patient. In the figure, the growth delay in xenografts for maximum tolerated treatment with the single chemotherapeutic agents that are in common clinical use against the disease is plotted against clinical complete response rate for that category of tumor. The correlation between these parameters is good. Testicular tumors are the most responsive in xenografts or in the clinic; small-cell lung cancer and breast tumors occupy an intermediate position; and the other three tumor types are unresponsive, either clinically or experimentally. This consistency of agreement between patient and xenograft responses to chemotherapeutic agents is encouraging for a variety of human tumor types tested. Similarly, studies of radiation response indicate that measurements of growth delay in xenografts rank tumors in the same order as clinical responsiveness: Response is greater in testicular teratoma than in pancreatic carcinoma, which is greater than in bladder carcinoma, for example.

SPHEROIDS: AN *IN VITRO* MODEL TUMOR SYSTEM

Mammalian cells in culture may be grown either as a monolayer attached to a glass or plastic surface or in suspension, in which case they are prevented from settling out and attaching to the surface of the culture vessel by continual gentle stirring. Most cells in suspension, or in "spinner culture," as it often is called, remain as single cells; at each mitosis the progeny cells separate, and although the cell concentration increases with time, it continues to consist of individual, separate cells.

Some cells, however, notably several rodent tumor cell lines, such as Chinese hamster V79 lung cells, mouse EMT6 mammary cells, RIF fibrosarcoma cells, and rat 9L brain tumor cells, do not behave in this way but instead grow as spheroids. At each successive division, the progeny cells stick together, and the result is a large spheric clump of cells that grows bigger and bigger with time. A photograph of a large spheroid consisting of about 8×10^4 cells is shown in Figure 20.9. Five days after the seeding of single cells into suspension culture, the spheroids have a diameter of about 200 μm; by 15 days, the diameter may exceed 800 μm. Oxygen and nutrients must diffuse into the spheroids from the surrounding tissue culture medium. In the center of a spheroid, there is a deficiency of oxygen and nutrients and a buildup of waste products because of diffusion limitations. Eventually, central necrosis appears and the mean cell cycle lengthens. Mature spheroids contain a heterogeneous population of cells resulting from many of the same factors, as in a tumor *in vivo*.

The spheroid system is simpler, more reproducible, less expensive, and easier to manipulate than animal tumors, and yet the cells can be studied in an environment that includes the complexities of cell-to-cell contact and nutritional stress from diffusion limitations that are characteristic of a growing tumor. Spheroids are irradiated intact and then separated into single cells by the use of trypsin and gentle agitation before being plated out into petri dishes to be assayed for the reproductive integrity of individual cells.

Mature spheroids consist of three populations of cells with varying radiosensitivity. Starting from the outside and working toward the center, they are

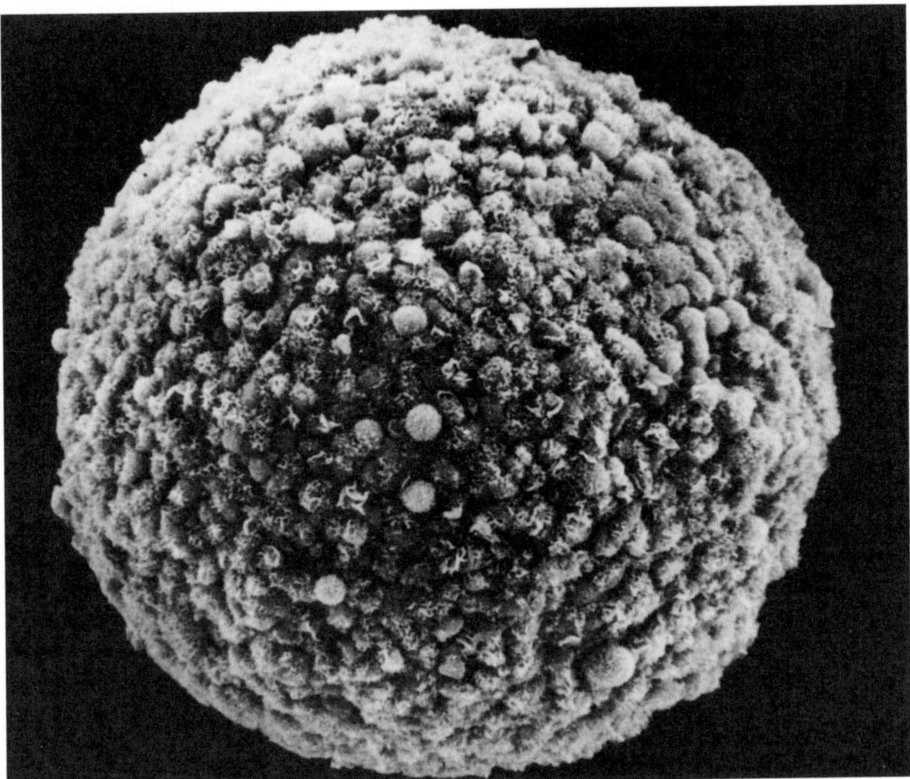

FIGURE 20.9 • Photograph of an 800-μm spheroid containing about 8×10^4 cells. (Courtesy of Dr. R.M. Sutherland.)

asynchronous, aerobic cycling cells, aerated noncycling G_1-like cells, and noncycling G_1-like hypoxic cells. Very large spheroids may contain about 20% hypoxic cells, similar to many animal tumors. By gently trypsinizing the spheroids for varying periods of time, the spheroid can be peeled like an onion and these three cell populations separated out. Using more sophisticated methods, such as centrifugal elutriation and flow cytometry, it is possible to separate many more cell subpopulations based on location in the spheroid, cell cycle, or other parameters. Figure 20.10 is a cross section through a large spheroid, showing clearly the development of a central necrotic area, which occurs when the spheroid's size is such that oxygen and other nutrients cannot diffuse into the center.

The spheroid system has been applied to a number of problems in radiobiology and in the study of pharmacologic agents, such as radiosensitizers or chemotherapeutic agents. A major problem in the application of these drugs to human tumors is the presence of resistant cells that are resting or noncycling, often located away from blood vessels. Drugs are required to diffuse in effective concentration to these cells through layers of growing, actively dividing cells, which may inactivate the drug through their metabolism. The spheroid system mimics many of these tumor characteristics and provides a rapid, useful, and economic method for screening sensitizers and chemotherapeutic agents because it is intermediate in complexity between single-cell *in vitro* culture and tumors in experimental animals.

SPHEROIDS OF HUMAN TUMOR CELLS

Many types of human tumor cells can be cultured as spheroids, with a wide spectrum of morphologic appearances and growth rates. In general, cells from disaggregated surgical specimens form spheroids if cultured in liquid suspension above a nonadhesive surface, which can be a thin layer of agar or agarose gel or the bottom of a culture dish not prepared for cell culture.

Only if the spheroid is formed and grown to a certain size can it be transferred to a spinner culture vessel and grown in the same way as

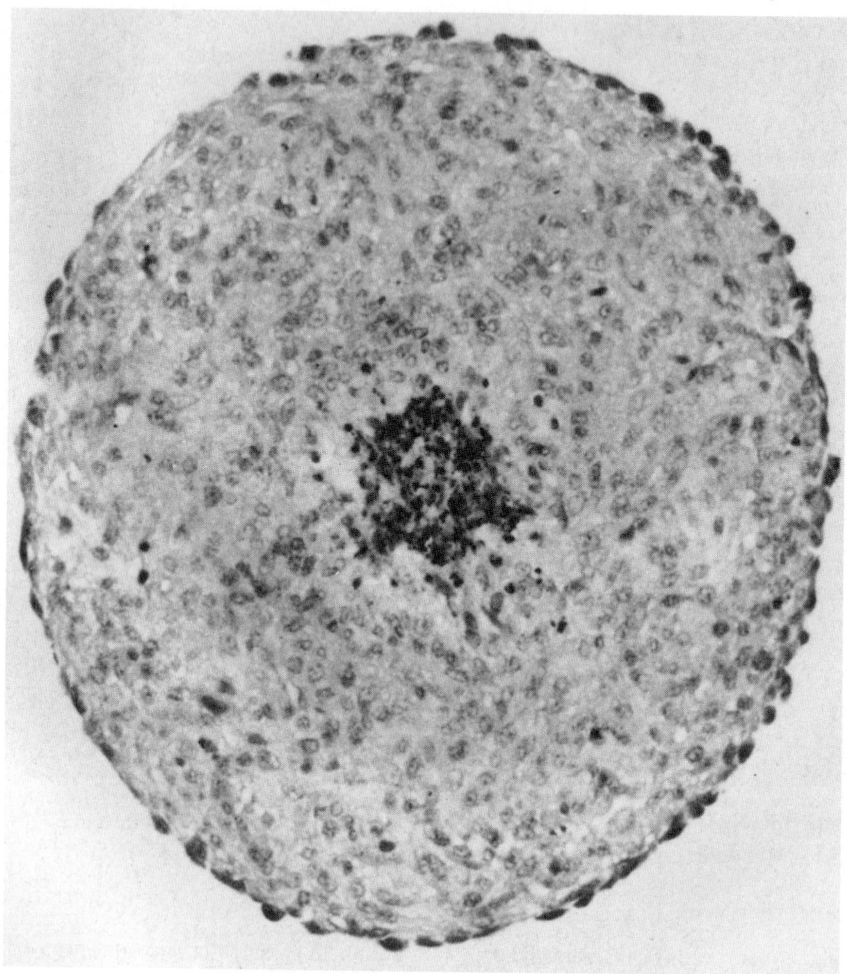

FIGURE 20.10 • Photomicrograph of a spheroid cross section. Note the area of central necrosis. The spheroid was grown for 15 days and was 520 μm in diameter; the viable rim had an average thickness of about 200 μm. (Courtesy of Dr R.M. Sutherland.)

spheroids of established rodent cell lines. Human tumors successfully grown as spheroids include thyroid cancer, renal cancer, squamous carcinoma, colon carcinoma, neuroblastoma, human lung cancer, glioma, lymphoid tumors, melanoma, and osteosarcoma. There appears to be no general pattern. One glioma line might form and grow as spheroids; another might not. The same applies to other tumor types. Thus, it seems that the capacity to form and grow as spheroids is not a general property of tumor cells. Many nontumor cells also form spheroids, but only the spheroids of lymphoid origin continue to grow to any size.

Morphologic studies of spheroids of human tumor cells show that they maintain many characteristics of the original tumor specimens taken from the patient and of the cells if grown as a xenograft in nude mice. Radiobiologic studies show that in addition to maintaining histologic characteristics of individual tumors, spheroids of human cells preserve characteristic radiosensitivity, because dose–response curves for spheroids are virtually identical to those for cells growing as xenografts in nude mice.

COMPARISON OF THE VARIOUS MODEL TUMOR SYSTEMS

In all transplantable systems described, the tumor is treated *in situ*, with all of the realism and complexities of the *in vivo* milieu, such as cell-to cell contact and the presence of hypoxic cells, factors that cannot be fully simulated in a petri dish. The tumor cure (TCD_{50}) and growth delay systems share the additional advantage that they are left *in situ* undisturbed after treatment. In the other techniques, the tumor must be removed, minced, and prepared into a single-cell suspension by the use of an enzyme, such as trypsin, before survival is assessed. Although this step does not appear to affect the assessment of the effects of radiation, it can result in artifacts in the case of other agents, such as chemotherapeutic drugs or hyperthermia, in which the cell membrane may be involved in the cellular response. The procedure of breaking up the tumor and partially dissolving the cell membrane with a digestive enzyme may influence results. For this reason, in the testing and evaluation of a new drug, one tumor system involving the determination of growth delay or TCD_{50} is always included. By the same token, these same systems are very expensive because they require a large number of animals for the amount of information produced. The determination of TCD_{50} is perhaps ideal for producing data relevant to clinical radiotherapy. It is certainly the most expensive; to produce a single TCD_{50} value for one of the lines in Figure 20.3, six to eight groups of up to ten animals must be kept and observed for weeks. The same information can be obtained in 10 days with one or two mice and six petri dishes using the *in vivo/in vitro* technique.

The dilution assay technique allows clonogenic cell survival to be assessed over a large range of doses and for tumors that cannot be grown in culture. It, too, is relatively expensive, because a whole group of recipient animals must be used and kept for weeks to obtain the same information obtained from one petri dish. Unquestionably, the most rapid and efficient technique is the *in vivo/in vitro* technique, which combines the realism of irradiation *in vivo* with the speed and efficiency of *in vitro* plating to assess clonogenic survival. The concomitant disadvantage is that any tumor that can be switched from petri dish to animal in alternate passages is so undifferentiated and anaplastic that it bears little resemblance to a spontaneous tumor in the human.

To some extent, the same criticism can be levied at all transplantable tumor systems. They are highly quantitative, but they are also very artificial. Having been passaged for many generations, they tend to be highly undifferentiated, and they grow as encapsulated tumors in a muscle or beneath the skin rather than in the tissue of origin. In addition, some have produced misleading results because they are highly antigenic, which, in general, human tumors are not.

In short, transplantable tumors in laboratory animals are model systems; they must be used with care, and the results must not be overinterpreted. Used with caution, these systems have provided invaluable quantitative data and helped to establish important radiobiologic principles. They also, however, have "led us up the garden path" on several occasions in the past (Fig. 20.11). For all of the reasons listed previously, they differ in important ways from spontaneous human tumors, and for the testing of drugs at the National Cancer Institute, they have been largely replaced by a battery of cells of human origin cultured *in vitro*.

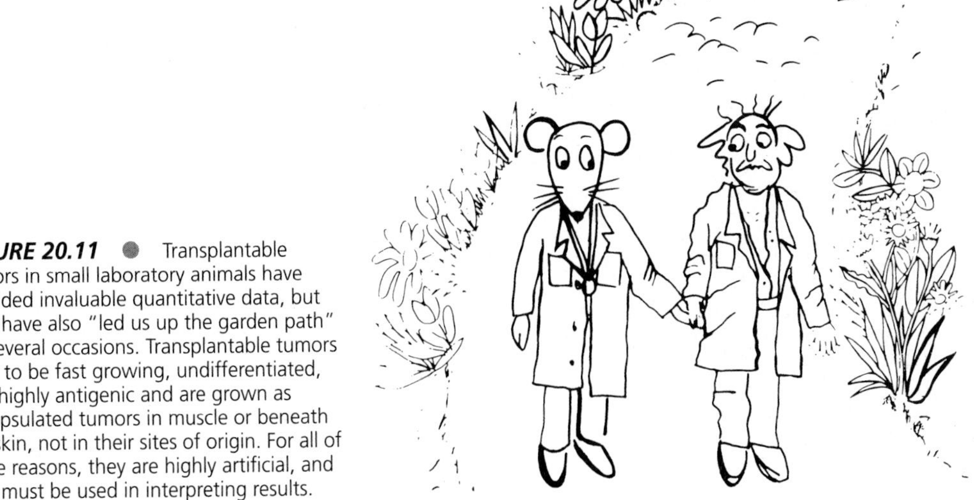

FIGURE 20.11 • Transplantable tumors in small laboratory animals have provided invaluable quantitative data, but they have also "led us up the garden path" on several occasions. Transplantable tumors tend to be fast growing, undifferentiated, and highly antigenic and are grown as encapsulated tumors in muscle or beneath the skin, not in their sites of origin. For all of these reasons, they are highly artificial, and care must be used in interpreting results.

Xenografts of human tumors so far have been used on a much more limited scale. Because they are grown in the absence of an immune response, it could be argued that they are the epitome of artificiality. They do, however, allow a comparison to be made of the intrinsic sensitivity to radiation or chemotherapeutic agents of fresh explants of human tumors. As *in vitro* culture techniques improve and better growth media are developed, xenografts may be less necessary.

Spheroids represent a most important intermediate model between monolayers of cells in culture and tumors *in vivo*. A number of important radiobiologic principles have been established using spheroids of rodent cells, in which the various populations of cells, aerated versus hypoxic or cycling versus noncycling, can be separated out. Human cell spheroids have only been used on a limited scale, but it is clear that the cells retain many of the characteristics of the tumor from which they were taken. Spheroids are much less expensive than xenografts in immunosuppressed animals and perform much the same function.

APOPTOSIS IN TUMORS

It is generally thought that irradiated cells die in attempting the next or a subsequent mitosis. This is not the only form of cell death, however. Programmed cell death, or *apoptosis*, also occurs in both normal tissues and tumors, spontaneously and as a result of irradiation.

In Chapter 21, it is pointed out that tumors grow much more slowly than would be predicted from the cell-cycle time of the individual cells and the fraction of cells actively dividing. One of the reasons for this "cell loss," as it is called, is random cell death resulting from apoptosis.

Studies with transplanted mouse tumors, as well as human tumors growing as xenografts in nude mice, have shown that the importance of apoptosis as a mechanism of cell death after x-irradiation varies substantially. Apoptosis was most important in lymphomas, essentially absent in sarcomas, and intermediate and very variable in carcinomas. In a mouse lymphoma, for example, 50 to 60% of the cells may show signs of dying an apoptotic death by 3 hours after irradiation, whereas in a sarcoma, there may be so few apoptotic cells that the process is of little significance. If a tumor responds rapidly to a relatively low dose of radiation, it generally means that apoptosis is involved, because the process peaks at 3 to 5 hours after irradiation.

Susceptibility to the induction of apoptosis also may be an important factor determining radiosensitivity, because programmed cell death appears to be a prominent early effect in radiosensitive mouse tumors and essentially absent in radioresistant tumors. It has been suggested that apoptosis is the dominant form of cell death in lymphoma cells treated with photodynamic therapy and that the process occurs more rapidly than after x-rays. Apoptosis is also involved in cell death by a range of cytotoxic drugs used in cancer therapy.

Summary of Pertinent Conclusions

- A wide range of tumors of different histologic types can be grown in laboratory animals and propagated by transplantation.
- Transplanted tumor systems can be highly quantitative, but in general the more quantitative the system, the more artificial it is, because the tumors are highly undifferentiated and encapsulated.
- The five assays in common use are tumor growth delay measurements, tumor cure (TCD_{50}) assay, tumor cell survival determined by the dilution assay technique, the production of lung colonies, and *in vivo* treatment followed by *in vitro* assay.
- In all five assays, the cells can be irradiated *in situ* with all the realism and complexity of *in vivo* conditions.
- If tumor cure (TCD_{50}) or growth delay is scored, the tumor is left undisturbed after treatment. This avoids artifacts involved in disaggregating the tumor, especially in the study of some chemicals or hyperthermia, in which cell membrane effects are important.
- The dilution assay technique, the lung colony assay, and the *in vivo/in vitro* assay all measure the cell-surviving fraction; that is, they are clonogenic assays. They require fewer animals and are therefore more efficient than the scoring of tumor cure or

(continued)

Summary of Pertinent Conclusions (Continued)

growth delay. All three assays require, however, that a single-cell suspension be prepared from the tumor, and this may result in artifacts.

- Transplantable tumors in small laboratory animals have been used to establish many radiobiologic principles; but they are highly artificial and must be used with care. They have "led us up the garden path" on several occasions.
- Many human tumor cells can be grown as xenografts in immune-deficient animals.
- Although the histologic characteristics of the human source tumor are maintained, the stroma is of mouse origin.
- Xenografts of human tumor cells are not much better than mouse tumors for studies in which the vascular supply is important.
- Human tumor cells undergo kinetic changes and selection if transplanted into immune-deficient mice.
- Xenografts generally maintain the chemotherapeutic response characteristics of the class of tumors from which they are derived. There is evidence, too, of individuality of response.
- Spheroids of established rodent cells can be grown in suspension culture (i.e., "spinner culture"). Oxygen and nutrients must diffuse into the spheroid from the surrounding culture medium. Oxygen deficiency and a buildup of waste products result, just as in a tumor.
- Mature spheroids contain a heterogeneous population of cells, much like a tumor, but are more quantitative and more economical to work with.
- Starting from the outside and working toward the center, spheroids consist of asynchronous aerated cells, noncycling G_1-like aerated cells, noncycling G_1-like hypoxic cells, and necrotic cells.
- Spheroids are intermediate in complexity between monolayer cell cultures *in vitro* and transplantable tumors in experimental animals.
- Many types of human tumor cells grow as spheroids and maintain many characteristics of the original tumor from the patient or of the same cells grown as xenografts.
- Programmed cell death, or apoptosis, occurs after irradiation in many animal tumors, as well as in human xenographs in nude mice.
- Apoptosis is most important in lymphomas, essentially absent in sarcomas, and intermediate and variable in carcinomas.
- Cells may show signs of dying an apoptotic death by 3 hours after irradiation.

BIBLIOGRAPHY

Acker H, Carlsson J, Durand R, Sutherland R (eds): *Spheroids in Cancer Research*. Berlin, Springer-Verlag, 1984

Andrews JR, Berry RJ: Fast neutron irradiation and the relationship of radiation dose and mammalian tumor cell reproductive capacity. *Radiat Res* 16:76–81, 1962

Barendsen GW, Broerse JJ: Experimental radiotherapy of a rat rhabdomyosarcoma with 15 MeV neutrons and 300 kV x-rays: I. Effects of single exposures. *Eur J Cancer* 5:373–391, 1969

Berry RJ: On the shape of x-ray dose-response curves for the reproductive survival of mammalian cells. *Br J Radiol* 37:948–951, 1964

Clifton KH, Briggs RC, Stone HB: Quantitative radiosensitivity studies of solid carcinomas *in vivo:* Methodology and effect of anoxia. *J Natl Cancer Inst* 36:965–974, 1966

Dertinger H, Guichard M, Malaise EP: Relationship between intercellular communication and radiosensitivity of human tumor xenografts. *Eur J Cancer Clin Oncol* 20:561–566, 1984

Fowler JF: Biological foundations of radiotherapy. In Turano L, Ratti A, Biagini C (eds): *Progress in Radiology*, vol 1, pp 731–737. Amsterdam, Excerpta Medica, 1967

Hermens AF, Barendsen GW: Cellular proliferation patterns in an experimental rhabdomyosarcoma in the rat. *Eur J Cancer* 3:361–369, 1967

Hermens AF, Barendsen GW: Changes of cell proliferation patterns in an experimental rhabdomyosarcoma in the rat. *Eur J Cancer* 5:173–189, 1969

Hewitt HB: Studies on the quantitative transplantation of mouse sarcoma. *Br J Cancer* 7:367–383, 1953

Hewitt HB, Chan DPS, Blake ER: Survival curves for clonogenic cells of a murine keratinizing squamous carcinoma irradiated in vivo or under hypoxic conditions. *Int J Radiat Biol* 12:535–549, 1967

Hewitt HB, Wilson CW: A survival curve for mammalian leukaemia cells irradiated *in vivo. Br J Cancer* 13:69–75, 1959

Hewitt HB, Wilson CW: Survival curves for tumor cells irradiated *in vivo. Ann NY Acad Sci* 95:818–827, 1961

Hill RP, Bush RS: A lung colony assay to determine the radiosensitivity of the cells of a solid tumor. *Int J Radiat Biol* 15:435–444, 1969

Hill RP, Bush RS, Yeung P: The effect of anemia on the fraction of hypoxic cells in an experimental tumor. *Br J Radiol* 44:299–304, 1971

Kerr JFR, Searle J: Apoptosis: Its nature and kinetic role. In Meyn RE, Withers HR (eds): *Radiation Biology in Cancer Research*, pp 367–384, New York, Raven Press, 1980

McNally NJ: Recovery from sublethal damage by hypoxic tumor cells *in vivo. Br J Radiol* 45:116–120, 1972

Pourreau-Schneider N, Malaise EP: Relationship between surviving fractions using the colony method, the LD50, and the growth delay after irradiation of human melanoma cells grown as multicellular spheroids. *Radiat Res* 85:321–332, 1981

Reinhold HS: Quantitative evaluation of the radiosensitivity of cells of a transplantable rhabdomyosarcoma in the rat. *Eur J Cancer* 2:33–42, 1966

Rockwell SC, Kallman RF: Cellular radiosensitivity and tumor radiation response in the EMT6 tumor cell system. *Radiat Res* 53:281–294, 1973

Rockwell SC, Kallman RF, Fajardo LF: Characteristics of a serially transplanted mouse mammary tumor and its tissue-culture-adapted derivative. *J Natl Cancer Inst* 49:735–749, 1972

Sparrow S. *Immunodeficient Animals for Cancer Research.* London, Macmillan, 1980

Steel GG: How well do xenografts maintain the therapeutic response characteristics of the source tumor in the donor patient? In Kallman RF (ed): *Rodent Tumors in Experimental Cancer Therapy*. New York, Pergamon, 1987

Steel GG, Courtenay VC, Beckjam MJ: The response to chemotherapy of a variety of human tumour xenografts. *Br J Cancer* 47:1–13, 1983

Stephens LC, Ang KK, Schultheiss TE, Milas L, Meyn R: Apoptosis in irradiated murine tumors. *Radiat Res* 127:308–316, 1991

Suit HD, Maeda M: Hyperbaric oxygen and radiobiology of the C3H mouse mammary carcinoma. *J Natl Cancer Inst* 39:639–652, 1967

Suit H, Wette R: Radiation dose fractionation and tumor control probability. *Radiat Res* 29:267–281, 1966

Suit HD, Wette R, Lindberg R: Analysis of tumor recurrence times. *Radiology* 88:311–321, 1967

Sutherland RM, Durand RE: Radiation response of multicell spheroids: An *in vitro* tumor model. *Curr Top Radiat Res Q* 11:87–139, 1976

Sutherland RM, McCredie JA, Inch WR: Growth of multicell spheroids in tissue culture as a model of nodular carcinomas. *J Natl Cancer Inst* 46:113–120, 1971

Sutherland RM, Sordat B, Bamat J, Gabbert H, Bourrat B, Mueller-Klieser W: Oxygenation and differentiation in multicellular spheroids of human colon carcinoma. *Cancer Res* 46:5320–5329, 1986

Tannock IF: The relation between cell proliferation and the vascular system in a transplanted mouse mammary tumour. *Br J Cancer* 22:258–273, 1968

Thomlinson RH, Craddock EA: The gross response of an experimental tumour to single doses of x-rays. *Br J Cancer* 21:108–123, 1967

Williams GT: Programmed cell death: Apoptosis and oncogenesis. *Cell* 65:1097–1098, 1991

Yuhas JM, Blake S, Weichselbaum RR: Quantitation of the response of human tumor spheroids to daily radiation exposures. *Int J Radiat Oncol Biol Phys* 10:2323–2327, 1984

Yuhas JM, Tarleton AK, Molzen KB: Multicellular tumor spheroid formation by breast cancer cells isolated from different sites. *Cancer Res* 38:2486–2491, 1978

CHAPTER 21

Cell, Tissue, and Tumor Kinetics

THE CELL CYCLE

Mammalian cells replicate and increase in number by mitosis. If growing cells are observed with a conventional light microscope, the only event that can be distinguished is the process of mitosis itself. For most of the cell cycle, the chromosomes are diffuse and not clearly seen, but for a short time before mitosis, they condense into discrete and recognizable entities. There is a brief flurry of activity as the chromosomes separate into two groups and move to the two poles of the cell; division then occurs to form two progeny cells. The average interval between successive mitoses, or divisions, is called the **cell cycle** or **mitotic-cycle time**.

Howard and Pelc were the first to further subdivide the mitotic cycle by the use of a labeled DNA precursor. This is described in Chapter 4 and is reviewed only briefly here. It is a simple matter to identify the proportion of cells synthesizing DNA (i.e., in S phase). The DNA precursor is made available to a growing population of cells, in which it is taken up and incorporated into the DNA of cells that are actively synthesizing DNA at that time. Cells that are not making DNA do not take up the label. The cell preparation then is fixed and stained and viewed through a microscope. The DNA precursor may be thymidine labeled with radioactive tritium, which may be identified later by autoradiography, or it may be 5-bromodeoxyuridine (BrdUrd), which may be identified later by the use of a specific stain or antibody.

These labeling techniques can be applied to cells growing *in vitro* in petri dishes or to tissues *in vivo* if, after the incorporation of the label, the tissue or tumor of interest is removed and sliced into sections a few microns thick.

By the use of these techniques, the cell cycle in all dividing mammalian cells may be divided as shown in Figure 21.1. After the cells pass through mitosis (M), there is a period of apparent inactivity, termed G_1 by Howard and Pelc simply because it was the first "gap" in activity observed in the cell cycle. After this period of inactivity, the cells actively synthesize DNA during the S phase. Between the S phase and the onset of the next division, or mitosis, there is another gap in activity, termed G_2.

QUANTITATIVE ASSESSMENT OF THE CONSTITUENT PARTS OF THE CELL CYCLE

Two relatively simple measurements can be made on a population of cells. First, it is possible to count

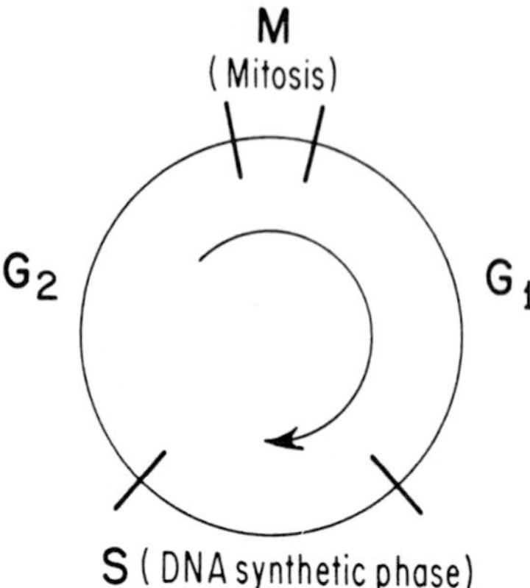

FIGURE 21.1 ● The phases of the cell cycle. Mitosis (M) is the only event that can be distinguished through the light microscope. The DNA synthetic phase (S) may be identified by the technique of autoradiography (Chapter 4). The intervals of apparent inactivity are labeled G_1 and G_2.

the proportion of cells that are seen to be in mitosis; this quantity is called the **mitotic index (MI)**. If it is assumed that all of the cells in the population are dividing and that all of the cells have the same mitotic cycle, then

$$MI = \lambda T_M/T_C$$

where T_M is the length of mitosis (i.e., the time taken for cells to complete division) and T_C is the total length of the mitotic cycle, or cell cycle.

The symbol λ is a correction factor to allow for the fact that cells cannot be distributed uniformly in time around the cycle because they double during mitosis (Fig. 21.2). The simplest assumption is that cells are distributed around the cycle exponentially in time, in which case λ has a value of 0.693. In any event, λ is a relatively small and unimportant correction factor.

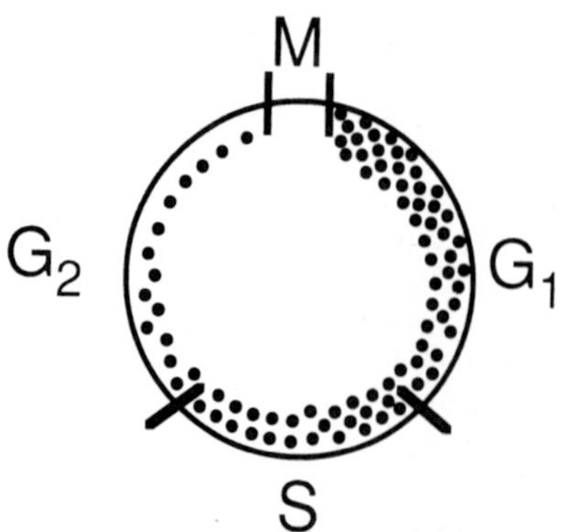

FIGURE 21.2 ● Diagram illustrating the fact that cells cannot be distributed uniformly in time around the cell cycle because they double in number during mitosis. The simplest assumption is that they are distributed as an exponential function of time.

The second relatively simple measurement requires that the cell population be fed for a brief time with a quantity of tritiated thymidine or 5-bromodeoxyuridine. In the jargon of cell kinetics, it is said to be **flash-labeled**. The cell population, whether on a petri dish or in a thin section cut from tissue, is then fixed, stained, and viewed through a microscope. A count is made of the proportion of labeled cells. This quantity is called the **labeling index (LI)**.

Given the assumption that all the cells are dividing with the same cell cycle, then

$$LI = \lambda T_S/T_C$$

where T_S is the duration of the DNA synthetic period and T_C is the total cell-cycle time.

In practice, these two quantities—the mitotic index and the labeling index—can be determined from a single specimen by counting the proportion of cells in mitosis and the proportion of cells that are labeled. This is a very important consideration in human studies, in which it is usually not practical to obtain a large number of serial specimens of tumor or normal-tissue material. Although these measurements yield ratios of the duration of mitosis and DNA synthesis as fractions of the total cell cycle, they do not give the absolute duration of any part of the cycle.

THE PERCENT LABELED MITOSES TECHNIQUE

A complete analysis of the cell cycle to obtain the length of each phase is only possible by labeling a cohort of cells in one phase of the cycle and observing the progress of this labeled cohort through a "window" in some other readily observable phase of the cycle. In practice, the easiest phase to label is S, and the easiest to observe is M.

As stated previously, the labeling can be achieved by using either tritiated thymidine, identifiable by autoradiography, or bromodeoxyuridine, identifiable by a specific stain or antibody. The basis of the technique, therefore, is to feed the population of cells a label that is taken up in S and then to observe the appearance of that label in mitotic cells as they move around the cycle from S to M. To avoid confusion, the technique involving tritiated thymidine is described in detail, partly because it is the original and classic technique and partly because pictures of autoradiographs show up well in black and white. The technique works equally well if bromodeoxyuridine is used. Bromodeoxyuridine-containing DNA can be stained and shows up well in color under a microscope, but does not reproduce well in black and white.

The **percent labeled mitoses technique** is laborious and time-consuming and requires a large number of serial samples. It is readily applicable *in vitro*, for which it is not difficult to obtain a large number of parallel replicate samples. It also may be applied *in vivo* for determining the cell-cycle parameters of normal tissue or tumors, provided a large number of sections from matched animals or tumors can be obtained at accurately timed intervals. The cell population first must be flash-labeled with tritiated thymidine. Theoretically, the labeled DNA precursor should be available to the cells for a negligibly short time; in practice, an exposure time of about 20 minutes is usually used. *In vitro* the thymidine is added to the growth medium; at the end of the flash-labeling period, it is simple to remove the radioactive medium and to add fresh medium. *In vivo*, the tritiated thymidine is injected intraperitoneally; it clearly cannot be removed after 20 minutes, so the exposure time is terminated by the injection of a massive dose of "cold" (i.e., nonradioactive) thymidine.

During the period in which tritiated thymidine is available, cells in S phase take up the radioactive label. After the label is removed, cells progress through their cell cycles. At regular intervals, usually of 1 hour, a specimen of the cell population must be removed, fixed, and stained and an autoradiograph prepared. This is continued for a total time longer than the cell cycle of the population under study. For each sample, the percentage of mitotic cells that carry a radioactive label must then be counted; this is the **percentage of labeled mitoses**. A photomicrograph of a cell preparation is shown in Figure 21.3. This is a particularly laborious process because only 1 or 2% of the cells are in mitosis in any case, and only a fraction of these will be labeled.

The basis for this type of experiment, if applied to an idealized population of cells that all have identical cell cycles, is illustrated in Figure 21.4, a plot of the percentage of labeled mitoses as a function of time. The cells that are in S while the radioactive thymidine is available take up the label. This labeled cohort of cells then moves through the cell cycle (as indicated by the circles at the top of Fig. 21.4) after the pool of radioactive thymidine has been

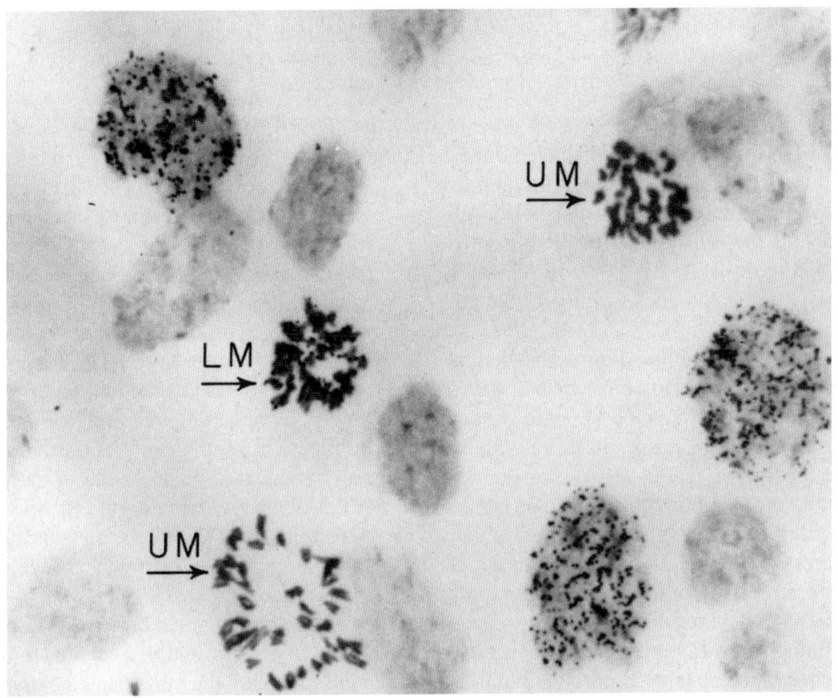

FIGURE 21.3 • Photomicrograph of a preparation of mouse corneal cells. The cell preparation was flash-labeled some hours before with tritiated thymidine, which was taken up by cells in S phase. By the time the autoradiograph was made, the cell marked *LM* had moved around the cycle into mitosis; this is an example of a labeled mitotic figure. Other cells in mitosis are unlabeled (*UM*). (Courtesy of Dr. M. Fry.)

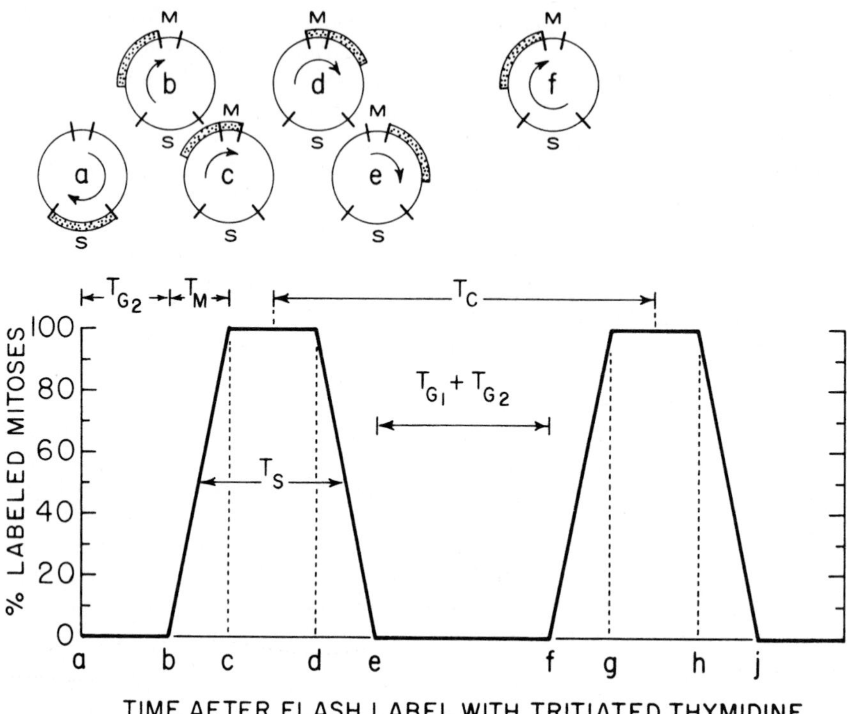

FIGURE 21.4 ● Percent labeled mitoses curve for an idealized cell population in which all of the cells have identical mitotic-cycle times. The cell population is flash-labeled with tritiated thymidine, which labels all cells in S. The proportion of labeled mitotic cells is counted as a function of time after labeling. The circles at the top of the figure indicate the position of the labeled cohort of cells as it progresses through the cycle. The length of the various phases (e.g., T_{G_2}, T_M) of the cycle (T_C) may be determined as indicated.

removed. Early samples contain no labeled mitotic figures, and the first labeled mitotic figure appears as the leading edge of the cohort of labeled cells reaches M. This point in time is labeled *b* on the time axis of Figure 21.4; the position of the labeled cohort is indicated above on the circle also marked *b*.

The percentage of mitotic figures labeled increases rapidly as the leading edge of the labeled cohort of cells passes through the M phase; when it reaches the end of the M phase, all mitotic figures are labeled (position *c* in Fig. 21.4). For the next few hours, all mitotic figures continue to be labeled until the trailing edge of the labeled cohort of cells reaches the beginning of mitosis (position *d*), after which the percentage of labeled mitoses rapidly falls and reaches zero when the trailing edge reaches the end of mitosis (position *e*). There is then a long interval during which no labeled mitotic figures are seen until the labeled cohort of cells goes around the entire cycle and comes up to mitosis again, after which the whole pattern of events is repeated.

All of the parameters of the cell cycle may be calculated from Figure 21.4. The time interval before the appearance of the first labeled mitosis, the length *ab*, is in fact the length of G_2 or T_{G_2}. The time it takes for the percent labeled mitoses curve to rise from 0 to 100% (*bc*) corresponds to the time necessary for the leading edge of the labeled cohort of cells to proceed through mitosis and is therefore equal to the length of mitosis, T_M. The duration of DNA synthesis (T_S) is the time taken for the cohort of labeled cells to pass the beginning of mitosis (*bd*). Likewise, it is the time required for the labeled cohort to pass the end of mitosis (*ce*). In practice, T_S usually is taken to be the width of the curve at the 50% level, as marked in Figure 21.4.

The total cycle (T_C) is the distance between corresponding points on the first and second wave (*bf*, *cg*, *dh*, or *ej*) or the distance between the centers of the two peaks as marked on the figure. The remaining quantity, T_{G_1}, usually is calculated by subtracting the sum of all the other phases of the cycle from the total cell cycle, or

$$T_{G_1} = T_C - (T_S + T_{G_2} + T_M)$$

Experimental data are never as clear-cut as the idealized picture in Figure 21.4. Points such as *b* and

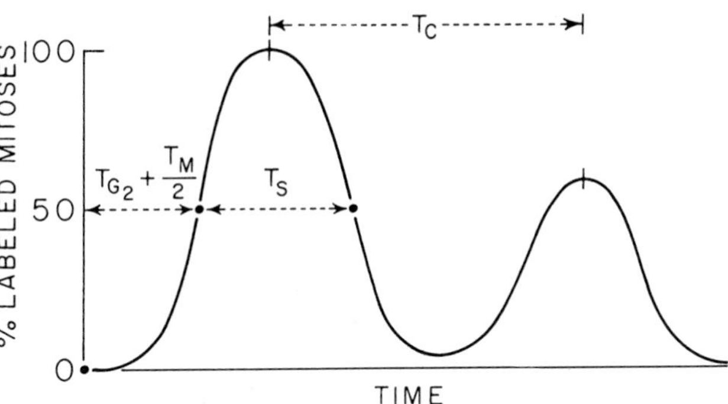

FIGURE 21.5 ● Typical percent labeled mitoses curve obtained in practice for the cells of a tissue or tumor. It differs from the idealized curve in Figure 21.4 in that the only points that can be identified with precision are the peaks of the curve and the 50% levels. The first peak is not perfectly symmetric, and the second peak is lower than the first because the cells of a population have a range of cell-cycle times.

e, at which the curve begins to rise and reaches zero, are poorly defined. A more typical experimental result is illustrated in Figure 21.5. The only points that can be defined with any certainty are the peaks of the curves and the 50% levels, and these may be used to give a rough estimate of the lengths of the various phases of the cycle. The S period (T_S) is given approximately by the width of the first peak, from the 50% level on the ascending portion of the wave to the corresponding point on the descending curve. The total cell cycle, T_C, is readily obtained as the time between successive peaks. In a separate experiment, the mitotic index may be counted, which is equal to $\lambda T_M/T_C$; because T_C is known, T_M may be calculated. The time from flash labeling to the point at which the curve passes the 50% level in Figure 21.5 is $T_{G_2} + 0.5\ T_M$; because T_M already is known, T_{G_2} may be calculated. The remaining quantity, T_{G_1}, is deduced by subtraction, because the total cycle time and all other phases are known.

A careful examination of an actual set of experimental data makes it plain that the first wave in the percent labeled mitoses curve is not symmetric; the downswing is shallower than the upswing. This observation, coupled with the fact that the second peak is much smaller than the first, indicates that the population is made up of cells with a wide range of cycle times. In many instances, particularly if the population of cells involved is an *in vivo* specimen of a tumor or normal tissue, the spread of cell-cycle times is so great that a second peak is barely discernible.

In practice, therefore, the constituent parts of the cycle are not simply read off the percent labeled mitoses curve. Instead, a complex computer program is used to try various distributions of cell-cycle times and to calculate the curve that best fits the experimental data. In this way, an estimate is obtained of the mean cell-cycle time and also of the range of cell-cycle times in the population.

EXPERIMENTAL MEASUREMENTS OF CELL-CYCLE TIMES *IN VIVO* AND *IN VITRO*

A vast number of cell-cycle measurements have been made. Only a few representative results are reviewed here to highlight the most important points.

Figure 21.6 shows the percent labeled mitoses data for two transplantable rat tumors with very different growth rates. The tumor represented in the upper panel has a gross doubling time of about 20 hours, which can be judged easily from the separation of the first and second waves of labeled mitotic cells.

For the tumor illustrated in the lower panel, there is no discernible second peak in the percent labeled mitoses curve because of the large range of cell-cycle times among the cells of the population. To obtain an estimate of the average cell cycle in this case, it is necessary to pool information from the percent labeled mitoses curve and from a knowledge of the labeling index. The width of the first wave of the percent labeled mitoses curve indicates that the length of the DNA synthetic phase (T_S) is about 10 hours. To obtain the average cell-cycle time (T_C), it is essential in this situation to know the labeling index. For this tumor, the labeling index is about 3.6%. The average cell cycle time (T_C) can then be calculated from the following equation:

$$LI = \lambda\, T_S/T_C$$

Therefore,

$$T_C = (0.693 \times 10)/(3.6/100) = 192.5 \text{ hours}$$

The absence of a second peak is a clue to the fact that there is a wide range of cell-cycle times for the cells of this population, so 192.5 hours is very much an average value.

A computer analysis makes it possible to estimate the distribution of cell-cycle times in a population. For example, Figure 21.7 shows the percent

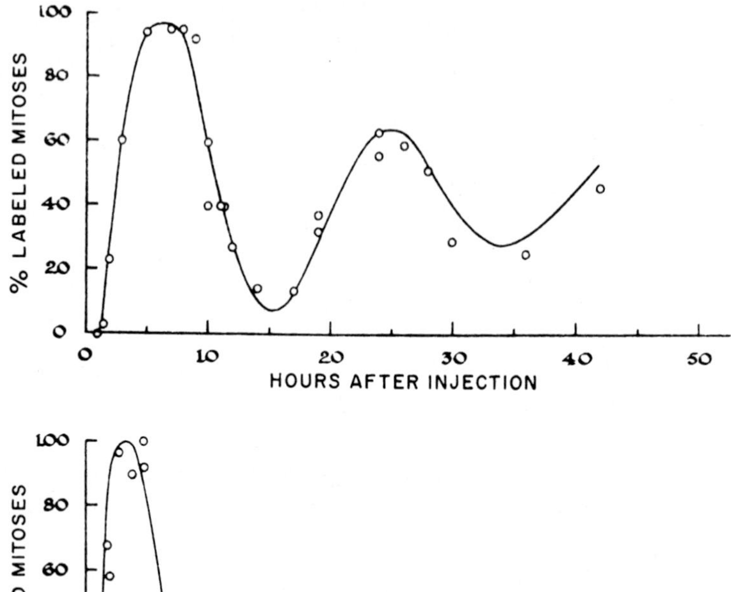

FIGURE 21.6 ● Percent labeled mitoses curve for two transplantable rat sarcomas with widely different growth rates. The tumor in the **upper panel** has a gross doubling time of 22 hours, compared with 192.5 hours for the tumor in the **lower panel**. (From Steel GG, Adams K, Barratt JC: Analysis of the cell population kinetics of transplanted tumours of widely differing growth rate. *Br J Cancer* 20:784–800, 1966, with permission.)

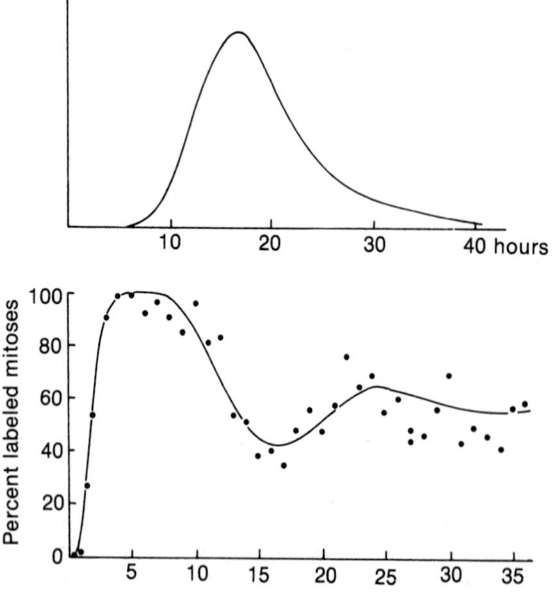

FIGURE 21.7 ● **Bottom:** Percent labeled mitoses curve for an EMT6 mouse tumor. (Data from Dr. Sara Rockwell.) **Top:** The distribution of cell-cycle times consistent with the damped labeled mitoses curve, obtained by computer analysis of the data and a mathematical model. (From Steel GG: The growth kinetics of tumors in relation to their therapeutic response. *Laryngoscope* 85:359–370, 1975, with permission.)

TABLE 21.1

The Constituent Parts of the Cell Cycle (in hours) for Some Cells in Culture and Tumors in Experimental Animals

Authors	Cell or Tissue	T_C	T_S	T_M	T_{G_2}	T_{G_1}
Bedford	Hamster cells *in vitro*	10	6	1	1	2
	HeLa cells *in vitro*	23	8	1	3	11
Steel	Mammary tumors in the rat					
	BICR/M1	19	8	~1	2	8
	BICR/A2	63	10	~1	2	50
Quastler and Sherman	Mouse intestinal crypt	18.75	7.5	0.5	0.5–1.0	9.5
Brown and Berry	Hamster cheek pouch epithelium	120–152	8.6	1.0	1.9	108–140
	Chemically induced carcinoma in pouch	10.7	5.9	0.4	1.6	2.8

labeled mitoses curve for a transplantable mouse tumor, together with an analysis of cell-cycle times based on a mathematical model. There is a wide range of cell-cycle times, from less than 10 to more than 40 hours, with a modal value of about 19 hours. This range of cycle times explains the damped labeled mitoses curve and the fact that the first peak is not symmetric.

Table 21.1 is a summary of the cell-cycle parameters for cell lines in culture and some of the tissues and tumors for which percent labeled mitoses curves have been shown in this chapter. The top row of Table 21.1 shows the data for Chinese hamster cells in culture. These cells are characterized by a short cell cycle of only 10 hours and a minimal G_1 period. The second row of the table gives the comparable figures for HeLa cells. From a comparison of these two *in vitro* cell lines, a very important point emerges. The cell cycles of the two cell lines differ by a factor of more than 2, nearly all of which results from a difference in the length of G_1. The other phases of the cycle are very similar in the two cell lines.

Also included in Table 21.1 are data for the cells of the normal cheek pouch epithelium in the hamster and a chemically induced carcinoma in the pouch. These are representative of a number of studies in which cells from a solid tumor have been compared with their normal-tissue counterparts. In general, it usually is found that the malignant cells have the shorter cycle time.

In reviewing the data summarized in Table 21.1, it is at once evident that although the length of the cell cycle varies enormously between populations, particularly *in vivo*, the lengths of G_2, mitosis, and S are remarkably constant. The vast bulk of the cell-cycle variation is accounted for by differences in the length of the G_1 phase.

PULSED FLOW CYTOMETRY

During the past several decades, classic autoradiography largely has been replaced by pulsed flow cytometry (Fig. 21.8). The conventional techniques of autoradiography give precise, meaningful answers, but they are laborious and so slow that information is never available quickly enough to act as a predictive assay to influence the treatment options of an individual patient. Techniques based on flow cytometry provide data that are available within a few days. Detailed cell kinetic data can be obtained by such techniques, including an analysis of the distribution of cells in the various phases of the cycle; but in practice, the measurement of most immediate relevance to clinical radiotherapy is the estimate of $\mathbf{T_{pot}}$, the **potential tumor doubling time**.

MEASUREMENT OF POTENTIAL TUMOR DOUBLING TIME (T_{pot})

T_{pot} is a measure of the rate of increase of cells capable of continued proliferation and therefore may determine the outcome of a radiotherapy treatment protocol delivered in fractions over an extended period of time. Tumors with a short T_{pot} may repopulate if fractionation is extended over too long a period. To measure T_{pot} precisely requires a

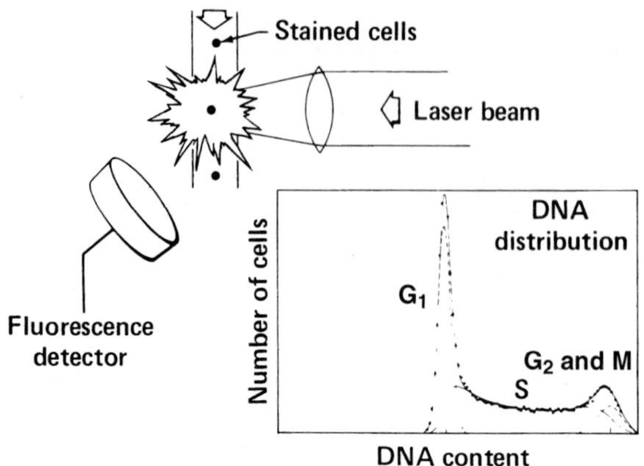

FIGURE 21.8 • The principles of DNA distribution analysis of flow cytometry. Suspensions of fluorescent-stained single cells flow one at a time through a light beam, with its wavelength adjusted to excite the fluorescent dye. The fluorescence stimulated in each cell is recorded as a measure of that cell's DNA content. Thousands of cells can be measured each second and the results accumulated to form a DNA distribution like that shown for asynchronously growing Chinese hamster ovary cells. (From Gray JW, Dolbeare F, Pallavicini MG, Beisker W, Waldman F: Cell cycle analysis using flow cytometry. *Int J Radiat Biol* 49:237–255, 1986, with permission.)

knowledge of T_S and the labeling index. T_{pot} can be calculated from the following:

$$T_{pot} = \lambda T_S/LI$$

where T_S is the length of the DNA synthetic period, LI is the labeling index (i.e., the fraction of cells synthesizing DNA at any time), and λ is a correction factor to allow for the nonlinear distribution in time of the cells as they pass through the cycle; this factor has a value between 0.67 and 1.

The labeling index can be determined from a single sample, but to measure T_S precisely, it is necessary to label the cell population with tritiated thymidine or bromodeoxyuridine, take a sample every hour for a time period about equal to the cell cycle, and count the proportion of labeled mitoses as a function of time, as previously described. This is out of the question in a clinical situation, but an estimate of T_{pot} can be made by flow cytometry from a single biopsy specimen taken 4 to 8 hours after the injection of a tracer amount of a thymidine analogue (bromodeoxyuridine or iododeoxyurine). The biopsy specimen is treated with fluorescent-labeled monoclonal antibody, which is used to detect the incorporation of the thymidine analogue into the DNA. The specimen is also stained with propidium iodide to determine DNA content. A single-cell suspension of the biopsy specimen is then passed through a flow cytometer, which simultaneously measures DNA content (red) and bromodeoxyuridine content (green). This is illustrated in Figure 21.9.

The labeling index is simply the proportion of cells that show significant green fluorescence. T_S can be calculated from the mean red fluorescence of S cells relative to G_1 and G_2 cells. The DNA content of cells in G_2 is double that in G_1. The method assumes that the red fluorescence of bromodeoxyuridine-labeled cells (i.e., the DNA content of cells in S phase) increases linearly with time (Fig. 21.10). If, for example, the biopsy specimen were obtained 6 hours after administration of bromodeoxyuridine, and the relative DNA content of cells labeled with bromodeoxyuridine (i.e., in S phase) were 0.75, midway between that characteristic of G_1 and that of G_2, T_S would be simply 12 hours. This method has been validated in a number of *in vitro* cell lines and also in animal tumor systems, in which it can be checked by conventional cell kinetic studies.

This technique gives an average value for T_{pot} of the cells in the biopsy specimen because the cells are disaggregated and made into single-cell suspensions. There is some evidence from animal experiments that individual cells may have much shorter T_{pot} values.

This technique to measure T_{pot} has proved to be practical as a predictive assay and has been used on a large number of patients entered in a clinical trial of altered fractionation patterns by the European Cooperative Radiotherapy Group. This is described in more detail in the chapter on predictive assays (Chapter 23).

THE GROWTH FRACTION

Central to an appreciation of the pattern of growth of solid tumors is the realization that at any given moment, not all of the tumor cells that are viable and capable of continued growth are actually proceeding through the cell cycle. The population consists of proliferating (P) cells and quiescent (Q) cells. The growth fraction (GF), a term introduced by Mendelsohn, is defined as the ratio of the number of proliferating cells to the total number of cells (P + Q), or

$$GF = P/(P + Q)$$

There are various ways to estimate growth fraction. One method consists of injecting tritiated

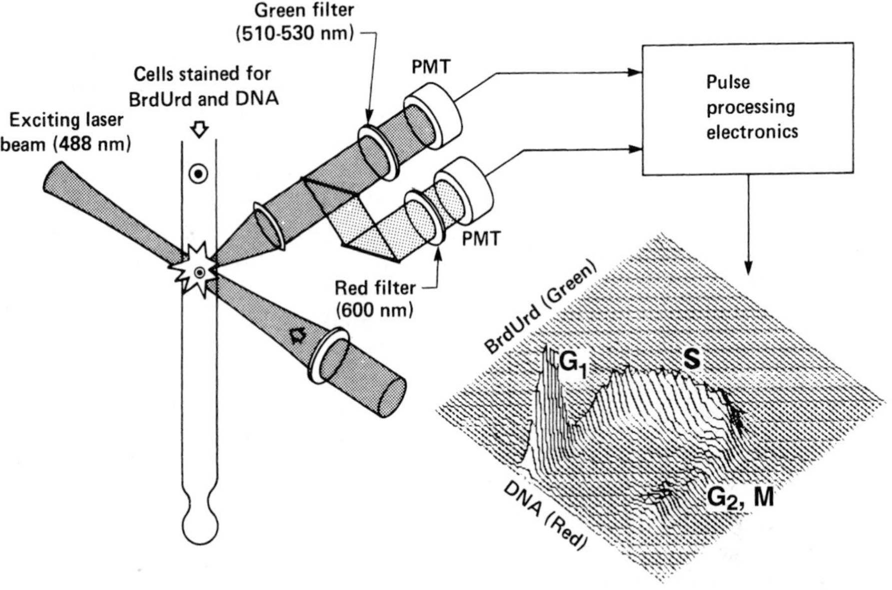

FIGURE 21.9 • The flow cytometric analysis of cellular bromodeoxyuridine (BrdUrd) and DNA content for cells stained with fluorescein (linked to BrdUrd) and propidium iodide (linked to DNA). The cells are processed one at a time through a blue (488-nm) laser beam that excites cellular BrdUrd content, and red fluorescence is recorded as a measure of cellular DNA content. The BrdUrd (green fluorescence) axis in the bivariate is logarithmic, with every seven channels representing a doubling of fluorescence intensity. (From Gray JW, Dolbeare F, Pallavicini MG, Beisker W, Waldman F: Cell cycle analysis using flow cytometry. *Int J Radiat Biol* 49:237–255, 1986, with permission.)

thymidine into an animal with a tumor and then, several cell generations later, preparing an autoradiograph from sections of the tumor. The growth fraction is given by the expression

$$\text{GF} = \frac{\text{fraction of cells labeled}}{\text{fraction of mitoses labeled}}$$

This method assumes that there are two distinct subpopulations, one growing with a uniform cell cycle, the other not growing at all.

Continuous labeling is an alternative way to provide an approximate measure of the proportion of proliferating cells. Tritiated thymidine is infused continuously for a time equal to the cell cycle minus the length of the S phase. The fraction of labeled cells then approximates to the growth fraction.

Table 21.2 is a summary of growth fractions measured for a variety of solid tumors in experimental animals, which frequently fall between 30 and 50%, even though the tumors vary widely in degree of differentiation, arise in different species, and are of varied histologic types. As a tumor outgrows its blood supply, areas of necrosis often develop that are accompanied by the presence of hypoxic cells, the proportion of which for many solid tumors is about 15%. This accounts for part, but not all, of the quiescent cell population.

CELL LOSS

The overall growth of a tumor is the result of a balance achieved between cell production from division and various types of cell loss. In most cases, tumors grow much more slowly than would be predicted from a knowledge of the cycle time of the individual cells and the growth fraction. The difference is a result of cell loss. The extent of the cell loss from a tumor is estimated by comparing the rate of production of new cells with the observed growth rate of the tumor. The discrepancy provides a measure of the rate of cell loss. If T_{pot} is the potential tumor doubling time, calculated from the cell-cycle time and the growth fraction, and T_d is the actual tumor doubling time, obtained from simple direct measurements on the diameter of the tumor mass, the **cell loss factor** (Φ) has been defined by Steel to be

$$\Phi = 1 - T_{pot}/T_d$$

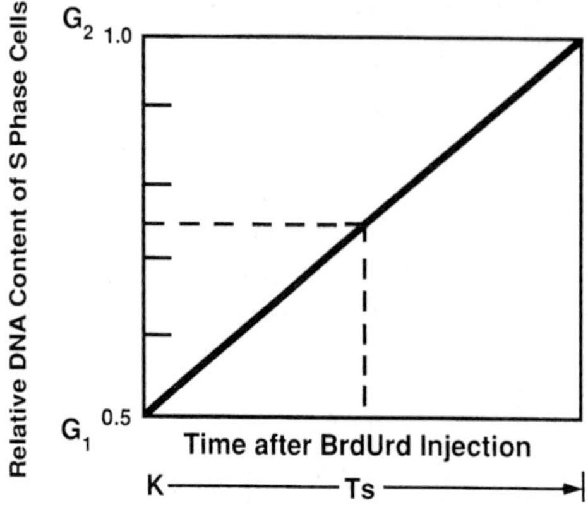

FIGURE 21.10 ● Graph illustrating the way T_S can be estimated by flow cytometry on cells from a single tumor biopsy specimen taken 4 to 8 hours after an injection of a thymidine analogue (bromodeoxyuridine or iododeoxyuridine). Cells in S phase are identified by the green fluorescence from an antibody to the thymidine analogue. The relative DNA content is measured by the red fluorescence owing to the incorporated propidium iodide. The DNA content in G_2 cells is double that in G_1. The length of the DNA synthetic phase (T_S) can be estimated by the relative DNA content of the S phase cells in relation to the time between the injection of the thymidine analogue and the biopsy.

The cell loss factor represents the *ratio of the rate of cell loss to the rate of new cell production*. It expresses the loss of growth potential by the tumor. A cell loss factor of 100%, for instance, indicates a steady state of neither growth nor regression.

Cells in tumors can be lost in a number of ways:

1. Death from inadequate nutrition: As the tumor outgrows its vascular system, rapid cell proliferation near capillaries pushes other cells into regions remote from blood supply, in which there is an inadequate concentration of oxygen and other nutrients. These cells die, giving rise to a progressively enlarging necrotic zone.
2. Apoptosis, or programmed cell death: This form of cell death is manifested by the occurrence of isolated degenerate nuclei remote from regions of overt necrosis.
3. Death from immunologic attack.
4. Metastasis, including all processes by which tumor cells are lost to other parts of the body, such as spread through the bloodstream and lymphatic system.
5. Exfoliation, which would not apply to most model tumors in experimental animals but which could be an important mechanism of cell loss from, for example, carcinoma of the gastrointestinal tract, in which the epithelium is renewed at a considerable rate.

There are limited data on the relative importance of these different processes in different tumor types, but it is clear that death from inadequate nutrition—by entry into necrotic areas—is often a major factor. It reflects the latent inability of the vascular system to keep up with the rate of cell production. There is still a great deal to be learned about the occurrence of cell loss from tumors, the mechanisms by which it occurs, and the factors by which it can be controlled. It is clear, however, that any understanding of the growth rate of tumors at the cellular level must include a consideration of this often dominant factor.

DETERMINATIONS OF CELL LOSS IN EXPERIMENTAL ANIMAL TUMORS

The cell loss factor has been estimated in a considerable number of tumors in experimental animals. Some of the results are listed in Table 21.3.

TABLE 21.2

Growth Fraction for Some Tumors in Experimental Animals

Tumor	Author	Growth Fraction, %
Primary mammary carcinoma in the mouse (G_3H)	Mendelsohn	35–77
Transplantable sarcoma in the rat (RIB_5)	Denekamp	55
Transplantable sarcoma in the rat (SSO)	Denekamp	47
Transplantable sarcoma in the rat (SSB_1)	Denekamp	39
Mammary carcinoma in the mouse (C_3H)	Denekamp	30
Chemistry induced carcinoma in the hamster cheek pouch	Brown	29

TABLE 21.3

Cell Loss Factor (Φ) for Some Tumors in Experimental Animals

Tumor	Author	Φ, %
Mouse sarcoma	Frindel	
3-day-old tumor		0
7-day-old tumor		10
20-day-old tumor		55
Rat carcinoma	Steel	9
Rat sarcoma	Steel	0
Mouse carcinoma	Mendelsohn	69
Hamster carcinoma	Brown	75
Rat sarcoma	Hermens	26
Hamster carcinoma	Reiskin	81–93
Mouse carcinoma	Tannock	70–92

Values for the cell loss factor vary from 0 to more than 90%. In reviewing the literature on this subject, Denekamp pointed out that sarcomas tended to have low cell loss factors, but carcinomas tended to have high cell loss factors. All the sarcomas investigated had cell loss factors less than 55%; most carcinomas had cell loss factors in excess of 70%. Therefore, cell loss appears to be a dominant factor in the growth of carcinomas and of considerably less importance for sarcomas. This pattern correlates with the importance of apoptosis as a mode of cell death. Apoptosis is quite common in carcinomas and rare in sarcomas. If this is found to be a general phenomenon, it might be attributed to the origin of carcinomas from continuously renewing epithelial tissues, in which the cell loss factor is 100%.

This difference between sarcomas and carcinomas also may account for their differing responses to radiation. In carcinomas, in which the production of new cells is temporarily stopped or reduced by a dose of radiation, cells continue to be removed from the tumor because of the high cell loss factor, and the tumor shrinks. In sarcomas, however, even if a large proportion of the cells are sterilized by a dose of radiation, they do not disappear from the tumor mass as quickly.

It would be simple, then, to explain why two tumors, one a carcinoma and one a sarcoma, containing the same number of cells and exposed to the same radiation dose, would appear to behave quite differently. The carcinoma might shrink dramatically soon after the radiation dose, whereas the sarcoma would not appear as affected by the radiation. In the long term, the "cure" rates of both tumors may well be identical, but in the short term, the carcinoma would be said to have "responded" to the radiation, whereas the sarcoma might be said to be unresponsive or resistant to radiation.

GROWTH KINETICS OF HUMAN TUMORS

The first quantitative study of the growth rate of human tumors was done by Collins and his colleagues in 1956. They observed the growth of pulmonary metastases from serial chest radiographs. It is now possible to gather from the literature information on the doubling time of more than 1,000 human tumors. Most of the data were obtained either by measurements from radiographs or by direct measurements of skin tumors or metastases in soft tissue. The doubling time of human tumors varies widely from patient to patient and is on the average very long; Tubiana and Malaise have estimated that the median value is about two months.

Tumors of the same histologic type arising in different patients differ widely in growth rate. By contrast, metastases arising in the same patient tend to have similar rates of growth. The latter observation is the basis for using patients with multiple skin or pulmonary metastases to test and compare new treatment modalities, such as high linear energy transfer radiations or hyperthermia. There is certainly a correlation between histologic type and growth rate. Tubiana and Malaise have collected values for the doubling time in 389 patients with pulmonary metastases, classified into five histologic categories. They can be arranged in order of doubling time as follows: embryonic tumors, 27 days; malignant lymphomas, 29 days; mesenchymal sarcomas, 41 days; squamous cell carcinomas, 58 days; and adenocarcinomas, 82 days. In addition, the degree of differentiation seems to be related to the doubling time, with poorly differentiated cancers generally progressing more rapidly.

In addition to growth rate measurements, studies of cell population kinetics also have been performed on a limited number of human tumors. Studies of this kind raise practical and ethical problems. The ethical problems stem from the fact that *in vivo* experiments require an injection of tritiated thymidine or bromodeoxyuridine, which limits such studies to patients who have short life expectancies and in whom the injection of the label does not raise any problems of possible genetic consequences. The practical problems arise because the percent labeled mitoses technique, which is the most satisfactory way to obtain the duration of the various phases of the cell cycle, requires a large number of sequential samples to be taken for several days after the injection of the label.

In mice or rats, the multiple samples are obtained from a large number of identical animals bearing transplanted tumors of the same size and type by sacrificing one or more animals each time. In humans, each spontaneous tumor is unique, so the multiple samples must be obtained by repeated biopsies at frequent intervals from the same tumor. This heroic procedure is uncomfortable and inconvenient for the patient and is only practical with large superficial skin tumors, which may not be truly representative of human tumors in general. Nevertheless, a surprisingly large number of human tumors have been studied in this way. The percent labeled mitoses curves obtained are similar to those for laboratory animals, although the second wave of labeled mitoses is rarely distinct and is usually altogether absent.

Tubiana and Malaise surveyed the field and reported 40 cases in which the cell cycle of solid tumors in humans had been evaluated with the percent labeled mitoses technique. The cell cycles observed were between 15 and 125 hours in 90% of the cases, with a modal value of 48 hours (Table 21.4). The duration of S (T_S) was less variable than the total cell cycle, with 90% of the values falling between 9.5 and 24 hours and a modal value of about 16 hours. As a first approximation, it can be assumed that T_S has a duration of about 16 hours and that the mean duration of the cell cycle is about three times the duration of T_S.

Although the percent labeled mitoses technique has been used on relatively few human tumors, the labeling index has been measured in many more after *in vitro* incubation of a fresh piece of excised tumor with tritiated thymidine. The rationale underlying this technique is that cells already synthesizing DNA *in vivo* are able to continue synthesis of DNA *in vitro*, but no new cells enter synthesis under the incubation conditions that normally are used.

The growth fraction, too, has been measured in only a limited number of human tumors by the method of continuous labeling. If a population of cells is labeled continuously during a period corresponding to the duration of the cell cycle less the duration of the DNA synthetic phase (i.e., $T_C - T_S$), all the actively proliferating cells should be labeled. This method of continuous labeling can be performed only with a small number of patients who are in no way representative. An alternative procedure is to estimate the growth fraction by assuming that the proportion of cells in cycle is about equal to three times the labeling index, an assumption based on the notion that the cell cycle is three times the length of the S phase. The growth fraction calculated in this way correlates well with the tumor doubling time: It is 0.9 in malignant lymphomas and embryonic tumors and less than 0.06 in adenocarcinomas. The relation between the growth rate and growth fraction appears to be much closer in human tumors than in animal tumors.

Of the various parameters that characterize tumor kinetics, the cell loss factor is, in general, the most difficult to evaluate. The cell loss factor for human tumors generally has been calculated by comparing the *observed tumor volume-doubling time* with the *potential doubling time*, which is the time required for the population of cells to double, assuming that all the cells produced are retained in the tumor. Tubiana and Malaise calculated a mean value of the cell loss factor for five histologic groups of human tumors, assuming the duration of S to be 16 hours. Their results suggest that in general, the mean cell loss factor exceeds 50%. Furthermore, it appeared to be higher if the tumor was growing quickly and if its growth fraction was high. In humans, the smallest cell loss factors seem to be associated with those histologic types of tumors that have the slowest rate of growth. The cell loss factor, therefore, tends to reduce the spread of growth rates that results from the differences in growth fraction of the various types of tumors.

TABLE 21.4

Individual Values for the Duration of the Cell Cycle (T_C) in Human Solid Tumors of Various Histologic Types

Authors	T_C, h
Frindel et al. (1968)	97, 51.5, 27.5, 48, 49.8
Bennington (1969)	15.5, 14.9
Young and de Vita (1970)	42, 82, 74
Shirakawa et al. (1970)	120, 144
Weinstein and Frost (1970)	217
Terz et al. (1971)	44.5, 31, 14, 25.5, 26
Peckham and Steel (1973)	59
Estevez et al. (1972)	37, 30, 48, 30, 38, 96, 48
Terz and Curutchet (1974)[a]	18, 19, 19.2, 120
Malaise et al. (unpublished data)[a]	24, 33, 48, 42
Muggia et al. (1972)	64
Bresciani et al. (1974)	82, 50, 67, 53, 58

[a] Measured by the mean grain count halving time.

From Tublana M, Malaise E: Growth rate and cell kinetics in human tumors: Some prognostic and therapeutic implications. In Symington T, Carter RL (eds): *Scientific Foundations of Oncology*, pp 126–136. Chicago, Year Book Medical Publishers, 1976, with permission.

TABLE 21.5

Volume-Doubling Times of Human Tumors

Authors	Site	Volume-Doubling Time, d	Range, d
Breuer	Lung metastases	40	4–745
Collins et al.	Lung metastases	40	11–164
Collins	Lung metastases from colon or rectum	96	34–210
Garland	Primary bronchial carcinoma	105	27–480
Schwartz	Primary bronchial carcinomas	62	17–200
Spratt	Primary skeletal sarcomas	75	21–366

Based on data from Steel GG: Cell loss from experimental tumors. *Cell Tissue Kinet* 1:193–207, 1968.

Steel has estimated independently the extent of cell loss in human tumors by comparing the potential doubling time with observed tumor growth rates. The relevant data on the volume-doubling time for six groups of human tumors are given in Table 21.5. They consist mostly of measurements of primary and secondary tumors of the lung. There are differences between individual series, which indeed may reflect significant differences in the growth rates of the various types of tumors, but if the results are all pooled, they yield an average median doubling time of 66 days, with 80% of the values falling in the range between 18 and 200 days. Taking the median values for the labeling index, doubling time, and S phase as suggested by Steel, the median cell loss factor in all human tumors studied is 77%. It thus would appear that for human tumors, cell loss is generally the most important factor determining the pattern of tumor growth.

The high rate of cell loss in human tumors largely accounts for the great disparity between the cell-cycle time of the individual dividing cells and the overall doubling time of the tumor. Although the tumor doubling time is characteristically 40 to 100 days, the cell-cycle time is relatively short, 1 to 5 days. This has important implications, which often are overlooked, in the use of cycle-specific chemotherapeutic agents or radiosensitizing drugs, for which it is the cell-cycle time that is relevant.

Because Bergonié and Tribondeau established a relation between the rate of cell proliferation and the response to irradiation in normal tissues, it might be supposed that this would be the same for tumors. It is of interest to note that the histologic groups of human tumors that have the most rapid mean growth rates and the highest growth fractions and cell turnover rates are indeed those that are the most radiosensitive. There is also a correlation between, on the one hand, the growth rate and the labeling index or the cell loss and, on the other hand, the reaction to chemotherapy. This is not surprising, because the majority of drugs act essentially on cells in S phase. It is remarkable, however, that the only human tumors in which it is possible to achieve cures by chemotherapy are the histologic types with high labeling indexes. Furthermore, a high level of cell loss appears to favor the response to chemotherapy, and in humans this occurs especially in tumors with high labeling indexes.

Summary of Pertinent Conclusions

- Mammalian cells proliferate by mitosis (M). The interval between successive mitoses is the cell-cycle time (T_C).
- In mitosis, the chromosomes condense and are visible. The DNA synthetic (S) phase can be identified by autoradiography. The first gap (G_1) separates mitosis from the S phase. The second gap (G_2) separates the S phase from the subsequent mitosis.
- Fast-growing cells in culture and some cells in self-renewal tissues *in vivo* have a T_C of 10 hours; stem cells in a resting normal tissue, such as the skin, have a cell-cycle time of 10 days.

(continued)

Summary of Pertinent Conclusions (Continued)

- Most of the difference in cell cycle between fast- and slow-growing cells is a result of differences in G_1, which varies from less than 1 hour to more than a week.
- The mitotic index (MI) is the fraction of cells in mitosis

$$MI = \lambda T_M / T_C$$

- The labeling index (LI) is the fraction of cells that take up tritiated thymidine (i.e., the fraction of cells in S)

$$LI = \lambda T_S / T_C$$

- The percent labeled mitoses technique allows an estimate to be made of the lengths of the constituent phases of the cell cycle. The basis of the technique is to label cells with tritiated thymidine or bromodeoxyuridine in S phase and time their arrival in mitosis.
- Flow cytometry allows a rapid analysis of the distribution of cells in the cycle. Cells are stained with a DNA-specific dye and sorted on the basis of DNA content.
- The bromodeoxyuridine–DNA assay in flow cytometry allows cells to be stained simultaneously with two dyes that fluoresce at different wavelengths: One binds in proportion to DNA content to indicate the phase of the cell cycle, and the other binds in proportion to bromodeoxyuridine incorporation to show if cells are synthesizing DNA.
- T_{pot}, the potential doubling time of a tumor, reflects the cell cycle of individual cells and the growth fraction, but ignores cell loss.
- T_{pot} may be the relevant parameter for estimating the effect of cell proliferation on a protracted radiotherapy protocol.
- T_{pot} can be estimated by means of flow cytometric analysis on cells from a single biopsy specimen taken 4 to 8 hours after an intravenous administration of bromodeoxyuridine.
- The growth fraction is the fraction of cells in active cell cycle (i.e., the fraction of proliferative cells).
- In animal tumors, the growth fraction frequently ranges from 30 to 50%.
- The cell loss factor (Φ) is the fraction of cells produced by cell division lost from the tumor.
- In animal tumors, Φ varies from 0 to more than 90%, tending to be small in small tumors and to increase with tumor size.
- The cell loss factor Φ tends to be large for carcinomas and small for sarcomas.
- The observed volume-doubling time of a tumor is the gross time for it to double overall in size as measured, for example, in serial radiographs.
- Tumors grow much more slowly than would be predicted from the cycle time of individual cells. One reason is the growth fraction, but the principal reason is the cell loss factor.
- The overall pattern of tumor growth may be summarized as follows. A minority of cells (the growth fraction) are proliferating rapidly; most are quiescent. The majority of the new cells produced by mitosis are lost from the tumor.
- In general, the cell-cycle time of malignant cells is appreciably shorter than that of their normal-tissue counterparts.
- In general, irradiation causes an elongation of the cell-cycle time in tumor cells and a shortening of the cell cycle in normal tissues.
- In 90% of human tumors, the cell-cycle time has a modal value of 48 hours (a range of 15 to 125 hours).
- In human tumors, T_S has a modal value of about 16 hours (a range of 9.5 to 24 hours).
- As a first approximation, the mean duration of the cell cycle in human tumors is about three times the duration of the S phase.
- Growth fraction is more variable in human tumors than in rodent tumors and correlates better with gross volume-doubling time.
- Cell loss factor for human tumors has been estimated by Tubiana and Malaise to have an average value for a range of tumors in excess of 50%. Steel's estimate for a median value for all human tumors studied is 77%.

BIBLIOGRAPHY

Begg AC, Hofland I, Van Clabekke M, Bartlelink H, Horiot JC: Predictive value of potential doubling time for radiotherapy of head and neck tumor patients: Results from the EORTC Cooperative Trial 22851. *Semin Radiat Oncol* 2:22–25, 1992

Begg AC, McNally NJ, Shrieve D, et al.: A method to measure the duration of DNA synthesis and the potential doubling time from a single sample. *Cytometry* 6:620–625, 1985

Begg AC, Moonen I, Hofland I, et al.: Human tumor cell kinetics using a monoclonal antibody against iododeoxyuridine: Intratumoral sampling variations. *Radiother Oncol* 11:337–347, 1988

Bergonié J: Interpretation of some results of radiotherapy in an attempt at determining a logical technique of treatment (Tribondeau L, trans). *Radiat Res* 11:587–588, 1959

Bresciani F: A comparison of the generative cycle in normal hyperplastic and neoplastic mammary gland of the C3H mouse. In *Cellular Radiation Biology*, pp 547–557. Baltimore, Williams & Wilkins, 1965

Breuer K: Growth rate and radiosensitivity of human tumours: 1. Growth rate of human tumours. *Eur J Cancer* 2:157–171, 1966

Brown JM: The effect of acute x-irradiation on the cell proliferation kinetics of induced carcinomas and their normal counterpart. *Radiat Res* 43:627–653, 1970

Brown JM, Berry RJ: Effects of x-irradiation on the cell population kinetics in a model tumor and normal tissue system: Implication for the treatment of human malignancies. *Br J Radiol* 42:372–377, 1969

Collins VP, Loeffler K, Tivey J: Observation on growth rates of human tumors. *AJR Am J Roentgenol* 6:988–1000, 1956

Denekamp J: The cellular proliferation kinetics of animal tumors. *Cancer Res* 30:393–400, 1970

Denekamp J: The relationship between the "cell loss factor" and the immediate response to radiation in animal tumours. *Eur J Cancer* 8:335–340, 1972

Dolbeare F, Beisker W, Pallavicini MC, Vanderlaan M, Cary JW: Cytochemistry for BrDUrd/DNA analysis: Stoichiometry and sensitivity. *Cytometry* 6:521–530, 1985

Dolbeare F, Gratzner H, Pallavicini M, Gray JW: Flow cytometric measurement of total DNA content and incorporated bromodeoxyuridine. *Proc Natl Acad Sci USA* 80:5573–5577, 1983

Frankfurt OS: Mitotic cycle and cell differentiation in squamous cell carcinomas. *Int J Cancer* 2:304–310, 1967

Frindel E, Malaise EP, Alpen E, Tubiana M: Kinetics of cell proliferation of an experimental tumor. *Cancer Res* 27:1122–1131, 1967

Frindel E, Malaise EP, Tubiana M: Cell proliferation kinetics in five human solid tumors. *Cancer* 22:611–620, 1968

Frindel E, Valleron AJ, Vassort F, Tubiana M: Proliferation kinetics of an experimental ascites tumor of the mouse. *Cell Tissue Kinet* 2:51–65, 1969

Gray JW: Cell-cycle analysis of perturbed cell populations: Computer simulation of sequential DNA distributions. *Cell Tissue Kinet* 9:499–516, 1976

Gray JW, Carver JH, George YS, Mendelsohn ML: Rapid cell cycle analysis by measurement of the radioactivity per cell in a narrow window in S-phase (RCSi). *Cell Tissue Kinet* 10:97–104, 1977

Gray JW, Dolbeare F, Pallavicini MG, Beisker W, Waldman F: Cell cycle analysis using flow cytometry. *Int J Radiat Biol* 49:237–255, 1986

Hermens AF, Barendsen CW: Cellular proliferation patterns in an experimental rhabdomyosarcoma in the rat. *Eur J Cancer* 3:361–369, 1967

Hoshima T, Yagashima T, Morovic J, Livin E, Livin V: Cell kinetic studies of in situ human brain tumors with bromodeoxyuridine. *Cytometry* 6:627–632, 1985

Howard A, Pelc SR: Synthesis of deoxyribonucleic acid in normal and irradiated cells and its relation to chromosome breakage. *Heredity* 6(suppl):261, 1952

Lesher S: Compensatory reactions in intestinal crypt cells after 300 roentgens of cobalt-60 gamma irradiation. *Radiat Res* 32:510–519, 1967

Mendelsohn ML: Autoradiography analysis of cell proliferation in spontaneous breast cancer of the C3H mouse: III. The growth fraction. *JNCI* 28:1015–1029, 1962

Mendelsohn ML: The growth fraction: A new concept applied to tumors. *Science* 132:1496, 1960

Mendelsohn ML: Principles, relative merits, and limitations of current cytokinetic methods. In Drewinko B, Humphrey RM (eds): *Growth Kinetics and Biochemical Regulation of Normal and Malignant Cells*, pp 101–112. Baltimore, Williams & Wilkins, 1977

Morstyn C, Hsu S-M, Kinsella T, Gratzuer H, Russo A, Mitchell J: Bromodeoxyuridine in tumors and chromosomes detected with a monoclonal antibody. *J Clin Invest* 72:1844–1850, 1983

Palekar SK, Sirsat SM: Replication time pattern of transplanted fibrosarcoma in the mouse. *Indian J Exp Biol* 5:173–175, 1967

Post J, Hoffman J: The replication time and pattern of carcinogen-induced hepatoma cells. *J Cell Biol* 22:341–350, 1964

Quastler H, Sherman FG: Cell population kinetics in the intestinal epithelium of the mouse. *Exp Cell Res* 17:420–438, 1959

Raashad AL, Evans CA: Radioautographic study of epidermal cell proliferation and migration in normal and neoplastic tissues of rabbits. *JNCI* 41:845–853, 1968

Refsum SB, Berdal P: Cell loss in malignant tumors in man. *Eur J Cancer* 3:235–236, 1967

Reiskin AB, Berry RJ: Cell proliferation and carcinogenesis in the hamster cheek pouch. *Cancer Res* 28:898–905, 1968

Reiskin AB, Mendelsohn ML: A comparison of the cell cycle in induced carcinomas and their normal counterpart. *Cancer Res* 24:1131–1136, 1964

Simpson-Herren L, Blow JG, Brown PH: The mitotic cycle of sarcoma 180. *Cancer Res* 28:724–726, 1968

Steel GG: Autoradiographic analysis of the cell cycle: Howard and Pelc to the present day. *Int J Radiat Biol* 49:227–235, 1986

Steel GG: Cell loss as a factor in the growth rate of human tumours. *Eur J Cancer* 3:381–387, 1967

Steel GG: Cell loss from experimental tumours. *Cell Tissue Kinet* 1:193–207, 1968

Steel GG: The growth kinetics of tumors in relation to their therapeutic response. *Laryngoscope* 85:359–370, 1975

Steel GG: The kinetics of cell proliferation in tumors. In Bond VP (ed): *Proceedings of the Carmel Conference on Time and Dose Relationships in Radiation Biology as Applied to Radiotherapy*, pp 130–149. BNL Report 50203 (C-57). Upton, NY, 1969

Steel GG, Adams K, Barratt JC: Analysis of the cell population kinectics of transplanted tumours of widely differing growth rate. *Br J Cancer* 20:784–800, 1966

Steel GG, Haynes S: The technique labeled mitoses: Analyses by automatic curve fitting. *Cell Tissue Kinet* 4:93–105, 1971

Tubiana M, Malaise E: Growth rate and cell kinetics in human tumors: Some prognostic and therapeutic implications. In Symington T, Carter RL (eds): *Scientific Foundations of Oncology*, pp 126–136. Chicago, Year Book Medical Publishers, 1976

CHAPTER 22

Time, Dose, and Fractionation in Radiotherapy

THE INTRODUCTION OF FRACTIONATION

The multifraction regimens commonly used in conventional radiation therapy are a consequence largely of radiobiologic experiments performed in France in the 1920s and 1930s. It was found that a ram could not be sterilized by exposing its testes to a single dose of radiation without extensive skin damage to the scrotum, whereas if the radiation was spread out over a period of weeks in a series of daily fractions, sterilization was possible without producing unacceptable skin damage (Fig. 22.1). It was postulated that the testes were a model of a growing tumor, whereas the skin of the scrotum represented a dose-limiting normal-tissue. The reasoning may be flawed, but the conclusion proved to be valid: Fractionation of the radiation dose produces, in most cases, better tumor control for a given level of normal-tissue toxicity than a single large dose.

THE FOUR Rs OF RADIOBIOLOGY

Now, more than 80 years later, we can account for the efficacy of fractionation based on more relevant radiobiologic experiments. We can appeal to the "four Rs" of Radiobiology:

Repair of sublethal damage
Reassortment of cells within the cell cycle
Repopulation
Reoxygenation

The basis of fractionation in radiotherapy can be understood in simple terms. Dividing a dose into a number of fractions spares normal tissues because of repair of sublethal damage between dose fractions and repopulation of cells if the overall time is sufficiently long. At the same time, dividing a dose into a number of fractions increases damage to the tumor because of reoxygenation and reassortment

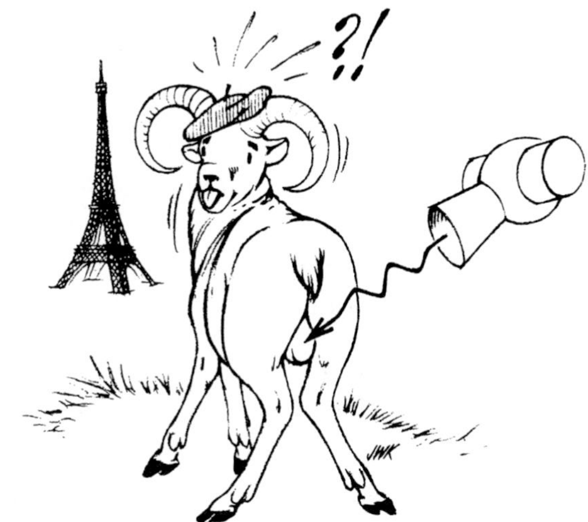

FIGURE 22.1 • Conventional multifraction radiotherapy was based on experiments performed in Paris in the 1920s and 1930s. Rams could not be sterilized with a single dose of x-rays without extensive skin damage, whereas if the radiation were delivered in daily fractions over a period of time, sterilization was possible without skin damage. The testes were regarded as a model of a growing tumor and skin as dose-limiting normal tissue.

of cells into radiosensitive phases of the cycle between dose fractions.

The advantages of prolongation of treatment are to spare early reactions and to allow adequate reoxygenation in tumors. Excessive prolongation, however, allows surviving tumor cells to proliferate during treatment.

THE STRANDQUIST PLOT AND THE ELLIS NOMINAL STANDARD DOSE SYSTEM

Early attempts to understand and account for fractionation gave rise to the well-known Strandquist plot, in which total dose was plotted as a function of the overall treatment time (Fig. 22.2). Because all treatments were given as three or five fractions per week, overall time in this plot contains, by implication, the number of fractions as well. It commonly was found in these plots that the slope of the isoeffect curve for skin was about 0.33; that is, the total dose for an isoeffect was proportional to $T^{0.33}$.

The most important contribution in this area, made by Ellis and his colleagues with the introduction of the **nominal standard dose (NSD)** system, was the recognition of the importance of separating overall time from the number of fractions. According to this hypothesis, total dose for the tolerance of connective tissue is related to the number of fractions (N) and the overall time (T) by the relation

$$\text{Total dose} = (\text{NSD})T^{0.11}N^{0.24}$$

The NSD system has been discussed extensively. It does enable predictions to be made of equivalent dose regimens, provided that the range of time and number of fractions are not too great and do not exceed the range over which the data are available. For example, in changing a treatment protocol from five to four fractions per week, the formula can be used to calculate the size of dose fractions needed to result in the same normal-tissue tolerance with the two different protocols. Of course, because the system is based ultimately on skin reaction data, it does not in any way predict *late effects*. An obvious

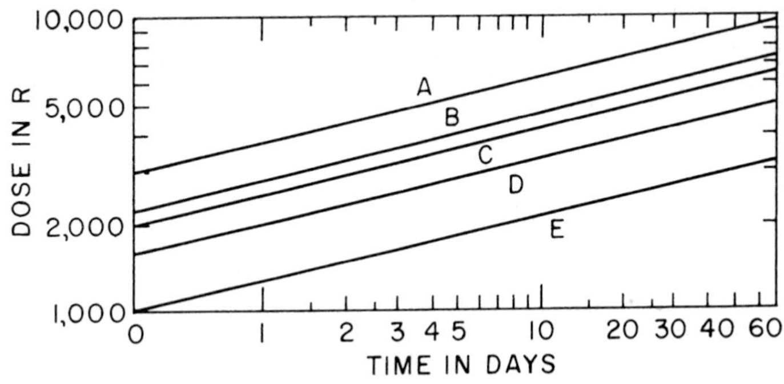

FIGURE 22.2 • Isoeffect curves relating the total dose to the overall treatment time for skin necrosis (A), cure of skin carcinoma (B), moist desquamation of skin (C), dry desquamation of skin (D), and skin erythema (E). (Adapted from Strandquist M: A study of the cumulative effect of fractionated x-ray treatment based on the experience mined at the Radium Hemmant with the treatment of 280 cases of carcinoma of the skin and lip. *Acta Radiol* 55[suppl]:1–300, 1944, with permission.)

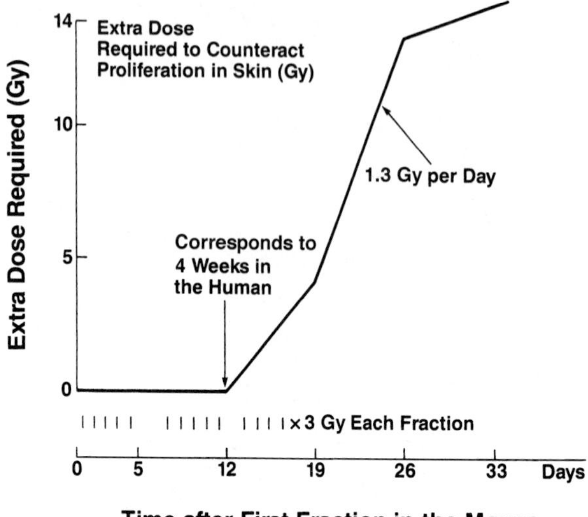

FIGURE 22.3 • The extra dose required to counteract proliferation in the skin of mice as a function of time after starting daily irradiation with 3 Gy (300 rad) per fraction. A delay followed by a rapid rise is typical of time factors in proliferating normal tissues. In mouse skin, the delay is about 2 weeks; in humans, it is about 4 weeks. (Adapted from Fowler JF: Fractionated radiation therapy after Strandquist. *Acta Radiol* 23:209–216, 1984, with permission; data from Denekamp J: Changes in the rate of repopulation during multifraction irradiation of mouse skin. *Br J Radiol* 46:381, 1973.)

weakness of the NSD system is that time is allowed for in terms of a single power function, in which the nominal single dose is proportional to $T^{0.11}$. In fact, biologic experiments with small animals have shown that this relationship is far from accurate. Proliferation does not affect the total dose required to produce a given biologic reaction at all until some time after the start of irradiation, but then the dependence in time is much greater than allowed for by the Ellis formula.

PROLIFERATION AS A FACTOR IN NORMAL TISSUES

Experimental evidence indicates that the total dose required to produce a given biologic effect is not a power function of time, as postulated by the Ellis NSD system, but turns out to be more complex. The extra dose required to counter proliferation and result in a given level of skin damage in mice does not increase at all until about 12 days into a fractionated regimen, but then it increases very rapidly as a function of time. The shape of the curve is roughly sigmoidal (Fig. 22.3). If similar data were available for humans, the effects of proliferation would not be seen until a longer period into a fractionation regimen because of the slower response of the human skin and the longer cell cycle of the individual cells. Figure 22.3 is not meant to be quantitative but to indicate that the shape of the curve relating extra dose to proliferation is sigmoidal. This illustrates immediately that the method of allowing for overall time in the NSD system is incorrect or at best a very crude approximation.

A further consideration is that all normal tissues are not the same. In particular, there is a clear distinction between tissues that are *early responding*, such as the skin, mucosa, and intestinal epithelium, and those that are *late responding*, such as the spinal cord. Figure 22.4 shows the extra dose required to

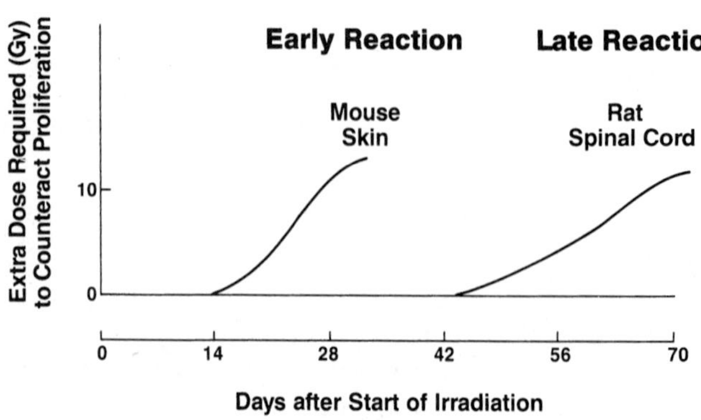

FIGURE 22.4 • The extra dose required to counteract proliferation only as a function of time after starting daily irradiation in rodents. The left curve represents a typical early reaction; the right curve represents a typical late reaction. The delays are much longer in humans. (Adapted from Fowler JF: The second Klaas Breur memorial lecture. La Ronde—radiation sciences and medical radiology. *Radiother Oncol* 1:1–22, 1983, with permission.)

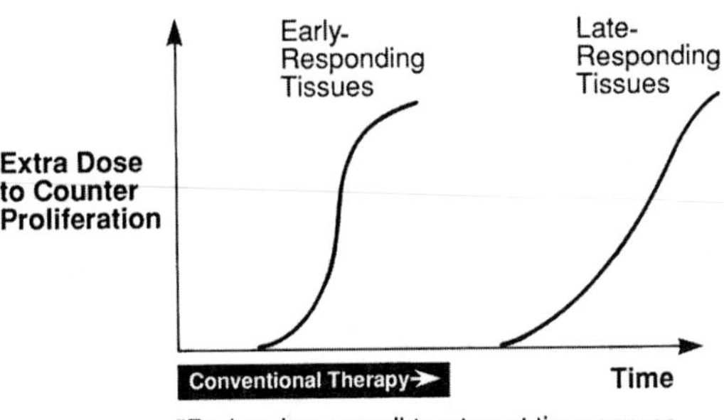

FIGURE 22.5 ● Highly speculative illustration attempting to extrapolate the experimental data for early- and late-responding tissue in rats and mice to principles that can be applied in clinical radiotherapy. The extra dose required to counter proliferation in early-responding tissues begins to increase after a few weeks into a fractionated regimen, certainly during the time course of conventional therapy. By contrast, conventional protocols are never sufficiently long to include the proliferation of late-responding tissues.

produce a given level of damage for a fractionated protracted regimen in the case of representative tissues from the early- and late-responding groups. This diagram compares mouse skin, representative of early-responding tissues, and rat spinal cord, representative of late-responding tissues. It is recognized that these may not be ideal examples, but suitable data for more relevant systems are simply not available; comparable quantitative data certainly are not available for humans. The point made by this figure is that the time after the start of a fractionated regimen at which extra dose is required to compensate for cellular proliferation is quite different for late- versus early-responding tissues. The other point made, of course, is that these are data from rodents and that in the case of humans, the time scales (although they are not known with any precision) are likely to be very much longer. In particular, the time at which extra dose is required to compensate for proliferation in late-responding tissues in humans is far beyond the overall time of any normal radiotherapy regimen.

Figure 22.5 is an attempt to convert the experimental laboratory data contained in Figure 22.4 into a general principle that can be applied to clinical practice. Early-responding tissues are triggered to proliferate within a few weeks of the start of a fractionated regimen so that the "extra dose to counter proliferation" increases with time, certainly during conventional radiotherapeutic protocols. By contrast, conventional radiotherapy extending to 6 or 8 weeks is never long enough to allow the triggering of proliferation in late-responding tissues. These considerations lead to the following important axiom:

> Prolonging overall time within the normal radiotherapy range has little sparing effect on late reactions but a large sparing effect on early reactions.

This has far-reaching consequences in radiotherapy. Early reactions, such as reactions of the skin or of the mucosa, can be dealt with easily by the simple expedient of prolonging the overall time. Although such a strategy overcomes the problem of the early reactions, it has no effect whatsoever on the late reactions.

THE SHAPE OF THE DOSE–RESPONSE RELATIONSHIP FOR EARLY- AND LATE-RESPONDING TISSUES

Clinical and laboratory data suggest that there is a consistent difference between early- and late-responding tissues in their responses to changing fractionation patterns. If fewer and larger dose fractions are given, late reactions are more severe, even though early reactions are matched by an appropriate adjustment in total dose. This dissociation can be interpreted as differences in repair capacity or shoulder shape of the underlying dose–response curves. The dose–response relationship for late-responding tissues is more curved than that for early-responding tissues. In terms of the linear-quadratic relationship between effect and dose, this translates into a larger α/β ratio for early effects than for late effects. The difference in the shapes of the dose–response relationships is illustrated in Figure 22.6. The α/β ratio is the dose at which cell killing by the linear (α) and quadratic (β) components are equal.

For early effects, α/β is large; as a consequence, α dominates at low doses, so that the dose–response curve has a marked initial slope and does not bend until higher doses. The linear and quadratic components of cell killing are not equal until about 10 Gy (1,000 rad). For late effects, α/β is small, so that the β term has an influence at low doses. The dose–response curve bends at lower doses to appear more curvy; the linear and quadratic components of cell killing are equal by about 2 Gy (200 rad).

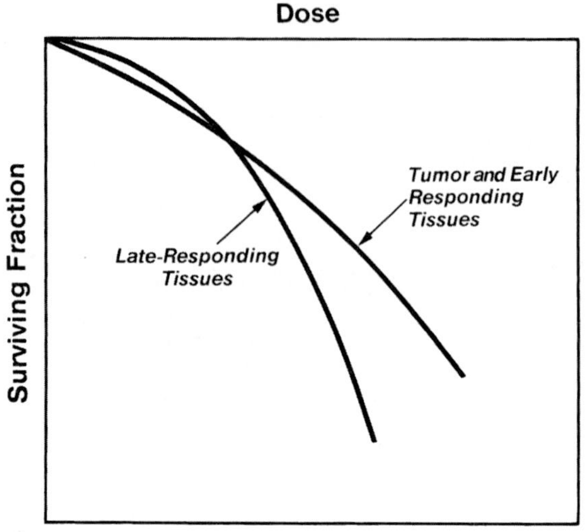

FIGURE 22.6 • The dose–response relationship for late-responding tissues is more curved than for early-responding tissues. In the linear-quadratic formulation, this translates into a larger α/β ratio for early effects than for late effects. The ratio α/β is the dose at which the linear (α) and the quadratic (β) components of cell killing are equal: that is, $\alpha D = \beta D^2$, or $D = \alpha/\beta$. (Based on the concepts of Withers.)

Dose–response curves for organ function must be distinguished clearly from those for clonogenic cell survival. The distinction is not a trivial one. Organ function obviously is related more to the proportion of functional cells remaining in an irradiated organ at a particular time than to the proportion of clonogenic (stem) cells. The dose–effect curves for clonogenic cells tend to be straight, with relatively small shoulders, whereas dose–effect relations for organ function tend to be more curved, with larger shoulders. It is, of course, the dose–response curves for organ function that are more relevant to the tolerance of normal tissues.

There are three pieces of information from clinical experience and animal studies that represent circumstantial evidence for the conclusion that the shape of the dose–response relationship differs for early- and late-responding tissues. First, if a fractionation scheme is changed in clinical practice from many small doses to a few large fractions and the total dose is titrated to produce equal early effects, the treatment protocol involving a few large fractions results in *more severe late effects*. There is an abundance of clinical evidence for the truth of this statement.

Second, clinical trials of hyperfractionation, in which two doses are delivered per day for 6 or 7 weeks, appear to result in greatly reduced late effects if the total dose is titrated to produce equal or possibly slightly more severe acute effects. Tumor control is the same or slightly improved. This important clinical observation has been made in a number of centers and again is compatible with the same difference in shape of dose–response curves between early- and late-responding tissues. Late-effect tissues are more sensitive to changes in fractionation patterns than are early-responding tissues.

Third, in experiments with small laboratory animals, the isoeffect curves (i.e., dose versus number of fractions to produce an equal biologic effect) are *steeper* for a range of late effects than for a variety of acute effects. The data are shown in Figure 22.7, in which early effects are represented by, for example, skin desquamation or jejunal crypt colonies, and late effects are represented by, for example, lung or spinal cord injury.

Table 22.1 is a summary of the values of α/β for a number of early- and late-responding tissues. The important result is that for early-responding tissues, α/β (i.e., the dose at which single- and multiple-event cell killing is about equal) occurs at the dose of about 10 Gy (1,000 rad). By contrast, α/β for late-responding tissues is about 2 Gy (200 rad). The values of α/β shown in Table 22.1 come from experiments in which the reciprocal of the total dose is plotted against the quadratic relationship in biologic systems in which it is possible to observe equal effects from various fractionation regimens, even though single-cell dose–survival curves cannot be generated (Fig. 18.28).

The parameters derived from curves reconstructed from multifraction experiments are specifically relevant to the end point measured in each experiment, whether it is a proportion of clonogenic cells or a stated reduction in organ function. The dose–response curve constructed from multifraction experimental data by making simple assumptions is a functional dose–response curve, deduced from data in which repair after each fractional dose is basically the quantity being measured. It is just such functional dose–response curves that are required to elucidate the relationship between tolerance dose in radiotherapy and size of dose per fraction, with overall time considered separately.

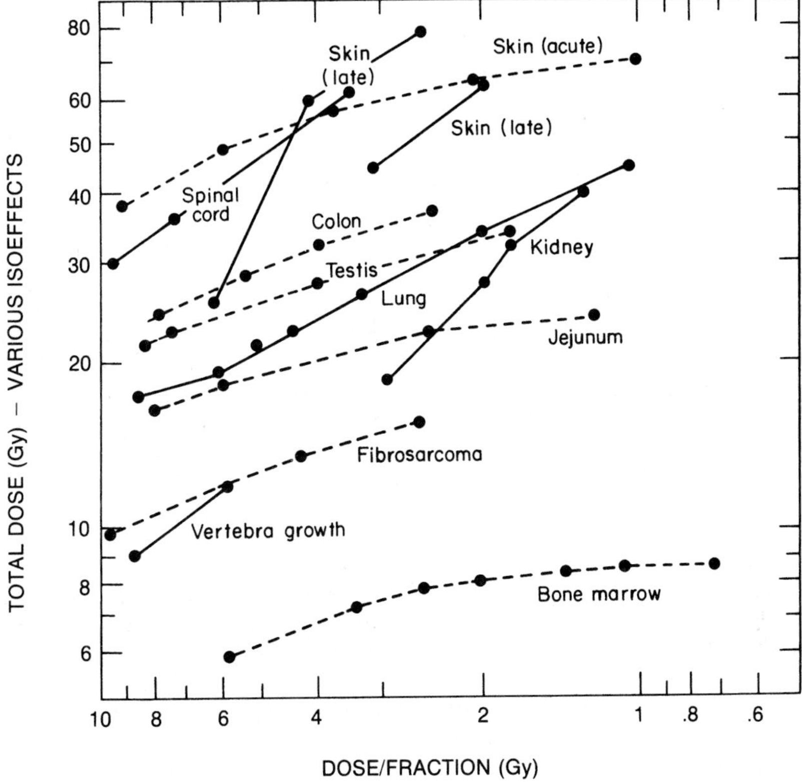

FIGURE 22.7 ● Isoeffect curves in which the total dose necessary for a certain effect in various tissues in laboratory animals is plotted as a function of dose per fraction. Late effects are plotted with solid lines, acute effects with dashed lines. The data were selected to exclude an influence on the total dose of regeneration during the multifraction experiments. The main point of the data is that the isodoses for late effects increase more rapidly with a decrease in dose per fraction than is the case for acute effects. (From Withers HR: Biologic basis for altered fractionation schemes. *Cancer* 55:2086–2095, 1985, with permission.)

TABLE 22.1

Ratio of Linear to Quadratic Terms from Multifraction Experiments

Reactions	α/β, Gy
Early	
Skin	9–12
Jejunum	6–10
Colon	10–11
Testis	12–13
Callus	9–10
Late	
Spinal cord	1.7–4.9
Kidney	1.0–2.4
Lung	2.0–6.3
Bladder	3.1–7

A POSSIBLE EXPLANATION FOR THE DIFFERENCE IN SHAPE OF DOSE–RESPONSE RELATIONSHIPS FOR EARLY- AND LATE- RESPONDING TISSUES

The radiosensitivity of a population of cells varies with the distribution of cells through the cycle. In general, cells are most resistant in late S phase; slowly growing cells with a long cycle, however, may have a second resistant phase in the early G_1 phase, which may be termed G_0 if the cells are out of cycle. Thus, two quite different cell populations may be radioresistant:

1. A population proliferating so fast that S phase occupies a major portion of the cycle.
2. A population proliferating so slowly that many cells are in early G_1 or not proliferating at all, so that many resting cells are in G_0.

It is thought that many late-responding normal tissues are resistant owing to the presence of many resting cells. This type of resistance applies particularly to small doses per fraction and disappears at larger doses per fraction.

If resistance results from the presence of many cells in S phase in a rapidly proliferating population, redistribution occurs through all the phases of the cell cycle, which can be considered a "self-sensitizing" activity. The fast proliferation itself is a form of resistance, because the new cells produced by division offset those killed by the dose fractions. This applies to *acutely responding tissues* and also to *tumors*. Proliferation occurring during a protracted, fractionated regimen helps to spare normal tissues but of course is a potential danger as far as the tumor is concerned. This is discussed subsequently in this chapter.

FRACTION SIZE AND OVERALL TREATMENT TIME: INFLUENCE ON EARLY- AND LATE-RESPONDING TISSUES

The difference in shape of the dose–response relationship for early- and late-responding tissues leads to an important axiom:

> Fraction size is the dominant factor in determining late effects; overall treatment time has little influence. By contrast, fraction size and overall treatment time both determine the response of acutely responding tissues.

It is remarkable that neither clinical radiation oncologists nor experimental radiobiologists came to recognize this simple fact before it was described by Withers in the 1980s.

ACCELERATED REPOPULATION

Treatment with any cytotoxic agent, including radiation, can trigger surviving cells (clonogens) in a tumor to divide faster than before. This is known as **accelerated repopulation**.

Figure 22.8 illustrates this phenomenon in a transplanted rat tumor. Figure 22.8**A** shows the overall growth curve for this tumor, together with the shrinkage and regrowth that occurs after a single dose of 20 Gy (2,000 rad) of x-rays. Figure 22.8**B** shows the proliferation of individual surviving cells (i.e., clonogenic cells), which, after treatment, are dividing with a cycle time of 12 hours. The important point to note is that during the time that the tumor is overtly shrinking and regressing, the surviving clonogens are dividing and increasing in number more rapidly than ever.

There is evidence for a similar phenomenon in human tumors. Withers and his colleagues surveyed the literature on radiotherapy for head and neck cancer and estimated the dose to achieve local control in 50% of cases as a function of the overall duration of fractionated treatment. The results are summarized in Figure 22.9. The analysis suggests that clonogen repopulation in this human cancer accelerates at about 28 days after the initiation of radiotherapy in a fractionated regimen. A dose increment of about 0.6 Gy (60 rad) per day is required to compensate for this repopulation. Such a dose increment is consistent with a 4-day clonogen doubling rate, compared with a median of about 60 days for unperturbed growth.

The conclusion to be drawn from this is that radiotherapy, at least for head and neck cancer and probably in other instances also, should be completed as soon after it has begun as is practicable. It may be better to delay initiation of treatment than to introduce delays during treatment. If overall treatment time is too long, the effectiveness of later dose fractions is compromised because the surviving clonogens in the tumor have been triggered into rapid repopulation.

The experimental data referred to here all relate to radiotherapy. It might be anticipated, however, that similar considerations would apply to chemotherapy or to a combination of radiotherapy and chemotherapy. There is evidence in some human malignancies that radiotherapy produces poorer results if preceded by a course of chemotherapy. It may be that accelerated repopulation, triggered by the chemotherapy, is the explanation.

MULTIPLE FRACTIONS PER DAY

We are now in a position to sum up the pros and cons of fractionation and prolongation of treatment in a much more sophisticated way than would have been possible at the beginning of this chapter. The advantages of prolongation of treatment are to spare early reactions and to allow adequate reoxygenation in tumors. Excessive prolongation, however, has two disadvantages: It can decrease deceptively the acute reactions without sparing late injury, and it allows the surviving tumor cells to proliferate during treatment. There are two separate strategies that use multiple treatments per day: hyperfractionation and accelerated treatment. The aims and objectives of these strategies are quite different.

Hyperfractionation

The basic aim of hyperfractionation is to further separate early and late effects. "Pure" hyperfractionation might be defined as keeping the same

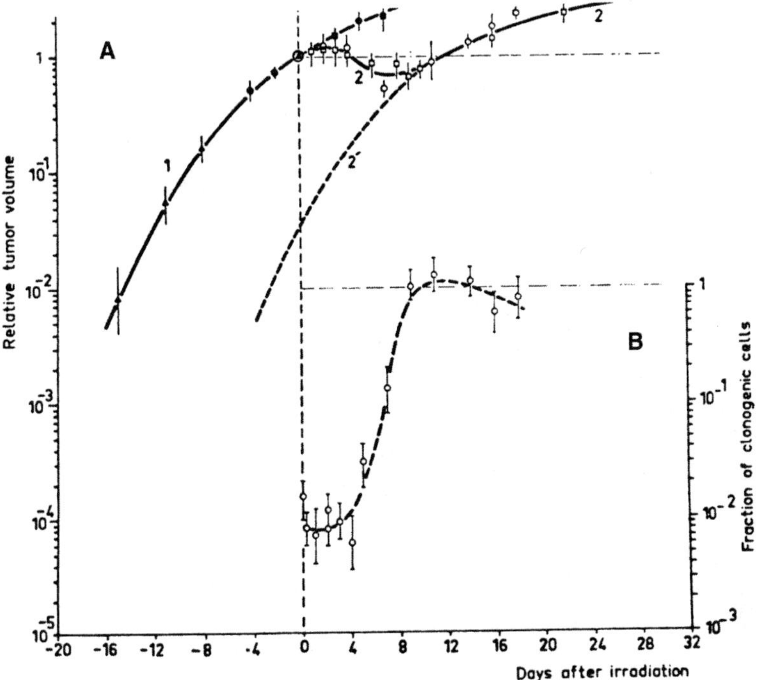

FIGURE 22.8 ● Accelerated repopulation. Growth curves of a rat rhabdomyosarcoma showing the shrinkage, growth delay, and subsequent recurrence following treatment with a single dose of 20 Gy (2,000 rad) of x-rays. **A:** Curve 1: Growth curve of unirradiated control tumors. Curve 2: Growth curve of tumors irradiated at time t = 0, showing tumor shrinkage and recurrence. **B:** Variation of the fraction of clonogenic cells as a function of time after irradiation, obtained by removing cells from the tumor and assaying for colony formation *in vitro*. The surviving clonogenic cells are dividing rapidly with a cell cycle of about 12 hours. (From Hermens AF, Barendsen GW: Changes of cell proliferation characteristics in a rat rhabdomyosarcoma before and after x-irradiation. *Eur J Cancer* 5:173–189, 1969, with permission.)

total dose as in a conventional regimen in the same overall time but delivering it in twice as many fractions by the expedient of treating twice per day. This would not be satisfactory, because the total dose would need to be increased if the dose per fraction is decreased. In practice, then, "impure" hyperfractionation involves an increase in the total dose and sometimes a longer overall time as well as many more fractions delivered twice per day. The intent is to further reduce late effects but achieve the same or better tumor control and the same or slightly increased early effects.

A large controlled clinical trial of hyperfractionation was conducted in the 1990s by the European Cooperative Group (EORTC 22791) in the treatment of head and neck cancer. A hyperfractionated schedule of 80.5 Gy delivered in 70 fractions (1.15 Gy twice per day) over a period of 7 weeks was compared with a conventional regimen of 70 Gy delivered in 35 fractions of 2 Gy over 7 weeks. Local tumor control at 5 years was increased from 40% with the conventional regimen to 59% with hyperfractionation, and this was reflected in improved survival. There was no increase reported in late effects or complications. It was concluded that hyperfractionation confers an unequivocal advantage in the treatment of oropharyngeal cancer.

The hyperfractionation results of the cooperative trial are summarized as follows:

- Comparing 80.5 Gy in 70 fractions (1.15 Gy twice per day), 7 weeks, with 70 Gy in 35 fractions, 7 weeks
- Local tumor control, at 5 years, increased from 40 to 59%, reflected also in improved survival
- No increase in side effects
- Unequivocal advantage for hyperfractionation in oropharyngeal cancer

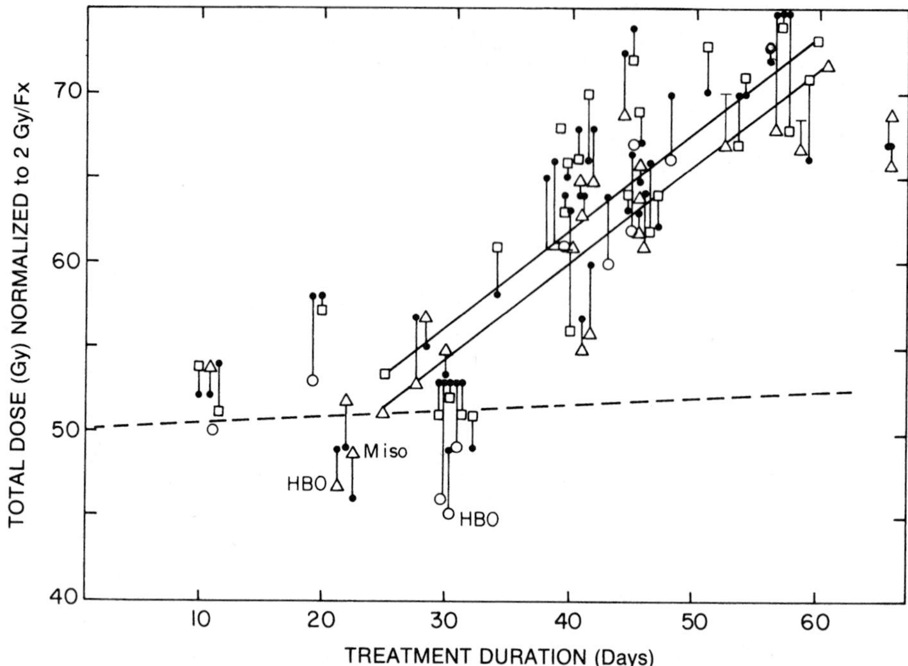

FIGURE 22.9 • Doses to achieve local control in 50% of cases (TCD_{50}), as a function of overall treatment time, for squamous cell tumors of the head and neck. The data points include many published results from the literature, including hyperbaric oxygen (HBO) trials and the trial of misonidazole (Miso). In those cases involving hypofractionation, the total dose was corrected to be relevant to a treatment schedule of 2 Gy per day. The dashed line shows the rate of increase in TCD_{50} predicted from a 2-month clonogen doubling rate. (From Withers HR, Taylor JMG, Maciejewski B: The hazard of accelerated tumor clonogen repopulation during radiotherapy. *Acta Oncol* 27:131–146, 1988, with permission.)

Two fractions per day may not be the limit of hyperfractionation: A further sparing of late effects by splitting the dose into more and more fractions of smaller and smaller size would occur as long as the dose fraction is still on the curved portion of the dose–response curve. In order not to prolong overall treatment time too much, these small doses per fraction would necessitate three or even four fractions per day.

Accelerated Treatment

The alternative strategy to hyperfractionation is **accelerated treatment**. "Pure" accelerated treatment might be defined as the same total dose delivered in half the overall time by the expedient of giving two or more fractions each day. In practice, it is never possible to achieve this because the acute effects become limiting. It is necessary either to interpose a rest period in the middle of the treatment or to reduce the dose slightly with acute effects as the limiting factor. The intent of this accelerated treatment strategy is to reduce repopulation in rapidly proliferating tumors. There should be little or no change in the late effects, because the number of fractions and the dose per fraction are unaltered.

A large prospective randomized clinical trial of accelerated treatment for head and neck cancer, except oropharynx, was carried out in the 1990s by the European Cooperative Group (EORTC 22851). The accelerated treatment consisted of 72 Gy in 45 fractions (three fractions of 1.6 Gy per day) over a total time of 5 weeks, with a rest of 2 weeks in the middle. The conventional control arm consisted of 35 fractions of 2 Gy, with a total dose of 70 Gy in 7 weeks. The results of this trial showed a 15% increase in locoregional control, which did not translate, however, into a survival advantage. As expected, acute effects were increased significantly, but the observed increase in late effects was decidedly not expected; some involved complications that proved lethal.

This EORTC trial and several other trials testing accelerated treatment show that attempting to keep the total dose as high as 66 to 72 Gy but shorten the overall time by as much as 2 to 3 weeks from a conventional 6 or 7 weeks leads to serious late complications. There are probably two reasons for this: First, the late effects observed are "consequential" late damage, that is, late damage developing out of the very severe acute effects. Second, there is incomplete repair between dose fractions if several fractions per day are given. This is especially likely for protocols involving three fractions per day, in which any unrepaired damage in the first interval accumulates in the second interval in each day, and also because intervals between fractions of only 4 hours were used in the early years of the EORTC trial.

This cooperative trial's results for accelerated treatment are summarized as follows:

- Head and neck cancer, except oropharynx
- Comparing 72 Gy in 45 fractions (1.6 Gy, three fractions per day), 5 weeks, with 70 Gy in 35 fractions, 7 weeks
- 15% increase in locoregional control, no survival advantage
- Increased acute effects (expected)
- Unexpected increase in late effects, including lethal complications
- Evidence that pure accelerated treatment must be used with extreme caution

Continuous Hyperfractionated Accelerated Radiation Therapy (CHART)

A unique and most interesting study of accelerated treatment was carried out in the 1990s at the Mount Vernon Hospital (United Kingdom) in association with the Gray Laboratory. This trial is known as **continuous hyperfractionated accelerated radiation therapy** (**CHART**). The protocol consisted of 36 fractions over 12 consecutive days, with three fractions delivered daily with an interfraction interval of 6 hours. The dose per fraction was 1.4 to 1.5 Gy, to a total dose of 50 to 54 Gy. By conventional standards, the total dose was very low, but it was delivered in a very short time. The strategy was based on a low dose per fraction to minimize late effects and a very short overall time to minimize tumor proliferation. The results of the CHART protocol showed good local tumor control with severe acute reactions. It was claimed that patients favored the protocol because treatment was concluded quickly. The incidence of late effects in general did not increase and by some measures actually decreased. The notable exception was damage to the spinal cord. Several myelopathies were recorded at total doses of 50 Gy (5,000 rad), the probable cause being that an interfraction interval of 6 hours is not sufficient for the full repair of sublethal damage in this tissue.

Characteristics of continuous hyperfractionated accelerated radiation therapy (CHART) included:

- Low dose/fractionation: 36 fractions
- Short overall time: 12 consecutive days
- No gap in treatment: three fractions per day at 6-hour intervals
- Three fractions per day: 1.4 to 1.5 Gy per fraction, 50 to 54 Gy total

CHART is the only one of the "new" fractionation schedules that results in a *lower* incidence of late complications. CHART's severe but tolerable acute reactions did not translate into late sequelae, probably because the total dose (50–54 Gy) was so low. Effectiveness in tumor control was not lost even at this low dose because the shortening of overall time was extreme, minimizing tumor cell proliferation. Compliance was also high with CHART because acute reactions did not peak and become uncomfortable until after the end of treatment.

The results of CHART can be summarized as follows:

- Good local tumor control owing to short overall time
- Acute reactions that are brisk but peak after treatment is completed
- Most late effects acceptable because of small dose per fraction
- Exception: spinal cord, with several myelopathies occurring at 50 Gy because the time between fractions (6 hours) was too short

Accelerated Hyperfractionated Radiation Therapy while Breathing Carbogen and with the Addition of Nicotinamide (ARCON)

The last experimental protocol that deserves mention is accelerated hyperfractionated radiation therapy while breathing carbogen and with the addition of nicotinamide (ARCON). The strategy was to accelerate treatment to avoid tumor proliferation, hyperfractionate (small doses per fraction) to minimize late effects, and add carbogen breathing to overcome chronic hypoxia and nicotinamide to overcome acute hypoxia. Clinical trials to test this complex but imaginative protocol are under way in Europe. Early results of a trial of ARCON in the Netherlands, involving advanced laryngeal cancer, showed spectacular results compared with historical controls. Results of a prospective randomized trial have yet to be published.

Characteristics of ARCON are summarized as follows:

- Accelerated treatment to overcome proliferation
- Hyperfractionated to spare normal tissues
- Carbogen breathing to overcome chronic hypoxia
- Nicotinamide to overcome acute hypoxia

The Time Interval between Multiple Daily Fractions

One thing the two strategies of hyperfractionation and accelerated treatment have in common is that both involve multiple fractions per day, and in this context it is important to ensure that the fractions are separated by a sufficient time interval for the effects of the doses to be independent—that is, for the repair of sublethal damage from the first dose to be complete before the next dose is delivered. With cells cultured *in vitro*, the half-time of repair is usually about 1 hour, although there is evidence that for cells of human origin cultured *in vitro*, it may vary widely from a few minutes to several hours. For normal tissues *in vivo*, it has been inferred from fractionation experiments that the repair of sublethal damage may be very much slower in late-responding tissues.

The most pertinent and remarkable evidence comes from twice-a-day trials by the Radiation Therapy Oncology Group (RTOG) that indicate that for a given total dose delivered in a given number of fractions, the incidence of late effects is worse for interfraction intervals less than 4 hours compared with interfraction intervals longer than 6 hours. These data imply that the repair of sublethal damage in late-responding tissues is slow, and so current wisdom dictates an interfraction interval of 6 hours or more if multiple fractions per day are used. Indeed, the CHART pilot study clearly indicated that even 6 hours is not sufficient for the spinal cord, a late-responding tissue in which, it appears, sublethal damage repair has a very slow component. This is radiobiology learned from the clinic.

LESSONS LEARNED FROM FRACTIONATION STUDIES

A number of lessons have been learned from the clinical trials that have been performed to test the usefulness of altered fractionation patterns:

First, hyperfractionation appears to confer an unequivocal benefit in the treatment of head and neck cancer, in terms of both local control and survival, without a significant increase in late sequelae. By contrast, caution is needed in the application of accelerated treatment, because the EORTC trials showed an unexpected increase in serious complications, both early and late. Particular caution is necessary if the spinal cord is in the treatment field for twice-a-day treatments, because repair of sublethal damage has a slow component in this tissue.

Second, late effects depend primarily on total dose and dose per fraction; overall time within the usual therapeutic range has little influence.

Third, overall treatment time affects both acute effects and tumor control. Gaps in treatment should be avoided because they lead to an increase in overall time with a concomitant decrease in tumor control.

The importance of overall treatment time is illustrated dramatically by the retrospective analysis by Overgaard of three consecutive trials of the Danish cooperative group. All three trials involved a total dose of 66 to 68 Gy (6,600–6,800 rad). The first trial was of a split-course regimen that extended over a total of 9.5 weeks. The 3-year local control was 32%. The second trial involved five fractions per week over a treatment time of 6.5 weeks, with a 3-year local control of 52%. The third trial included six fractions per week, reducing the overall treatment time to 5.5 weeks and improving the 3-year local control to 62%. There was no change in late effects, but as would be expected, the acute reactions became brisker as the overall time was shortened. The protocols and results of these three trials are illustrated in Figure 22.10. These most interesting data must be viewed with some caution, because the three treatment arms were not in a single randomized study but come from different trials over a period of years, the initial purpose of which was to investigate the usefulness of hypoxic-cell radiosensitizers. They indicate strongly, nevertheless, that in the case of relatively rapidly growing tumors, such as head and neck cancer, overall treatment time can be a dominant factor in determining outcome (Table 22.2).

One of the major lessons to be learned from fractionation studies is that local control is lost if overall treatment time is prolonged. Since it first was proposed independently in the 1980s by Withers and by Fowler, it is now well documented for head and neck cancer that local control is reduced by about 1.4% (range 0.4–2.5%) for each day that the overall treatment time is prolonged. This does not differ much from the other way of expressing the same problem—namely, that (after the first 4 weeks of a fractionated schedule) the first 0.61 Gy of each day's dose fraction is required to overcome proliferation from the previous day. An equally solid estimate can be made from data for carcinoma of

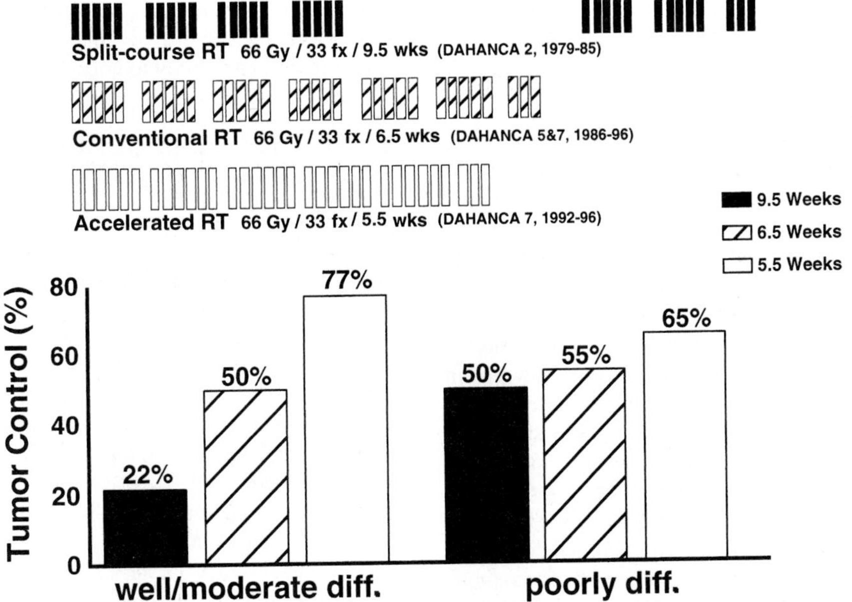

FIGURE 22.10 • **Top:** Overview of the fractionation schedules used in the three Danish head and neck trials. **Bottom:** Relationship among histopathologic grading, overall treatment time, and local tumor control from the three trials. Only the well-differentiated and moderately differentiated tumors were significantly influenced by overall treatment time. (Adapted from Overgaard J, Sand Hansen H, Overgaard M, et al.: Importance of overall treatment time for the outcome of radiotherapy in head and neck carcinoma: Experience from the Danish Head and Neck Cancer Study. In *Proceedings of ICRO/ÖGRO 6, 6th International Meeting on "Progress in Radio-Oncology," Salzburg, Austria, 13–17 May 1998*, pp 743–752. Bologna, Monduzzi Editore S.p.A., 1998, with permission.)

the cervix, in which a mean of 0.5% local control (range 0.3–1.1%) is lost for each day that the overall time is prolonged.

Rapid proliferation does not occur for carcinoma of the breast or prostate, so overall treatment time is not so critical. Although the potential tumor doubling time (T_{pot}) has not proved useful as a predictive assay for individual patients (Chapter 23), mean T_{pot} values for groups of patients are in accord with the importance, or otherwise, of overall treatment time. For example, the T_{pot} for prostate cancer is about 40 days and for noninflammatory breast cancer about 14 days; in both cases, overall treatment time has not been found to be critical. This can be contrasted with head and neck cancer, in which the mean T_{pot} can be as short as 4 days and, as we have seen, overall treatment time is an important factor governing tumor control.

TABLE 22.2

Importance of Overall Treatment Time

Total Dose, Gy	Dose, Gy	Comment	Overall Time, Weeks	3-Year Local Control
66–68	2	Split course	9.5	32%
66–68	2	5fr/wk	6.5	52%
66–68	2	6fr/wk	5.5	62%

Note: DAHANCA trials show improved locoregional control with shorter overall time—no increase in late effects.

HYPOFRACTIONATION: RENEWED INTEREST

For the past 3 decades, the trend in radiotherapy, particularly in the United States, has been to increase the number of fractions more and more to exploit the difference in shape of the dose–response relationship between early- and late-responding tissues as described in detail previously. However, the most dramatic recent trend in fractionation is the exact opposite, namely, a renewed interest in dose fractions larger than 2 Gy for curative radiotherapy. Three lines of research all point in this direction.

First, evidence has accumulated to show that in the special case of prostate cancer, the α/β ratio is low, in the region of 2 to 3—more similar to late-responding normal tissues than to tumors. This essentially removes the basic rationale for a multifraction regimen of 35 or more fractions. The implication is that an external-beam regimen consisting of a smaller number of larger-dose fractions, or alternatively high-dose-rate brachytherapy delivered in a limited number of fractions, should result in good local tumor control without increased normal-tissue damage.

Second, the outcome of several large fractionation trials, mainly involving head and neck tumors, and particularly the CHART trial, have clearly demonstrated the importance of "acceleration," that is, shortening the overall treatment time, to improve local control. On the other hand, the demonstration that the half-times of late normal-tissue repair are long severely limits the strategy of using multiple treatments per day to maintain a large number of treatments in a short overall time. The only alternative is a smaller number of larger-dose fractions.

Third, the development of **Intensity Modulated Radiation Therapy (IMRT)**, tomotherapy, and proton/light-ion beams results in greatly improved dose distributions, with more limited doses to normal tissues for comparable tumor doses. This suggests the attractive possibility of increasing the dose per fraction, since the need to spare late responding normal tissues by fractionation is reduced, because of the lower dose to these tissues.

All of this means that acceleration by hypofractionation—a smaller number of larger-dose fractions—emerges as an interesting alternative. Disasters from the past involving unacceptable late normal-tissue damage limit enthusiasm for this strategy in many quarters. All of the strategies outlined previously need to be approached cautiously and the perceived benefits proven by careful clinical trials. Treatment regimens involving fewer fractions would clearly be more convenient for patients and result in significant economies in health-care systems. However, it would be folly to espouse such strategies at the expense of either local tumor control or increased toxicity to normal tissues.

USING THE LINEAR-QUADRATIC CONCEPT TO CALCULATE EFFECTIVE DOSES IN RADIOTHERAPY

It is often useful in practice to have a simple way to compare different fractionation regimens and to assign them a numeric score. For many years, the NSD and TDF systems developed by Ellis and colleagues were used widely. They proved useful for assessing modest changes in fractionation but fell into dispute when extrapolated beyond the data range on which they were based.

The linear-quadratic model is now more widely used and has received greater acceptance. This section was suggested by Dr. Jack Fowler; the format is based on tutorials he has given at the American Society of Therapeutic Radiology and Oncology and at the European Society of Therapeutic Radiology and Oncology in the 1990s.

Use of the linear-quadratic model, with appropriate values for the parameters α and β, emphasizes the difference between early- and late-responding tissues and the fact that it is never possible to match two different fractionation regimens to be equivalent for both. Calculations of this sort, although a useful guide for residents in training or for research purposes, are not to be considered a substitute for clinical judgment and experience. They are presented only as examples.

Figure 22.11 illustrates the familiar way in which biologic effect as a function of dose varies with the number of fractions in which the radiation is delivered—always assuming that the fractions are spaced sufficiently to allow full repair of sublethal radiation damage. For a multifraction regimen, the shoulder of the curve has to be repeated many times, and as a consequence, the effective dose–response relationship is a straight line from the origin through the point on the single-dose survival curve for that dose fraction (typically 2 Gy). This is discussed in Chapter 3. For the linear portion of the curve, α represents the $\log_e$ of the cells killed per gray. As the curve bends, the quadratic component of cell killing is represented by β, which is the $\log_e$ of the cells killed per gray squared. This is illustrated in Figure 22.12. The ratio α/β has the dimensions of dose and is the dose at which the linear and quadratic components of cell killing are equal.

For a single acute dose D, the biologic effect is given by

$$E = \alpha D + \beta D^2 \quad (1)$$

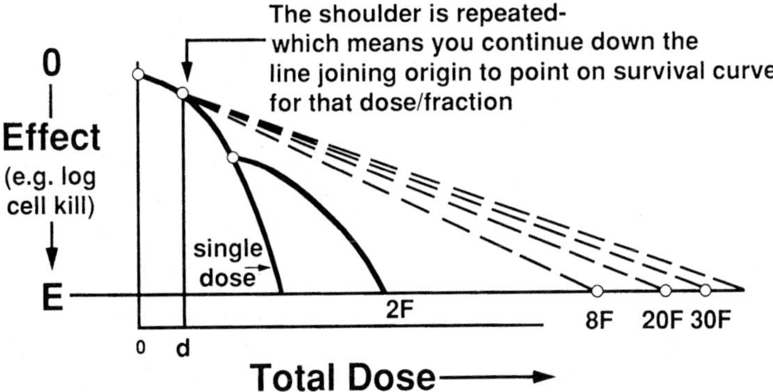

FIGURE 22.11 • Graph illustrating that if the dose–response relationship is linear-quadratic in form for graded single doses, the effective dose–response curve for a multifraction regimen approaches an exponential function of dose for many doses. The effective dose–response relationship is a straight line from the origin through the point on the single-dose survival curve corresponding to the daily dose fraction (typically 2 Gy). (Based on the concepts of Fowler, 1989, and Barendsen, 1982.)

For n well separated fractions of dose d, the biologic effect is given by

$$E = n(\alpha d + \beta d^2) \qquad (2)$$

As suggested by Barendsen, this equation may be rewritten as

$$E = (nd)(\alpha + \beta d)$$

$$= (\alpha)(nd)\left(1 + \frac{d}{\alpha/\beta}\right) \qquad (3)$$

but nd equals D, the total dose, so

$$E = \alpha(\text{total dose})\ (\text{relative effectiveness})$$

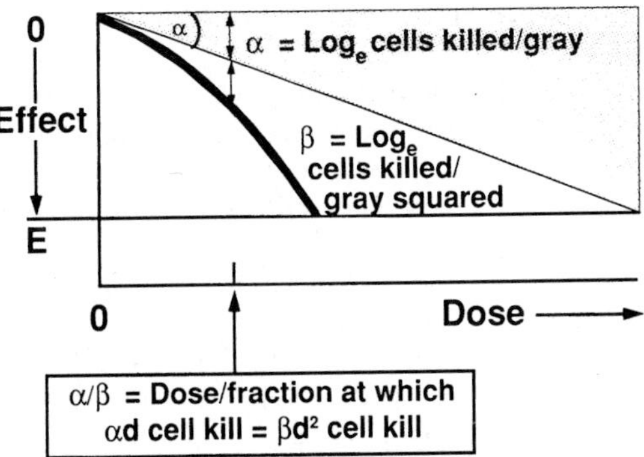

FIGURE 22.12 • Graph illustrating the linear-quadratic nature of the radiation cell survival curve, $S = e^{-\alpha D - \beta D^2}$, in which S is the fraction of cells surviving a dose D, α is the number of logs of cell kill per Gy from the linear portion of the curve, and β is the number of logs of cell kill per $(Gy)^2$ from the quadratic component. The linear and quadratic components of cell kill are equal at a dose $D = \alpha/\beta$.

in which the quantity $1 + [d/(\alpha/\beta)]$ is called *relative effectiveness*. If this equation is divided through by α, we have

$$\frac{E}{\alpha} = (\text{total dose}) \times (\text{relative effectiveness})$$

$$= (nd) \times \left(1 + \frac{d}{\alpha/\beta}\right) \qquad (4)$$

The quantity E/α is the **biologically effective dose** and is the quantity by which different fractionation regimens are intercompared. In words, the final equation is

Biologically effective dose

$$= (\text{total dose}) \times (\text{relative effectiveness})$$

$$\frac{E}{\alpha} = (nd) \times \left(1 + \frac{d}{\alpha/\beta}\right) \qquad (5)$$

Choice of α/β

For calculating the examples that follow, α/β is assumed to be 3 Gy for late-responding tissues and 10 Gy for early-responding tissues. The reader, of course, may substitute other values that seem more appropriate. It should be noted that parts of schedules can be added—that is, $(\text{partial effect})_1$ and $(\text{partial effect})_2$—as in the concomitant boost. It also should be noted that although it is permissible to compare biologically effective doses for late effects (in Gy_3) of one schedule with another and permissible to compare biologically effective doses for early effects (in Gy_{10}) of one schedule with another, it is clearly not permissible or meaningful to compare early with late effects.

Model Calculations

1. Conventional treatment: 30 fractions of 2 Gy given one fraction per day, 5 days per week, for an overall treatment time of 6 weeks (this is written as 30F × 2 Gy/6 weeks)

$$\text{Early effects: } \frac{E}{\alpha} = (nd)\left(1 + \frac{d}{\alpha/\beta}\right)$$
$$= 60\left(1 + \frac{2}{10}\right)$$
$$= 72 \text{ Gy}_{10}$$
$$\text{Late effects: } \frac{E}{\alpha} = 60\left(1 + \frac{2}{3}\right)$$
$$= 100 \text{ Gy}_{3}$$

Comment: The subscripts to the biologically effective dose are a reminder that this figure is not in gray and specify the particular values of α/β used in the calculation.

2. Hyperfractionation: 70 fractions of 1.15 Gy given twice daily, 6 hours apart, 5 days per week, for an overall treatment time of 7 weeks; that is, 70F × 1.15 Gy twice daily/7 weeks

$$\text{Early effects: } \frac{E}{\alpha} = (nd)\left(1 + \frac{d}{\alpha/\beta}\right)$$
$$= 80.5\left(1 + \frac{1.15}{10}\right)$$
$$= 89.8 \text{ Gy}_{10}$$
$$\text{Late effects: } \frac{E}{\alpha} = 80.5\left(1 + \frac{1.15}{3}\right)$$
$$= 111.4 \text{ Gy}_{3}$$

Comment: This treatment is much "hotter," that is, more effective, than the conventional 60 Gy for both early and late effects.

3. A one-fraction-a-day control schedule frequently used to compare with hyperfractionation: 35 fractions of 2 Gy given once a day for 5 days a week, for an overall treatment time of 7 weeks; that is, 35F × 2 Gy/7 weeks

$$\text{Early effects: } \frac{E}{\alpha} = (nd)\left(1 + \frac{d}{\alpha/\beta}\right)$$
$$= 70\left(1 + \frac{2}{10}\right)$$
$$= 84 \text{ Gy}_{10}$$
$$\text{Late effects: } \frac{E}{\alpha} = 70\left(1 + \frac{2}{3}\right)$$
$$= 116.7 \text{ Gy}_{3}$$

Comment: This "control" schedule is not as effective as the hyperfractionation because it is less effective by 7% for early effects, which includes tumor control (84 versus 89.8 Gy_{10}), but hotter for late effects by 5% (116.7 versus 111.4 Gy_{3}).

4. Concomitant boost: 30 fractions of 1.8 Gy given once a day, 5 days a week, and at the same time (concomitant) a boost to a smaller field of 12 fractions of 1.5 Gy once a day; overall treatment time 6 weeks; that is, ([30F × 1.8 Gy] + [12F × 1.5 Gy])/6 weeks (this protocol is much favored at the University of Texas M. D. Anderson Hospital and Tumor Institute; by giving the boost concomitantly, a prolongation of overall time is avoided)

$$\text{Early effects: } \frac{E}{\alpha} = (nd)\left(1 + \frac{d}{\alpha/\beta}\right)$$
$$= 54\left(1 + \frac{1.8}{10}\right) + 18\left(1 + \frac{1.5}{10}\right)$$
$$= 84.4 \text{ Gy}_{10}$$
$$\text{Late effects: } \frac{E}{\alpha} = 54\left(1 + \frac{1.8}{3}\right) + 18\left(1 + \frac{1.5}{3}\right)$$
$$= 113.4 \text{ Gy}_{3}$$

Comment: The Gy_{10} and Gy_{3} values should be compared with the comparable figures for the previous schedules given. The concomitant boost is hotter than the conventional schedule for both early and late effects. Compared with hyperfractionation, however, this concomitant boost is almost the same for late effects but less effective for early effects, including tumor control.

5. CHART: 36 fractions of 1.5 Gy given three fractions a day, 6 hours apart, for 12 consecutive days, with an overall treatment time of 12 days; that is, 36F × 1.5 Gy (3F/day)/12 days.

Early effects including tumor:

$$\frac{E}{\alpha} = (nd)\left(1 + \frac{d}{\alpha/\beta}\right)$$
$$= 54\left(1 + \frac{1.5}{10}\right)$$
$$= 62.1 \text{ Gy}_{10}$$
$$\text{Late effects: } \frac{E}{\alpha} = 54\left(1 + \frac{1.5}{3}\right)$$
$$= 81.0 \text{ Gy}_{3}$$

Comment: Direct comparison of CHART with the previous examples in terms of Gy_{10} and Gy_3 is meaningless because CHART has an overall time of only 12 days compared with 6 or 7 weeks for the other schedules.

Allowance for Tumor Proliferation

Calculations Suggested by Fowler

The correction proposed here for tumor proliferation is a crude approximation and should not be taken too seriously. It assumes, among other things, that the rate of cellular proliferation remains constant throughout the overall treatment time.

The number of clonogens (N) at time t is related to the initial number of clonogens (N_0) by the expression

$$N = N_0 e^{\lambda t} \quad (6)$$

in which λ is a constant related to the potential doubling time of the tumor, T_{pot}, by the expression

$$\lambda = \frac{\log_{e^2}}{T_{pot}} = \frac{0.693}{T_{pot}} \quad (7)$$

The decrease in the number of clonogens because of cell killing by the fractionated radiation regimen is balanced to some extent by cell division of the surviving clonogens. The biologic effect in equation 2 now becomes

$$E = n(\alpha d + \beta d^2) - 0.693\frac{t}{T_{pot}} \quad (8)$$

The biologically effective dose E/α becomes

$$\frac{E}{\alpha} = (nd)\left(1 + \frac{d}{\alpha/\beta}\right) - \frac{0.693}{\alpha}\frac{t}{T_{pot}} \quad (9)$$

or, in words,

$$\text{Biologically effective dose} = (\text{total dose}) \times (\text{relative effectiveness}) - \frac{\log_{e^2}}{\alpha}(\text{no. of cell doublings}) \quad (10)$$

The time t is the time in days available for proliferation. Rapid proliferation in tumors appears not to start up until about 21 to 28 days after treatment begins in head and neck tumors. Therefore, $t = T - 21$ or $t = T - 28$ is a suitable value, where T is overall time. The start-up time is called T_K for "kick-off" time, and $t = T - T_K$.

It is now necessary to assume a value for α, the initial slope of the cell survival curve, as well as for T_{pot}, the potential doubling time of the tumor. A reasonable value for α is 0.3 ± 0.1/Gy. T_{pot} may have a value of 2 to 25 days, with a median value of about 5 days.

For typical 6-week (39-day) schedules referred to earlier, proliferation may reduce the biologically effective dose by

$$\frac{E}{\alpha} = \frac{0.693}{0.3} \times \frac{(39-21)}{5} = 8.3\ Gy_{10}$$

Note that because we are concerned with tumor proliferation, the reduction in biologically effective dose is in Gy_{10}; that is, an early-effect α/β value is used. By the same token, proliferation during a 7-week protocol (i.e., 46 days) would decrease the biologically effective dose by

$$\frac{E}{\alpha} = \frac{0.693}{0.3} \times \frac{(46-21)}{5} = 11.6\ Gy_{10}$$

CHART calls for three fractions per day over 12 days, and so rapid proliferation has not started in head and neck tumors by the time the treatment is completed in this very short schedule; that is, T_K is greater than T, so t must be set at zero.

Table 22.3 summarizes the effect of tumor proliferation on the biologically effective doses characteristic of the various treatment regimens discussed earlier.

Based on the assumptions made, hyperfractionation results in the largest biologically effective dose and therefore may be expected to result in the best tumor control, followed closely by the concomitant boost schedule. CHART is a less effective schedule based on a T_{pot} of 5 days. It is necessary to assume a very fast-growing tumor, with a T_{pot} of 3 days or less, for CHART to become the most effective schedule.

It must be emphasized again that calculations of this sort should be used only as a guide for residents in training, because they do not in any way replace clinical judgment. It is useful, however, to have a yardstick by which new fractionation schemes may be judged.

Pragmatic Approach of Peters and Colleagues

Changing dose per fraction often results in a change in overall treatment time. This may be an important issue with the advent of IMRT, especially in the case of head and neck cancer, which may be rapidly growing. For example, with conventional treatment planning, a shrinking-field technique may be used, with typically 50 Gy being given to known sites of disease and potential routes of regional spread, followed by a boost of 10 to 20 Gy using a one- or two-phase cone down, with all treatments being given in 2-Gy fractions. However, owing to the complexity of IMRT, a single plan can be utilized with

TABLE 22.3

Effect of Tumor Proliferation on Biologically Effective Doses Characteristic of Various Treatment Regimens

Protocol	E/α Early, i.e., Tumor, Gy_{10}	Proliferation Correction, Gy_{10}	Corrected for Time, Gy_{10}
Conventional protocol: 30F × 2 Gy/6 wk (39 d)	72	−8.3	63.7
Hyperfractionation: 70F × 1.15 Gy/7 wk (46 d)	89.8	−11.6	78.2
Concomitant boost: (30F × 1.8 Gy) + (12F × 1.5 Gy)/6 wk (39 d)	84.4	−8.3	76.1
Chart: 36F × 1.5 Gy/12 d	62.1	0	62.1

This correction for time assumes $T_p = 5$ days; $T_K = 21$ days; and $\alpha = 0.3$ ln per Gy.

differential dose per fraction to areas of different risk on the same day, in place of the shrinking-field technique. This shortens the overall treatment time and raises the question, What total dose given in 35 fractions over 7 weeks is equivalent to 50 Gy in 25 fractions over 5 weeks, or 60 Gy in 30 fractions over 6 weeks? Given that the α/β ratio for squamous cell carcinoma of the head and neck is usually considered high, the correction factor for overall treatment time becomes more important than the correction factor for fraction size. Some groups, notably Lester Peters and colleagues at the Peter McCallam Cancer Institute in Melbrourne, Australia, have taken the pragmatic approach that between 5 and 7 weeks after the start of a fractionated regimen, the dose equivalent of regeneration with protraction of treatment is about 0.5 Gy per day, rounded down to 3 Gy per week. Thus, the equivalent of 50 Gy in 5 weeks is 56 Gy in 7 weeks at 1.6 Gy per fraction, while the equivalent of 60 Gy in 6 weeks is 63 Gy in 7 weeks at 1.8 Gy per fraction.

Obviously there is considerable room for debate concerning the actual numeric values chosen, but in the case of rapidly growing squamous cell tumors of the head and neck, it would be wrong to simply ignore the time factor, since it is more important than the correction for fraction size. For other tumor types, the dose equivalent of regeneration is almost certainly different and in most cases less. For some tumors, such as low to intermediate prostate cancer, it may be negligible. There is a general lack of data regarding accelerated tumor cell regeneration, both in regard to its magnitude and in regard to the length of the lag time before it sets in.

Summary of Pertinent Conclusions

- The "four Rs" of Radiobiology are:

  Repair of sublethal damage
  Reassortment of cells within the cell cycle
  Repopulation
  Reoxygenation

- The basis of conventional fractionation may be explained as follows: Dividing a dose into a number of fractions spares normal tissues because of the repair of sublethal damage between dose fractions and cellular repopulation. At the same time, fractionation increases tumor damage because of reoxygenation and reassortment.
- The Strandquist plot is the relation between total dose and overall treatment time. In this context, "time" includes the number of fractions. On a double log plot, the slope of the line for skin is often close to 0.33.
- The Ellis NSD system made the important contribution of separating the effects of number of fractions and overall time. The time correction was a power function ($T^{0.11}$) that is far from accurate.
- The extra dose required to counteract proliferation in a normal tissue irradiated in a fractionated regimen is a sigmoidal function of time. No extra dose is required until some weeks into a fractionated schedule.

(continued)

Summary of Pertinent Conclusions
(Continued)

- The delay before an extra dose is required to counteract the effects of proliferation is much longer for late-responding tissues and is beyond the overall time for conventional radiotherapy schedules.
- Prolonging overall time within the normal radiotherapy range has little sparing effect on late reactions but a large sparing effect on early reactions.
- The dose–response relationship for late effects is more curvy than for early effects. The ratio α/β is about 10 Gy (1,000 rad) for early effects and about 3 Gy (300 rad) for late-responding tissues. Consequently, late-responding tissues are more sensitive to changes in fractionation pattern.
- Fraction size is the dominant factor in determining late effects; overall treatment time has little influence. By contrast, fraction size and overall treatment time both determine the response of acutely responding tissues.
- Accelerated repopulation refers to the triggering of surviving cells (clonogens) to divide more rapidly as a tumor shrinks after irradiation or treatment with any cytotoxic agent.
- Accelerated repopulation starts in head and neck cancer in humans about 4 weeks after initiation of fractionated radiotherapy. About 0.6 Gy (60 rad) per day is needed to compensate for this repopulation.
- This phenomenon mandates that treatment be completed as soon as practical once it has started; it may be better to delay the start than to introduce interruptions during treatment.
- The basic aim of hyperfractionation is to further separate early and late effects. The overall treatment time remains conventional at 6 to 8 weeks, but because two fractions per day are used, the total number of fractions is 60 to 80. The dose must be increased because the dose per fraction is decreased. Early reactions may be increased slightly, tumor control improved, and late effects greatly reduced.
- In accelerated treatment, to reduce repopulation in rapidly proliferating tumors, conventional doses and number of fractions are used, but because two doses per day are given, the overall treatment time is halved. In practice, the dose must be reduced or a rest interval allowed because acute effects become limiting.
- Hyperfractionation has been shown in randomized clinical trials of head and neck cancer to improve local tumor control and survival with no increase in acute or late effects.
- Accelerated treatment: the EORTC trial of 72 Gy in 45 fractions (three fractions per day) over 5 weeks, showed an increase in local tumor control, but no increase in survival. There was an unexpected increase in late effects, some of which were lethal. The late effects were probably "consequential" late effects, developing out of the severe acute effects. Incomplete repair between fractions also may have been a problem because the time interval between fractions was too short.
- CHART stands for continuous hyperfractionated accelerated radiation therapy. The protocol consists of 36 fractions over 12 days (three fractions per day) to a total dose of 50.4 to 54 Gy. Tumor control was maintained because of the extreme acceleration of treatment time; late effects were not increased and even may have decreased because of the low dose; and acute effects were severe, but their peak occurred after completion of treatment, so patient compliance was not prejudiced.
- ARCON involves accelerated treatment to overcome tumor cell proliferation, hyperfractionation to spare late-responding normal tissues, carbogen breathing to overcome chronic hypoxia, and nicotinamide to overcome acute hypoxia.
- Overall treatment time is a very important factor for fast-growing tumors. In head and neck cancer, local tumor control is decreased by about 1.4% (range 0.4–2.5%) for each day that the overall treatment time is prolonged. The corresponding figure for carcinoma of the cervix is about 0.5% (range 0.3–1.1%) per day. Such rapid proliferation is not seen in breast or prostate cancer.

(continued)

Summary of Pertinent Conclusions* *(Continued)

- The linear-quadratic concept may be used to calculate the biologic effectiveness of various radiotherapy protocols involving different numbers of dose fractions. The useful formula is

(Biologically effective dose)

= (total dose) × (relative effectiveness)

$$\frac{E}{\alpha} = (nd) \times \left(1 + \frac{d}{\alpha/\beta}\right)$$

- An approximate allowance can be made for tumor cell proliferation when comparing protocols involving different overall treatment times. There are two approaches.

1. Fowler has suggested corrections based on the T_{pot} value for different tumors.
2. Peters and colleagues have suggested a pragmatic approach in the case of fast-growing squamous cell carcinomas of the head and neck, where corrections for overall time may be more important than number of fractions. They assume that between 5 and 7 weeks after the start of a fractionated regimen, the dose equivalent of regeneration with protraction of treatment is about 0.5 Gy per day, rounded down to 3 Gy per week. The correction will be different for other tumors and probably negligible for prostate cancer.

BIBLIOGRAPHY

Begg AC, Hofland I, Van Glabekke M, Bartlelink H, Horiot JC: Predictive value of potential doubling time for radiotherapy of head and neck tumor patients: Results from the EORTC Cooperative Trial 22851. *Semin Radiat Oncol* 2:22–25, 1992

Begg AC, McNally NJ, Shrieve D, et al.: A method to measure the duration of DNA synthesis and the potential doubling time from a single sample. *Cytometry* 6:620–625, 1985

Begg AC, Moonen I, Hofland I, et al.: Human tumor cell kinetics using a monoclonal antibody against iododeoxyuridine: Intratumoral sampling variations. *Radiother Oncol* 11:337–347, 1988

Bentzen SM. High-tech in radiation oncology: Should there be a ceiling? *Int J Radiat Oncol Biol Phys* 58:320–330, 2004

Bentzen SM, Saunders MI, Dische S: Repair halftimes estimated from observations of treatment-related morbidity after CHART or conventional radiotherapy in head and neck cancer. *Radiother Oncol* 53:219–226, 1999

Bentzen SM, Saunders MI, Dische S, Bond SJ: Radiotherapy-related early morbidity in head and neck cancer: Quantitative clinical radiobiology as deduced from the CHART trial. *Radiother Oncol* 60:123–135, 2001

Brenner DJ: Hypofractionation for prostate cancer radiotherapy—what are the issues? *Int J Radiat Oncol Biol Phys* 57:912–914, 2003

Brenner DJ: Toward optimal external-beam fractionation for prostate cancer. *Int J Radiat Oncol Biol Phys* 48:315–316, 2000

Brenner DJ, Hall EJ: Fractionation and protraction for radiotherapy of prostate carcinoma. *Int J Radiat Oncol Biol Phys* 43:1095–1101, 1999

Denekamp J: Changes in the rate of repopulation during multifraction irradiation of mouse skin. *Br J Radiol* 46:381, 1973

Dische S, Saunders M, Barrett A, Harvey A, Gibson D, Parmar M: A randomised multicentre trial of CHART versus conventional radiotherapy in head and neck cancer. *Radiother Oncol* 44:123–136, 1997

Douglas BG, Fowler JF: The effect of multiple small doses of x-rays on skin reactions in the mouse and a basic interpretation. *Radiat Res* 66:401–426, 1976

Ellis F: Dose time and fractionation: A clinical hypothesis. *Clin Radiol* 20:1–7, 1969

Ellis F: Nominal standard dose and the ret. *Br J Radiol* 44:101–108, 1971

Fowler J, Chappell R, Ritter M: Is alpha/beta for prostate tumors really low? *Int J Radiat Oncol Biol Phys* 50:1021–1031, 2001

Fowler JF: Dose-response curves for organ function in cell survival. *Br J Radiol* 56:497–500, 1983

Fowler JF: The second Klaas Breur memorial lecture. La Ronde—radiation sciences and medical radiology. *Radiother Oncol* 1:1–22, 1983

Fowler JF: 40 years of radiobiology: Its impact on radiotherapy. *Phys Med Biol* 29:97–113, 1984

Fowler JF: Fractionated radiation therapy after Strandqvist. *Acta Radiol* 23:209–216, 1984

Fowler JF: What next in fractionated radiotherapy? *Br J Cancer* 49(suppl VI):285S–300S, 1984

Fowler JF: Potential for increasing the differential response between tumors and normal tissues: Can proliferation rate be used? *Int J Radiat Oncol Biol Phys* 12:641–646, 1986

Fowler JF: The linear-quadratic formula and progress in fractionated radiotherapy. *Br J Radiol* 62:679–694, 1989

Fowler JF, Lindstrom M: Loss of local control with prolongation in radiotherapy. *Int J Radiat Oncol Biol Phys* 23:457–467, 1992

Hansen O, Overgaard J, Hansen HS, et al.: Importance of overall treatment time for the outcome of radiotherapy of advanced head and neck carcinoma: Dependency on tumor differentiation. *Radiother Oncol* 43:47–51, 1997

Hendry JH, Bentzen SM, Dale RG, et al.: A modelled comparison of the effects of using different ways to compensate for missed treatment days in radiotherapy. *Clin Oncol* 8:297–307, 1996

Hermens AF, Barendsen GW: Changes of cell proliferation characteristics in a rat rhabdomyosarcoma before and after x-irradiation. *Eur J Cancer* 5:173–189, 1969

Horiot J-C, Bontemps P, van den Bogaert W, et al.: Accelerated fractionation (AF) compared to conventional fractionation (CF) improves loco-regional control in the radiotherapy of advanced head and neck cancers: results of the EORTC 22851 randomised trial. *Radiother Oncol* 44:111–121, 1997

Horiot J-C, Le Fur R, N'Guyen T, et al.: Hyperfractionation versus conventional fractionation in oropharyngeal carcinoma: Final analysis of a randomized trial of the EORTC cooperative group of radiotherapy. *Radiother Oncol* 25: 231–241, 1992

Kaanders JHAM, Pop LAM, Marres HAM, et al.: Accelerated radiotherapy with carbogen and nicotinamide (ARCON) for laryngeal cancer. *Radiother Oncol* 48:115–122, 1998

Overgaard J: Advances in clinical applications of radiobiology: Phase III studies of radiosensitizers and novel fractionation schedules. In Johnson JT, Didolkar MS (eds): *Head and Neck Cancer*, vol III, pp 863–869. Amsterdam, Elsevier Science Publishers, 1993

Overgaard J, Hjelm-Hansen M, Johnsen LV, Andersen AP: Comparison of conventional and split-course radiotherapy as primary treatment in carcinoma of the larynx. *Acta Oncol* 27:147–152, 1988

Overgaard J, Sand Hansen H, Andersen AP, et al.: Misonidazole combined with split-course radiotherapy in the treatment of invasive carcinoma of larynx and pharynx: Final report from the DAHANCA 2 study. *Int J Radiat Oncol Biol Phys* 16:1065–1068, 1989

Overgaard J, Sand Hansen H, Overgaard M, et al.: Importance of overall treatment time for the outcome of radiotherapy in head and neck carcinoma: Experience from the Danish Head and Neck Cancer Study. In *Proceedings of ICRO/ÖGRO 6, 6th International Meeting on "Progress in Radio-Oncology," Salzburg, Austria, 13–17 May 1998*, pp 743–752. Bologna, Monduzzi Editore S.p.A., 1998

Overgaard J, Sand Hansen H, Overgaard M, et al.: Randomized double-bind phase III study of nimorazole as a hypoxic radiosensitizer of primary radiotherapy in supraglottic larynx and pharynx carcinoma: Results of the Danish Head and Neck Cancer Study DAHANCA protocol 5-85. *Radiother Oncol* 46:135–146, 1998

Overgaard J, Sand Hansen H, Sapru W, et al.: Conventional radiotherapy as the primary treatment of squamous cell carcinoma of the head and neck: A randomized multicenter study of 5 versus 6 fractions per week—preliminary report from the DAHANCA 6 and 7 trial. *Radiother Oncol* 40:S31, 1996

Parsons JT, Boom FJ, Million RR: A reevaluation of split-course technique for squamous cell carcinoma of the head and neck. *Int J Radiat Oncol Biol Phys* 6:1645–1652, 1980

Peters LJ, Ang KK: The role of altered fractionation in head and neck cancers. *Semin Radiat Oncol* 2:180–194, 1992

Peters LJ, Ang KK, Thames HD: Accelerated fractionation in the radiation treatment of head and neck cancer. *Acta Oncol* 27:185–194, 1988

Peters LJ, Withers HR, Thames HD: Radiobiological bases for multiple daily fractionation. In Kaercher KH, Kogelnik HD, Reinartz G (eds): *Progress in RadioOncology* 11: 317–323. New York, Raven Press, 1982

Ronde LA: Radiation sciences and medical radiology. *Radiother Oncol* 1:1–22, 1983

Saunders MI, Dische S: Continuous hyperfractionated accelerated radiotherapy in non-small-cell carcinoma of the bronchus. In McNally NJ (ed): *The Scientific Basis of Modern Radiotherapy*, pp 47–51. BIR Report 19. London, British Institute of Radiology, 1989

Saunders MI, Dische S, Barrett A, et al.: Randomised multicentre trials of CHART vs. conventional radiotherapy in head and neck cancer and non-small-cell lung cancer: An interim report. *Br J Cancer* 73:1455–1462, 1996

Saunders MI, Dische S, Hong A, et al.: Continuous hyperfractionated accelerated radiotherapy in locally advanced carcinoma of the head and neck region. *Int J Radiat Oncol Biol Phys* 17:1287–1293, 1989

Strandquist M: A study of the cumulative effect of fractionated x-ray treatment based on the experience mined at the Radium Hemmant with the treatment of 280 cases of carcinoma of the skin and lip. *Acta Radiol* 55(suppl):1–300, 1944

Thames HD Jr, Withers HR: Test of equal effect per fraction and estimation of initial clonogen number in microcolony assays of survival after fractionated irradiation. *Br J Radiol* 53:1071–1077, 1980

Thames HD, Peters LJ, Withers HR, Fletcher GH: Accelerated fractionation vs. hyperfractionation: Rationales for several treatments per day. *Int J Radiat Oncol Biol Phys* 9: 127–138, 1983

Thames HD, Withers HR, Peters LJ, Fletcher GH: Changes in early and late radiation responses with altered dose fractionation: Implications for dose-survival relationships. *Int J Radiat Oncol Biol Phys* 8:219–226, 1982

Withers HR: Biologic basis for altered fractionation schemes. *Cancer* 55:2086–2095, 1985

Withers HR: Cell cycle redistribution as a factor in multifraction irradiation. *Radiology* 114:199–202, 1975

Withers HR: Response of tissues to multiple small dose fractions. *Radiat Res* 71:24–33, 1977

Withers HR, Peters LJ, Kogelnik HD: The pathobiology of late effects of irradiation. In Meyn RE, Withers HR (eds): *Radiation Biology in Cancer Research,* pp 439–448. New York, Raven Press, 1980

Withers HR, Peters LJ, Taylor JMG, et al.: Late normal tissue sequelae from radiation therapy for carcinoma of the tonsil: Patterns of Fractionation Study of Radiobiology. *Int J Radiat Oncol Biol Phys* 33:563–568, 1995

Withers HR, Taylor JMG, Maciejewski B: The hazard of accelerated tumor clonogen repopulation during radiotherapy. *Acta Oncol* 27:131–146, 1988

Withers HR, Thames HD, Peters LJ, Fletcher GH: Normal tissue radioresistance in clinical radiotherapy. In Fletcher GH, Nervi C, Withers HR (eds): *Biological Bases and Clinical Implications of Tumor Radioresistance*, pp 139–152. New York, Masson, 1983

Withers HR, Thames HE Jr, Flow BL, Mason HA, Hussey DH: The relationship of acute to late skin injury in 2 and 5 fraction/week gamma-ray therapy. *Int J Radiat Oncol Biol Phys* 4:595–601, 1978

CHAPTER 23

Predictive Assays

In the routine day-to-day practice of radiotherapy, treatment schedules are designed for the "average" patient with a given type of malignancy at a given site. Although much "lip service" is rendered to the subject, in practice little is done to tailor a treatment schedule to the individual case. The eventual goal of predictive assays is to choose a treatment protocol that is optimal for each individual patient and that might give a better chance of cure than the conventional therapy. In particular, such assays may one day be used to select patients suitable for new experimental protocols. This chapter is included only after much thought, because although a wide variety of assays are being explored, none are suitable to be used routinely in the clinic. The potential, however, is so great that the resident in training should be aware of the basic ideas.

INDIVIDUAL RADIOSENSITIVITY OF NORMAL TISSUES

Among any group of patients given the same radiation treatment, some show more severe normal-tissue reactions than others, and a small proportion suffer unacceptable late sequelae. There is a powerful incentive to find ways to prospectively identify radiosensitive individuals, both to minimize patient suffering and to avoid potential lawsuits.

A number of research groups have addressed the feasibility of predicting normal-tissue tolerance from laboratory measurements of the radiosensitivity of cells taken from biopsies or blood samples. Figure 23.1 shows the results of one of the more convincing studies. Fibroblasts were grown out of skin biopsies and the fraction of cells surviving a dose of 2 Gy (SF_2) determined by a colony assay. The results show a significant correlation with late radiation damage to the skin, though, interestingly enough, not with acute reactions. The measurement of fibroblast cell survival takes many weeks and is therefore too slow to be used as a predictive assay. Other efforts to identify rapid and reliable alternatives to fibroblast colony formation, such as chromosome damage, micronucleus formation, and the comet assay for DNA damage, have failed to get to first base.

A more likely possibility in the future would be to screen potential radiation therapy patients for mutations in genes that may be involved in radiosensitivity or radioresistance. An obvious first candidate is the *ATM* gene. Ataxia-telangiectasia (AT) heterozygotes are at risk of late effects following radiation therapy because it is known that AT homozygotes are extremely radiosensitive and cells from AT heterozygotes are slightly more radiosensitive than normal. There is also some evidence that mutations in *BRCA1* or *BRCA2* confer radiosensitivity. Other genes have been identified that influence radiosensitivity in experimental systems, but

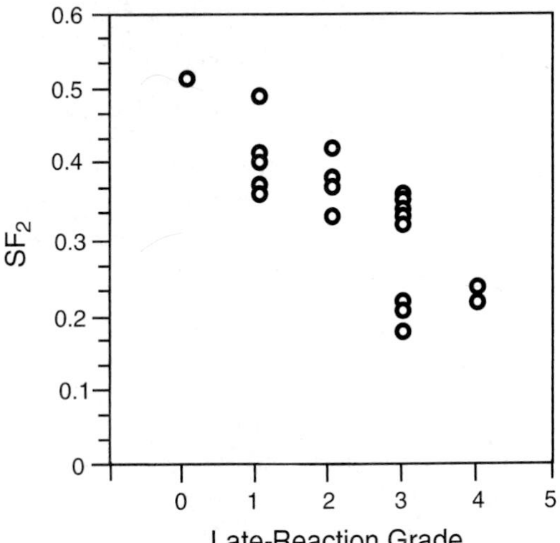

FIGURE 23.1 • Data for 20 patients showing the correlation between late reaction to radiation therapy and the *in vitro* radiosensitivity of fibroblasts obtained from skin biopsies. SF_2 is the fraction of cells surviving an acute dose of 2 Gy (200 rad). The correlation is significant with a probability of 0.0001. (Redrawn from the data of Geara FB, Peters LJ, Ang KK, et al.: Prospective comparison of *in vitro* normal cell radiosensitivity and normal tissue reactions in radiotherapy patients. *Int J Radiat Oncol Biol Phys* 27:1173–1179, 1993, with permission.)

their importance in patients is unknown. It remains an attractive speculation that someday, rapid and inexpensive genetic tests will be available to prospectively identify patients who are radiosensitive and likely to suffer unacceptable late effects if given a standard course of radiation therapy.

PREDICTIVE ASSAYS FOR TUMORS

Radiobiologic determinants of tumor response to radiotherapy fall into three broad categories:

1. Intrinsic cellular radiosensitivity
2. Oxygen status
3. Proliferative potential

Predictive assays have been developed to address each.

Intrinsic Cellular Radiosensitivity

Clonogenic cell survival, assessed by the single-cell plating techniques described in Chapter 3, has long been considered the gold standard for judging the cellular response to anticancer agents, including radiation. The formation of a microscopic colony from a single cell requires sustained cell division and is the ultimate proof of reproductive integrity. Cells taken directly from human tumor biopsy specimens, however, do not grow readily and usually are characterized by a poor plating efficiency (often about 1%). It is not easy to obtain a repeatable or accurate estimate of the cell-surviving fraction to a dose of, say, 2 Gy (200 rad).

The possibility of a predictive assay for intrinsic cellular radiosensitivity derives from the many attempts that have been made to correlate the *in vitro* radiosensitivity of cell lines derived from human tumors with the clinical responsiveness of tumors of the same histologic group. The most extensive studies are those of Deacon, Peckham, and Steel in the United Kingdom and of Malaise and Fertil in France.

The conclusion from these studies is that the steepness of the initial slope of the survival curve (rather than the final slope) correlates with clinical responsiveness. This initial region of the survival curve is best characterized by SF_2. The characteristics of the survival curve at higher doses, designated by the final D_0, or β in the linear-quadratic formula, did *not* correlate with clinical outcome.

Malaise and his colleagues divided tumors into six histologic groups: From the most radioresistant to the most radiosensitive, these are glioblastomas, melanomas, squamous cell carcinomas, adenocarcinomas, lymphomas, and oat-cell carcinomas. The order of SF_2 correlates with clinical responsiveness. This is illustrated in Figure 23.2. But most important, Malaise and his colleagues demonstrated

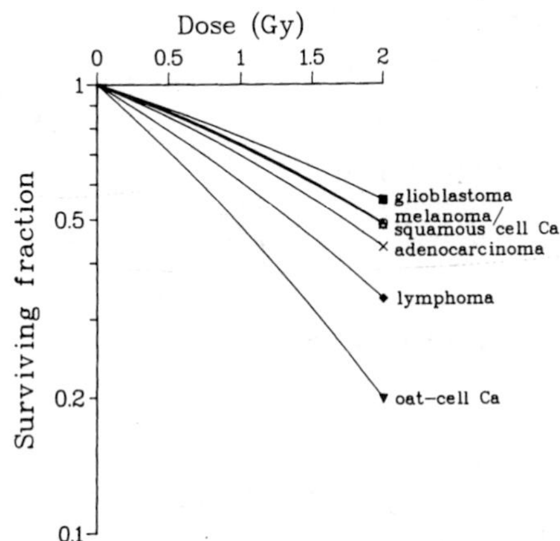

FIGURE 23.2 • Initial portion of the mean representative survival curves for cells from each of six histologic groups of human tumors, showing also the surviving fraction at 2 Gy (SF_2). (Data from Malaise EP, Fertil B, Chavaudra N, Guichard M: Distribution of radiation sensitivities for human tumor cells of specific histological types: Comparison of *in vitro* to *in vivo* data. *Int J Radiat Oncol* 12:617–624, 1986.)

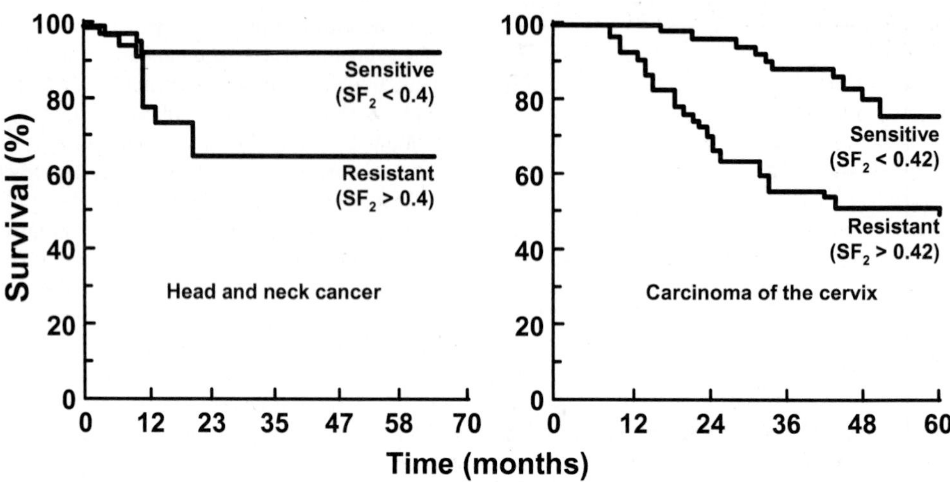

FIGURE 23.3 ● Examples in which radiosensitivity, measured by the fraction of cells surviving a dose of 2 Gy (SF_2), predicted for patient survival. Patients in whom the tumors were "radiosensitive," defined by $SF_2 < 0.4$, showed a better survival than those in whom the tumors were "radioresistant," defined by $SF_2 > 0.4$. (Left panel adapted from Björk-Eriksson T, West C, Karlsson E, Mercke C: Tumor radiosensitivity (SF_2) is a prognostic factor for local control in head and neck cancers. *Int J Radiat Oncol Biol Phys* 46:13–19, 2000. Right panel adapted from West CM, Davidson SE, Roberts SA, Hunter RD: The independence of intrinsic radiosensitivity as a prognostic factor for patient response to radiotherapy of carcinoma of the cervix. *Br J Cancer* 76:1184–1190, 1997.)

widely diverse sensitivities within each histologic group, such that the most sensitive glioblastoma had a radiosensitivity similar to the most resistant lymphoma.

These findings are of significant radiobiologic interest because they contradict the widely held view that clinical responsiveness is not related to inherent cellular radiosensitivity. It is, however, not of much use to the clinical radiotherapist, who does not need *in vitro* measurements to tell him or her that lymphomas are more radiosensitive than glioblastomas. What the radiotherapist needs is information on the individual patient. These data from Malaise and his colleagues indicate that individual responsiveness may be predicted if a suitable assay were available.

Growth in Soft Agar: The Courtenay Assay

Although cell lines derived from human tumors can be studied using standard *in vitro* plating assays (described in Chapter 3), fresh explants from tumor biopsy specimens are much more difficult to grow. Conventional cell culture techniques using cells attached to plastic dishes prove unsuitable. Many cells do not grow at all, and those that do have very low plating efficiencies. More success has been achieved by growing fresh explants of tumor biopsy specimens in soft agar, using the so-called Courtenay technique. In this technique, cells do not attach to the surface of the petri dish but grow as spheres or clumps in a semisolid agar gel, supplemented with growth factors. Using this technique, West and her colleagues at the Christie Hospital in Manchester, England, analyzed prospectively for intrinsic radiosensitivity over 128 patients with stage I–III carcinoma of the cervix who were to receive radical radiotherapy. They found that survival of patients with SF_2 greater than the median value (0.42) was significantly poorer than those with SF_2 below the median value. Their data are shown in Figure 23.3. A similar study was performed by Björk-Eriksson and colleagues with 156 patients with primary carcinomas of the head and neck. Again, survival of patients with SF_2 above the median value (0.4) was significantly poorer than those with SF_2 values below the median value. These data are also shown in Figure 23.3. These findings suggest that intrinsic radiosensitivity (measured as SF_2) is a significant prognostic factor for both local control and survival.

The two principal disadvantages of colony assay system use are, first, the poor success rate in growing human tumor cells from biopsies, and second, the time that it takes, which may be as long as 4 weeks.

Various surrogates for the clonal assay have been tried that give results in a week or less. These include colorimetric assays, such as the tetrazolium-based (MTT) assay. This assay was adopted by the National Cancer Institute to screen large numbers of potential anticancer drugs. It measures cell growth rather than colonogenicity.

Another technique that measures growth in a few days is the cell adhesive matrix assay. Cells are plated into 24-well microtest plates coated with a special formulation of fibronectin and fibrinopeptides to encourage cell attachment. The staining density of irradiated wells, compared with controls, is the end point observed; this is not, of course, related to the reproductive integrity of individual cells.

The various studies of tumor cell radiosensitivity have been useful in confirming that this is a factor that directly influences local control and patient survival. However, they have very limited clinical utility as a predictive assay; they have certainly not found widespread use!

Oxygen Status

New modalities aimed at overcoming the perceived problem of hypoxic cells did not enjoy great success when applied indiscriminately to large groups of patients. This was true for neutrons and hypoxic-cell sensitizers, both of which were introduced initially on the premise that the curability of human tumors by x-rays was limited by the presence of hypoxic cells that are resistant to killing with x-rays. It would be desirable to have available assays that would identify which individual patients have tumors containing hypoxic cells.

Labeled Nitroimidazoles

One successful approach has been based on nitroimidazoles labeled with a radioactive material. In regions of low oxygen tension, the nitroimidazole undergoes bioreduction, and radioactive material becomes covalently linked to cellular molecules, which can be detected.

Early studies used misonidazole tagged with a β-emitter radionuclide assayed by autoradiography. The test could not be used prospectively as a predictive assay in individual patients because β-rays cannot be detected outside the body, but by taking sections of tumors excised from patients previously given the labeled drug, it was shown that only a minority of tumors contain hypoxic cells.

Throughout the 1980s and 1990s, a considerable effort was devoted to the development of nuclear-medicine markers of tissue hypoxia that could be detected by single-photon emission computed tomographic (SPECT) scanning or by positron emission tomography (PET). The research collaboration at the Cross Cancer Institute in Edmonton selected iodinated azomycin arabinoside for SPECT studies; the research group at the University of Washington in Seattle selected fluoromisonidazole for positron emission tomographic studies. Preliminary clinical investigations of iodinated azomycin arabinoside in 51 patients and fluoromisonidazole in 37 patients have been reported. There appears to be reasonable consistency between the two different approaches, and overall, between one third and one half of the tumors show significant hypoxia.

These data suggest that the oxygenation status of solid human tumors is, on average, significantly higher than that found in rodent tumors and that their radiobiologic hypoxic fractions may be significantly lower. The result is consistent with the higher median pO_2 values measured for human relative to rodent tumors by the Eppendorf pO_2 probe. Figure 23.4 shows a SPECT image of a small-cell lung cancer 18 hours after the administration of iodinated azomycin arabinoside, which is labeled with iodine-123. The label is not attached as well as in the case of β-emitters, resulting in uptake of released iodine in the thyroid. A hypoxic area, however, shows up clearly in the small-cell lung cancer. This represents a noninvasive test that can be performed on individual patients prospectively. The results could be used to "select" those patients likely to benefit from, for example, a hypoxic-cell cytotoxin or radiosensitizer.

Oxygen Probes

Oxygen probes, that is, electrodes implanted directly into tumors to measure oxygen concentration by a polarographic technique, have a long and checkered history (see Chapter 6). The situation has improved, however, as a consequence of technical developments of considerable interest and importance. One of the long-standing problems is that the implantation of a rigid probe crushes tissue, compresses vessels, and causes damage, thereby altering the oxygen tension, the very quantity being measured. The breakthrough was the development of the Eppendorf probe, a commercially available polarographic electrode that moves quickly through tissue under computer control and has a very fast response time of about 1 second. These properties circumvent any significant effect on the recorded local tissue pO_2 brought about by the compression of vessels in the vicinity of the electrode and the oxygen consumption of the cathode. The probe moves under computer control, making a measurement of pO_2 every second as it moves along a track through the tumor in steps of about 1 mm.

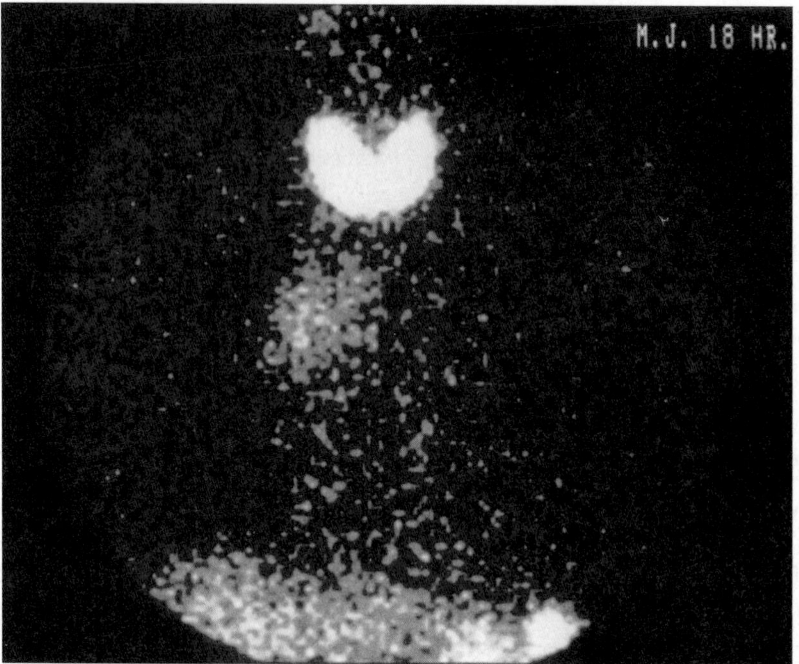

FIGURE 23.4 • Single-photon emission computed tomographic image of a human small-cell lung cancer 18 hours after administration of iodinated azomycin arabinoside, which is labeled with iodine-123. Note the "bow-tie" uptake of released iodine in the thyroid and the uptake in the tumor, indicating the presence of hypoxic cells. (Courtesy of Dr. J.D. Chapman, Fox Chase Cancer Center.)

A prospective clinical trial was conducted in the 1990s at the University of Mainz in Germany to investigate the usefulness of this new generation of oxygen probes. Patients with locally advanced carcinoma of the uterine cervix were treated with a combination of external-beam radiotherapy and three high-dose-rate brachytherapy insertions. Before treatment, measurements of oxygen concentration were made in each patient, 25 to 30 measurements along each of two tracks through the tumor.

Patients whose tumors exhibited median pO_2 values of less than 10 mm Hg had significantly lower survival and recurrence-free survival rates compared with patients with tumors in which the pO_2 was greater than or equal to 10 mm Hg. Figure 23.5 shows the data for recurrence-free survival. This dramatic result appears to confirm that oxygen-probe measurements represent a practical predictive assay to identify hypoxic tumors that may benefit from alternate treatment strategies, such as radiosensitizers or bioreductive drugs. They compete with radiolabeled nitroimidazoles detected by SPECT imaging, although they do suffer the disadvantages that an invasive procedure is involved and they are useful only for accessible tumors.

The obvious and straightforward interpretation of these data is that the presence of hypoxic cells makes tumors intransigent to cure by radiation because of the oxygen effect. A similar study, however, showed that survival was poorer in similar patients with low pO_2 values even if surgery was used instead of radiotherapy. The implication is that hypoxia is a measure of tumor aggression. This is discussed in more detail in Chapter 6.

Proliferative Potential

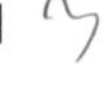

An increasing volume of data suggests overall treatment time to be a very important factor determining the outcome of head and neck cancer treated by radiation. Higher doses are required to achieve tumor control when overall time is lengthened. This is illustrated in the CHART study, three fractions per day for 12 days; the European Cooperative Radiotherapy Group (EORTC) trial of accelerated fractionation; the DAHANCA (Danish Head and Neck Cancer Study Group) study, six versus five fractions per week; and the Polish study of seven versus five fractions per week. These data strongly suggest, but do not prove conclusively, that tumor cell

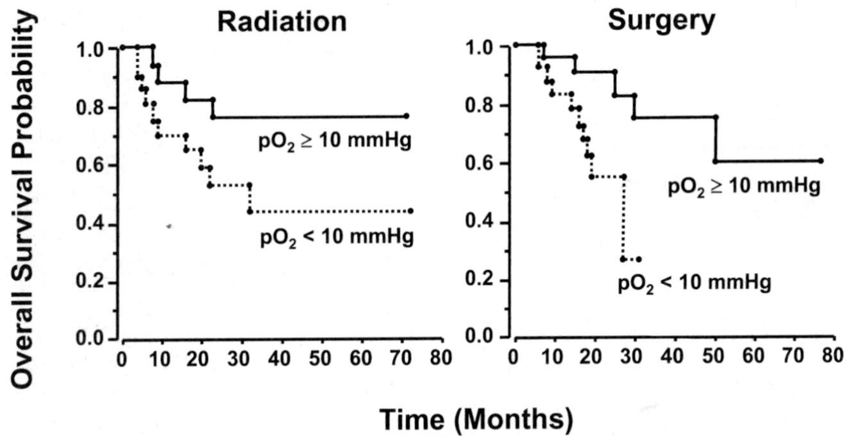

FIGURE 23.5 ● Recurrence-free survival in patients with advanced carcinoma of the cervix treated either by a combination of external-beam radiotherapy and high-dose-rate brachytherapy or by surgery. The patients were divided into two groups on the basis of pretreatment oxygen-probe measurements that indicated mean pO_2 values of less than, or of greater than or equal to 10 mm Hg. The natural interpretation of the radiotherapy trial is that hypoxia compromises the efficacy of radiation. The fact that poorer survival is seen after surgery when tumors are hypoxic suggests that hypoxia results in more aggressive tumors. (Left panel adapted from Höckel M, Schlenger K, Aral B, Mitze M, Schaffer U, Vaupel P: Association between tumor hypoxia and malignant progression in advanced cancer of the uterine cervix. *Cancer Res* 56:4509–4515, 1996; right panel adapted from Höckel M, Knoop C, Schlenger K, et al.: Intratumoral pO_2 predicts survival in advanced cancer of the uterine cervix. *Radiother Oncol* 26:45–50, 1993, with permission.)

repopulation during treatment is an important factor determining outcome.

Strategies to achieve shorter overall treatment times, such as giving two or three fractions per day or treating Saturdays and Sundays as well as weekdays, represent inconvenient, labor-intensive, and therefore expensive forms of treatment. They should be reserved, therefore, for patients likely to benefit, so what is required is a pretreatment cell kinetic parameter that can be measured quickly and easily to pick out fast-growing tumors. Methods available for measuring tumor proliferation are described in Chapter 21.

Some years ago, it appeared that the potential tumor doubling time (T_{pot}) was just such a parameter. T_{pot} is a measure of tumor growth that includes the cell-cycle time and the growth fraction but excludes the effect of cell loss. T_{pot} can be estimated by flow cytometry from a single tumor biopsy taken several hours after an injection of bromodeoxyuridine.

A number of studies have been carried out attempting to correlate T_{pot} with outcome of radiation therapy. The largest was an EORTC multicenter analysis of over 470 head and neck cancer patients treated with radiotherapy; in this study T_{pot} was not a significant predictor of outcome. This same study showed that labeling index was superior to T_{pot} as a predictor, but the correlation is weak. These studies should not be interpreted as showing that proliferation is unimportant as a determinant of radiotherapy outcome—far from it—but rather that T_{pot} and labeling index are not appropriate measures of it.

CONCLUSION

The development of reliable and useful predictive assays has been slow and their application disappointing. They have certainly not found a place in routine radiotherapy. For the most part, they are restricted to a few research-oriented institutions, and even then a given laboratory usually specializes in the test that particularly interests it—radiosensitivity, oxygen status, or tumor proliferation—with no one, it appears, measuring them all.

The potential for predictive assays is enormous, if only they could be developed. For example:

- Patients with an unusually radioresistant tumor may benefit from the addition of chemotherapy or even switching to an alternative such as surgery.
- Patients with tumors showing a fast rate of proliferation may be candidates for accelerated fractionation.

- Patients with tumors containing hypoxic regions could be assigned to treatments that include hypoxic sensitizers or hypoxic cytotoxins such as ARCON or tirapazamine.

In the past, the trial of new strategies in radiotherapy has been hampered significantly by the heterogeneity of patient populations, and that continues to be the case. Clinical trials require greatly increased numbers of patients in each arm of the protocol if the new agent or technique benefits only a subset of the patients entered in the trial. Reliable predictive assays could improve this situation, but at the present time, they are simply not available.

Summary of Pertinent Conclusions

- The aim of predictive assays is to identify patients whose tumors or normal tissues show unusual intrinsic sensitivity to radiation or whose tumors are intransigent to conventional treatment because of the presence of hypoxic cells or a rapid proliferative potential. In short, the aim is to individualize therapy.

Radiosensitivity of Normal Tissues

- It is possible that conventional protocols are designed to avoid problems in the normal tissues of a radiosensitive minority, thus underdosing the average patient.
- Pilot studies with patients on radiotherapy indicate a correlation between the radiosensitivity of normal-tissue fibroblasts cultured *in vitro* and late reactions in the same patients from whom the cells were taken.
- In the future, radiosensitive subsets of patients may be identified by genetic analysis rather than by measurements of radiosensitivity from biopsy samples.

Predictive Assays for Tumors

- Predictive assays for tumors fall into three categories: intrinsic radiosensitivity, oxygen status, and proliferative potential.

Intrinsic Radiosensitivity

- Intrinsic cellular radiosensitivity can be measured by clonogenic assays of cells from human tumors grown *in vitro*. One of the problems is that clonogenic assays take too long to realistically be used prospectively as a predictive assay.
- The initial region of the survival curve correlates best with clinical results: either the SF_2, the fraction of cells surviving 2 Gy, or α, the linear component or initial slope.
- Tumors have been divided into six histologic groups: From the most radioresistant to the most radiosensitive, they are glioblastomas, melanomas, squamous cell carcinomas, adenocarcinomas, lymphomas, and oat-cell carcinomas. The order of SF_2 values correlates with clinical responsiveness, but these data come from cell lines and do not allow predictions for individual patients.
- West and her colleagues found a lower probability of local tumor control in patients with carcinoma of the cervix treated with radiotherapy if the SF_2 (measured by the Courtenay assay) was greater than 0.42.
- Björk-Eriksson and colleagues found a similar result for head and neck cancer; that is, survival was poorer in patients for which the SF_2 was above the mean value of 0.4.
- Assays for radiosensitivity based on clonogenic survival have been useful in demonstrating that local control and patient survival correlate with the sensitivity of individual tumor cells. However, such assays have very limited clinical usefulness for two reasons: (1) Human tumor cells are difficult to grow in cell culture from biopsy specimens, and (2) the assay takes many weeks, which delays the start of therapy.
- Various surrogates for a clonal assay have been devised that give a result in a week or less, such as colorometric assays that mirror overall growth, but none have found widespread acceptance.
- Nonclonogenic assays have been developed based on cell growth in multiwell dishes. Growth is assessed by density of stain. These are rapid and easy but have not found clinical usefulness.

Oxygen Status

- The oxygen status of a tumor may be assessed by deposited labeled nitroimidazoles

(continued)

Summary of Pertinent Conclusions
(Continued)

in the tumor or by polarographic oxygen probes.

- Compounds labeled with the short-lived γ-emitting isotope iodine-123 also can be used in regions of low oxygen tension; the compound is covalently linked and the isotope deposited. The presence of hypoxia can be visualized by SPECT imaging.
- Eppendorf probes have a very fast response and can be moved quickly through a tumor under computer control to obtain an oxygen profile.
- A clinical trial in Germany of patients with advanced carcinoma of the cervix treated with radiotherapy has shown lower survival and lower recurrence-free survival in patients whose tumors exhibited median pO_2 values less than or equal to 10 mm Hg as measured by the Eppendorf probe.
- Although this evidence initially was interpreted to show that radioresistance resulting from hypoxia is important, later studies indicate that hypoxia leads to more aggressive and malignant tumors.

Proliferative Potential

- There is strong evidence that lengthening overall treatment time leads to a poorer outcome of radiotherapy, at least in head and neck cancers. This implies that repopulation during treatment is important, but at the present time, there is no robust reliable method to prospectively predict which tumors will respond poorly because of rapid repopulation.
- T_{pot} can be measured in individual patients by flow cytometry on a single tumor biopsy specimen taken some hours after an injection of bromodeoxyuridine. However, it has not been shown to correlate with the outcome of radiotherapy.
- Labeling index was shown to be superior to T_{pot} as a predictor, but the correlation is weak.

Conclusion

- Predictive assays are in a developmental stage; they have not yet proved their worth, but show some promise in selecting groups of patients that may benefit from altered treatment protocols: accelerated treatment, hyperfractionation, bioreductive drugs, neutrons, and so on.

BIBLIOGRAPHY

Begg AC, Haustermans K, Hart AAM, et al.: The value of pretreatment cell kinetic parameters as predictors for radiotherapy outcome in head and neck cancer: A multicenter analysis. *Radiother Oncol* 50:13–23, 1999

Begg AC, Hofland I, Moonen L, et al.: The predictive value of cell kinetic measurements in a European trial of accelerated fractionation in advanced head and neck tumors: An interim report. *Int J Radiat Oncol Biol Phys* 19:1449–1453, 1990

Begg AC, McNally NJ, Shrieve DC, Karcher H: A method to measure the duration of DNA synthesis and the potential doubling time from a single sample. *Cytometry* 6:620–626, 1985

Björk-Eriksson T, West C, Karlsson E, Mercke C: Tumor radiosensitivity (SF_2) is a prognostic factor for local control in head and neck cancers. *Int J Radiat Oncol Biol Phys* 46:13–19, 2000

Brock W, Campbell H, Goepfert H, Peters LJ: Radiosensitivity testing of human tumor cell cultures: A potential method of predicting the response to radiotherapy. *Cancer Bull* 39:98–102, 1987

Cater DB, Silver IA: Quantitative measurements of oxygen tension in normal tissues and in the tumors of patients before and after radiotherapy. *Acta Radiol* 53:233–256, 1960

Chapman JD, Peters LJ, Withers HR (eds): *Prediction of Tumor Treatment Response*. New York, Pergamon Press, 1989

Deacon J, Peckham MJ, Steel GG: The radioresponse of human tumors and the initial slope of the cell survival curve. *Radiother Oncol* 2:317–323, 1984

Fertil B, Malaise EP: Intrinsic radiosensitivity of human cell lines is correlated with radiosensitivity of human tumors: Analysis of 101 published survival curves. *Int J Radiat Oncol Biol Phys* 11:1699–1707, 1985

Geara FB, Peters LJ, Ang KK, et al.: Intrinsic radiosensitivity of normal human fibroblasts and lymphocytes after high- and low-dose-rate irradiation. *Cancer Res* 52:6348–6352, 1992

Geara FB, Peters LJ, Ang KK, et al.: Prospective comparison of in vitro normal cell radiosensitivity and normal tissue reactions in radiotherapy patients. *Int J Radiat Oncol Biol Phys* 27:1173–1179, 1993

Groshar D, McEwan AJB, Parliament MB, et al.: Imaging tumor hypoxia and tumor perfusion. *J Nucl Med* 34:885–888, 1993

Höckel M, Knoop C, Schlenger K, et al.: Intratumoral pO_2 predicts survival in advanced cancer of the uterine cervix. *Radiother Oncol* 26:45–50, 1993

Höckel M, Schlenger K, Aral B, Mitze M, Schaffer U, Vaupel P: Association between tumor hypoxia and malignant progression in advanced cancer of the uterine cervix. *Cancer Res* 56:4509–4515, 1996

Höckel M, Terris DJ, Vaupel P: The role of oxygen tension distribution on the radiation response of human breast carcinoma. *Adv Exp Med Biol* 345:485–492, 1994

Johansen J, Bentzen SM, Overgaard J, Overgaard M: Evidence for a positive correlation between in vitro radiosensitivity of normal human skin fibroblasts and the occurrence of subcutaneous fibrosis after radiotherapy. *Int J Radiat Biol* 66:407–412, 1994

Kiltie AE, Ryan AJ, Swindell R, et al.: A correlation between residual radiation-induced DNA double-strand breaks in cultured fibroblasts and late radiotherapy reactions in breast cancer patients. *Radiother Oncol* 51:55–65, 1999

Koh WJ, Bergman KS, Rasey JS, et al.: Evaluation of oxygenation status during fractionated radiotherapy in human nonsmall cell lung cancers using [F-18]fluoromisonidazole positron emission tomography. *Int J Radiat Oncol Biol Phys* 33:391–398, 1995

Koh WJ, Rasey JS, Evans ML, et al.: Imaging of hypoxia in human tumors with [F-18]fluoromisonidazole. *Int J Radiat Oncol Biol Phys* 22:1–13, 1992

Loncaster J, Cooper RA, Logue JP, Davidson SE, West CML: Vascular endothelial growth factor (VEGF) expression is a prognostic factor for radiotherapy outcome in advanced carcinoma of the cervix. *Br J Cancer* 83:620–625, 2000

Loncaster J, Harris A, West CML: CA IX expression, a potential new intrinsic marker of hypoxia: Correlations with tumour oxygen measurements and prognosis in locally advance carcinoma of the cervix. *Cancer Res* 61:6394–6399, 2001

Malaise EP, Fertil B, Chavaudra N, Guichard M: Distribution of radiation sensitivities for human tumor cells of specific histological types: Comparison of *in vitro* to *in vivo* data. *Int J Radiat Oncol* 12:617–624, 1986

Mitchell JB: Potential applicability of nonclonogenic measurements to clinical oncology. *Radiat Res* 114:401–414, 1988

Parliament MB, Chapman JD, Urtasun RC, et al.: Noninvasive assessment of human tumor hypoxia with 123I-iodoazomycin arabinoside: Preliminary report of a clinical study. *Br J Cancer* 65:90–95, 1992

Peacock J, Ashton A, Bliss J, et al.: Cellular radiosensitivity and complication risk after curative radiotherapy. *Radiother Oncol* 55:173–178, 2000

Peters LJ, Brock WA, Johnson T, Meyn RE, Tofilon PJ, Milas L: Potential methods for predicting tumor radiocurability. *Int J Radiat Oncol Biol Phys* 12:459–467, 1968

Rasey JS, Koh WJ, Evans ML, et al.: Quantifying regional hypoxia in human tumors with positron emission tomography of [18F]fluoromisonidazole: A pretherapy study of 37 patients. *Int J Radiat Oncol Biol Phys* 36:417–428, 1996

Russell NS, Grummels A, Hart AA, et al.: Low predictive value of intrinsic fibroblast radiosensitivity for fibrosis development following radiotherapy for breast cancer. *Int J Radiat Biol* 73:661–670, 1998

Urtasun RC, McEwan AJ, Parliament MB, et al.: Measurement of hypoxia in human tumors by SPECT imaging of iodoazomycin arabinoside. *Br J Cancer* 74:209–212, 1996

Vaupel P, Schlenger K, Knoop C, Hockel M: Oxygenation of human tumors: Evaluation of tissue oxygen distribution in breast cancers by computerized O_2 tension measurements. *Cancer Res* 51:3316–3322, 1991

Weiss C, Fleckenstein W: Local tissue pO_2 measured with thick needle probes. *Funktionsanal Biol Systeme* 15:155–166, 1986

West CM: Intrinsic radiosensitivity as a predictor of patient response to radiotherapy. *Br J Radiol* 68:827–837, 1995

West CM, Davidson SE, Burt PA, Hunter RD: The intrinsic radiosensitivity of cervical carcinoma: Correlations with clinical data. *Int J Radiat Oncol Biol Phys* 31:841–846, 1995

West CM, Davidson SE, Elyan SAG, et al.: Lymphocyte radiosensitivity is a significant prognostic factor for morbidity in carcinoma of the cervix. *Int J Radiat Oncol Biol Phys* 51:10–15, 2000

West CM, Davidson SE, Hendry JH, Hunter RD: Prediction of cervical carcinoma response to radiotherapy. *Lancet* 338:818, 1991

West CM, Davidson SE, Roberts SA, Hunter RD: The independence of intrinsic radiosensitivity as a prognostic factor for patient response to radiotherapy of carcinoma of the cervix. *Br J Cancer* 76:1184–1190, 1997

West CM, Davidson SE, Roberts SA, Hunter RD: Intrinsic radiosensitivity and prediction of patient response to radiotherapy for carcinoma of the cervix. *Br J Cancer* 68:819–823, 1993

West CM, Elyan SA, Berry P, Cowan R, Scott D: A comparison of the radiosensitivity of lymphocytes from normal donors, cancer patients, individuals with ataxia-telangiectasia (A-T) and A-T heterozygotes. *Int J Radiat Biol* 68:197–203, 1995

West CM, Loncaster JA, Cooper RA, Wilks DP, Bromley M: Tumor vascularity: A histological measure of angiogenesis and hypoxia. *Cancer Res* 61:2907–2910, 2001

Wilson GD, Dische S, Saunders MI: Studies with bromodeoxyuridine in head and neck cancer and accelerated radiotherapy. *Radiother Oncol* 36:189–197, 1995

CHAPTER 24

Alternative Radiation Modalities

The early recognition that x-rays could produce local tumor control in some patients and not in others led to the notion that other forms of ionizing radiations might be superior.

Neutrons first were introduced in a speculative way, not based on any particular hypothesis. The later use of neutrons and the introduction of protons, negative π-mesons, and heavy ions all were based clearly on a putative advantage, either of physical dose distribution or radiobiologic properties. In the case of neutrons, they give up their energy to produce recoil protons, α-particles, and heavier nuclear fragments. Consequently, their biologic properties differ from those of x-rays: reduced oxygen enhancement ratio (OER), little or no repair of sublethal damage, and less variation of sensitivity through the cell cycle.

The use of neutrons following World War II was based squarely on the premise that the presence of hypoxic cells limits the curability of human tumors by x-ray therapy, so the lower OER characteristic of neutrons might confer an advantage. An alternative rationale for neutrons, proposed at a later date, was that their relative biologic effectiveness (RBE) is larger for slow-growing tumors, possibly giving them an advantage in a limited number of specific human tumors.

Protons have radiobiologic properties similar to those of x-rays, and their introduction into radiotherapy was based entirely on the superiority of the physical dose distribution possible with charged particles. Negative π-mesons and heavy ions were introduced with the hope of combining the radiobiologic advantages attributed to neutrons with the dose distribution advantage characteristic of protons.

Neutrons have been shown to be superior to x-rays in a limited number of situations, specifically for the treatment of prostatic cancer, salivary gland tumors, and possibly soft-tissue sarcomas. A number of controlled clinical trials have been performed for a wide variety of cancer sites, but a gain was apparent only in these few circumstances. For almost 50 years, protons generated in facilities originally intended for physics research have found a small but important niche for the treatment of uveal melanoma and tumors such as chordomas, which are located close to the spinal cord and therefore benefit greatly from the localized dose distribution. The wider use of protons for broad-beam radiotherapy is being tested now that custom-built facilities are available, but no advantage has been proved yet in controlled clinical trials. Negative π-mesons and heavy ions have been used to treat hundreds of patients, but prospective randomized trials have never been completed to prove their superiority over conventional x-rays. Negative π-mesons have completely disappeared from the scene, but high-energy carbon ions are enjoying a renaissance in Europe and Japan.

The casual reader may be content with this overview of alternative radiation modalities and may not wish to proceed further in this chapter. Interest in high linear energy transfer (LET) radiations for radiotherapy largely has waned, but protons are very much in vogue. In this chapter, neutrons and protons are considered in turn.

FAST NEUTRONS

Rationale

Neutrons were first used for cancer therapy at the Lawrence Berkeley Laboratory in California in the 1930s (Fig. 24.1). This first clinical trial of neutrons was not based on any radiobiologic rationale but was prompted largely by the availability of a new and unique beam. It is said that it received some impetus when the mother of the Lawrence brothers (E.O. Lawrence was the inventor of the cyclotron and the director of what was to become the Lawrence Berkeley Laboratory) contracted cancer, which was judged by her physician to be incurable by conventional means. She was treated with neutrons and lived for many years, although from a retrospective review of the case, it is probable that she did not have cancer in the first place. This early effort at Berkeley was hampered because the complexities of the relationship between RBE and dose for high-LET radiations were not understood at the time. Consequently, a number of patients were overdosed seriously before the trial was terminated by the entry of the United States into World War II. In reviewing their experience many years later, Dr. Robert Stone, the radiotherapist in charge of the study, concluded in his famous Janeway Lecture of 1948 that:

> neutron therapy as administered by us resulted in such bad late sequelae in proportion to a few good results that it should not be continued.

The Hammersmith Neutron Experience

The renewed interest in neutrons in the years following World War II originated at the Hammersmith Hospital in London, where neutrons were generated by the Medical Research Council's 60-inch cyclotron. In this machine, 16-MeV deuterons

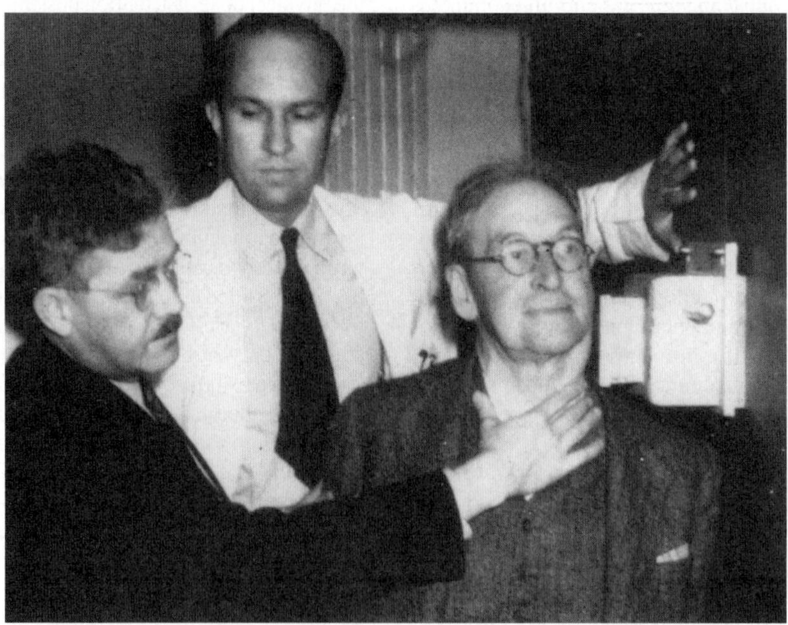

FIGURE 24.1 • The first patient treated with neutrons in the 1930s at the Lawrence Berkeley Laboratory of the University of California. On the left is Dr. Robert Stone, the radiotherapist, and in the center is Dr. John Lawrence, the physician brother of the inventor of the cyclotron, E.O. Lawrence. (Courtesy of the University of California.)

incident on a beryllium target produced neutrons with a modal value of 6 MeV. The Hammersmith cyclotron was suggested and conceived by Gray, based on the notion that a lowered OER would be advantageous to radiotherapy. The machine suffered from the limitations of poor depth doses (equivalent to 250-kVp x-rays) and a fixed horizontal beam.

A prospective randomized clinical trial to compare neutrons with x-rays was started in 1971. Advanced tumors of the head and neck were chosen because the poor depth–dose characteristics made neutrons suitable only for treating relatively superficial lesions. The trial involved patients with tumors of the salivary glands, buccal cavity, hypopharynx, and larynx. The neutron treatments delivered in only 12 fractions were clearly superior as judged by local control of the primary tumor, but the gain was achieved at the expense of a higher complication rate.

The United States Neutron Experience

Because of the limitations associated with low-energy cyclotrons, interest at a number of centers in the United States turned to the use of large cyclotrons that accelerate deuterons to energies of 22 to 50 MeV. Several such machines had been built for high-energy physics research and were converted for part-time neutron therapy. In addition, neutrons were produced at the Fermilab in Batavia, Illinois, by bombarding a beryllium target with 67-MeV protons.

All of these machines had adequate dose rates and quite good depth doses. Unfortunately, they had other disadvantages: All had fixed horizontal beams, and all were located in physics installations rather than in large, busy hospitals, so that the availability of a sufficient number of patients was a problem. A number of controlled clinical trials were performed for a variety of tumor sites, and they showed no advantage for neutrons over x-rays. Neutrons, however, appeared to be superior for salivary gland tumors, soft-tissue sarcomas, and prostate cancer.

Enthusiasm for neutron therapy waned just at a time when technology became available that allowed machines to be built that are suitable for clinical use. A new generation of hospital-based cyclotrons using the $p^+ \rightarrow$ Be reaction had adequate dose rates, good percentage depth doses, and a full isocentric mount, similar to a conventional Linac. A few centers operate such machines in the United States, Europe, and Japan, but neutrons have never become mainstream in radiotherapy.

BORON NEUTRON-CAPTURE THERAPY

The basic idea behind boron neutron-capture therapy (BNCT) is elegant in its simplicity. It has appealed to physicians, and particularly to physicists, for the best part of half a century. The idea is to deliver to the cancer patient a boron-containing drug that is taken up only in tumor cells and then to expose the patient to a beam of low-energy (thermal) neutrons that themselves produce little radiobiologic effect but that interact with the boron to produce short-range, densely ionizing α-particles. Thus, the tumor is intensely irradiated, but the normal tissues are spared. There are two problems inherent in this idea that have so far proved intractable:

1. How does one find a "magic" drug that can distinguish malignant cells from normal cells? (The skeptic might add that searching for such a drug has been the Holy Grail of cancer research and that if one were found, the obvious strategy would be to attach an alkylating agent or an α-emitting radionuclide to it; combining its use with neutrons would be a distant third.)
2. The low-energy neutrons necessary for BNCT are poorly penetrating in tissue and consequently result in percentage depth doses that are extremely poor by today's standards.

A number of nuclides have high propensities for absorbing low-energy or thermal neutrons; that is, they have a high neutron-capture cross section. Boron is the most attractive of these because it is readily available in a nonradioactive form, its chemistry is such that it can be incorporated into a wide variety of compounds, and if it interacts with low-energy neutrons, it emits short-range, high-LET α-particles.

Boron Compounds

For BNCT to be successful, the compounds used should have high specificity for malignant cells, with concomitantly low concentrations in adjacent normal tissues and in blood. In the early days, the compounds used were not specially synthesized for BNCT, but were already available. In the brain, which is the site for which BNCT largely has been used, some selectivity is obtained because compounds do not penetrate normal brain tissue to the same degree as brain tumors, in which the blood–brain barrier is absent or severely compromised.

Critical to the success of BNCT is the requirement that boron compounds be developed that target tumor versus normal cells selectively, achieve a sufficient concentration within the tumor, and produce tumor to normal-tissue ratios of 3 or 4 to 1. This, of course, is a tall order.

Two classes of compounds have been proposed:

1. Low-molecular-weight agents that simulate chemical precursors required for tumor cell proliferation, have the ability to traverse the cell membrane and be retained intracellularly. Two boron compounds have been identified and used clinically, known as BSH and BPA. Both have been used to treat brain tumors, and the latter also has been listed for cutaneous melanoma.
2. High-molecular-weight agents such as monoclonal antibodies and bispecific antibodies have been developed that contain boron. These are highly specific, but very small amounts reach brain tumors following systemic administration. Boron-containing conjugates of epidermal growth factor, the receptor for which is overexpressed on some tumors (including glioblastoma), also have been developed.

If the blood–brain barrier is disrupted temporarily, these high-molecular-weight compounds may have some utility, or direct intracerebral delivery may be required. They have not yet proved effective in clinical use.

Neutron Sources

During fission within the core of a nuclear reactor, neutrons are "born" that have a wide range of energies. Neutron beams can be extracted from the reactor by the application of suitable techniques and the use of appropriate moderators. Thermal neutrons, or room-temperature neutrons (0.025 eV), react best with boron to produce densely ionizing α-particles. Unfortunately, thermal neutrons are attenuated rapidly by tissue; the half-value layer is only about 1.5 cm. Consequently, it is not possible to treat to depths of more than a few centimeters without heavily irradiating surface normal tissues. Nevertheless, most clinical trials have utilized neutrons of this energy.

Current interest in the United States focuses on the use of epithermal neutron beams (1–10,000 eV), which have a somewhat greater depth of penetration. These can be obtained by using moderators or filters to slow the fast neutrons into the epithermal range and filtering out the residual thermal neutrons. These epithermal neutrons do not themselves interact with the boron but are degraded to become thermal neutrons in the tissue by collisions with hydrogen atoms. Even so, the peak in dose occurs at a depth of only 2 to 3 cm, with a rapid falloff beyond this depth. Thus, the very high surface doses are avoided but the depth doses are still poor.

The need for a nuclear reactor as a source of neutrons is a serious limitation and would preclude BNCT facilities in densely populated urban areas. If BNCT were shown to have a clear therapeutic advantage, then it would be essential to design and build compact proton accelerators as sources of neutrons. Some research has been performed in this area, and it is clear that appropriate accelerators could be produced commercially if the demand were there.

Clinical Trials

A number of clinical trials have been performed over the years, beginning in the 1950s and 1960s. Results are tantalizing but never definitive. A number of patients have been treated with BNCT in the United States, but the results are largely anecdotal. The concept of BNCT is as attractive as ever, but it continues to be difficult to convert to a practical treatment modality, even for shallow tumors.

PROTONS

Protons are attractive for radiotherapy because of their physical dose distribution; their radiobiologic properties are unremarkable. The RBE of protons is indistinguishable from that of 250-kV x-rays, which means that they are 10 to 15% more effective than cobalt-60 γ-rays or megavoltage x-rays generated by a linear accelerator. The OER for protons also is indistinguishable from that for x-rays, namely about 2.5 to 3. These biologic properties are consistent with the physical characteristics of high-energy proton beams; they are sparsely ionizing, except for a very short region at the end of the particles' range, just before they stop. In the entrance plateau, the average LET is about 0.5 keV/μm, rising to a maximum of 100 keV/μm over a few microns as the particles come to rest. This high-LET component is restricted, however, to such a tiny length of track and represents such a small proportion of the energy deposited that, for high-energy protons, it does not have any significant effect.

The dose deposited by a beam of monoenergetic protons increases slowly with depth, but reaches a sharp maximum near the end of the particles' range in the **Bragg peak**. The beam has sharp edges, with little side-scatter, and the dose falls to zero after the Bragg peak, at the end of the particles' range. The possibility of precisely confining the high-dose region to the tumor volume and minimizing the dose to surrounding normal tissue is obviously attractive

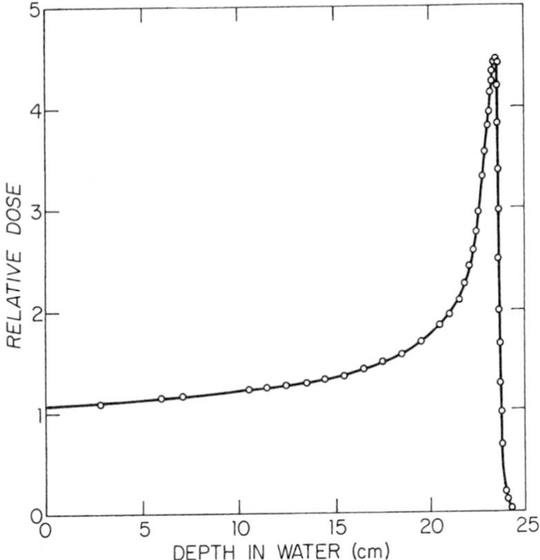

FIGURE 24.2 • Depth–dose curve for 187-MeV protons from the Uppsala synchrocyclotron. The dose reaches a sharp peak at a depth of about 23 cm. (Adapted from Larsson B: Pre-therapeutic physical experiments with high energy protons. *Br J Radiol* 34:143–151, 1961, with permission.)

to the radiotherapist. Protons and helium ions come closest to realizing this dream at modest cost.

Proton beams ranging in energy from 150 to 200 MeV are of interest in radiotherapy because this corresponds to a range in tissue of 16 to 26 cm. Intense proton beams in this energy range are produced readily by cyclotrons, many of which were built initially for high-energy physics research.

Figure 24.2 shows the depth–dose curve for the 187-MeV proton beam from the synchrocyclotron at Uppsala, Sweden. The sharply defined Bragg peak occurs at a depth in tissue that depends on the initial energy of the particles.

The early medical use of proton beams involved treatment of the pituitary, first in patients with advanced breast cancer and later in patients with diabetic retinopathy, Cushing's disease, and acromegaly. Protons were used for these applications to exploit their well-defined beam, which made it possible to give a huge dose to the pituitary without causing unacceptable damage to nearby structures. These treatments have been performed for many years at both Berkeley and Harvard, although the two institutions adopted very different strategies. At Harvard, an attempt was made to use a narrow pencil beam of protons of just the right range for the Bragg peak to fall exactly in the pituitary; in this way, a huge local dose could be delivered to the gland with minimal irradiation of surrounding tissues. This would appear to be a very elegant approach to the problem, but it is fraught with difficulty because the exact location of the Bragg peak can vary considerably with small inhomogeneities in the tissue traversed. For this reason, the Berkeley group favored the use of the plateau portion of a very high-energy beam that passed right through the patient's head; the Bragg peak was not within the patient at all. Multiple beams then were used in a pseudorotation technique, converging on the pituitary, to obtain good dose localization.

The way the Bragg peak can be spread out to encompass a tumor of realistic size is illustrated in Figure 24.3. In this figure, curve A shows the narrow Bragg peak of the primary beam of the 160-MeV proton beam at the Harvard cyclotron. Beams of lower intensity and shorter range, shown in curves B, C, D, and E, are readily obtainable by passing the beam through a rotating wheel with plastic sectors of varying thickness. The composite curve, S, which is the sum of all the individual Bragg peaks of the beams of varying range, results in a uniform dose over 2.8 cm. The spread-out Bragg peak, of course, can be made narrower or broader than this, as necessary.

Many researchers consider protons to be the treatment of choice for choroidal melanoma. Figure 24.4 shows the dose distribution that is achieved at the Harvard cyclotron, which allows very high doses to be delivered to small tumors without unacceptable damage to nearby normal tissues. Protons have found a small but important place in the treatment of ocular tumors and also some specialized tumors close to the spinal cord.

Broad-beam radiotherapy, with the Bragg peak spread out to cover a large tumor, has been in progress at Uppsala since 1957, and a comparable U.S. effort began at Harvard in 1961 and at Loma Linda University in 1990. Table 24.1 lists the current proton therapy facilities worldwide, as well as light- and heavy-charged-particle facilities, together with the number of patients treated. It is instructive to note that by 2005, about 40,000 patients had already been treated with protons worldwide.

Most of the proton machines used in the past were built initially for physics research and were located in physics laboratories. There is much current interest in the development of hospital-based proton facilities producing beams sufficiently penetrating to make possible the treatment of any cancer sites in the human; such facilities would include a gantry with an isocentric mount and would feed several treatment rooms. The first machine of this kind was built at Loma Linda University in California, where a 250-MeV cyclotron produces a proton beam that can be directed into any one of four treatment rooms. The layout of the facility is shown in

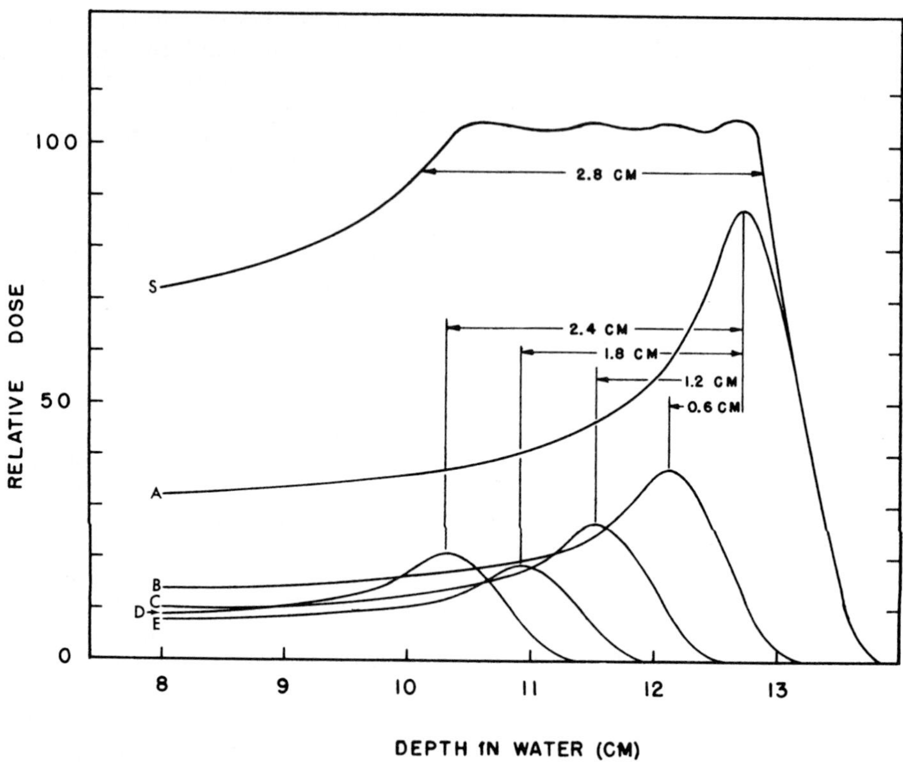

FIGURE 24.3 • The way the Bragg peak for a proton beam can be spread out. Curve A is the depth–dose distribution for the primary beam of 160-MeV protons at the Harvard cyclotron, which has a half-width of only 0.6 cm. Beams of lower intensity and shorter range, as illustrated by curves B, C, D, and E, can be added to give a composite curve S, which results in a uniform dose over 2.8 cm. The broadening of the peak is achieved by passing the beam through a rotating wheel with sectors of varying thickness. (Adapted from Koehler AM, Preston WM: Protons in radiation therapy. Comparative dose distributions for protons, photons, and electrons. *Radiology* 104:191–195, 1972, with permission.)

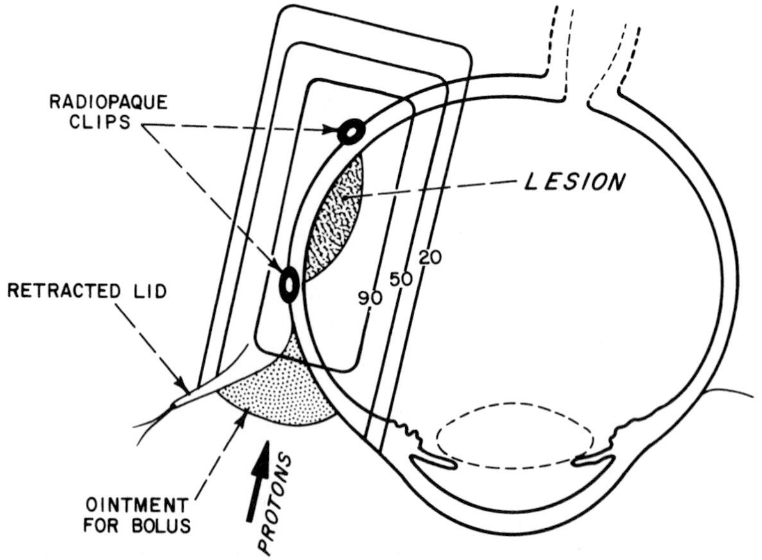

FIGURE 24.4 • Dose distribution used for the treatment of choroidal melanoma at the Harvard cyclotron. Note the sharp edges to the beam and rapid falloff of dose outside the treatment volume. (Courtesy of Dr. Herman Suit.)

TABLE 24.1

Worldwide Charged-Particle Patient Totals, July 2004

Who	Where	What	Date First RX	Date Last RX	Recent Patient Total	Date of Total
Berkeley 184	CA, USA	p	1954	1957	30	
Berkeley	CA, USA	He	1957	1992	2,054	
Uppsala	Sweden	p	1957	1976	73	
Harvard	MA, USA	p	1961	2002	9,116	
Dubna	Russia	p	1967	1996	124	
ITEP, Moscow	Russia	p	1969		3,748	June 04
Los Alamos	NM, USA	π^-	1974	1982	230	
St. Petersburg	Russia	p	1975		1,145	Apr 04
Berkeley	CA, USA	ion	1975	1992	433	
Chiba	Japan	p	1979		145	Apr 02
TRIUMF	Canada	π^-	1979	1994	367	
PSI (SIN)	Switzerland	π^-	1980	1993	503	
PMRC (1), Tsukuba	Japan	p	1983	2000	700	
PSI (72 MeV)	Switzerland	p	1984		4,066	June 04
Dubna	Russia	p	1999		191	Nov 03
Uppsala	Sweden	p	1989		418	Jan 04
Clatterbridge	England	p	1989		1,287	Dec 03
Loma Linda	CA, USA	p	1990		9,282	July 04
Louvain-la-Neuve	Belgium	p	1991	1993	21	
Nice	France	p	1991		2,555	Apr 04
Orsay	France	p	1991		2,805	Dec 03
iThemba LABS	South Africa	p	1993		446	Dec 03
MPRI (1)	IN, USA	p	1993	1999	34	
UCSF - CNL	CA, USA	p	1994		632	June 04
HIMAC, Chiba	Japan	C ion	1994		1,796	Feb 04
TRIUMF	Canada	p	1995		89	Dec 03
PSI (200 MeV)	Switzerland	p	1996		166	Dec 03
G.S.I. Darmstadt	Germany	C ion	1997		198	Dec 03
H. M. I., Berlin	Germany	p	1998		437	Dec 03
NCC, Kashiwa	Japan	p	1998		270	June 04
HIBMC, Hyogo	Japan	p	2001		359	June 04
PMRC (2), Tsukuba	Japan	p	2001		492	July 04
NPTC, MGH	MA, USA	p	2001		800	July 04
HIBMC, Hyogo	Japan	C ion	2002		30	Dec 02
INFN-LNS, Catania	Italy	p	2002		77	June 04
WERC	Japan	p	2002		14	Dec 03
Shizuoka	Japan	p	2003		69	July 04
MPRI (2)	IN, USA	p	2004		21	July 04
				Total pions	1,100	
				Total ions	4,511	
				Total protons	39,612	
				Total all particles	45,223	

Adapted from *Particles* 34 (July 2004):12. (*Particles* is a newsletter for those interested in proton, light-ion, and heavy-particle radiotherapy, published by the Particle Therapy Cooperative Group [http:ptcog.mgh.harvard.edu].)

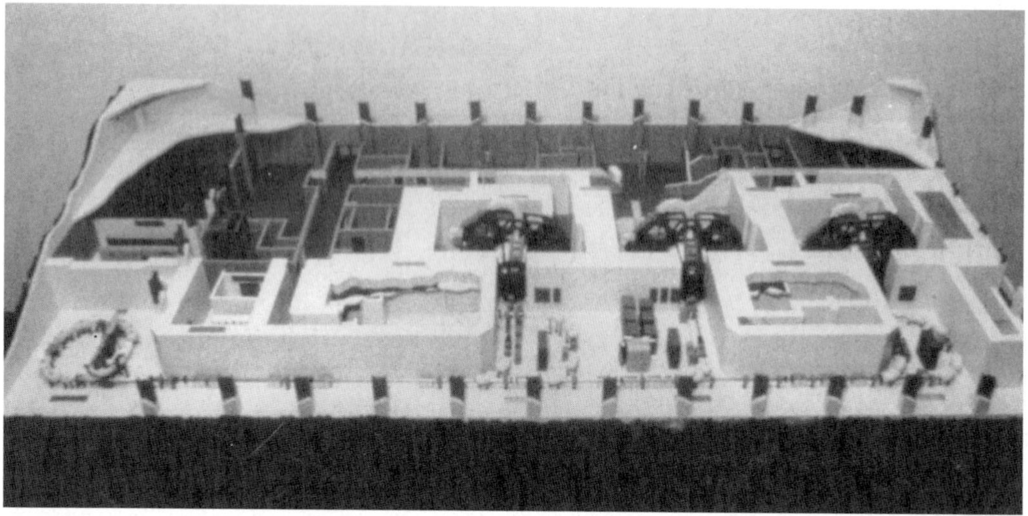

FIGURE 24.5 • Model of the proton facility at Loma Linda. Protons are accelerated to energies up to 250 MeV in a large cyclotron. The protons then can be directed into any one of four treatment rooms. This arrangement minimizes "idle" time, because while one patient is being treated in one room, the next two patients can be set up in adjoining treatment rooms. This sort of facility sets the scene for the future: a large radiation therapy facility with multiple treatment rooms in the context of a cancer center. (Courtesy of Drs. James Slater and John Archambeau, Loma Linda University, Loma Linda, California.)

Figure 24.5. The intention is to treat a broad spectrum of human cancers, not just the limited sites for which the dose distributions possible with protons already have proved their worth.

An even more impressive facility has been completed at the Massachusetts General Hospital in Boston. Whereas formerly they used a fixed horizontal beam from a cyclotron in the Harvard Physics Department, they now have a new facility constructed within the hospital. Similar facilities are being built or are in the planning stage at several locations in the United States, Europe, and Japan. Such facilities set the scene for the future. Figure 24.6 shows a typical dose distribution that can be obtained with intensity-modulated proton therapy compared with intensity modulated photon therapy.

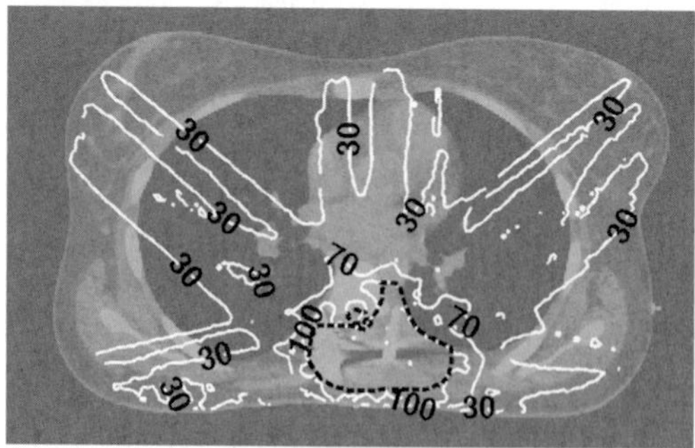

Photon IMRT

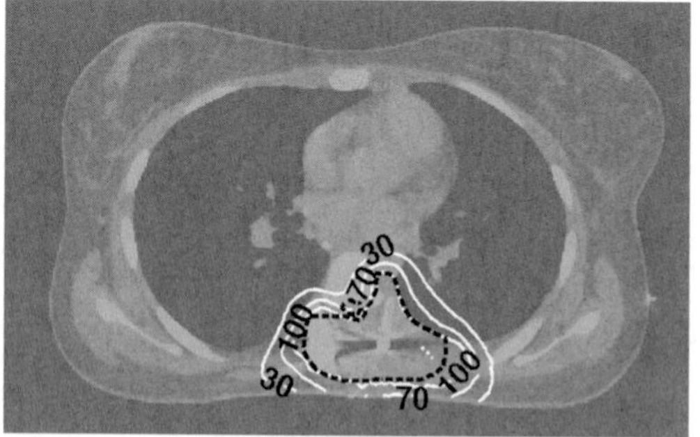

Proton IMRT

FIGURE 24.6 • Treatment planning comparison of a seven-field intensity-modulated photon treatment plan (left) with an intensity-modulated proton (three scanned pencil beams) plan (right) for a patient with an epithelioid sarcoma involving the paravertebral tissues adjacent to the fifth through seventh vertebrae. The 30%, 70%, and 100% isodose lines are shown. The dashed line outlines the target volume. Although dose to the target volume is similar, note the significantly higher integral dose to the lungs and heart with the intensity-modulated photon plan, which may be associated with an increase in acute and late normal-tissue toxicity. Treatment comparison plans were prepared by Alexei V. Trofimov, Ph.D., at the Northeast Proton Therapy Center using the KonRad radiation treatment planning system originally designed at DKFZ (Deutsches Krebsforschungszentrum), Heidelberg, Germany. For further illustrations and discussion, see Weber DC, Trofimov AV, DeLaney TF, Bortfeld T: A treatment planning comparison of intensity modulated photon and proton therapy for paraspinal sarcomas. *Int J Radiat Oncol Biol Phys* 58:1596–1606, 2004. (Courtesy of Dr. Thomas DeLaney, Massachusetts General Hospital, Boston.)

It is striking that with protons, the dose can be confined to the target volume, with much less irradiation of normal structures. With photons, a large fraction of the lungs are exposed to low doses of radiation.

CARBON ION RADIOTHERAPY

There is a sufficient renaissance of interest in heavy-ion radiotherapy to merit a brief description. The early work in this field centered at Berkeley, where a large body of radiobiologic data was accumulated and some patients treated with various heavy ions; however, the facility closed some years ago. Interest has been rekindled largely in Europe and Japan, with attention focused on high-energy carbon ions.

Depth–Dose Profiles

The characteristic depth–dose profile of heavy ions, which they share with protons (i.e., the increase in dose with depth of penetration), makes them attractive as a modality for the radiotherapy of deep-seated tumors.

Figure 24.7 shows the depth–dose profiles for carbon-12 (^{12}C) ions of two different energies compared with that for cobalt-60 (^{60}Co) γ-rays. In the case of carbon ions, dose is almost constant until close to the end of the range, when there is a sharp increase in dose in the Bragg peak. The depth at which the peak occurs depends on the energy. The peak is much too narrow to cover any tumor of realistic dimensions, and so the Bragg peak must be "spread out" to the required dimension by varying the energy of the beam. For carbon ions produced by a synchrotron, this can be achieved by varying the energy from pulse to pulse. Any required field size can be achieved from the narrow pencil beam that emerges from the synchrotron by "scanning" the beam, that is, deflecting the beam with magnetic fields so that voxel by voxel it conforms to the desired shape and size.

RBE Considerations

For carbon ions, there is the additional factor, which may be exploited to advantage, of an increase in relative biologic effectiveness (RBE) toward the end of the particle range. The rapid change of RBE with depth is shown in the top panel of Figure 24.8. This is a classic case of "good news—bad news." In principle, it is good news because the effectiveness of the dose is increased toward the end of the track, which is located in the tumor volume, exaggerating the change of effective dose with depth; the bad news is that one does not know the correct RBE to use, since RBE values must come from *in vitro* or animal experiments. Consequently, there is an element of uncertainty in these data.

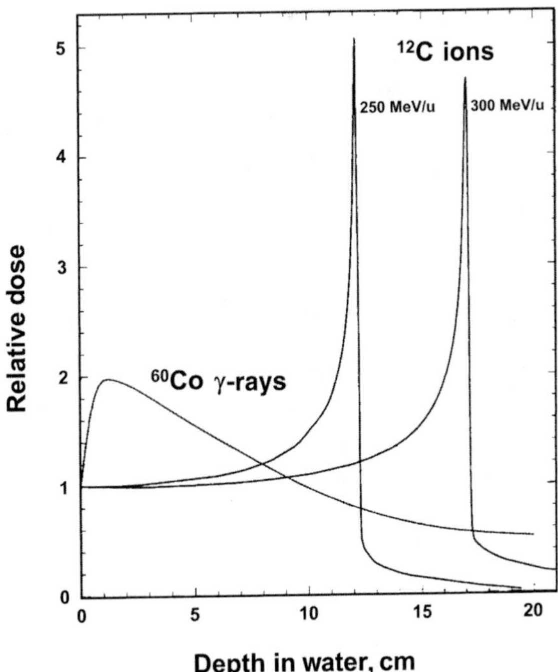

FIGURE 24.7 • Comparison of the depth–dose profiles of carbon ions of two different energies with that of ^{60}Co γ-rays. (Adapted from Kraft G: Tumor therapy with heavy charged particles. *Progress in Particle and Nuclear Physics* 45:S473–S544, 2000.)

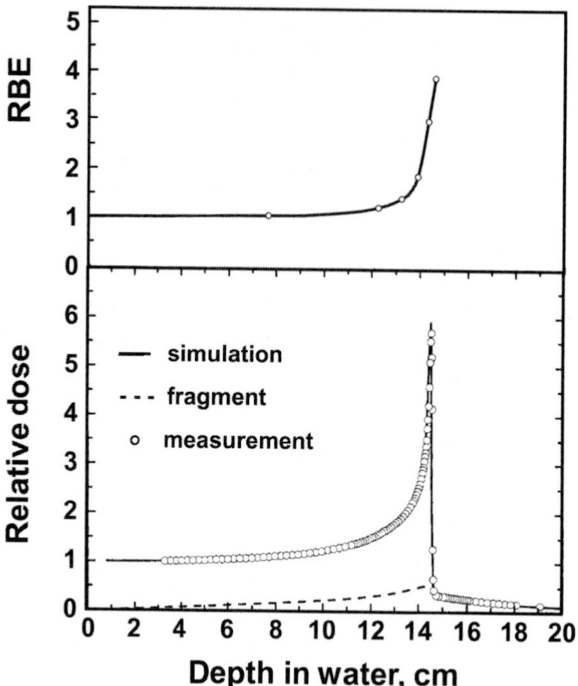

FIGURE 24.8 • **Top**: Measured relative biologic effectiveness as a function of distance from the Bragg peak for 270-MeV/u carbon ions. Note the rapid increase in RBE dose to the peak. (Data taken from Blakely EA, Tobias CA, Ngo FQH, Curtis SB: Physical and cellular radiobiological medical research with accelerated heavy ions at the Bevalac (eds.: Pirncello MD, Tobias CA), *LBL* 11220: 73–88, 1980.) **Bottom:** Measured depth–dose profile for 270-MeV/u carbon ions, including the contribution from nuclear fragments in the "tail" beyond the Bragg peak. (Redrawn from Kraft G: Tumor therapy with heavy charged particles. *Progress in Particle and Nuclear Physics* 45:S473–S544, 2000.)

Scattering and Fragmentation

Compared with protons, carbon ions have less lateral scattering, leading to sharper beam edges, but there is a "tail" of lighter fragments beyond the Bragg peak. This is illustrated in the lower panel of Figure 24.8. Carbon ions do not therefore share the proton advantage that dose stops sharply at the end of the range of the primary particle.

PET Verification of Treatment Plans

There is a unique opportunity to verify the treatment plan in the case of carbon ions. The basis is as follows: When a beam of carbon ions penetrates a thick absorber, a small fraction of the ions will undergo nuclear fragmentation—that is, they will break up. A frequent process is the stripping of one or two neutrons, converting the stable ^{12}C to the positron-emitting isotopes ^{11}C and ^{10}C. These isotopes travel with *almost* the same velocity as the main beam and stop in *almost* the same place. They have short half-lives, and as they annihilate, they emit γ-rays that can be detected as in a conventional PET scanner. As a consequence, the location of the spread-out Bragg peak, and therefore the high-dose treatment volume, is visualized.

Summary of Pertinent Conclusions

Neutrons

- Neutrons are indirectly ionizing. In tissue, they give up their energy to produce recoil protons, α-particles, and heavier nuclear fragments.
- Biologic properties of neutrons differ from those of x-rays in several ways: reduced OER, little or no repair of sublethal damage or potentially lethal damage, and less variation of sensitivity through the cell cycle.
- The rationale for the use of neutrons in radiotherapy has changed over the years. The earlier rationale was the reduced OER to overcome the problem of hypoxic cells. The revised rationale is based on a higher neutron RBE for slowly growing tumors.

(continued)

Summary of Pertinent Conclusions (Continued)

- An advantage has been proved in clinical trials for neutrons in the treatment of salivary gland and prostate tumors and soft-tissue sarcomas, but not for the majority of cancer sites tested.
- A new generation of hospital-based cyclotrons, generating neutrons by the $p^+ \rightarrow$ Be reaction, are now available, but enthusiasm for neutrons has waned.

Boron Neutron-Capture Therapy

- The principle of boron neutron-capture therapy (BNCT) is to deliver a drug containing boron that localizes only in tumors and then to treat with low-energy thermal neutrons that interact with boron to produce α-particles.
- Boron is a suitable substance because it has a large cross section for thermal neutrons and emits short-range densely ionizing α-particles if bombarded by thermal neutrons. Its chemistry is such that it can be incorporated into a wide range of compounds.
- Many attempts have been made to synthesize boron-containing compounds that are selectively localized in tumors relative to normal tissues, with limited success. They fall into two categories:
  1. Low-molecular-weight agents that simulate chemical precursors needed for tumor cell proliferation
  2. High-molecular-weight agents such as monoclonal antibodies and bispecific antibodies
- Thermal neutrons are poorly penetrating in tissue, with a half-value layer of only 1.5 cm.
- Epithermal neutrons are somewhat more penetrating. They are degraded to thermal neutrons by collisions with hydrogen atoms in tissue. The peak dose is at 2 to 3 cm, and the high surface dose is avoided.
- Results of clinical trials of the efficacy of BNCT are tantalizing but not definitive.
- The concept of BNCT is very attractive, but there are formidable practical difficulties in making it a treatment modality even for relatively shallow tumors.

Protons

- Protons result in excellent physical dose distributions.
- Protons have biologic properties similar to those of x-rays.
- There is an established place for protons in the treatment of choroidal melanoma or tumors close to the spinal cord, in which a sharp cutoff of dose is important.
- Hospital-based high-energy cyclotrons with isocentric mounts are now being used to treat a broader spectrum of cancer patients with protons. Their efficacy has yet to be proved in clinical trials, but they offer the obvious physical advantage of good dose distributions with reduced dose to normal structures.

Carbon Ion Radiotherapy

- The use of high-energy carbon ions has experienced a renaissance in Europe and Japan.
- For carbon ions, as for protons, the narrow Bragg peak must be spread out to cover a tumor of realistic dimensions by varying the energy of the beam.
- Inevitably, the RBE varies across the spread-out Bragg peak. In theory, this could be an advantage for carbon ions because it further exaggerates tumor dose relative to normal tissue. In practice, it is a complication because one must estimate RBE values from experiments in model systems.
- A unique attraction of carbon ion therapy is that the target volume can be visualized by PET as some ^{12}C ions decay to radioactive ^{11}C and ^{10}C.

BIBLIOGRAPHY

Asbury AK, Ojeann RG, Nielson SL, Sweet WH: Neuropathologic study of fourteen cases of malignant brain tumor treated by boron-10 slow neutron capture radiation. *J Neuropathol Exp Neurol* 31:278–303, 1972

Barth RF, Soloway AH, Fairchild RG: Boron neutron capture therapy of cancer. *Cancer Res* 50:1061–1070, 1990

Batterman JJ: *Clinical Application of Fast Neutrons: The Amsterdam Experience*. Amsterdam, Rodipi, 1981

Blakely EA, Tobias CA, Ngo FQH, Curtis SB: Physical and cellular radiobiological medical research with accelerated heavy ions at the Bevalac (eds.: Pirncello MD, Tobias CA), *LBL* 11220:73–88, 1980

Broerse JJ, Barendsen GW, van Kersen GR: Survival of cultured human cells after irradiation with fast neutrons of different energies in hypoxic and oxygenated conditions. *Int J Radiat Biol* 13:559–572, 1968

Catterall M: Results of neutron therapy: Differences, correlations, and improvements. *Int J Radiat Oncol Biol Phys* 8:2141–2144, 1982

Catterall M, Sutherland L, Bewley DK: First results of a clinical trial of fast neutrons compared with x or gamma rays in treatment of advanced tumors of the head and neck. *Br Med J* 2:653–656, 1975

Catterall M, Vonberg DD: Treatment of advanced tumors of head and neck with fast neutrons. *Br Med J* 3:137–143, 1974

D'Angio GJ, Aceto M, Nisce LZ, et al.: Preliminary clinical observations after extended Bragg peak helium ion irradiation. *Cancer* 34:6–11, 1974

Drake CG: Arteriovenous malformations of the brain. *N Engl J Med* 309:308–310, 1983

Field, SB, Hornsey S: RBE values for cyclotron neutrons for effects on normal tissues and tumors as a function of dose and dose fractionation. *Eur J Cancer* 7:151–169, 1971

Fowler JF, Morgan RL, Wood CAP: Pretherapeutic experiments with fast neutron beam from the Medical Research Council Cyclotron: I. The biological and physical advantages and problems of neutron therapy. *Br J Radiol* 36:77–80, 1963

Hall EJ: Radiobiology of heavy particle radiation therapy: Cellular studies. *Radiology* 108:119–129, 1973

Hall EJ, Graves RG, Phillips TL, Suit HD (eds): Particle accelerators in radiation therapy. *Int J Radiat Oncol Biol Phys* 8:2041–2207, 1982

Hatanaka H: A revised boron-neutron capture therapy for malignant brain tumors: 11. Interim clinical result with the patients excluding previous treatments. *J Neurol* 209:81–94, 1975

Hatanaka H, Amano K, Kanemitsu H, Ikeuchi 1, Yoshizaki T: Boron uptake by human brain tumors and quality control of boron compounds. In Hatanaka H (ed): *Boron Neutron Capture Therapy for Tumors*, pp 77–106. Niigata, Japan, Nishimura Co, 1986

Javid M, Brownell GL, Sweet WH: The possible use of neutron-capture isotopes such as boron-10 in the treatment of neoplasms: 11. Computation of the radiation energy and estimates of effects in normal and neoplastic brain. *J Clin Invest* 31:603–610, 1952

Kjellberg RN, Hanamura T, Davis KR, Lyons SL, Adams RD: Bragg-peak proton-beam therapy for arteriovenous malformations of the brain. *N Engl J Med* 309:269–274, 1983

Koehler AM, Preston WM: Protons in radiation therapy. Comparative dose distributions for protons, photons, and electrons. *Radiology* 104:191–195, 1972

Kraft G: Tumor therapy with heavy charged particles. *Progress in Particle and Nuclear Physics* 45:S473–S544, 2000

Laramore GE, Krall JM, Thomas FJ, Griffin TW, Maor MH, Hendrickson FR: Fast neutron radiotherapy for locally advanced prostate cancer: Results of an RTOG randomized study. *Int J Radiat Oncol Biol Phys* 11:1621–1627, 1985

Larsson B: Pre-therapeutic physical experiments with high energy protons. *Br J Radiol* 34:143–151, 1961

Locher GL: Biological effects and therapeutic possibilities of neutrons. *AJR* 36:1–13, 1936

Particles 34 (July 2004):12. *Particles* is a newsletter for those interested in proton, light-ion, and heavy-particle radiotherapy, published by the Particle Therapy Cooperative Group (http:ptcog.mgh.harvard.edu).

Raju MR: *Heavy Particle Radiotherapy*. New York, Academic Press, 1980

Sweet WH: The use of nuclear disintegration in the diagnosis and treatment of brain tumor. *N Engl J Med* 245:875–878, 1951

Weber DC, Trofimov AV, DeLaney TF, Bortfeld T: A treatment planning comparison of intensity modulated photon and proton therapy for paraspinal sarcomas. *Int J Radiat Oncol Biol Phys* 58:1596–1606, 2004

Withers HR, Thames HD, Peters LJ: Biological bases for high RBE values for late effects of neutron irradiation. *Int J Radiat Oncol Biol Phys* 8:2071–2076, 1982

CHAPTER 25

Radiosensitizers and Bioreductive Drugs

Radiosensitizers are chemical or pharmacologic agents that increase the lethal effects of radiation if administered in conjunction with it. Many compounds that modify the radiation response of mammalian cells have been discovered over the years, but most offer no practical gain in radiotherapy because they do not show a *differential effect* between tumors and normal tissues. There is no point in employing a drug that increases the sensitivity of tumor and normal cells to the same extent.

With this all-important criterion of a differential effect, only two types of sensitizers have found practical use in clinical radiotherapy:

1. **Halogenated pyrimidines** sensitize cells to a degree dependent on the amount of the analogue incorporated. In this case, a differential effect is based on the premise that tumor cells cycle faster and therefore incorporate more of the drug than the surrounding normal tissues.
2. **Hypoxic-cell sensitizers** increase the radiosensitivity of cells deficient in molecular oxygen but have no effect on normally aerated cells. In this case, a differential effect is based on the premise that hypoxic cells occur only in tumors and not in normal tissues.

These two classes of sensitizers are discussed in turn. The basic strategy of all radiosensitizers is illustrated in Figure 25.1. The aim is to move the tumor control curve to lower doses by sensitizing tumor cells but not affecting the normal-tissue complication curve, or at least not altering it as much. The outcome would be to increase the tumor control probability for a given level of normal-tissue complications.

THE HALOGENATED PYRIMIDINES

The combining size (the van der Waals radius) of an atom of chlorine, bromine, or iodine is very similar to that of the methyl group CH_3. The halogenated pyrimidines 5-iododeoxyuridine and 5-bromodeoxyuridine consequently are very similar to the normal DNA precursor thymidine, having a halogen substituted in place of the methyl group.

The similarity is so close that they are incorporated into the DNA chain in place of thymidine. This substitution "weakens" the DNA chain, making the cells more susceptible to damage by γ-rays or ultraviolet light. These substances are effective as sensitizers only if they are made available to cells for several cell generations so that an appreciable quantity of the analogue actually may be incorporated

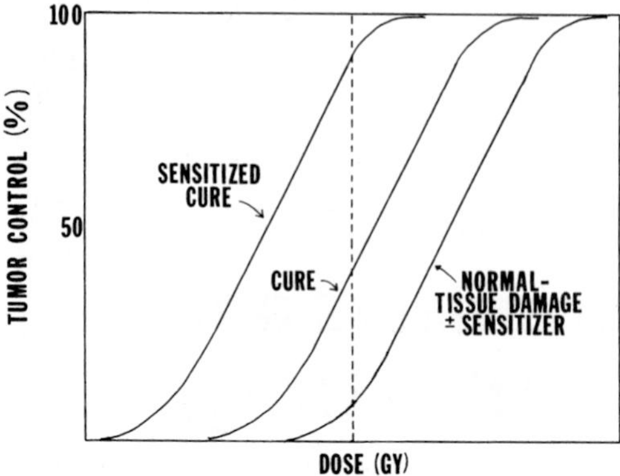

FIGURE 25.1 • The basic strategy of all radiosensitizers. The addition of the drug is expected to move the tumor control curve to the left but not affect the normal-tissue complication curve, or at least not alter it as much. For halogenated pyrimidines, this expectation is based on the premise that tumor cells are cycling more rapidly than cells of the dose-limiting normal tissues, so that they incorporate more sensitizer. For hypoxic-cell radiosensitizers, this expectation is based on the premise that hypoxic cells are present only in tumors, not in normal tissues, and these drugs preferentially sensitize hypoxic cells. (Based on an idea by Dr. Ged Adams.)

into the DNA. As the percentage of thymidine bases replaced increases, so does the extent of radiosensitization.

The effectiveness of the halogenated pyrimidines as sensitizers was first shown in bacteria, but a similar effect has been demonstrated amply in mammalian cells both *in vitro* and *in vivo*. Figure 25.2 shows the sensitization of hamster cells to x-rays and to fluorescent light by the incorporation of bromodeoxyuridine and iododeoxyuridine. Although there is little to choose between the bromine or the iodine analogues as far as sensitization to x-rays is concerned, bromodeoxyuridine is a much more efficient sensitizer for fluorescent light. This turns out to be an important difference in the clinical application of these drugs. One of the unpleasant side effects of bromodeoxyuridine in some patients is a rash, caused by phototoxicity from the interaction of light with the drug. This is much less of a problem with the iodine analogue, as might be predicted from Figure 25.2.

The use of halogenated pyrimidines as an adjunct to radiotherapy began in the 1970s. The rationale was that tumor cells may be cycling more rapidly than the normal cells in surrounding tissues, so that more drug could be incorporated in the tumor cell DNA, resulting in "selective"

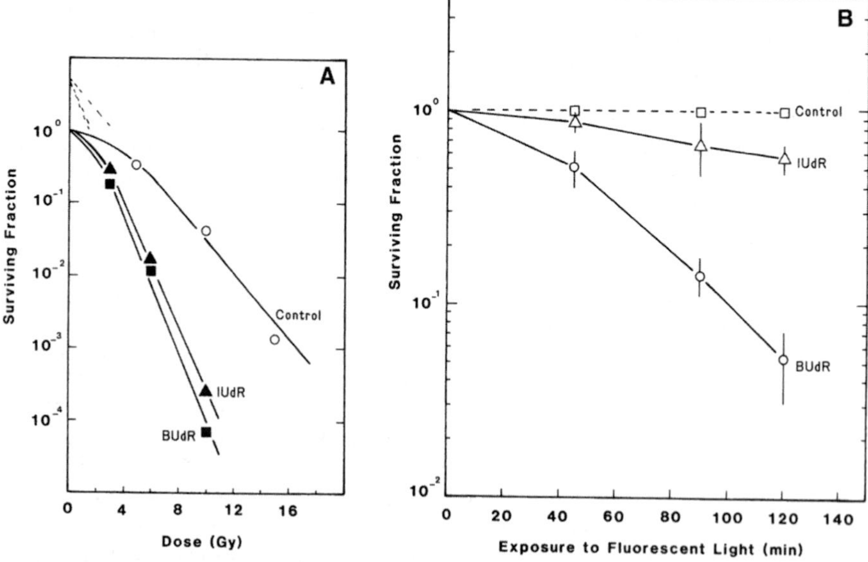

FIGURE 25.2 • Survival curves for bromodeoxyuridine (BUdR)- and iododeoxyuridine (IUdR)-substituted cells exposed to x-rays (**A**) and fluorescent light (**B**). Both halogenated pyrimidines sensitize equally to x-rays, and there is little to choose between them on this count. Iododeoxyuridine, however, has little effect with fluorescent light; thus, it is preferred clinically because it avoids the light-induced rash produced by bromodeoxyuridine. (From Mitchell J, Morstyn G, Russo A, et al.: Differing sensitivity to fluorescent light in Chinese hamster cells containing equally incorporated quantities of BUdR versus IUdR. *Int J Radiat Oncol Biol Phys* 10:1447–1451, 1984, with permission.)

radiosensitization. It was perhaps unfortunate that head and neck tumors were among those treated in this early study at Stanford University, because they are surrounded by actively proliferating normal tissues. The choice of tumors in the head and neck was determined partly by the need to deliver the analogue by an intra-arterial infusion into the main vessel supplying the neoplasm to be treated because the liver tends to dehalogenate the circulating drug. Tumor responses were reported to be good, but normal-tissue damage was unacceptable.

Consequently, these sensitizers were not used for a number of years, until several centers began an evaluation in more suitable tumor sites, in which the proximity of actively proliferating normal tissues is not such a problem. Among the tumors evaluated were high-grade glioblastomas and large unresectable sarcomas.

Because the all-important differential effect between tumor and normal tissues is based on the greater uptake of the halogenated pyrimidines in the malignant cells, the most appropriate tumors are those characterized by a high growth fraction and high labeling index, both indicators of cell division. In the future, measurements of these quantities in individual patients may be used as a basis for choosing suitable cases.

RADIOSENSITIZING HYPOXIC CELLS

As described in Chapter 20, a great deal of experimental work through the years had established that at least in transplanted tumors in animals, tumor control by x-rays frequently is limited by the presence of foci of hypoxic cells that are intransigent to killing by x-rays, which may result in tumor regrowth. Among the methods suggested to overcome this problem are treatment in hyperbaric oxygen chambers and the introduction of high linear energy transfer radiations, such as neutrons and heavy ions. Chemical sensitizers address the same problem. High linear energy transfer radiations are discussed in Chapter 7. This chapter addresses hyperbaric oxygen, chemical radiosensitizers, and the latest approach, namely, hypoxic cytotoxins.

Hyperbaric Oxygen

Following the identification of hypoxia as a possible source of tumor resistance, a major effort was made to solve the problem by the use of hyperbaric oxygen. Patients were sealed in chambers filled with pure oxygen raised to a pressure of three atmospheres. Churchill Davidson at St. Thomas' Hospital in London pioneered this work, but it was taken up by researchers on both sides of the Atlantic. The clinical trials that were performed involved small numbers of patients and were difficult to interpret because unconventional fractionation schemes were used; that is, a few large fractions were used because of the time and effort involved in the technical procedures. Patient compliance was also a problem because of the feeling of claustrophobia from being sealed in a narrow tube. There was also the serious risk of fire, because tissue is highly flammable in pure oxygen (as evidenced by the accident when the crew of a space capsule died in an oxygen fire on the ground), though in practice an accident of this nature never happened during the treatment of several thousand patients. The largest multicenter trials performed by the Medical Research Council in the United Kingdom showed a significant benefit both in local control and in survival for patients with carcinoma of the uterine cervix and advanced head and neck cancer, but not for patients with bladder cancer. The data generated a great deal of debate. An overview of the trials showed a 6.6% improvement in local control, with a suggestion, too, of an increase in late normal-tissue damage. Hyperbaric oxygen fell into disuse, partly because it is cumbersome and difficult in practice, and partly because of the promise of drugs that would achieve the same end by simpler means.

The notion of improving tumor oxygenation by breathing 100% oxygen rather than air has been revived in recent years by experiments involving carbogen. If pure oxygen is breathed, it tends to lead to vasoconstriction, a closing down of some blood vessels, which of course defeats the object of the exercise. This is avoided if 5% carbon dioxide is added to the oxygen, a mixture called *carbogen.* Breathing carbogen at atmospheric pressure, then, is a relatively simple attempt to overcome chronic hypoxia, that is, diffusion-limited hypoxia. The use of carbogen in combination with nicotinamide is described subsequently in this chapter.

Improving the Oxygen Supply to Tumors

A group at the Princess Margaret Hospital in Toronto showed convincingly that a blood transfusion prior to radiotherapy led to a significant improvement in local tumor control probability in patients with carcinoma of the uterine cervix. A number of other studies have shown that hemoglobin levels can influence the success of radiation therapy.

Tumor oxygenation also can be improved by the use of artificial blood substances such as *perfluorocarbons.* Because smoking can decrease tumor oxygenation, it is clearly advisable for patients to give up smoking, at least during radiotherapy.

Hypoxic-Cell Radiosensitizers

Spurred largely by the efforts of radiation chemists (most notably, Adams), a search was under way in the early 1960s for compounds that mimic oxygen in their ability to sensitize biologic materials to the effects of x-rays. Instead of trying to "force" oxygen into tissues by the use of high-pressure tanks, the emphasis shifted to oxygen substitutes that diffuse into poorly vascularized areas of tumors and achieve the desired effect by chemical means. The vital difference between these drugs and oxygen, on which their success depends, is that the sensitizers are not rapidly metabolized by the cells in the tumor through which they diffuse. Because of this, they can penetrate further than oxygen and reach all of the hypoxic cells in the tumor, including those most remote from a blood supply. In the early 1960s, many simple chemical compounds were found to have the ability to sensitize hypoxic microorganisms. These studies were guided by the hypothesis, now known to be correct, that sensitizing efficiency is related directly to the electron affinity of the compounds.

Adams and his colleagues listed properties that would be essential for a clinically useful hypoxic-cell sensitizer. First, it has to selectively sensitize hypoxic cells at a concentration that would result in acceptable toxicity to normal tissues. Second, it should be chemically stable and not subject to rapid metabolic breakdown. Third, it must be highly soluble in water or lipids and must be capable of diffusing a considerable distance through a nonvascularized cell mass to reach the hypoxic cells, which in a tumor may be located as far as 200 μm from the nearest capillary. Fourth, it should be effective at the relatively low daily doses of a few gray (a few hundred rad) used in conventional fractionated radiotherapy. The first candidate compound that appeared to satisfy these criteria was misonidazole.

Misonidazole

Figure 25.3 illustrates the numbering of the basic ring structure of the nitroimidazoles. The side chain determines position 1, and the position of the nitro group (NO_2) leads to the classification of the drug as a 2-nitroimidazole, 4-nitroimidazole, and so on. In general, 2-nitroimidazoles have a higher electron affinity than 5-nitroimidazoles, the class that includes metronidazole, which was briefly tried as a radiosensitizer. Misonidazole is a 2-nitroimidazole; its structure is shown in Figure 25.4.

Misonidazole produces appreciable sensitization with cells in culture (Fig. 25.5). Hypoxic cells in the presence of 10 mM of misonidazole have a radiosensitivity approaching that of aerated cells.

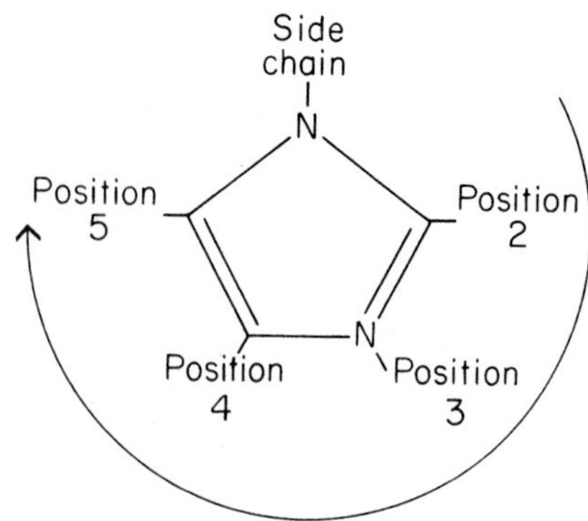

FIGURE 25.3 • Method of numbering the basic ring structure of the nitroimidazoles. The side chain determines position 1. If the nitro group (NO_2) is in the second position, the drug is a 2-nitroimidazole. If the NO_2 group is in the fifth position, the drug is a 5-nitroimidazole. In general, 2-nitroimidazoles are more efficient radiosensitizers of hypoxic cells.

Misonidazole also has a dramatic effect on tumors in experimental animals. This is illustrated in Figure 25.6, which shows the proportion of mouse mammary tumors controlled as a function of x-ray dose delivered in a single fraction. If x-rays are used alone, the dose required to control half of the tumors is 43.8 Gy (4,380 rad). This falls to 24.1 Gy (2,410 rad) if the radiation is delivered 30 minutes after the administration of misonidazole (1 mg/g body weight). This corresponds to an enhancement ratio of 1.8. Dramatic results, such as those shown in Figure 25.6 in which an enhancement ratio of 1.8 was obtained, are rather misleading; they represent single-dose treatments, in contrast to the multifraction regimens common in conventional radiotherapy. Most animal tumors reoxygenate to some extent between irradiations, so in a multifraction regimen, the enhancement ratio for a hypoxic-cell sensitizer is usually much less than for a single-dose treatment.

After encouraging results in laboratory studies, misonidazole was introduced into a large number of clinical trials, involving many different types of human tumors, in Europe and the United States. In general, the results have been disappointing. Of the 20 or so randomized prospective controlled clinical trials performed in the United States by the Radiation Therapy Oncology Group (RTOG), none yielded a statistically significant advantage for misonidazole, although a number indicated a slight benefit. The only trial that shows a clear advantage for misonidazole was the head and neck trial performed in Denmark, the largest single trial performed with the sensitizer. If patients of all categories are compared in this trial, the addition

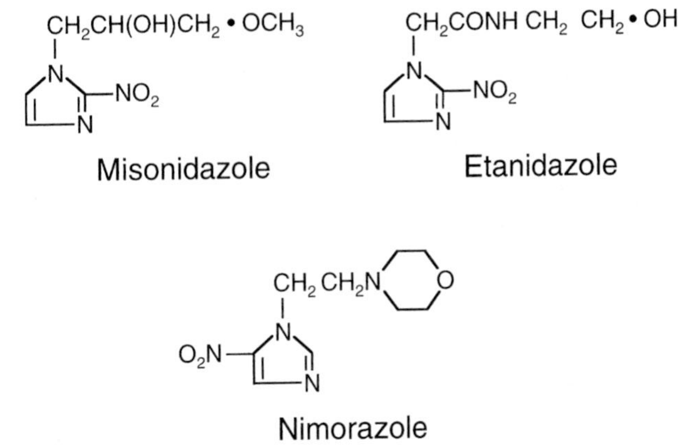

$CH_2CH(OH)CH_2 \bullet OCH_3$

N, NO_2, N

Misonidazole

$CH_2CONH\ CH_2\ CH_2 \bullet OH$

N, NO_2, N

Etanidazole

$CH_2\ CH_2N$ O

O_2N, N, N

Nimorazole

FIGURE 25.4 ● The structure of misonidazole, etanidazole, and nimorazole, the three compounds used most widely in clinical trials. Misonidazole and etanidazole are 2-nitroimidazoles; nimorazole is a 5-nitroimidazole. Misonidazole and etanidazole are equally active as radiosensitizers, but etanidazole is less neurotoxic because it has a shorter half-life and is hydrophilic. Nimorazole is less active but very much less toxic than either misonidazole or etanidazole, so that larger doses are tolerable.

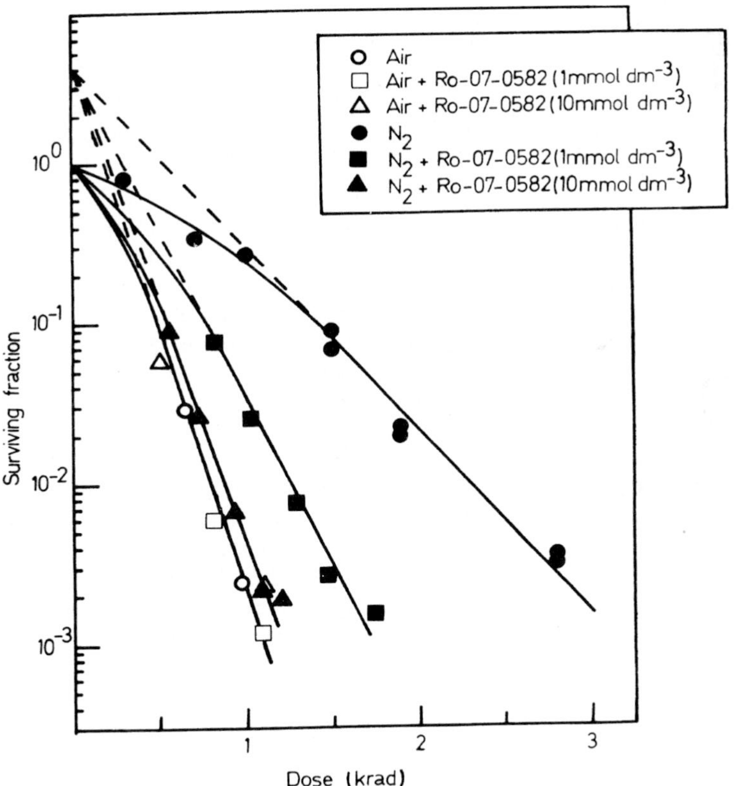

FIGURE 25.5 ● Survival data for aerated and hypoxic Chinese hamster cells x-irradiated in the presence of various concentrations of misonidazole (Ro-07-0582). At a concentration of 10 mM of this drug, the radiosensitivity of hypoxic cells approaches that of aerated cells. The response of aerated cells is not affected by the drug at all. (From Adams GE, Flockhart IR, Smithen CE, Stratford IJ, Wardman P, Watts ME: Electron-affinic sensitization. VII. A correlation between structures, one-electron reduction potentials, and efficiencies of nitroimidazoles as hypoxic cell radiosensitizers. *Radiat Res* 67:9–20, 1976, with permission.)

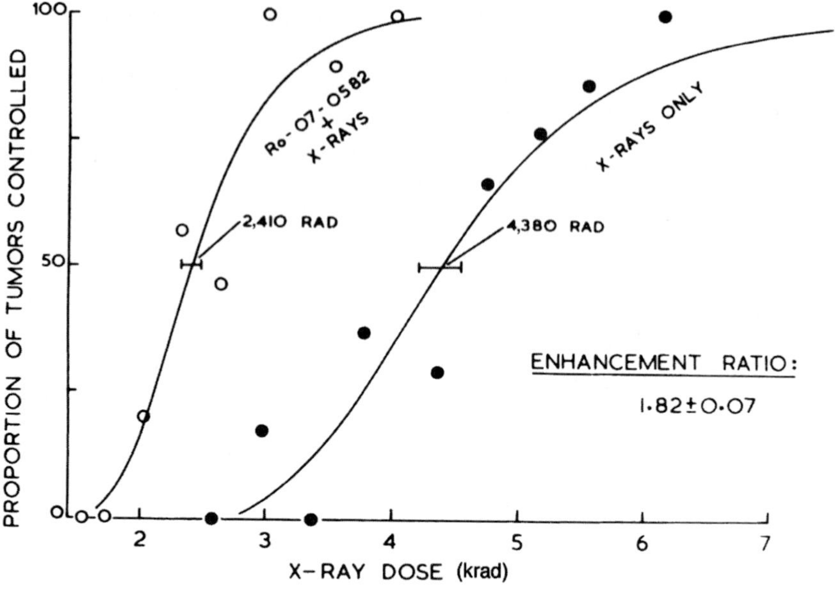

FIGURE 25.6 • Proportion of mouse mammary tumors controlled at 150 days as a function of x-ray dose for a single treatment. The right curve represents x-rays only; the left curve refers to x-rays delivered after the administration of 1 mg/g body weight of misonidazole (Ro-07-0582). The enhancement ratio is the ratio of x-ray doses in the absence or presence of the drug that results in the control of 50% of the tumors; it has a value of 1.8. (From Sheldon PW, Foster JL, Fowler JF: Radiosensitization of C3H mouse mammary tumours by a 2-nitroimidazole drug. *Br J Cancer* 30:560–565, 1974, with permission.)

of misonidazole to the radiotherapy schedule conferred no significant advantage. If the patients are categorized into a number of subgroups, however, males with high hemoglobin levels and cancer of the pharynx showed a great benefit from the addition of misonidazole. Tumor control at three years was about double in the group receiving the drug, compared with those patients receiving radiotherapy alone. This interesting result is shown in Figure 25.7. Other subgroups, including patients with cancer of the larynx, showed no benefit from the addition of the sensitizer.

When misonidazole was used in the clinic, the dose-limiting toxicity was found to be peripheral neuropathy that progressed to central nervous system toxicity if drug administration was not stopped. This toxicity prevented use of the drug at adequate dose levels throughout multifraction regimens. The disappointing results obtained with misonidazole in the clinic must be attributed largely to the fact that doses were limited to inadequate levels because of this toxicity.

Etanidazole and Nimorazole

Spurred by the promise of misonidazole in the laboratory compared with its failure in the clinic, efforts were made to find a better drug. The compound chosen for the next series of clinical trials in the United States was etanidazole, a 2-nitroimidazole, the structure of which also is shown in Figure 25.4.

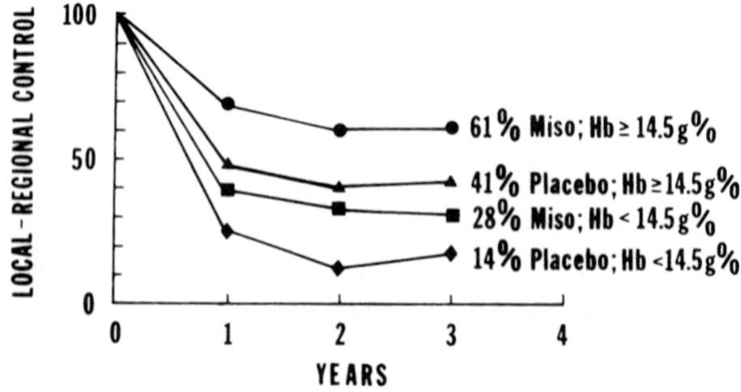

FIGURE 25.7 • Some results from the Danish head and neck cancer trial of misonidazole. Misonidazole produced a significant improvement of tumor control by radiotherapy only for males with tumors of the pharynx and depended on hemoglobin status. (Data from Dr. Jens Overgaard.)

This compound equals misonidazole as a sensitizer but is less toxic, so that doses could be increased by a factor of 3. The lower neurotoxicity is a function of a shorter half-life *in vivo* plus a lower partition coefficient, so that it penetrates poorly into nerve tissue and does not cross the blood–brain barrier. Controlled clinical trials by the RTOG in the United States and a multicenter consortium in Europe showed no benefit when etanidazole was added to conventional radiation therapy.

Nimorazole is a 5-nitroimidazole (structure also shown in Fig. 25.4); it is less effective as a radiosensitizer than either misonidazole or etanidazole, but it is much less toxic, so that very large doses could be given. In a Danish head and neck cancer trial, this compound produced a significant improvement in both locoregional control and survival compared with radiotherapy alone in patients with supraglottic and pharyngeal carcinoma. It is surprising that nimorazole has not been used elsewhere.

The development of nitroimidazoles is illustrated by the following:

Metronidazole

↓

Misonidazole: more active, toxic; benefit in subgroups

↓

Etanidazole: less toxic, no benefit

↓

Nimorazole: less active, much less toxic; benefit in head and neck cancer

Overgaard's Meta-Analysis of Clinical Trials Addressing the Problem of Hypoxia

For over three decades, an enormous effort has been expended in an attempt to overcome the perceived problem of hypoxia. Dozens of clinical trials have been performed, most of which have been inconclusive or have shown results with borderline significance. Overgaard and colleagues performed a meta-analysis in which the results of all the trials were combined and analyzed together. They identified 10,602 patients treated in 82 randomized clinical trials involving hyperbaric oxygen, chemical sensitizers, carbogen breathing, or blood transfusions. Tumor sites included the bladder, uterine cervix, central nervous system, head and neck, and lung.

Overall, local tumor control was improved by 4.6%, survival by 2.8%, and the complication rate increased by only 0.6%, which was not statistically significant. The largest number of trials involved head and neck tumors, which also showed the greatest benefit. It also was concluded that the problem of hypoxia may be marginal in most adenocarcinomas and most important in squamous cell carcinomas.

Nicotinamide and Carbogen Breathing

Hypoxic-cell radiosensitizers, such as the nitroimidazoles, were designed primarily to overcome chronic hypoxia, that is, diffusion-limited hypoxia resulting from the inability of oxygen to diffuse further than about 100 μm through respiring tissue. As explained in Chapter 6, however, there is another form of hypoxia known as *acute hypoxia*, in which local regions of hypoxia are caused by the intermittent closing down of blood vessels. Nicotinamide, a vitamin B_3 analogue, prevents these transient fluctuations in tumor blood flow that lead to the development of acute hypoxia, at least in mouse tumors.

A combination of nicotinamide to overcome acute hypoxia and carbogen breathing to overcome chronic hypoxia is the basis of the ARCON trials under way at a number of European centers. The trials are also accelerated and hyperfractionated to avoid tumor proliferation and damage to late-responding normal tissues. Here, briefly, is a summary of the ARCON treatment:

Accelerated, to overcome proliferation
Hyperfractionated, to spare late-responding normal tissues
Carbogen breathing, to overcome chronic hypoxia
Nicotinamide, to overcome acute hypoxia

HYPOXIC CYTOTOXINS

An alternative approach to designing drugs that preferentially *radiosensitize* hypoxic cells is to develop drugs that selectively *kill* hypoxic cells. It was pointed out at an early stage that the greater reductive environment of tumors might be exploited by developing drugs that are reduced preferentially to cytotoxic species in the hypoxic regions of tumors. Three classes of agents in this category are known:

1. Quinone antibiotics
2. Nitroaromatic compounds
3. Benzotriazine di-N-oxides

Mitomycin C is an example of the first class and has been used as a chemotherapy agent, active against hypoxic cells, for many years. The aerated–hypoxic differential, however, is relatively small for these compounds. Examples of the second class of compounds include dual-function agents developed by Adams and his group at the Medical Research

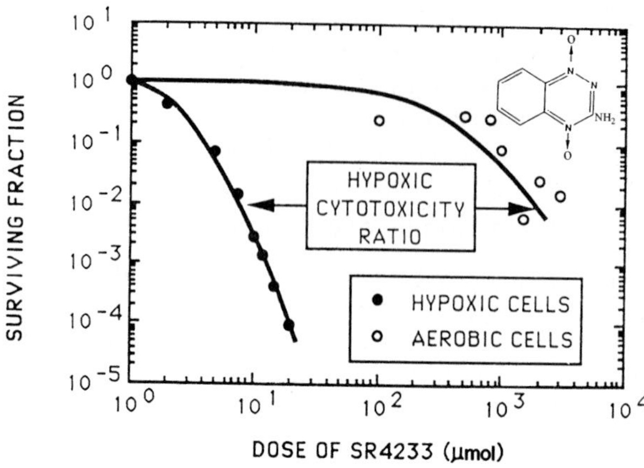

FIGURE 25.8 • Dose–response curves for Chinese hamster cells exposed for 1.5 hours to graded concentrations of SR 4233 (tirapazamine) under aerated and hypoxic conditions. Cells deficient in oxygen are killed preferentially. The hypoxic cytotoxicity ratio (defined as the ratio of drug concentrations under aerated and hypoxic conditions required to produce the same cell survival) is variable between different cell lines. For the Chinese hamster cells shown, the ratio is about 100; for cells of human origin, the ratio is somewhat smaller, closer to 20. Tirapazamine is an organic nitroxide synthesized by Stanford Research International. Its structure is shown in the **inset**. (Courtesy of Dr. J. Martin Brown.)

Council radiobiology unit in England. Normal-tissue toxicity prevented the trial of these compounds in the clinic. The lead compound of the third class, tirapazamine, shows highly selective toxicity toward hypoxic cells both *in vitro* and *in vivo*.

Tirapazamine

Figure 25.8 shows survival curves for Chinese hamster cells treated with graded concentrations of tirapazamine. Note the hypoxic/oxic cytotoxicity ratio of about 100. This compound is believed to be activated by the enzyme cytochrome P450. The hypoxic/oxic cytotoxicity ratio is not as large (about 20) in cell lines of human origin, presumably reflecting a different spectrum, or different levels, of enzymes.

Figure 25.9 shows the results of an experiment in which a transplanted mouse carcinoma was treated with x-rays alone, tirapazamine alone, or a combination of the two, with the drug injected 30 minutes prior to each irradiation. The irradiation schedule consisted of 2.5-Gy fractions given twice daily. Following treatment, the tumors were removed and the cells assayed for clonogenic survival. The effect of x-rays plus tirapazamine is evidently much greater than additive (what would be expected from independent cell killing of the two agents). The effect was even more dramatic when the study was conducted entirely *in vivo*, scoring regrowth delay (Fig. 25.10). Tumors were treated with x-rays alone, tirapazamine alone, or a combination of both agents. The radiation schedule consisted of eight 2.5-Gy (250-rad) fractions designed to mimic as

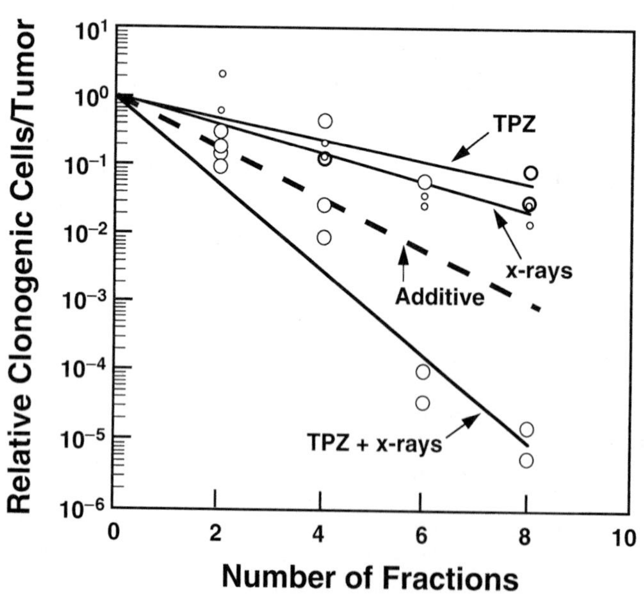

FIGURE 25.9 • Response of SCCVII mouse carcinomas to tirapazamine (TPZ) alone, radiation alone, or a combination of both. The radiation or drug treatment was given every 12 hours for up to eight fractions and the mice sacrificed for clonogenic cell survival 12 hours after the last dose. The additive line is the survival expected for independent cell killing by x-rays and tirapazamine, assuming a homogeneous tumor cell population. The actual killing observed is clearly greater than this. (Adapted from Brown JM, Lemmon MJ: Potentiation by the hypoxic cytotoxin SR4233 of cell killing produced by fractionated irradiation of mouse tumors. *Cancer Res* 50:7745–7749, 1990, with permission.)

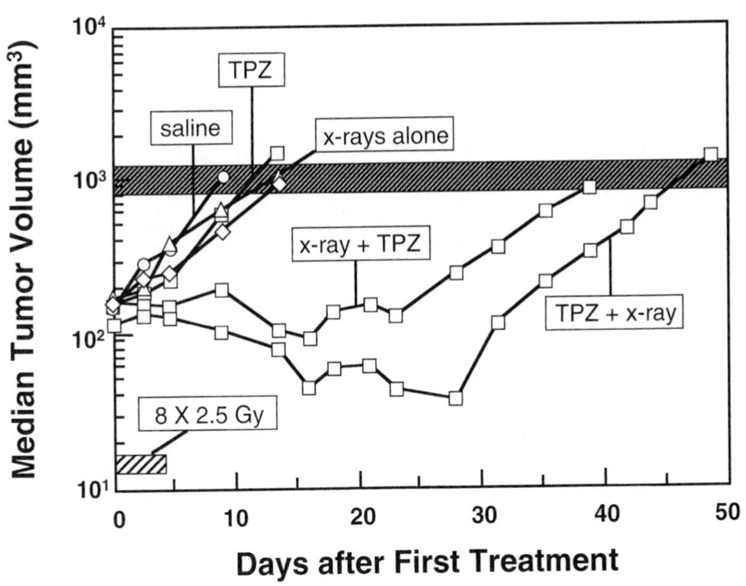

FIGURE 25.10 • Tumor volume as a function of time after various treatments of a SCCVII transplantable mouse carcinoma. Tirapazamine or radiation alone had little effect. The combination of tirapazamine and x-rays caused significant growth delay, with radiation following the drug causing a slightly greater effect. (Adapted from Brown JM, Lemmon MJ: Tumor hypoxia can be exploited to preferentially sensitize tumors to fractionated irradiation. *Int J Radiat Oncol Biol Phys* 20:457–461, 1991, with permission.)

far as possible a clinical radiation therapy protocol. The combination of drug and radiation is highly effective, with the time sequence of drug before radiation slightly more effective than the reverse. In parallel experiments using the same x-ray and drug protocols, skin reactions were scored, and no radiosensitization or additive cytotoxicity was observed by the addition of the tirapazamine to the radiation treatments. This substantiates the tumor selectivity of the radiation enhancement.

Similar results were obtained in four different mouse tumors that differed significantly in their hypoxic fractions. The observed interaction between x-rays and tirapazamine results largely from the selective hypoxic toxicity of the drug. This does not totally explain the observations, however. It appears that tirapazamine can act as an aerobic radiosensitizer of cells exposed to the drug under hypoxic conditions before or after the aerobic irradiation. This latter mechanism would be important for intermittent or acute hypoxia, that is, where a given region of a tumor cycles between aerated and hypoxic conditions.

Clinical Trials with Tirapazamine

In spite of the extensive laboratory data *in vitro* and *in vivo* showing the greater-than-additive effect of the combination of x-rays with tirapazamine, little has been done clinically to combine tirapazamine with radiation therapy, except for one RTOG phase II trial. The reason may be the side effects of nausea and severe muscle cramping.

The situation adding tirapazamine to chemotherapy protocols is more advanced. A phase III trial has been completed comparing cisplatin alone with cisplatin combined with tirapazamine for advanced (stages IIB and IV) non–small-cell lung cancer. There was a doubling of response rates and an increased survival rate in patients receiving the drug combination. The systemic cisplatin toxicity was not increased by the tirapazamine, but the tirapazamine-associated nausea and muscle cramping were reported.

MARKERS OF HYPOXIC CELLS

A major development in the past two decades has been the synthesis of radioactive-labeled nitroimidazoles for use as markers of hypoxic cells. The technique is as follows: A dose of misonidazole (or one of its analogues) carrying a radioactive label is administered. The drug is quickly excreted without being broken down from tissues that are well aerated, but under conditions of reduced oxygen tension, the drug is metabolized and broken down.

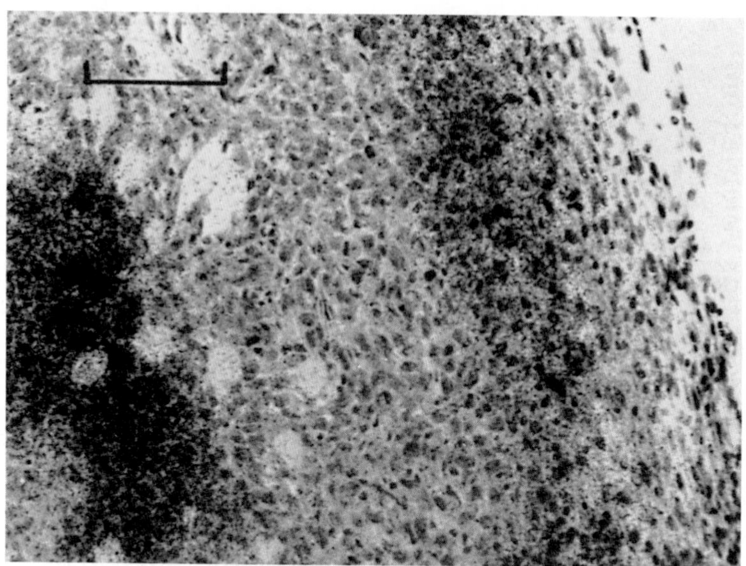

FIGURE 25.11 ● Autoradiograph of a section of a human small-cell lung carcinoma from a patient who received radioactive-labeled misonidazole the previous day. There are areas of intense labeling (many grains in the emulsion), suggesting the presence of hypoxic regions in the tumor. In areas deficient in oxygen, the misonidazole undergoes anaerobic metabolism and is broken down, and the radioactive label is deposited. (Courtesy of Drs. J.D. Chapman and R. Urtasun.)

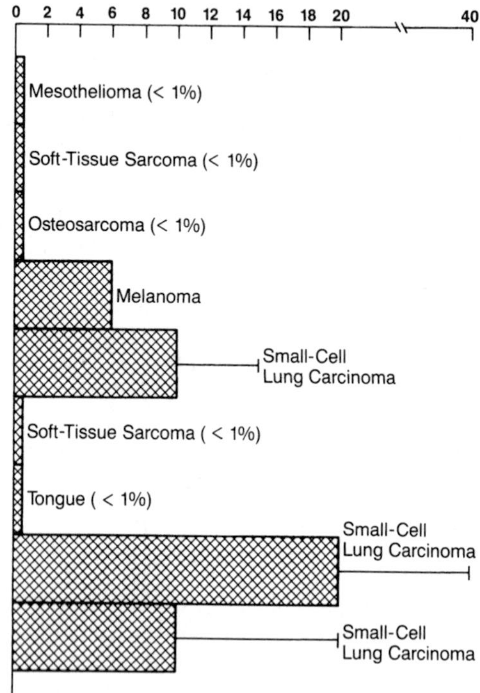

FIGURE 25.12 ● Summary of the labeling levels found in the first nine patients to be administered radioactive-labeled misonidazole. Only four of the nine patients show levels of labeling commensurate with the presence of hypoxic cells. (Courtesy of Drs. J.D. Chapman and R. Urtasun.)

Chapman and Urtasun in Edmonton, Canada, performed a study in which patients were given a nitroimidazole labeled with tritiated thymidine 22 hours before a tumor was removed surgically. Figure 25.11 is a section of a human small-cell lung carcinoma showing the density of grains over a region of the tumor, indicating the presence of hypoxic cells. The interesting result of the study is that only four of nine patients had tumors with a significant proportion of hypoxic cells (Fig. 25.12). In this small group of patients, biased inasmuch as only accessible tumors could be studied, only melanoma and small-cell lung cancer appeared to contain a proportion of hypoxic cells that would prejudice the outcome of radiotherapy. Until recently, it was possible to use only β-emitting isotopes as labels, which can be detected only by autoradiography when the tumor is removed and sectioned. More recently, Chapman has successfully labeled a nitroimidazole by attaching a radionuclide (iodine-123) using a sugar molecule. The presence of hypoxia then may be detected by single-photon emission computed tomography imaging, which of course is noninvasive. This exciting development opens up the possibility of screening patients prospectively to select those in whom hypoxia is a problem for inclusion in protocols involving hypoxic-cell sensitizers or bioreductive drugs. This topic is discussed further in Chapter 23.

Summary of Pertinent Conclusions

Halogenated Pyrimidines

- If the methyl group in thymidine is replaced by a halogen and incorporated into DNA, it results in radiosensitization.
- The halogenated pyrimidine must be incorporated into DNA for sensitization to occur. Consequently, cells must be grown in the presence of the analogue for several cell cycles. The extent of radiosensitization increases with the amount incorporated.
- For a sensitizer to be useful, there must be a differential effect between tumors and normal tissues. The halogenated pyrimidines require the tumor to be cycling faster than the dose-limiting normal tissues.
- Iododeoxyuridine is preferred to bromodeoxyuridine because it is an equally effective radiosensitizer but a less effective photosensitizer. Rash therefore is reduced in patients.
- Gliomas are suitable for clinical studies because they are rapidly growing and surrounded by slowly growing or nongrowing normal tissue.

Radiosensitizing Hypoxic Cells

- Hypoxic-cell radiosensitizers increase the radiosensitivity of hypoxic cells but not aerated cells. The differential effect on tumors is based on the presence of hypoxic cells in tumors but not in normal tissues.
- Sensitization is a free-radical process. The sensitizer mimics oxygen by "fixing" damage produced by free radicals.
- Misonidazole, the first compound used widely, sensitizes cells in culture as well as in both animal and human tumors.
- Doses of misonidazole that can be used clinically are limited to suboptimal levels by peripheral neuropathy. Only 1 of 30 or so clinical trials showed an advantage for misonidazole.
- Etanidazole is less toxic than misonidazole, and three times larger doses are tolerated. However, clinical trials in Europe and the United States showed no advantage of combined radiotherapy and etanidazole over radiotherapy alone.
- Nimorazole is less active as a radiosensitizer, but so much less toxic than either misonidazole or etanidazole that much larger doses can be given. A benefit was shown for adding nimorazole to conventional radiotherapy for head and neck cancer (Danish head and neck trial).
- A meta-analysis of all 82 trials of hyperbaric oxygen and hypoxic-cell radiosensitizers showed a 4.6% gain in local tumor control.

Hypoxic Cytotoxins

- Bioreductive drugs are compounds that are reduced intracellularly to form cytotoxic agents.
- Bioreduction is favored under hypoxia; this is a rationale for selectivity in solid tumors.
- Mitomycin C is active against hypoxic cells in a wide range of tumors. The hypoxic/oxic cytotoxicity ratio is quite small.
- Tirapazamine is an organic nitroxide. It shows a large hypoxic/oxic cytotoxicity ratio. The compound is active in many animal tumors and has undergone several clinical trials in conjunction with radiation or chemotherapy agents.
- Tirapazamine was designed to be used as an adjunct to irradiation, with the radiation killing the aerobic cells and the drug targeted to kill the hypoxic cells. It has found more use as an adjunct to chemotherapy agents.

Markers of Hypoxic Cells

- Nitroimidazoles labeled with a radionuclide can be used as markers of hypoxic cells. The drug is quickly excreted from aerobic tissues without breaking down. In areas of hypoxia, the drug undergoes bioreduction, and the radionuclide is deposited.
- Nitroimidazoles labeled with a β-emitter have been available for some time. By autoradiography on sections of a tumor surgically removed about a day after administration of a labeled drug, hypoxic areas can be identified. Only a minority of human tumors (notably melanomas and small-cell lung carcinomas) showed an appreciable proportion of hypoxic cells.
- Nitroimidazoles now can be labeled with iodine-123. Hypoxic regions of a tumor can be visualized by single-photon emission computed tomography scanning. This is a noninvasive procedure that can be used as a predictive assay in individual patients. In the few patients tested to date, about 40% show the presence of hypoxic areas.
- The availability of methods to detect significant areas of hypoxia will allow selection of patients who may benefit from methods of overcoming hypoxia (e.g., radiosensitizers, hypoxic cytotoxins, neutrons).

BIBLIOGRAPHY

Adams GE: Chemical radiosensitization of hypoxic cells. *Br Med Bull* 29:48–53, 1973

Adams GE: Hypoxic cell sensitizers for radiotherapy. In Becker FF (ed): *Cancer*, vol 6, pp 181–223. New York, Plenum Press, 1977

Adams GE: Redox, radiation and reductive bioactivation. *Radiat Res* 132:129–139, 1992

Adams GE, Bremner J, Stratford IJ, et al.: Nitroheterocyclic compounds as radiosensitizers and bioreductive drugs. *Radiother Oncol* 20(suppl 1):85–91, 1991

Adams GE, Clarke ED, Flockhart IR, et al.: Structure-activity relationships in the development of hypoxic cell radiosensitizers: 1. Sensitization efficiency. *Int J Radiat Biol* 35:133–150, 1979

Adams GE, Clarke ED, Gray P, et al.: Structure-activity relationships in the development of hypoxic cell radiosensitizers: 11. Cytotoxicity and therapeutic ratio. *Int J Radiat Biol* 35:151–160, 1979

Adams GE, Dewey DW: Hydrated electrons and radiobiological sensitization. *Biochem Biophys Res Commun* 12:473–477, 1963

Adams GE, Flockhart IR, Smithen CE, Stratford IJ, Wardman P, Watts ME: Electron-affinic sensitization. VII. A correlation between structures, one-electron reduction potentials, and efficiencies of nitroimidazoles as hypoxic cell radiosensitizers. *Radiat Res* 67:9–20, 1976

Alper T: The modification of damage caused by primary ionization of biological targets. *Radiat Res* 5:573–585, 1956

Ash DV, Peckham MJ, Steel GG: The quantitative response of human tumours to radiation and misonidazole. *Br J Cancer* 40:883–889. 1979

Bagshaw MA, Doggett RL, Smith KC: Intra-arterial 5-bromodeoxyuridine and x-ray therapy. *AJR Am J Roentgenol* 99:889–894, 1967

Baker MA, Zeman EM, Hirst VK, Brown JM: Metabolism of SR 4233 by Chinese hamster ovary cells: Basis for selective hypoxic toxicity. *Cancer Res* 48:5947–5952, 1988

Brown JM: Evidence for acutely hypoxic cells in mouse tumours, and a possible mechanism of reoxygenation. *Br J Radiol* 52:650–656, 1979

Brown JM, Goffinet DR, Cleaber JE, Kallman RF: Preferential radiosensitization of mouse sarcoma relative to normal skin by chronic intra-arterial infusion of halogenated pyrimidine analogs. *J Natl Cancer Inst* 47:75–89, 1971

Brown JM, Lemmon MJ: Potentiation by the hypoxic cytotoxin SR4233 of cell killing produced by fractionated irradiation of mouse tumors. *Cancer Res* 50:7745–7749, 1990

Brown JM, Lemmon MJ: Tumor hypoxia can be exploited to preferentially sensitize tumors to fractionated irradiation. *Int J Radiat Oncol Biol Phys* 20:457–461, 1991

Brown JM, Siim BG: Hypoxia-specific cytotoxins. *Semin Rad Oncol* 6:22–36, 1996

Bush RS: The significance of anemia in clinical radiation therapy. *Int J Radiat Oncol Biol Phys* 12:2047–2050, 1986

Chapman JD, Urtasun RC, Franko AJ, Raleigh JA, Meeker BE, McKinnon SA: The measurement of oxygenation status of individual tumors. In *Prediction of Response in Radiation Therapy: The Physical and Biological Basis. Proceedings of the American Association of Physical Medicine Symposium*, no. 7, pp 49–60, 1989

Chapman JD, Whitmore GF (eds): Chemical modifiers of cancer treatment. *Int J Radiat Oncol Biol Phys* 10:1161–1813, 1984

Churchill-Davidson I: The oxygen effect in radiotherapy: Historical review. *Front Radiat Ther Oncol* 1:1–15, 1968

Cole S, Stratford IJ, Bowler J, et al.: A toxicity and pharmacokinetic study in man of the hypoxic cell radiosensitizer RSU 1069. *Br J Radiol* 59:1238–1240, 1986

Coleman CN: Hypoxia in tumours: A paradigm for the approach to biochemical and physiological heterogeneity. *J Natl Cancer Inst* 80:310–317, 1988

Coleman CN: Hypoxic cell radiosensitizers: Expectations and progress in drug development. *Int J Radiat Oncol Biol Phys* 11:323–329, 1985

Dische S: Chemical sensitizers for hypoxic cells: A decade of experience in clinical radiotherapy. *Radiother Oncol* 3:97–115, 1988

Dische S, Gray AJ, Zanelli GD: Clinical testing of the radiosensitizer Ro-07-0582: 11. Radiosensitization of normal and hypoxic skin. *Clin Radiol* 27:159–166, 1976

Foster JL, Conroy PM, Searle AJ, Willson RL: Metronidazole (Flagyl): Characterization as a cytotoxic drug specific for hypoxic tumor cells. *Br J Cancer* 33:485–490, 1976

Gatenby RA, Kessler HB, Rosenblum JS, et al.: Oxygen distribution in squamous cell carcinoma metastases and its relationship to outcome of radiation therapy. *Int J Radiat Oncol Biol Phys* 14:831–838, 1988

Gray AJ, Dische S, Adams GE, Flockhart IR, Foster JL: Clinical testing of the radiosensitizer Ro-07-0582: 1. Dose, tolerance, serum and tumor concentrations. *Clin Radiol* 27:151–157, 1976

Gray C, Khalil AA, Nordsmark M, Horsman MR, Overgaard J: The relationship between carbon monoxide breathing, tumour oxygenation and local tumour control in the C3H mammary carcinoma *in vivo*. *Br J Cancer* 69:50–57, 1994

Hall EJ, Astor M, Geard C, Biaglow J: Cytotoxicity of Ro-07-0582: Enhancement by hyperthermia and protection by cysteamine. *Br J Cancer* 35:809–815, 1977

Hall EJ, Roizin-Towle L: Hypoxic sensitizers: Radiobiological studies at the cellular level. *Radiology* 117:453–457, 1975

Hirst DG: Anemia: A problem or an opportunity in radiotherapy? *Int J Radiat Oncol Biol Phys* 12:2009–2017, 1986

Horsman MR: Nicotinamide and other benzamide analogs as agents for overcoming hypoxic cell radiation resistance in tumours. *Acta Oncol* 34:571–587, 1995

Horsman MR: Nicotanimide and the hypoxia problem. *Radiother Oncol* 22:79–80, 1991

Horsman MR, Chaplin DJ, Overgaard J: Combination of nicotinamide and hyperthermia to eliminate radioresistant chronically and acutely hypoxic tumor cells. *Cancer Res* 50:7430–7436, 1990

Jenkins TC, Naylor MA, O'Neill P, Threadgill MD, et al.: Synthesis and evaluation of 1-(3-[2haloethyl-amino]propyl)-2-nitroimidazoles as pro-drugs of RSU 1069 and its analogues, which are radiosensitizers and bioreductively activated cytotoxins. *J Med Chem* 33:2603–2610, 1990

Jette DC, Wiebe LI, Flanagan RJ, Lee J, Chapman JD: Iodoaz omycin riboside (1-[58-iodo-58deoxyribofuranosyl]-2-nitroimidazole): A hypoxic cell marker: 1. Synthesis and *in vitro* characterization. *Radiat Res* 105:169–179, 1986

Kinsella T, Mitchell J, Russo A, et al.: Continuous intravenous infusions of bromodeoxyuridine as a clinical radiosensitizer. *J Clin Oncol* 2:1144–1150, 1984

Kinsella T, Mitchell J, Russo A, Morstyn G, Glatstein E: The use of halogenated thymidine analogs as clinical radiosensitizers: Rationale, current status, and future prospects for non-hypoxic cell sensitizers. *Int J Radiat Oncol Biol Phys* 10:1399–1406, 1984

Kinsella T, Russo A, Mitchell J, et al.: A phase I study of intravenous iododeoxyuridine as a clinical radiosensitizer. *Int J Radiat Oncol Biol Phys* 11:1941–1946, 1985

Kjellen E, Joiner MC, Collier JM, et al.: A therapeutic benefit from combining normobaric carbogen or oxygen with nicotinamide in fractionated x-ray treatments. *Radiother Oncol* 22:81–91, 1991

Laderoute K, Wardman P, Rauth AM: Molecular mechanisms for the hypoxia-dependent activation of 3-amino-1,2,4-benzotriazine-1,4-dioxide (SR 4233). *Biochem Pharmacol* 37:1487–1495, 1988

Lin AJ, Cosby LA, Shansky CW, Sartorelli AC: Potential bioreductive alkylating agents: 1. Benzoquinone derivatives. *J Med Chem* 15:1247–1252, 1972

Lorimore SA, Adams GE: Oral (PO) dosing with RS 1069 or RB 6145 maintains their potency as hypoxic cell radiosensitizers and cytotoxins but reduces systemic toxicity compared with parenteral (IP) administration in mice. *Int J Radiat Oncol Biol Phys* 21:387–395, 1991

Mitchell J, Kinsella T, Russo A, et al.: Radiosensitization of hematopoietic precursor cells (CFUc) in glioblastoma patients receiving intermittent intravenous infusions of bromodeoxyuridine (BUdR). *Int J Radiat Oncol Biol Phys* 9:457–463, 1983

Mitchell J, Morstyn G, Russo A, et al.: Differing sensitivity to fluorescent light in Chinese hamster cells containing equally incorporated quantities of BUdR versus IUdR. *Int J Radiat Oncol Biol Phys* 10:1447–1451, 1984

Mitchell J, Russo A, Kinsella T, Glatstein E: The use of non-hypoxic cell sensitizers in radiobiology and radiotherapy. *Int J Radiat Oncol Biol Phys* 12:1513–1518, 1986

Mohindra JK, Rauth A: Increased cell killing by metronidazole and nitrofurazone of hypoxic compared to aerobic mammalian cells. *Cancer Res* 36:930–936, 1976

Morstyn G, Hsu SM, Kinsella T, Gratzner H, Russo A, Mitchell JB: Bromodeoxyuridine in tumors and chromosomes detected with a monoclonal antibody. *J Clin Invest* 72:1844–1850, 1983

Nordsmark M, Overgaard M, Overgaard J: Pretreatment oxygenation predicts radiation response in advanced squamous cell carcinoma of the head and neck. *Radiother Oncol* 41:31–40, 1996

Overgaard J: Clinical evaluation of nitroimidazoles as modifiers of hypoxia in solid tumors. *Oncol Res* 6:507–516, 1994

Overgaard J, Horsman MR: Modification of hypoxia induced radioresistance in tumours by the use of oxygen and sensitizers. *Semin Radiat Oncol* 6:10–21, 1996

Overgaard J, Sand-Hansen H, Andersen AP, et al.: Misonidazole combined with split-course radiotherapy in the treatment of invasive carcinoma of larynx and pharynx: Final report from the DAHANCA 2 study. *Int J Radiat Oncol Biol Phys* 16:1065–1068, 1989

Overgaard J, Sand-Hansen H, Lindelov B, et al.: Nimorazole as a hypoxic radiosensitizer in the treatment of superglottic larynx and pharynx carcinoma. First report from the Danish Head and Neck Cancer Study (DAHANCA) Protocol 5-85. *Radiother Oncol* 20(suppl 1):143–150, 1991

Overgaard J, Sand-Hansen H, Overgaard M, et al.: The Danish Head and Neck Cancer Study Group (DAHANCA) randomized trials with radiosensitizers in carcinoma of the larynx and pharynx. In Dewey WC, Eddington M, Fry RJM, Hall EJ, Whitmore GF (eds): *Radiation Research: A Twentieth-Century Perspective*, vol II, pp 573–577. New York, Academic Press, 1992

Parliament MB, Chapman JD, Urtasun RC, et al.: Noninvasive assessment of human tumor hypoxia with 123I-iodoazomycin arabinoside: Preliminary report of a clinical study. *Br J Cancer* 65:90–95, 1992

Rasey JS, Koh WJ, Grierson JR, Granbaum Z, Krohn KA: Radiolabelled fluoromisonidazole as an imaging agent for tumor hypoxia. *Int J Radiat Oncol Biol Phys* 17:985–991, 1989

Roizin-Towle LA, Hall EJ, Flynn M, Bigalow JE, Varnes ME: Enhanced cytotoxicity of melphalan by prolonged exposure to nitroimidazoles: The role of endogenous thiols. *Int J Radiat Oncol Biol Phys* 8:757–760, 1982

Rose CM, Millar JL, Peacock JH, Phelps TA, Stephens TC: Differential enhancement of melphalan cytotoxicity in tumour and normal tissue by misonidazole. In Brady LW (ed): *Radiation Sensitizers*, pp 250–257. New York, Masson, 1980

Sheldon PW, Foster JL, Fowler JF: Radiosensitization of C3H mouse mammary tumours by a 2-nitroimidazole drug. *Br J Cancer* 30:560–565, 1974

Stratford IJ, Adams GE: Effect of hyperthermia on differential cytotoxicity of a hypoxic cell radiosensitizer, Ro-07-0582, on mammalian cells *in vitro*. *Br J Cancer* 35:307–313, 1977

Stratford IJ, Stephens MA: The differential hypoxic cytotoxicity of bioreductive agents determined *in vitro* by the MTT assay. *Int J Radiat Oncol Biol Phys* 16:973–976, 1989

Sutherland RM: Selective chemotherapy of noncycling cells in an *in vitro* tumour model. *Cancer Res* 34:3501–3503, 1974

Thomlinson RH, Dische S, Gray AJ, Errington LM: Clinical testing of the radiosensitizer Ro-07-0582: 111. Response of tumors. *Clin Radiol* 27:167–174, 1976

Urtasun RC, Band P, Chapman JD, Feldstein ML, Mielke B, Fryer C: Radiation and high dose metronidazole (Flagyl) in supratentorial glioblastomas. *N Engl J Med* 294:1364–1367, 1976

Urtasun RC, Band P, Chapman JD, Rabin HR, Wilson AF, Fryer CG: Clinical phase I study of the hypoxic cell radiosensitizer Ro-07-0582, a 2-nitroimidazole derivative. *Radiology* 122:801–804, 1977

Urtasun RC, Chapman JD, Raleigh JA, Franko AJ, Koch CJ: Binding of 3H-misonidazole to solid human tumors as a measure of tumor hypoxia. *Int J Radiat Oncol Biol Phys* 12:1263–1267, 1986

Wong TW, Whitmore GF, Gulyas S: Studies on the toxicity and radiosensitizing ability of misonidazole under conditions of prolonged incubation. *Radiat Res* 75:541–555, 1978

Zeman EM, Brown JM, Lemmon MJ, Hirst VK, Lee WW: SR 4233: A new bioreductive agent with high selective toxicity for hypoxic mammalian cells. *Int J Radiat Oncol Biol Phys* 12:1239–1242, 1986

Zeman EM, Hirst VK, Lemmon MJ, Brown JM: Enhancement of radiation induced tumour cell killing by the hypoxic cell toxin SR 4233. *Radiother Oncol* 12:209–218, 1988

CHAPTER 26

Gene Therapy

The initial concept of gene therapy was to replace the defective or aberrant gene in monogenic diseases—that is, diseases where there was one gene involved. It is a paradox, therefore, that two thirds of all patients who have so far received gene therapy have been treated for cancer—a complex disease likely involving multiple genes, most of which might have to be targeted to reverse the course of the disease. This development is clearly motivated by need and market pressure rather than by any scientific rationale.

VIRAL VECTORS

Gene therapy is a catchall term that covers a number of quite different new approaches to cancer treatment. Common to them all is the need for a means to introduce a gene into the cells of a tumor. At the present time, viral vectors are the most obvious choice and the most commonly used. The various types of viruses have different pros and cons, as summarized here.

Retroviruses are convenient to work with but infect only dividing cells. This is a severe limitation. **Adenoviruses** infect both dividing and quiescent cells, but the downside to their use is that they evoke an immune response, which can make their repeated use difficult. The **herpesvirus** is attractive because it is a much bigger virus, which allows more to be packaged into it, but it is also potentially more pathogenic and difficult to control.

In most instances, the virus is used simply to deliver a gene of interest to the cells, in which case, in the interest of safety, the virus is engineered so that it is not replication competent. In a few instances, the virus is designed to be cytotoxic, in which case some means is sought to selectively limit its activity to tumor cells only.

There are at least six quite different approaches to gene therapy:

1. Suicide-gene therapy
2. Cytotoxic virus targeted to p53-deficient cells
3. Molecular immunology (cancer vaccines)
4. Tumor-suppressor gene therapy
5. Radiation-inducible gene linked to a cytotoxic agent
6. Targeting signal transduction pathways

These six approaches are described very briefly in turn.

SUICIDE-GENE THERAPY

Suicide-gene therapy is based on the strategy of transducing into cells a gene that converts an inert prodrug into a toxic agent. It is axiomatic that

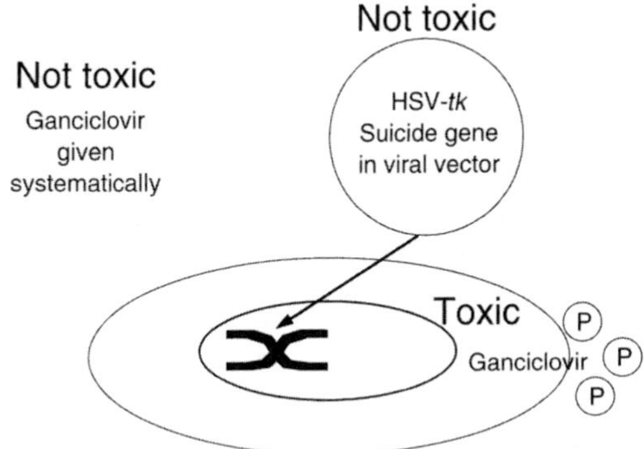

FIGURE 26.1 • The principle of suicide-gene therapy. The thymidine kinase gene from the herpes simplex virus (HSV-*tk*), contained in a viral vector (adenovirus, so that dividing and nondividing cells can be infected), is injected into the tumor. Ganciclovir is administered systemically. This is a prodrug that is in itself nontoxic. In cells containing the thymidine kinase gene, the prodrug is activated to become a toxic agent.

alone, both the gene product and the prodrug are essentially nontoxic. The theoretical advantage of suicide-gene therapy compared with chemotherapy as an adjunct to radiotherapy is that following direct intratumoral injection, the therapeutic molecules are produced locally within the tumor, thereby avoiding the systemic toxicity so often observed, for example, with traditional chemoradiotherapy.

The most widely used system involves the combination of the herpes simplex virus thymidine kinase gene (HSV-*tk*) packaged into an adenovirus plus ganciclovir (GCV). The virus containing the gene is injected into the tumor; the ganciclovir is administered systemically. HSV-*tk* phosphorylates ganciclovir, converting it to a nucleoside analogue that inhibits DNA synthesis, leading to cell death. The idea is illustrated in Figure 26.1. More cells are killed than are transduced initially; that is, there is a substantial "bystander effect," resulting from several causes: (1) Gap junctions between cells transport the toxic agent to cells not themselves transduced; (2) as cells die and are lysed, the toxic agent is released and spreads to other cells; and (3) an induced immune response kills more tumor cells, even some remote from the injection site.

More than 30 clinical trials have been performed for human malignancies as diverse as brain tumors, mesotheliomas, liver metastases, and peritoneal metastases. Although local treatments are tolerated well, attempts at systemic delivery of the HSV-*tk* to target metastatic disease is limited by liver damage caused by hepatotropism of the adenovirus.

Tumor growth reductions by HSV-*tk* plus ganciclovir are sometimes impressive, but cure rates are low, pointing to the need to use this new form of therapy as an adjuvant to radiation or chemotherapy. In fact, the combined therapy may have a greater-than-additive effect, because HSV-*tk* plus ganciclovir can radiosensitize cells in a manner similar to that shown for other nucleoside analogues.

An alternative suicide-gene system involves cytosine deaminase (CD). CD is expressed in bacteria (b-CD) and in yeast (y-CD) and converts 5-fluorocytosine (5-FC) to 5-fluorouracil (5-FU), which is widely used as a chemotherapy agent. As before, the gene is introduced into tumor cells in a viral vector, and the 5-fluorocytosine, itself nontoxic, is administered systemically.

It was recognized from the outset that these suicide-gene strategies cannot realistically be expected to offer much hope of producing tumor "cures" as a single modality. For one thing, the efficiency of gene delivery is too low and tumor specificity too poor. Moreover, most detectable tumors contain at least a billion cells, all (or at least most) of which need to be eradicated to achieve a long-term cure, and this is a tall order for any current gene therapy strategy.

Nevertheless, suicide-gene therapy is a logical candidate to be combined with radiation therapy because the target cells are the same (making cell kill at least additive if not synergistic), while the normal-tissue toxicities are different. There have been a number of attempts to pursue this strategy, notably the combining of the two suicide-gene systems with conventional radiotherapy.

Because the CD/5-FC system appears to induce DNA strand breaks, while the HSV-*tk*/GCV system can inhibit repair of double-strand breaks, it was hypothesized that used simultaneously, the two systems would be most effective. This proved to be the case *in vitro* and in some animal tumor systems. The safety and efficacy of combining the two systems has been evaluated in several phase I/II clinical trials using a replication-competent adenovirus containing the b-CD/HSV-*tk* fusion gene combined with conventional-dose radiotherapy in intermediate to high risk prostate cancer patients.

CYTOTOXIC VIRUS TARGETED TO p53-DEFICIENT CELLS

A novel strategy to differentially treat tumors (both primary and metastatic) that are characterized by mutant *p53* involves the use of an adenovirus that replicates only within *p53*-mutant cells, killing them through cell lysis. The basic biology involved in this strategy is interesting.

Two of the principal checks on normal cell growth are provided by Rb and p53. Rb, first discovered in retinoblastoma, is involved in cell-cycle regulation. It prevents cells from entering S phase until the appropriate growth signal is received. The protein p53, on the other hand, detects damage to DNA and initiates cell suicide by apoptosis. Cells become cancerous, it is thought, if one or both of these sentinel proteins are inactivated. The adenovirus also can cause uncontrolled division, because it is equipped with the two genes *Ela* and *Elb*; *Ela* targets Rb, and *Elb* targets and inactivates p53. It follows that a virus with the *Ela* gene deleted or inactivated would grow only in Rb-deficient cells, and a virus with the *Elb* gene deleted or inactivated would grow only in p53-deficient cells. To date, only the latter idea has been exploited, namely, to produce a virus that replicates only in cells deficient in p53. To the extent that mutant *p53* is a hallmark of cancer, this strategy preferentially targets cancer cells with a cytotoxic virus and spares normal cells.

Designing a therapeutic modality that can distinguish between normal and malignant cells has been the Holy Grail of cancer research for decades. Although there is still some debate as to the extent to which these viruses proliferate and kill cells with normal p53, in early clinical trials the systemic inoculation of this vector has produced significant growth suppression of primary head and neck cancer. Again, because only partial responses are evoked, the treatment must be combined with standard radiation or chemotherapy regimens.

MOLECULAR IMMUNOLOGY (CANCER VACCINES)

The basis of this approach is to provoke or stimulate a cellular immune response to the invading cancer that is effective against metastatic lesions. Vaccines can be engineered genetically to express cytokines or other molecules known to be important in the generation of immune responses or, alternatively, one of the relatively few known tumor-specific antigens. Vaccination with tumor cells expressing cytokines, such as IL-2, GM-CSF or IFN-g, has been shown to induce an immunologic response in some animal model systems, resulting in growth arrest (and occasionally cures) of local or metastatic tumors.

This approach is not without its problems. First, the molecular requirements for the generation of an immune response that would be capable of causing tumor rejection are not known precisely. Also, in general, antitumor activity is only effective against small tumor burdens. A strategy, still in the development stage but showing some promise, is to combine molecular immunology with suicide-gene therapy. The notion here is to use the suicide-gene technique to cause rapid necrosis and generate large quantities of tumor antigen in combination with an immune-gene strategy to enhance the immune response to the liberated antigen.

TUMOR-SUPPRESSOR GENE THERAPY

The closest strategy to real gene therapy is to replace, with a correct copy, a gene, the mutation of which either initiates or substantially alters the malignant phenotype. The goal of such treatment may be to modify cell growth, invasiveness, or metastatic potential as much as to kill the cell.

The gene *p53* has received a great deal of attention as a target for gene therapy. This is logical, because *p53* is the most commonly mutated gene in human cancer and can influence transcription, cell-cycle checkpoints, DNA repair, apoptosis, and angiogenesis.

In several model tumor systems, transduction of cells with wild-type *p53* can inhibit growth and angiogenesis or initiate apoptosis. Phase I/II trials have been conducted combining *p53* gene therapy with radiotherapy in patients with nonmetastatic non-small-cell lung cancer, with results described as "encouraging"!

The factors that greatly limit the field of tumor-suppressor gene therapy are the paucity of known target genes that are causative of the malignant phenotype, or at least necessary to maintain it, and the fact that more than one genetic change is needed for carcinogenesis.

As with most forms of gene therapy, eradication of treated tumors is a rarity, even in model experimental systems. This is because of the technical difficulty of transducing a sufficiently large proportion of cells within the tumor. The problem is mitigated, but not solved, by an apparent "bystander effect," whereby more cells die than actually are transduced. As might be expected, expression of wild-type *p53* in tumor cells can sensitize them to the effects of irradiation, making an additional case for the combined approach to therapy.

RADIATION-INDUCIBLE GENE LINKED TO A CYTOTOXIC AGENT

The principle here is to combine the physics of radiation-targeting technology with the molecular aspects of gene therapy. The general principle is illustrated in Figure 26.2. Specifically, a chimeric gene is created that can be activated by radiation and inserted into the genome of a nonreplicating adenovirus. The chimeric gene involves the human cDNA sequence that encodes tumor necrosis factor (TNF) α and parts of the early-growth-response

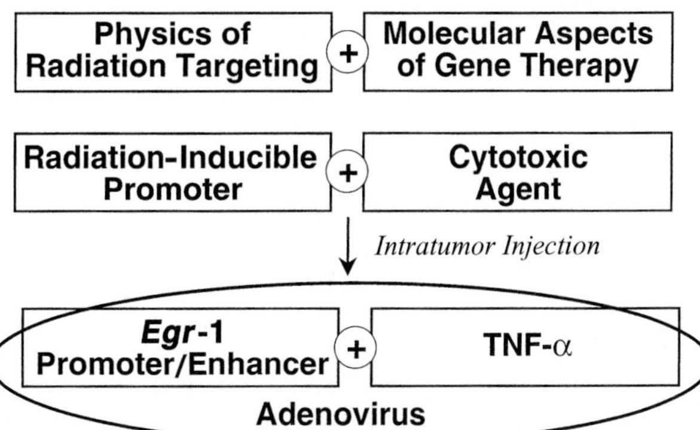

FIGURE 26.2 • Illustrating the general principle of radiation-targeting gene therapy. The idea is to combine the physics of radiation targeting with the molecular aspects of gene therapy. A radiation-inducible promoter ahead of a cytotoxic agent and contained in an adenovirus is injected into the tumor. The promoter is turned on only in the radiation field, thus targeting the therapy.

gene (*Egr*-1) promoter/enhancer, which is activated by a dose of radiation of about 0.5 Gy (50 rad). The adenovirus is injected into the tumor, but the TNF-α is activated only in the target volume delineated by the radiation field. By this means, total-body toxicity is avoided. Released in the tumor, the TNF-α causes vascular destruction as well as apoptosis in tumor cells. The principle is illustrated in Figure 26.3. The key to the success of this strategy is to have radiation-inducible promoters/enhancers, such as members of the early-growth-response gene family. These generally respond to a variety of stimuli, including ionizing radiation. The sequences that trigger this radiation response consist of 10 base-pair motifs known as *CArG elements*, located within the "entrance" regions of the promoter. These elements are activated by reactive oxygen intermediates, the triggering stimuli produced by radiation. *Egr*-1 transcripts return to basal levels within 3 hours after irradiation.

Radiogenetic therapy, as it now is called, has shown promise in one model system consisting of human laryngeal tumor cells growing as a xenograft in the hind limbs of immunodeficient nude mice. This single demonstration of the technique may be just a preview of things to come. There is the potential to use a much more radiation-specific promoter than *Egr*-1 with a more effective toxic agent than TNF-α. The basic idea is the synthesis of the well-developed physics of radiation-targeting technology with the molecular aspects of gene therapy.

TARGETING SIGNAL TRANSDUCTION PATHWAYS

A hallmark of the malignant cell is the dysregulation of growth and signal transduction pathways that often result in resistance to radiotherapy. Several potential targets have been identified:

1. The epidermal growth factor receptor (EGFR) mediates growth regulation in a wide spectrum of human cancers, and tumors expressing high levels of EGFR appear to be radioresistant.
2. Raf-1 is a kinase that plays an important role in cell proliferation, differentiation, survival, and angiogenesis and is therefore a prime target for novel cancer therapies.
3. NFκB is a cellular transcription factor that plays a central role in the cellular stress response.

Because EGFR, Raf-1, and NFκB signaling are disrupted in a wide spectrum of human cancers, they all represent attractive targets for therapy.

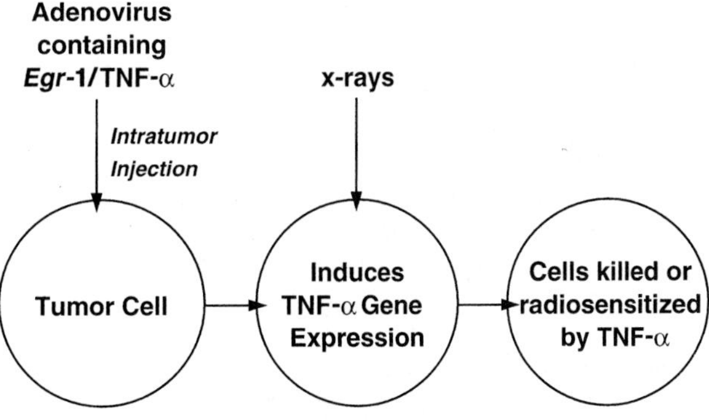

FIGURE 26.3 • The principle of the specific form of radiation-inducible gene therapy, or radiogenetic therapy, developed by Weichselbaum and colleagues. The radiation-inducible gene is the *Egr*-1 gene, which if exposed to radiation activates tumor necrosis factor (TNF) α, which is cytotoxic to tumor cells.

Competing with gene therapy in this area is the development of monoclonal antibodies and low-molecular-weight chemical inhibitors.

TARGETING GENE THERAPY

In an attempt to make gene therapy more specific and improve tumor cell killing relative to normal-tissue toxicity, a number of possibilities have been explored to target the toxic agent used in gene therapy to particular cells.

For example, many tumors contain regions of hypoxia, and a hypoxia-inducible factor has been identified that binds to DNA at specific hypoxia-responsive elements to up-regulate transcription of certain genes. Put simply, a hypoxia-sensitive element can be added to the gene therapy construct so that the prodrug is converted to a cytotoxic agent only in regions of hypoxia, which, it is assumed, occur only in tumors.

Alternatively, tumor-specific promoters can be used. The clearest example is prostate cancer, in which prostate-specific antigen can be used. There are published reports, too, of specific promoters for hepatoma, breast cancer, and gastric carcinoma. The field is in its infancy, but there is great potential.

CONCLUSION

The variety of strategies described in this chapter, lumped together under the heading of gene therapy, all have made significant and impressive progress in the treatment of localized and even metastatic cancer in animal models. Some progress has been made in the treatment of cancer in the human, the real problem, but progress is less impressive to date. Significant problems remain to be solved, but the field bears watching.

All strategies discussed share a common problem, namely, the difficulty of transducing therapeutic genes into a sufficiently large proportion of tumor cells. For example, a 99% efficiency of infection gives just 2 logs of cell kill; 9 or 10 logs are needed to sterilize the tumor. A mitigating phenomenon is the "bystander effect," whereby more cells are killed than are transduced initially. Bystander effects may act locally via cell-to-cell communication or systemically through an immune-mediated response. In the latter case, a local therapy may induce a systemic antitumor response and have an effect on distant metastases.

It would appear logical to combine one or another of the new gene therapy approaches with standard radiation therapy or chemotherapy. The guiding principle must be to combine modalities that have additive or synergistic effect as far as tumor cell killing is concerned, but for which the limiting normal-tissue toxicities are different. The rationale for combining gene therapy with, for example, standard radiotherapy is that a small increment in cell killing from the gene therapy could translate into a large increase in tumor control, because the radiation alone already results in a tumor control on the steep portion of the tumor control–dose relationship.

Summary of Pertinent Conclusions

- *Gene therapy* is a catchall term for several very different approaches to cancer therapy.
- All forms of gene therapy rely on vectors to transport a therapeutic agent into cells.
- Viruses are most commonly used as vectors:

  Retroviruses are convenient, but they infect only dividing cells.

  Adenoviruses infect both dividing and nondividing cells but invoke an immune response, which can hamper repeat applications.

  Herpesviruses are bigger, allowing a larger package to be inserted, but are potentially more dangerous.
- Suicide-gene therapy is based on transducing cells with a gene that converts a prodrug into a cytotoxic agent.
- The herpes simplex virus thymidine kinase gene (HSV-*tk*) plus ganciclovir is an example of suicide-gene therapy. The steps involved are as follows:

  1. The virus containing the gene is injected into the tumor; the ganciclovir is administered systemically.
  2. The thymidine kinase gene phosphorylates the ganciclovir, converting it to a cytotoxic agent within the tumor.
  3. There is a substantial bystander effect; that is, more cells are killed than transduced initially.

(continued)

Summary of Pertinent Conclusions (Continued)

- Suicide-gene therapy has produced growth delay and some cures in animal models.
- An alternative suicide-gene system involves cytosine deaminase, which converts 5-fluorocytosine (nontoxic) to 5-fluorouracil (toxic) within the cell.
- A fusion gene has been produced that combines the two systems in a single viral vector.
- Because of the limited efficiency of gene delivery, suicide-gene therapy needs to be combined with conventional radiotherapy.
- Phase I/II clinical trials have shown promise.
- A cytotoxic virus can be constructed that is engineered to replicate and kill only in cells with mutant *p53*.
- To the extent that mutant *p53* is a hallmark of cancer, this treatment differentiates between normal cells and cancer cells.
- Growth arrest has been observed in model animal tumors and in early clinical trials by targeting mutant *p53*.
- Molecular immunology seeks to provoke a cellular immune response against the cancer by injecting a vaccine genetically engineered to express immune stimulatory molecules or tumor-specific antigens.
- Molecular immunology shows some promise in animal models but is generally only effective against small tumor burdens.
- Tumor-suppressor gene therapy is the replacement, with a correct copy, of the mutated gene that initiates or contributes significantly to the malignant phenotype.
- The gene *p53* has received the most attention of any gene because it is so commonly mutated in human cancers.
- Phase I/II clinical trials show some promise in the treatment of non-small-cell lung cancer.
- Tumor-suppressor gene therapy is limited by a lack of information on the target genes that are essential for maintaining the malignant phenotype and the fact that multiple genetic changes are involved.
- Radiation-activated genes combine the physics of radiation-targeting technology with molecular gene therapy.
- The principle of radiation-activated genes is to link a radiation-inducible promoter to a cytotoxic agent; the cytotoxic agent is "turned on" only in the carefully delineated radiation field.
- In the practical case used in a model animal tumor system, the *Egr*-1 radiation-inducible promoter is linked to tumor necrosis factor (TNF) α and packaged in an adenovirus in order to infect the tumor cells.
- There is the potential to use a more radiation-specific promoter gene and a more effective toxic agent.
- There is the possibility of including a promoter that is specific for a particular tumor, for example, prostate or breast cancer.
- Several gene therapy strategies have made progress in achieving growth reduction in animal model systems and in some human cancers, advancing to phase II trials.
- Several forms of gene therapy claim a "bystander effect"; that is, more cells are killed than are transduced initially.
- A problem common to all strategies is to transduce a sufficiently large proportion of tumor cells; growth reduction is common, but cures are rare.
- It is logical to combine gene therapy with radiation therapy or chemotherapy. The hypothesis is that a small increase in cell killing from gene therapy could translate into a large increase in tumor control by conventional therapies.
- The guiding principle of combination therapy must be to combine modalities that have an additive or synergistic effect on tumor cell kill, but for which normal-tissue toxicities are different.

BIBLIOGRAPHY

Barba D, Hardin J, Sadelin M, Gage FH: Development of antitumor immunity following thymidine kinase-based killing of experimental brain tumors. *Proc Natl Acad Sci USA* 91:4348–4352, 1994

Bischoff JR, Kirn DH, Williams A, et al.: An adenovirus mutant that replicates selectively in p53 deficient human tumor cells. *Science* 274:373–376, 1996

Brach MA, Hass R, Sherman ML, Gunji H, Weichselbaum R, Kufe D: Ionizing radiation induces expression and binding activity of the nuclear factor kappa B. *J Clin Invest* 88:691–695, 1991

Brand K, Arnold W, Bartels T, et al.: Liver-associated toxicity of the *HSV-tk*/GCV approach and adenoviral vectors. *Cancer Gene Ther* 4:9–16, 1997

Bruno MC, Benedetti S, Ottolenghi S, et al.: The bystander effect: Association of U87 cell death with ganciclovir-mediated apoptosis of nearby cells and the lack of effect in athymic mice. *Hum Gene Ther* 6:763–772, 1995

Caruso M, Pham-Nguyen K, Kwong Y-L, et al.: Adenovirus-mediated interleukin-12 gene therapy for metastatic colon cancer. *Proc Natl Acad Sci USA* 93:11302–11306, 1996

Chen S-H, Chen XHL, Wang Y, et al.: Combination gene therapy for liver metastases of colon carcinoma *in vivo*. *Proc Natl Acad Sci USA* 2:2577–2581, 1995

Chen S-H, Kosai KI, Xu B, et al.: Combination suicide and cytokine gene therapy for hepatic metastases of colon carcinoma: Sustained antitumor immunity prolongs animal survival. *Cancer Res* 56:3758–3762, 1996

Chen S-H, Shine HD, Goodman JC, Grossman RG, Woo SLC: Gene therapy for brain tumors: Regression of experimental gliomas by adenovirus-mediated gene transfer *in vivo*. *Proc Natl Acad Sci USA* 91:3054–3057, 1994

Chinnaiyan AM, Prasad U, Shankar S, et al.: Combined effect of tumor necrosis factor-related apoptosis-inducing ligand and ionizing radiation in breast cancer therapy. *Proc Natl Acad Sci USA* 97:1754–1759, 2000

Criswell T, Leskov K, Miyamoto S, Luo G, Boothman DA: Transcription factors activated in mammalian cells after clinically relevant doses of ionizing radiation. *Oncogene* 22:5813–5827, 2003

Culver KW, Ram Z, Wallbridge S, Ishii H, Oldfield EH, Blaese RM: *In vivo* gene transfer with retroviral vector-producer cells for treatment of experimental brain tumors. *Science* 256:1550–1552, 1992

Datta R, Rubin E, Sukhatme V, et al.: Ionizing radiation activates transcription of the EGR1 gene via CArG elements. *Proc Natl Acad Sci USA* 89:10149–10153, 1992

Datta R, Taneja N, Sukhatme VP, Querish SA, Weichselbaum R, Kufe DW: Reactive oxygen intermediates target CC(A/T)6GG sequences to mediate activation of the early growth response 1 transcription factor gene by ionizing radiation. *Proc Natl Acad Sci USA* 90:2419–2422, 1992

Dranoff G, Jaffee E, Lazenby A, et al.: Vaccination with irradiated tumor cells engineered to secrete murin granulocyte-macrophage colony-stimulating factor stimulates potent, specific, and long lasting anti-tumor immunity. *Proc Natl Acad Sci USA* 90:3539–3543, 1993

Elshami AA, Kucharczuk JC, Zhang HB, et al.: Treatment of pleural mesothelioma in an immunocompetent rat model utilizing adenoviral transfer of the herpes simplex virus thymidine kinase gene. *Hum Gene Ther* 7:141–148, 1996

Fearon ER, Pardoll DM, Itaya T, et al.: Interleukin-2 production by tumor cells bypasses T helper function in the generation of an antitumor response. *Cell* 60:397–403, 1990

Freeman SM, Abboud CN, Whartenby KA, et al.: The 'bystander effect': Tumour regression when a fraction of the tumour mass is genetically modified. *Cancer Res* 53: 5274–5283, 1993

Freeman SM, Ramesh R, Shastri M, Munshi A, Jensen AK, Marrogi IAJ: The role of cytokines in mediating the bystander effect using *HSV-TK* xenogeneic cells. *Cancer Lett* 92:167–174, 1995

Freytag SO, Khil M, Stricker H, et al.: Phase I study of replication-competent adenovirus-mediated double suicide gene therapy for the treatment of locally recurrent prostate cancer. *Cancer Res* 62:4968–4976, 2002

Freytag SO, Stricker H, Pegg J, et al.: Phase I study of replication-competent adenovirus-mediated double-suicide gene therapy in combination with conventional-dose three-dimensional conformal radiation therapy for the treatment of newly diagnosed, intermediate- to high-risk prostate cancer. *Cancer Res* 63:7497-7506, 2003

Fujiwara T, Cai DW, Gerges RN, Mukhopadhyay T, Grimm EA, Roth JA: Therapeutic effect of a retroviral wild-type of *p53* expression vector in an orthotopic lung cancer model. *J Natl Cancer Inst* 86:1458–1462, 1994

Gagandeep S, Brew R, Green B, et al.: Prodrug-activated gene therapy: Involvement of an immunological component in the "bystander effect." *Cancer Gene Ther* 3:83–88, 1996

Gallardo D, Drazan KE, McBride WH: Adenovirus-based transfer of wild-type *p53* gene increases ovarian tumor radiosensitivity. *Cancer Res* 56:4891–4893, 1996

Gansbacher B, Zier K, Daniels B, Cronin K, Bannerji R, Gilboa E: Interleukin 2 gene transfer into tumor cells abrogates tumorigenicity and induces protective immunity. *J Exp Med* 172:1217–1224, 1990

Gjerset RA, Turla ST, Sobol RE, et al.: Use of wild-type *p53* to achieve complete treatment sensitization of tumor cells expressing endogenous mutant *p53*. *Mol Carcinog* 14:275–285, 1995

Hall SJ, Chen SH, Woo SLC: The promise and reality of cancer gene therapy. *Am J Hum Genet* 61:785–789, 1997

Hallahan DE, Mauceri HJ, Seung LP, et al.: Spatial and temporal control of gene therapy using ionizing radiation. *Nat Med* 1:786–791, 1995

Hamel W, Magnelli L, Chiarugi VP, Israel MA: Herpes simplex virus thymidine kinase/ganciclovir-mediated apoptotic death of bystander cells. *Cancer Res* 56:2697–2702, 1996

Harris JD, Gutierrez AA, Hurst HC, Sikora K, Lemoine NR: Gene therapy for cancer using tumor-specific prodrug activation. *Gene Ther* 1(3):170–175, 1994

Heise C, Sampson-Johannes A, Williams A, McCormick F, Von Hoff DD, Kirn DH: ONYX-015, an Elb gene-attenuated adenovirus, causes tumor-specific cytolysis and antitumoral efficacy that can be augmented by standard chemotherapeutic agents. *Nat Med* 3:639–645, 1997

Huber BE, Austin EA, Good SS, Knick VC, Tibbels T, Richards CA: *In vivo* antitumour activity of 5-fluorocytosine on human colorectal carcinoma cells genetically modified to express cytosine deaminase. *Cancer Res* 53:4619–4626, 1993

Huber BE, Austin EA, Richards CA, Davis ST, Good SS: Metabolism of 5-fluorocytosine to 5-fluorouracil in human colorectal tumor cells transduced with the cytosine deaminase gene: Significant antitumor effects when only a small percentage of tumor cells express cytosine deaminase. *Proc Natl Acad Sci USA* 91:8302–8306, 1994

Kim JH, Kim SH, Brown SL, Freytag SO: Selective enhancement by an antiviral agent of the radiation-induced cell killing of human glioma cells transduced with *HSV-tk* gene. *Cancer Res* 54:6053–6056, 1994

Lammering G, Hewit TH, Valerie K, et al.: Anti-erbB receptor strategy as a gene therapeutic intervention to improve radiotherapy in malignant human tumours. *Int J Radiat Biol* 79:561–568, 2003

Lammering G, Lin PS, Contessa JN, et al.: Adenovirus-mediated overexpression of dominant negative epidermal growth factor receptor-CD533 as a gene therapeutic approach radiosensitizes human carcinoma and malignant glioma cells. *Int J Radiat Oncol Biol Phys* 51:775–784, 2001

Lesoon-Wood LA, Kim WH, Kleinman HK, Weintraub BD, Mixson AJ: Systemic gene therapy with *p53* reduces growth and metastases of a malignant human breast cancer in nude mice. *Hum Gene Ther* 6:395–405, 1995

Lowe SW, Bodis S, McClatchey A, et al.: p53 status and the efficacy of cancer therapy *in vivo*. *Science* 266:807–810, 1994

Manome Y, Abe M, Hagen MF, Fine HA, Kufe DW: Enhancer sequences of the *DF3* gene regulate expression of the herpes-simplex virus thymidine kinase gene and confer sensitivity of human breast-cancer cells to ganciclovir. *Cancer Res* 54(20):5408–5413, 1994

Mauceri HJ, Hanna NN, Wayne JD, Hallahan DE, Hellman S, Weicselbaum RR: Tumor necrosis factor alpha (TNF-alpha) gene therapy targeted by ionising radiation selectively damages tumor vasculature. *Cancer Res* 56(19):4311–4314, 1996

Melillo G, Musso T, Sicz A, Taylor LS, Cox GW, Varesio L: A hypoxic-responsive element mediates a novel pathway of activation of the inducible nitric oxide synthase promoter. *J Exp Med* 182(6):1683–1693, 1995

Mesnil M, Piccoli C, Tiraby G, Willecke K, Yamasaki H: Bystander killing of cancer cells by herpes simplex virus thymidine kinase gene is mediated by connexins. *Proc Natl Acad Sci USA* 93:1831–1835, 1996

Moolten FL: Tumor chemosensitivity conferred by inserted herpes thymidine kinase genes: Paradigm for a prospective cancer control strategy. *Cancer Res* 46:5276–5281, 1986

Nguyen DM, Spitz FR, Yen N, Cristiano RJ, Roth JA: Gene therapy for lung cancer: Enhancement of tumor suppression by a combination of sequential systemic cisplatin and adenovirus-mediated *p53* gene transfer. *J Thorac Cardiovasc Surg* 112:1372–1377, 1996

Pope IM, Poston GJ, Kinsella AR: The role of the bystander effect in suicide gene therapy. *Eur J Cancer* 33(7):1005–1016, 1997

Porgador A, Banneji R, Watanabe Y, Feldman M, Gilboa E, Eisenbach L: Antimetastatic vaccination of tumor-bearing mice with two types of IFN-γ gene-inserted tumor cells. *J Immunol* 150:1458–1470, 1993

Porgador A, Gansbacher B, Bannerji R, et al.: Anti-metastatic vaccination of tumor-bearing mice with IL-2-gene-inserted tumor cells. *Int J Cancer* 53:471–477, 1993

Qian C, Idoate M, Bilbao R, et al.: Gene transfer and therapy with adenoviral vector in rats with diethylnitrosamine-induced hepatocellular carcinoma. *Hum Gene Ther* 8:349–358, 1997

Roth JA, Nguyen D, Lawrence DD, et al.: Retrovirus-mediated wild-type p53 gene transfer to tumors of patients with lung cancer. *Nat Med* 2:985–991, 1996

Sakamoto KM, Bardeleben C, Yates KE, Raines MA, Golde DW, Gasson JC: 5′ upstream sequence and genomic structure of the human primary response gene, *EGR-1/RIS8*. *Oncogene* 6:867–871, 1991

Schuur ER, Henderson G, Kmetec, LA, Miller JD, Lamparski HG, Henderson DR: Prostate-specific antigen expression is regulated by an upstream enhancer. *J Biol Chem* 271(12):7043–7051, 1996

Seung LP, Mauceri HJ, Beckett MA, Hallahan DE, Hellman S, Weichselbaum RR: Genetic radiotherapy overcomes tumor resistance to cytotoxic agents. *Cancer Res* 55:5561–5565, 1995

Soldatenkov VA, Dritschilo A, Wang FH, Olah Z, Anderson WB, Kasid U: Inhibition of Raf-1 protein kinase by antisense phosphorothioate oligodeoxyribonucleotide is associated with sensitization of human laryngeal squamous carcinoma cells to gamma radiation. *Cancer J Sci Am* 3:13–20, 1997

Swisher SG, Roth JA, Nemunaitis J, et al.: Adenovirus-mediated p53 gene transfer in advanced non-small-cell lung cancer. *J Natl Cancer Inst* 91:763–771, 1999

Tanaka T, Kanai F, Okabe S, et al.: Adenovirus-mediated prodrug gene therapy for carcinoembryonic antigen-producing human gastric carcinoma cells *in vitro*. *Cancer Res* 56(6): 1341–1345, 1997

Teh BS, Aguilar-Cordova E, Kernen K, et al.: Phase I/II trial evaluating combined radiotherapy and *in situ* gene therapy with or without hormonal therapy in the treatment of prostate cancer—a preliminary report. *Int J Radiat Oncol Biol Phys* 51:605–613, 2001

Teh BS, Ayala G, Aguilar L, et al.: Phase I-II trial evaluating combined intensity-modulated radiotherapy and in situ gene therapy with or without hormonal therapy in treatment of prostate cancer—interim report on PSA response and biopsy data. *Int J Radiat Oncol Biol Phys* 58:1520–1529, 2004

Tong XW, Block A, Chen SH, et al.: *In vivo* gene therapy of ovarian cancer by adenovirus-mediated thymidine kinase gene transduction and ganciclovir administration. *Gynecol Oncol* 61:175–179, 1996

Vieweg J, Rosenthal FM, Bannerji R, et al.: Immunotherapy of prostate cancer in the Dunning rat model: Use of cytokine gene modified tumor vaccines. *Cancer Res* 54:1760–1765, 1994

Vile RG, Nelson JA, Castleden S, Chong H, Hart IR: Systemic gene therapy of murine melanoma using tissue specific expression of the *HSV-tk* gene involves an immune component. *Cancer Res* 54:6226–6234, 1994

Wang GL, Semenza GL: Characterisation of hypoxia-inducible factor 1 and regulation of DNA binding activity by hypoxia. *J Biol Chem* 268(29):21513–21518, 1993

Wang GL, Semenza GL: General involvement of hypoxia-inducible factor 1 in transcriptional response to hypoxia. *Proc Natl Acad Sci USA* 90(9):4304–4308, 1993

Wang GL, Semenza GL: Purification and characterisation of hypoxia-inducible factor. 1. *J Biol Chem* 270(3):1230–1237, 1995

Weichselbaum RR, Hallahan DE, Beckett MA, et al.: Gene therapy targeted by radiation preferentially radiosensitizes tumor cells. *Cancer Res* 54:4266–4269, 1994

Weichselbaum RR, Hallahan DE, Fuks Z, Kufe D: Radiation induction of immediate early genes: Effectors of the radiation-stress response. *Int J Radiat Oncology Biol Phys* 30:229–234, 1994

Weichselbaum RR, Hallahan DE, Sukhatme VP, Kufe DW: Gene therapy targeted by ionizing radiation. *Int J Radiat Oncology Biol Phys* 24:565–567, 1992

Xu M, Kumar D, Srinivas S, et al.: Parenteral gene therapy with *p53* inhibits human breast tumors *in vivo* through a bystander mechanism without evidence of toxicity. *Hum Gene Ther* 8:177–185, 1997

Yee D, McGuire SE, Brunner N, et al.: Adenovirus-mediated gene transfer of herpes simplex virus thymidine kinase in an ascites model of human breast cancer. *Hum Gene Ther* 7:1251–1257, 1996

CHAPTER 27

Chemotherapeutic Agents from the Perspective of the Radiation Biologist

> *Alice:* There's no use trying—one can't believe impossible things.
>
> *The Queen:* I dare say you haven't had much practice. Why, sometimes I've believed as many as six impossible things before breakfast.
>
> —*Alice in Wonderland* (Lewis Carroll)

This chapter is included after much thought and some equivocation. It was written in response to numerous requests that chemotherapeutic agents be compared and contrasted with radiation from the perspective of the experimental biologist. Many of the techniques and concepts used in chemotherapy were developed initially by radiation biologists, including quantitative tumor assay systems, the concept of cell cycle, sensitivity changes through the cell cycle, and, particularly, population kinetics. The term **growth fraction**, for example, was coined by a radiation biologist but never assumed the importance in radiotherapy that it has in chemotherapy.

The study of chemotherapeutic agents in the laboratory, as well as in the clinic, is vastly more complicated than the study of ionizing radiations. For example, **dose** is more difficult to define or to measure, and time of drug exposure is a critical parameter. Variations in sensitivity through the cell cycle are more dramatic for chemicals than for radiation, assuming essentially an all-or-nothing effect for some agents; there are many more factors involving the milieu that can influence cellular response.

The term **chemotherapy** was coined by Paul Erhlich around the turn of the 20th century to describe the use of chemicals of known composition for the treatment of parasites. Erhlich synthesized an organic arsenic compound that was effective against trypanosome infections and rabbit syphilis. This was the first synthetic chemical effective in the treatment of parasitic disease and was rather optimistically named *salvarsan*, which roughly translates to "the savior of mankind." The next milestone was the discovery and clinical use of penicillin in the early years of World War II. Alkylating agents had been developed as military weapons by both belligerents in World War I, but it was an explosion in Naples harbor and the exposure of seamen to these agents during World War II that led to the observation that these agents cause marrow and lymphoid hypoplasia. As a result, they were first tested in humans with Hodgkin's disease in 1943 at Yale University.

It has long been known beyond doubt that a single chemotherapeutic drug, used in the appropriate schedule, can cure patients with certain rapidly proliferating cancers. The initial demonstration of this was the use of methotrexate to cure patients with choriocarcinoma and, later, the use of cyclophosphamide for Burkitt's lymphoma.

The next major step forward was the use of combination chemotherapy in the treatment of acute lymphocytic leukemia in the early 1960s and, subsequently, in the treatment of Hodgkin's disease, diffuse histiocytic lymphoma, and testicular cancer in the mid-1970s. These trials verified that multiple non-cross-resistant drugs with different dose-limiting normal-tissue toxicities could be used effectively in combination to cure tumors that were not curable with a single agent. The principle of combination therapy then was extended to combined-modality treatment, in which chemotherapy was used in conjunction with surgery or radiotherapy, or both, to cure tumors such as pediatric sarcomas.

Today, a wide variety of antineoplastic agents are used routinely in clinical oncology. Drug-induced cures are claimed for choriocarcinoma, acute lymphocytic leukemia of childhood, other childhood tumors, Hodgkin's disease, certain non-Hodgkin's lymphomas, and some germ-cell tumors of the testes. Other evidence suggests that chemotherapeutic agents given in an "adjuvant" setting for clinically inapparent micrometastatic disease may prolong disease-free survival and possibly effect cure of breast cancer and osteogenic sarcoma.

There are about 13 types of cancer for which cures are claimed by chemotherapy; this accounts for about 10% of all cancers. For comparison, the proportion of cancer patients cured by radiation therapy often is claimed to be about 12.5%. This comes from the so-called $1/2 \times 1/2 \times 1/2$ rule; that is, one half of all cancer patients receive radiation therapy, one half of those treated are treated with intent to cure, and one half of those treated definitively are cured.

The bad public image of chemotherapy relates in large part from the toxicity to normal tissue resulting from multidrug protocols used to induce remissions and achieve tumor cure. "The dose makes the poison" was the advice of Paracelcus, the 16th-century German-Swiss physician and alchemist who established the role of chemistry in medicine. In other words, anything powerful enough to help also has the power to harm. In the past, the lack of tumor-specific agents carried the burden of damage to self-renewing normal tissues, such as the gut and bone marrow. There is hope that the situation is improving with the development of targeted therapy such as, for example, cetuximab (Erbitux) for cancers of the colon and rectum. (This is discussed later in this chapter.)

BIOLOGIC BASIS OF CHEMOTHERAPY

Most anticancer drugs work by affecting DNA synthesis or function, and they usually do not kill resting cells unless such cells divide soon after exposure to the drug. Consequently, the effectiveness of anticancer drugs is limited by the growth fraction of the tumor—that is, by the fraction of cells in active cycle. Rapidly growing neoplasia with a short cell cycle, a large proportion of cells in S phase, and therefore a large growth fraction, are more responsive to chemotherapy than large tumor masses in which the growth fraction is small. There is a strong tendency for growth fraction to decrease as tumor size increases, at least in experimental animal tumors.

Agents that are mainly effective during a particular phase of the cell cycle, such as S phase or M phase, are said to be **cell-cycle specific**, or **phase specific**. Those whose action is independent of the position of the cell in the cycle are said to be **cell-cycle nonspecific** or **phase nonspecific**. Figure 27.1 illustrates two contrasting cell-cycle-specific drugs. *Cis*-platinum compounds produce interstrand cross-links and thus inhibit DNA synthesis; this occurs in S phase. Taxanes bind to microtubules and, by enhancing their stability and preventing disassembly, adversely affect their function. They act as mitotic inhibitors, blocking cells in the G_2/M phase of the cell cycle.

Agents that are most effective against cells in S phase are relatively ineffective against cell populations that turn over slowly and have large proportions of dormant cells. On the other hand, the action of alkylating agents and other drugs interacting primarily with macromolecular DNA is largely independent of the phase of the cell cycle, and they

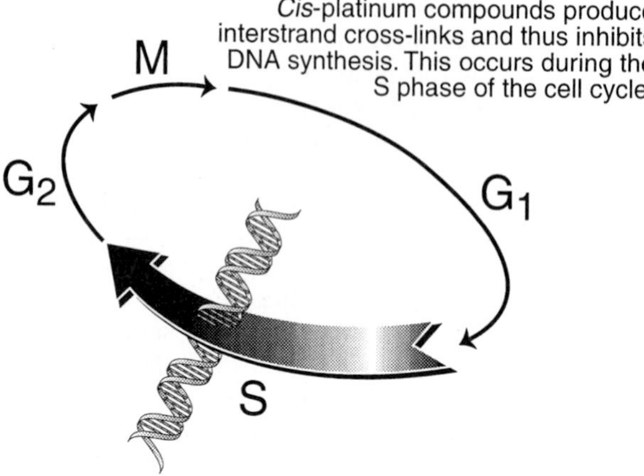

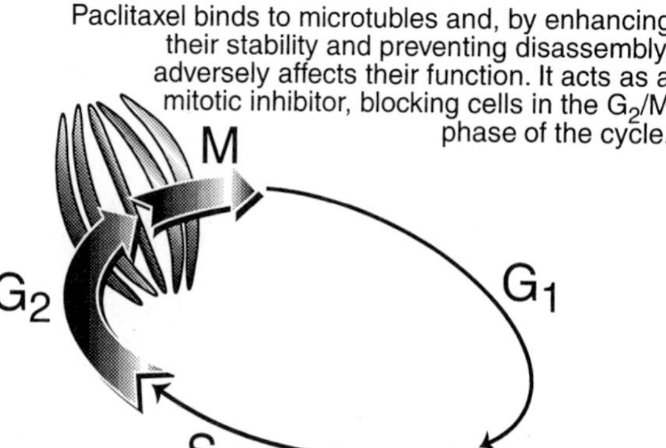

FIGURE 27.1 • Two contrasting chemotherapy agents that are both cell-cycle specific but produce their effects at quite different phases. **Top:** *Cis*-platinum compounds produce DNA interstrand cross-links that inhibit DNA synthesis; this occurs in the S phase. **Bottom:** Taxanes bind to microtubules and, by enhancing their stability and preventing disassembly, adversely affect their function. Taxanes act as mitotic inhibitors, blocking cells in the G_2/M phase of the cycle and, if the concentration is sufficient, killing them in this phase.

may be effective against tumors with relatively low proliferative activity.

The other side of the coin is that the selective normal-tissue toxicity of anticancer drugs is reflected in cytotoxic effects on stem cells of the intestinal epithelium or hematopoietic stem cells, which have high growth fractions.

Although many clinical oncologists claim that their thinking has been influenced by research on tumor growth kinetics, it is hard to point to clear advances in treatment that may be attributed to anything more than inspired clinical experimentation. This may be because the study of growth kinetics in human tumors is still in its infancy.

CLASSES OF AGENTS AND THEIR MODE OF ACTION

Many of the classical chemotherapeutic agents fall into one of three classes: alkylating agents, antibiotics, or antimetabolites. However, many of the newer and most widely used agents do not fall into any of these classes. This includes the platinum compounds, procarbazine, the vinca alkaloids, the taxanes, and the newest of all, the topoisomerase inhibitors and "targeted therapy" agents that target a specific pathway that may be elevated or vulnerable in some tumor cells.

An attempt to summarize the classification of chemotherapeutic drugs is presented in Table 27.1. A few of the most commonly used agents are described briefly, with emphasis on their characteristics and mechanism of action and comments on the extent to which they interact with radiation. A thorough discussion of their clinical usefulness is outside the scope of this book.

The effectiveness of at least some chemotherapeutic agents is dependent on the presence or absence of molecular oxygen, in much the same way as x-rays. This is not surprising, at least for drugs whose action is mediated by free radicals.

Alkylating Agents

The alkylating agents are highly reactive compounds with the ability to substitute alkyl groups for hydrogen atoms of certain organic compounds, including DNA. There are five classes of alkylating agents:

1. Nitrogen mustard derivatives, such as cyclophosphamide, chlorambucil, and melphalan.

TABLE 27.1

Chemotherapeutic Agents

Compound Class Chemotherapeutic Agent	Diseases for which Drugs Are Useful (Indications)	Unique/Major Toxicity	Targeted Pathway/Receptor (Mechanism of Action)	Synergy with Radiation
Alkylating agents				
Busulfan (Myleran)—BSF	Regular-dose therapy in CML (FDA approved) and polycythemia vera. High-dose therapy in bone-marrow transplant.	Myelosuppression. Pulmonary toxicity especially with TBI when used in high doses for bone-marrow transplant.	DNA alkylation, i.e., interstrand cross-links.	
Carboplatin (Paraplatin)—Carbo, CBDCA	FDA approved for ovarian cancer, and used extensively in testicular cancer; squamous cell cancers of the head, neck, and cervix; and lung cancer.	Myelosuppression, especially thrombocytopenia, is dose limiting.	Produces intra- and interstrand cross-links in DNA via association bonds with the platinum molecule, leading to DNA strand breakage during replication.	
Carmustine (BiCNU)—BCNU, Bischloronitrosourea	FDA approved for brain tumors, multiple myeloma, Hodgkin's disease, and lymphoma.	Myelosuppression, especially thrombocytopenia, which is slow in onset and cumulative, is dose limiting. Interstitial lung disease, including fibrosis, is rare but can occur with any dose. **Weak synergy with RT.**	Cell-cycle-independent mechanism. **Penetrates blood–brain barrier.**	+
Chlorambucil (Leukeran)	FDA approved for chronic lymphocytic leukemia (CLL) and low-grade lymphomas. Also used for Waldenström's macroglobulinemia, multiple myeloma, hairy cell leukemia, and rarely in some solid tumors.	Myelosuppression is dose limiting and universal, and it can be cumulative.	Cell-cycle independent.	
Cyclophosphamide (Cytoxan, Neosar)—CTX, CPM, Cy [prototypical alkylator]	FDA approved for many malignancies and used for even more. Most commonly used for breast carcinoma, non-Hodgkin's lymphoma, ovarian carcinoma, and testicular cancer.	Myelosuppression is dose limiting, with leukopenia being most significant. Hemorrhagic cystitis common with doses over 2 g/m^2.	Cell-cycle independent.	
Dacarbazine (DTIC-Dome)—DTIC, DIC, Imidazole Carboxamide	FDA approved for the treatment of malignant melanoma and Hodgkin's disease, and also used for adult sarcomas and neuroblastoma.	Myelosuppression is dose limiting. Nausea and vomiting are severe without aggressive antiemetic therapy. **Strong synergy with RT.**	Methylates guanine bases preferentially; non-cell-cycle dependent.	+++
Ifosfamide (Ifex)	FDA approved for the treatment of recurrent germ-cell tumors. Used for many other tumor types, including adult sarcomas, lymphoma, Hodgkin's disease, breast cancer, and ovarian cancer.	Myelosuppression, hemorrhagic cystitis, and CNS toxicity are all fairly common and can be dose limiting. Hemorrhagic cystitis can largely be prevented by coadministration of the uroprotective agent mesna.	Non-cell-cycle dependent.	
Lomustine (CeeNU)—CCNU	FDA approved for primary brain tumors and Hodgkin's disease. Also used in melanoma, multiple myeloma, other lymphomas, and breast cancer.	Myelosuppression especially thrombocytopenia, is dose limiting and tends to be cumulative. Pulmonary fibrosis can occur with long-term administration. **Weak synergy with RT.**	Cell-cycle independent. Penetrates blood–brain barrier.	+

(continued)

TABLE 27.1

(Continued)

Compound Class Chemotherapeutic Agent	Diseases for which Drugs Are Useful (Indications)	Unique/Major Toxicity	Targeted Pathway/Receptor (Mechanism of Action)	Synergy with Radiation
Mechlorethamine (Mustargen)—Nitrogen Mustard, HN2	FDA approved for a variety of hematologic malignancies and solid tumors, but generally used less in the last decade. Still used for Hodgkin's disease and topically for cutaneous T-cell lymphoma.	This drug is a powerful vesicant, so optimal extravasation precautions and rapid infusion are a must. Myelosuppression is expected and also often dose limiting. Secondary leukemia.	Cell-cycle independent.	
Melphalan (Alkeran)—L-PAM, L-phenylalanine mustard, L-sarcolysin	Used primarily for multiple myeloma, but also FDA approved for ovarian carcinoma. Could also be useful in high-dose chemotherapy/transplant settings and in regional perfusion of extremities for melanoma and sarcoma.	Myelosuppression is expected and is dose limiting. Recovery can be prolonged, and effects can be cumulative. Secondary leukemia.	Cell-cycle independent.	
Oxaliplatin (Eloxatin)	FDA approved for metastatic colorectal cancer in combination with 5-fluorouracil/leucovorin. Has been used as a single agent in this disease and is being studied in other malignancies.	Neurotoxicity, in the form of a transient neuropathy with each dose and a persistent, cumulative typical sensory poly-neuropathy, is very common and dose limiting.	Disrupts DNA via intra- and interstrand cross-links with two strong platinum association bonds in the molecule, which induces apoptosis beyond a certain level of DNA damage in malignant cells.	
Procarbazine (Matulane)—N-methylhydrazine	FDA approved for Hodgkin's disease and might also be useful in non-Hodgkin's lymphoma, multiple myeloma, brain tumors, melanoma, and lung cancer.	Myelosuppression is expected and dose limiting, but anemia is uncommon. Hives and photosensitivity sometimes occur. Dietary restrictions.	Cell-cycle independent. **Penetrates blood–brain barrier.**	
Temozolomide (Temodar)	FDA approved for treatment of recurrent high-grade astrocytomas. Used commonly for other gliomas and also for metastatic melanoma.	Myelosuppression is expected and dose limiting.	**Penetrates blood–brain barrier.**	
Atypical alkylating agents Cisplatin (Platinol)—cDDP, DDP, Cisplatinum, Cis-diamminedi-chloroplatinum (II)	Used for almost every class of solid tumor and lymphoma. FDA approved for testicular and ovarian cancers and transitional cell carcinoma.	Nephrotoxicity is dose limiting for an individual dose, while neurotoxicity, especially painful peripheral neuropathy, is dose limiting for cumulative doses. Cumulative ototoxicity is also common. **Intermediate synergy with RT.**	Produces intra- and interstrand cross-links in DNA via association bonds with the platinum molecule, leading to DNA strand breakage during replication.	++
Antibiotics Bleomycin (Blenoxane)—Bleo	FDA approved for germ-cell tumors, Hodgkin's disease, and squamous cell cancers. Used off-label for melanoma, ovarian cancer, and Kaposi's sarcoma. Also used as a sclerosing agent for malignant pleural or pericardial effusions.	Pulmonary toxicity, including reversible and irreversible fibrosis, is dose limiting. **Strong synergy with RT.**	Causes DNA strand breaks directly in normal and neoplastic cells.	+++

Dactinomycin (Cosmegen)—Actinomycin D, ACT-D	FDA approved for Wilms' tumor, Ewing's sarcoma, rhabdomysarcoma, uterine carcinoma, germ-cell tumors, and sarcoma botryoides, and also used for other sarcomas, melanoma, acute myeloid leukemia, ovarian cancer, and trophoblastic neoplasms.	This drug is a moderate vesicant. Myelosuppression is dose limiting. Nausea, vomiting, skin erythema, acneiform lesions, and hyperpigmentation are common. **Strong synergy with RT.**	Inhibits transcription by complexing with DNA.	+++
Doxorubicin (Adriamycin, Rubex)—Adria, Hydroxydaunorubicin	FDA approved for a variety of cancers and used for many more. Most commonly used for breast carcinoma, adult sarcomas, pediatric solid tumors, Hodgkin's disease, non-Hodgkin's lymphomas, and ovarian cancer.	Doxorubicin is a potent vesicant, and extravasation precautions are a must. Myelosuppression is universal and usually dose limiting with each individual cycle. Cardiotoxicity is common and can be dose limiting, though usually subclinical. Chronic, cumulative cardiomyopathy is expected when total dose exceeds 400–500 mg/m^2. **Strong synergy with RT. Recall skin reactions that correspond to prior RT treatment fields may develop, can be severe. Concurrent RT or initiation of RT within 2 weeks of administration of doxorubicin should be avoided.**	Intercalating agent.	++++
Mitomycin C (Mutamycin)	FDA approved for adenocarcinomas of the stomach and pancreas. Also used commonly in breast cancer and lung cancer.	Mitomycin C is a vesicant; extravasation precautions are a must. Myelosuppression is expected and is dose limiting, with a white blood cell nadir at 4 weeks and full recovery at 6–7 weeks. **Strong synergy with RT.**	Inhibits DNA and RNA synthesis.	+++
Antimetabolites 5-Fluorouracil (Adrucil, Efudex)—5-FU	FDA approved for colon, rectum, gastric, pancreas, and breast carcinomas and used for a wide range of other neoplasms in combination regimens. Used for intrahepatic arterial infusion for liver metastases from GI tumors and also used topically for various cutaneous neoplasms and disorders.	GI toxicities, primarily mucositis for bolus injection and diarrhea for prolonged infusions, are dose limiting. **Rare patients with dyhydropyrimidine dehydrogenase deficiency have excessive GI toxicity.** Dermatitis and other cutaneous toxicities, including hand-foot syndrome, are common. **Intermediate synergy with RT.**	Inhibitor of thymidylate synthase; partially cell-cycle dependent.	++
Capecitibine (Xeloda) [Antimetabolite prodrug]	FDA approved for metastatic breast cancer and metastatic colorectal cancer. Used also in head and neck squamous cell cancer.	Myelosuppression and palmar-plantar erythrodysesthesia are dose limiting. Diarrhea, fatigue, stomatitis, and hyperbilirubinemia are uncommon. **Intermediate synergy with RT.**		++
Cytarabine (Cytosar-U)—AraC, Cytosine Arabinoside	Acute myelogenous leukemia (AML), acute lymphoblastic lymphoma (ALL), and non-Hodgkin's lymphoma. Intrathecal use in acute leukemia.	Myelosuppression, often severe and prolonged, is dose limiting. Neurologic toxicity, mostly central with ataxia being predominant, is common and usually mild, but it is dose dependent and could leave permanent dysfunction. It is more common with intrathecal administration.	Incorporated into DNA during replication, leading to strand termination; S phase specific. **Penetrates blood–brain barrier.**	

(continued)

TABLE 27–1

(Continued)

Compound Class Chemotherapeutic Agent	Diseases for which Drugs Are Useful (Indications)	Unique/Major Toxicity	Targeted Pathway/Receptor (Mechanism of Action)	Synergy with Radiation
Fludarabine (Fludara)—FAMP	FDA approved for the treatment of CLL. Also used for low-grade lymphomas and for AML.	Neurotoxicity, including cortical blindness, confusion, somnolence, coma, and demyelinating lesions, is dose limiting, but the lower doses conventionally used rarely produce these side effects.	Only partially cell-cycle dependent.	
Gemcitibine (Gemzar)	FDA approved for advanced pancreatic adenocarcinoma, NSCLC, and metastatic breast cancer; extensively used in bladder cancer also.	Myelosuppression, including anemia, is mild but dose limiting. **Strong synergy with RT even at low doses of drug.**	A nucleoside analogue that exhibits cell-cycle-dependent and S-phase-specific cytotoxicity, likely due to inhibition of DNA synthesis.	++++
Hydroxyurea (Hydrea)—Hydrocarbamide	FDA approved for CML; commonly used for other myeloproliferative disorders and also used occasionally for metastatic melanoma, refractory ovarian carcinoma, and squamous cell carcinoma of the cervix and head and neck.	Myelosuppression is common and dose limiting. Other toxicities include rash, headache, fever, and hyperuricemia. Nausea and vomiting are uncommon. Liver toxicity and serious neurologic toxicity are rare. **Weak synergy with RT.**	Inhibitor of ribonucleotide reductase, which converts nucleotides to the deoxyribose forms for DNA synthesis; cell-cycle dependent. **Penetrates blood–brain barrier.**	+
Methotrexate (Mexate, Folex, others)—MTX, Amethopterin	FDA approved for a wide spectrum of malignant and nonmalignant diseases. Most often used for acute leukemias, lymphomas, breast cancer, bladder cancer, squamous cell cancers, and sarcomas.	Myelosuppression is expected and is usually dose limiting. Renal toxicity is uncommon and usually reversible, but can be severe. **Encephalopathy is rare with moderate to low-dose therapy but is more common with high doses, intrathecal administration, or concomitant CNS radiation. It can be severe and permanent. Drug should be administered prior to rather than concurrently or following brain RT when feasible to lessen risk of leukoencephalopathy. Weak synergy with RT.**	Interferes with nucleotide synthesis by inhibiting dihydrofolate reductase; cell-cycle dependent. **Penetrates blood–brain barrier at high intravenous doses.**	+
Corticosteroids				
Prednisone (Deltasone, others)	FDA approved for a wide variety of malignant and nonmalignant conditions. Used in oncology for lymphoid malignancies, for palliative care, and for management of side effects/toxicities.	Toxicity is mostly in the form of constitutional symptoms, including mood changes (depressive, anxious, or euphoric), insomnia, indigestion, enhanced appetite, weight gain, acne, and cushingoid features. Other side effects may be more serious but are less common. Hyperglycemia and increased stomach acid predisposing to ulceration occur acutely, while osteopenia, cataracts, skin atrophy, and adrenal insufficiency occur with prolonged use.		
Enzymes				
l-Asparaginase (Elspar)—Colaspase	FDA approved for ALL; also used in AML, late-stage chronic myelogenous leukemia (CML), chronic lymphocytic leukemia (CLL), and non-Hodgkin's lymphomas.	Hypersensitivity can be life threatening, requiring anaphylaxis precautions and a 2-unit test dose. Coagulopathy is common and requires monitoring. Lethargy, somnolence, fatigue, depression, and confusion are seen, as are pancreatitis and fever.	Cleaves the amino acid asparagine, which is an essential amino acid required by rapidly proliferating cells.	

Monoclonal antibodies				
Trastuzumab (Herceptin)	FDA approved for HER2/neu overexpressing metastatic or locally advanced breast cancer; has shown clinical benefit as a single agent and in conjunction with paclitaxel-based chemotherapy.	Common toxicities include acute fever, chills, nausea, vomiting, and headache. Trastuzumab seems to worsen leukopenia, anemia, and diarrhea when given with chemotherapy compared with chemotherapy alone. Also, trastuzumab could have uncommon acute cardiotoxicity, which might add to the more common anthracycline-induced cardiotoxicity; therefore, the use of trastuzumab with doxorubicin is not indicated by the FDA.	Directed against the HER2/neu growth factor receptor overexpressed on many invasive breast carcinomas; mechanism of action for clinical activity in breast cancer is unknown, but could be complement-mediated cell lysis, antibody-dependent cellular cytotoxicity, or induction of apoptosis.	
Steroidal progestational agents				
Megestrol acetate (Megace)—Megestrol	FDA approved for treatment of breast and endometrial carcinoma. Also used for renal cell carcinoma and for appetite stimulation in HIV disease and cancer patients.	Toxicities are similar to those of other progestins as noted previously. They include menstrual changes, hot flashes, edema, weight gain, fatigue, acne, hirsutism, anxiety, depression, sleep disturbance, and headache. Urinary frequency can occur also. Nausea, vomiting, diarrhea, skin rash or allergy, jaundice, and thrombophlebitis are uncommon.		
Targeted therapy				
Cetuximab (Erbitux)	Colorectal cancer, head and neck cancer.	**Self-limiting sterile, nonsuppurative acne like skin rash is common. Resolves with cessation of drug. Hypersensitivity reactions are less common. Strong synergy with RT.**	**Blocks EGFR receptor dimerization and tyrosine kinase phosphorylation, which inhibits tyrosine kinase pathway signal transduction.**	+++
Imatinib mesylate (Gleevec)	FDA approved for treatment of CML in the frontline setting, in accelerated phase, and in blast crisis. It is also approved for treatment of recurrent inoperable or metastatic gastrointestinal stromal tumors.	There is no definite dose-limiting toxicity of imatinib. Myelosuppression is significant in chronic myelogenous leukemia (CML) but mild in gastrointestinal stromal tumors. Hepatotoxicity is common but usually mild. Liver function tests should be monitored closely during therapy. Fluid retention is common but usually mild, as are nausea, vomiting, and diarrhea. Rash and fever are uncommon.	Specific receptor tyrosine kinase inhibitor, which selectively inhibits the tyrosine kinases of the bcr-abl, c-kit, and PDGF receptors.	
Rituximab (Rituxan)	FDA approved for relapsed or refractory low-grade or follicular, CD20-positive, B-cell lymphomas.	Fever, chills, and malaise are common during administration, even with premedication with acetaminophen and diphenhydramine. Other infusion-related symptoms include nausea, vomiting, flushing, urticaria, angioedema, hypotension, dyspnea, bronchospasm, fatigue, headache, rhinitis, and pain at disease sites. These symptoms are generally self-limited, improve with slowing of the infusion, and resolve after infusion. Short-lived myelosuppression, abdominal pain, and myalgia are uncommon. Arrhythmias and angina pectoris are rare.	Directed against the B-cell surface antigen CD20.	

(continued)

TABLE 27–1

(Continued)

Compound Class Chemotherapeutic Agent	Diseases for which Drugs Are Useful (Indications)	Unique/Major Toxicity	Targeted Pathway/Receptor (Mechanism of Action)	Synergy with Radiation
Taxanes				
Docetaxel (Taxotere)—RP-56976	FDA approved for metastatic breast cancer and first- and second-line non-small-cell lung cancer. Clinical experience increasing in ovarian cancer and other epithelial neoplasms.	Myelosuppression is universal and dose limiting. Alopecia is also universal. Edema and fluid accumulation, including pleural effusions and ascites, are common and can be dose limiting. Fluid accumulation is partially preventable with corticosteroid treatment before and after each cycle of docetaxel. Mild sensory or sensorimotor neuropathy is common.	Inhibits the mitotic spindle apparatus by stabilizing tubulin polymers, leading to death of mitotic cells.	
Paclitaxel (Taxol, Onxol)	FDA approved for salvage therapy in ovarian cancer and for breast cancer in both the metastatic and adjuvant setting. Used also in lung cancer, head and neck cancers, and bladder cancer.	Paclitaxel is an irritant or mild vesicant when extravasated into subcutaneous tissue. Myelosuppression, predominantly neutropenia, is expected and is dose limiting. Shorter infusions of the same dose produce less neutropenia. Mucositis is also very common, particularly with longer infusions. Peripheral neuropathy is common, usually mild, and increases with cumulative dose. Acute neuromyopathy is also common and occurs for several days after each dose. Hypersensitivity reactions to paclitaxel, including urticaria, wheezing, chest pain, dyspnea, and hypotension, are common but are reduced in frequency and severity by premedication with corticosteroids and H1 and H2 histamine receptor blockers (recommended regimen is dexamethasone 20 mg PO 12 and 6 hours prior to paclitaxel and diphenhydramine 50 mg and cimetidine 300 mg IV 30 minutes prior to paclitaxel). **Weak synergy with RT.**	Inhibits depolymerization of tubulin in the spindle apparatus, thereby inducing apoptosis in dividing cells.	+
Topoisomerase inhibitors Etoposide (Vespid)—VP-16, Epipodophyllotoxin; also available as Etoposide Phosphate (Etopophos)	FDA approved for germ-cell tumors and SCLC. Also used for lymphomas, AML, brain tumors, non-SCLC, and as high-dose therapy in the transplant setting for breast cancer, ovarian cancer, and lymphomas.	Myelosuppression, primarily leukopenia, is universal and dose limiting. Nausea and vomiting are common with PO administration but rare when the drug is given IV. Stomatitis and diarrhea are rare with normal doses but common with high doses. Secondary AML has been reported after etoposide.	Partially cell-cycle dependent. Topoisomerase II inhibitor	
Irinotecan (Camptosar)—CPT-11	Irinotecan is FDA approved for refractory or recurrent metastatic colon cancer, and it has now been used in other malignancies, including lung cancer, ovarian cancer, and lymphoma.	Myelosuppression, primarily neutropenia, is common and dose limiting. Diarrhea is also common and can be dose limiting.	Partly cell-cycle dependent. Topoisomerase I inhibitor	

Vinca alkaloids			
Vinblastine (Velban, Velsar, others)—VLB, Vincaleukoblastine	FDA approved for multiple hematologic and solid neoplasms. Most often used for Hodgkin's disease, non-Hodgkin's lymphoma, germ-cell tumors, and breast cancer.	Vinblastine is a soft-tissue vesicant, requiring extravasation precautions during administration. Myelosuppression, especially leukopenia, is expected and dose limiting.	Inhibitor of tubulin polymerization and thereby mitosis; G_2 phase specific
Vincristine (Oncovin, Vincasar)—Leurocristine, VCR	FDA approved for Hodgkin's disease and other lymphomas, acute leukemias, rhabdomyosarcoma, neuroblastoma, and Wilms' tumor. Used for many other neoplasms as well.	Vincristine is a vesicant and should be administered with extravasation precautions. Neurotoxicity is dose limiting in the form of peripheral neuropathy, which is related to total cumulative dose.	Inhibitor of tubulin polymerization and thereby mitosis; G_2 phase specific.
Vinorelbine (Navelbine)—5'-noranhydrovinblastine, NVB	FDA approved for the treatment of relapsed metastatic breast cancer and for NSCLC as a single agent or combined with a platinating agent.	Vinorelbine is a mild vesicant, requiring exravasation precautions. Myelosuppression, mostly leukopenia, is expected and dose limiting. Neurotoxicity in the form of neuropathy is less common and milder than that seen with vincristine. Tumor pain during administration has been reported.	Inhibitor of tubulin polymerization and thereby mitosis; G_2 phase specific.
LHRH (Luteinizing hormone-release hormone) Goserelin acetate (Zoladex)	FDA approved for advanced prostate cancer and used also in metastatic breast cancer.	Toxicity is mild. Endocrine side effects are most prominent and include hot flashes, diminished libido, impotence, gynecomastia, amenorrhea, and breakthrough vaginal bleeding.	Inhibits pituitary–gonadal axis function; causes steroid hormone withdrawal from dependent tissues, including prostate cancer and breast cancer cells.
Leuprolide acetate (Leupron)—Leuprorelin Acetate	FDA approved for the treatment of hormone-dependent advanced prostate cancer. Also used for breast cancer and endometriosis.	Usually well tolerated, but side effects can affect many systems, including endocrine (hot flashes, impotence, gynecomastia, breast tenderness, diminished libido, amenorrhea, atrophic vaginitis, increased cholesterol).	Gonadotropin-releasing hormone agonist, which shuts down the pituitary release of gonadotropins, resulting in a dramatic decrease in gonadal estrogens and androgens, and growth inhibition of hormone-dependent neoplasms.
Nonsteroidal antiandrogens Bicalutamide (Casodex)	FDA approved for stage D2 prostate cancer, in combination with a luteinizing hormone- releasing hormone (LHRH) agonist agent.	Constitutional symptoms predominate, including hot flashes, decreased libido, depression, weight gain, edema, gynecomastia, early disease-site pain (flare reaction), and constipation.	
Tamoxifen (Nolvedex)	FDA approved for the treatment of breast cancer, generally in postmenopausal patients or those with estrogen receptor-positive tumors. The same dose has been approved for chemoprevention of breast cancer in high-risk individuals. Higher doses are used for melanoma and pancreatic cancer.	Tamoxifen is usually very well tolerated. Constitutional symptoms are most prevalent and usually dose limiting. Hot flashes, sweating, mood changes, weight gain or loss, and stomach upset are most common.	Cytostatic effects on estrogen-dependent and nondependent malignant cells.
Nonsteroidal aromatase inhibitors Anastrazole (Arimidex)	As adjuvant therapy of breast cancer and for treatment of postmenopausal women with breast carcinoma who have progressed on tamoxifen therapy.	The drug is very well tolerated. Asthenia, headache, and hot flashes occur in less than 15% of women. Thrombophlebitis has been reported.	Blocks estrogen production selectively.
Cytoprotectants Amifostine (Ethyol)—WR-2721, Ethiofos	FDA approved for pretreatment with cisplatin. Useful as a bone-marrow, kidney, and nerve cytoprotectant. Useful with other alkylators. Also FDA approved as a radiation protectant to reduce xerostomia.	Transient hypotension is dose limiting. Nausea, vomiting, and somnolence are common.	Free-radical scavenger.

+ indicates the degree of synergy with radiation.

Compiled by Christopher Schultz, M.D., 2005.

2. Ethylenimine derivatives, such as thiotepa.
3. Alkyl sulfonates, such as busulfan.
4. Triazine derivatives, such as dacarbazine.
5. Nitrosoureas, including BCNU (carmustine), CCNU (lomustine), and methyl CCNU.

Most of these drugs contain more than one alkylating group and therefore are considered **polyfunctional alkylating agents**. The nitrosoureas and dacarbazine have mechanisms and cytotoxicity over and above their ability to alkylate nucleic acids. As a class, alkylating agents are considered cell-cycle nonspecific.

Nitrogen mustard is the prototype for three other useful alkylating agents: cyclophosphamide, chlorambucil, and melphalan. Nitrogen mustard given intravenously interacts rapidly with cells *in vivo*, producing its primary effect in seconds or minutes. By contrast, cyclophosphamide (Cytoxan) is inert until it undergoes biotransformation in the liver. Disappearance of injected cyclophosphamide from the plasma is biexponential, with an average half-life of 4 to 6.5 hours. Like all useful alkylating agents, cyclophosphamide produces toxicity in rapidly proliferating normal tissues. Chlorambucil (Leukeran) is an aromatic derivative of nitrogen mustard and is the slowest acting alkylating agent in general use. Melphalan (Alkeran, L-PAM) is a phenylalanine derivative of nitrogen mustard.

The nitrosoureas are a group of lipophilic alkylating agents that undergo extensive biotransformation *in vivo*, leading to a variety of biologic effects, including alkylation, carbamylation, and inhibition of DNA repair. The multiple mechanisms of action may explain why the nitrosoureas generally lack cross-resistance with other alkylating agents. These compounds are very lipid-soluble and readily cross the blood–brain barrier. They disappear from plasma rapidly, but their metabolites may persist for days.

Antibiotics

The clinically useful antibiotics are natural products of various strains of the soil fungus *Streptomyces*. They produce their tumoricidal effects by directly binding to DNA, and so their major inhibiting effects are on DNA and RNA synthesis. As a class, these drugs behave as cell-cycle-nonspecific agents. Doxorubicin (Adriamycin) and daunorubicin (also known as daunomycin) are closely related anthracycline antibiotics. After intravenous injection, both drugs undergo extensive bioreduction in the liver to active and inactive metabolites, are bound extensively in tissues, and persist in plasma for prolonged periods. Neither drug crosses the blood–brain barrier to any appreciable extent. Both doxorubicin and daunorubicin are highly toxic drugs, producing a variety of severe reactions; the major limiting toxicity, however, is cardiac damage.

Dactinomycin (Actinomycin D) inhibits DNA-primed RNA synthesis by intercalating with the guanine residues of DNA; at higher concentrations, it also inhibits DNA synthesis. The net effect is cell-cycle-nonspecific cytotoxicity. Dactinomycin must be administered intravenously. Its important longer plasma half-life is about 36 hours, and the drug is extensively bound to tissues.

Bleomycin sulfate (Blenoxane) affects cells by directly binding to DNA, resulting in reduced synthesis of DNA, RNA, and proteins. It also can lead to single-strand DNA breaks. Drugs acting by intercalation appear to augment the cytotoxic effects of bleomycin, as do x-rays and chemicals that generate superoxide radicals. Bleomycin is considered cell-cycle nonspecific. It is more damaging to nonproliferating cells than to most proliferating cells.

Mitomycin C (Mutamycin) is an extremely toxic antitumor antibiotic. Unlike most other antibiotics, it is activated *in vivo* to a bifunctional or trifunctional alkylating agent. It is cell-cycle nonspecific and is considerably more toxic to hypoxic than to aerated cells. Mitomycin C almost always is administered intravenously; it is cleared rapidly from the plasma, with a half-life of 10 to 15 minutes, primarily by metabolism in the liver. It does not appear to cross the blood–brain barrier. The major toxicity of mitomycin C is myelosuppression.

Antimetabolites

The antimetabolites are analogues of normal metabolites required for cell function and replication. They may interact with enzymes and damage cells by any of these modes of action

1. *Substituting* for a metabolite normally incorporated into a key molecule.
2. *Competing* successfully with a normal metabolite for occupation of the catalytic site of a key enzyme.
3. *Competing* with a normal metabolite that acts at an enzyme regulatory site, thereby altering the catalytic rate of the enzyme.

Methotrexate is a folic acid antagonist. It works by competing for the folate-binding site of the enzyme dihydrofolate reductase. This results in decreased synthesis of thymidine and purine nucleotides. The cytotoxicity of methotrexate can be reversed by leucovorin, which is converted readily to other forms of reduced folate within the cell and which then can act as methyl donors for a variety of biochemical reactions. The use of high-dose methotrexate with leucovorin rescue is based on the pharmacology of the two drugs, with the possibility of a differential effect between tumors and normal tissues in their ability to transport the two drugs across cell membranes. How true this differential effect turns out to be is another matter.

5-Fluorouracil

5-Fluorouracil (5-FU) is a structural analogue of the DNA precursor thymine. It works primarily as an irreversible inhibitor of the enzyme thymidylate synthetase, but only after intracellular conversion to the active metabolite. It also is degraded by the liver and some other tissues. As a single agent, 5-fluorouracil is most useful in the treatment of carcinoma of the breast and gastrointestinal tract. The degradative enzymes are found in high concentrations in the gut but not in colonic carcinomas, and it has been suggested that this may explain in part the susceptibility of colon cancer to 5-fluorouracil.

Nucleoside Analogues

A variety of nucleoside analogues have been synthesized and tested for antineoplastic properties. They are transported readily into rapidly dividing cells and activated by the single metabolic step of phosphorylation. Two analogues of cytosine are useful in cancer chemotherapy.

Cytarabine (cytosine arabinoside) is an analogue of deoxycytidine in which the sugar moiety is altered. The active form of cytarabine is the triphosphate that functions as a competitive inhibitor of DNA polymerase. Cytarabine is cell-cycle specific and in clinical practice almost always is used in combination with other drugs in the treatment of acute myeloid leukemia.

-Azacytidine contains a single nitrogen substitution in the pyrimidine ring of cytidine. It undergoes a sequence of biotransformations similar to cytarabine, with the ultimate formation of an active triphosphate. The major biochemical effect of 5-azacytidine is believed to be the inhibition of the processing of large-molecular-weight species of RNA, with less important effects on DNA and protein synthesis. Like cytarabine, it is cell-cycle specific.

Vinca Alkaloids

Some of the most useful antineoplastic agents are produced from plants. Vincristine sulfate (Oncovin) and vinblastine sulfate (Velban) are alkaloids produced from the common periwinkle plant. The clinically useful alkaloids are large, complex molecules that exert their major antitumor effect by binding to cellular microtubular proteins and inhibiting microtubule polymerization. Because these are essential compounds of the mitotic spindle of dividing cells, this binding leads to mitotic arrest.

Taxanes

The toxicity of products of the yew tree has been known for thousands of years. For example, essentially every rural village in England has a huge spreading yew tree, dating from medieval times when the archer's weapon, the long bow, was fabricated from the wood of the yew—but the tree always is found in the walled-in church cemetery, because the leaves or bark are toxic to browsing livestock. This toxicity is caused by a class of compounds known as taxanes. For those who see chemotherapy for cancer as simply the latest round in the never-ending battle between plants and animals, taxanes do indeed provide the perfect example.

Paclitaxel is the prototype of a new class of antineoplastic agents, the taxanes, that targets the microtubules. It is a natural product, isolated from the bark of the western yew, *Taxus brevifolia*. Docetaxel is a largely synthetic derivative.

Taxanes are potent microtubule-stabilizing agents and promoters of microtubule assembly. This is in contrast to agents such as the vinca alkaloids and colchicine that bind to tubulin, the subunit of microtubules, and inhibit microtubule formation. The taxanes block or prolong the transit time of cells in the G_2/M phase of the cell cycle. The inability of these cells to pass through the G_2 and M phases of the cycle results from the inability of these cells to form a competent mitotic spindle or to disassociate a drug-treated spindle.

In addition to multiple *in vitro* studies from the early 1970s on, human studies have demonstrated the ability of taxanes to increase the mitotic index in a variety of normal tissues *in vivo*, while the two taxanes in clinical use, Taxol (paclitaxel) and Taxotere (docetaxel), have demonstrated significant levels of activity in a broad range of human tumors. The taxanes are of particular interest to radiobiologists because of the way in which they interact with radiation (described later).

Miscellaneous Agents

Procarbazine

Procarbazine is a hydrazine derivative that must undergo biotransformation before it can exert its cytotoxic effects. The precise mechanism of action is not clear, because it interferes with a wide variety of biochemical processes. Procarbazine is well absorbed from the gastrointestinal tract and is cleared from the plasma with a half-life of about 10 minutes. The drug freely crosses the blood–brain barrier. It is used primarily in the treatment of advanced Hodgkin's disease.

Hydroxyurea

Hydroxyurea first was synthesized as long ago as 1869 and was found to be bone-marrow suppressive in 1928. It was not used in the treatment of cancer until the 1960s. It acts as an inhibitor of ribonucleotide reductase, an enzyme essential to DNA synthesis, and is consequently specifically cytotoxic to cells in the S phase of the cell cycle. In experimental biology, hydroxyurea is used to synchronize cells, because in addition to killing S phase cells, it causes survivors to pile up at a block at the G_1/S interface. Clinically, hydroxyurea is used primarily in the treatment of chronic myeloid leukemia.

Cis-Platinum

Structurally, *cis*-platinum (*cis*-dichlorodiammineplatinum) is an inorganic complex formed by an atom of platinum surrounded by chlorine and ammonium ions in the *cis* position of the horizontal plane. *Cis*-platinum bears a resemblance to the bifunctional alkylating agents based on nitrogen mustard. It inhibits DNA synthesis to a greater extent than it does the synthesis of RNA or protein. It binds to DNA, causing both interstrand and intrastrand cross-linking.

Cis-platinum is cell-cycle nonspecific. Its isomer, *trans*-platinum, is much less cytotoxic, presumably because of the different way that it cross-links to DNA. There is some evidence that *cis*-platinum is more toxic to hypoxic than to aerated cells—that is, that it is a hypoxic-cell radiosensitizer, though not as powerful in this regard as the nitroimidazoles.

Topoisomerase Inhibitors

DNA topoisomerases are nuclear enzymes that reduce twisting and supercoiling that occur in selected regions of DNA as a result of transcription, replication, and repair recombination. Little is known of the actual mechanism by which they kill cells.

Top I inhibitors, thus far consisting primarily of camptothecin analogues, interact with the enzyme–DNA complex and prevent the resealing of DNA strand breaks, leading to cell death in cells actively replicating.

Top II inhibitors prevent religation of DNA cleaved by Top II and lead to cell death. Etoposide, a semisynthetic podophyllotoxin derivative, is a prime example.

Targeted Therapy

Achieving tumor response with traditional chemotherapeutic agents, such as the alkylating agents, *cis*-platinum, and 5-FU (5-fluorouracil), for example, inevitably involved substantial toxicity to self-renewal normal tissues, such as the gastrointestinal tract and the blood-forming organs. There is some promise that the situation is much more favorable in the case of the new generation of targeted therapeutic agents that, in combination with radiotherapy, enhance tumor control with little if any increase in normal-tissue toxicity. Cetuximab (Erbitux) might be regarded as a model for this class of pathway-targeting agents.

Cetuximab (Erbitux)

There appears to be a strong correlation between both locoregional control and overall survival and the level of Epidermal Growth Factor Receptor (EGFR) expression in advanced head and neck squamous carcinoma. Because high levels of EGFR predict for a poor outcome, EGFR is an attractive target for cancer therapy.

Cetuximab (brand name Erbitux) is a recombinant human/mouse chimeric monoclonal antibody produced in mammalian cell culture. Cetuximab specifically binds to EGFR, blocking phosphorylation and activation of receptor-associated kinases, resulting in inhibition of cell growth, induction of apoptosis, and decreased matrix metalloproteinase and vascular endothelial growth factor.

Studies using cetuximab with a xenograft tumor in mice (Fig. 27.2) indicate that while the antibody alone produces a modest tumor growth delay, there is a substantial interaction with radiation. These promising preclinical results led to a phase III trial that demonstrated that the addition of cetuximab to high-dose radiotherapy in patients with locoregionally advanced squamous cell carcinoma of the head and neck produced a statistically significant prolongation in overall survival. Median survival increased from 28 to 54 months. There was a minimal enhancement of toxicity in the form of worse skin reactions.

Other agents that target specific pathways include trastizumab (Herceptin), imatinib mesylate (Gleevec), and rituximab (Rituxan) (see Table 27.1).

DOSE–RESPONSE RELATIONSHIPS

Dose–response relationships have been produced for a wide range of chemotherapeutic agents

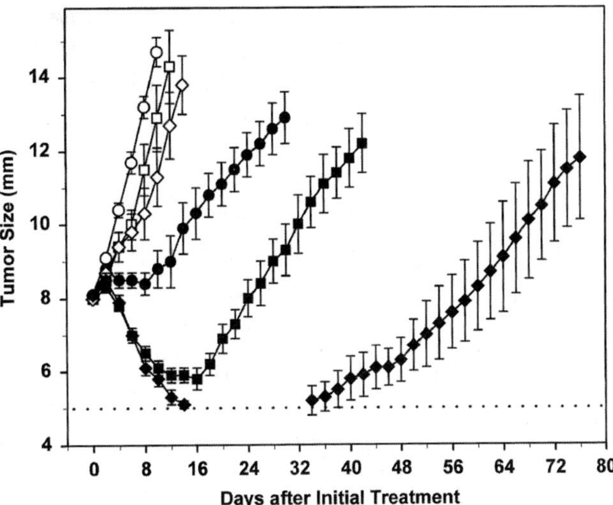

FIGURE 27.2 • The effect of C225 (cetuximab) on the radioresponse of A431 tumor xenografts: *open circles*, no treatment; *open squares*, treated with a single injection of C225; *open diamond*, treated with three injections of C225; *closed circles*, 18 Gy of local tumor irradiation; *closed squares*, single dose of C225 plus 18 Gy of local tumor irradiation; *closed diamonds*, three doses of C225 plus 18 Gy. (Redrawn from Milas L, Mason K, Hunter N, et al.: *In vivo* enhancement of tumor radioresponse by C225 antiepidermal growth factor receptor antibody. *Clinical Cancer Research* 6:701–708, 2000.)

using techniques developed initially for radiation, although much less effort has been expended on fitting data to models than has been the case for ionizing radiations. From even a cursory examination of the data, however, it is evident that—with some clear exceptions—the shape of the survival curve is unremarkable and reminiscent of that of survival curves for ionizing radiations. If surviving fraction is plotted on a log scale against drug dose on a linear scale, the dose–response curve has an initial shoulder followed by a region that becomes steeper and straighter (Fig. 27.3). The antibiotics doxorubicin (Adriamycin), bleomycin, and dactinomycin (Actinomycin D) are clear exceptions. For these agents, the dose–response curve appears to have no shoulder, and the curve is concave upward. A dose–response curve with this shape usually is associated with a variation of sensitivity within the population (i.e., nonuniform sensitivity of cells). This has never been demonstrated experimentally, however. For example, synchronously dividing cells likewise show the same upwardly concave dose–response curve. This shape therefore must remain unexplained at the present time.

Dose–response curves indicate that, at best, anticancer drugs kill by first-order kinetics; that is, a given dose of the drug kills a constant fraction of a population of cells, regardless of its size. This assumes, of course, that the growth fraction and the proportion of sensitive to resistant cells remains the same. This leads to the conclusion that the chance of eradicating a cancer is greatest if the population size is small, or that there is an inverse relationship between curability and the tumor cell burden at the initiation of chemotherapy. This conclusion has been arrived at from long and bitter clinical experience, but in fact, it is an inevitable consequence of the shape of the simplest dose–response relationship.

Another characteristic of chemotherapy agents is that the sensitivity to cell killing varies enormously among cell types. Radiosensitivity varies, too, of course, but not to the same extent as chemosensitivity. Dose–response curves for several cell lines exposed to paclitaxel are shown in Figure 27.4, illustrating the wide range of sensitivities.

SUBLETHAL AND POTENTIALLY LETHAL DAMAGE REPAIR

Studies with radiation led to the concepts of sublethal damage repair and potentially lethal damage repair, which are discussed in some detail in Chapter 5. These are still largely operational terms, although a notable exception is mitomycin C, in which the gene for repair of DNA damage has been identified and cloned. Sublethal damage repair is demonstrated by an increase in survival if a dose of radiation (or other cytotoxic agent) is divided into two or more fractions separated in time. There is a tendency for the extent of sublethal damage repair to correlate with the shoulder of the acute dose–response curve, but this is not always true. Repair of potentially lethal damage is manifest as an increase in survival if cells are held in a nonproliferative state for some time after treatment.

Similar studies have been performed with a variety of chemotherapeutic agents. The results are not as clear-cut as for radiation, and there is much greater variability between different cell lines.

Potentially lethal damage repair is a significant factor in the antibiotics bleomycin and doxorubicin. Data for bleomycin are shown in Figure 27.5.

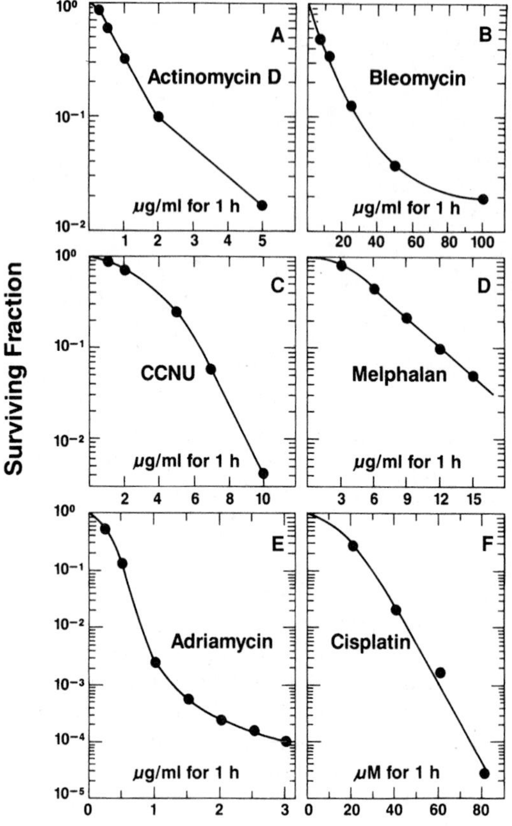

FIGURE 27.3 • Dose–response relationships *in vitro* for six commonly used chemotherapeutic agents. Note the diverse shapes. Many have shapes similar to survival curves for x-rays, except that drug concentration replaces absorbed dose. The antibiotics bleomycin (graph B), Adriamycin (doxorubicin) (graph E), and actinomycin D (graph A) have dose–response relationships that are concave upward. **A:** Dose–response relationship for dividing CHO cells treated for 1 hour with graded doses of actinomycin D. (Adapted from Barranco SC, Fluorney DR: Modification of the response to actinomycin-D-induced sublethal damage by simultaneous recovery from potentially lethal damage in mammalian cells. *Cancer Res* 36:1634–1640, 1976, with permission.) **B:** Dose–response relationship for plateau-phase CHO cells treated for 1 hour with graded doses of bleomycin. (Adapted from Barranco SC, Novak JKJ, Humphrey RM: Response of mammalian cells following treatment with bleomycin and 1,3-BTS(2 chloroethyl)-1-nitrosourea during plateau phase. *Cancer Res* 33:691–694, 1973, with permission.) **C:** Dose–response relationship for CHO cells treated for 1 hour with graded doses of CCNU. (Adapted from Barranco SC: *In vitro* responses of mammalian cells to drug-induced potentially lethal and sublethal damage. *Cancer Treat Rep* 60:1799–1810, 1976, with permission.) **D:** Dose–response relationship for human lung cancer cells exposed for 1 hour to graded doses of melphalan. (Unpublished data, courtesy of Dr. Laurie Roizin-Towle.) **E:** Dose–response relationship for V79 Chinese hamster cells exposed for 1 hour to graded doses of Adriamycin (doxorubicin). (Adapted from Belli JA, Piro AJ: The interaction between radiation and Adriamycin damage in mammalian cells. *Cancer Res* 37:1624–1630, 1975, with permission.) **F:** Dose–response relationship for V79 Chinese hamster cells exposed for 1 hour to graded doses of *cis*-platinum (cisplatin). (Unpublished data, courtesy of Dr. Laurie Roizin-Towle.)

Potentially lethal damage repair is also seen after treatment with dactinomycin. Sublethal damage repair is essentially absent with all of these drugs.

No potentially lethal or sublethal damage repair is seen with nitrosourea, even though the dose–response curves for single doses have substantial shoulders. The breakdown products of the nitrosoureas are known to inhibit DNA repair, and this may be a contributing factor.

Studies of repair of sublethal damage with drugs are complicated, because if a split-dose study is performed, decisions must be made about the equivalence of drug concentration and time. It frequently is assumed that biologic response is determined by an *integral dose* (i.e., the product of concentration and time), but this has not been checked and confirmed in all cases. There appears to be no correlation between the existence of a shoulder on the dose–response curve for single doses and the appearance of sublethal damage repair, as evidenced by an increase in survival in a split-dose experiment. It is possible that the presence of a shoulder in a survival curve does not have the same meaning for chemically induced damage as it does for radiation-induced damage. The presence of a shoulder on a survival curve for a chemotherapeutic agent may reflect more about drug concentrations and the time required for entry of the drug into the cells and interaction with a target molecule than it does about the accumulation and repair of sublethal damage.

THE OXYGEN EFFECT AND CHEMOTHERAPEUTIC AGENTS

The importance of the oxygen effect for cell killing by radiation is discussed in Chapter 6. It has been known for more than half a century that the presence or absence of molecular oxygen has a dramatic influence on the proportion of cells surviving a given dose of x-rays. Only in more recent years has the influence of oxygen on the cytotoxicity resulting from chemotherapeutic agents been studied. It is certainly more complicated than for ionizing radiations.

Some agents, such as bleomycin, are more toxic to oxygenated cells than to chronically hypoxic

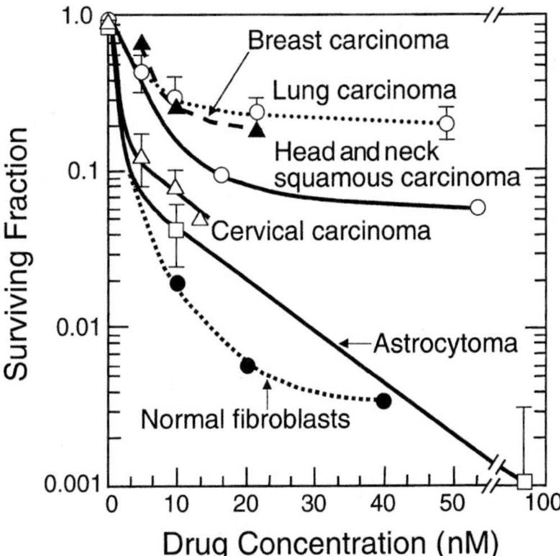

FIGURE 27.4 • Illustrating the wide variability in sensitivity to taxanes. All the data refer to cells of human origin exposed for 24 hours. (Data for the cervical carcinoma line and the astrocytoma line from Geard CR, Jones JM, Schiff PB: Taxol and radiation. *J Natl Cancer Inst Monogr* 15:89–94, 1993; data for the head and neck squamous carcinoma line from Leonard CE, Chan DC, Chou TC, Kumar R, Bunn PA: Paclitaxel enhances *in vitro* radiosensitivity of squamous carcinoma cell lines of the head and neck. *Cancer Res* 56:5198–5204, 1996; data for the lung carcinoma line [A545] from Liebmann JE, Hahn SM, Cook JA, et al.: Glutathione depletion by L-buthionine sulfoximine antagonizes taxol cytotoxicity. *Cancer Res* 53:2066–2070, 1993; data for the breast carcinoma line [MCF-7] from Liebmann JE, Cook JA, Lipschultz C, et al.: Cytotoxic studies of paclitaxel (Taxol) in human tumour cell lines. *Br J Cancer* 68:1104–1109, 1993.)

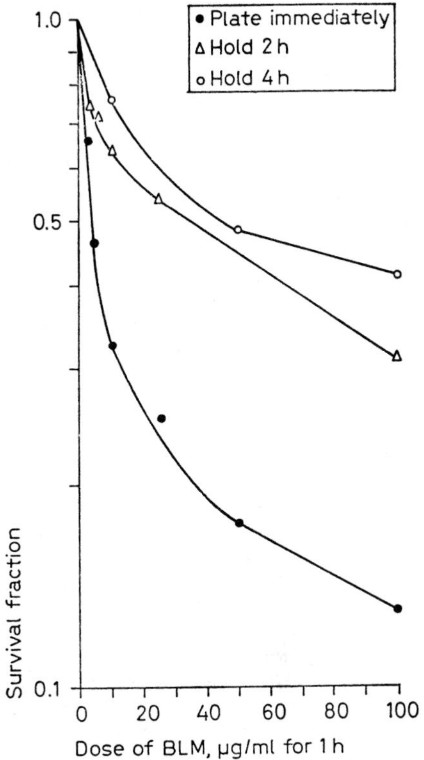

FIGURE 27.5 • Potentially lethal damage repair (PLDR) in cultured Chinese hamster cells treated with bleomycin. An increase in survival is observed, interpreted as PLDR, when cells are held in depleted medium for 2 to 4 hours after the drug treatment. (From Barranco SC, Humphrey RM: Response of mammalian cells to bleomycin-induced potentially lethal and sublethal damage. *Prog Biochem Pharmacol* 11:78–92, 1976, with permission.)

cells. Dose–response curves for cells exposed to graded concentrations of bleomycin in the presence or absence of oxygen are shown in Figure 27.6**B**. At high concentrations of the drug, there is an extra log of cell killing if oxygen is present, compared with hypoxic conditions. Other examples of agents that are more toxic to aerated than to hypoxic cells are procarbazine, dactinomycin, and vincristine. It should come as no surprise to those familiar with x-rays that oxygen is a factor in the response of cells to any chemotherapeutic agent in which the mechanism of cell killing is mediated by free radicals.

By contrast, agents such as mitomycin C are substantially more toxic to hypoxic than to aerated cells (Fig. 27.6**A**), because the drug undergoes bioreduction in the absence of oxygen. The same is true, of course, of tirapazamine, which is discussed in Chapter 25.

A third group of drugs, including 5-fluorouracil, methotrexate, *cis*-platinum, and the nitrosoureas, appears to be equally cytotoxic to aerated or hypoxic cells. This oversimplified classification only holds true if the level or duration of the hypoxia is not sufficient to disturb the movement of cells through the cell cycle. Table 27.2 is a summary of the classification of antineoplastic agents based on the effect of the presence or absence of molecular oxygen.

RESISTANCE TO CHEMOTHERAPY AND HYPOXIC CYTOTOXINS

Tumor cells protect themselves from changes in the microenvironment resulting from a decrease in both nutrients and oxygen by reducing macromolecular synthesis and inducing genes that promote angiogenesis and tissue remodeling. This is discussed in some detail in Chapter 6. The ability of malignant cells to survive fluctuations in oxygen tension is important in the context of cancer therapy, because it is well documented that tumors that are hypoxic are aggressive and respond poorly to all forms of treatment.

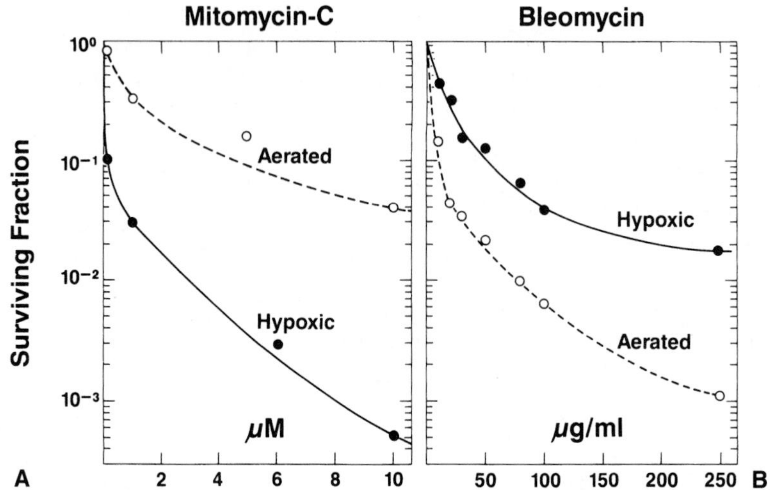

FIGURE 27.6 ● Molecular oxygen can be either a sensitizer or a protector, depending on the particular chemotherapeutic agent. **A:** Survival curves for EMT6 cells treated for 1 hour with graded doses of mitomycin C under aerated or hypoxic conditions. In the absence of oxygen, the cells are substantially more sensitive. (Data from Teicher BA, Lazo JS, Sartorelli AC: Classification of antineoplastic agents by their selective toxicities toward oxygenated and hypoxic tumor cells. *Cancer Res* 41:73–81, 1981.) **B:** Survival curves for Chinese hamster cells in culture exposed for 4 hours to graded doses of bleomycin under aerated or hypoxic conditions. In the absence of molecular oxygen, the cells are more resistant. (Adapted from Roizin-Towle L, Hall EJ: Studies with bleomycin and misonidazole on aerated and hypoxic cells. *Br J Cancer* 37:254–260, 1978, with permission.)

The shortage of oxygen in hypoxic cells renders them refractory to killing by ionizing radiations that require oxygen to "fix" the damage produced in DNA by the hydroxyl radicals; it is equally true that cells may be refractory to killing by "radiation-mimetic drugs" that operate via a free-radical mechanism. Cessation of cell division and loss of apoptotic potential (cell suicide), however, in hypoxic cells are likely to be more important reasons why hypoxic cells are resistant to chemotherapy.

TABLE 27.2

Classification of Antineoplastic Agents Based on Cellular Oxygenation

Preferential Toxicity to Aerobic Cells	Preferential Toxicity to Hypoxic Cells	Minimal or No Selectivity Based on Cellular Oxygenation
Bleomycin	Mitomycin-C	5-Fluorouracil[a]
Procarbazine	Doxorubicin	Methotrexate[a]
Streptonigrin	Misonidazole, metronidazole	Cisplatin
	Etanidazole	
	Tirapazamine	
	RB6145	
Dactinomycin	5-thio-D-glucose, 2-deoxy-D-glucose	BCNU, CCNU

[a] These conclusions are based on experiments in which hypoxic cells were still capable of DNA synthesis and cellular replication. These agents have cytotoxic effects primarily on cells in the S phase of the cell cycle. Thus, in hypoxic cells that are blocked in their progression through the cell cycle or cycling slowly, agents such as these that act on the S phase of the cell cycle would be expected to be relatively nonoctotoxic.

Based on Teicher BA, Lazo, JS, Sartorelli AC: Classification of antineoplastic agents by their selective toxicities toward oxygenated and hypoxic tumor cells. *Cancer Res* 412:73–81, 1981, with permission.

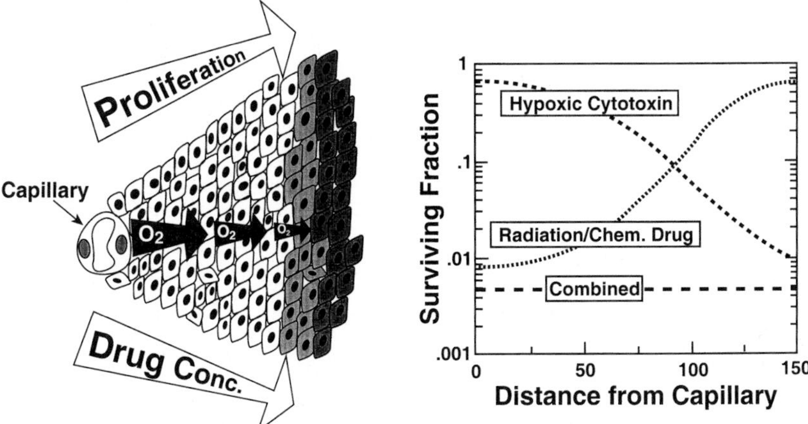

FIGURE 27.7 ● Illustrating why the microenvironment in a tumor may lead to resistance to chemotherapy agents and how the addition of a hypoxic cytotoxin may remedy the situation. **Left:** Oxygen diffuses from a capillary, but the concentration falls with distance because of respiration in the mass of tumor cells. This leads to a region of hypoxia and a region of anoxia. Chemotherapeutic agents must also diffuse through a tumor from capillaries. The effect of the agent decreases with distance from the capillary because the drug concentration falls because of metabolism, proliferation decreases with distance from a capillary because of lack of oxygen, and cells that are not dividing are resistant to many chemotherapeutic agents. **Right:** The fraction of cells surviving a treatment with radiation or most chemotherapeutic agents rises with distance from a capillary because both are less effective in hypoxic nondividing cells. This can be balanced by the addition of a hypoxic cytotoxin, such as tirapazamine, which only becomes effective in regions of reduced oxygen concentration. Consequently, the fraction of cells surviving a hypoxic cytotoxin decreases with distance from a capillary; that is, more cells are killed because cells are more hypoxic. (Adapted from Brown JM, Siim BG: Hypoxia-Specific Cytotoxins in Cancer Therapy. *Semin Radiat Oncol* 6:22–36, 1996, with permission.)

Hypoxic cells located remote from capillaries are least likely to be killed by radiation but most likely to be killed by a hypoxic cytotoxin. This is illustrated in Figure 27.7.

The most effective way to partly circumvent the problem introduced by hypoxia in reducing the efficacy of chemotherapy is to introduce a bioreductive drug or hypoxic cytotoxin that is most effective at reduced oxygen concentrations. This is described in more detail in Chapter 25. Mitomycin C and its derivatives have been used for this purpose for many years. A more recently developed drug is tirapazamine, which already has been used successfully in combination with *cis*-platinum in the therapy of advanced lung cancer.

DRUG RESISTANCE

The biggest single problem in chemotherapy is drug resistance, which either may be evident from the outset or may develop during prolonged exposure to a cytostatic drug. Cells resistant to the drug take over, and the tumor as a whole becomes unresponsive. The development of resistance can be demonstrated readily for cells in culture. Figure 27.8 shows a substantial resistance to doxorubicin developing as cells are grown continuously in a low concentration of the drug for a period of weeks.

Underlying this problem of drug resistance are genetic changes that can sometimes be seen in chromosome preparations. Figure 27.9 shows two illustrations involving gene amplification or the presence of multiple minute chromosome fragments.

Drug resistance is an important factor that occurs readily—a phenomenon quite alien to the radiobiologist. Radiation-resistant cells can be produced and isolated, but it is a difficult and time-consuming process. For instance, cells continuously irradiated at low dose rates occasionally do spawn radioresistant clones. By contrast, resistance to chemotherapeutic agents is acquired quickly, uniformly, and inevitably.

If a resistant clone can arise by a chance mutation of a gene responsible for one of the important steps in drug action, then the probability of it occurring would be expected to increase rapidly as the tumor increases in size. The average mutation rate for mammalian genes is about 10^{-5} to 10^{-6} per division, so that in a tumor containing 10^{10} cells that go through many divisions, a mutation is

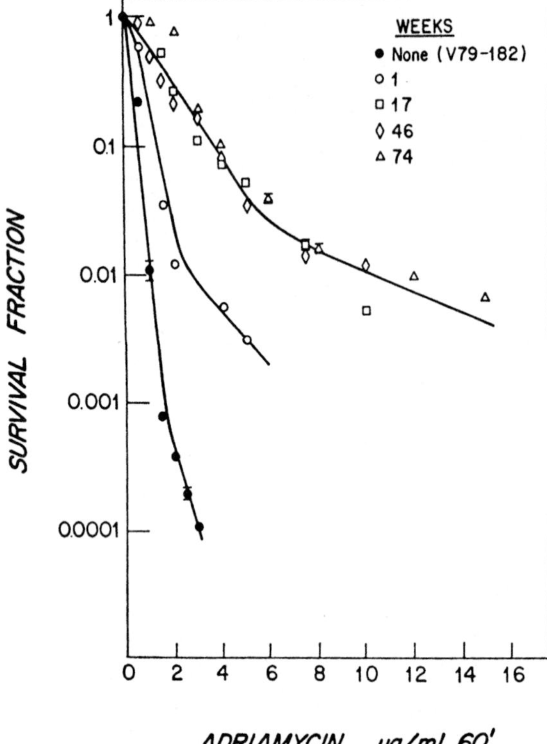

FIGURE 27.8 • Change in survival response to doxorubicin (Adriamycin) of Chinese hamster cells grown in culture and exposed continuously to a low concentration of the drug (0.05 μg/ml) for prolonged periods of time, namely 1, 17, 46, or 74 weeks. The closed circles show the survival response for the parent cell line. A dramatic resistance to the drug develops by 17 weeks; that is, prolonged exposure at a low concentration renders the cells resistant to subsequent high concentrations. (From Belli JA: Radiation response and Adriamycin resistance in mammalian cells in culture. *Front Radiat Ther Oncol* 13:9–20, 1979, with permission.)

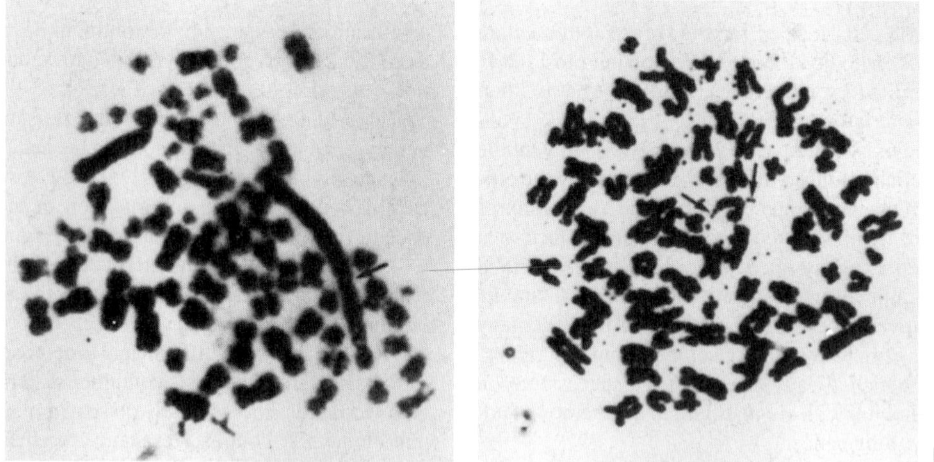

FIGURE 27.9 • Most forms of drug resistance probably have a genetic basis. A few extreme examples can be seen in chromosome changes. **A:** The arrow indicates an elongated chromosome, which on banding shows the features of an extended homogeneously staining region. This karyotype was observed in the human breast cancer cell line (MCF-7), which is resistant to methotrexate. (From Cowan KH, Goldsmith ME, Levine R, et al.: Dihydrofolate reductase gene amplification and possible rearrangement in estrogen-responsive methotrexate-resistant human breast cancer cells. *J Biol Chem* 257:15079–15086, 1982, with permission.) **B:** Small-cell lung carcinoma line derived from a patient treated with methotrexate. These cells are very resistant to the drug and contain numerous double minute chromosomes. A pair is indicated by arrows. (From Curt GA, Carney DN, Cowan KH, et al.: Unstable methotrexate resistance in human small-cell carcinoma associated with double minute chromosomes. *N Engl J Med* 308:199–202, 1983, with permission.)

almost certain to occur, especially in the presence of a powerful mutagen, which most chemotherapeutic agents are.

The usual strategy to overcome the problem of induced resistance is to use a battery of different drugs, applied sequentially and cyclically, that produce their cytotoxicity by diverse mechanisms. By this strategy, cells that develop resistance to drug A are killed by drug B, and so on.

The bigger problem is pleiotropic resistance, the phenomenon by which the development of resistance to one drug results in cross-resistance to other drugs, even those with different mechanisms of action. There are four interesting points to be made:

1. Multidrug resistance in tumor cells is caused by extrusion of the drugs; that is, cells pump the drugs out as fast as they get in. This is mediated by increased expression of the product of the multiple drug resistance gene (*mdr*), a p-glycoprotein expressed in the cell membrane. This membrane protein is a polypeptide of 1,280 amino acids composed of two similar domains, each containing six potential transmembrane segments and two putative adenosine triphosphate-binding regions. Its structure is similar to that of various transporters of ions, amino acids, peptides, or proteins in bacterial, yeast, and animal cells. Indeed, it has been reported that the multiple drug resistance gene in human tumor cells shows considerable homology to the gene in yeast that extrudes an attractant that is important in the reproductive cycle. The *mdr* gene has been mapped to human chromosome 7. Resistance by this means can be reversed by calcium channel-blocking drugs, such as verapamil. This has been shown to be an important mechanism of resistance to doxorubicin in Chinese hamster ovary cells in culture, and there appears to be expression of this same gene for resistance in cells from some human solid tumors that have acquired resistance.
2. Glutathione is a naturally occurring thiol in all cells. Elevated levels of glutathione have been observed in resistant cells, especially those made resistant by treatment with melphalan. Drugs are available that block the synthesis of glutathione and that can be used to lower the levels of this compound in tumors and normal tissues. The best-known example is buthionine sulfoximine. Use of buthionine sulfoximine has been shown to reduce cross-resistance, particularly between melphalan and *cis*-platinum in tumor-bearing mice. The use of buthionine sulfoximine would not be advisable in combination with doxorubicin or *cis*-platinum, because an increase in specific normal-tissue toxicity (lung or kidney, respectively) would be expected.
3. A marked increase in DNA repair has been noted in some cells resistant to melphalan or *cis*-platinum. In principle, drugs could be used to block repair; aphidicolin has been used in experimental systems, but no suitable drugs are available for clinical use.
4. A debatable issue is whether cells that have acquired resistance to chemotherapeutic agents are also resistant to radiation. The consensus is that they are not. There may be some data from clinical experience to suggest that they are, but the laboratory data show rather clearly that acquiring resistance to a drug does not necessarily result in radioresistance. This is illustrated in Figure 27.10, in which cells that have acquired extreme resistance to melphalan show a normal response to radiation. Radioresistance and chemoresistance may occur together, but radiation rarely induces chemoresistance and vice versa.

The evolving story of drug resistance has an impact on the development and screening of new drugs. In the past, the initial screening for new agents consisted of fast-growing, highly drug-sensitive mouse tumors. Tests against specific patterns or types of drug resistance were not included. The screening systems, therefore, were weighted heavily in favor of producing more of the same types of drugs. This has changed, and the screening of new drugs for activity is performed using a battery of cells of human origin cultured *in vitro*.

COMPARISON OF CHEMOTHERAPEUTIC AGENTS WITH RADIATION

The title of this chapter includes the words "from the perspective of the radiation biologist." This limited and specialized viewpoint must be kept in mind in what follows. A number of important differences are evident in the response of cells to chemotherapeutic agents versus ionizing radiation:

1. There is a much greater variation of sensitivity to chemotherapeutic agents than there is to radiation. In the case of x-rays, the variation of D_0 from the most sensitive to the most resistant known mammalian cells may be a factor of about 4. By contrast, the response of a variety of cell lines to a given chemotherapeutic agent may differ by orders of magnitude. A particular cell line may be exquisitely sensitive to one drug and extremely resistant to another. A different cell line

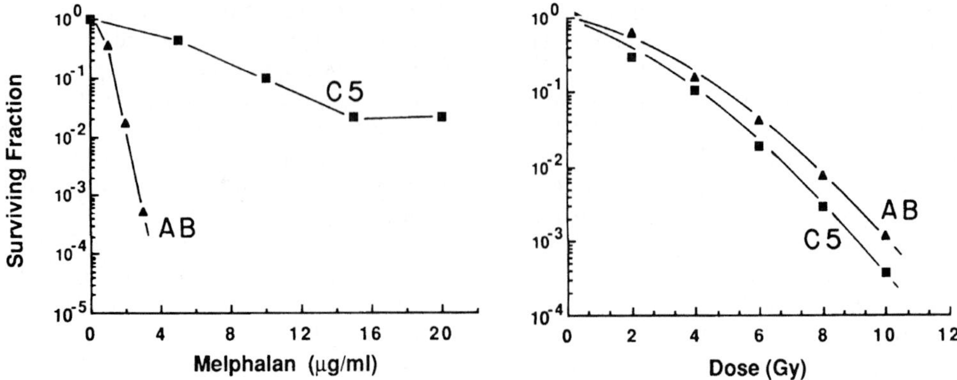

FIGURE 27.10 ● Chinese hamster pleiotropic multidrug-resistant cells are not necessarily resistant to radiation. The parental ovary cell line is designated AB. The multidrug-resistant cell line C5 was isolated by Dr. Victor Ling by exposing the parental line to the mutagen ethyl methane sulfonate, after which surviving cells were grown for an extended period of time in increasing concentrations of colchicine. A clone was isolated that is resistant to colchicine and to a variety of chemotherapeutic agents. **Left:** C5 cells are resistant to melphalan, compared with the parental line (AB). They are also resistant to other agents, such as daunorubicin. **Right:** The radiation responses of the parental and the chemotherapy-resistant cell lines are virtually indistinguishable. (From Mitchell JB, Gamson J, Russo A, et al.: Chinese hamster pleiotropic multidrug resistant cells are not radioresistant. *Natl Cancer Inst Monogr* 6:187–191, 1988, with permission.)

may have a different order of sensitivity to various drugs, as well as a quite different absolute sensitivity. Different clones derived from a common stock may exhibit quite different sensitivity to a given agent. This variability is shown in Figure 27.11, which gives the response of one cell line to nine different cytotoxic agents, and in Figure 27.12, which shows the widely different response to Me CCNU of three permanent clones derived from a common astrocytoma cell line.

2. The sensitivity of a given cell line to a given drug may be manipulated to a much greater extent than for radiation.
3. Repair of sublethal and potentially lethal damage is more variable and less predictable for drugs than for radiation.
4. The oxygen effect is more complex for drugs than for ionizing radiations. For radiation, the presence or absence of molecular oxygen has an important influence on the proportion of cells surviving a given dose of low linear energy transfer radiation, in which about two thirds of the damage is caused by indirect action (i.e., mediated by free radicals). As the linear energy transfer of the radiation increases and the balance shifts from indirect to direct action, the importance of oxygen decreases. For very high linear energy transfer radiations (above about 200 keV/μm) the biologic effect for a given dose is independent of the presence or absence of molecular oxygen. Under no circumstances is oxygen protective in the case of ionizing radiations.

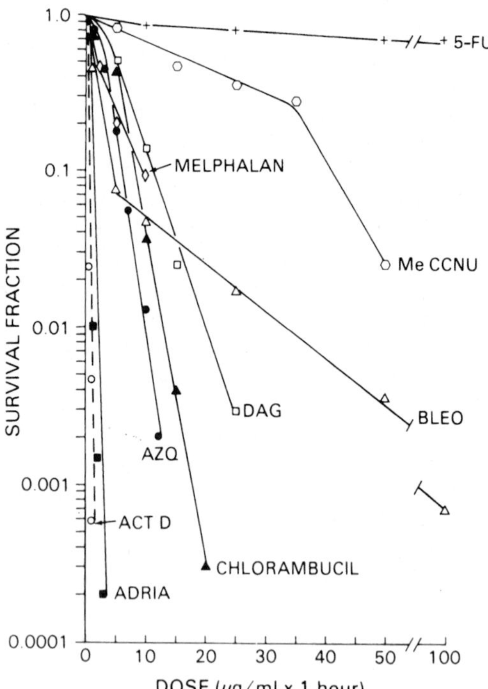

FIGURE 27.11 ● Comparison of dose–response curves of a stomach cancer cell line in culture exposed for 1 hour to graded doses of nine anticancer drugs. There is a wide variation in sensitivity and in the shape of the various curves. (From Barranco SC, Townsend CM Jr, Quraishi MA, et al.: Heterogeneous responses of an *in vitro* model of human stomach cancer to anticancer drugs. *Invest New Drugs* 1(2):117–127, 1983, with permission.)

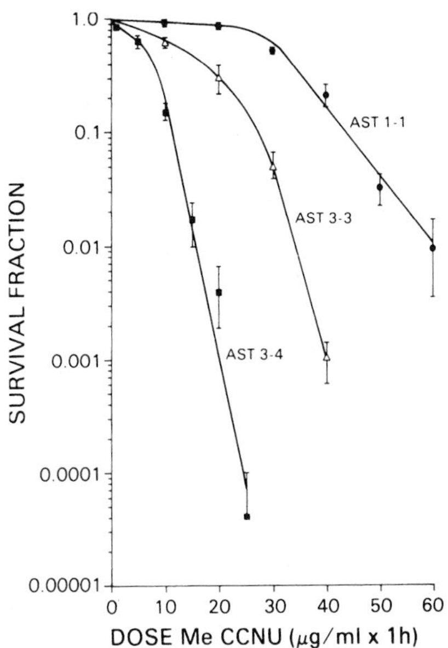

FIGURE 27.12 ● Dose–response data for three permanent clones derived from a common astrocytoma cell line exposed to the anticancer drug Me CCNU. Note the great variation in sensitivity. (From Rubin NH, Casantelli C, Maerk BG, Boerwinkle WR, Barranco SC: *In vitro* cellular characteristics and survival responses of human astrocytoma clones to chloroethyl-nitrosoureas and idanhydrogalactical. *Invest New Drugs* 1:129–137, 1983, with permission.)

For drugs in which the biologic effect involves free radicals, the presence or absence of oxygen is important in the same way as for low linear energy transfer ionizing radiations. The new factor in the case of drugs is that there is a whole class of antineoplastic agents that undergo bioreduction in the absence of oxygen, so that they are more effective in hypoxic cells. There is no parallel for ionizing radiations.

Other agents do not depend primarily on free radicals for their biologic effects, nor do they undergo bioreduction under hypoxic conditions; consequently, the effect of a given treatment is independent of the presence or absence of molecular oxygen, a property these agents have in common with very densely ionizing radiations.

5. Resistance to drugs develops more quickly and more regularly than it does to radiation. Acquired resistance to drugs does not necessarily involve resistance to x-rays as well.
6. Drug resistance may be caused by changes in thiol levels or by molecular changes observable at the chromosome level that result in the activation of a gene that functions to pump the drug out of the cells.

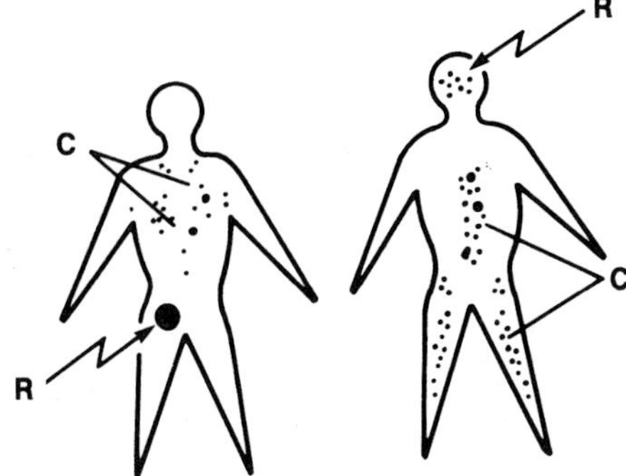

FIGURE 27.13 ● Spatial cooperation. **Left:** In some instances, radiation may be used to treat a large primary tumor, with chemotherapy added to cope with systemic disease in the form of disseminated metastases. **Right:** In other situations, chemotherapy may be used as the primary treatment, with radiation added to treat "sanctuary" sites that the cytotoxic drug cannot reach.

ADJUNCT USE OF CHEMOTHERAPEUTIC AGENTS WITH RADIATION

The initial rationale for the combination of radiation and chemotherapeutic agents was what usually is known as "spatial cooperation" (Figure 27.13). Radiation may be more effective for controlling the localized primary tumor, because it can be aimed and large doses given, but it is ineffective against disseminated disease. Chemotherapy, on the other hand, may be able to cope with micrometastases, whereas it could not control the larger primary tumor. In other situations, chemotherapy is the primary treatment modality, and radiation is used only to treat "sanctuary" sites not reached by the drug.

Although spatial cooperation was the original rationale, it is no longer the only one. Radiation and chemotherapeutic agents are combined in an attempt to achieve better local control. A specific example is the integrated use of taxanes and x-rays for the treatment of breast cancer. This is based on laboratory experiments *in vitro*. The initial hypothesis for the mechanism of interaction is that cell-cycle alterations induced by paclitaxel leave cells in a state in which they are more sensitive to radiation. This is illustrated in Figure 27.14, which shows survival curves for astrocytoma cells of human origin cultured *in vitro* and exposed to graded doses of γ-rays, either alone or following a 24-hour treatment with 10 nM paclitaxel. This drug treatment alone kills about 95% of the cells and accumulates the survivors in the radiosensitive G_2/M phase of the cell cycle (Fig. 27.14, **inset**).

Inasmuch as the cell killing resulting from the combination of drug and radiation is greater than

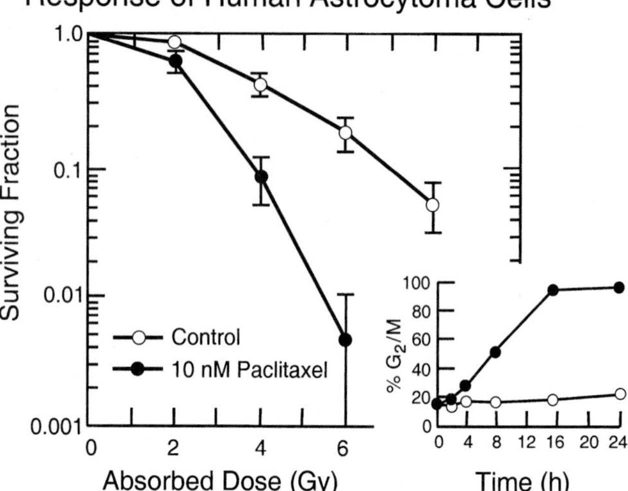

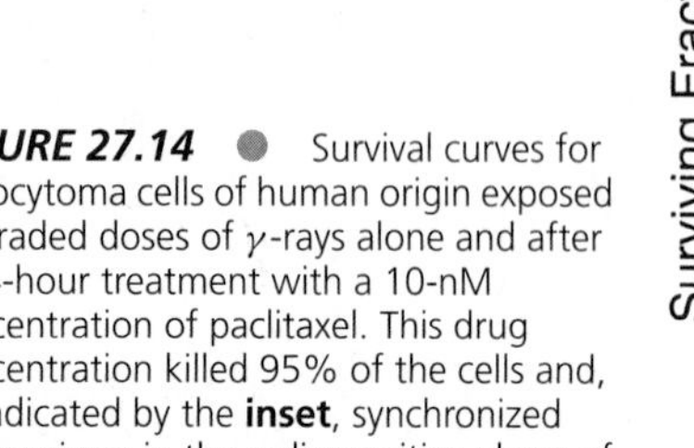
FIGURE 27.14 ● Survival curves for astrocytoma cells of human origin exposed to graded doses of γ-rays alone and after a 24-hour treatment with a 10-nM concentration of paclitaxel. This drug concentration killed 95% of the cells and, as indicated by the **inset**, synchronized the survivors in the radiosensitive phase of the cell cycle. (Data from Tishler RB, Geard CR, Hall EJ, Schiff PB: Taxol sensitizes human astrocytoma cells to radiation. *Cancer Res* 52:3495–3497, 1992.)

the sum of the two separately, the interaction may be described as "synergistic." For this to occur, the drug must accumulate some cells in G_2/M, which is a radiosensitive phase of the cycle, without killing them. Although similar results have been obtained for several cell lines, there are a significant number of reports in the literature in which the interaction between radiation and paclitaxel was shown to be purely additive. Additivity is observed in any cell line in which the G_2/M arrested cells are doomed to die as a consequence of the drug alone. Even an additive interaction, however, may be therapeutically useful. For example, in animal tumors *in vivo*, the paclitaxel-induced death of G_2/M cells can lead to tumor shrinkage and reoxygenation, which result in an enhanced response to subsequent irradiation.

Although the initial rationale for the combination of taxanes and radiation was based on classic radiobiologic considerations regarding the cell-cycle dependence of radiosensitivity, there are other possible explanations for a synergistic effect if the two agents are used together. For example, the contribution of *p53* to paclitaxel-dependent cytotoxicity is in marked contrast with its role for DNA-damaging agents such as radiation. Cells with a mutant *p53* phenotype are more sensitive to paclitaxel treatment than are nontransformed or wild-type *p53* cells. This finding offers an explanation for the effectiveness of paclitaxel as a cytotoxic agent alone, as well as for the efficacy of its combination with radiation. In this theory, paclitaxel and radiation act as non-cross-resistant agents; radiation is more effective against wild-type *p53* cells in a tumor population, and paclitaxel is relatively more cytotoxic to cells with a mutant *p53* phenotype.

In general, a therapeutic gain requires differential effects between tumor and normal tissue. One or more of the following tumor characteristics may be exploited to achieve this difference:

1. Genetic instability of tumor cells
2. Rapid proliferation of some tumor cells
3. Cell age distribution of tumor cell populations
4. Hypoxia (characteristic of larger tumors)
5. pH (often low in tumors)
6. Elevation of specific pathways in tumors (for example, EGFR)

The goal of combining the two modalities of radiation and cytotoxic drugs is to increase local tumor control, relapse-free survival and overall survival, and to alter the pattern of relapse. Three obvious strategies are (1) to start chemotherapy after the completion of the local treatment (*adjuvant chemotherapy*), (2) to start chemotherapy before the local treatment (*induction chemotherapy*), or (3) to give chemotherapy during local treatment (*concurrent chemotherapy*). Most cytotoxic agents do not provide enough differential sensitization of tumors compared with normal tissues; consequently, the probability of dose-limiting or life-threatening toxicity to critical tissues may be increased.

Integrating surgery, chemotherapy, and radiotherapy has been found to increase materially the cure rate of a dozen or more experimental animal tumors. Emerging principles include the following:

1. The lower the initial body burden of the tumor, the better.
2. A maximally effective drug regimen should begin as soon as possible after surgery, with maximum practicable doses.
3. Concurrent chemotherapy may lead to improved local control, but at the price of increased local toxicity.

Improving local control can improve overall survival rates and avoid uncontrolled local growth and the possible need for mutilating surgery. For example, induction chemotherapy prior to radiation therapy has a proven benefit in larynx preservation. For this reason alone, aggressive use of combined modalities to improve local control is warranted.

It often has been said that "you can only kill the sensitive cells once." There is no point in using a battery of different agents that all target the same subpopulation of sensitive cells. Rather, the *heterogeneity* of the tumor cell population should be acknowledged and exploited. One agent should be effective against cycling cells, another against resting cells, and a third perhaps against hypoxic cells; in other words, the strategy should be to combine agents that specifically attack the different subpopulations in the tumor.

A problem to be avoided is the triggering of "accelerated repopulation." This refers to triggering surviving clonogens to divide and repopulate even more rapidly as a tumor shrinks after treatment with a cytotoxic agent. It is a phenomenon described in Chapter 22. It may be one of the reasons why radiotherapy after induction chemotherapy has shown disappointing results.

ASSAYS FOR SENSITIVITY OF INDIVIDUAL TUMORS

A great deal of effort has been expended to develop ways to assess which agents are likely to be effective for a particular tumor. The long-term goal would be to mimic the testing of a bacterial infection for sensitivity to a wide range of antibiotic drugs to select the one most suitable and effective.

One approach is to take biopsy specimens from a tumor in a patient, grow the cells *in vitro*, and subject the cells to a battery of chemotherapeutic agents in the petri dish. This approach has the advantages of not being too expensive to be practical and of providing answers quickly enough to influence the treatment and modify the protocol of the individual from whom the cells were taken. It suffers, of course, from the obvious disadvantages of focusing attention solely on the question of inherent cellular sensitivity and not addressing the questions of drug access, hypoxia, or any of the more complex factors involved as determinants of overall tumor response.

A different approach is to grow cells from human tumors as xenografts in immune-suppressed mice. This is a difficult and limited technique beset with problems, some of which are discussed in Chapter 20. Human tumor cell xenografts, however, maintain many characteristics of the clinical response of the donor tumors. Indeed, there is a good correlation between clinical remission in donor patients and growth delay in xenografts established from transplanted cells. The method of establishing xenografts and then performing the necessary growth delay experiments is sufficiently slow and time-consuming that the technique cannot be expected ever to provide realistic input into deciding treatment strategy in individual patients, although it can provide guidance on the sensitivity of broad categories of human tumors to a battery of chemotherapeutic agents.

SECOND MALIGNANCIES

Late effects are the key to the acceptance of combined treatments. The induction of second malignancies is one of the unfortunate late effects of treatment with radiation or cytotoxic drugs. In a large series of 3,000 patients with Hodgkin's disease treated with a combination of radiotherapy and chemotherapy, 114 developed second malignancies. The greatest relative risk was leukemia, but the greatest in number were solid tumors.

Radiation is a relatively weak carcinogen; chemotherapeutic agents vary widely. There is a choice of many chemotherapeutic agents, and the variable potential for producing a second malignancy must be a factor influencing the choice of drug in patients who are likely to be long-term survivors.

Table 27.3 compares radiation, bleomycin, ultraviolet radiation, and benzopyrene in terms of the number of DNA lesions per cell necessary to kill 63% of the cell population, that is, to allow 37% to survive. Radiation is characterized by a relatively small number of double-strand breaks, only about 40 per cell on average, at a dose that allows 37% of the cells to survive. At the other extreme, ultraviolet light produces one million dimers, and benzopyrene produces 100,000 lesions for the same level of survival. These interesting figures show that radiation is a weak carcinogen, because it is efficient at killing cells; the same is true of bleomycin. By contrast, benzopyrene produces many more DNA lesions for a given level of cell killing and is therefore a powerful carcinogen; ultraviolet light is in the same category.

It is an interesting speculation, supported by these data, that the factor that determines whether an agent is a powerful or a weak carcinogen is the number of DNA lesions required, on average, to kill a cell. If the number is small, the agent is an efficient cytotoxic agent but is likely to be a weaker carcinogen. If the number is large, there will be many DNA lesions in cells that are not killed, and some of these lesions may involve the transformation to a neoplastic state.

TABLE 27.3

Lesions Produced for a Given Level of Cell Killing by Various Cytotoxic Agents

Agent	D_{37}	DNA Lesion	Number of Lesions per Cell per D_{37}
X-rays	100 rad	SSB	1,000
		DSB	40
Bleomycin	5.5 $\mu g \times 1$ h	SSB	150
		DSB	30
Ultraviolet light	10 J/m^2	TT dimer	1,000,000
		SSB	100
Benzopyrene	—	Adduct	100,000

SSB, single-strand DNA break; DSB, double-strand DNA break.
Courtesy of Dr. John Ward, University of California at San Francisco.

Summary of Pertinent Conclusions

- Single chemotherapeutic agents have been used successfully to cure a few rapidly proliferating tumors.
- Combinations of drugs are used routinely for the treatment of a variety of malignancies.
- Most anticancer drugs work by affecting DNA synthesis or function.
- Inevitably, many traditional anticancer drugs are toxic to stem cells of the intestinal epithelium and hematopoietic stem cells because they have a high growth fraction. Some of the new targeted therapy drugs (e.g., cetuximab) have the potential to increase tumor response with minimal effect on normal-tissue toxicity.
- Agents that are mainly effective during a particular phase of the cell cycle, such as the S phase or M phase, are said to be cell-cycle specific, or phase specific.
- Agents whose action is independent of the position of the cell in the cycle are said to be cell-cycle nonspecific, or phase nonspecific.
- Many classically used chemotherapeutic agents fall into one of several classes:

  Alkylating agents, which are highly active, with the ability to substitute alkyl groups for hydrogen atoms in DNA, include nitrogen mustard derivatives, cyclophosphamide, chlorambucil, melphalan, and the nitrosoureas (BCNU and CCNU).

  Antibiotics, which bind to DNA and inhibit DNA and RNA synthesis, include dactinomycin, doxorubicin, daunorubicin, and bleomycin.

  Antimetabolites, which are analogues of the normal metabolites required for cell function and replication, include methotrexate, 5-fluorouracil, cytarabine, and 5-azacytidine.

- Many of the newer and widely used drugs do not fall into any of these classes, including the vinca alkaloids, the taxanes, procarbazine, hydroxyurea, platinum complexes, topoisomerase inhibitors, and "targeted therapy" agents that target a specific pathway elevated in some tumors (Erbitux, Herceptin, Gleevac, and Rituxan).
- Dose–response relationships for many chemotherapeutic agents resemble those for radiation, with drug concentration replacing absorbed dose; that is, there is an initial shoulder followed by an exponential relationship between surviving fraction and dose. The exceptions are doxorubicin, bleomycin, dactinomycin, and taxanes, which have dose response curves that are concave upward.

(continued)

Summary of Pertinent Conclusions (Continued)

- At best, traditional anticancer drugs kill cells by first-order kinetics; that is, a given dose kills a constant fraction of cells. Consequently, the chance of eradicating a cancer is greatest if the population size is small (i.e., there is an inverse relationship between curability and tumor cell burden) at the initiation of chemotherapy.
- Studies of sublethal damage and potentially lethal damage are more confusing and less clear-cut for drugs than for radiation.
- Potentially lethal damage repair is a significant factor for bleomycin and doxorubicin, but sublethal damage repair is essentially absent. Neither potentially lethal nor sublethal damage repair is reported for the nitrosoureas.
- The oxygen effect is more complex for drugs than for radiation.
- Some drugs (e.g., bleomycin) are more toxic to aerated than to hypoxic cells. For these drugs, free radicals are involved in the mechanism of cell killing, as is the case for x-rays.
- Some drugs (such as mitomycin C) are more toxic to hypoxic than to aerated cells because they undergo bioreduction. This also applies to tirapazamine, as discussed in Chapter 25.
- Other drugs (including 5-fluorouracil, methotrexate, *cis*-platinum, and the nitrosoureas) appear to be equally cytotoxic to aerated and hypoxic cells.
- The effectiveness of chemotherapeutic agents decreases with distance from a capillary because the drug concentration falls off because of metabolism and because cells are not proliferating because they are hypoxic.
- The addition of a hypoxic cytotoxin to other chemotherapeutic agents may alleviate this problem. As the effectiveness of conventional agents falls off with distance from a capillary, hypoxic cytotoxins become more effective because they only function in low oxygen concentrations.
- Drug resistance is the biggest single problem in chemotherapy. For example, cells exposed continuously to low levels of doxorubicin become very resistant to subsequent treatments with this drug.
- The usual strategy to overcome resistance is to use a battery of drugs that produce cytotoxicity by diverse mechanisms.
- Pleiotropic resistance occurs if the development of resistance to one drug results in cross-resistance to other drugs with a different mechanism of action.
- Underlying acquired resistance are genetic changes.
- Resistance may be associated with the following: decreased drug accumulation and the expression of p-glycoproteins in the cell membrane from gene amplification; elevated levels of glutathione; marked increase in DNA repair.
- Radioresistance and chemoresistance may occur together, but radiation rarely induces chemoresistance, and vice versa.
- The adjunct use of chemotherapy with radiation may involve sequential or concurrent treatments.
- The extent to which chemotherapeutic agents show synergy with radiation varies widely. Some interact strongly (e.g., doxorubicin, gemcitibine), others less so, and some not at all. See Table 27.1.
- Some agents penetrate the blood–brain barrier (e.g., BCNU, temozolomide, cytosine arabinoside, hydroxyurea), others only at high intravenous doses (e.g., methotrexate), while many do not cross the blood–brain barrier at all. See Table 27.1.
- A therapeutic gain requires a differential between tumor and normal tissue. This may be achieved by exploiting one or more of the following tumor characteristics: genetic instability; rapid proliferation; cell age distribution; hypoxia; pH; elevated specific pathways (e.g., EGFR).
- Sensitive cells can be killed only once. Tumor heterogeneity should be exploited by using a combination of drugs effective against different cell subpopulations.
- Sensitivity of individual tumors to chemotherapeutic agents with or without radiation may be assessed by the following: *in vitro* clonogenic assays; xenografts in nude mice; micronuclei in treated cells.

BIBLIOGRAPHY

Barranco SC: *In vitro* responses of mammalian cells to drug-induced potentially lethal and sublethal damage. *Cancer Treat Rep* 60:1799–1810, 1976

Barranco SC, Fluorney DR: Modification of the response to actinomycin-D-induced sublethal damage by simultaneous recovery from potentially lethal damage in mammalian cells. *Cancer Res* 36:1634–1640, 1976

Barranco SC, Humphrey RM: Response of mammalian cells to bleomycin-induced potentially lethal and sublethal damage. *Prog Biochem Pharmacol* 11:78–92, 1976

Barranco SC, Novak JKJ, Humphrey RM: Response of mammalian cells following treatment with bleomycin and 1,3-BTS(2 chloroethyl)-1-nitrosourea during plateau phase. *Cancer Res* 33:691–694, 1973

Barranco SC, Townsend CM Jr, Quraishi MA, et al.: Heterogeneous responses of an *in vitro* model of human stomach cancer to anticancer drugs. *Invest New Drugs* 1(2):117–127, 1983

Belli JA: Radiation response and Adriamycin resistance in mammalian cells in culture. *Front Radiat Ther Oncol* 13:9–20, 1979

Belli JA, Piro AJ: The interaction between radiation and Adriamycin damage in mammalian cells. *Cancer Res* 37:1624–1630, 1975

Bissery MC, Vrignaud P, Lavelle F: Preclinical profile of docetaxel (Taxotere): Efficacy as a single agent and in combination. *Semin Oncol* 22(suppl 13):3–16, 1995

Boice JD, Greene MH, Killen JY, et al.: Leukemia and preleukemia after adjuvant treatment of gastrointestinal cancer with semustine (methyl CCNU). *N Engl J Med* 309:1079–1084, 1983

Bonadonna G, Valagussa P: Dose-response effect of CMF in breast cancer. *Proc Am Soc Clin Oncol* 21:413, 1980

Bonner JA, Giralt J, Harari PM, et al.: Cetuximab prolongs survival in patients with locoregionally advanced squamous cell carcinoma of head and neck: A phase III study of high dose radiation therapy with or without cetuximab. *Journal of Clinical Oncology, 2004 ASCO Annual Meeting Proceedings* (Post-Meeting Edition) 22, 14S (July 15 Supplement), 5507, 2004

Brown JM, Siim BG: Hypoxia-specific cytotoxins in cancer therapy. *Semin Radiat Oncol* 6:22–36, 1996

Carney DN, Winkler CF: *In vitro* assays of chemotherapeutic sensitivity. In DeVita VT Jr, Hellman S, Rosenberg SA (eds): *Important Advances in Oncology*, vol 1. Philadelphia, Lippincott, 1984

Chabner BA: The oncologic end game. *J Clin Oncol* 4:625–638, 1986

Chabner BA, Sponzo R, Hubbard S, et al.: High-dose intermittent intravenous infusion of procarbazine. *Cancer Chemother Rep* 57:361–363, 1973

Chan HSL, Haddad G, Thorner PS, et al.: P-glycoprotein expression as a predictor of the outcome of therapy for neuroblastoma. *N Engl J Med* 325:1608–1614, 1991

Cowan KH, Goldsmith ME, Levine R, et al.: Dihydrofolate reductase gene amplification and possible rearrangement in estrogen-responsive methotrexate-resistant human breast cancer cells. *J Biol Chem* 257:15079–15086, 1982

Curt GA, Carney DN, Cowan KH, et al.: Unstable methotrexate resistance in human small-cell carcinoma associated with double minute chromosomes. *N Engl J Med* 308:199–202, 1983

Debenham PG, Kartner H, Simonovitch L, et al.: DNA-mediated transfer of multiple drug resistance and plasma membrane glycoprotein expression. *Mol Cell Biol* 2:881–889, 1982

DeVita VT: Cell kinetics and the chemotherapy of cancer: 111. *Cancer Chemother Rep* 2:23–33, 1971

DeVita VT Jr: The James Ewing lecture: The relationship between tumor mass and resistance to chemotherapy: Implications for surgical adjuvant treatment of cancer. *Cancer* 51:1207–1220, 1983

DeVita VT, Henney JE, Hubbard SM: Estimation of the numerical and economic impact of chemotherapy in the treatment of cancer. In Burchenal JH, Oettgen HS (eds): *Cancer Achievements, Challenges, and Prospects for the 1980s*, pp 857–880. New York, Grune & Stratton, 1981

DeVita VT, Henney JE, Stonehill E: Cancer mortality: The good news. In Jones SE, Salmon SE (eds): *Adjuvant Therapy of Cancer* II, pp xv–xx. New York, Grune & Stratton, 1979

DeVita VT, Oliverio VT, Muggia FM, et al.: The Drug Development Program and Clinical Trials Programs of the Division of Cancer Treatment, National Cancer Institute. *Cancer Clin Trials* 2:195–216, 1979

DeVita VT, Serpick AA, Carbone PP: Combination chemotherapy in the treatment of advanced Hodgkin's disease. *Ann Intern Med* 73:881–895, 1970

Durand RE: The influence of microenvironmental factors during cancer therapy. *In Vivo* 8:691–702, 1994

Elkiind MM, Kano E, Sutton-Gilbert H: Cell killing by actinomycin D in relation to the growth cycle of Chinese hamster cells. *J Cell Biol* 42:366–377, 1969

Endicott JA, Ling V: The biochemistry of p-glycoprotein-mediated drug resistance. *Annu Rev Biochem* 58:137–171, 1989

Erlich E, McCall AR, Potkul RK, Walter S, Vaughan A: Paclitaxel is only a weak radiosensitizer of human cervical carcinoma cell. *Gynecol Oncol* 60:251–254, 1996

Fine RL, Patel J, Allegra CJ, et al.: Increased phosphorylation of a 20,000 M.W. protein in pleiotropic drug-resistant MCH-7 human breast cancer lines. *Proc Am Assoc Cancer Res* 26:345, 1985

Frei E: The clinical use of actinomycin. *Cancer Chemother Rep* 58:49–54, 1974

Frei E III, Canellos GP: Dose: A critical factor in cancer chemotherapy. *Am J Med* 69:585–594, 1980

Frei E III, Freireich EJ, Gehan E, et al.: Studies of sequential and combination antimetabolite therapy in acute leukemia: 6-Mercaptopurine and methotrexate. *Blood* 18:431–454, 1961

Geard CR, Jones JM, Schiff PB: Taxol and radiation. *J Natl Cancer Inst Monogr* 15:89–94, 1993

Gottesman MM, Pastan I: The multidrug transporter, a double-edged sword. *J Biol Chem* 263:12163–12166, 1988

Gottesman MM, Schoenlien PV, Currier SJ, Bruggemann EP, Pastan I: In Pretlow TG, Pretlow TP (eds): *Biochemical and Molecular Aspects of Selected Cancers*, pp 339–371. San Diego, CA, Academic Press, 1991

Graeber TG, Osmanian C, Jacks T, et al.: Hypoxia medicated selection of cells with diminished apoptotic potential in solid tumors. *Nature* 379:88–91, 1996

Grandis JR, Melhem MF, Gooding WE, et al.: Levels of TGF-alpha and EGFR protein in head and neck squamous cell carcinoma and patient survival. *J Natl Cancer Inst* 90:824–832, 1998

Green SL, Giaccia AJ: Tumor hypoxia and the cell cycle: Implications for malignant progression and response to therapy. *The Cancer Journal* 4:218–223, 1998

Hamburger AW, Salmon SE: Primary bioassay of human tumor stem cells. *Science* 197:461–463, 1977

Hennequin C, Giocanti N, Favaudon V: Interaction of ionizing radiation with paclitaxel (Taxol) and docetaxel

(Taxotere) in HeLa and SQ20B cells. *Cancer Res* 56:1842–1850, 1996

Hockel M, Schlenger K, Aral B, Mitze M, Schaffer U, Vaupel P: Association between tumor hypoxia and malignant progression in advanced cancer of the uterine cervix. *Cancer Res* 56:4509–4515, 1996

Hu G, Liu W, Mendelsohn J, Ellis LM, Radinsky R, Andreeff M, Deisseroth AB: Expression of epidermal growth factor receptor and human papillomavirus E6/E7 proteins in cervical carcinoma cells. *J Natl Cancer Inst* 89:1271–1276, 1997

Hutchinson DJ: Cross-resistance and collateral sensitivity studies in cancer chemotherapy. In Haddow A, Weinhouse S (eds): *Advances in Cancer Research*, vol 7, pp 235–350. New York, Academic Press, 1983

Hyde SC, Emsley P, Hartshorn MJ, et al.: Structural model of ATP binding proteins associated with cystic fibrosis, multidrug resistance and bacterial transport. *Nature* 346:362–365, 1990

Iihara K, Shiozaki H, Tahara H, et al.: Prognostic significance of transforming growth factor-alpha in human esophageal carcinoma. Implication for the autocrine proliferation. *Cancer* 71:2902–2909, 1993

Jain RK: Barriers to drug delivery in solid tumors. *Sci Am* 271:58–65, 1994

Juranka PF, Zastawny RL, Ling V: P-glycoprotein: Multidrug-resistance and a superfamily of membrane associated transport proteins. *FASEB J* 3:2583–2592, 1989

Klijin JG, Berns PM, Schmitz PI, Foekens JA: The clinical significance of epidermal growth factor receptor (EGF-R) in human breast cancer: A review on 5232 patients. *Endocr Rev* 13:3–17 (Review), 1992

Lee IP, Dixon RL: Mutagenicity, carcinogenicity, and teratogenicity of procarbazine. *Mutat Res* 55:1–14, 1978

Leonard CE, Chan DC, Chou TC, Kumar R, Bunn PA: Paclitaxel enhances *in vitro* radiosensitivity of squamous carcinoma cell lines of the head and neck. *Cancer Res* 56:5198–5204, 1996

Liebmann JE, Cook JA, Fisher J, Teague D, Mitchell JB: *In vitro* studies of Taxol as a radiation sensitizer in human tumor cells. *J Natl Cancer Inst* 86:441–446, 1994

Liebmann JE, Cook JA, Lipschultz C, Teague D, Fisher J, Mitchell JB. Cytotoxic studies of paclitaxel (Taxol) in human tumour cell lines. *Br J Cancer* 68:1104–1109, 1993

Liebmann JE, Hahn SM, Cook JA, Lipschultz C, Mitchell JB, Kaufman DC. Glutathione depletion by L-buthionine sulfoximine antagonizes taxol cytotoxicity. *Cancer Res* 53:2066–2070, 1993

Ling V, Kartner N, Sudo T, Siminovitch L, Riodan JR: Multidrug-resistance phenotype in Chinese hamster ovary cells. *Cancer Treat Rep* 67:869–874, 1983

Ling V, Thompson LH: Reduced permeability in CHO cells as a mechanism of resistance to colchicine. *J Cell Physiol* 83:103–116, 1976

Lokcshwar BL, Ferrell SM, Block NL: Enhancement of radiation response of prostatic carcinoma by taxol: Therapeutic potential for late-stage malignancy. *Anticancer Res* 15:93–98, 1995

Madoc-Jones H, Mauro F: Interphase action of vinblastine and vincristine: Differences in their lethal action through the mitotic cycle of cultured mammalian cells. *J Cell Physiol* 72:185–196, 1968

Mendelsohn J: Epidermal growth factor receptor inhibition by a monoclonal antibody as anticancer therapy. *Clin Cancer Res* 3:2703–2707, 1997

Milas L, Hunter NR, Mason KA, et al.: Role of reoxygenation in induction of enhancement of tumor radioresponse by paclitaxel. *Cancer Res* 55:3564–3568, 1995

Milas L, Mason K, Hunter N, et al.: *In vivo* enhancement of tumor radioresponse by C225 antiepidermal growth factor receptor antibody. *Clinical Cancer Research* 6:701–708, 2000

Milas L, Milas MM, Mason KA: Combination of taxanes with radiation: Preclinical studies. *Semin Radiat Oncol* 9(suppl 1):12–26, 1999

Milross CG, Mason KA, Hunter NR, et al.: Relationship of mitotic arrest and apoptosis to antitumor effect of paclitaxel. *J Natl Cancer Inst* 88:1308–1314, 1996

Mitchell JB, Gamson J, Russo A, et al.: Chinese hamster pleiotropic multidrug resistant cells are not radioresistant. *Natl Cancer Inst Monogr* 6:187–191, 1988

Mote PA, Davey MW, Davey RA, Oliver L: Paclitaxel sensitizes multidrug resistant cells to radiation. *Anticancer Drugs* 7:182–188, 1996

Piccart MJ, Core M, ten Bokkel Huinink W, et al.: Docetaxel: An active new drug for treatment of advanced epithelial ovarian cancer. *J Natl Cancer Inst* 87:676–681, 1995

Rave-Frank M, Mcdon H, Jaschke A, Tanzer A, Boghun O, Fictkau R: The effect of paclitaxel on the radiosensitivity of gynecological tumor cells. *Strahlenther Onkol* 173:281–286, 1997

Roizin-Towle L, Hall EJ: Studies with bleomycin and misonidazole on aerated and hypoxic cells. *Br J Cancer* 37:254–260, 1978

Rowinsky EK, Donehower RC: Paclitaxel (Taxol). *N Engl J Med* 332:1004–1014, 1995

Rubin NH, Casantelli C, Maerk BG, Boerwinkle WR, Barranco SC: *In vitro* cellular characteristics and survival responses of human astrocytoma clones to chloroethylnitrosoureas and idanhydrogalactical. *Invest New Drugs* 1:129–137, 1983

Saito Y, Mitsuhashi N, Takahashi T, et al.: Cytotoxic effect of paclitaxel (taxol) either alone or in combination with irradiation in two rat yolk sac tumour cell lines with different radiosensitivities *in vitro*. *Int J Radiat Biol* 73:225–231, 1998

Salmon SE: Application of the human tumor stem cell assay in the development of anticancer therapy. In Burchenal JF, Oettgen HS (eds): *Cancer Achievements, Challenges, and Prospects for the 1980s*. New York, Grune & Stratton, 1981

Salmon SE, Hamburger AW, Soehnlen BJ, et al.: Quantitation of differential sensitivity of human tumor stem cells to anticancer drugs. *N Engl J Med* 298:1321–1327, 1978

Sartorelli AC: Approaches to the combination chemotherapy of transplantable neoplasms. *Prog Exp Tumor Res* 6:228–288, 1965

Schiff PB, Fant S, Horwitz SB: Promotion of microtubule assembly *in vitro* by Taxol. *Nature* 277:665–667, 1979

Schiff PB, Horwitz SB: Taxol stabilizes microtubules in mouse fibroblast cells. *Proc Natl Acad Sci USA* 77:1561–1565, 1980

Siemann DW, Keng PC: Characterization of radiation resistant hypoxic cell subpopulations in KHT sarcomas: (ii) Cell sorting. *Br J Cancer* 58:296–300, 1988

Skipper HE: Reasons for success and failure in treatment of murine leukemias with the drugs now employed in treating human leukemias. In *Cancer Chemotherapy*, vol 1, pp 1–166. Ann Arbor, MI, University Microfilms International, 1978

Skipper HE, Hutchison DJ, Schabel FM Jr, et al.: A quick reference chart on cross-resistance between anticancer agents. *Cancer Treat Rep* 56:493–498, 1972

Skipper HE, Schabel FM Jr, Wilcox WS: Experimental evaluation of potential anticancer agents: XII. On the criteria and kinetics associated with "curability" of experimental leukemia. *Cancer Chemother Rep* 35:1–111, 1964

Tannock I: Cell kinetics and chemotherapy: A critical review. *Cancer Treat Rep* 62:1117–1133, 1978

Tannock IF: The relation between cell proliferation and the vascular system in a transplanted mouse mammary tumour. *Br J Cancer* 22:258–273, 1968

Teicher BA, Lazo JS, Sartorelli AC: Classification of antineoplastic agents by their selective toxicities toward oxygenated and hypoxic tumor cells. *Cancer Res* 41:73–81, 1981

Tishler RB, Geard CR, Hall EJ, Schiff PB: Taxol sensitizes human astrocytoma cells to radiation. *Cancer Res* 52:3495–3497, 1992

Tishler RB, Schiff PB, Geard CR, Hall EJ: Taxol: A novel radiation sensitizer. *Int J Radiat Oncol Biol Phys* 22:613–617, 1992

Trent JM, Buick RN, Olson S, et al.: Cytologic evidence for gene amplification in methotrexate resistant cells obtained from a patient with ovarian adenocarcinoma. *J Clin Oncol* 2:8–15, 1984

Wahl AF, Donaldson KL, Fairchild C, et al.: Loss of normal p53 function confers sensitization to Taxol by increasing G_2/M arrest and apoptosis. *Nat Med* 2:72–79, 1996

Wani MC, Taylor HL, Wall ME, et al.: Plant antitumor agents: VI. The isolation and structure of Taxol, a novel antileukemic and antitumor agent from *Taxus brevifolia. J Am Chem Soc* 93:2325–2327, 1971

Weinstein JM, Magin RL, Cysyk RL, et al.: Treatment of solid L1210 murine tumors with local hyperthermia and temperature-sensitive liposomes containing methotrexate. *Cancer Res* 40:1388–1396, 1980

CHAPTER 28

Hyperthermia

In Greek mythology, Prometheus, a demigod, stole fire from Olympus and taught humans how to use it. For this act he was chained to a rock by Zeus, the king of the gods, and a vulture fed daily on his liver.

The use of hyperthermia for the treatment of cancer is certainly not new. The very first medical text known today contains a case study describing a patient with a breast tumor treated with hyperthermia. The case is cited in the Edwin Smith Surgical Papyrus, an Egyptian papyrus roll, which is said to date from more than 3,500 years ago and to be a copy of an even older text. Later, heat was used in all cultures as one of the most prominent medical therapies for almost any disease, including cancer. Thus, Hippocrates (470–377 BC), in one of his aphorisms, states:

> Those who cannot be cured by medicine can be cured by surgery. Those who cannot be cured by surgery can be cured by fire [hyperthermia]. Those who cannot be cured by fire, they are indeed incurable.

The attempt in modern times to exploit elevated temperatures to treat cancer has a longer history than the use of ionizing radiations. In 1866, 30 years before Röntgen discovered "a new kind of ray," the German physician W. Busch described a patient with a sarcoma in the face that disappeared after a prolonged infection with erysipelas, an infectious disease normally characterized by high fever. This and similar cases led the New York surgeon William B. Coley to believe that the bacteria causing erysipelas may be effective against cancer. He extracted a toxin (Coley's toxin, or mixed bacterial toxin), with which he treated a number of patients.

Although it is difficult to evaluate the direct role of heat in this combined total-body hyperthermia and unspecific immunotherapy, the work by Coley initiated a number of other studies using local hyperthermia applied to patients and to tumors in experimental animals. In 1898, Westermark, a Swedish gynecologist, published a paper describing a marked regression of large carcinomas of the uterine cervix after local hyperthermia, although the treatments involved were poorly controlled and the cases largely anecdotal. The use of hyperthermia, either alone or in combination with radiation, has been attempted at irregular intervals over the years but has never found a permanent place in the management of cancer. Historical reviews of the early clinical use of hyperthermia can be found in several excellent articles (e.g., by Dewey and colleagues, 1977, and by Overgaard, 1984).

Interest in hyperthermia flourished in the 1970s and 1980s, when laboratory experiments *in vitro* and *in vivo* laid a firm foundation for understanding the biology of hyperthermia and clinical evidence of tumor regression following heat treatments looked very promising. In the 21st century, enthusiasm has waned in the United States, but clinical investigations continue in Europe.

METHODS OF LOCAL HEATING

The major problem in the development of clinical hyperthermia for cancer therapy has been the design of equipment to heat designated tumor volumes accurately and uniformly. Methods of local heating include (1) shortwave diathermy, (2) radiofrequency capacitative heating, (3) microwaves, (4) ultrasound, and (5) interstitial implants.

Most of the work with cells cultured *in vitro*, as well as much of the early animal experimentation, involves heating by hot-water baths. The simplest and most reliable way to heat a petri dish or a tumor transplanted into the leg of a mouse is to immerse it totally in a thermostatically controlled bath of water. Water temperature can be controlled within a fraction of a degree, and temperature measurement involves no problem, although even in this simplest of situations, the tumor may not be at the same temperature as the skin.

If localized hyperthermia is achieved by microwaves, radiofrequency-induced currents, or ultrasound, there are serious technical problems and limitations. In the case of microwaves, good localization can be achieved at shallow depths, but at greater tumor depths, even if the frequency is lowered to allow deeper penetration, the localization is much poorer and surface heating limits therapy. If ultrasound is used, the presence of bone or air cavities causes distortions of the heating pattern, but adequate penetration and good uniform temperature distributions can be achieved in soft tissues, particularly with ultrasound in focused arrays. In practice, then, tumors such as recurrent chest wall nodules can be treated adequately with microwaves, and it should theoretically be possible to heat deep-seated tumors below the diaphragm with focused ultrasound, regional microwave devices, or interstitial techniques.

In all cases, however, present methods of heating pose a problem, though significant progress has been made as a result of the clever application of focused arrays. For example, the use of multiphased arrays allows uniformity of temperature to the edge of the field. The picture is complicated, and it is unlikely that one simple answer to all the complex problems will be found. This is the area, then, in which engineering developments are needed and a breakthrough in basic science would be welcome.

One method of producing localized hyperthermia that suffers from fewer problems is the use of implanted microwave or radiofrequency sources. Good temperature distributions can be achieved and maintained if radiofrequency-induced currents or microwaves are applied to an array of wires actually implanted in the tumor and surrounding tissues. The "wires" used are frequently radioactive sources, so that heat and radiation can be combined. Alternatively, microwave coaxial antennae can be inserted into the catheters used to hold the radioactive iridium-92 wires; in this way, deep-tumor volumes are heated from the inside out. Some of the most promising results have been obtained in this way for the small fraction of patients with cancer for whom an interstitial implant is practical.

THERMAL ABLATION

Thermal ablation is a form of hyperthermia in which short exposures of a few minutes are used at very high temperatures of 50°C to 70°C to ablate nodules in the liver, kidney, or prostate. The heating is produced by RF or microwave antennae and is sufficiently intense to overcome blood flow. Thermal ablation has been proposed as an alternative to surgery. This will not be discussed further in this chapter and is not the form of hyperthermia combined with radiotherapy or chemotherapy.

CELLULAR RESPONSE TO HEAT

Heat kills cells in a predictable and repeatable way. Figure 28.1 shows a series of survival curves for

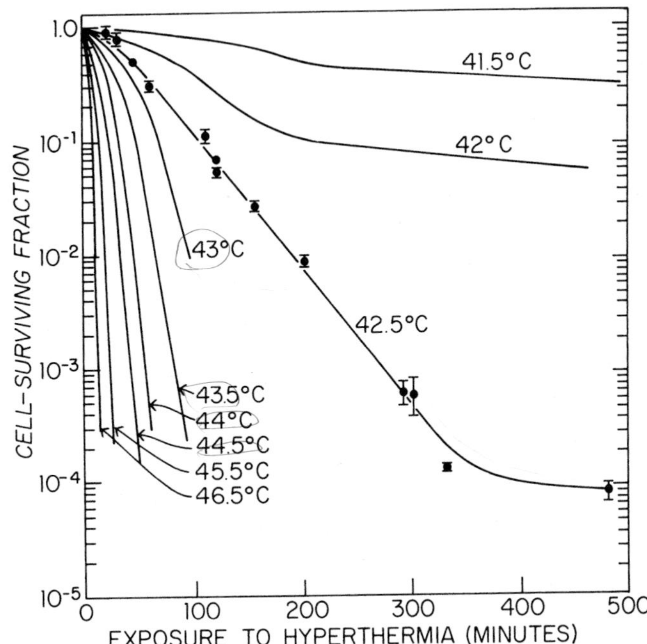

FIGURE 28.1 ● Survival curves for mammalian cells in culture (Chinese hamster ovary line) heated at different temperatures for varying lengths of time. (Adapted from Dewey WC, Hopwood LE, Sapareto LA, Gerweck LE: Cellular responses to combinations of hyperthermia and radiation. *Radiology* 123:463–474, 1977, with permission.)

cells exposed for various periods of time to a range of temperatures from 41.5°C to 46.5°C. The cell survival curves for heat are similar in shape to those obtained for x-rays (i.e., an initial shoulder followed by an exponential region), except that the time of exposure to the elevated temperature replaces the absorbed dose of x-rays. For lower temperatures, the picture is complicated, because the survival curves flatten out after a protracted exposure to hyperthermia, indicating the development of a resistance or tolerance to the elevated temperature. This is discussed subsequently. The similarity in the shape of the cell survival curves for heat and x-rays is misleading. It is important, therefore, not to draw conclusions for heat based on the interpretation of radiation dose–response curves, because the amount of energy involved in cell inactivation is a thousand times greater for heat than for x-rays. This reflects the different mechanisms involved in cell killing by heat and x-rays.

Families of survival curves similar to those in Figure 28.1 have been obtained for many different cell types, and it is clear that cells differ widely in their sensitivity to hyperthermia. As with ionizing radiations, there is no consistent difference between normal and malignant cells, in spite of numerous individual reports claiming that tumor cells are inherently more sensitive to heat than their normal-tissue counterparts.

Survival data for cells exposed to various levels of hyperthermia (taken from Fig. 28.1) are replotted in Figure 28.2, with $1/D_0$ on the ordinate and $1/T$ on the abscissa. T is the absolute temperature; D_0 is the reciprocal of the slope of the exponential region of the survival curve (i.e., the time at a given temperature that is necessary to reduce the fraction of surviving cells to 37% of their former value). This type of presentation is known as an **Arrhenius plot**; its slope gives the activation energy of the chemical process involved in the cell killing. The dramatic *change* of slope that occurs at a temperature of about 43°C, which means that the activation energy is different above and below this temperature, may reflect different mechanisms of cell killing (i.e., different targets for cytotoxicity above and below 43°C). On the other hand, it may equally well be a manifestation of thermotolerance: Below 43°C, thermotolerance can develop gradually during the heating; above 43°C, it cannot. On this basis, the intrinsic heat sensitivity is that observed above 43°C; cell survival for continuous heating below this temperature is an expression of heat sensitivity modified by the induction, development, and decay of thermotolerance.

The similarity of the activation energy for protein denaturation to the activation energy for heat cytotoxicity, calculated from the Arrhenius analysis, led to the hypothesis that the target for heat cell killing may be a protein. The structural chromosomal proteins, nuclear matrix and cytoskeleton repair enzymes, and membrane components all have been identified as possible targets that are denatured by hyperthermia.

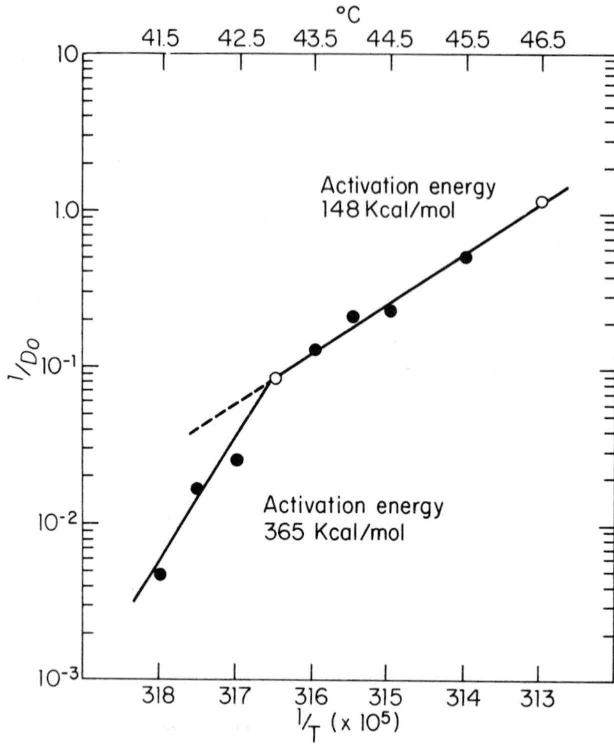

FIGURE 28.2 • An Arrhenius plot for heat inactivation of mammalian cells in culture. The reciprocals of the D_0 values obtained for Fig 28.1 are plotted versus the reciprocal of the absolute temperature. (Adapted from Dewey WC, Hopwood LE, Sapareto LA, Gerweck LE: Cellular responses to combinations of hyperthermia and radiation. *Radiology* 123:463–474, 1977, with permission.)

The Arrhenius plot for a given cell line can be modified by a number of things. For example, altering the pH of the cells *raises* the curves, and the break point occurs at a *higher* temperature.

Sensitivity to Heat as a Function of Cell Age in the Mitotic Cycle

The age–response function for heat complements that for x-rays (Fig. 28.3). The phase of the cycle most *resistant* to x-rays, late in the DNA synthetic phase (late S), is most *sensitive* to hyperthermia treatment. On this basis, cycling tumor cells should be killed selectively by hyperthermia compared with the slowly turning over normal tissues responsible for late effects that are in a G_1 or G_0 state.

Effect of pH and Nutrient Deficiency on Sensitivity to Heat

Cells in an acid pH environment appear to be more sensitive to killing by heat. This is certainly true of cells treated with heat soon after their environmental pH is altered by adjusting the buffer. The intracellular pH (pH_i) of cells in an acidic environment is slightly higher than the extracellular pH (pH_e). The pH dependence of cytotoxicity at elevated temperatures, however, is affected by pH history. Cells can adapt to pH changes and avoid the pH_i heat sensitivity shown for low pH.

Cells deficient in nutrients are certainly heat sensitive. This can be demonstrated with cells in culture, in which sensitivity to heat increases progressively as cells have their energy supply compromised, either by depriving them of glucose or by the use of a drug that uncouples oxidative phosphorylation.

These conclusions about pH and nutrients, obtained under controlled conditions with cells in culture, led to the speculation that cells in tumors that are nutritionally deprived and at acid pH because of their location remote from a blood capillary may be particularly sensitive to heat. Because of their environment, it is likely that these cells are out of cycle and possibly hypoxic, also. This conclusion certainly correlates with the observation that large necrotic tumors often shrink dramatically after a heat treatment. In this context, also, heat and x-rays appear to be complementary in their action, because the cells that are most resistant to x-rays (out of cycle and hypoxic because of their remoteness from a capillary) show enhanced sensitivity to heat. A further complicating factor here is that regions of a tumor in which the vasculature is poorly developed tend to be at an elevated

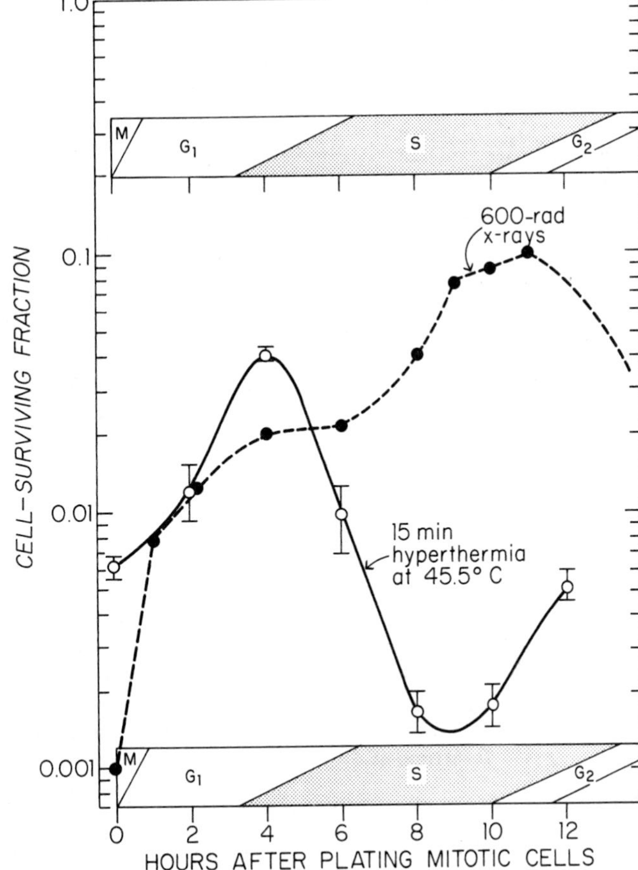

FIGURE 28.3 ● Comparison of the fraction of cells surviving heat or x-irradiation delivered at various phases of the cell cycle. The heat treatment consisted of 15 minutes at 45.5°C, and the x-ray dose was 600 rad (6 Gy). (Adapted from Westra A, Dewey WC: Variation in sensitivity to heat shock during the cell cycle of Chinese hamster cells *in vitro*. *Int J Radiat Biol* 19:467–477, 1971, with permission.)

temperature because the cooling effect of blood flow is reduced.

RESPONSE OF ORGANIZED TISSUES TO HEAT

Normal tissues respond to heat in a way that is substantially different from their more familiar response to x-rays. The principal difference is that after irradiation, cells die only in attempting the next or a subsequent mitosis (except in very unusual circumstances), whereas heated cells die by apoptosis, so that heat damage is expressed *early*. In addition, heat affects differentiating as well as dividing cells. The familiar delay between exposure to x-rays and the subsequent response of a cell renewal tissue is because moderate doses of x-rays kill the dividing stem cells and leave the differentiated cells functional. The response is delayed for a time that is related to the natural lifetime of the mature differentiated cells and the time it takes for stem cells to progress through the process of differentiation and become functional. This delay is absent in the case of heat because all cells are affected, differentiated or dividing; the damage to the tissue is expressed immediately.

As a result of these considerations, experimental assay systems based on clonogenic survival may seriously underestimate the effect of hyperthermia.

THERMOTOLERANCE

The development of a transient and nonhereditary resistance to subsequent heating by an initial heat treatment has been described variously as induced thermal resistance, thermal tolerance, or, most commonly, **thermotolerance.** In 1975, Henle and Leeper and Gerner and Schneider independently showed that the resistance induced in cells by one heat exposure exceeded anything that could be expected from repair of sublethal damage or progression into a resistance phase of the cycle.

Figure 28.4 illustrates the phenomenon of thermotolerance. If heating at 44°C is interrupted after

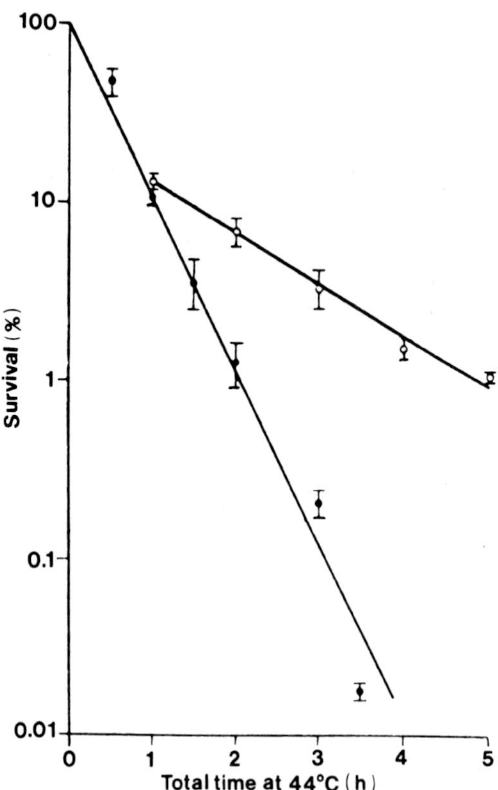

FIGURE 28.4 ● Thermotolerance in HeLa cells. Closed circles indicate cell survival to single heat exposures; open circles indicate response of cells treated at 44°C for 1 hour, returned to 37°C for 2 hours, and given second graded doses of 44°C for graded times. (From Gerner EW, Schneider MJ: Induced thermal resistance in HeLa cells. *Nature* 256:500–502, 1975, with permission.)

1 hour and resumed some 2 hours later, the dose–response curve is much shallower (i.e., the cells have become more resistant) than if heating had been continued. Operationally, there are two ways in which heating can induce thermotolerance. First, at lower temperatures of around 39°C to 42°C, thermotolerance is induced during the heating period after an exposure of 2 or 3 hours. This phenomenon is already apparent by the change of slope in the survival curves of Figure 28.1. Second, at temperatures above 43°C, thermotolerance cannot be produced during the heating, and it takes some time to develop after the heating has been stopped. It then decays slowly.

Thermotolerance is a substantial effect; the slope of a survival curve may be altered by a factor of 4 to 10, which translates into a difference in cell killing of several orders of magnitude. It is a factor to be reckoned with in fractionated hyperthermia.

For cells in culture, the time taken for cells that have become thermotolerant to revert to their normal sensitivity (i.e., the decay of thermotolerance) may be as long as 160 hours. Groups led by Overgaard and by Urano have shown that thermotolerance can be induced in transplantable mouse tumors and that this thermotolerance also decays very slowly, requiring something on the order of 120 hours before the decay is complete.

There is evidence from the work of Field and Law and their colleagues at Hammersmith that in normal-tissue systems, such as gut, skin, and cartilage, the appearance of thermotolerance may not reach a maximum until 1 or 2 days after heating, depending on the initiating treatment. It may take as long as 1 or 2 weeks to decay completely.

Thermotolerance is a serious problem in the clinical use of hyperthermia. Figure 28.5 illustrates why by contrasting heat and radiation. The top graph shows the familiar pattern for a multifraction regimen of x-rays given in daily doses, in which the shoulder must be repeated each time and each dose produces about the same amount of cell killing. The bottom graph shows a strikingly different pattern for hyperthermia. The first heat dose kills a substantial fraction of cells, but subsequent daily treatments are comparatively ineffective because of the development of thermotolerance, which occurs a few hours after the first treatment and may take as much as a week to decay. Because of the problems and uncertainties involved, Field advises, "The best way to deal with thermotolerance is to avoid it." This advice generally has been followed in the clinical use of hyperthermia, which imposes a limit of one or at most two heat treatments per week.

HEAT-SHOCK PROTEINS

If cells are exposed to heat, proteins of a defined molecular weight (mainly 70 or 90 kDa) are produced. The appearance of these **heat-shock proteins** tends to coincide with the development of thermotolerance, and their disappearance coincides with the decay of thermotolerance. Although the correlation is clear, it is not known if the heat-shock proteins are involved in the mechanism producing thermotolerance or if they are an independent manifestation of the heat insult. In fact, although they have been given the name *heat-shock proteins*, they are also produced after treatment with other agents, including arsenite and ethanol. Proteins of roughly the same molecular weight are found in cells of many species and first were discovered, in fact, in the fruit fly *Drosophila*. They appear to be a ubiquitous cellular response to stress.

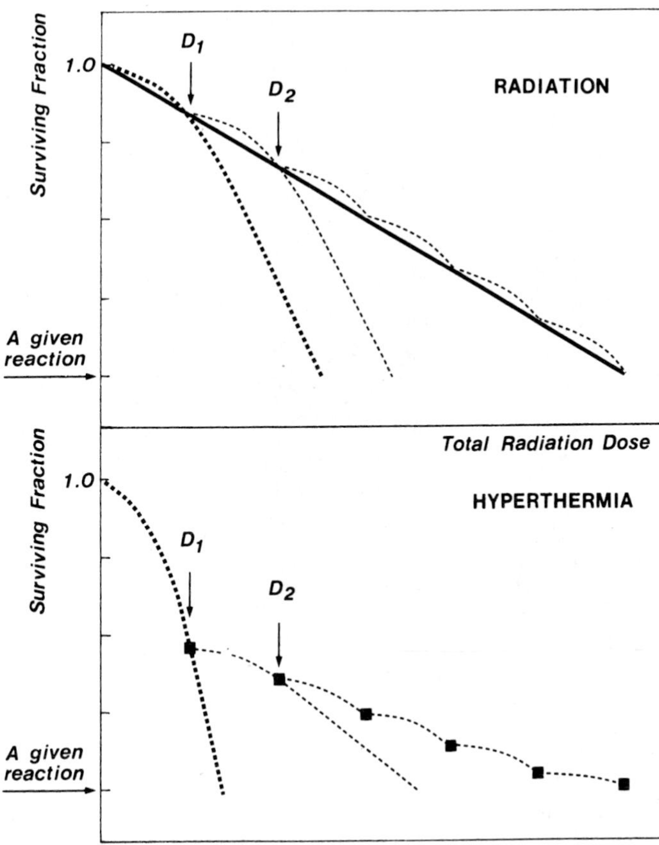

FIGURE 28.5 • Why thermotolerance is such a problem in a daily fractionated regimen. **Top:** X-rays. Each dose in a fractionated regimen has about the same effect (i.e., kills the same proportion of cells). The shoulder of the curve must be reexpressed for each dose fraction. **Bottom:** Hyperthermia. The first heat treatment results in a substantial biologic effect but also triggers the development of thermotolerance, which may take as long as a week to decay. Subsequent daily heat treatments would be relatively ineffective because of the acquired thermoresistance of the cells. (From Urano M: Kinetics of thermotolerance in normal and tumor tissues: A review. *Cancer Res* 46:474–482, 1986, with permission.)

Heat-shock proteins are identified by gel electrophoresis, in which they show up as clearly defined bands of specific molecular weights. Methionine labeled with sulfur-75 is used to label the protein in the treated cells, which then are run on a polyacrylamide gel in an electrical field. The proteins move a distance that depends on their molecular weight, with smaller proteins going farther. This separates out the various proteins in the cell (Fig. 28.6). After a treatment of 45°C for 20 minutes, proteins that are present only in small quantities before heat treatment are synthesized some hours later. Comparison with the control indicates a molecular weight of about 70 to 110 kDa. The time of appearance of these proteins coincides with the development of thermotolerance.

HYPOXIA AND HYPERTHERMIA

The response of hypoxic cells constitutes a vital difference between x-rays and hyperthermia. Hypoxia protects cells from killing by x-rays. By contrast, hypoxic cells are not more resistant than aerobic cells to hyperthermia; indeed, the evidence suggests that under some conditions, they may be slightly more sensitive to hyperthermia.

Cells made acutely hypoxic and then treated with heat have a sensitivity similar to aerated cells. Cells subject to *chronic hypoxia* (i.e., deprived of oxygen for prolonged periods) show a slightly enhanced sensitivity to heat. This increased sensitivity probably does not result from hypoxia *per se* but may be a consequence of the lowered pH and the nutritional deficiency that cells suffer as a result of prolonged hypoxia. Of utmost importance in a practical situation is that hypoxic cells in tumors are often both nutrient deficient and at a lowered pH.

HEAT AND TUMOR VASCULATURE

Tumors in general have a less organized and less efficient vasculature than most normal tissues. All

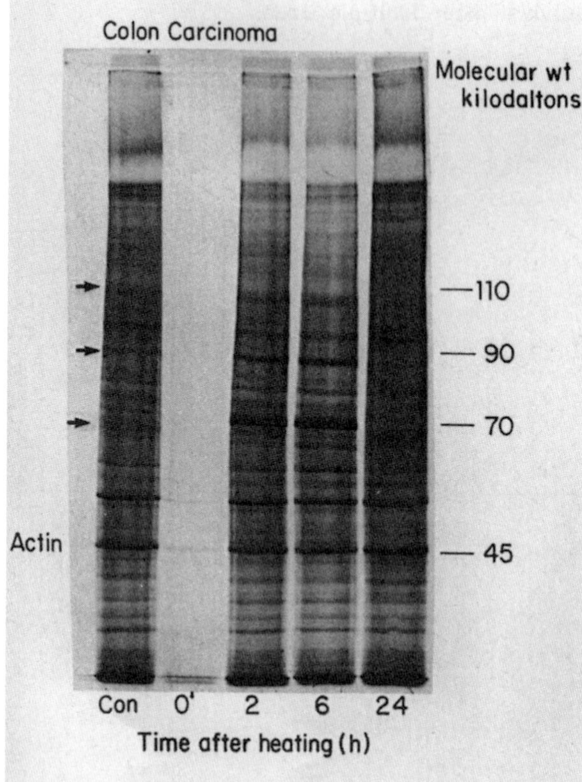

FIGURE 28.6 • Autoradiograph of cells labeled with methionine labeled with sulfur-35 in a polyacrylamide gel, to illustrate the synthesis of heat-shock proteins in cells derived from human colon carcinoma. The left column shows the normal pattern of protein synthesis in untreated cells. The other columns show patterns of protein synthesis at various times (0, 2, 6, and 24 hours) after a heat treatment of 20 minutes at 45°C. Immediately after treatment (0 hours), protein synthesis is completely shut down. At 2 and 6 hours after heat treatment, proteins of molecular weight 70, 90, and 110 kDa are overexpressed, as evidenced by the dark bands. These are the heat-shock proteins, whose appearance coincides with the development of thermotolerance. (Courtesy of Dr. Laurie Roizin-Towle.)

functional capillaries in tumors are open and used to capacity, even under ordinary conditions; in normal tissues, many capillaries are closed under ambient conditions. Consequently, although blood flow may be greater in tumors (particularly those that are small) compared with normal tissues at physiologic temperatures, the capacity of tumor blood flow to increase during heating appears to be rather limited in comparison with normal tissues. It is well documented that in normal tissues, heat induces a prompt increase in blood flow accompanied by dilation of vessels and an increase in permeability of the vascular wall. As a result, heat dissipation by blood flow is slower in tumors than in normal tissues, and so it often is found that the temperature within a tumor is higher than in the surrounding normal tissues. In a practical situation, therefore, the difference in intrinsic sensitivity between normal and malignant tissues becomes a moot point, because the tumor is often hotter anyway.

A postulated mechanism for selective solid-tumor heating is shown in Figure 28.7. Lest it be thought that this is a function of the artificial "encapsulated" nature of most transplanted tumors in experimental animals, it should be noted here that differential heating of tumors relative to normal tissues frequently has been observed in humans in clinical trials of hyperthermia. It may be one of the reasons why excessive normal-tissue damage has seldom been observed in clinical studies with heat.

There is, however, more to the story of heat and tumor vasculature. For reasons that are not fully understood, heat appears to preferentially damage the fragile vasculature of tumors; as a consequence, the heat-induced change in blood flow in at least transplantable tumors in animals is quite different from that in normal tissues. The relative change in blood flow in the skin and muscle of rats, as well as in various transplanted tumors, is summarized graphically in Figure 28.8. After hyperthermia, tumor blood flow in most cases goes *down*; blood flow in representative normal tissues goes *up* by a factor of 8 to 10. This further exacerbates the difference in blood flow and further increases the temperature of the tumor compared with the surrounding normal tissues.

There is a complex interplay in tumors between hyperthermia, blood flow, and cell killing; this is illustrated in Figure 28.9. If a tumor is heated to an elevated temperature, there is direct cell killing, but there is also a reduction in blood flow. This causes

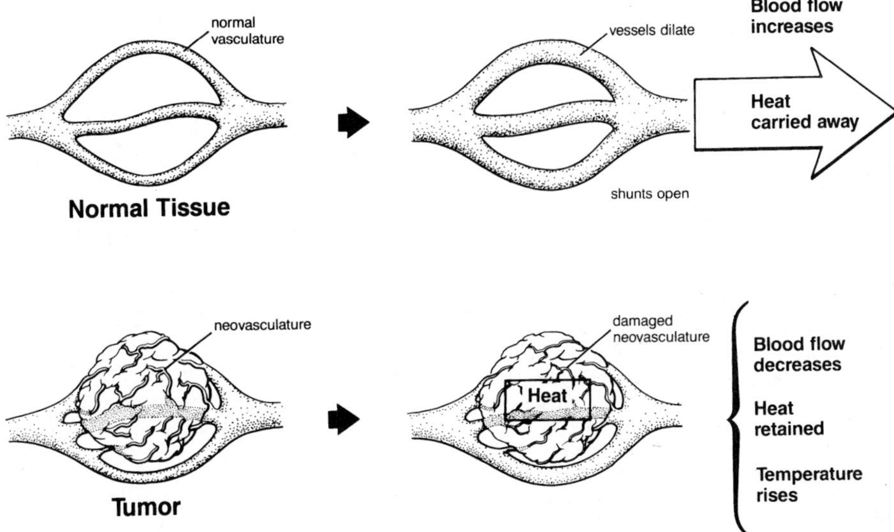

FIGURE 28.7 • Possible mechanism explaining why tumors get hotter than surrounding normal tissues. Normal tissues have a relatively high ambient blood flow, which increases in response to thermal stress, thereby dissipating heat. Tumors, with relatively poor blood flow and unresponsive neovasculature, are incapable of augmenting flow (i.e., shunting blood) and act as a heat reservoir. (Idea courtesy of Dr. F.K. Storm.)

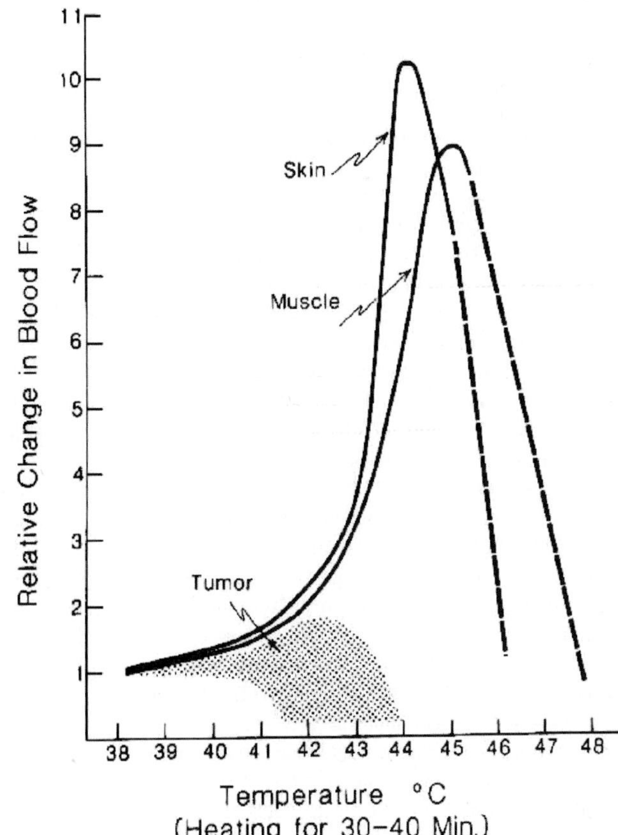

FIGURE 28.8 • Relative changes in blood flow in the skin and muscle of a rat and in various animal tumors at different temperatures. In general, blood flow increases in normal tissues during hyperthermia and decreases in tumors, often leading to differential tumor heating. (From Song CW: Effect of local hyperthermia on blood flow and microenvironment: A review. *Cancer Res* 44(suppl):4721S–4730S, 1984, with permission.)

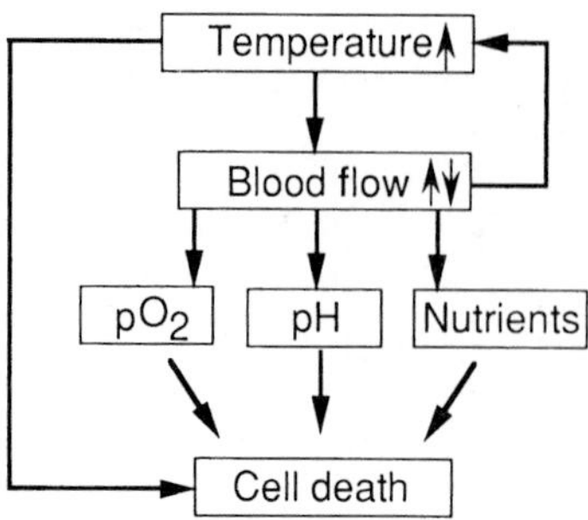

FIGURE 28.9 ● The complex interplay between hyperthermia and blood flow. An elevated temperature leads to direct cell killing, but it also causes a reduction in blood flow in tumors; this, in turn, causes changes in pH, pO_2, and nutrients, leading to enhanced cell killing. The reduction in blood flow also further elevates the temperature in the tumor, because heat is not being carried away. By contrast, mild hyperthermia causes an increase in blood flow with a concomitant increase in tumor pO_2. (Based on the ideas of Dr. Chang Song.)

the tumor to get even hotter, because the reduced blood flow carries less heat away; at the same time, the pH, pO_2, and nutrient status of the cells are affected, leading to enhanced cell killing.

HYPERTHERMIA AND TUMOR OXYGENATION

Early studies with transplanted tumors in rodents showed that heat caused vascular damage. It was concluded, therefore, that care was needed in combining heat and radiation, because the oxygen status of the tumor would be compromised by heating. However, it turns out that tumor vasculature in spontaneous human tumors is considerably more resistant to thermal damage than in transplanted tumors in mice, and in any case, much of the early work with mice utilized thermal doses far in excess of those that can be achieved clinically.

It is now recognized from animal studies that mild hyperthermia (41–41.5°C) can actually promote tumor reoxygenation, with the degree of reoxygenation correlating with the level of the radiosensitivity of the tumor. Song reviewed 22 different studies and concluded that mild hyperthermia of animal tumors increases tumor oxygenation, which can last as long as 24 hours. This also has been confirmed in a clinical study of patients with soft-tissue sarcomas and breast cancer. Brizel and colleagues showed that one heat treatment led to reoxygenation within 24 to 48 hours, whereas there was no measurable reoxygenation during a week of standard radiation therapy.

Jones and colleagues reported that mild hyperthermia (41–41.5°C at 90% of the measured points for 1 hour) significantly increased the pO_2 in hypoxic, but not oxic, human tumors. Such increases in tumor oxygenation significantly improved tumor response to radiotherapy, as will be described later.

TEMPERATURE MEASUREMENT

The control and measurement of temperature in tissues, if heating is achieved by an external source, is not a trivial problem. If microwaves, shortwave diathermy, or radiofrequency-induced currents are used, accurate temperature measurements cannot be made with metal thermometers, such as thermocouples or thermistors, because of direct heating of the electrically conducting components and the perturbations of the electromagnetic field. These initial problems were solved largely by the development of nonmetallic, temperature-sensitive crystal and fiberoptic probes.

It was recognized from an early date that the clinical development of hyperthermia would be impeded until it was possible to replace invasive methods of measuring temperature at a limited number of points with a noninvasive technology that would provide a detailed temperature distribution. The solution was very slow in coming, but the problem has now been largely solved by the use of magnetic resonance imaging. While hyperthermia is being applied, the patient is wheeled into an MRI scanner, and proton resonance frequency shifts are measured as a means to determine temperature. The method is totally noninvasive and yields a three-dimensional temperature distribution. The application of this technology should make it possible to correlate elevated temperature with tumor response and thus greatly facilitate the interpretation of future clinical trials of hyperthermia.

THERMAL DOSE

The temperature distribution in a tumor during hyperthermia treatment is almost always nonuniform. This nonuniformity stems from two spatially varying sources: power deposition, which produces heat, and tumor blood perfusion, which carries the heat away.

It has been demonstrated by both *in vitro* and *in vivo* experiments that hyperthermia cytotoxicity is dependent on both temperature and time, so that some time-integrated temperature descriptor is the best concept of thermal dose.

The quantity that has emerged as the most widely used measure of thermal dose is **CEM 43°C T_{90}**, the number of cumulative equivalent minutes at 43°C exceeded by 90% of the monitored points within the tumor.

Because in practice the tumor temperature may fluctuate up and down during a typical treatment, some method is needed to convert the varying times at various temperatures to equivalent minutes at 43°C. Probably the best method proposed is to use the relationship between treatment time and temperature for a biologic isoeffect (the Arrhenius plot, shown for cells in culture in Figure 28.2). This has been confirmed in principle for a variety of normal tissues and tumors. A marked change of slope occurs somewhere between 42°C and 43°C. Above this transition temperature, the slope is consistent for a variety of cells and tissues. It generally is agreed that a 1°C rise of temperature is equivalent to a reduction of time by a factor of 2. Consequently, above this transition temperature,

$$\frac{t_2}{t_1} = 2^{T_1 - T_2}$$

in which t_1 and t_2 are the heating times at temperatures T_1 and T_2, respectively, to produce equal biologic effect.

For temperatures below the transition temperature, an increase in temperature by 1°C requires that time be decreased by a factor of 4 to 6:

$$\frac{t_2}{t_1} = (4 \text{ to } 6)^{T_1 - T_2}$$

CEM 43°C T_{90}—the thermal dose—may be calculated from one or the other of these expressions or a combination of both; that is, the heat dose associated with a changing temperature may be calculated as the sum of equivalent heating times at 43°C for each temperature.

Although the concept of thermal dose is attractive, there are problems in its implementation:

- Nonuniformity of temperature occurs throughout the tumor.
- The concept relates only to cell killing by heat and does not include radiosensitization.
- Thermotolerance complicates the situation for multiple heat treatments unless they are well separated in time.

In spite of these limitations, the use of this measure of thermal dose has been shown in a prospective randomized trial of superficial tumors to result in improved local tumor control when hyperthermia was used as an adjunct to radiotherapy.

THE INTERACTION BETWEEN HEAT AND RADIATION

The biologic effect of a combination of heat and radiation may be a consequence of:

1. The independent but additive cytotoxic effects of the heat and radiation, with their complementary patterns of sensitivity through the cell cycle and the greater sensitivity to heat of nutritionally deprived cells at low pH.
2. The interaction between heat and radiation, in the form of sensitization of the radiation cytotoxicity by heat, resulting from the inhibition of repair of radiation-induced damage.

In a practical situation in the clinic, the interaction is most likely to be the independent and additive cytotoxic effects (as described in the first point listed) because of the modest heat levels that can be achieved and the time interval usually used between hyperthermia and radiation treatment. Of course, both may occur simultaneously, in which case the combination of hyperthermia and x-rays results in a greater cytotoxicity than can be accounted for by the addition of the cytotoxic effects of the agents alone; that is, the interaction between the two modalities is *synergistic*, or supra-additive. This interaction has been studied with cells in culture and with experimental animal systems.

In the case of cells cultured *in vitro*, the shape of the x-ray survival curve is changed by the addition of heat. For *acute hyperthermia* (i.e., brief exposures to temperatures of about 45°C, which lead to a substantial amount of cell killing), the principal effect of hyperthermia is a steepening (i.e., reduced D_0) of the x-ray survival curve. The change in the shoulder of the curve is minimal. On the other hand, if a more modest level of hyperthermia is used (40–43°C, which involves little or no cell killing), the principal effect observed is a removal of the shoulder from the x-ray survival curve, and then heat treatment after irradiation is the more effective sequence. These differences between higher and lower temperatures, associated with the break in the Arrhenius plot at around 43°C, may reflect different critical targets or simply be a consequence of the fact that thermotolerance can develop during the treatment at lower temperatures.

Heat inhibits the repair of radiation-induced single-strand breaks and radiation-induced chromosome aberrations. This inability to repair molecular damage translates into the inability to repair both sublethal damage and potentially lethal damage produced by radiation. Repair of sublethal damage does not occur if hyperthermia is applied during the interval between the two doses of x-rays.

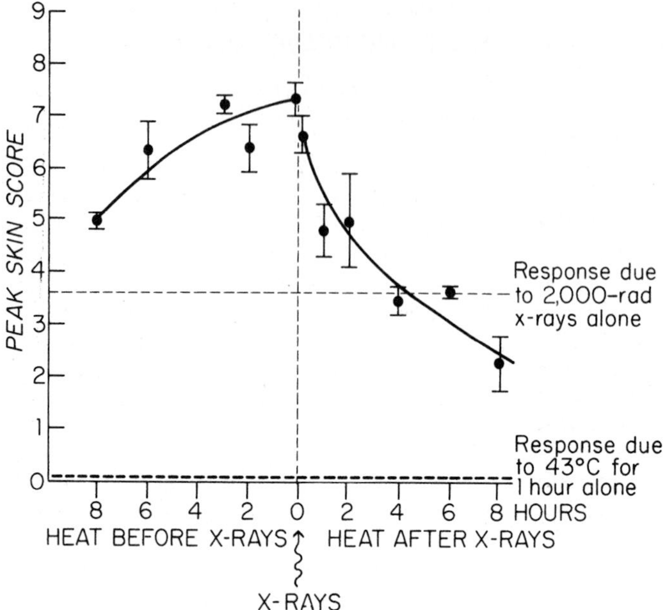

FIGURE 28.10 • Response of mouse skin to the effect of combined heat and x-rays. The heat treatment was 43°C for 1 hour, and the x-ray dose was 20 Gy (2,000 rad). Heat was given before or after irradiation, and the time interval between the two was varied. (Adapted from Field SB, Hume S, Law MP, Morris C, Myers R: The response of tissues to combined hyperthermia and X rays. Presented at the International Symposium on Radiological Research Needed for the Improvement of Radiotherapy, Vienna, November 22–26, 1976, with permission.)

If heat and radiation are combined, an important consideration is sequencing. The effect of the sequence of heating and radiation for mouse skin is shown in Figure 28.10. Heating at 43°C for 1 hour was applied before or after a single 20-Gy (2,000-rad) dose of x-rays. There was a marked variation in the normal-tissue response after a given dose of x-rays, depending on the time interval between heat and irradiation and on the order in which the two treatments were given. Heating before radiation was more effective than heating after radiation in causing damage in mouse skin. It appeared that the heating before radiation increased skin blood flow, thereby increasing oxygenation in the skin and enhancing radiation damage.

If hyperthermia is used in the clinic as an adjunct to radiotherapy, their effects are probably not interactive at all. Because the daily doses used in conventional fractionated radiotherapy are small (2 Gy) and the levels of heating achieved are modest, the cytotoxicity of heat and radiation at the cellular level are more probably independent but additive. However, an increase in blood flow and consequent increase in oxygenation by modest heating may enhance the response of tumors to radiotherapy.

THERMAL ENHANCEMENT RATIO (TER)

In the case of either normal tissues or transplantable tumors in experimental animals, the extent of the interaction of heat and radiation is expressed in terms of the **thermal enhancement ratio (TER)**, defined as the ratio of doses of x-rays required to produce a given level of biologic damage with and without the application of heat.

The TER has been measured for a variety of normal tissues, including skin, cartilage, and intestinal epithelium. The data form a consistent pattern of increasing TER with increasing temperature, up to a value of about 2 for a 1-hour heat treatment at 43°C. The TER is more difficult to measure in transplanted tumors in laboratory animals, because the direct cytotoxic effect of the heat tends to dominate. Heat often can control experimental tumors with acceptable damage to normal tissues, because cell killing by heat is strongly enhanced by nutritional deprivation and increased acidity, conditions that are typical of the poorly vascularized parts of solid tumors. Thus, a moderate heat treatment, which can be tolerated by well-vascularized normal tissues, destroys a large proportion of the cells of many solid tumors in experimental animals. In those cases in which thermal radiosensitization has been studied, typical TER values are 1.4 at 41°C, 2.7 at 42.5°C, and 4.3 at 43°C, with heat applied for 1 hour.

HEAT AND THE THERAPEUTIC-GAIN FACTOR

The **therapeutic-gain factor** can be defined as the ratio of the TER in the tumor to the TER in normal tissues. There is no advantage to using heat plus lower doses of x-rays if there is no therapeutic gain compared with the use of higher doses of x-rays alone.

The question of a therapeutic-gain factor is complicated in the case of heat, because the tumor and normal tissues are not necessarily at the same temperature. If the statement is made that heat preferentially damages tumor cells compared with normal tissue, it is implied that they both are at the same temperature. In a practical situation, however, this is not always the case. For example, if a poorly vascularized tumor is treated with microwaves, it may reach a *higher* temperature than the surrounding normal tissue, because less heat is carried away by the flow of blood. In addition, the overlying skin can be cooled actively by a draft of air or even a cold-water pack. In these circumstances, the normal tissues may be at a significantly *lower* temperature than the tumor, which therefore exaggerates the differential response in a favorable direction.

With these reservations in mind, there are still good reasons for believing that the effects of heat, alone or in combination with x-rays, may be greater on tumors than on normal tissues, for reasons discussed previously.

MECHANISMS OF ACTION OF HYPERTHERMIA

Hyperthermia induces effects in both the nucleus and the cytoplasm. It is unclear whether heat effects in the nucleus, such as loss of polymerase activities, inhibition of DNA synthesis, and chromosomal aberrations, are direct effects of heat within the nucleus or secondary to the effects on the membranes, intracellular structures, and cytoskeleton. Heat killing appears to be associated with degradation or denaturation of proteins, in particular, nuclear protein (as judged by the inactivation energies from the Arrhenius plots), which is different from that for radiation killing, which clearly involves primarily damage to DNA. In addition, hyperthermia at relatively modest temperatures may increase the metabolic rate in cells, which then causes production of toxic free radicals.

Although the intermediate steps may be different, the ultimate cytotoxic effect of both heat and radiation occurs at the DNA level, especially for cells treated in the S phase of the cell cycle. For cells *in vitro*, heat induces chromosomal aberrations in the S phase, and for a given level of cell killing induced by heat alone or heat plus radiation, the frequency and types of chromosomal aberrations correspond closely to those resulting from radiation alone; that is, one aberration corresponds to 37% survival. In organized tissues, however, heat damage occurs more rapidly than radiation damage, because differentiated cells are killed as well as dividing cells. Also, cells tend to die in apoptosis.

The events associated with heat radiosensitization involve DNA damage and the inhibition of its repair. Hyperthermia has little effect on the amount of radiation-induced DNA damage in terms of single- or double-strand breaks. The role of heat appears to be to block the process of repair of these radiation-induced lesions.

HEAT AND CHEMOTHERAPEUTIC AGENTS

The cell-killing potential of some but not all chemotherapeutic agents is enhanced substantially by a temperature elevation of even a few degrees. This is illustrated for cisplatin (*cis*-platinum) in Figure 28.11. There is also a striking synergism in

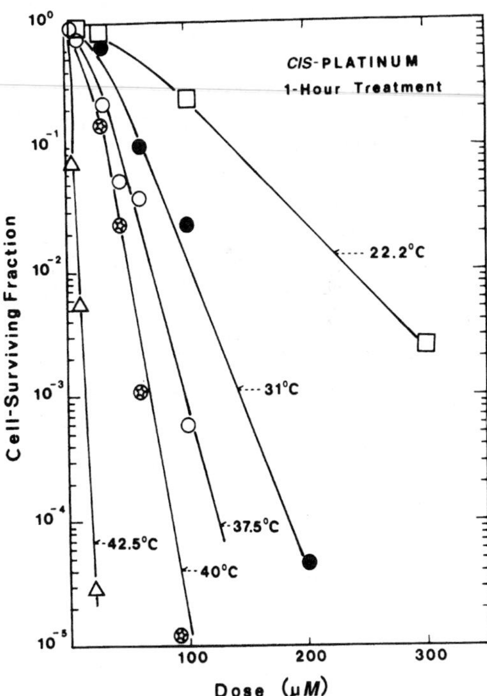

FIGURE 28.11 • Effect of elevated temperatures on the cytotoxicity of cisplatin (*cis*-platinum) in V79 hamster cells *in vitro*. Cells were heated for 1 hour at the temperatures indicated. (From Roizin-Towle L, Hall EJ, Capuano L: Interaction of hyperthermia and cytotoxic agents. *Natl Cancer Inst Monogr* 61:149–151, 1982, with permission.)

cytotoxicity if hyperthermia (42–43°C) is combined with either bleomycin or doxorubicin. It is probable that at least part of the cell's sensitization to bleomycin at 43°C is related to the inhibition of a repair mechanism. No such explanation can account for the sensitization to doxorubicin, but it has been shown clearly that the drug gets into the cells more easily at 43°C than at 37°C, possibly because of a change in the properties of the plasma membrane at the higher temperature. Once thermotolerance develops, however, less doxorubicin gets into the cells.

Whatever the mechanisms involved, the synergism between heat and drugs may prove very useful in the chemotherapy of solid tumors. The addition of local hyperthermia to a chemotherapy schedule would have the obvious advantage of "targeting" and localizing the principal effect of the drug, allowing greater tumor cell killing for a given systemic toxicity. This would help to overcome one of the principal problems and limitations of chemotherapy. It is surprising that more has not been done in this area in view of the substantial potential benefits. Table 28.1 lists drugs that are potentiated by heat and those that are not. There are several different mechanisms that may be involved, some of which are listed in Table 28.2.

The possibility of combining chemotherapy with whole-body hyperthermia at temperatures above 41°C has been investigated but proved to be too toxic. On the other hand, preliminary studies have demonstrated the feasibility of using fever-range whole-body temperatures (39–40°C) in combination with anticancer drugs, which proved to be both safe and effective.

TABLE 28.1

Interaction of Heat and Chemotherapeutic Agents

Effect	Drug
Potentiated by heat	Melphalan
	Cyclophosphamide
	BCNU
	Cis DDP
	Mitomycin C
	Bleomycin
	Vincristine
Unaffected by heat	Hydroxyurea
	Methotrexate
	Vinblastine
Complex interaction	Doxorubicin

From Kano E: Hyperthermia and drugs. In Overgaard J (ed): *Hyperthermic Oncology*, pp 277–282. London, Taylor & Francis, 1985, with permission.

TABLE 28.2

Mechanisms of Interaction of Hyperthermia and Drugs

Mechanism	Drug
Increased rate of alkylation	Thiotepa
	Nitrosoureas
	Mitomycin C
Single-strand DNA breaks	Bleomycin
Inhibition of repair	Methylmethane sulphonate
	Lonidamine
	Bleomycin
Altered drug uptake[a]	Doxorubicin +/–
	Bleomycin –
	Melphalan +/–
	Thiotepa –
	Cyclo-phosphamide –
	Methyl-CCNU –
	Fluorouracil +
	Methotrexate +/–
	Cisplatin +/–
	Dactinomycin +/–
Common membrane target	Polyene antibiotics
	Local anesthetics
	Alcohols
Energy metabolism	Several
Production of oxygen radicals	Several

Other mechanisms for the interaction of drugs and heat have been suggested, including increased ability of an agent to penetrate membranes and prolongation by drugs of the heat-sensitive cell-cycle phases.
[a]+, a reported increase from hyperthermia; –, a reported decrease.
Based on Dahl O: Hyperthermia and drugs. In Watmough DJ, Ross WM (eds): *Hyperthermia*. Glasgow, Blackie and Son, pp 121–153, 1986, with permission.

Low-Temperature Liposomes

Liposomes consist of a lipid membrane that can be filled with a cytotoxic chemotherapeutic agent such as doxorubicin (or in some cases *cis*-platinum).

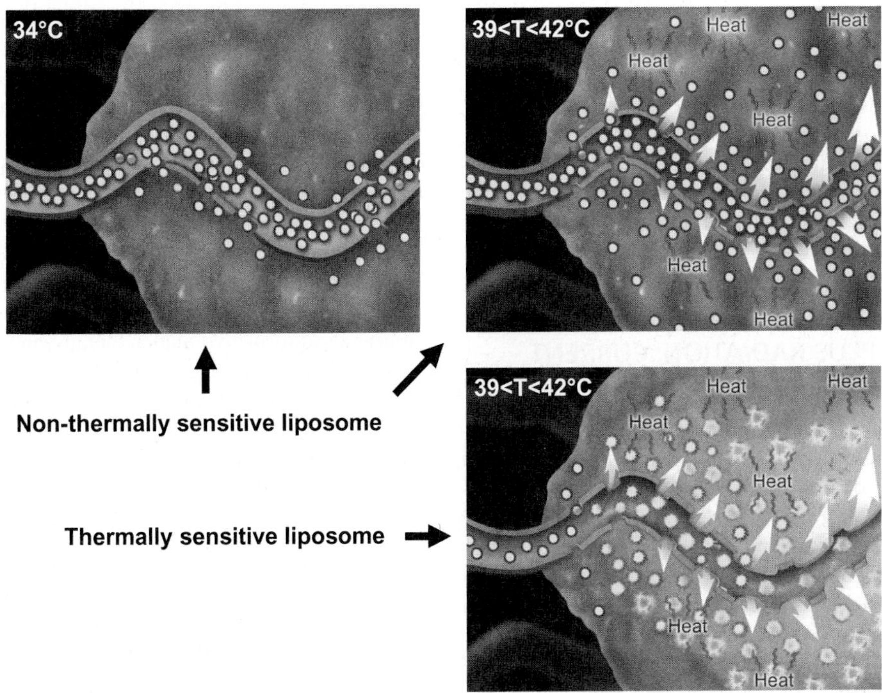

FIGURE 28.12 • **Top left:** Liposomes extravasate very slowly out of tumor vessels under normothermic conditions. **Top right:** The effect of hyperthermia on microvessel pore size. When tumors are subjected to mild heating, pores open up between tumor endothelial cells, permitting liposomes to extravasate out. They extravasate out at about 2 to 5 times faster than at normothermic conditions. **Bottom:** In the case of a thermally sensitive liposome, enhanced extravasation and drug release occur both inside and outside the vessels. This yields another factor of 5 increase in drug delivery over what can be achieved with heat and non-thermally sensitive liposomes. (Illustration prepared by Dr. Mark Dewhirst, Duke University Medical Center.)

Liposomes tend to get trapped in the chaotic disorganized blood vessels of a tumor. As a consequence of a modest hyperthermia treatment (41–42°C), liposomes "extravasate" (i.e., leave the vasculature) into the tumor interstitium, the membrane melts, and the chemotherapeutic agent is deposited in the tumor. This hyperthermia-triggered drug release in the tumor results in a large therapeutic effect. The mechanism is illustrated in Figure 28.12.

HUMAN APPLICATIONS

Hyperthermia has been widely used as a form of cancer therapy. Its use in the treatment of human tumors dates back many thousands of years. In 1891, Coley noted that the regression of an inoperable "round cell sarcoma of the neck" was associated with a febrile bout of erysipelas. At this stage, it was not clear whether the shrinkage of the tumor was caused by fever or was a direct effect of the bacterial toxins. In 1953, Nauts, Fowler, and Bogatko repeated Coley's work, and 25 of their 30 selected patients with soft-tissue sarcoma, lymphosarcoma, or carcinoma of the cervix and breast were alive and disease free at 10 years. The earlier results of Coley with the highly pyrogenic agents never were equaled with lesser agents or systemic hyperthermia, however, perhaps because the fever rather than the toxin was the tumoricidal agent. Because the immune system undoubtedly was influenced by Coley's toxins, one can speculate that in those patients in whom permanent cures were obtained, the cures could be the result of immune stimulation rather than direct thermal effect on the tumor alone.

HYPERTHERMIA ALONE

It generally is agreed, based on a considerable body of data, that local hyperthermia has no role in the curative treatment of tumors. Regardless of treatment schedules, the complete response rate to heat alone does not exceed about 10% and seems to be of short duration. Local tumors can be sterilized only at high temperatures, which cause significant damage to surrounding normal tissues. This is in agreement with experimental studies in the laboratory that suggest that tumor cells in a well-vascularized area under normal conditions have about the same sensitivity as normal tissues.

Nevertheless, local hyperthermia has been shown to be useful in palliation, in the relief of pain. Treatment with heat alone, therefore, plays a limited role in cancer and is now usually recommended only in patients who have limited life expectancies or if conventional therapy is contraindicated.

HEAT PLUS RADIATION: CURRENT STATUS OF CLINICAL STUDIES

Hyperthermia has been used extensively as an adjuvant to radiation in the treatment of local and regional cancer, and this is the area in which it appears to offer the biggest advantage. The protocol that has emerged from the clinic is of the sequential application of radiation and heat, with one or two applications of heat interspersed with a normal multifraction course of radiotherapy.

The radiosensitizing effect of heat is most evident if the heat and radiation are applied simultaneously, but the effect is generally of the same magnitude in both tumors and normal tissues and does not improve the therapeutic ratio unless the tumor is heated to a higher temperature than the normal tissue. On the other hand, the hyperthermic cytotoxic mechanism predominates if heat follows radiation in a sequential procedure. The heat-sensitive cells are those found in a nutritionally deprived, chronically hypoxic and acidic environment, conditions that are found in tumors but not generally seen in normal tissues. In addition, as a result of heat killing of the hypoxic radioresistant tumor cells, the actual radiation dose necessary to effectively control the tumor should be reduced. Thus, not only do we see a preferential enhancement occurring in tumors, but the overall radiation damage to normal tissues also is decreased because the radiation dose is decreased. Consequently, a therapeutic gain should result.

A sequential administration of radiation and heat has several other advantages over a simultaneous treatment. The aim of giving heat is to improve the already existing radiotherapy treatment. If heat is combined with radiation in a simultaneous protocol, it has to be given with each radiation fraction. Thermotolerance then becomes a problem. This can be overcome by increasing the fraction interval, but that would be expected to reduce the effectiveness of the radiation alone. With sequential heat and radiation treatment, the heat can be administered once or twice, without interfering with the normal radiotherapy protocol. Last but not least, the sequential application of the two modalities is much more practical; to heat and irradiate simultaneously would be very difficult indeed.

There is abundant evidence from phase I and II trials that heat may enhance radiotherapy to a significant degree; these data were chronicled in some detail in previous editions of this book. In addition, a number of randomized phase III multicenter trials have been conducted that must replace the more extensive but less convincing data from the past. The results of these trials are summarized in Table 28.3. Some show a benefit for the addition of hyperthermia as an adjuvant to radiation therapy, and some do not. The trials involving advanced breast cancer and neck nodes with full-dose radiation therapy do not show any benefit from the use of hyperthermia. It may be that heating techniques were inadequate in these sites. Three trials show a clear and significant advantage for the addition of hyperthermia to standard radiation therapy. These may be summarized as follows:

Superficial Localized Breast Cancer

An international collaborative hyperthermia group combined the results of five randomized controlled clinical trials conducted in the United Kingdom, Europe, and Canada, in which external-beam radiation therapy alone was compared with radiation therapy plus hyperthermia. Hyperthermia was induced using various externally applied electromagnetic applicators, aiming at a tumor temperature of 42.5°C or 43°C. In fact, the minimum temperature rarely exceeded 41°C because of difficulties in heating. Not all trials demonstrated an advantage for the combined treatment, but the pooled data showed a significant improvement in complete tumor response. The greatest effect was seen in patients with recurrent lesions in previously treated areas, in whom further irradiation was limited to low doses.

Interestingly, heating at moderate temperatures (41–41.5°C) significantly increased the response rates of the locally advanced breast cancer to a combined treatment of Taxol and radiotherapy. The pO_2 in tumors was observed to be significantly increased 24 hours after heating, indicting that the increase in response rate was due to a heat-induced improvement of tumor oxygenation.

Recurrent or Metastatic Malignant Melanoma

Within the framework of the European Society for Hyperthermic Oncology, a multicenter randomized trial showed improved local control at 2 years and survival at 5 years for patients with recurrent malignant melanoma. The patients received three

TABLE 28.3

Results of Six Randomized Clinical Trials Comparing the Response of Thermoradiotherapy versus Radiotherapy Alone

		Response					
		Complete Response, %		Local Control, 2 y, %		Survival, 5 y (actuarial), %	
Site	Number of Lesions	HT + RT	RT	HT + RT	RT	HT + RT	RT
Head and neck[a] (stage III & IV)	65	46	12	25	8		
Head and neck[b] (stage IV nodes)	44	83	41	69	24	53	0
Melanoma[c]	134	62	32	46	28		
Breast[d] (primary and recurrent)	396	59	41	45	29		
Breast[d] (recurrent, previously irradiated)	210	57	31				
Glioma[e] (interstitial HT + RT and RT)	64			Survival = 91 wk	Survival = 76 wk; P = 0.014		
Pelvic tumors[f]			P = 0.005			3 yr Survival	P = 0.014
Overall	360	56	39			32	24
			P = 0.013				P = 0.01
Cervix[f] (68 Gy)	115	83	57			52	27
Bladder[f] (66 Gy)	102	74	51			NS	
Rectum[f] (56 Gy)	143	21	15			NS	

All differences significant to $P < 0.05$.
HT + RT, thermoradiotherapy; RT, radiotherapy.
[a] Datta NR, Bose AK, Kapoor HK, Gupta S, Head and neck cancers: Results of thermoradiotherapy versus radiotherapy. *Int J Hypertherm* 6:479–486, 1990.
[b] Valdagni R, Amichetti M: Report of long-term follow-up in a randomized trial comparing radiation therapy and radiation therapy plus hyperthermia to metastatic lymph nodes in stage IV head and neck patients. *Int J Radiat Oncol Biol Phys* 28:163–169, 1994.
[c] Overgaard J, Gonzalez Gonzalez D, Hulshof MCCM, et al.: Randomized trial of hyperthermia as adjuvant to radiotherpy for recurrent or metastatic malignant melanoma. *Lancet* 345:540–543, 1995.
[d] Vernon CC, Hand JW, Field SB, et al.: Radiotherapy with or without hyperthermia in the treatment of superficial localized breast cancer. Results from five randomized controlled trials. *Int J Radiat Oncol Biol Phys* 35:731–744, 1996.
[e] Sneed PK, Stauffer PR, Diederich CJ, et al.: Survival benefit of hyperthermia in a prospective randomized trial of brachytherapy boost ± hyperthermia for glioblastoma multiforme. 38th Am. Soc. Therap. Radiol. Oncol., Los Angeles, CA, October, 1996 (Abs 1).
[f] van der Zee J, Gonzalez Gonzalez D, Vernon CC, et al.: Therapeutic gain by hyperthermia added to radiotherapy. ICRO/OGRO 6, 6th Int. Meeting on Progress in Radio-Oncology, Salzburg, Austria, May 13–17, 1998.

fractions of 8 or 9 Gy (800 or 900 rad) within a period of 8 days, either alone or combined with hyperthermia aiming at 43°C for 60 minutes.

Hyperthermia and Implants

The dose-rate effect was described in detail in Chapter 5. In short, if x- or γ-rays are delivered at low dose rates, the biologic effectiveness of a given dose is reduced because of the repair of sublethal damage that takes place during the protracted treatment time. Because heat inhibits the repair of sublethal damage, it is logical to predict that the effectiveness of low-dose-rate irradiation would be enhanced by the simultaneous application of heat. This has been investigated in detail *in vitro* and confirmed *in vivo*, with TER values approaching 2. These reports inspired the use of hyperthermia and low-dose-rate irradiation in implants in patients. Independent of the method used to produce the heating, some remarkable results have been obtained with interstitial heating combined with brachytherapy. The reason for this superior response is likely to be the relatively homogeneous heating distribution, in general far better than can be achieved by external heating.

In a randomized clinical study for local glioblastoma, interstitial heating given before and after brachytherapy following conventional radiotherapy significantly improved both local control and patient survival.

POSTSCRIPT ON HYPERTHERMIA

Research in hyperthermia has dropped out of the limelight in recent years, despite the demonstration in several clinical trials summarized previously that it can enhance the effect of radiation therapy in a number of sites. At the present time, there is more enthusiasm for hyperthermia in Europe than in the United States. The position can be summed up as follows:

1. The biologic properties of hyperthermia make it an attractive modality for the treatment of cancer, suggesting a useful differential between effects on tumors and effects on normal tissues.
2. It is still difficult to achieve uniform heating of a volume deep within the body, despite considerable ingenuity displayed in designing heating systems. The basic laws of physics make the desired end difficult to achieve.
3. The clinical value of hyperthermia in the routine treatment of cancer is still not clear, despite its proven efficacy in a few specific instances. It should be noted that the situations in which hyperthermia appears to be effective involve either combination with external-beam radiotherapy for the treatment of superficial tumors—in which adequate heating is not so difficult—or combination with brachytherapy, in which heating is induced by implanted electrodes, inevitably involving all the complications and limitations of accessibility.
4. Recent evidence suggests that modest hyperthermia (41–41.5°C), which is easier to achieve, may be useful to improve oxygenation and thus sensitize tumors to radiotherapy.

Summary of Pertinent Conclusions

- Localized hyperthermia using external devices can be induced by shortwave diathermy, radiofrequency capacitative heating, microwaves, ultrasound, and interstitial implants.
- The best heat distributions can be obtained by implanting microwave or radiofrequency sources.
- Heat kills: Survival curves for heat are similar in shape to those for radiation, except that time at the elevated temperature replaces absorbed dose.
- The inactivation energy is different above and below a break temperature of about 43°C; that is, change of sensitivity with temperature is more rapid below than above this temperature.
- Above the break point, the heating time required to produce a given level of cell killing is halved for every 1°C temperature rise; below the break point, the time must be reduced by a factor of 4 to 6 for each 1°C temperature rise.
- Different cells have very different sensitivities to heat. No consistent difference in inherent sensitivity exists between normal and malignant cells.
- The age–response function for heat complements that for x-rays. S phase cells that are resistant to x-rays are sensitive to heat.
- Cells at low pH and nutritionally deprived (more likely to be in tumors) are more sensitive to heat, although cells can adapt to pH changes and lose their sensitivity to heat.
- Hypoxia does not protect cells from heat as it does from x-rays.
- Heat damage in normal tissues and tumors is expressed more rapidly than x-ray damage because heat kills differentiated as well as dividing cells and because cells can die in interphase rather than at the next (or subsequent) mitosis, as in the case of x-rays.

(continued)

Summary of Pertinent Conclusions (Continued)

- Thermotolerance is the induced resistance to a second heat exposure by prior heating.
- Thermotolerance can be induced during a heat exposure at temperatures below about 42.5°C but develops some hours after heating for temperatures above 42.5°C.
- The development of thermotolerance may be monitored by the appearance of heat-shock proteins.
- Thermotolerance is a complication in fractionated clinical hyperthermia. With our present state of knowledge, the best way to deal with it may be to avoid it.
- Heat preferentially damages tumor vasculature. After heating, blood flow goes down in tumors but increases in normal tissues. This may result in an enhanced temperature differential between tumors and normal tissues. There is good evidence for this in transplantable animal tumors, but it is less clear in spontaneous human tumors.
- Mild hyperthermia (41–41.5°C) can promote tumor reoxygenation; this has been shown in animal experiments and in clinical studies.
- Temperature measurement *in vivo* is difficult but improving with multiple nonmetallic thermometers. The most successful noninvasive technique involves magnetic resonance imaging.
- Thermal dose is expressed in terms of CEM 43°C T_{90}, the cumulative equivalent minutes at 43°C exceeded by 90% of the monitored points within the tumor.
- Delivered simultaneously, hyperthermia interacts with radiation in a more-than-additive way and inhibits the repair of sublethal damage.
- Hyperthermia induces effects in both the nucleus and the cytoplasm. Probable mechanisms for heat killing include damage to the plasma membrane and inactivation of proteins, but these mechanisms may be different above and below the break temperature in the Arrhenius plot.
- The thermal enhancement ratio (TER) is the ratio of radiation doses with and without heat to produce the same biologic effects. TER values of 2 to 4 can be obtained in tumors and normal tissues in experimental animals.
- The therapeutic-gain factor is the ratio of the TER in the tumor to the TER in normal tissues.
- In a clinical situation, in which modest levels of hyperthermia are attained and small daily doses of radiation are delivered, the cytotoxic effects of the two modalities are probably independent and additive. However, tumor pO_2 may be increased by mild hyperthermia, thereby improving tumor response to radiotherapy.
- Heat radiosensitization involves DNA damage and the inhibition of its repair.
- Hyperthermia potentiates some chemotherapeutic agents. Local hyperthermia "targets" their action.
- Many thousands of patients have been treated with hyperthermia.
- The general consensus is that hyperthermia alone is of limited use, except for palliation or retreatment of recurrent tumors.
- Several clinical studies have shown that the combination of hyperthermia and radiation produces more complete and partial tumor responses than radiation alone.
- Several phase III randomized trials show a clear and significant benefit for the addition of hyperthermia to standard radiation therapy. The sites include superficial localized breast cancer, recurrent or metastatic malignant melanoma, and nodal metastases from head and neck cancer.
- Trials involving advanced breast cancer and neck nodes with full-dose radiation therapy did not show any benefit from the addition of hyperthermia.
- Biologic properties of heat appear favorable for its use in cancer therapy. Physical devices to produce uniform heating at a depth are not well developed, and adequate thermometry is also difficult.
- Microwaves provide good localization at shallow depths, but localization is poor at greater depths, at which low frequencies are needed.

(continued)

Summary of Pertinent Conclusions (Continued)

- With ultrasound, deep heating can be achieved with focused arrays, but bones or air cavities cause distortions.
- In practice, breast tumors, including recurrences and melanomas, can be heated adequately with microwaves, and deep-seated tumors below the diaphragm can be heated adequately with ultrasound. In any other site, present methods of heating pose a problem.
- The combination of interstitial implants of radioactive sources with hyperthermia generated by radiofrequency power applied to the implanted sources appears to be particularly promising, because a good radiation dose distribution is combined with a good heat distribution.

BIBLIOGRAPHY

Breasted JH: The Edwin Smith surgical papyrus. In Licht S (ed): *Therapeutic Heat and Cold*, 2nd ed, p 196. New Haven, CT, Waverly Press, 1930

Brizel DM, Scully SP, Harrelson JM, et al.: Radiation therapy and hyperthermia improve the oxygenation of human soft tissue sarcomas. *Cancer Res* 56:5347–5350, 1996

Bull JMC: An update on the anticancer effects of a combination of chemotherapy and hyperthermia. *Cancer Res* 44(suppl):4853S–4859S, 1984

Coley WB: The treatment of malignant tumors by repeated inoculation of erysipelas: With a report of ten original cases. *Am J Med Sci* 105:487, 1893

Corry PM, Spanos WJ, Tilchen EJ, Barlogie B, Barkley HT, Armour EP: Combined ultrasound and radiation therapy treatment of human superficial tumors. *Radiology* 145:165–169, 1982

Cosset JM, Dutreix J, Haie C, Gerbaulet A, Janoray P, Dewars JA: Interstitial thermoradiotherapy: A technical and clinical study of 29 implantations performed at the Institut Gustave-Roussy. *Int J Hypertherm* 1:3–13, 1985

Crile G: The effects of heat and radiation on cancers implanted on the feet of mice. *Cancer Res* 23:372–380, 1963

Dahl O: Hyperthermia and drugs. In Watmough DJ, Ross WM (eds): *Hyperthermia*. Glasgow, Blackie and Son, 121–153, 1986

Datta NR, Bose AK, Kapoor HK, Gupta S: Head and neck cancers: Results of thermoradiotherapy versus radiotherapy. *Int J Hypertherm* 6:479–486, 1990

Dewey WC, Hopwood LE, Sapareto LA, Gerweck LE: Cellular responses to combinations of hyperthermia and radiation. *Radiology* 123:463–474, 1977

Dewhirst MW, Prosnitz L, Thrall D, et al.: Hyperthermic treatment of malignant diseases: Current status and a view toward the future. *Semin Oncol* 24:616–625, 1997

Emami BH, Perez CA, Leybovich L, Straube W, Vongerichten D: Interstitial thermoradiotherapy in treatment of malignant tumours. *Int J Hypertherm* 3:107–118, 1987

Field SB, Hume S, Law MP, Morris C, Myers R: The response of tissues to combined hyperthermia and X rays. Presented at the International Symposium on Radiological Research Needed for the Improvement of Radiotherapy, Vienna, November 22–26, 1976

Field SB, Morris CC: The relationship between heating time and temperature: Its relevance to clinical hyperthermia. *Radiother Oncol* 1:179–186, 1983

Gellerman J, Wlodarczyk W, Hildebrandt B, Ganter H, et al.: Noninvasive magnetic resonance thermography of recurrent rectal carcinoma in a 1.5 Tesla hybrid system. *Cancer Res* 65:5872–5880, 2005

Gerner EW, Boon R, Conner WG, Hicks JA, Boon MLM: A transient thermotolerant survival response produced by single thermal doses in HeLa cells. *Cancer Res* 36:1035–1040, 1976

Gerner EW, Schneider MJ: Induced thermal resistance in HeLa cells. *Nature* 256:500–502, 1975

Gerweck LE, Nygaard TG, Burlett M: Response of cells to hyperthermia under acute and chronic hypoxic conditions. *Cancer Res* 39:966–972, 1979

Gonzalez Gonzalez D, van Dijk JDP, Blank LECM, Rumke PH: Combined treatment with radiation and hyperthermia in metastatic malignant melanoma. *Radiother Oncol* 6:105–113, 1986

Griffin RJ, Okajima K, Barrios B, Song CW: Mild temperature hyperthermia combined with carbogen breathing increases tumor partial pressure of oxygen (pO_2) and radiosensitivity. *Cancer Res* 56:5590–5593, 1996

Hahn GM, Li GC: Thermotolerance and heat shock proteins in mammalian cells. *Radiat Res* 92:452–457, 1982

Hahn GM, Shiu C: Adaptation to low pH modifies thermal and thermo-chemical responses of mammalian cells. *Int J Hyperther* 2:379–387, 1986

Hall EJ, Roizin-Towle L: Biological effects of heat. *Cancer Res* (Suppl) 44:4708S–4713S, 1984

Henle KJ: Sensitization to hyperthermia below 43°C induced in Chinese hamster ovary cells by step-down heating. *J Natl Cancer Inst* 64:1479–1483, 1980

Henle KJ, Kramuz JE, Leeper DB: Induction of thermotolerance in Chinese hamster ovary cells by high (45°) or low (40°) hyperthermia. *Cancer Res* 38:570–574, 1978

Henle KJ, Leeper DB: Combinations of hyperthermia (40°, 45°C) with radiation. *Radiology* 121:451–454, 1976

Hiraoka M, Jo S, Dodo Y, et al.: Clinical results of radiofrequency hyperthermia combined with radiation in the treatment of radioresistant cancers. *Cancer* 54:2898–2904, 1984

Hornback NB, Shupe RE, Shidnia H, Marshall CU, Lauer T: Advanced state IIIB cancer of the cervix treatment by hyperthermia and radiation. *Gynecol Oncol* 23:160–167, 1986

Horsman MR, Overgaard J: Can mild hyperthermia improve tumour oxygenation? *Int J Hypertherm* 13:141–147, 1997

Iwata K, Shakil A, Hur HJ, et al.: Tumor pO_2 can be increased markedly by mild hyperthermia. *Br J Cancer* 74(suppl):217s–221s, 1996

Jones EL, Prosnitz, LR, Dewhirst MW, Marcom PK, Hardenbergh H, Marks LB, Brizel DM, Vujaskovic Z: Thermochemoradiotherapy improves oxygenation in locally advanced breast cancer. *Clinical Cancer Res* 10:4287–4293, 2004

Kano E: Hyperthermia and drugs. In Overgaard J (ed): *Hyperthermic Oncology*, pp 277–282. London, Taylor & Francis, 1985

Kapp DS, Cox RS: Thermal treatment parameters are most predictive of outcome in patients with single tumor nodules per treatment field in recurrent adenocarcinoma of the breast. *Int J Radiat Oncol Biol Phys* 33:887–899, 1995

Kong G, Anyarambhatia G, Petros WP, Braum RD, Colvin OM, Needham D, Dewhirst MW: Efficacy of liposomes and hyperthermia in a human tumor xenograft model: Importance of triggered drug release. *Cancer Res* 60:6950–6957, 2001

Kong G, Braun RD, Dewhirst MW: Characterization of the effect of hyperthermia on nanoparticle extravasation from tumor vasculature. *Cancer Res* 61:3027–3032, 2001

Lam K, Astraham M, Langholtz B, et al.: Interstitial thermoradiotherapy for recurrent or persistent tumors. *Int J Hypertherm* 4:259–266, 1988

Law MP, Ahier RG, Field SB: The response of the mouse ear to heat applied alone or combined with x-rays. *Br J Radiol* 51:132–138, 1978

Leopold KA, Dewhirst M, Tucker JA, et al.: Relationships among tumor temperature, treatment time, and histopathological outcome using preoperative hyperthermia with radiation in soft tissue sarcomas. *Int J Radiat Oncol Biol Phys* 22:989–998, 1992

Li GC, Hahn GM: A proposed operational model of thermotolerance based on effects of nutrients and the initial treatment temperature. *Cancer Res* 40:4501–4508, 1980

Lindholm CE, Kjellen E, Nilsson P, Hertzman S: Microwave-induced hyperthermia and radiotherapy in human superficial tumours: Clinical results with a comparative study of combined treatment versus radiotherapy alone. *Int J Hypertherm* 3:393–411, 1987

MacFall JR, Prescott DM, Charles HC, et al.: 1H MRI Phase Thermometry *in vivo* in canine brain, muscle and tumor tissue. *Med Phys* 23:1775–1782, 1996

MacFall J, Prescott DM, Fullar E, et al.: Temperature dependence of canine brain tissue diffusion coefficient measured *in vivo* with magnetic resonance echo-planar imaging. *Int J Hyperthermia* 11:73–86, 1995

Nauts HC, Fowler GA, Bogatko FA: A review of the influence of bacterial infection and of bacterial products (Corey's toxins) on malignant tumors in man. *Acta Med Scand* 276:1–103, 1953

Oleson JR, Dewhirst MW, Harrelson JM, Leopold KA, Samulski TV, Tso CY: Tumor temperature distributions predict hyperthermia effect. *Int J Radiat Oncol Biol Phys* 16:559–570, 1989

Oleson J, Heusinkveld A, Manning M: Hyperthermia by magnetic induction: II. Clinical experience with concentric electrodes. *Int J Radiat Oncol Biol Phys* 9:549–566, 1983

Oleson JR, Samulski TV, Leopold KA, et al.: Sensitivity of hyperthermia trial outcomes to temperature and time: Implications for thermal goals of treatment. *Int J Radiat Oncol Biol Phys* 25:289–297, 1993

Overgaard J: Historical perspectives of hyperthermia. In Overgaard J (ed): *Introduction to Hyperthermic Oncology*, vol 2. New York, Taylor & Francis, 1984

Overgaard J, Gonzalez Gonzalez D, Hulschof MC, Arcangeli G, Dahl O, Mella O, Bentzen SM: Hyperthermia as an adjuvant to radiation therapy of recurrent or metastatic malignant melanoma: A multicentre randomized trial by the European Society for Hyperthermic Oncology. *Int J Hypertherm* 12:3–20, 1996

Overgaard J, Gonzalez Gonzalez D, Hulschof MC, et al.: Randomized trial of hyperthermia as adjuvant to radiotherapy for recurrent or metastatic malignant melanoma. *Lancet* 345:540–543, 1995

Overgaard J, Overgaard M: Hyperthermia as an adjuvant to radiotherapy in the treatment of malignant melanoma. *Int J Hypertherm* 3:483–501, 1987

Perez CA, Kuske RR, Emani B, Fineberg B: Irradiation alone or combined with hyperthermia in the treatment of recurrent carcinoma of the breast in the chest wall: A nonradomized comparison. *Int J Hypertherm* 2:179–187, 1986

Robinson JE, Wizenburg MJ: Thermal sensitivity and the effect of elevated temperatures on the radiation sensitivity of Chinese hamster cells. *Acta Radiol* 13:241–248, 1974

Roizin-Towle L, Hall EJ, Capuano L: Interaction of hyperthermia and cytotoxic agents. *Natl Cancer Inst Monogr* 61:149–151, 1982

Sapareto SA, Dewey WC: Thermal dose determination in cancer therapy. *Int J Radiat Oncol Biol Phys* 10:787–800, 1984

Sherar M, Liu FF, Pintilie M, et al.: Relationship between thermal dose and outcome in thermoradiotherapy treatments for superficial recurrences of breast cancer: Data from a phase III trial. *Int J Radiat Oncol Biol Phys* 39:371–380, 1997

Sneed PK, Stauffer PR, Diederich CJ, et al.: Survival benefit of hyperthermia in a prospective randomized trial of brachytherapy boost ± hyperthermia for glioblastoma multiforme. *Int J Radiat Oncol Biol Phys* 40:287–295, 1998

Song CW: Effect of local hyperthermia on blood flow and microenvironment: A review. *Cancer Res* 44(suppl):4721S–4730S, 1984

Song CW, Park HJ, Griffin RJ. Improvement of tumor oxygenation by mild hyperthermia. *Review Radiat Res* 155:515–528, 2001

Song CW, Shakil A, Griffin RJ, Okajima K. Improvement of tumor oxygenation status by mild temperature hyperthermia alone or in combination with carbogen. *Seminar Oncol* 24:626–635, 1997

Song CW, Shakil A, Osborn JL, Iwata K: Tumour oxygenation is increased by hyperthermia at mild temperatures. *Int J Hyperthermia* 12:367–373, 1996

Steeves RA, Severson SB, Paliwal BR, Anderson S, Robins HI: Matched-pair analysis of response to local hyperthermia and megavoltage electron therapy for superficial human tumors. *Endocuriether Hyperther Oncol* 2:163–170, 1986

Subjeck JR, Sciandra JJ, Chao CF, Johnson RJ: Heat shock proteins and biological response to hyperthermia. *Br J Cancer* 45(suppl V):127–131, 1982

Urano M: Kinetics of thermotolerance in normal and tumor tissues: A review. *Cancer Res* 46:474–482, 1986

Urano M, Kenton A, Kahn J: The effect of hyperthermia on the early and late appearing mouse foot reactions and on the radiation carcinogenesis: Effect on early and late appearing reactions. *Int J Radiat Oncol Biol Phys* 15:159–166, 1988

Valdagni R, Amichetti M: Report of long-term follow-up in a randomized trial comparing radiation therapy and radiation therapy plus hyperthermia to metastatic lymph nodes in stage IV head and neck patients. *Int J Radiat Oncol Biol Phys* 28:163–169, 1994

Valdagni R, Kapp DS, Valdagni C: N3 (TNM-UICC) metastatic neck nodes managed by combined radiation therapy and hyperthermia: Clinical results and analysis of treatment parameters. *Int J Hyperthermia* 2:189–200, 1986

van der Zee J, Gonzalez Gonzalez D, Vernon CC, et al.: Therapeutic gain by hyperthermia added to radiotherapy. ICRO/OGRO 6, 6th Int. Meeting on Progress in Radio-Oncology, Salzburg, Austria, May 13–17, 1998

Vernon CC, Hand JW, Field SB, et al.: Radiotherapy with or without hyperthermia in the treatment of superficial localized breast cancer: Results from five randomized controlled trials. *Int J Radiat Oncol Biol Phys* 35:731–744, 1996

Vora N, Shaw S, Forell B, et al.: Primary radiation combined with hyperthermia for advanced (stage III–IV) and inflammatory carcinoma of breast. *Endocuriether Hyperther Oncol* 2:101–106, 1986

Westra A, Dewey WC: Variation in sensitivity to heat shock during the cell cycle of Chinese hamster cells *in vitro. Int J Radiat Biol* 19:467–477, 1971

Glossary

A: Symbol for mass number.
absolute risk: The risk of an adverse health effect that is independent of other causes of that same health effect.
absorbed dose (D): The energy imparted per unit mass by ionizing radiation to matter at a specific point. The SI unit of absorbed dose is joule per kilogram (J/kg). The special name for this unit is gray (Gy). The previously used special unit of absorbed dose, the rad, was defined to be an energy absorption of 100 erg/g. Thus, 1 Gy = 100 rad.
absorption: Removal of x-rays from a beam.
accelerated fractionation: Reduction in overall treatment time; a schedule in which the average rate of dose delivery exceeds the equivalent of 10 Gy (1,000 rad) per week in 2-Gy (200-rad) fractions.
accelerator (linear): A machine, often called a *linac*, that produces high-energy x-rays for the treatment of cancer.
acentric ring: A circular piece of a chromosome lacking a centromere.
acidic fibroblast growth factor (FGF): A mitogen for many types of cells of mesodermal origin, including endothelial cells, chondrocytes, and fibroblasts. In presence of heparin, induces blood vessel growth.
action level: Concentration of radon in a house above which it is recommended that some action be taken to reduce that radon level; currently, the action level is 4 pCi/L in the United States.
activation: The process of making a material radioactive by bombardment with neutrons, protons, or other nuclear particles. See **activation analysis**.
activation analysis: Identifying and measuring chemical elements in a sample of material. First, the sample is made radioactive by bombardment with neutrons, charged particles, or γ-rays. Then the newly formed radioactive atoms in the sample give off characteristic nuclear radiations, such as γ-rays, which tell the types and quantities of atoms present. Activation analysis is usually more sensitive than chemical analysis.
activity: Quantity of a radionuclide that describes the rate at which decays occur in an amount of a radionuclide. The SI unit of radioactivity is the becquerel (Bq), which replaced the old unit, the curie (Ci). One becquerel corresponds to one disintegration of a radionuclide per second.
acute radiation syndrome (ARS): Biologic changes and symptoms, including death, that occur within weeks after a high-intensity total-body irradiation.
acyclovir: A nucleoside analogue of guanosine that blocks DNA replication when incorporated into an elongating polynucleotide. Used under the trade name Zovirax as a treatment for herpes.
additive: A situation in which the effect of a combination is the sum of the effects of the separate treatments (i.e., independent cell kill).
adenoma: A benign tumor of epithelial origin, such as a polyp of the colon.
adenovirus: One of a group of viruses responsible for upper respiratory and other infections in humans, other mammals, and birds. Adenoviruses are useful as a vector in gene therapy because they infect both dividing and nondividing cells, but the downside to their use is that they evoke an immune response, which makes their repeated use difficult.
adjuvant therapy: A treatment method used in addition to the primary therapy. Radiation therapy often is used as an adjuvant to surgery or chemotherapy.
ALARA (as low as reasonably achievable): The principle of limiting the radiation dose of exposed persons to levels as low as are reasonably achievable, economic and social factors being taken into account.
alleles: Alternate forms of a gene or DNA sequence on the two homologous chromosomes of a pair.
alopecia: Hair loss.

alpha/beta ratio (α/β ratio): The ratio of the parameters α and β in the linear-quadratic model; used to quantify the fractionation sensitivity of tissues.

alpha fetoprotein (AFP): A 70-kDa glycoprotein synthesized in embryonic development by the yolk sac. High levels of this protein in the amniotic fluid are associated with neural tube defects such as spina bifida. Lower than normal levels may be associated with Down's syndrome.

alpha particle (α-particle): A positively charged particle emitted by radioactive materials. It consists of two neutrons and two protons bound together; hence, it is identical with the nucleus of a helium atom. It is the least penetrating of the three common types of radiation—α, β, and γ—and it is stopped by a sheet of paper. It is not dangerous to plants, animals, or humans unless the α-emitting substance has entered the organisms. α-Particles are ejected from a nucleus during the decay of some radioactive elements; for example, an α-particle is emitted if either of the radon progeny polonium-218 or polonium-214 decays.

alpha ray (α-ray): A stream of α-particles. Used loosely as a synonym for α-particles.

***Alu* sequence:** An interspersed DNA sequence of approximately 300 bp found in the genome of primates that is cleaved by the restriction enzyme *Alu* I. *Alu* sequences are composed of a head-to-tail dimer, with the first monomer approximately 140 bp and the second approximately 170 bp. In humans, they are dispersed throughout the genome and are present in 300,000 to 600,000 copies, constituting some 3 to 6% of the genome. See **SINES**.

Ames test: A procedure devised by Bruce Ames to test carcinogenic properties of chemicals by their ability to induce mutations in the bacterium *Salmonella*.

amino acid: Any of the 20 subunit building blocks that are covalently linked to form proteins.

ampicillin: An antibiotic that prevents bacterial growth.

amplify: To increase the number of copies of a DNA sequence by inserting into a cloning vector that replicates within a host cell *in vivo* or *in vitro* by the polymerase chain reaction.

analogue: A chemical compound structurally similar to another, but differing by a single functional group (e.g., 5-bromodeoxyuridine is an analogue of thymidine).

anaphase: Stage of cell division in which chromosomes begin moving to opposite poles of the cell.

anemia: Having too few red blood cells. Symptoms of anemia include feeling tired, weak, and short of breath.

aneuploidy: A condition in which the chromosome number is not an exact multiple of the haploid set.

angiography: The radiographic visualization of blood vessels following introduction of contrast material.

angioplasty: Reconstruction of blood vessels.

angstrom (Å): A unit of length equal to 10^{-10} m.

anneal: The pairing of complementary DNA or RNA sequences via hydrogen bonding to form a double-stranded polynucleotide.

anode: Positive side of the x-ray tube; contains the target.

anorexia: Poor appetite.

antibiotic: A class of natural and synthetic compounds that inhibit the growth of or kill microorganisms.

antibiotic resistance: The ability of a microorganism to disable an antibiotic or prevent transport of the antibiotic into the cell.

antibody: Protein (immunoglobulin) produced in response to an antigenic stimulus with the capacity to bind specifically to the antigen.

antiemetic: A drug used to control nausea and vomiting.

antigen: Any foreign substance that elicits an immune response by stimulating the production of antibodies.

antiparallel: Describing molecules in parallel alignment, but running in opposite directions. Most commonly used to describe the opposite orientations of the two strands of a DNA molecule.

antisense RNA: A complementary RNA sequence that binds to a naturally occurring (sense) mRNA molecule, thus blocking its translation.

apoptosis: A mode of rapid cell death after irradiation in which the cell nucleus displays characteristic densely staining globules and at least some of the DNA is subsequently broken down into internucleosomal units. Sometimes postulated to be a "programmed," and therefore potentially controllable, process. Plays an important part in embryogenesis and in tissue regeneration following an insult and can eliminate cells whose DNA has been damaged and not repaired with a high fidelity.

Arrhenius plot: Probably the most common life–stress relationship when the stress is thermal. In hyperthermia research, a plot of $1/D_0$ versus 1/T, where D_0 is the reciprocal of the slope of the cell survival curve and T is the absolute temperature. Named after the Swedish physical chemist.

asexual reproduction: Production of offspring in the absence of any sexual process.

atomic mass: See **atomic weight**.

atomic mass unit (amu): One sixteenth the mass of a neutral atom of the most abundant isotope of oxygen, ^{16}O. See **atomic weight, mass number**.

atomic number (Z): The number of protons in the nucleus of an atom and also its positive charge.

atomic weight (at. wt.): The mass of an atom relative to other atoms. The present-day basis for the scale of atomic weights is oxygen; the commonest isotope of this element arbitrarily has been assigned an atomic weight of 16. The unit of the scale is 1/16 the weight of the ^{16}O atom, or roughly the mass of one proton or one neutron. The atomic weight of any element is approximately equal to the total number of protons and neutrons in its nucleus. Compare **atomic number**.

autoimmune disease: The production of antibodies that results from an immune response to one's own molecules, cells, or tissues. Such a response results from the inability of the immune system to distinguish self from non-self. Diseases such as arthritis, scleroderma, systemic lupus erythematosus, and perhaps diabetes are considered autoimmune diseases.

autoradiography: Use of a photographic emulsion to detect the distribution of a radioactive label in a tissue specimen.

autosomes: Chromosomes other than the sex chromosomes. In humans, there are 22 pairs of autosomes.

B lymphocyte: A white blood cell responsible for production of antibodies involved in the humoral immune response.

background radiation: The radiation in the natural environment, including cosmic rays and radiation from the naturally radioactive elements, both outside and inside the bodies of humans and animals. Also called *natural radiation*. The term also may mean radiation that is unrelated to a specific experiment.

bacteriophage: A virus that infects bacteria. Altered forms are used as vectors for cloning DNA.

bacterium: A single-celled prokaryotic organism.

basal cells: Cells at the base of the wall of the lung airways. These cells divide to replenish the other cells in the lung wall and often are considered the key cells that, if damaged, can lead to lung cancer.

base pair: A pair of complementary nitrogenous bases in a DNA molecule—adenine–thymine and guanine–cytosine. Also, the unit of measurement for DNA sequences.

basic fibroblast growth factor (FGF): A mitogen for many types of cells of mesodermal or neuroectodermal origin. Has a variety of angiogenic properties.

B-DNA: See **double helix**.

beam: A stream of particles or electromagnetic radiation moving in a single direction.

becquerel (Bq): Unit of radioactivity, corresponding to one radioactive disintegration per second. See **activity**.

benign: Describing a slow-growing, not malignant, tumor that does not spread to other parts of the body. If completely removed, benign lesions do not tend to recur. Incompletely removed tumors may recur but do not spread. Although benign, these tumors may cause permanent damage to some structures in the brain.

beta particle (β-particle): An elementary particle emitted from a nucleus during radioactive decay, with a single electrical charge and a mass equal to 1/1,837 that of a proton. A negatively charged β-particle is identical to an electron. A positively charged β-particle is called a *positron*. β-Radiation may cause skin burns, and β-emitters are harmful if they enter the body. β-Particles, however, are stopped easily by a thin sheet of metal.

BeV: One billion electron volts. Also written GeV.

bilateral: On both sides of the body.

biochemistry: Chemical reactions that sustain life.

biologic half-life: See **half-life, biologic**.

biologic therapy: Treatment to stimulate or restore the ability of the immune system to fight infection and disease. Also called *immunotherapy*.

biologically effective dose (BED): In fractionated radiotherapy, the quantity by which different fractionation regimens are compared.

biopsy: The removal of a small portion of a tumor to allow a pathologist to examine it under a microscope and provide a diagnosis of tumor type.

biotechnology: Commercial or industrial processes that utilize biologic organisms or products.

blob: A concentration of about 12 ion pairs in a region about 7 nm in diameter.

blood count: The number of red blood cells, white blood cells, and platelets in a sample of blood.

body burden: The amount of radioactive material present in a human or an animal. See **background radiation**, **whole-body counter**.

bone marrow: Spongy tissue in the cavities of large bones where the body's blood cells are produced.

bone seeker: A radioisotope that tends to accumulate in the bones; for example, the strontium-90 isotope, which behaves chemically like calcium.

brachytherapy: Internal radiation treatment achieved by implanting radioactive material directly into the tumor or very close to it. Sometimes called *internal radiation therapy*.

breeder reactor: A nuclear reactor that produces fissionable fuel as well as consuming it, especially one that creates more than it consumes. The new fissionable material is created by neutron capture in fertile materials. The process by which this occurs is known as *breeding*.

Bremsstrahlung x-rays: X-rays resulting from interaction of the projectile electron with a target nucleus; braking radiation.

5-bromodeoxyuridine (BrdU or BrdUrd): A mutagenically active analogue of thymidine in which the methyl group at the 6′ position in thymine is replaced by bromine.

by-product material: Any radioactive material (except source material or fissionable material) obtained during the production or the use of source material or fissionable material. By-product material includes fission products and many other radioisotopes produced in nuclear reactors.

bystander effect: Induction of biologic effects in cells that are not directly traversed by a charged particle but are in close proximity to cells that are.

cancer: A general name for more than 100 diseases in which abnormal cells grow out of control; a malignant tumor.

carcinogen: A physical or chemical agent capable of causing cancer, such as radon progeny, cigarette smoke, or asbestos.

carcinogenesis: Process that leads to the formation of a cancer. It involves several stages (resulting from successive alterations of the genome). The first stage is *initiation* (which may, for instance, be due to the mutation of a proto-oncogene into an oncogene). For a normal cell to be "transformed" (i.e., for it to become preneoplasic), its genome has to undergo several modifications: appearance of an oncogene, inactivation of both copies of a suppressor gene, immortalization (i.e., acquisition of an unlimited capacity to proliferate), changes affecting the apoptosis system, and so on. A transformed cell can give rise to an invasive cancer at the end of the second stage, known as *promotion*, which is associated with the proliferation of the descendants of the initiated cell and the escape of one of them from the control of the normal surrounding cells and of the body.

carcinogenic: Having the potential (as, for example, smoke or alcohol) to contribute to the development of cancer (same as **oncogenic**).

carcinoma: A malignant tumor derived from epithelial tissue, which forms the skin and outer cell layers of internal organs.

CAT scan: Computerized axial tomography, often called a *CT scan*, which provides three-dimensional x-ray images of some part of the body. It is useful for diagnosing cancer and for planning radiation therapy treatments.

catalyst: A substance that promotes a chemical reaction by lowering the activation energy of a chemical reaction, but itself remains unaltered at the end of the reaction.

cataract: An opacification in the normally transparent lens of the eye.

cathode: Negative side of the x-ray tube; contains the filament and focusing cup.

Cdc2 (also known as Cdk1): Kinase that associates with cyclin B to regulate entry into mitosis. Complex is activated by Cdc25-mediated dephosphorylation. Also associates with cyclin A during M phase.

Cdc25C: Phosphatase that activates the cyclin B–Cdc2 complex.

Cdk2: Kinase that associates with cyclin E during the G_1/S transition and cyclin A during S phase. Inhibited by p21 and p27.

Cdk4: Kinase that associates with cyclin D_1. Complex can phosphorylate pRb to allow cells to progress through G_1. Inhibited by p16, p21, and p27.

Cdks (cyclin-dependent kinases): Proteins that complex with their cyclin regulatory subunits to phosphorylate proteins necessary for progression through the cell cycle.

cDNA (copy DNA): DNA synthesized from an RNA template using reverse transcriptase.

cDNA library: A library composed of complementary copies of cellular mRNAs (i.e., the exons without the introns).

cell cycle: Sum of the phases of growth of an individual cell type; divided into G_1 (gap 1), S

(DNA synthesis), G_2 (gap 2), and M (mitosis); the cycle of cellular events from one mitosis to the next.

cell loss factor (Φ): The rate of cell loss from a tumor as a proportion of the rate at which cells are being added to the tumor by mitosis.

cell-cycle time: The time between one mitosis and the next.

cells: The body's tiny functioning units, which can be observed under a microscope. Each cell plays a specialized role in the body. Groups of cells are organized together to form tissues. Tissues are organized to form organs in the body.

cellular oncogene (proto-oncogene): A normal gene that if mutated or improperly expressed contributes to the development of cancer.

centimorgan: A unit of distance between genes on chromosomes. One centimorgan represents a value of 1% crossing over between two genes.

central nervous system (CNS): The brain and spinal cord.

centriole: A cytoplasmic organelle composed of nine groups of microtubules, generally arranged in triplets. Centrioles function in the generation of cilia and flagella and serve as foci for the spindles in cell division.

centromere: The chromosome constriction to which the spindle fiber attaches. The position of the centromere determines whether chromosomes are metacentric (X shaped; e.g., chromosomes 1, 3, 16, 19, 20) or acrocentric (inverted V shaped; e.g., chromosomes 13–15, 21, 22, Y). During mitosis, the identical chromatids of each chromosome are separated by shortening of the spindle fibers attached to opposite poles of the dividing cell.

c-*Erb*-B2(*HER2/neu*): A gene closely related to the epidermal growth factor receptor, which is amplified in a variety of cancers, including that of the breast.

cervix: The lower part of the uterus, which projects out into the vagina.

c-*fos*: An early-response gene induced by mitogenic stimuli. Forms complexes in the nucleus that act as transcription factors. Recognizes AP-1 sites if complexed with c-*jun*.

chain reaction: A reaction that stimulates its own repetition. In a fission chain reaction, a fissionable nucleus absorbs a neutron and fissions, releasing additional neutrons. These, in turn, can be absorbed by other fissionable nuclei, releasing still more neutrons. A fission chain reaction is self-sustaining if the number of neutrons released in a given time equals or exceeds the number of neutrons lost by absorption in nonfissioning material or by escape from the system.

characteristic x-rays: X-rays produced following ionization of inner-shell electrons; characteristic of the target element.

charged particle: An ion; an elementary particle that carries a positive or negative electrical charge.

chemotherapist: A physician who specializes in the use of drugs to treat cancer, now called a *medical oncologist.*

chemotherapy: A treatment for cancers that involves administering chemicals toxic to malignant cells.

chromatid: Each of the two progeny strands of a duplicated chromosome joined at the centromere during mitosis and meiosis.

chromatin: The complex of DNA, RNA, histones, and nonhistone proteins that make up chromosomes.

chromatography: Technique for the separation of a mixture of solubilized molecules by their differential migration over a substrate.

chromosomal aberration: Any change resulting in the duplication, deletion, or rearrangement of chromosomal material.

chromosomal instability: An effect of irradiation in which chromosomal aberrations continue to appear through many cell generations.

chromosomal mutation: See **chromosomal aberration**.

chromosomal polymorphism: Alternate structures or arrangements of a chromosome that are carried by members of a population.

chromosome: In prokaryotes, an intact DNA molecule containing the genome; in eukaryotes, a DNA molecule complexed with RNA and proteins to form a threadlike structure containing genetic information arranged in a linear sequence.

chromosome banding: Technique for the differential staining of mitotic or meiotic chromosomes to produce a characteristic banding pattern or selective staining of certain chromosomal regions such as centromeres, the nucleolus organizer regions, and GC- or AT-rich regions.

chromosome map: A diagram showing the location of genes on chromosomes.

chronic: Persisting for a long time.

chronic hypoxia: Persistent low oxygen concentrations, such as exists in viable tumor cells close to regions of necrosis.

c-*jun*: An early-response gene induced by mitogenic stimuli and stress responses. Forms complexes in the nucleus that act as transcription factors. Recognizes AP-1 sites if complexed with c-*fos*.

classical scattering: Scattering of x-rays with no loss of energy.

clinical trials: Medical research studies conducted with volunteers. Each study is designed to answer scientific questions and to find better ways to prevent or treat disease.

clone: Genetically identical cells or organisms all derived from a single ancestor by asexual or parasexual methods; for example, a DNA segment that has been enzymatically inserted into a plasmid or chromosome of a phage or bacterium and replicated to form many copies.

cloned library: A collection of cloned DNA molecules representing all or part of an individual's genome.

clonogenic cells: Cells that have the capacity to produce an expanding family of descendants (usually at least 50). Also called colony-forming cells or clonogens.

c-*myc*: An early-response gene induced by mitogenic stimuli, as well as TGF-β. Is highly overexpressed as a result of translocations in Burkitt's lymphomas. Gene is amplified in certain cancers, as is its relative, N-*myc*.

cobalt-60: A radioactive substance used as a radiation source to treat cancer.

code: See **genetic code**.

codon: A group of three nucleotides that specifies the addition of one of the 20 amino acids during translation of mRNA into a polypeptide.

colchicine: An alkaloid compound that inhibits spindle formation during cell division. Used in the preparation of karyotypes to collect a large population of cells inhibited at the metaphase stage of mitosis.

collective dose: Usually refers to the collective effective dose obtained by multiplying the average effective dose by the number of persons exposed to that given dose. Expressed in person-sieverts. The old unit was the man-rem.

colon: Large intestine.

colony: A group of identical cells derived from a single ancestor cell.

combination chemotherapy: The use of more than one drug to treat cancer.

complementarity: Chemical affinity between nitrogenous bases as a result of hydrogen bonding. Responsible for the base pairing between the strands of the DNA double helix.

complementary nucleotides: Members of the pairs adenine–thymine, adenine–uracil, and guanine–cytosine, which have the ability to hydrogen-bond to each other.

complementation: Identification of whether a (radiosensitive) phenotype in different mutants is due to the same gene. Studied by means of cell fusion.

complementation test: A genetic test to determine whether two mutations occur within the same gene. If two mutations are introduced into a cell simultaneously and produce a wild-type phenotype (i.e., they complement each other), they are often nonallelic. If a mutant phenotype is produced, the mutations are noncomplementing and are often allelic.

Compton effect: Scattering of x-rays resulting in ionization and loss of energy. The energy lost by the photon is given to the ejected electron as kinetic energy.

concomitant boost: The practice of adding an extra dose to a smaller field on the later days of a fractionated regimen.

concordance: Pairs or groups of individuals identical in their phenotype. In twin studies, a condition in which both twins exhibit or fail to exhibit a trait under investigation.

conduction: Transfer of heat by molecular agitation.

conductor: Material that allows heat or electrical current to flow.

connective tissue: The tissues of the body that bind together and support various structures of the body. Examples are bone, cartilage, and muscle.

consequential late effects: Late effects that develop as a consequence of severe early effects.

contrast agent: A chemical used to highlight disease processes on x-ray tests, contrasting them against the background of normal tissues.

control group: A group of people subject to the same conditions as another group under study, except that the control group is not exposed to the specific factor being investigated in the study group.

cosmic rays: Radiation of many sorts, but mostly protons and heavier atomic nuclei with very high energies originating outside the earth's atmosphere. Cosmic radiation is part of the natural background radiation. Some cosmic rays are more energetic than any human-made forms of radiation.

cosmid: A vector designed to allow cloning of large segments of foreign DNA

(25,000–45,000 bp). Cosmids are hybrids composed of the cos sites of lambda inserted into a plasmid. In cloning, the recombinant DNA molecules are packaged into phage protein coats, and after infection of bacterial cells, the recombinant molecule replicates and can be maintained as a plasmid.

covalent bond: A nonionic chemical bond formed by the sharing of electrons.

critical: Capable of sustaining a chain reaction. See **criticality**.

critical assembly: An assembly of sufficient fissionable material and moderator to sustain a fission chain reaction at a very low power level, permitting study of the assembly's components for various fissionable materials in different geometric arrangements.

critical mass: The smallest mass of fissionable material that supports a self-sustaining chain reaction under stated conditions.

criticality: The state of a nuclear reactor if it is sustaining a chain reaction.

cross section (σ): A measure of the probability that a nuclear reaction will occur. Usually measured in barns, it is the apparent or effective area presented by a target nucleus or particle to an oncoming particle or other nuclear radiation, such as a photon of γ-radiation.

crossing over: The exchange of chromosomal material (parts of chromosomal arms) between homologous chromosomes by breakage and reunion. The exchange of material between nonsister chromatids during meiosis is the basis of genetic recombination.

CT scan (CAT scan, CT x-ray): A three-dimensional x-ray. CT stands for *computerized tomography*.

cure: An outcome of treatment that leaves the patient disease free, with no likelihood of recurrence.

curie (Ci): Old unit of radioactivity, corresponding to 3.7×10^{10} radioactive disintegrations per second. Now replaced by the becquerel.

cyclic adenosine monophosphate (cAMP): An important regulatory molecule in both prokaryotic and eukaryotic organisms.

cyclin A: Regulatory protein that associates with Cdk2 during the S phase of the cell cycle.

cyclin B: Regulatory protein that associates with Cdc2 to regulate entry into mitosis.

cyclin E: Protein that associates with Cdk2 during late G_1 phase and is thought to regulate entry into S phase.

cyclin D_1: One of three cyclin D family members (also D_2, D_3). Associates with Cdk5 or Cdk6 to regulate through the G_1 phase of the cell cycle. Is induced by a variety of mitogens.

cyclins: Proteins that complex with Cdks to regulate progression through the cell cycle.

cyst: A cavity, usually filled with a liquid, sometimes associated with benign or malignant tumors.

cytogenetics: Study that relates the appearance and behavior of chromosomes to genetic phenomena.

cytokines: Polypeptides originally defined as being released from lymphocytes and involved in maintenance of the immune system. These factors have pleiotropic effects on not only hematopoietic cells but on many other cell types as well.

D_0: A parameter in the multitarget equation: the radiation dose that reduces survival to e^{-1} (i.e., 0.37) of its previous value on the exponential portion of the survival curve.

Dalton: A unit of measurement equal to the mass of a hydrogen atom, 1.67×10^{-24} g; 1/Avogadro's number.

daughter: A nuclide formed by the radioactive decay of another nuclide, which in this context is called the *parent*. Replaced by *progeny*.

decay, radioactive: The spontaneous transformation of one nuclide into a different nuclide or into a different energy state of the same nuclide. The process results in a decrease, with time, of the original radioactive atoms in a sample. Radioactive decay involves the emission from the nucleus of α-particles, β-particles (electrons), or γ-rays; the nuclear capture or ejection of orbital electrons; or fission. Also called *radioactive disintegration*. See **half-life**, **radioactive series**.

decay series (decay chain): A series of radioactive atoms, each the progeny of the one before and the parent of the one after; the series ends if any progeny is not radioactive.

deletion: A segment of a chromosome that is missing as a result of two breaks and the loss of the intervening piece.

denature: To induce structural alterations that disrupt the biologic activity of a molecule. Often refers to breaking hydrogen bonds between base pairs in double-stranded nucleic acid molecules to produce single-stranded polynucleotides or altering the secondary and tertiary structure of a protein, destroying its activity.

dermatitis: A skin rash.

deterministic effect: An effect for which the severity of the effect in affected individuals varies with the dose, and for which a threshold usually exists.

deuterium (^2H, D): An isotope of hydrogen whose nucleus contains one neutron and one proton and therefore is about twice as heavy as the nucleus of normal hydrogen, which contains only a single proton. Deuterium often is referred to as *heavy hydrogen*; it occurs in nature as 1 atom to every 6,500 atoms of normal hydrogen. It is nonradioactive. Compare **tritium**. See **heavy water**.

deuteron: The nucleus of deuterium. It contains one proton and one neutron.

dicentric chromosome: A chromosome having two centromeres.

dideoxynucleotide (*did*N): A deoxynucleotide that lacks a 3′ hydroxyl group and is thus unable to form a 3′–5′ phosphodiester bond necessary for chain elongation. Dideoxynucleotides are used in DNA sequencing and the treatment of viral diseases.

differential diagnosis: A list of the most likely diagnoses for a particular set of symptoms and x-ray findings. The use of different imaging techniques often narrows the differential diagnosis to the most likely disease present.

differentiation: The process of complex changes by which cells and tissues attain their adult structure and functional capacity.

digest: To cut DNA molecules with one or more restriction endonucleases.

diploid: A condition in which each chromosome exists in pairs; having two of each chromosome.

direct action: Ionization or excitation of atoms within DNA leading to free radicals, as distinct from the reaction with DNA of free radicals formed in nearby water molecules.

disjunction: The separation of chromosomes at the anaphase stage of cell division.

diuretics: Drugs that help the body get rid of excess water and salt.

dizygotic twins: Twins produced from separate fertilization events; two ova fertilized independently. Also known as *fraternal twins*.

DNA (deoxyribonucleic acid): An organic acid composed of four nitrogenous bases (adenine, thymine, cytosine, and guanine) linked via sugar and phosphate units. DNA is the genetic material of most organisms and usually exists as a double-stranded molecule in which two antiparallel strands are held together by hydrogen bonds between adenine–thymine and cytosine–guanine base pairs.

DNA fingerprint: A unique pattern of DNA fragments identified by Southern hybridization or by polymerase chain reaction.

DNA polymerase: An enzyme that catalyzes the synthesis of DNA from deoxyribonucleotides and a template DNA molecule.

DNA polymorphism: One or two or more alternate forms of a chromosomal locus that differ in nucleotide sequence or have variable numbers of repeated nucleotide units.

DNA sequencing: Procedures for determining the nucleotide sequence of a DNA fragment.

DNase (deoxyribonucleosidase): An enzyme that degrades or breaks down DNA into fragments or constitutive nucleotides.

dominance: The expression of a trait in the heterozygous condition.

dominant gene: A gene whose phenotype is expressed if it is present in a single copy.

dominant-acting oncogene: A gene that stimulates cell proliferation and contributes to oncogenesis when present in a single copy.

dose: General term for the quantity of radiation. See **absorbed dose**, **equivalent dose**, **effective dose**, **collective dose**.

dose rate: The radiation dose delivered per unit time and measured, for instance, in grays per hour.

dose-modifying factor (DMF): A ratio indicating the dose without to the dose with the agent for the same level of effect. (Similarly, *dose-reduction factor* or *sensitizer enhancement ratio*).

dose-rate effect: Decreasing radiation response with decreasing radiation dose rate.

dosimetrist: A person who plans and calculates the proper radiation dose for treatment.

double helix: The model for DNA structure proposed by James Watson and Francis Crick, involving two antiparallel, hydrogen-bonded polynucleotide chains wound into a right-handed helical configuration, with 10 base pairs per full turn of the double helix. Often called *B-DNA*.

double minutes: Chromosome fragments that are the result of chromosome duplication and in which oncogenes may be amplified. A common cytologic feature of tumor cells.

double trouble: The situation in which a hot spot within a treatment field receives not only a higher dose but also a higher dose per fraction, which means that the biologic effectiveness of the dose is also greater.

doubling dose: Applied to hereditary effects, the dose required to double the spontaneous mutation incidence; put another way, the dose required to produce an incidence of mutations equal to the spontaneous rate.

doubling time: The time it takes for a cell population or tumor volume to double its size.

***Drosophila melanogaster*:** The fruit fly, whose common use in genetic studies was introduced by Thomas Hunt Morgan in the early 1900s.

early-response gene: A gene such as c-*fos*, c-*jun*, or c-*myc*, whose mRNA levels are induced dramatically following mitogenic stimuli or stress.

early responses: Radiation-induced normal-tissue damage that is expressed in weeks to a few months after exposure. Generally due to damage to parenchymal cells. The α/β ratio tends to be large.

ED_{50} (effect dose 50%): Radiation dose that produces a specified effect in the normal tissues of 50% of animals.

edema: Abnormal accumulation of fluid (e.g., pulmonary edema, a buildup of fluid in the lungs).

effective dose: The radiation dose allowing for the fact that some types of radiation are more damaging than others, and some parts of the body are more sensitive to radiation than others. It is defined as the sum over specified tissues of the products of the equivalent dose in a tissue and the weighting factor for that tissue.

effective dose equivalent: Quantity obtained by multiplying the dose equivalent to a tissue by the appropriate risk weighting factor for that tissue. Expressed in sieverts.

electromagnetic radiation: Radiation consisting of associated and interacting electrical and magnetic waves that travel at the speed of light, such as light, radio waves, γ-rays, and x-rays. All electromagnetic radiation can be transmitted through a vacuum.

electron (e): An elementary particle with a unit negative electrical charge and a mass 1/1,837 that of the proton. Electrons surround the positively charged nucleus and determine the chemical properties of the atom. Positive electrons, or *positrons*, also exist.

electronvolt (eV): The amount of energy gained by a particle of charge e (-1.6×10^{-19} C) if it is accelerated by a potential difference of 1 V $1\ \text{eV} \approx 1.6 \times 10^{-19}$ J.

electrophoresis: The technique of separating charged molecules in a matrix to which an electrical field is applied.

electroporation: A process whereby high-voltage pulses of electricity are used to open pores in the cell membrane, through which foreign DNA can pass.

Ellis formula: The relation between dose, overall time, and number of fractions in radiotherapy.

endonuclease: An enzyme that cleaves at internal sites in the substrate molecule.

epidermal growth factor (EGF): Protein that promote growth of epidermal cells and can stimulate or inhibit the proliferation and differentiation of a wide variety of cells.

epithelium: A thin layer of cells in the skin, mucous membrane, or any duct that replaces worn-out cells by cell division.

equivalent dose: A quantity used for radiation protection purposes that takes into account the different probability of effects that occur with the same absorbed dose delivered by radiations with different radiation weighting factor values. It is defined as the product of the average absorbed dose in a specified organ or tissue and the radiation weighting factor values. If dose is in grays, equivalent dose is in sieverts.

erb-B (EGFR/HER1): Membrane receptor that binds epidermal growth hormone.

error-free repair: DNA repair whereby the molecule is reconstituted with a high fidelity (i.e., without loss of information).

erythropoietin: Cytokine that stimulate late erythroid progenitors to form small colonies of erythrocytes.

***Escherichia coli* (*E. coli*):** A bacterium found in the human colon that is used widely as a host for molecular cloning experiments.

ethidium bromide: A fluorescent dye that is used to stain DNA and RNA and that intercalates between nucleotides and fluoresces if exposed to ultraviolet light.

eukaryote: An organism whose cells posses a nucleus and other membrane-bounded vesicles, including all members of the protist, fungi, plant, and animal kingdoms.

evolution: The origin of plants and animals from preexisting types. Descent with modifications.

excision repair: Repair of DNA lesions by removal of a polynucleotide segment and its replacement with a newly synthesized, corrected segment.

exon: DNA segment of a gene that is transcribed and translated into protein.

exonuclease: An enzyme that breaks down nucleic acid molecules by breaking the phosphodiester bonds at the 3′ or 5′ terminal nucleotides.

exponential growth: Growth according to an exponential equation.

exponential survival curve: A survival curve without a threshold or shoulder region that is a straight line on a semilogarithmic plot.

exposure (X): (Often used in its more general sense and not as the specially defined radiation quantity). A measure of the quantity of x- or γ-radiation based on its ability to ionize the air through which it passes. The SI unit of exposure is coulomb per kilogram (C/kg). The previously used special unit of exposure was the röntgen (R).

expression library: A library of cDNAs whose encoded proteins are expressed by specialized vectors.

expression vector: A plasmid or phage-carrying promoter region designed to cause expression of cloned DNA sequences.

external radiotherapy: Radiation therapy that uses a machine located outside the body to aim high-energy rays at cancer cells. Sometimes called *external-beam radiotherapy*.

extrapolated total dose (ETD): Calculated isoeffect dose when the dose rate is very low or when fraction size is very small.

extrapolation number: A parameter in the multitarget equation: the point on the survival scale to which the straight part of the curve back-extrapolates.

familial trait: A trait transmitted through and expressed by members of a family.

fast neutrons: Neutrons with energy greater than approximately 100,000 eV. Compare **thermal neutrons**.

fibroblast: A precursor cell of connective tissue that is relatively easy to maintain in cell culture.

field: A term used in radiation oncology to describe or define an area through which x-rays are directed toward the tumor.

field-size effect: The dependence of normal-tissue damage on the size of the irradiated area; also known as *volume effect*.

film badge: An assembly containing a packet of unexposed photographic film and a variety of filters (absorbers); when the film is developed, the dose and type of radiation to which the wearer was exposed can be estimated.

fingerprint: The pattern of ridges and whorls on the tip of a finger. The pattern obtained by enzymatically cleaving a protein or nucleic acid and subjecting the digest to two-dimensional chromatography or electrophoresis.

FISH (fluorescence *in situ* hybridization): The process whereby fluorescent dyes are attached to specific regions of the genome, thus aiding the identification of chromosomal damage.

fission: The splitting of a heavy nucleus into two approximately equal parts (which are nuclei of lighter elements), accompanied by the release of a relatively large amount of energy and generally one or more neutrons. Fission can occur spontaneously, but usually it is caused by nuclear absorption of γ-rays, neutrons, or other particles.

fission products: The nuclei (fission fragments) formed by the fission of heavy elements plus the nuclides formed by the fission fragments' radioactive decay.

flanking region: The DNA sequences extending on either side of a specific locus or gene.

flexible tissues: Nonhierarchical cell populations in which function and proliferation take place in the same cells.

flow cytometry: Analysis of cell suspensions in which a dilute stream of cells is passed through a laser beam. DNA content and other properties are measured by light scattering and fluorescence following staining with dyes or labeled antibodies.

founder effect: A form of genetic drift. The establishment of a population by a small number of individuals whose genotypes carry only a fraction of the different kinds of alleles in the parental population.

fractionation: The daily dose of radiation based on the total dose divided into a particular number of daily treatments.

fragile site: A gap or nonstaining region of a chromosome that can be induced to generate chromosome breaks.

frameshift mutation: A mutational event leading to the insertion of one or more base pairs in a gene, shifting the codon reading frame in all codons following the mutational site.

free radical: A fragment of an atom or molecule that contains an unpaired electron which therefore make it very reactive.

fusion, thermonuclear: The reaction that occurs when two or more light nuclei coalesce to form a heavier nucleus with the release of energy.

fusion gene: A hybrid gene created by joining portions of two different genes (to produce a new protein) or by joining a gene to a different promoter (to alter or regulate gene transcription).

gamete: A specialized reproductive cell with a haploid number of chromosomes.

gamma rays (γ-rays): High-energy, short-wavelength electromagnetic radiation. γ-Radiation frequently accompanies α- and β-emissions and always accompanies fission. γ-Rays are very penetrating and are stopped best or shielded against by dense materials, such as lead or depleted uranium. γ-Rays are indistinguishable from x-rays except for their source: γ-rays originate inside the nucleus, x-rays from outside.

gastrointestinal (GI): Having to do with the digestive tract, which includes the mouth, esophagus, stomach, and intestines.

gene: The fundamental physical unit of heredity whose existence can be confirmed by allelic variants and that occupies a specific chromosomal locus; a DNA sequence coding for a single polypeptide.

gene amplification: The presence of multiple copies of a gene and one of the mechanisms by which proto-oncogenes are activated to result in neoplasia.

gene expression: The process of producing a protein from its DNA- and mRNA-coding sequences.

gene mutation: See **point mutation**.

gene pool: The total of all genes possessed by reproductive members of a population.

genetic burden: Average number of recessive lethal genes carried in the heterozygous condition by an individual in a population. Also called *genetic load*.

genetic code: The three-letter code that translates nucleic acid sequence into protein sequence.

genetic counseling: Analysis of risk for genetic defects in a family and the presentation of options available to avoid or ameliorate possible risks.

genetic disease: A disease that has its origin in changes to the genetic material, DNA. Usually refers to diseases that are inherited in a Mendelian fashion, although noninherited forms of cancer also result from DNA mutation.

genetic drift: Random variation in gene frequency from generation to generation, most often observed in small populations.

genetic effects of radiation: Radiation effects that can be transferred from parent to offspring; any radiation-caused changes in the genetic material of sex cells. Now called *hereditary effects*.

genetic engineering: The manipulation of an organism's genetic endowment by introducing or eliminating specific genes. A broad definition of genetic engineering also includes selective breeding and other means of artificial selection.

genetic polymorphism: The stable coexistence of two or more discontinuous genotypes in a population. If the frequencies of two alleles are carried to equilibrium, the condition is called *balanced polymorphism*.

genetically significant dose: The dose that, if given to every member of a population, should produce the same hereditary harm as the actual doses received by the individuals. Expressed in sieverts, this dose takes into account the childbearing potential of those receiving the dose.

genetics: The branch of biology that deals with heredity and the expression of inherited traits.

genome: The genetic complement contained in the chromosomes of a given organism, usually the haploid chromosome state.

genomic library: A library composed of fragments of genomic DNA.

genotype: The structure of DNA that determines the expression of a trait (phenotype).

GeV: One billion electronvolts. Also written BeV.

GI: Gastrointestinal.

giga: A prefix that multiplies a basic unit by 1 billion (10^9).

gonads: The ovaries or testes.

grade: In reference to tumors, the aggressiveness of the cell type, from very low aggressiveness with slow growth pattern to very aggressive with rapid spread. Tumor grading classifications vary according to type of tumor.

graft-versus-host disease (GVHD): In transplants, reaction by immunologically competent cells of the donor against the antigens present on the cells of the host. In human bone-marrow transplants, often a fatal condition.

granulocyte colony-stimulating factor (G-CSF): Cytokine that stimulates differentiation of progenitors into granulocytes.

granulocyte-macrophage colony-stimulating factor (GM-CSF): Cytokine that stimulates differentiation of progenitors into granulocytes, macrophages, and eosinophils.

gray (Gy): The special name for the SI unit of absorbed dose, kerma, and specific energy imparted equal to 1 J/kg. The previous unit of absorbed dose, rad, has been replaced by the gray. One gray equals 100 rad.

ground state: The state of a nucleus, an atom, or a molecule at its lowest (normal) energy level.

growth delay: Extra time required for an irradiated tumor to reach a given size, compared with an unirradiated control.

growth factor: A serum protein that stimulates cell division when it binds to its cell-surface receptor.

growth-factor receptor: A membrane-spanning protein that selectively binds its growth factor and then transduces a signal for cell division to other molecules in the cytoplasm and nucleus.

growth fraction: Proportion of viable cells in active cell division.

growth hormone (GH): Secreted by the anterior pituitary gland, a harmone that acts mainly on the growth of bone and muscles. Can be secreted by lymphocytes in response to phorbol ester treatment and may be involved in lymphocyte growth. Also known as *somatotropin*.

half-life ($t_{1/2}$): The time taken for the activity of a radionuclide to decay to half its initial value.

half-life, biologic: The time required for a biologic system, such as a human or an animal, to eliminate by natural processes half the amount of a substance, such as a radioactive material, that has entered it.

haploid: Having only one of each type of chromosome, as is usually the case in gametes (oocytes and spermatozoa).

heat shock: A transient response following exposure of cells or organisms to elevated temperatures. The response involves activation of a small number of loci, inactivation of previously active loci, and selective translation of heat-shock mRNA. Appears to be a nearly universal phenomenon, observed in organisms ranging from bacteria to humans.

heavy water (D_2O): Water containing significantly more than the natural proportion (1 in 6,500) of heavy hydrogen (deuterium) atoms to ordinary hydrogen atoms. Heavy water is a moderator in some nuclear reactors because it slows down neutrons effectively and also has a low cross section for absorption of neutrons.

helicase: An enzyme that participates in DNA replication by unwinding the double helix near the replication fork.

hematocrit: The percentage of blood made up of red blood cells.

hematology: The study of blood and its disorders.

hemizygous: Describing a condition in which a gene is present in a single dose. Usually applied to genes on the X chromosome in heterogametic males.

hemoglobin (Hb): An iron-containing, conjugated respiratory protein occurring chiefly in the red blood cells of vertebrates. Carries oxygen to the tissues.

hemophilia: A sex-linked trait in humans associated with defective blood-clotting mechanisms.

herpesvirus: One of a group of viruses causing herpes in man and other primates. These viruses are potentially useful as vectors in gene therapy because they are large and can accommodate a large insert, but they are seldom used in practice because they are potentially more pathogenic and difficult to control.

heterochromatin: The heavily staining, late-replicating regions of chromosomes that are condensed in interphase. Thought to be devoid of structural genes.

heterozygote: An individual with different alleles at one or more loci. Such individuals produce unlike gametes and therefore do not breed true.

hierarchical tissues: Cell populations comprising a lineage of stem cells, proliferating cells, and mature cells. The mature cells do not divide.

high-dose-rate (HDR) remote brachytherapy: A type of internal radiation in which each treatment is given in a few minutes with the radioactive source in place. The source of radioactivity is removed between treatments.

histones: Proteins complexed with DNA in the nucleus. They are rich in the basic amino acids arginine and lysine and function in the coiling of DNA to form nucleosomes.

HLA: Cell-surface proteins, produced by histocompatibility loci, that are involved in the acceptance or rejection of tissue and organ grafts and transplants.

homogeneously staining region: Segment of mammalian chromosomes that stains lightly with Giemsa following exposure of cells to a selective agent. These regions arise in conjunction with gene amplification and are regarded as the structural locus for the amplified gene.

homologous chromosomes: Chromosomes that have the same linear arrangement of genes; a pair of matching chromosomes in a diploid organism.

homologue: Any member of a set of genes or DNA sequences from different organisms whose nucleotide sequences show a high degree of one-to-one correspondence.

homozygote: An individual with identical alleles at one or more loci. Such individuals produce identical gametes and therefore breed true.

hormesis: The phenomenon whereby a physical or chemical agent has one effect at high doses and the reverse effect at low doses. It probably results from the activation of defense mechanisms. Hormesis is observed with several drug molecules that are toxic at high doses, but which can have a beneficial protective effect at low doses.

hormones: Factors synthesized in endocrine glands that if released act to regulate and modulate the functions of multicellular organisms.

Human Genome Project: A project coordinated by the National Institutes of Health (NIH) and the Department of Energy (DOE) to determine the entire nucleotide sequence of the human chromosomes.
hybrid: The offspring of two parents differing in at least one genetic characteristic.
hybridization: The hydrogen bonding of complementary DNA or RNA sequences to form a duplex molecule.
hybridoma: A somatic cell hybrid produced by the fusion of an antibody-producing cell and a cancer cell, specifically a myeloma. The cancer cell contributes the ability to divide indefinitely, and the antibody cell confers the ability to synthesize large amounts of a single antibody.
hydrogen bond: An electrostatic attraction between a hydrogen atom bonded to a strongly electronegative atom such as oxygen or nitrogen and another atom that is electronegative or contains an unshared electron pair.
hyperbaric oxygen (HBO): The use of high oxygen pressures (two or three atmospheres) to enhance oxygen availability in radiotherapy.
hyperdiploid: Additional chromosomes; the modal number is 47 or more.
hyperfractionated radiation: Division of the total dose of radiation into smaller doses usually given more than once a day.
hyperthermia: The use of heat to treat cancer.
hypodiploid: Loss of chromosomes with modal number 45 or less.
hypofractionation: The use of dose fractions substantially larger than the conventional level of ~2 Gy (~200 rad).
hypopharynx: Part of the lower throat beside and behind the larynx (voice box).
hypoxia: Low oxygen tension; usually the very low levels required to make cells maximally radioresistant. Sometimes used to mean *anoxia* (literally, the complete absence of oxygen).
ICRP: International Commission on Radiological Protection.
identical twins: See **monozygotic twins**.
IFNα: Cytokine that is produced in response to viral infection and that protects cells from viruses and causes growth arrest of normal and tumor cells.
IFNβ: Cytokine that is produced in response to viral infection and that protects cells from viruses and causes growth arrest of normal and tumor cells.
IFNγ: Cytokine that is produced in response to viral infection and that activates macrophages, protects cells from viruses, and causes growth arrest of normal and tumor cells.
IL-1: Cytokine involved in the regulation of immune and inflammatory responses.
IL-2: Cytokine that stimulates growth of T cells. Also stimulates B cell growth and differentiation, generation of lymphokine-activated killer cells, activation of macrophages, and production of other cytokines.
IL-3: Cytokine that induces the proliferation of hematopoietic cells, particularly erythroid and myeloid cells. Produced by activated T cells and mast cells.
IL-4: Cytokine that has general effects on hematopoietic cells, including the activation, growth, and differentiation of B cells. Also induces growth of mast cells and T cells.
IL-5: Cytokine that induces eosinophil differentiation, as well as B cell activation, growth, and differentiation.
IL-6: Cytokine that regulates B cell differentiation, T cell activation, killer cell induction, and other physiologic responses. Induced by cytokines, ultraviolet irradiation, and other stimuli. Many effects similar to IL-1 and TNF.
IL-7: Cytokine that promotes the growth of B and T cell progenitors.
IL-8: One of an extended family of cytokines that act as chemoattractants for neutrophils, T cells, and basophils.
IL-9: Cytokine that stimulates proliferation of T cells and enhances mast cell activity and growth.
IL-10: Cytokine that enhances IL-2 and IL-4 proliferative response of T cells. Also acts to inhibit cytokine production by a variety of different cells.
IL-11: Cytokine that together with other cytokines stimulates the growth of a variety of hematopoietic progenitors.
IL-12: Cytokine that promotes growth of T and natural killer cells and enhances cytotoxic T cell responses.
immortalization: Term used to describe the change as cells from somatic tissues that are only able to perform a limited number of cell divisions undergo a "crisis" and become capable of unlimited cell divisions.
immortalizing oncogene: A gene that upon transfection enables a primary cell to grow indefinitely in culture.
immune system: The body's defense system, which protects it from foreign substances, such as bacteria and viruses that are harmful to it.

immunoglobulin: The class of serum proteins having the properties of antibodies.

implant: A quantity of radioactive material placed in or near a cancer.

***in situ* hybridization:** A technique for the cytologic localization of DNA sequences complementary to a given nucleic acid or polynucleotide.

***in vitro*:** Literally, in glass; outside the living organism; occurring in an artificial environment.

***in vivo*:** Literally, in the living; occurring within the living body of an organism.

inbreeding: Mating between closely related organisms.

incomplete repair: Increased damage from fractionated radiotherapy if the time interval between doses is too short to allow complete recovery of sublethal damage.

indirect action: Damage to DNA by free radicals formed through the ionization of nearby water molecules.

inducible response: A response to irradiation that is modified by a small dose of radiation given shortly before.

infusion: Slow or prolonged intravenous delivery of a drug or fluid.

initial slope: The steepness of the initial part of the oxic cell survival curve.

initiating agent: Something that causes initial "latent" damage to the DNA. The cell requires more damage from a second "promoting agent" before the damage is expressed as cancer. Radiation usually is considered an initiating agent.

initiation codon: The mRNA sequence AUG, which codes for methionine and initiates translation.

intercalating agent: A compound that inserts between bases in a DNA molecule, disrupting the alignment and pairing of bases in the complementary strands (e.g., acridine dyes).

interferon: One of a family of proteins that act to inhibit viral replication in higher organisms. Some interferons may have anticancer properties.

interphase: That portion of the cell cycle between divisions.

interphase death: The death of irradiated cells before they reach mitosis.

interstitial implant: The placement of fine tubes in a gridlike pattern through tissues containing a cancer; these tubes are filled later with radioactive sources for brachytherapy.

intracavitary implant: The placement of a small tube within a body cavity, such as the bronchus or vagina; this tube later is filled with radioactive sources for brachytherapy.

intraoperative radiation: A type of radiation used to deliver a large dose of radiation therapy to the tumor bed and surrounding tissue at the time of surgery.

intravenous (IV): Into a vein.

intron: A portion of DNA that is located between coding regions in a gene and which is transcribed, but which does not appear in the mRNA product.

inverse square law: A physical law stating that the intensity of x- or γ-radiation from a point source emitting uniformly in all directions is inversely proportional to the square of the distance from the source.

inversion: Two breaks occurring in the same chromosome with rotation of the intervening segment. If both breaks are on the same side of the centromere, it is called a *paracentric* inversion. If they are on opposite sides, it is called a *pericentric* inversion.

ion: An electrically charged atom or group of atoms.

ion pair: A closely associated positive ion and negative ion (usually an electron) having charges of the same magnitude and formed from a neutral atom or molecule by radiation.

ionization: The process of adding one or more electrons to, or removing one or more electrons from, atoms or molecules, thereby creating ions. High temperatures, electrical discharges, or nuclear radiations can cause ionization.

ionization chamber: A device for detection of ionizing radiation or for measurement of radiation dose and dose rate.

ionizing radiation: Any radiation displacing electrons from atoms or molecules, thereby producing ions. Examples of ionizing radiation are α-, β-, and γ-radiation, x-rays and shortwave ultraviolet light. Ionizing radiation may produce severe skin or tissue damage. See **radiation burn**, **radiation illness**.

ipsilateral: On the same side of the body (opposite of contralateral).

irradiation: Exposure to radiation, as in a nuclear reactor.

isobars: Atoms having the same number of nucleons but different numbers of protons and neutrons.

isochromosome: A chromosome that consists of identical copies of one chromosome arm with loss of the other arm. Thus, an isochromosome for the long arm of chromosome 17 (i[17][q10]) contains two copies of the long arm (separated by the centromere) with loss of the short arm of the chromosome.

isoeffect plots: Graphs of the total dose for a given effect (e.g., ED_{50}) plotted, for instance, against dose per fraction or dose rate.

isomers: Atoms having the same number of protons and neutrons but a different nuclear energy state.

isotopes: Forms of a chemical element that have the same number of protons and electrons but differ in the number of neutrons contained in the atomic nucleus. Unstable isotopes undergo a transition to a more stable form with the release of radioactivity.

isotropic: Having equal intensity in all directions.

Karnofsky score: A measure of the patient's overall physical health following treatment, judged by his or her level of activity.

karyotype: Arrangement of chromosomes from a particular cell according to a well-established system such that the largest chromosomes are first and the smallest ones are last. Normal female karyotype is 46,XX; normal male karyotype is 46,XY.

kerma: The sum of the initial kinetic energies of all the charged ionizing particles liberated by uncharged ionizing particles per unit mass of a specified material. Kerma is measured in the same unit as absorbed dose. The SI unit of kerma is joule per kilogram, and its special name is gray (Gy). Kerma can be quoted for any specified material at a point in free space or in an absorbing medium.

kilobase (kb): A unit of length consisting of 1,000 nucleotides.

kilovolt (kV): A unit of electrical potential difference equal to 1,000 V.

labeling index (LI): Proportion or percentage of cells in the population (S phase) that take up tritiated thymidine or other precursors, such as bromodeoxyuridine; that is, the proportion synthesizing DNA.

late responses: Radiation-induced normal-tissue damage that in humans is expressed months to years after exposure. Generally results from damage to connective tissue cells. The α/β ratio tends to be small (<5 Gy).

latency period: The time between an injury occurring and the effects of the injury expressing themselves as disease.

$LD_{50/30}$: Radiation dose to produce lethality in 50% of animals by 30 days; similarly, $LD_{50/7}$, and so on.

leader sequence: That portion of an mRNA molecule from the 5′ end to the beginning codon. May contain regulatory or ribosome-binding sites.

leading strand: During DNA replication, the strand synthesized continuously 5′ to 3′ toward the replication fork.

leakage radiation: All radiation coming from within the source assembly except for the useful beam.

LET: Linear energy transfer.

lethal dose (LD): A dose of ionizing radiation sufficient to cause death. Median lethal dose (MLD, or LD_{50}) is the dose required to kill, within a specified period of time, half the individuals in a large group of organisms similarly exposed. The $LD_{50/60}$ for humans is about 4 Gy (400 rad).

lethal gene: A gene whose expression results in death.

leucine zipper: A secondary protein structure in which projecting leucine residues on two polypeptide changes interdigitate to form a stable dimer.

leukemia: A malignant cancer of the blood-forming tissues (bone marrow or lymph nodes), generally characterized by an overproduction of white blood cells.

leukocyte: White blood cell.

lifetime risk: The risk of dying of some particular cause over the whole of a person's life.

ligase: An enzyme that catalyzes a reaction that links two DNA molecules by the formation of a phosphodiester bond.

ligation: The process of joining two or more DNA fragments.

linear accelerator: A machine creating high-energy radiation to treat cancers. See **accelerator**.

linear energy transfer (LET): The rate of energy loss along the track of an ionizing particle, usually expressed in keV/μm.

linear-quadratic (LQ) model: Model in which the effect (E) is a linear-quadratic function of dose (d): $E = \alpha d + \beta d^2$. For cell survival: $S = \exp(-\alpha d - \beta d^2)$.

linkage: Condition in which two or more nonallelic genes tend to be inherited together. Linked genes have their loci along the same chromosome, do not assort independently, but can be separated by crossing over.

local invasion: The spread of cancer from an original site to the surrounding tissues.

localized tumors: Tumors that are contained in one particular site and have not spread.

locally multiply damaged site (LMDS): Any of a wide variety of complex lesions, including base damage as well as double-strand breaks, produced by "spurs" and "blobs" from a high-LET track.

log-phase culture: A cell culture growing exponentially.

long terminal repeat (LTR): Sequence of several hundred base pairs found at the ends of retroviral DNAs.

lymph node: A collection of lymphocytes within a capsule and connected to other lymph nodes by fine lymphatic vessels; a common site for certain cancer cells to grow after traveling along lymphatic vessels.

lymphatic system: A network of fine lymphatic vessels that collects tissue fluids from all over the body and returns these fluids to the blood. Accumulations of lymphocytes, called *lymph nodes*, are situated along the course of lymphatic vessels.

lymphocyte: A type of white blood cell that helps protect the body against invading organisms by producing antibodies and regulating the immune system response.

lymphoma: A type of cancer beginning in an altered lymphocyte. There are two broad categories of lymphomas, Hodgkin's disease and non-Hodgkin's lymphoma.

lysis: The destruction of the cell membrane.

macrophage: A type of white blood cell assisting in the body's fight against bacteria and infection by engulfing and destroying invading organisms.

macrophage colony-stimulating factor (M-CSF): Cytokine that stimulates formation of macrophages from pluripotent hematopoietic cells.

magnetic resonance imaging (MRI): A method of taking pictures of body tissue using magnetic fields.

mammogram: An x-ray of the breast used to detect cancer, sometimes before it can be detected by palpation. Women older than 50 years are advised to have a mammogram every year; women in their 40s, every 2 years.

mapping: Determining the physical location of a gene or genetic marker on a chromosome.

mass number (A): The sum of the neutrons and protons in a nucleus. It is the nearest whole number to an isotope's atomic weight. For instance, the mass number of the uranium-235 isotope is 235. Compare **atomic number**.

mean: Arithmetic average.

median: The value in a group of numbers below and above which there are an equal number of data points or measurements.

medical oncologist: A doctor specializing in using chemotherapy to treat cancer.

mega: A prefix that multiplies a basic unit by 1 million (10^6).

meiosis: The process in gametogenesis or sporogenesis during which one replication of the chromosomes is followed by two nuclear divisions to produce four haploid cells.

melanoma: A type of cancer that begins in the pigment-containing cells of a skin mole or the lining of the eye.

Mendelian: Referring to diseases that are caused by mutations in single genes located on either the autosomes or the sex chromosomes and that show a simple, predictable pattern of inheritance.

meningioma: A type of brain tumor that is relatively common and usually benign.

messenger RNA (mRNA): The class of RNA molecules that copies the genetic information from DNA, in the nucleus, and carries it to ribosomes, in the cytoplasm.

metacentric chromosome: A chromosome with a centrally located centromere, producing chromosome arms of equal lengths.

metaphase: The stage of cell division in which the condensed chromosomes lie in a central plane between the two poles of the cell and in which the chromosomes become attached to the spindle fibers.

metastasis: The ability of cancerous cells to invade surrounding tissues, enter the circulatory system, and establish new malignancies in body tissues distant from the site of the original tumor.

metastatic cancer: An advanced stage of cancer in which cells from the original (primary) site have spread (metastasized) to other organs.

methionine: The amino acid encoded by the sequence AUG.

methylate: The addition of one or more methyl groups (CH_3) to a molecule.

MeV: One million (10^6) electronvolts.

micro (μ): A prefix that divides a basic unit by 1 million (10^{-6}).

microinjection: Introducing DNA into a cell using a fine microcapillary pipette.

micrometer (μm): A unit of length equal to 1×10^{-6} m. Previously called a *micron*.

micron: See **micrometer**.

migration coefficient: An expression of the proportion of migrant genes entering the population per generation.

millimeter (mm): A unit of length equal to one thousandth of a meter.

minimal medium: A medium containing only those nutrients that support the growth and reproduction of wild-type strains of an organism.

misrepair (error-prone repair): Reconstitution with a loss of information (e.g., deletion due to the loss of a fragment of the molecule or mutation or translocation).

missense mutation: A mutation that alters a codon to that of another amino acid, causing an altered translation product to be made.

mitochondrion: Found in the cells of eukaryotes, a cytoplasmic, self-reproducing organelle that is the site of ATP synthesis.

mitogen: A substance (e.g., phytohemagglutinin) that stimulates mitosis in nondividing cells.

mitogen-activated protein (MAP) kinase: A family of two protein kinases of 42 and 44 kDa (ERK1 and ERK2) and 38 kDa that act to induce certain early-response genes.

mitosis: The replication of a cell to form two progeny cells with identical sets of chromosomes.

mitotic death: Cell death associated with a postirradiation mitosis.

mitotic delay: Delay of entry into mitosis, or accumulation in G_2, as a result of treatment.

mitotic index (MI): Proportion or percentage of cells in mitosis at any given time.

molecule: A group of atoms held together by chemical forces. The atoms of the molecule may be identical, as in H_2, S_2, and S_8, or different, as in H_2O and CO_2. A molecule is the smallest unit of matter that can exist by itself and retain all its chemical properties.

monoclonal antibodies: Immunoglobulin molecules of single-epitope specificity that are secreted by a clone of B cells.

monosomic: Describing an aneuploid condition in which one member of a chromosome pair is missing; having a chromosome number of $2n - 1$.

monozygotic twins: Twins produced from a single fertilization event; the first division of the zygote produces two cells, each of which develops into an embryo. Also known as identical twins.

morbidity: Sickness, side effects, and symptoms of a treatment or disease.

mRNA (messenger RNA): An RNA molecule transcribed from DNA and translated into the amino acid sequence of a polypeptide.

mtDNA: Mitochondrial DNA.

mucositis: Inflammation of the lining of areas such as the mouth.

multifactorial: Referring to diseases known to have a genetic component but whose transmission patterns cannot be described as simple Mendelian.

multitarget equation: Model that assumes the presence of a number of critical targets in a cell, all of which require inactivation to kill the cell. Survival is given by $S = 1 - [1 - \exp(D/D_0)]^n$.

mutagen: Any agent that causes an increase in the rate of mutation.

mutant: A cell or organism carrying an altered or mutant gene.

mutation: A relatively stable change in the DNA of the cell nucleus. Mutations in the germ cells of the body (ova and sperm) may lead to inherited effects in the offspring. Mutations in the somatic cells of the body may lead to effects in the individual (e.g., cancer).

mutation component (MC): This allows for the observation that only a proportion of mutations lead to a disease.

mutation rate: The frequency with which mutations take place at a given locus or in a population.

***myc*:** A nuclear oncogene involved in immortalizing cells.

myeloma: A tumor of the cells of the bone marrow.

nano (n): A prefix that divides a basic unit by 1 billion (10^{-9}).

nanometer (nm): A unit of length equal to 1×10^{-9} m.

nasopharynx: Part of the breathing passage behind the nasal cavity.

natural radioactivity: See **background radiation**.

natural selection: Differential reproduction of some members of a species resulting from variable fitness conferred by genotypic differences.

natural uranium: Uranium as found in nature, containing 0.7% of the isotope ^{235}U, 99.3% of ^{238}U, and a trace of ^{234}U.

neutrino (ν): An electrically neutral elementary particle with a negligible mass. It interacts very weakly with matter and hence is difficult to detect. It is produced in many nuclear reactions (e.g., in β decay) and has high penetrating power. Neutrinos from the sun usually pass right through the earth.

neutron (n): An uncharged elementary particle that has a mass slightly greater than that of the proton and that is found in the nucleus of every atom heavier than hydrogen. A free neutron is unstable and decays with a half-life of about 13 minutes into an electron, a proton, and a neutrino. Neutrons sustain the fission chain reaction in a nuclear reactor.

nondisjunction: An accident of cell division in which the homologous chromosomes (in meiosis) or the sister chromatids (in mitosis) fail to separate and migrate to opposite poles; responsible for defects such as monosomy and trisomy.

nonsense mutation: A mutation that alters a codon to one that encodes no amino acid; for example, UAG (amber codon), UAA (ochre codon), or UGA (opal codon). Leads to premature termination during the translation of mRNA.

nonstochastic effect: An effect the severity of which increases with increasing dose, after a threshold region. Now called **deterministic effect**.

normal distribution: A probability function that approximates the distribution of random variables. The normal curve, also known as a *Gaussian* or *bell-shaped curve*, is the graphic display of the normal distribution.

Northern blotting: A procedure in which RNA fragments are transferred from an agarose gel to a nitrocellulose filter, from which the RNA is then hybridized to a radioactive probe.

NSD: Nominal standard dose in the Ellis formula.

nuclear reactor: A structure in which nuclear fission may be sustained in a self-supporting chain reaction. In thermal reactors, the fission is produced by fission neutrons, and in fast reactors by fast neutrons.

nuclease: An enzyme that breaks bonds in nucleic acid molecules.

nucleic acid: A class of organic acids that play a role in protein synthesis, in the transmission of hereditary traits, and in the control of cellular activities.

nucleon: Proton or neutron.

nucleoside: A purine or pyrimidine base covalently linked to a ribosome or deoxyribose sugar molecule.

nucleotide: A buiding block of DNA and RNA, consisting of a nitrogtenous base, a five-carbon sugar, and a phosphate group.

nucleotide pair: The pair of nucleotides (A and T or G and C) in opposite strands of the DNA molecule that are hydrogen-bonded to each other.

nucleus (of a cell): The membrane-bounded region of a eukaryotic cell that contains the chromosomes.

nucleus (of an atom): The small, positively charged core of an atom. It is only about 1/10,000 the diameter of the atom but contains nearly all the atom's mass. All nuclei contain both protons and neutrons, except the nucleus of ordinary hydrogen, which consists of a single proton.

nuclide: A general term applicable to all atomic forms of the elements. The term often is used incorrectly as a synonym for *isotope*, which properly has a more limited definition. Whereas isotopes are the various forms of a single element (hence are a family of nuclides) and all have the same atomic number and number of protons, nuclides comprise all the isotopic forms of all the elements. Nuclides are distinguished by their atomic number, atomic mass, and energy state.

occupationally exposed: Exposed to radiation as a direct result of occupational duties.

oligonucleotide: A DNA polymer composed of only a few nucleotides.

oncogene: A gene that contributes to cancer formation when mutated or inappropriately expressed.

oncogenic: Having the potential to cause cancer (same as **carcinogenic**).

oncologist: A physician specializing in the study and treatment of cancer.

oncology: The study of cancer.

1 4-3-3: A protein that interacts with *raf* to promote translocation to the cell membrane, in which *raf*, in turn, interacts with *ras*.

open reading frame: A long DNA sequence, uninterrupted by a stop codon, that encodes part or all of a protein.

organ or tissue weighting factor (W_T): A factor that indicates the ratio of the risk of stochastic effects attributable to irradiation of a given organ or tissue to the total risk if the whole body is uniformly irradiated. Organs that have a large tissue weighting factor are those susceptible to radiation-induced carcinogenesis (such as the breast or thyroid).

oxidative stress: Formation of reactive oxygen species (ROS) in and outside cells, such as those resulting from the lysis of water molecules induced by ionizing radiation. This stress can not only activate several enzyme systems, but can also modify the transcription of genes. These reactions are known collectively as oxidative stress.

oxygen enhancement ratio (OER): The ratio of the radiation dose given under anoxic conditions to produce a given effect relative to the radiation dose given under fully oxygenated conditions to produce the same effect.

p15: G_1 inhibitor induced in epithelial cells by TGF-β. Inhibits cyclin D_1–Cdk4 and cyclin D_1–Cdk6 complexes.

p16: G_1 inhibitor of epithelial cells. Inhibits cyclin D_1–Cdk4 and cyclin D_1–Cdk6 complexes. Gene is deleted in familial melanomas and other tumor types.

p21 (WAF1): Inhibitor of Cdc2, Cdk4, and Cdk6. Induced through p53 pathway.

p27: Cell-cycle inhibitor induced in epithelial cells by TGF-β. Inhibits cyclin E–Cdk2 complex.

p53: Considered the guardian of the genome. Mediates cellular responses to DNA-damaging agents such as ionizing radiation at the G_1 checkpoint. Induces p21. The gene *p53* on chromosome 17 is mutated in colon, breast, esophageal, and a variety of other human cancers. Binds DNA; can act as transcription factor.

palindrome: A word, number, verse, or sentence that reads the same backward or forward. In nucleic acids, a sequence in which the base pairs read the same on complementary strands ($5' \rightarrow 3'$). For example: $5'$ GAATTC $3'$, $3'$ CTTAAG $5'$. These often occur as sites for restriction endonuclease recognition and cutting.

palliative care: Treatment to relieve, rather than cure, symptoms caused by cancer. Palliative care can help people live more comfortably.

palpate: To examine by carefully feeling with the fingers.

paracentric inversion: A chromosomal inversion that does not include the centromere.

parent: Radioactive atom that disintegrates to a different atom, its progeny.

particle: A minute constituent of matter, generally one with a measurable mass. The primary particles involved in radioactivity are α-particles, β-particles, neutrons, and protons.

pathologist: A specialist who attempts to describe the nature of a disease by analyzing samples obtained from tissues, organs, or body fluids.

pathology: The study of diseased tissues, both by gross and by microscopic examination of tissues removed during surgery and postmortem.

pedigree: In human genetics, a diagram showing the ancestral relationships of a given genotype manifest in a specific mutant phenotype associated with a trait.

penetrance: The frequency (expressed as a percentage) with which individuals of a given genotype manifest at least some degree of a specific mutant phenotype associated with a trait.

peptide bond: The covalent bond between the amino group of one amino acid and the carboxyl group of another amino acid.

pericentric inversion: A chromosomal inversion that involves both arms of the chromosome and thus involves the centromere.

phage: See **bacteriophage**.

pharynx: Medical term for the throat from the nasal and oral cavities above to the larynx and esophagus below.

phosphodiester bond: In nucleic acids, the covalent bond between a phosphate group and adjacent nucleotides, extending from the $5'$ carbon of one pentose (ribose or deoxyribose) to the $3'$ carbon of the pentose in the neighboring nucleotide. Phosphodiester bonds form the backbone of nucleic acid molecules.

photodynamic therapy: Cancer treatment using light to activate a photosensitizing agent, thereby releasing cytotoxic free radicals.

photoelectric effect: Absorption of an x-ray by ionization.

photon: The carrier of a quantum of electromagnetic energy. Photons have an effective momentum but no mass or electrical charge.

pico (p): A prefix that divides a basic unit by 1 trillion (10^{-12}). Same as *micromicro*.

picocuries per liter (pCi/L): A unit of measurement of the activity concentration of a radioactive material; measures, for example, how many radioactive disintegrations of radon occur every second in a liter of air.

plaque: A clear spot on a lawn of bacteria or cultured cells on which cells have been lysed by viral infection and replication.

plasmid (p): A circular DNA molecule, capable of autonomous replication, which typically carries one or more genes encoding antibiotic resistance proteins.

plateau-phase cultures: Cell cultures grown to confluence so that proliferation is markedly reduced (also called stationary phase).

platelet-derived growth factor (PDGF): A protein that induces growth fibroblasts and is involved in wound healing. Also acts on some epithelial and endothelial cells and on mesenchymal cells.

platelets: Special blood cells that help stop bleeding.

plating efficiency: The proportion or percentage of *in vitro* plated cells that form colonies.

pleiotropy: Condition in which a single mutation simultaneously affects several characters.

ploidy: Relates to the number of sets of chromosomes in a cell. Diploid cells have two sets of chromosomes, a chromosome complement twice that found in the gametes.

Tetraploid cells have four sets of chromosomes.

point mutation: A mutation that can be mapped to a single locus. At the molecular level, a mutation that results in the substitution of one nucleotide for another.

polar body: A cell that is produced at either the first or second meiotic division in females and which contains almost no cytoplasm as a result of an unequal cytokinesis.

polyacrylamide gel electrophoresis: Electrophoresis through a matrix composed of a synthetic polymer, used to separate small DNA or RNA molecules (up to 1,000 nucleotides) or proteins.

polyclonal antibodies: A mixture of immunoglobulin molecules secreted against a specific antigen, each recognizing a different epitope.

polymerase: An enzyme that catalyzes the addition of multiple subunits to a substrate molecule.

polymerase chain reaction (PCR): A procedure that enzymatically amplifies a DNA sequence through repeated replication by DNA polymerase.

polymorphism: The existence of two or more discontinuous, segregating phenotypes in a population.

polypeptide: A molecule made up of amino acids joined by covalent peptide bonds. This term is used to denote the amino acid chain before it assumes its functional three-dimensional configuration.

polyploid: A cell or individual having more than two sets of chromosomes.

population: A local group of individuals that belong to the same species and that are actually or potentially interbreeding.

positron (β^+): An elementary particle with the mass of an electron but charged positively. It is the "antielectron." It is emitted in some radioactive disintegrations and is formed by the interaction of high-energy γ-rays with matter.

potential doubling time (T_{pot}): Tumor doubling time, taking into account the cell-cycle time and the growth fraction, but ignoring cell loss.

potentially lethal damage (PLD): Cellular damage that is repaired during the interval between treatment and assay, especially under suboptimal growth conditions.

pRb: A protein of ~110 kDa that regulates cell-cycle progression through G_1. Phosphorylated by cyclin D–Cdk complexes to release G_1 transcription factors. Inactivated in hereditary retinoblastoma and sporadic tumors of the bone, breast, esophagus, and other tissues.

precursor: In a radioactive decay chain, a member of the decay chain that occurs before a particular atom in question.

pre-mRNA: The initial mRNA transcript prior to any mRNA processing.

primary cell: A cell or cell line that is taken directly from a living organism and that is not immortalized.

primary tumor: The place in which a cancer originates, which is referred to regardless of the site of its eventual spread. Thus, prostate cancer that spreads to the bone is still prostate cancer and is not referred to as bone cancer.

primer: A short DNA or RNA fragment annealed to single-stranded DNA.

primordial: Existing at the beginning of the universe, or at the beginning of the earth.

prion: An infectious pathogenic agent devoid of nucleic acid and composed mainly of a protein, PrP, with a molecular weight of 27,000 to 30,000 Da. Prions are known to cause scrapie, a degenerative neurologic disease in sheep, and are thought to cause similar diseases in humans, such as kuru and Creutzfeldt–Jakob disease.

probability: Ratio of the frequency of a given event to the frequency of all possible events.

probe: A single-stranded DNA (or RNA) that has been labeled radioactively and is used to identify complementary sequences.

prodromal phase: Signs and symptoms in the first 48 hours following irradiation of the central nervous system.

progeny: Formerly called a "daughter" in a radioactive decay chain.

prognosis: The predicted or likely outcome.

prokaryotes: Organisms lacking nuclear membranes, meiosis, and mitosis. Bacteria and blue-green algae are examples of prokaryotic organisms.

promoter: A region of DNA extending 150 to 300 bp upstream from the transcription start site that contains binding sites for RNA polymerase and a number of proteins that regulate the rate of transcription of the adjacent gene.

promoter site: Region having a regulatory function and to which RNA polymerase binds prior to the initiation of transcription.

promoting agent: Something that acts on earlier cellular damage caused by an initiating agent; can cause the earlier damage to be expressed as cancer. Tobacco smoke usually is considered a promoting agent.

prophylactic: Preventive measure or medication.

prostate: A gland at the base of the bladder in males for the production of seminal fluids. Cancer of this gland is common in elderly men.

protein: A molecule composed of one or more polypeptides, each composed of amino acids covalently linked together.

protein kinase: An enzyme that adds phosphate groups to a protein molecule at serine, threonine, or tyrosine residues.

protein kinase C (PKC): A family of protein kinases involved in mitogenic signaling. Activated by second messengers, including diacylglycerol and Ca^{2+} (some isoforms). Can be activated directly by the phorbol ester class of tumor promoters. Can induce early-response genes through *raf*.

protocol: A standardized combination of therapies developed specifically for particular tumors.

proton: An elementary particle that is a component of all nuclei and that has a single positive electrical charge and a mass approximately 1,837 times that of the electron. The nucleus of an ordinary or light hydrogen atom. The atomic number of an atom is equal to the number of protons in its nucleus.

proto-oncogene: A gene generally active in the embryo and fetus and during proliferation processes. A mutation can result in the permanent activation of a proto-oncogene, which then becomes an oncogene.

pulsed-field gel electrophoresis (PFGE): Process whereby current is alternated between pairs of electrodes set at angles to one another to separate very large DNA molecules of up to 10 million nucleotides.

purines: Organic bases with carbon and nitrogen atoms in two interlocking rings; components of nucleic acids and other biologically active substances.

pyrimidines: Nitrogenous bases composed of a single ring of carbon and nitrogen atoms; components of nucleic acids.

quality factor: The factor by which absorbed dose is to be multiplied to obtain a quantity that expresses on a common scale, for all ionizing radiations, the irradiation incurred by exposed persons. Largely replaced by radiation weighting factor.

quasithreshold dose (D_q): Point of extrapolation of the exponential portion of a multitarget survival curve to the level of zero survival: $D_q = D_0 \ln(n)$.

rad: The old unit of absorbed dose, equivalent to an energy absorption of 10^{-2} J/kg. Replaced by the gray (Gy). See **absorbed dose**.

radiation: The emission and propagation of energy through matter or space by means of electromagnetic disturbances (x-rays) that display both wavelike and particle-like behavior; in this context the "particles" are known as *photons*. Also, the energy so propagated. The term has been extended to include streams of fast-moving particles, such as α- and β-particles, free neutrons, and cosmic radiation. Nuclear radiation is that emitted from atomic nuclei in various nuclear reactions, including α-, β-, and γ-radiation and neutrons.

radiation (ionizing): Any electromagnetic or particulate radiation capable of producing ions, directly or indirectly, by interaction with matter. Examples are x-rays, photons, charged atomic particles and other ions, and neutrons.

radiation absorbed dose: See **rad**.

radiation accidents: Accidents resulting in the spread of radioactive material or in the exposure of individuals to radiation.

radiation burn: Radiation damage to the skin. β-Burns result from skin contact with or exposure to emitters of β-particles. See **beta particle, ionizing radiation**.

radiation chemistry: The branch of chemistry that is concerned with the chemical effects, including decomposition, of energetic radiation or particles on matter.

radiation dose: The amount of radiation absorbed by an irradiated object. This unit is the gray (Gy), defined to be 1 J/kg.

radiation illness: An acute organic disorder that follows exposure to relatively large doses of ionizing radiation. It is characterized by nausea, vomiting, diarrhea, blood cell changes, and (in later stages) hemorrhage and loss of hair.

radiation oncologist: A physician specializing in the treatment of tumors by radiation therapy.

radiation protection: Legislation and regulations to protect the public and workers against radiation. Also, measures to reduce exposure to radiation.

radiation quality: Relative penetrability of an x-ray beam determined by its average energy; usually measured by HVL (half value layer) or kVp (peak kilovoltage).

radiation shielding: Reduction of radiation by interposing a shield of absorbing material between any radioactive source and a person, laboratory area, or radiation-sensitive device.

radiation sterilization: Using radiation to make a plant or animal sterile. Also, radiation to kill all forms of life, especially bacteria, in food or surgical equipment.

radiation therapy: Treatment of disease with any type of radiation. Often called *radiotherapy*.

radiation warning symbol: An officially prescribed symbol, a magenta trefoil on a yellow background, that should be displayed whenever a radiation hazard exists.

radiation weighted dose: New name proposed by ICRP for equivalent dose.

radiation weighting factor (W_R): A factor used for radiation protection purposes that accounts for differences in biologic effectiveness between different radiations. The radiation weighting factor is independent of the tissue weighting factor.

radioactive decay: See **decay**, **radioactive**.

radioactive half-life: Time for a radioisotope to decay to one half its activity.

radioactive isotope: One of the forms of an element, differing in atomic weight and possessing an unstable nucleus that emits ionizing radiation.

radioactive series: A succession of nuclides, each in turn transforming by radioactive disintegration into the next nuclide until a stable nuclide is reached. The first member is called the *parent*, the intermediate members are called *progeny*, and the final, stable member is called the *end product*.

radioactive tracer: A small quantity of a radioactive isotope, either with or without a carrier, used to follow biologic, chemical, or other processes by detection, determination, or localization of the radioactivity.

radioactive waste: Unwanted radioactive materials in any form. Often categorized in the nuclear power industry into low-level, intermediate-level, and high-level waste.

radioactivity: A property of all unstable elements that regularly decay to an altered state by releasing energy in the form of photons (γ-rays) or particles (e.g., electrons, α-particles).

radiobiology: The body of knowledge and the study of the principles, mechanisms, and effects of ionizing radiation on living matter.

radiogenic: Of radioactive origin; produced by radioactive transformation.

radioisotope: A radioactive isotope; an unstable isotope of an element that decays or disintegrates spontaneously, emitting radiation. More than 1,300 natural and artificial radioisotopes have been identified.

radiologist: A physician with special training in reading diagnostic x-rays and performing specialized x-ray procedures.

radiology: The science that investigates all forms of ionizing radiation in the diagnosis and treatment of disease.

radionuclide: A radioactive nuclide.

radioprotector: A chemical compound that reduces the biologic consequences of radiation.

radioresistance: A relative resistance of cells, tissues, organs, or organisms to the harmful action of radiation.

radioresponsiveness: A general term indicating the overall level of clinical response to radiotherapy.

radiosensitivity: (1) A relative susceptibility of cells, tissues, organs, or organisms to the effects of radiation. (2) The radiation dose required to produce a defined level of cell inactivation, usually indicated by the surviving fraction at 2 Gy (i.e., SF_2) or by the parameters of the linear-quadratic or multitarget equations.

radiosensitizer: In general, any agent that increases the sensitivity of cells to radiation. Most commonly applied to electron-affinic chemicals that mimic oxygen in fixing free-radical damage.

radiotherapy: The treatment of disease with ionizing radiation. Often termed *radiation therapy*.

radium (Ra): A radioactive metallic element with atomic number 88. As found in nature, the most common isotope has an atomic weight of 226. It occurs in minute quantities associated with uranium in pitchblende, carnotite, and other minerals. The uranium decays to radium in a series of α- and β-emissions. By virtue of being an α- and γ-emitter, radium is used as a source of luminescence and as a radiation source in medicine and radiography.

radon (Rn): Colorless, odorless, naturally occurring radioactive gas; a radioactive element and the heaviest gas known. Its atomic number is 86 and its atomic weight varies from 200 to 226. Rn-222 is the progeny of radium in the uranium radioactive series.

radon daughter: Any atom that is below radon-222 in the uranium decay chain; often specifically refers to polonium-218 and polonium-214, as these have the most biologic significance; now referred to as *radon progeny*.

raf: A protein kinase that is activated by GTP-bound *ras*. Acts to transduce mitogenic signaling by phosphorylation of MAP kinases.

ras: A family of 21-kDa proteins (H-, K-, and N-*ras*) found to be activated by point mutations at codons 12, 13, and 61 in a variety of tumors. Involved in mitogenic signaling, coupling growth signals from growth factor receptors to *raf* activation, and downstream stimulation of early-response genes. Binds GTP in its activated state. Is found at the inner face of the cell membrane.

RBE: See **relative biologic effectiveness**.

reading frame: A series of triplet codons beginning from a specific nucleotide.

reassortment (redistribution): Return toward a more even cell age distribution, following the selective killing of cells in certain phases of the cell cycle.

recessive: Term describing an allele that is not expressed in the heterozygous condition.

recessive gene: Gene whose phenotype is expressed only when both copies of the gene are mutated or missing.

recessive-acting oncogene (anti-oncogene): A single copy of this gene is sufficient to suppress cell proliferation; the loss of both copies of the gene contributes to cancer formation.

reciprocal translocation: A chromosomal aberration in which nonhomologous chromosomes exchange parts.

recombinant DNA: The process of cutting and recombining DNA fragments as a means to isolate genes or to alter their structure and function.

recovery: An increase in cell survival as a function of time during or after irradiation. See **repair**.

recurrence: The return of a cancer after all detectable traces had been removed by primary therapy; recurrences may be local (near the primary site) or distant (metastatic).

relapse: Recurrence of a disease following treatment.

relative biologic effectiveness (RBE): A factor used to compare the biologic effectiveness of different types of ionizing radiation. It is the inverse ratio of the amount of absorbed radiation required to produce a given effect to a standard (or reference) radiation required to produce the same effect.

relative risk: Situation in which the risk of a disease resulting from some injury is expressed as some percentage increase of the normal rate of occurrence of that disease; in contrast to an absolute risk, in which the risk of a disease resulting from an injury does not depend on the normal rate of occurrence of that disease.

rem: Old unit of equivalent or effective dose. It is the product of absorbed dose (in rad) and the radiation weighting factor. One rem is one hundredth of a sievert.

remediation: Reducing a home's indoor radon level.

remission, complete: Condition in which no cancerous cells can be detected and the patient appears to be free of disease.

remission, partial: Generally means that by all methods used to measure the existence of a tumor, there has been at least a 50% regression of the disease following treatment.

remote brachytherapy: See **high-dose-rate (HDR) remote brachytherapy**.

reoxygenation: The process by which surviving hypoxic clonogenic cells become better oxygenated during the period after irradiation of a tumor.

repair: Restoration of the integrity of damaged macromolecules.

repair saturation: Explanation of the shoulder on cell survival curves on the basis of the reduced effectiveness of repair after high radiation doses.

reproductive death: The loss of the proliferative ability of a cell. Commonly restricted to those cells having an indefinite capacity to divide.

reproductive integrity: Ability of cells to divide many times and thus be "clonogenic."

resection: Surgical removal. In relation to cancer resection, the pathologist often indicates if the outer margins of the resection had no cancer cells present or were "negative."

restriction endonuclease: Nuclease that recognizes specific nucleotide sequences in a DNA molecule and cleaves or nicks the DNA at that site. Derived from a variety of microorganisms, those enzymes that cleave both strands of the DNA are used in the construction of recombinant DNA molecules.

restriction fragment length polymorphism (RFLP): Differences in nucleotide sequence between alleles that result in restriction fragments of varying lengths.

retrovirus: A member of a class of RNA viruses that utilizes the enzyme reverse transcriptase to reverse-copy its genome into a DNA intermediate, which integrates into the host cell chromosome. Many naturally occurring cancers of vertebrate animals are caused by retroviruses. They are convenient to work with as a vector in gene therapy, but infect only dividing cells, which is a severe limitation.

reverse transcriptase (RNA-dependent DNA polymerase): An enzyme isolated from retrovirus-infected cells that synthesizes a complementary cDNA strand from an RNA template.

reversion: A mutation that restores the wild-type phenotype.

ribosomal RNA: See **rRNA**.

RNA (ribonucleic acid): An organic acid composed of repeating nucleotide units of adenine, guanine, cytosine, and uracil, whose ribose components are linked by phosphodiester bonds.

RNA polymerase: An enzyme that catalyzes the formation of an RNA polynucleotide strand using the base sequence of a DNA molecule as a template.

Robertsonian translocation: A form of chromosomal aberration that involves the fusion of long arms of acrocentric chromosomes at the centromere.

röntgen (R): A unit of exposure to ionizing radiation named after Wilhelm Röntgen, the German scientist who discovered x-rays in 1895. It is that amount of γ- or x-rays required to produce ions carrying one electrostatic unit of electrical charge (either positive or negative) in 1 cm^3 of dry air under standard conditions.

rRNA: The RNA molecules that are the structural components of the ribosomal subunits. In prokaryotes, these are the 16S, 23S, and 5S molecules; in eukaryotes, they are the 18S, 28S, and 5S molecules.

***Saccharomyces cerevisiae*:** Brewer's yeast.

sarcoma: A type of cancer derived from connective bone or fat tissue. Examples include fibrosarcoma, osteogenic sarcoma, and liposarcoma.

satellite DNA: DNA that forms a minor band if genomic DNA is centrifuged in a cesium salt gradient. This DNA usually consists of a short sequence repeated many times in the genome.

scan: A diagnostic test usually involving the movement or scanning of a detector to produce a picture. Examples include ultrasound, nuclear medicine, computer-assisted tomographic, and magnetic resonance scans.

scattered radiation: Radiation that, during passage through matter, is changed in direction (the change is usually accompanied by a decrease in energy).

SCE: See **sister chromatid exchange**.

Scheimpflug imaging system: An imaging system that gives an objective and quantitative assessment of the severity of an ocular cataract. Named after the Austrian army officer Theodor Scheimpflug (1865–1911).

secondary cancer: Cancer arising from a primary cancer; metastatic cancer.

segregation: The separation of homologous chromosomes into different gametes during meiosis.

selectable marker: A gene whose expression makes it possible to identify cells that have been transformed or transfected with a vector containing the marker gene. It is usually a gene for resistance to an antibiotic.

selection: The force that brings about changes in the frequency of alleles and genotypes in populations through differential reproduction.

semiconservative replication: A model of DNA replication in which a double-stranded molecule replicates in such a way that the progeny molecules are composed of one parental (old) and one newly synthesized strand.

sensitizing agent: A substance that increases the biologic effectiveness of a given dose of radiation.

sex chromosome: A chromosome, such as the X or Y in humans, that is involved in sex determination.

sex linkage: The pattern of inheritance resulting from genes located on the X chromosome.

sexual reproduction: Reproduction through the fusion of gametes, which are the haploid products of meiosis.

SF_2: Surviving fraction at 2 Gy (200 rad).

sickle-cell anemia: A genetic disease in humans caused by an autosomal recessive gene, usually fatal in the homozygous condition. Caused by an alteration in the amino acid sequence of the β chain of globin.

side effects: Symptoms directly related to treatment, such as the side effect of nausea resulting from radiation treatment over the stomach. Side effects are considered acute if they occur during treatment and subside when treatment is complete. Those symptoms persisting over a longer period of time are considered chronic.

sievert (Sv): Unit of equivalent dose or effective dose. It is equal to the dose in gray multiplied by a weighting factor. One sievert equals 100 rem.

SINES: Short interspersed repetitive sequences found in the genomes of higher organisms, such as the 300-bp *Alu* sequence.

sister chromatid exchange (SCE): A crossing over event that can occur in meiotic and mitotic cells. Involves the reciprocal exchange of chromosomal material between sister chromatids (joined by a common centromere). Such exchanges can be detected cytologically after BrdUrd incorporation into the replicating chromosomes.

slow repair: Long-term recovery that takes place on a time scale of weeks to months.

solid tumor: A cancer originating in an organ or tissue other than bone marrow or the lymph system.

somatic: Pertaining to the body; pertaining to all cells except the germ cells.

somatic cell: Any cell other than a germ cell that composes the body of an organism and that possesses a set of multiploid chromosomes.

somatic effects of radiation: Effects of radiation limited to the exposed individual, as distinguished from genetic effects, which also affect subsequent, unexposed generations. Large radiation doses can be fatal. Smaller doses may make the individual noticeably ill, may produce temporary changes in blood cell levels detectable only in the laboratory, or may produce no detectable effects.

somatic mutation: A mutational event occurring in a somatic cell. Such mutations are not hereditary.

SOS response: The induction of enzymes to repair damaged DNA in *Escherichia coli*. The response involves activation of an enzyme that cleaves a repressor, activating a series of genes involved in DNA repair.

Southern blotting: A procedure in which DNA restriction fragments are transferred from an agarose gel to a nitrocellulose filter, where the denatured DNA is then hybridized to a radioactive probe.

spatial cooperation: The use of radiotherapy and chemotherapy to treat disease in different anatomic sites.

species: A group of actually or potentially interbreeding individuals isolated reproductively from other such groups.

specific activity: The radioactivity of a radioisotope of an element per unit weight of the element in a sample; the activity per unit mass of a pure radionuclide; the activity per unit weight of any sample of radioactive material.

spheroid: Clump of cells grown together in tissue culture suspension.

spindle fibers: Cytoplasmic fibrils formed during cell division that are involved in the separation of chromatids at anaphase and their movement toward opposite poles in the cell.

split-dose (SLD) recovery: Decrease in radiation effect if a single radiation dose is split into two fractions separated by times up to a few hours. Also called *Elkind recovery* or *recovery from sublethal damage*.

spontaneous mutation: A mutation that is not induced by a mutagenic agent.

spore: A unicellular body or cell that is encased in a protective coat and that is produced by some bacteria, plants, and invertebrates. Capable of survival in unfavorable environmental conditions and can give rise to a new individual upon germination. In plants, spores are the haploid products of meiosis.

spur: A concentration of about 3 ion pairs in a volume about 4 nm in diameter. See **locally multiply damage site**.

stable isotope: An isotope that does not undergo radioactive decay. Compare **radioisotope**.

stage: The anatomic extent of a cancer. Cancer may exist in the organ of origin and extend locally, or it may spread to regional tissues, then to local lymph nodes, and then to distant areas as metastases.

standard deviation: A quantitative measure of the amount of variation in a sample of measurements from a population.

standard error: A quantitative measure of the amount of variation in a sample of measurements from a population.

stathmokinetic method: Study of cell proliferation using agents that block cells in mitosis.

stem cells: Cells capable of self-renewal and of differentiation to produce all the various types of specialized cells in a lineage.

sterility: The condition of being unable to reproduce; the condition of being free from contaminating microorganisms.

sticky end: A single-stranded nucleotide sequence produced if a restriction endonuclease cleaves off-center in its recognition sequence.

stochastic effects: Effects the probability of which, rather than their severity, is a function of radiation dose without threshold. (More generally, *stochastic* means random in nature.)

strain: A group with common ancestry that has physiologic or morphologic characteristics of interest for genetic study or domestication.

stringency: Reaction conditions, such as temperature, salt, and pH, that dictate the annealing of single-stranded DNA/DNA, DNA/RNA, and RNA/RNA hybrids. At high stringency, duplexes form only between strands with perfect one-to-one complementarity; lower stringency allows annealing between strands with less than a perfect match between bases.

sublethal damage (SLD): Nonlethal cellular injury that can be repaired or accumulated with further dose to become lethal.

submetacentric chromosome: A chromosome with the centromere placed so that one arm of the chromosome is slightly longer than the other.

suppressor genes: Genes that oppose the continuous proliferation of cells. Also know as *tumor suppressor genes*.

supra-additivity (synergism): A biologic effect caused by a combination of effects that is greater than would be expected from the addition of the effects of the component agents.

survival curve: Curve obtained by plotting the number or the percentage of organisms surviving against the dose of radiation.

symbiont: An organism coexisting in a mutually beneficial relationship with another organism.

syndrome: A group of signs or symptoms that occur together and characterize a disease or abnormality.

synergism: Two or more agents reacting together to produce a result greater than the sum of the individual agents.

systemic: Having a widespread effect on the body as a whole, rather than just on local tissue.

***Taq* polymerase:** A heat-stable DNA polymerase isolated from the bacterium *Thermus aquaticus* and used in PCR.

target cell: A stem cell whose death contributes to a reduction in growth or tissue function.

target theory: (1) A theory based on the idea that death of a cell is caused by the inactivation of specific targets within the cell. (2) The idea that the shoulder on cell survival curves is a result of the number of unrepaired lesions per cell.

targeted radiotherapy: Treatment of disseminated cancer by means of drugs that localize in tumors and carry therapeutic amounts of radioactivity.

TBI: Total-body irradiation.

telocentric chromosome: A chromosome in which the centromere is located at the end of the chromosome.

telomerase: A reverse transcriptase that polymerizes TTAGGG repeats to offset the degradation of chromosome ends that occurs with successive cell divisions.

telomeres: Long arrays of TTAGGG repeats that cap and protect the ends of chromosomes. Each time a normal somatic cell divides, the terminal end of the telomere is lost.

telophase: The stage of cell division in which the progeny chromosomes reach the opposite poles of the cell and re-form nuclei. Telophase ends with the completion of cytokinesis.

temperature-sensitive mutation: A conditional mutation that produces a mutant phenotype at one temperature range and a wild-type phenotype at another temperature range.

template: An RNA or single-stranded DNA molecule on which a complementary nucleotide strand is synthesized.

teratocarcinoma: Embryonal tumors that arise in the yolk sac or gonads and are able to undergo differentiation into a wide variety of cell types. These tumors are used to investigate the regulatory mechanisms underlying development.

termination (stop) codon: Any of three mRNA sequences (UGA, UAG, UAA) that do not code for an amino acid and thus signal the end of protein synthesis.

therapeutic index (therapeutic ratio): Tumor response for a fixed level of normal-tissue damage.

therapeutic-gain factor: In hyperthermia, the ratio of the thermal enhancement ratio in the tumor to the thermal enhancement ratio in normal tissue. For high linear energy transfer radiations, the therapeutic-gain factor is the ratio of the relative biologic effectiveness in the tumor to the relative biologic effectiveness in normal tissue.

thermal dose: A function of temperature and heating time that is thought to relate well to biologic effect. It is defined to be the cumulative equivalent minutes at 43°C.

thermal enhancement ratio (TER): The ratio of radiation doses, with and without heat, to produce the same biologic effects.

thermal neutrons: Neutrons in thermal equilibrium with their surrounding medium. Thermal neutrons are those that have been slowed down by a moderator to an average speed of about 2,200 m/s at room temperature from the much higher initial speeds that they had when expelled by fission.

thermoluminescent dosimeter (TLD): A dosimeter containing a crystalline solid for measuring radiation dose, plus filters (absorbers) to help characterize the types of radiation encountered. If heated, TLD crystals that have been exposed to ionizing radiation give off light proportional to the energy they received from the radiation.

thermotolerance: The induced resistance to a second heat exposure by prior heating.

thorium series: Radioactive decay chain starting with thorium-232; one member of the chain is radon-220. This chain is of much less significance than the uranium decay chain containing radon-222.

threshold: A level (e.g., of radiation dose) below which there is no observable effect. There is no threshold for induction of cancer by radiation: All levels of radiation are considered harmful.

threshold dose: The minimum dose of radiation that produces a detectable biologic effect.

thymidine kinase (*tk*): An enzyme that allows a cell to utilize an alternate metabolic pathway for incorporating thymidine into DNA Used as a selectable marker to identify transfected eukaryotic cells.

thymine dimer: A pair of adjacent thymine bases in a single polynucleotide strand between which chemical bonds have formed. This lesion, usually the result of damage caused by exposure to ultraviolet light, inhibits DNA replication unless repaired by the appropriate enzyme system.

time–dose relationships: The dependence of isoeffective radiation dose on the duration (and number of fractions) in radiotherapy.

tolerance: The maximum radiation dose or intensity of fractionated radiotherapy that the therapist judges to be acceptable, usually expressed in dose units. Actual values depend on fractionation, field size, concomitant treatments, and so on.

topoisomerase: A class of enzymes that converts DNA from one topologic form to another. During DNA replication, these enzymes facilitate the unwinding of the double-helical structure of DNA.

totipotent: Referring to the ability of a cell or embryo part to give rise to all adult structures. This capacity usually is restricted progressively during development.

trait: Any detectable phenotypic variation of a particular inherited character.

transcription: Transfer of genetic information from DNA by the synthesis of an RNA molecule copied from a DNA template.

transfection: The uptake and expression of foreign DNA by cultured eukaryotic cells.

transformation: In higher eukaryotes, the conversion of cultured cells to a malignant phenotype. In prokaryotes, the natural or induced uptake and expression of a foreign DNA sequence.

transforming growth factor alpha (TGF-α): Functional and structural analogue of epidermal growth factor. Induces the growth of epithelial cells as well as fibroblasts and keratinocytes. May be involved in tumor-associated neovascularization.

transforming growth factor beta (TGF-β): A cytokine that regulates many of the biologic processes essential for embryo development and tissue homeostasis and which therefore plays a role in the healing of a tissue and carcinogenesis. The effects of TGF-β may differ, depending on the tissue involved. For instance, TGF-β inhibits the proliferation of epithelial cells, but stimulates that of fibroblasts.

transforming oncogene: A gene that upon transfection converts a previously immortalized cell to the malignant phenotype.

transgenic: A vertebrate organism in which a foreign DNA gene (a transgene) is stably incorporated into its genome early in embryonic development. The transgene is present in both somatic and germ cells, is expressed in one or more tissues, and is inherited by offspring in a Mendelian fashion.

transient hypoxia: Low oxygen concentrations associated with the transient closing and opening of blood vessels. Sometimes called *acute* or *cyclic hypoxia.*

translation: The process of converting the genetic information of mRNA on ribosomes into polypeptides.

translocation: The movement or reciprocal exchange of large chromosomal segments, typically between two different chromosomes.

trisomy: The condition in which a cell or organism possesses two copies of each chromosome, except for one, which is present in three copies. The general form for trisomy is therefore $2n + 1$.

tritium (^{3}H, T): A radioactive isotope of hydrogen with two neutrons and one proton in the nucleus. It is human-made and heavier than deuterium (heavy hydrogen). Tritium is used in industrial thickness gauges and as a label in chemical and biologic experiments. Its nucleus is a triton.

tRNA (transfer RNA): A small ribonucleic acid molecule that contains a three-base segment (anticodon) that recognizes a codon in mRNA, a binding site for a specific amino acid, and recognition sites for interaction with the ribosome and the enzyme that links it to its specific amino acid.

tumor: An abnormal growth of cells or tissues. Tumors may be benign (noncancerous) or malignant (cancerous).

tumor bed effect (TBE): Slower rate of tumor growth after irradiation, resulting from stromal injury in the irradiated "vascular bed."

tumor cord: Sleeve of viable tumor growing around a blood capillary.

tumor necrosis factor (TNF): Two proteins, TNF-α and TNF-β, involved in immune response control and inflammation. Induced by cytokines, ultraviolet radiations, and other agents.

UNSCEAR: United Nations Scientific Commission on Effects of Atomic Radiation.

uranium (U): A radioactive element with atomic number 92 and, as found in natural ores, an average atomic weight of approximately 238. The two principal natural isotopes are ^{235}U (0.7% of natural uranium), which is fissionable, and ^{238}U (99.3% of natural uranium), which is fertile. Natural uranium also includes a minute amount of ^{234}U.

uranium series (sequence): The series of nuclides resulting from the radioactive decay of the uranium isotope ^{238}U. The end product of the series is the lead isotope ^{206}Pb. The series includes radium and radon.

variance: A statistical measure of the variation of values from a central value, calculated as the square of the standard deviation.

vector: An autonomously replicating DNA molecule into which foreign DNA fragments are inserted and then propagated in a host cell.

viability: The measure of the number of individuals in a given phenotypic class that survive, relative to another class (usually wild-type).

viral oncogene: A viral gene that contributes to malignancies in vertebrate hosts.

virulent phage: A bacteriophage that infects and lyses the host bacterial cell.

virus: An infectious particle that is composed of a protein capsule and a nucleic acid core and that is dependent on a host organism for replication.

volume effect: Dependence of radiation damage to normal tissues on the volume of tissue irradiated.

volume-doubling time: Time taken for a tumor to double in volume.

waste, radioactive: Equipment and materials (from nuclear operations) that are radioactive and have no further use. Wastes are generally classified as high level: radioactivity concentrations of hundreds to thousands of curies per gallon or cubic foot; low level: in the range of 1 μCi (microcurie) per gallon or cubic foot; or intermediate: between these extremes.

wavelength: Distance between similar points on a sine wave; length of one cycle.

Western blot: Similar to a Southern blot (for DNA) or a Northern blot (for RNA), except that protein is used.

white blood cells: The blood cells that fight infection.

whole-body counter: A device used to identify and measure the radioactivity in the body (body burden) of humans and animals. It uses heavy shielding (to keep out background radiation), ultrasensitive scintillation detectors, and electronic equipment.

wild type: The most commonly observed phenotype or genotype, designated as the norm or standard.

X chromosome: The female sex chromosome.

xenografts: Transplants between species; usually applied to the transplantation of human tumors into immune-deficient mice and rats.

xerostomia: Dryness of the mouth caused by malfunctioning salivary glands.

X-linkage: See **sex linkage**.

X-linked disease: A genetic disease caused by a mutation on the X chromosome. In X-linked recessive conditions, a normal female "carrier" passes on the mutated X chromosome to an affected son.

x-ray: A penetrating form of electromagnetic radiation emitted either if the inner orbital electrons of an excited atom return to their normal state (these are characteristic x-rays) or if a metal target is bombarded with high-speed electrons. X-rays are always extranuclear in origin.

x-ray crystallography: A technique to determine the three-dimensional structure of molecules through diffraction patterns produced by x-ray scattering by crystals of the molecule under study.

Y chromosome: Sex chromosome in species in which the male is heterogametic (XY).

yeast artificial chromosome (YAC): A vector that is used to clone DNA fragments of up to 400,000 bp and that contains the minimum chromosomal sequences needed to replicate in yeast.

Z: The symbol for atomic number; the number of protons in the nucleus.

zinc fingers: A structural motif of DNA-binding proteins in which fingerlike loops of amino acids are stabilized by interactions with zinc atoms.

zygote: The diploid cell produced by the fusion of haploid gametic nuclei.

Index

Page numbers followed by *f* indicate figure and page numbers followed by *t* indicate table.

I

Q

R

T